Visit our website

to find out about other books from Mosby and our sister companies in Harcourt Health Sciences

Register free at
www.harcourt-international.com

and you will get

- **the latest information on new books, journals and electronic products in your chosen subject areas**

- **the choice of e-mail or post alerts or both, when there are any new books in your chosen areas**

- **news of special offers and promotions**

- **information about products from all Harcourt Health Sciences' companies including W. B. Saunders, Churchill Livingstone, and Mosby**

You will also find an easily searchable catalogue, online ordering, information on our extensive list of journals...and much more!

Visit the Harcourt Health Sciences' website today!

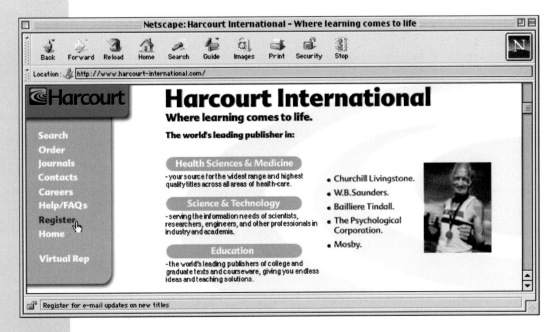

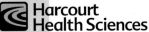

Comprehensive Clinical Hepatology

John G. O'Grady MD FRCPI
Consultant Hepatologist
Institute of Liver Studies
King's College School of Medicine
London
UK

John R. Lake MD
Professor of Medicine and Surgery
Director, Gastroenterology Division
Director, Liver Transplantation Program
University of Minnesota Medical School
Minneapolis
USA

Peter D. Howdle MD FRCP
Professor of Clinical Education,
University of Leeds
Consultant Gastroenterologist
St. James's University Hospital
Leeds
UK

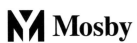 Mosby

London   Edinburgh   New York   Philadelphia   St Louis   Sydney   Toronto   2000

MOSBY
An imprint of Harcourt Publishers Limited

©Harcourt Publishers Limited 2000

M is a registered trademark of Harcourt Publishers Limited

The right of John G O'Grady, John R Lake, and Peter D Howdle
to be identified as authors of this work has been asserted by them
in accordance with the Copyright, Designs and Patents Act 1988

First published 2000

ISBN 07234 3106X

British Library Cataloguing in Publication Data
A catalogue record for this book is available from the British Library

Library of Congress Cataloging in Publication Data
A catalog record for this book is available from the Library of
Congress

Note
Medical knowledge is constantly changing. As new information
becomes available, changes in treatment, procedures, equipment
and the use of drugs become necessary. The editors/authors/con-
tributors and the publishers have taken care to ensure that the information given in this text is accurate and up to date. However,
readers are strongly advised to confirm that the information, especially with regard to drug usage, complies with the latest legislation
and standards of practice.

Reproduction by Prospect Litho, Basildon, UK.
Printed and bound by Grafos SA Arte sobre papel, Barcelona, Spain

Commissioning Editor: Sue Hodgson
Project Manager: Philip Dauncey
Production Controller: Mark Sanderson
Senior Designer: Ian Spick
Illustration Manager: Mick Ruddy

The
Publisher's
policy is to use
**paper manufactured
from sustainable forests**

Foreword

I am delighted to be writing this foreword for what is clearly an exciting new text in hepatology. The authors' aim was to provide a fresh and innovative look at the broad spectrum of modern hepatology. Being privy to the proofs of some of the chapters, I have little doubt that they will succeed. It is a multi-authored text but the editors, through their own substantial contributions to hepatology, are in a position to achieve the desired clinically focused approach with a consistent structure for each chapter. The inclusion of a substantial amount of illustrative material of a very high quality is also going to facilitate the consistency of presentation throughout the volume. For the internist, for the trainee fellow in gastroenterology and hepatology in the USA, and the specialist registrar in the UK or their equivalent in other parts of the world, it will surely be an encouragement to have a single volume on clinical liver disease available and with the blessing of only limited referencing to key papers and reviews. A great plus too for this new volume, is that liver transplantation is properly included as a part of modern day practice of hepatology. There will be no need for them to consult a separate volume.

It is an exciting time in hepatology with all the new advances in the treatment as well as in our understanding of the viral hepatitis infections, of autoimmune conditions, and of the major complications of liver disease: ascites, portal hypertention, and encephalopathy. With all the work currently going on, there must be a good anticipation that the tough kernel of temporary liver support for acute liver failure, and for acute episodes of chronic decompensation, will be finally cracked. The prospects of gene therapy with correction of genetic liver disorders, both congenital and acquired as in hepatocellular carcinoma, offer further challenges and excitement to those interested in liver disorders.

In applying these scientific advances to the bedside, the clinically orientated hepatologist will have an essential part to play. At present the number of hepatologists in training is far too small for current practice, let alone future developments. Fortunately, the American Association for the Study of Liver Diseases has already recognized this with its current proposals to extend and enhance the training programme for its fellows in hepatology. One hopes that the UK and other countries will see the necessity of such an approach. This new volume could perhaps mark the beginning of this process.

Professor Roger Williams CBE, MD, FRCS, FRCPE, FRACP, FMedSci, FACP (Hon)

Preface

Hepatology has emerged as a fascinating discipline and is no longer considered a minor component of the practice of gastroenterology. Liver disease always produced an array of challenging clinical scenarios that were complex but ultimately led to the demise of the patient. This position has been transformed by a number of developments including therapeutic advances and liver transplantation. The therapeutic advances have been disease specific, such as antiviral therapy, as well as generic to the complications of end-stage liver disease, for example TIPS or variceal ablation by banding. There is still momentum in this development process and it is feasible that extracorporeal liver assist systems may further alter the management of both acute and chronic liver failure over the forthcoming years. These major advances have been complemented by a huge number of modifications to investigative and management strategies that are largely unheralded but have undoubtedly contributed to the success associated with the modern management of liver disease.

Few doubt that liver transplantation has been the single biggest revolution in the practice of hepatology. The obvious benefit has been the prolonged life span for a substantial proportion of patients with liver disease. The impact of liver transplantation has extended much further into the therapy of liver disease than the management of end-stage disease. Patients with chronic liver disease need to be considered potential candidates for liver transplantation at an early stage and management strategies should be devised that deliver these patients to transplantation in the optimal condition. Surveillance programs are needed to detect complications that transform an ideal candidate for transplantation into a high risk or unsuitable candidate, such as hepatocellular carcinoma in cirrhosis and cholangiocarcinoma in primary sclerosing cholangitis.

Liver transplantation has spawned a new composite specialty incorporating facets of surgical implantation and maintenance of graft function with the implications of immunosuppression and the possibility of recurrence of the liver disease in its original or a modified form. The dramatic increase in the population of liver graft recipients means that more and more clinicians will be exposed to these patients and will need insight into the clinical problems that they pose.

The philosophy of this textbook is to integrate the diverse elements of hepatology in a way that facilitates the clinical management of patients with liver disease. It has been a goal of the editors to treat liver transplantation in the spirit of this philosophy rather than solely as a discrete section at the end of the book as in other textbooks. This has been our interpretation of 'comprehensive'. The practice points are intended to bring out subtleties of clinical expertise or valuable vignettes that can be lost in standard didactic descriptions of liver diseases. The references are deliberately selective in order to highlight the most appropriate sources of further reading against the ever expanding background of printed and electronic information.

The other guiding philosophical principle of this textbook has been the global nature of hepatology. The authors have been drawn from all continents and the editorial process has endeavored to harmonize differences of emphasis that may exist in different parts of the world. The presentation is highly illustrated to facilitate learning. The end product should be attractive to a wide range of clinicians, both in terms of seniority and discipline, who are involved in the management of patients with liver disease.

JGO, JRL, and PDH   2000

Acknowledgements

I would like to acknowledge the immense support of Professor Bernard Portmann for histopathology, and Drs. John Karani and Pauline Kane for Radiology.

JGO

My sincere apreciation to the authors who have so graciously shared their special knowledge and expertise with us. My special thanks also to my wife, Mamiko, and daughters Katrina, Chelsea and Natalie who have provided me unconditional support and love throughout my career.

JRL

I would like to thank Dr. Kris Miloszewski, Consultant Physician; Drs. Ashley Guthrie, Henry Irving and Maria Sheridan, Consultant Radiologists; and Dr. Judy Wyatt, Consultant Histopathologist; of St. James's University Hospital, Leeds, UK for being very willing to provide additional material to illustrate a number of chapters.

PDH

Contents

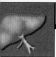

Contributors

Vincente Arroyo
Professor of Medicine
Director Institute for Digestive Diseases
Hospital Universitari Villarroel
Barcelona, Spain

Alistair J Baker
Pediatric Hepatologist
King's College Hospital
London, UK

Eleanor Barnes
Research Fellow
Royal Free and University College Medical
School
London, UK

Nathan M Bass
Professor of Medicine and Attending
Physician
Division of Gastroenterology
University of California
San Francisco
California, USA

Ramón Bataller
Research Fellow
Hospital Clinic Villarroel
Barcelona, Spain

Henri Bismuth
Professor of Surgery
University of Paris
Hopital Paul Brousse
Paris, France

Robert S Brown Jr
Associate Professor of Clinical Medicine
and Pediatrics
Chief of Clinical Hepatology
Medical Director
Columbia College of Physicians
& Surgeons
New York, USA

Henry Lik-Yuen Chan
Research Fellow
Prince of Wales Hospital
Hong Kong, China

Anil Dhanwan
Pediatric Hepatologist
King's College Hospital
London, UK

Rolland C Dickson
Assistant Professor of Medicine
Mayo Clinic
Jacksonville, Florida, USA

Geoffrey Dusheiko
Professor of Medicine
Royal Free and University College
Medical School
London, UK

Jean Crawford Emond
Professor of Surgery
Columbia College of Physicians & Surgeons
Director Center for Liver Disease
New York Presbyterian Hospital
New York, USA

Gregory T Everson
Professor of Medicine
University of Colorado
Denver, Colorado, USA

Guangsheng Fan
Assistant Professor
Division of Gastroenterology
University of Minnesota Medical School
Minneapolis, Minnesota, USA

José Figueiro
Surgeon
University of Paris
Hopital Paul Brousse
Paris, France

Peter J Friend
Professor of Transplantation
John Radcliffe Hospital
Oxford, UK

Pere Ginès
Senior Specialist
Hospital Clinic Villarroel
Barcelona, Spain

Peter C Hayes
Professor of Hepatology
Royal Infirmary of Edinburgh
Edinburgh, UK

J Michael Henderson
Staff Surgeon and Chairman
Cleveland Clinic Foundation
Cleveland, Ohio, USA

Michael A Heneghan
Associate in Medicine
Division of Gastroenterology
Duke University Medical Center
Durham, North Carolina, USA

Shaukat Iftikhar
Instructor of Clinical Medicine
Division of Gastroenterology
Tulane University School of Medicine
New Orleans, Louisiana, USA

Philip J Johnson
Professor and Chairman
Chinese University of Hong Kong
Hong Kong, China

John Karani
Consultant Radiologist
King's College Hospital
London, UK

Deirdre A Kelly
Consultant Paediatric Hepatologist
University of Birmingham
Birmingham, UK

Lawrence S Kim
South Denver Gastroenterology
Eaglewood, Colorado, USA

Milan Kinkhabwala
Assistant Professor of Surgery
New York Presbyterian Hospital
New York, USA

Johannes Koch
Assistant Clinical Professor of Medicine
and Radiology
Director of Endoscopy
San Francisco General Hospital
San Francisco, California, USA

Steven D Lidofsky
Associate Professor of Medicine and
Pharmacology
University of Vermont
Burlington, Vermont, USA

Anna Suk-Fong Lok
Professor of Internal Medicine
University of Michigan Medical Center
Ann Arbor, Michigan, USA

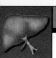

Martin Lombard
Consultant Physician and Honorary
Senior Lecturer
Royal Liverpool University Hospital
Liverpool, UK

Geoffrey W McCaughan
Professor
Royal Prince Alfred Hospital and
University of Sydney
Sydney, Australia

Michael P Manns
Professor of Medicine and Gastroenterology
Medical School of Hannover
Hannover, Germany

Kevin Moore
Senior Lecturer & Honorary Consultant
Gastroenterologist
Royal Free and University College
Medical School
London, UK

Richard H Moseley
Chief of Medicine
VA Medical Center, and
Associate Professor of Medicine
University of Michigan Medical Center
Ann Arbor, Michigan, USA

Andrea R Mueller
Surgeon
Charité Virchon Clinic
Berlin, Germany

Kevin D Mullen
Professor of Medicine
Case Western Reserve University
Cleveland, Ohio, USA

James Neuberger
Professor and Consultant Physician
The Queen Elizabeth Hospital
Birmingham, UK

Peter Neuhaus
Professor of Surgery
Charité Virchon Clinic
Berlin, Germany

Suzanne Norris
Consultant Hepatologist
Kings College Hospital
London, UK

Carlos V Paya
Consultant in Infectious Diseases
Mayo Clinic
Rochester, Minnesota, USA

Klaus-Peter Platz
Surgeon
Charité Virchon Clinic
Berlin, Germany

Bernard C Portmann
Consultant Histopathologist
Institute of Liver Studies
Kings College School of Medicine
London, UK

Richard G Quist
Fellow
Division of Gastroenterology
University of California
San Francisco
California, USA

Fredric Regenstein
Chief of Clinical Hepatology
Clinical Professor of Medicine
and Surgery
Tulane University School of Medicine
New Orleans, Louisiana, USA

Andrew Rhodes
Consultant in Intensive Care Medicine
St. George's Hospital
London, UK

Didier Samuel
Professor of Hepatology
University of Paris
Hopital Paul Brousse
Paris, France

Syed Hasnain Ali Shah
Visiting Specialist Registrar
Department of Medicine
Royal Infirmary of Edinburgh
Edinburgh, UK

Nick Sheron
Senior Lecturer in Medicine
University School of Medicine
Southampton General Hospital
Southampton, UK

Irene G Sia
Infectious Disease Fellow
Mayo Clinic
Rochester, Minnesota, USA

Clifford J Steer
Professor of Medicine and Genetics, Cell
Biology and Development
University of Minnesota Medical School
Minneapolis, Minnesota, USA

Christian P Strassburg
Fellow in Gastroenterology
Medical School of Hannover
Hannover, Germany

M Stuart Tanner
Professor of Pediatrics
University of Sheffield
The Sheffield Children's Hospital
Sheffield, UK

Federico G Villamil
Director of Hepatology
Medical Director, Liver Transplantation
Associate Professor of Medicine
Fundacion Favalord
Unidad de Higado
Buenos Aires, Argentina

David Vogt
Staff Surgeon and Chairman
Cleveland Clinic Foundation
Cleveland, Ohio, USA

George Webster
Clinical Research Fellow
Royal Free and University College Medical
School
London, UK

Julia A Wendon
Senior Lecturer and Consultant Physician
Institute of Liver Studies
King's College School of Medicine
London, UK

Simon Whalley
Research Fellow
Royal Free and University College Medical
School
London, UK

Russell H Wiesner
Medical Director of Liver Transplantation
Mayo Clinic
Rochester, Minnesota, USA

Steven L Zacks
Clinical Assistant Professor of Medicine
University of North Carolina
Durham, North Carolina, USA

Fernanda G Zingale
Hepatology Fellow
Hepatology and Liver Transplantation Unit
Fundacion Favalord
Unidad de Higado
Buenos Aires, Argentina

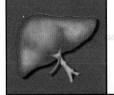

Section 1 Normal Structure and Function

Chapter 1

Anatomy of the Normal Liver

Bernard C Portmann

INTRODUCTION

This introductory chapter illustrates the gross anatomy, blood supply and internal structures of the normal liver. The aim is to emphasize those morphologic aspects that are likely to assist the interpretation of both imaging data and basic pathologic changes observed in the diseased liver. Reference is also made to the morphologic location of the various functions carried out by the liver. The discussion is preceded by a brief account of the development of the liver, in particular the development of both the hepatic vasculature and the intrahepatic bile duct, the latter exemplified by the formation and subsequent involution of the embryonal ductal plate.

DEVELOPMENT OF THE LIVER

The primitive liver appears in the 3-week-old embryo as an endodermal outgrowth from the ventral wall of the foregut, near the yolk sac, in that part destined to become the duodenum. This liver primordium rapidly develops into a diverticulum whose actively proliferating endodermal cells form solid cords; these invade the mesenchyme of the septum transversum which will later form the capsule and connective tissue framework of the liver. The anastomosing cords of primitive cells spread between the vitelline veins and their capillaries so that they enmesh, penetrate, and transform into the primitive sinusoids. Thus in the 4-week-old embryo, an intimate relation between hepatocytes and sinusoids already anticipates the pattern that is characteristic of the adult liver. The caudal part of the hepatic diverticulum remains independent from the invading sheets of primitive hepatocytes to form the epithelial primordium of the cystic duct and gallbladder.

The liver cell plates of the fetal liver are several cells in thickness, and remain so until after birth. The plate is two cells thick by 5 months after birth, the single cell pattern characteristic of the adult liver being established by about 5 years of age. The production of α-fetoprotein by the primitive liver cells starts as early as 4 weeks. Hemopoiesis commences within the liver at about 6 weeks, and by the 12th week the liver is the main site of hemopoiesis in the body, activity which subsides in the 5th month when the bone marrow starts functioning, and which normally ceases within a few weeks of birth.

The hepatic venous system

The vascular arrangement of the fetal liver is given in Figure 1.1.

Initially the hepatic sinusoidal plexus is essentially fed by the paired and symmetrically placed vitelline veins which drain into the sinus venosus (Fig. 1.1a). As the liver rapidly grows, the laterally placed right and left umbilical veins which carry the oxygenated blood and nutrients from the placenta become incorporated to supply the hepatic sinusoidal plexus, a connection which is established by the 5th week (Fig. 1.1b). With the placenta taking over from the yolk sac, the left umbilical vein becomes the principle source of placental blood while the right one disappears. The original vitelline veins give way to a single portal vein, whereas the newly developed ductus venosus provides a bypass channel directly connecting the umbilical vein to the inferior vena cava (Fig. 1.1c). This definitive vascular pattern of the fetal liver is already established in the 7-week embryo (Fig. 1.1d). At birth, blood flow ceases in the umbilical vein, the proximal end of the ductus venosus closes, and the expanding portal vein now takes over the supply of the whole liver, including the left lateral segments (Fig. 1.1e). The obliterated segment of the umbilical vein between the umbilicus and the left portal vein branch regresses to form the ligamentum teres; the ductus venosus becomes a fibrous cord or ligamentum venosum running in and encircling the right side of the caudate lobe.

The duct system and hepatic ductal plate

Bile canaliculi are first identified between the liver cell sheets in the embryo at the 6th week , while bile production begins at 12 weeks. The extrahepatic biliary tree arises from elongation of the original liver diverticulum, which initially forms a solid cord of epithelium continuous at its caudal end with the duodenum and at its cephalic end with the primitive hepatic sheets. Vacuolation later produces a lumen first in the common bile duct, and subsequently in the hepatic duct, cystic duct, and gallbladder.

The intrahepatic ducts in contrast begin to form at about 9–10 weeks, from the hepatocytes in direct contact with the mesenchyme which surrounds the developing and branching portal veins. These first appear as a single layer of flattened cells ensheathing the primitive portal tracts and strongly expressing cytokeratin 19, similar to adult biliary epithelial cells. A second layer then forms showing similar phenotypic change, and with the development of slit-like lumens from 12 weeks onwards, the ductal plate is formed taking the form of a double-cylinder surrounding the developing portal tracts (Fig. 1.2).

Further remodeling of the plate occurs by a subtle interplay of epithelial resorption and mesenchymal ingrowing; the primitive ductal plate thus changes from a circular structure to a network of tubules which then become separated from the parenchyma and incorporated into the portal mesenchyme. Excessive proliferation and arrest or aberrant remodeling of the embryonal ductal plate are likely explanations for various fibrocystic disorders such as autosomal recessive (infantile) polycystic disease, congenital hepatic fibrosis, Caroli's disease, and autosomal dominant (adult) polycystic disease.

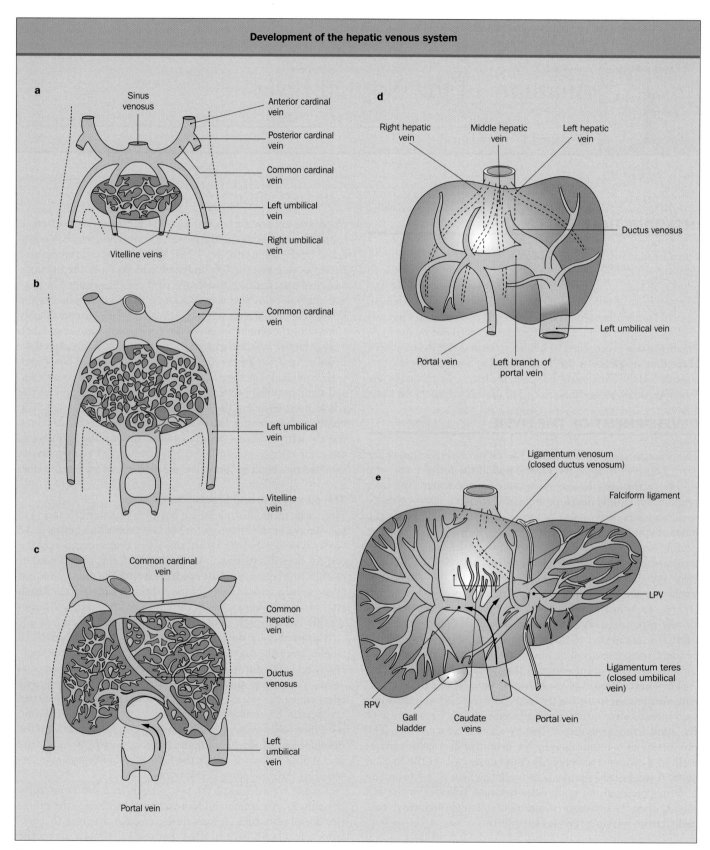

Development of the hepatic venous system

Figure 1.1 Development of the hepatic venous system.
(a) Proliferation of the primitive hepatic plates (brown) into the vitelline vein network to form the primitive sinusoidal plexus which drains into the sinus venosus. (b) Incorporation of the umbilical vessels. (c) Development on the inferior aspect of the liver of a derivation channel – the ductus venosus – that drains directly into the inferior vena cava; partial and total regression of the left and right umbilical veins respectively. (d) The definitive vascular pattern of the fetal liver already established in the 7th week embryo (about 17mm long). (e) Scheme of the hepatic circulation at birth after both closure of the ductus venosus through a sphincter mechanism and cessation of blood flow in the umbilical vein. LPV, left branch of portal vein; RPV, right branch of portal vein.

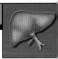

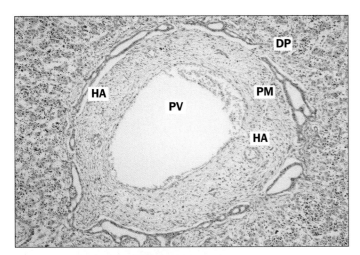

Figure 1.2 The embryonal ductal plate highlighted in a stillborn fetus with autosomal recessive polycystic kidney disease. Note the persistent ductal plate (DP) encircling the portal mesenchyme (PM) with a centrally placed portal vein branch (PV). HA, hepatic arteriole.

GROSS ANATOMY OF THE LIVER

The liver – the largest solid organ in the body with a median weight of approximately 1600g in men and 1400g in women – lies in the right upper quadrant of the abdomen essentially under the protection of the rib cage. Its high location and intimate relationship with neighboring organs are of major importance to clinicians examining patients with liver disease and taking percutaneous needle biopsies (Fig. 1.3):

- Both the right kidney and the right colonic flexure lie in close contact with the inferolateral-lateral surface of the right lobe; the stomach imprints the inferior aspect and margin of the left lobe which extends to variable degrees into the left hypochondrium as far as the left mid-clavicular line.
- The lung and pleural sac overlie the dome of the right lobe for some distance laterally, a disposition which is responsible for respectively dullness and flatness to percussion.
- Only the anterior edge of the liver comes into contact with the anterior abdominal wall below the costal margin and the xiphisternum, where it can be palpated during inspiration.
- The entire liver is covered by the fibrous capsule of Glisson, except posteriorly where it lies in direct contact with the diaphragm, the so-called 'bare area' which is surrounded by reflections of the peritoneum – the coronary and left and right triangular ligaments (Fig. 1.4b and c).

Anatomic landmarks seen on external examination are illustrated in Figure 1.4. On the upper surface, the falciform ligament running anteroposteriorly attaches the liver to the diaphragm and to the anterior abdominal wall. Visually it divides the organ into two uneven lobes, the right lobe being about six times the size of the left; these have no functional significance (Fig. 1.4a). The anterior portion of the falciform ligament – the round ligament (ligamentum teres) – runs within the fissure of the umbilical vein and connects the left branch of the portal vein to the umbilicus (Fig. 1.4b); it contains small vestigial veins that re-open and even become varicose when intrahepatic portal venous block develops secondary to liver cirrhosis. Posteriorly the falciform ligament

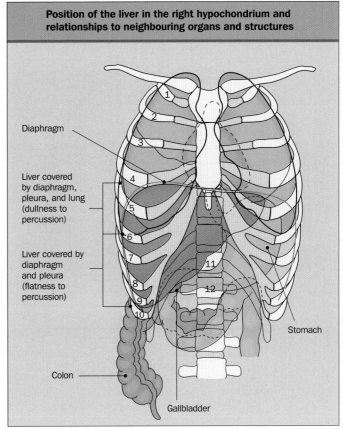

Figure 1.3 Position of the liver in the right hypochondrium and relationships to neighboring organs and structures.

merges with the coronary ligaments surrounding the bare areas (Fig. 1.4c).

On the inferior surface, the caudate lobe bulges posteriorly between the fossa for the ductus venosus and the vena cava. The quadrate lobe lies anteriorly, lined by the gallbladder to its right and the fissure of the umbilical vein to its left (Fig. 1.4b)

Between caudate and quadrate lobes is the porta hepatis. In this deep fissure the portal vein and hepatic artery enter, and bile ducts leave the liver contained in the peritoneal fold of the hepatoduodenal ligament. At that level the Glisson's capsule is reflected inwardly to form the fibrous sheaths that invest the portal vessels and ducts throughout the liver, down to their smallest ramifications, the so-called portal tracts.

Vessels and functional anatomy of the liver
The liver receives 75% of its blood through the portal vein (PV) that carries blood from the entire capillary system of the digestive tract, spleen, pancreas, and gallbladder, and 25% through the hepatic artery (HA), the second major branch of the celiac axis. Functionally, the liver is divided into two roughly equal parts ('true' lobes) on the basis of its blood supply and bile drainage. The line of demarcation between right and left hepatic arterial and portal venous inflow is located along a plane that passes some 4cm to the right of the falciform ligament, joining the tip of the gallbladder to the grove of the vena cava (Fig. 1.4a). The recognition of this plane of demarcation between true left and right lobes is of major importance in staging primary hepatic tumors. The liver can be further divided into eight functional segments

Anterosuperior view

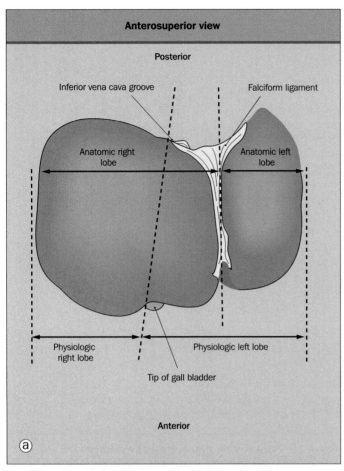

Posterior

Inferior vena cava groove

Falciform ligament

Anatomic right lobe

Anatomic left lobe

Physiologic right lobe

Physiologic left lobe

Tip of gall bladder

Anterior

(a)

Posteroinferior view

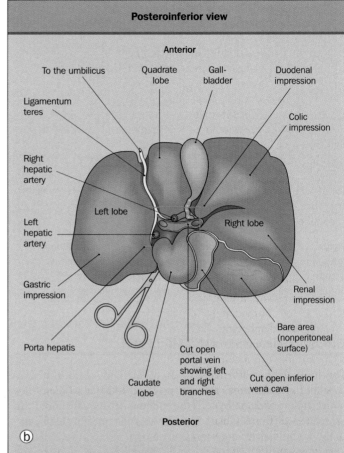

Anterior

To the umbilicus

Quadrate lobe

Gall-bladder

Duodenal impression

Ligamentum teres

Colic impression

Right hepatic artery

Left lobe

Right lobe

Left hepatic artery

Gastric impression

Renal impression

Porta hepatis

Bare area (nonperitoneal surface)

Caudate lobe

Cut open portal vein showing left and right branches

Cut open inferior vena cava

Posterior

(b)

Posterior aspect with the vena cava cut opened

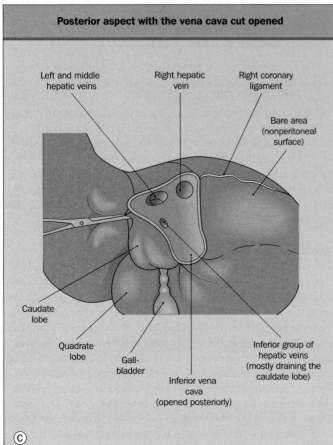

Left and middle hepatic veins

Right hepatic vein

Right coronary ligament

Bare area (nonperitoneal surface)

Caudate lobe

Quadrate lobe

Gall-bladder

Inferior vena cava (opened posteriorly)

Inferior group of hepatic veins (mostly draining the cauldate lobe)

(c)

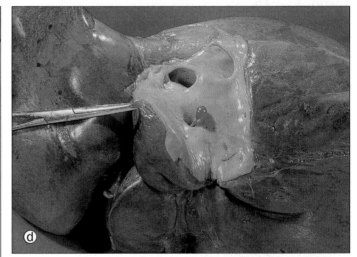

(d)

Figure 1.4 External appearances and surface markings of the liver.
(a) Anterosuperior view. (b) Posteroinferior view. (c & d) Posterior aspect with
the inferior vena cava cut opened to show the outlets of the hepatic veins.

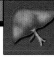

based on vascular distribution as illustrated in Figure 1.5, which follows the terminology of Couinaud, the one favored by most surgeons and radiologists.

The right lobe is divided into anteromedial and posterolateral sectors, each of which has superior and inferior segments, while the left lobe has medial (segment IV) and lateral sectors, the latter divided into anterior (III) and posterior (II) segments. The caudate lobe (or segment I) has its own venous supply and drainage and can be regarded as a separate lobe. The segments do not have surface landmarks or intersegmental septa, but attempts at identifying their boundaries (or fissures) is an essential step prior to any hepatic resection, and during split or reduction procedures of donor livers for transplantation. Important to the surgeon is that the left branches of both afferent vessels supply first the two lateral segments before forming a returning loop to supply the medial segment IV (see Fig. 1.5). This vascular arcade, which is located at the point of attachment of the obliterated umbilical vein, is liable to injury during resection of the left lateral segments.

The venous drainage from the liver operates through the hepatic veins which emerge from the posterior surface of the liver and open immediately into the inferior vena cava just before it pierces the diaphragm. There are three main hepatic veins: the left, the middle and the right, the first two usually joining to form a short stalk with a common outlet (Fig. 1.4c). Inferior vein(s) drain directly the posterior segment of the right lobe and the caudate lobe into the vena cava, allowing the caudate lobe to escape injury and to undergo hypertrophy when the main hepatic veins are occluded (Budd–Chiari syndrome). The hepatic veins are situated in the fissures between the main segments. The main left vein drains the two lateral segments of the left lobe (segments II and III); the middle vein drains segment IV and the anteromedial

sector of the right lobe (segments V and VIII); the right vein drains the remainder of the right lobe (segments VI and VII).

Intrahepatic organization

From the porta hepatis the hepatic artery and portal vein enter the liver invested by a sheath of connective tissue which incorporates bile duct branches. The vessels run parallel, and ramify by dichotomy to form a complex vascular tree in which the terminal branches develop in all directions before emptying into the sinusoids. In addition small perpendicular branches arise along the course of these vessels. A second system – the hepatic vein – runs in the opposite direction with terminal hepatic venules collecting the blood from the sinusoids and forming, by successive unions, larger and larger channels leading to the main hepatic veins. These two tree-like systems interdigitate in such a way that their thin terminal branches run at right angles to each other and remain constantly separated from each other by a layer of parenchyma of about 0.5mm in thickness. A three-dimensional representation of this organization is best illustrated by the stereoscopic reconstruction of Hans Elias (Fig. 1.6).

The various vascular relationships are shown with arterioles and portal venules opening into the sinusoids after piercing the parenchymal limiting plate that ensheathes the portal tract. A similar limiting plate surrounds the hepatic venules which contains fenestrations for the sinusoid outlets. Between supplying and draining vessels the sinusoids draw a complex network tunneling the interconnected liver cell plates (liver muralium), an intimate relationship between blood and cell surface that is essential to the high metabolic activity of the liver. Within the thickness of the plates the bile canaliculi form an anastomosing polygonal network, constantly separated by a half-cell thick layer of cytoplasm from the hepatic sinusoids. The canaliculi drain their content into periportal cholangioles or canals of Hering, which connect canaliculi to the smallest interlobular bile ducts.

Two aspects are of clinical and diagnostic relevance:
- The hepatic arteries give rise to terminal branches feeding the peribiliary plexi; this explains the development of ischemic cholangitis following arterial flow obstruction, for example in the liver allograft and after arterial chemoembolization.
- Inlet venules arise at right angles along the course of the portal vein to feed the parenchyma adjacent to the large portal tracts. In cases of peripheral occlusive venopathy (hepatoportal fibrosis), these venules dilate to produce thin-walled paraportal collateral channels, a diagnostic feature of noncirrhotic portal hypertension.

Functional organization of the liver

Basically there are two different concepts regarding the three-dimensional organization and functional unit of the liver:
- The Kiernan's or classic lobule is organized around a central venule, a terminal tributary of the hepatic vein, and is traditionally represented as hexagonal in outline, the boundaries of which are well-defined by thin interlobular septa of connective tissue in a few species only (Fig. 1.7). In humans, such liver lobules must be delineated by an imaginary line with the portal tracts lying in between the 'corners' of adjacent lobules. This lobular concept has been the basis for describing as centrilobular or perilobular (peripheral) the structural alterations occurring around the hepatic venule or portal tracts respectively. Although convenient for descriptive purposes, the liver

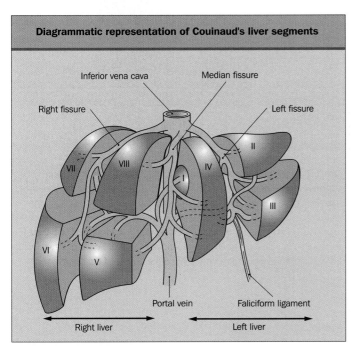

Diagrammatic representation of Couinaud's liver segments

Inferior vena cava   Median fissure

Right fissure   Left fissure

II

VII   VIII   IV

I

III

VI   V

Portal vein   Faliciform ligament

Right liver   Left liver

Figure 1.5 Diagrammatic representation of Couinaud's liver segments. The anterosuperior view is shown, with divisions of the portal and hepatic veins. The divisions of the hepatic artery and bile duct (not shown) closely follow those of the portal vein. The segments are indicated as I: caudate lobe; II, III, and IV left lobe; V, VI, VII, and VIII right lobe.

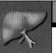

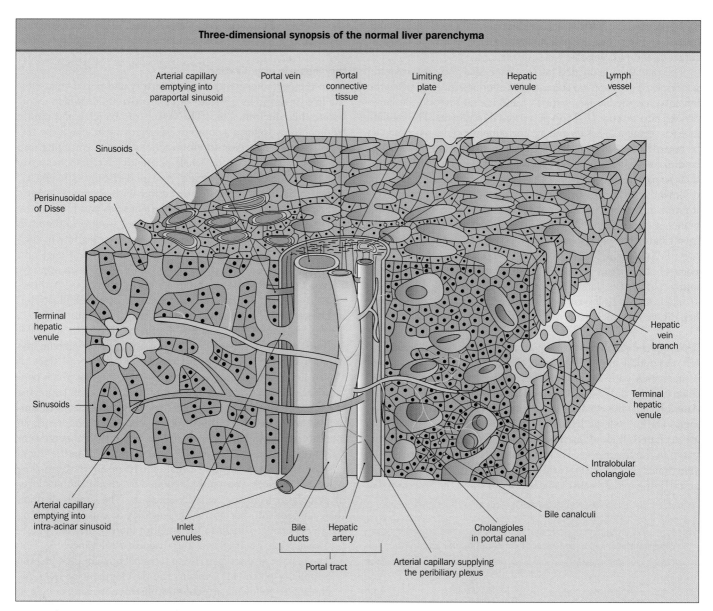

Three-dimensional synopsis of the normal liver parenchyma

Arterial capillary emptying into paraportal sinusoid

Portal vein

Portal connective tissue

Limiting plate

Hepatic venule

Lymph vessel

Sinusoids

Perisinusoidal space of Disse

Terminal hepatic venule

Sinusoids

Arterial capillary emptying into intra-acinar sinusoid

Inlet venules

Bile ducts

Hepatic artery

Portal tract

Arterial capillary supplying the peribiliary plexus

Cholangioles in portal canal

Bile canalculi

Intralobular cholangiole

Terminal hepatic venule

Hepatic vein branch

Figure 1.6 Three-dimensional synopsis of the normal liver parenchyma. Note the inlet venules pearcing the limiting plate to supply portal blood to the parenchyma disposed alongside larger portal tracts and the peribiliary plexus supplied by the hepatic artery. (Modified from Hans Elias, 1949.)

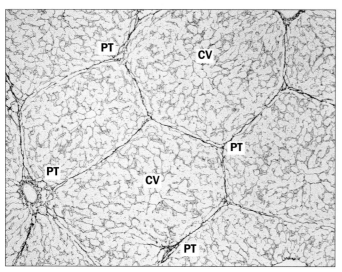

Figure 1.7 Light microscopy of a pig liver showing the traditional hexagonal lobule (Kiernan) outlined by thin fibrous septa. CV, 'central' venule; PT, portal tracts. (Silver stain for reticulin.)

lobule cannot be regarded as a microcirculatory unit, for each lobule is supplied by several terminal hepatic arterioles and portal venules, which also feed portions of adjacent lobules as evidenced in Figure 1.8.

- The liver acinus elegantly demonstrated using injection techniques (Fig. 1.8) is arranged around the terminal branches of the afferent vessels as a pear-shaped cuff of parenchyma lying between and draining into terminal hepatic venules, which in this model become peripheral. The diagrammatic representation of the liver simple acinus, the arbitrary zonation of the liver parenchyma within its boundaries, and the relationships with the classic lobule are illustrated in Figure 1.9.

Three or more simple acini form a complex acinus (Fig. 1.8), a sleeve of parenchyma surrounding the preterminal portal vein and hepatic arterial branches. Several complex acini in turn form part of larger units or acinar agglomerates.

MICROSCOPIC ANATOMY AND ULTRASTRUCTURE

The hepatocyte

Hepatocytes occupy some 80–88% of the total liver volume in humans. The individual hepatocyte is a polyhedral and highly polarized epithelial cell approximately 30–40mm in diameter. The cells are arranged in plates, which appear as 'cords' while seen in two-dimensions under the microscope (Fig. 1.10).

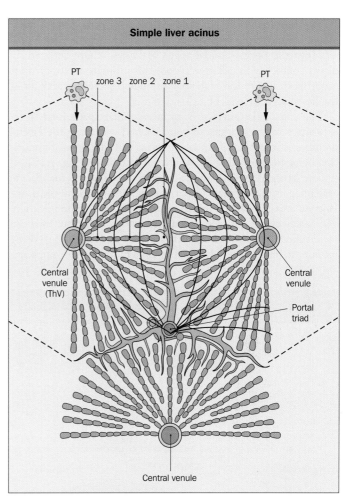

Figure 1.9 Liver simple acinus. Diagrammatic representation with the zonal arrangement of the hepatocytes and two neighboring classic lobules outlined by a discontinuous line. Blood becomes progressively poorer in oxygen and nutrients from zone 1 to zone 3, which thus represents the microcirculatory periphery. The most peripheral portions of zones 3 from adjacent acini form the perivenular area, the so-called centrilobular zone of the 'classic lobule'. PT, portal tract; ThV, terminal hepatic venule (central venule of 'classic lobule'); 1, 2, 3: microcirculatory zones; 1', 2', 3': microcirculatory zones of a neighboring acinus.

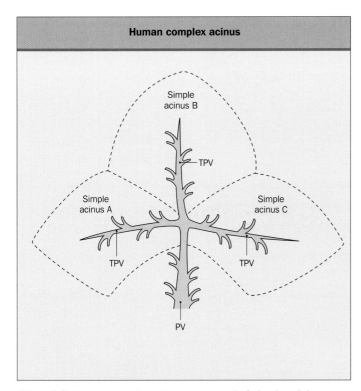

Figure 1.8 Human complex acinus composed of simple acini demonstrated by India ink injection. Three terminal portal venules (TPV) branch out from a preterminal parent stem (PV); each of them irrigates a simple acinus (A, B, and C). (Courtesy of AM Rappaport.)

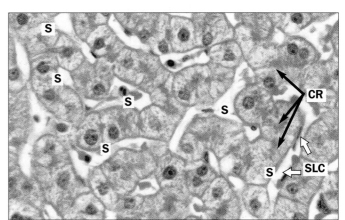

Figure 1.10 Light microscopy of liver cell plates cut longitudinally. Note the centrally placed nuclei, well demarcated sinusoidal membranes with intimately associated sinusoidal lining cells (SLC), intervening sinusoids (S), and the intercellular membranes with canalicular regions (CR) outlined by basophilic cytoplasmic condensation.

The basolateral or sinusoidal surface area is considerably increased due to the presence of numerous microvilli which project into the perisinusoidal space of Disse, where they are in direct contact with cell-free blood; this intimate relationship is essential to secure the high absorption and secretory activity of the hepatocyte (Fig. 1.11).

The canalicular surface is an intercellular space formed by apposition of the margins of a groove half way along the lateral membrane with that of the neighboring cell, the lines of apposition being held together by junctional complexes (Fig. 1.12).

The lateral domain is the flat region of the lateral membrane extending from the canaliculus to the margin of the sinusoidal surface, an area specialized in cell attachment and communication. The canaliculi are not seen in conventional histology, but they can be outlined by histochemical ATPase staining (Fig. 1.13a), or by immunostaining using polyclonal carcinoembryonic antigen; accu-mulation of lipofuscin or hemosiderin at the canalicular pole of the hepatocyte also outlines negatively stained canaliculi (Fig. 1.13b).

The nucleus is large, occupying 5–10% of the cell volume, surrounded with one or more prominent nucleoli. About 25% of hepatocytes are binucleated. Hepatocyte nuclei show a variation in size that reflects polyploidy with corresponding increased DNA content. This increases with age and in pathologic situations.

The marked functional diversity is matched by a great variety of cytoplasmic organelles as listed below and illustrated in Figs 1.11 & 1.14.

The endoplasmic reticulum – a complex network of parallel membranes and cisternae – comprises:
- the rough endoplasmic reticulum (RER), which is more developed in acinar zone 1, has attached polyribosomes, which are sites of protein synthesis including both cell constituent proteins and secretory plasma proteins;

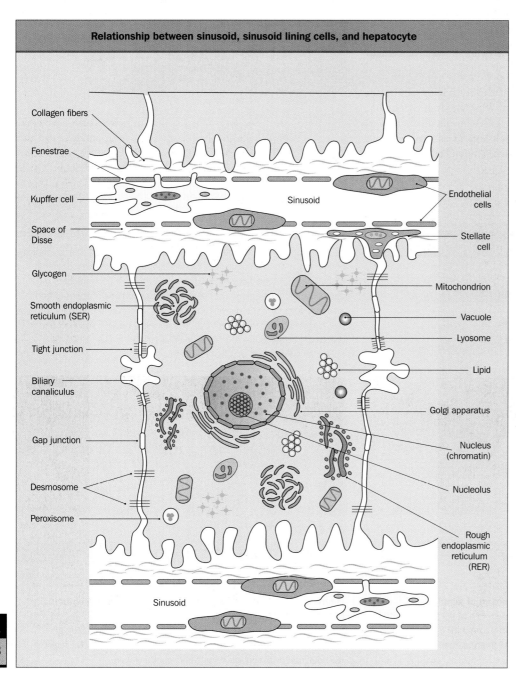

Relationship between sinusoid, sinusoid lining cells, and hepatocyte

Collagen fibers
Fenestrae
Kupffer cell
Space of Disse
Glycogen
Smooth endoplasmic reticulum (SER)
Tight junction
Biliary canaliculus
Gap junction
Desmosome
Peroxisome
Sinusoid
Endothelial cells
Stellate cell
Mitochondrion
Vacuole
Lyosome
Lipid
Golgi apparatus
Nucleus (chromatin)
Nucleolus
Rough endoplasmic reticulum (RER)
Sinusoid

Figure 1.11 Relationship between sinusoid, sinusoid lining cells and hepatocyte. The sketch illustrates the various hepatocyte organelles. Note Kupffer cells of which cytoplasmic processes are anchored in endothelial fenestrae.

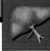

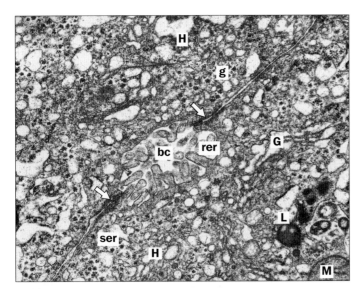

Figure 1.12 Electron micrograph of bile canaliculi (bc), intercellular membranes, and junctional complex. Note appearances of various organelles within the two adjacent hepatocytes (H). Open arrows, tight junctions; G, golgi apparatus; g, glycogen; ser, smooth endoplasmic reticulum; rer, rough endoplasmic reticulum; M, mitochondrion; L, lysosome (× 18000). (Courtesy of P Biloulac-Sage).

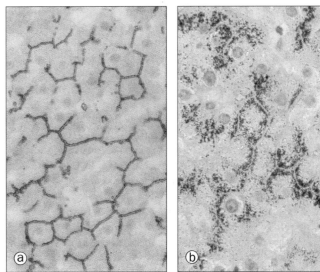

Figure 1.13 Bile canaliculi in light microscopy. (a) Histochemical demonstration of ATPase in pericanalicular cytoplasm. (b) Canalicular network outlined in iron overload due to pericanalicular accumulation of hemosiderin. (Perls' stain.)

- the smooth endoplamic reticulum (SER) of which cisternae are in continuity with those of the RER; here proteins are collected and transported to the Golgi apparatus, where they are packaged in vesicles prior to their export from the cell; the SER is the site of metabolism of xenobiotics, the SER harboring the cytochrome P450 oxidation system whose induction is expressed by a proliferation of SER membranes (see Chapter 29). Other cell functions associated with SER include metabolism of fatty acids, phospholipids and triglycerides, and synthesis of cholesterol and possibly of bile acid.

The mitochondria are particularly numerous in the hepatocytes, their inner membranes and cristae being concerned with the oxidative phosphorylation and fatty acid oxidation whereas their matrix contains the enzymes involved in the citric acid and urea cycles.

The lysosomes, first recognized in the liver, are membrane-bound vesicles that are involved in the digestion and catabolism of various exogenous and endogenous substances, a function that is reflected in their heterogeneous content – for example autophagic vacuoles, storage products, lipofuscin, hemosiderin, and copper complexes. They are rich in acid hydrolase, for example acid phosphatase, which can be used for their histochemical identification; they are involved in a number of storage disorders (see Chapter 22).

The peroxisomes (microbodies) are membrane-bound ovoid bodies that contain oxidases and use molecular oxygen for the production of H_2O_2. This is in turn hydrolysed by peroxisomal catalase, an enzyme that can be used for the ultrastructural identification of these organelles. Peroxisomes are involved in the

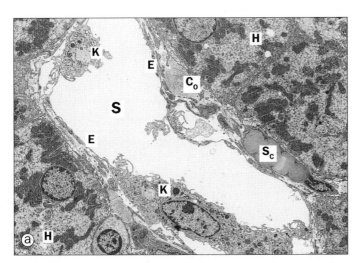

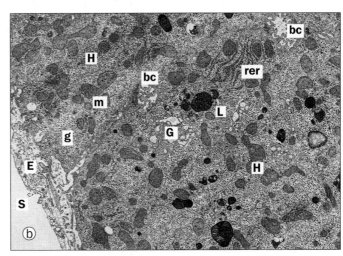

Figure 1.14 Electron micrograph of a sinusoid with its lining cells (a), and hepatocytes with organelles (b). H, hepatocyte; bc, bile canaliculus; m, mitochondrion; L, lyosome; G, golgi apparatus; g, glycogen; rer, rough endoplasmic reticulum; S, sinusoidal lumen; E, endothelial cell; K, Kupffer cell; Sc, hepatic stellate cell; Co, collagen in Disse space. (a) (×2600). (b) (×6400). (Courtesy of P Bioulac-Sage.)

metabolism of fatty acid and alcohol; they proliferate following administration of hypolipidemic drugs, such as clofibrate. The cytoskeleton comprises:

- The microfilaments (6nm) composed of filaments of actin and myosin which, associated in bundles, form a three-dimensional meshwork throughout the cytoplasm; they are attached to the plasma membrane, extend into the microvilli, and are particularly abundant in the pericanalicular ectoplasm, being attached to the junctional complex on either side of the canaliculus; they play a major role in bile secretion and flow regulation, as exemplified by intrahepatic cholestasis produced by drugs that cause depolymerization of the pericanalicular actin belt, in particular cytochalasin B and norethandrolone.
- The intermediate filaments (8–10nm) are a family of self-assembling protein fibers that act as an intracellular scaffold with a role in integrating cytoplasmic space and organelle movement; like in other epithelial cells in the body they react as cytokeratins, more specifically hepatocyte cytokeratins 8 and 18, in contrast to cytokeratins 7 and 19 which characterize biliary epithelium; intermediate filaments contribute to the formation of Mallory bodies as a result of depolymerization in alcoholic and other liver diseases.
- The microtubules (20nm) are hollow, unbranched structures that play a role in cell division (formation of mitotic spindle), in the movement of transport vesicles, and in the transport and export of proteins and lipoproteins.

Glycogen is abundant, reflecting a principal function of the liver in the synthesis of glycogen from glucose, or lactic and pyruvic acid, and its breakdown and release as glucose in the circulation. When depletion occurs, glycogen starts disappearing from the perivenular region. In electron microscopy it appears as dense β particles, 15–30nm in diameter, and α particles, aggregates of the smaller particles arranged in rosettes.

Cells of the hepatic sinusoid

Sinusoids with an average diameter of about 10mm, which may distend to about 30μm, are lined by endothelial cells which delineate the space of Disse running underneath their fenestrated cell process at the sinusoidal surface of the hepatocytes; perisinusoidal cells lie in the space of Disse, the Kupffer cells and liver-associated lymphocytes lie on the luminal aspect of the endothelium (see Figs 1.11 & 1.14).

The endothelial cells form an attenuated cytoplasmic sheet perforated by numerous holes (fenestrae), which constitute the sieve plate. They seem to form no intercellular junctions and do not lie on a basement membrane, a unique configuration that allows free passage of solutes from the sinusoidal lumen into the space of Disse. Unlike vascular endothelium, they do not bind *Ulex europaeus* or express FVIII-related antigen or CD34 in normal human liver, but their membrane is immunoreactive for intercellular adhesion molecule-1 (ICAM-1). The natural ligand for this adhesion molecule, leukocyte function-associated antigen-1 (LFA-1), is present on Kupffer cells. In pathologic situations such as capillarization of the sinusoids in the cirrhotic liver and in benign and malignant hepatocellular neoplasms, they do acquire CD34 immunoreactivity.

The Kupffer cells are members of the mononuclear-phagocytic system forming the largest part of the fixed tissue macrophages in the body. Irregularly stellate in shape, they float freely in the lumen of the sinusoids, anchored by their process to the endothelial cells. Their major function is the clearance of particles, immune complexes, injured red cells, and endotoxins. Their release of mediators, including interleukins 1 and 6, tumor necrosis factor-α (TNF-α), interferons, and eicosanoids, constitutes part of the host response to infection and explains some of the clinical manifestations of endotoxemia. They are immunoreactive to CD68 and express class II histocompatibility antigens, in particular human leukocyte antigen-DR (HLA-DR).

The hepatic stellate cells (perisinusoidal, fat-storing or Ito cells) lie in the space of Disse, their long cytoplasmic processes surrounding the sinusoids. Their nucleus and perykayon is often embedded within recesses between hepatocytes; their cytoplasm contains many small lipid droplets that are rich in vitamin A. Beside their role in the storage of vitamin A, they represent resting fibroblasts which are a major source of extracellular matrix in the normal and diseased liver. Their phenotypic transformation into transitional myofibroblasts in acute and chronic liver disease is associated with the acquisition of α-smooth muscle actin reactivity. Stellate cells are a potential source of hepatocyte growth factor and their contractility has led to a speculative role in controlling sinusoidal blood flow. They are not obvious in conventional light microscopy, but they become evident in semi-thin sections due to their microvesicular fatty cytoplasm (Fig. 1.15).

Liver-associated lymphocytes initially described as pit cells in the rat liver are now well-recognized in human liver. They seem to be recruited from the peripheral blood to the liver sinusoids where they acquire natural and lymphokine-activated killer cell activity.

Other constituent tissues
Extracellular matrix
The connective tissue represents only 5–10% of the normal liver weight, a figure largely below that of the rest of the body, of which 30% of the total proteins is collagen. The components of the extracellular matrix are the structural proteins, of which collagen is the most important, the matrix glycoproteins, and the proteoglycans.

Type I, III, IV, V, and VI collagens are found in the normal liver. Type I and III, which represent more than 95% of the total

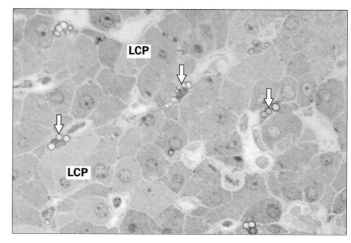

Figure 1.15 Hepatic stellate cells. Semi-thin section of a 2-year-old child liver showing a two cell-thick plate arrangement with nuclei disposed toward the sinusoidal border of the hepatocytes and well-identifiable stellate cells due to their microvesicular cytoplasm (arrowed). LCP: liver cell plate.

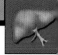

collagen weight, are mainly located in Glisson's capsule and its intrahepatic extension supporting the portal vein, hepatic artery, and bile-duct branches – the portal tracts. Some extension of the capsular tissue accompanies the major hepatic vein branches, but there is no fibrous coat around the terminal hepatic venules which lie in direct contact with perivenular hepatocyte plate (Fig. 1.16a).

Discrete strands of collagen are also present in the space of Disse. Type V collagen is closely associated with smooth muscle cells within vessel walls, and may also form core fibrils upon which growth of large fibrils of type I collagen is initiated. Type VI forms microfilaments which serve as a flexible network that anchors blood vessels and nerves into the surrounding connective tissue. Type IV differs in that its terminal propeptides are not removed, but serve to cross-link the molecule into a three-dimensional lattice. It is an essential component of the vascular and bile duct basement membranes.

The matrix glycoproteins are highly cross-linked and insoluble. They have well-defined domains that interact with cell surface receptors and other components of the extracellular matrix. Laminin is a major component of basement membranes where it interacts with type IV collagen; both components are normally present in small amounts in the space of Disse, where increased deposition is associated with so-called capillarization of the sinusoids. Fibronectin mediates cell adhesion to collagen.

The proteoglycans are macromolecules that consist of a central proteinic core to which proteoglycans and oligosaccharides are attached. They are classified according to the type of glycosaminoglycan. In the liver heparan sulfate is the most abundant, and is present in the portal tracts, in basement membrane, and on the surface of hepatocytes.

The extracellular matrix in the normal liver is considered of major importance in regulating and modulating hepatocyte function in the acinus; it serves to provide cohesiveness between cells, induces cell polarization, allows intercellular communication, and affects gene expression and cellular differentiation.

The extracellular matrix in the acini is confined to the space of Disse. It is of unusually low density and thus invisible ultrastructurally, but visualized in light microscopy after impregnation with a silver method – the so-called reticulin network (Fig. 1.16b).

Lymphatics

The liver is the largest single source of lymph in the body, producing 15–20% of the total volume. Hepatic lymph has a high protein and cell content and is formed mainly by drainage from the perisinusoidal space of Disse into the first-order lymphatic plexus of the portal tracts. Traced towards the portal hepatis, the plexus, composed of flattened endothelial tubes with a primarily periarterial distribution, progressively enlarges, and in larger tracts becomes associated with portal vein and bile duct tributaries. Large collectors are thickened at the porta hepatis due to the acquisition of a muscle layer. They mainly drain into the hepatic nodes, located along the hepatic artery, and celiac nodes. Other efferent routes include: via the falciform ligament and epigastric vessels to the parasternal nodes; from the liver surface to the left gastric nodes; and from the bare area to the posterior mediastinal nodes. In conditions such as portal hypertension there follows a great increase in production of hepatic lymph, with a protein content identical to that of the plasma, indicating unrestricted passage of protein into the space of Disse. There ensues a considerable enlargement of the capsular plexus due to important anastomoses between intrahepatic and capsular lymphatics, with lymph exudating from the capsular plexus to form protein-rich ascites.

Nerve supply

There are two main separate but intercommunicating nerve plexuses around the hepatic artery and portal vein that distribute with the branches of these vessels. These include preganglionic parasympathetic fibers derived from both vagi and sympathetic fibers with cell bodies in the celiac ganglia. Immunohistochemical studies of human liver using antibodies to common neural proteins such as protein gene product (PGP) 9.5 have demonstrated nerve fibers, not only around vessels and bile ducts in the portal tracts, but into the acini, running along the sinusoids. There is evidence that sympathetic nerves play a role in carbohydrate metabolism, and possibly in regulating sinusoidal blood flow.

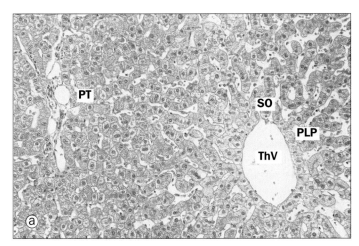

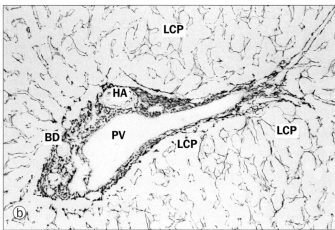

Figure 1.16 Liver histology at low magnification. (a) A terminal portal tract (PT) and a terminal hepatic venule (ThV) are shown, the latter in direct contact with the perivenular hepatocyte limiting plate (PLP). Note two sinusoidal outlets (SO). (b) Silver impregnation to show the reticulin network (black) and a small amount of type I collagen (gold brown) supporting portal vessels and bile duct. HA, hepatic arteriole; PV, portal venule; BD, bile duct; LCP, spaces occupied by liver cell plates.

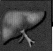
Light microscopy as seen in biopsy specimens

Referring to the three-dimensional model of Elias (see Fig. 1.6) it is easy to extrapolate that the liver cell plates appear as single cell thick anastomosing 'cords' in conventional light microscopy (see Fig. 1.10). These are two-cell thick up to the age of 5 years (see Fig. 1.15), a pattern which in adults reappears as an indication of liver regeneration, sometimes associated with an acinar or rosette arrangement. Hepatocytes appear as polygonal cells with clearly outlined cell margins and centrally placed nuclei which contain one or two nucleoli. There are occasional binucleated cells. Variation in nuclear size increases with increasing age, a pleomorphism that is more marked in acinar zone 2. The cytoplasm is granular and eosinophilic, but slightly basophilic aggregates of RER can be identified in a perinuclear and pericanalicular distribution (see Fig. 1.10). At low magnification relatively regularly spaced portal tracts and hepatic venules are expected (see Fig. 1.16a), but the boundaries between acini or acinar zones are not evident. Thus the sleeve of parenchyma surrounding the portal tracts is referred to as periportal parenchyma or acinar zone 1, the one surrounding the hepatic venules as perivenular parenchyma or acinar zone 3, intermediate areas between these zones being considered as acinar zone 2. Appearances of the portal areas depend on their size and the plane along which they are cut (Fig. 1.17a–c).

However, at any level the size of the arteriole roughly matches that of the bile duct. The portal venules are of variable shape and size, and they are thin-walled, their lumen being generally much larger than that of the corresponding arterial branch. Large tracts (Fig. 1.17c) may show a considerable amount of collagen (Fig. 1.17d), especially around the bile duct, and this can easily be misinterpreted as fibrotic liver.

Intrahepatic and extrahepatic biliary passages

The bile canaliculi, as already described, form a complicated anastomosing network running half-way within the thickness of the liver cell plates. They drain into periportal cholangioles or terminal ductules, also known as canals of Hering, which have a basement membrane and are lined by three to six cells with a variable bile duct or liver cell phenotype. These unite in the smallest portal tracts to form the interlobular bile ducts which are lined by a single layer of flattened cuboid cells (Fig. 1.17a) and by subsequent anastomoses will increase in size from 15–20μm

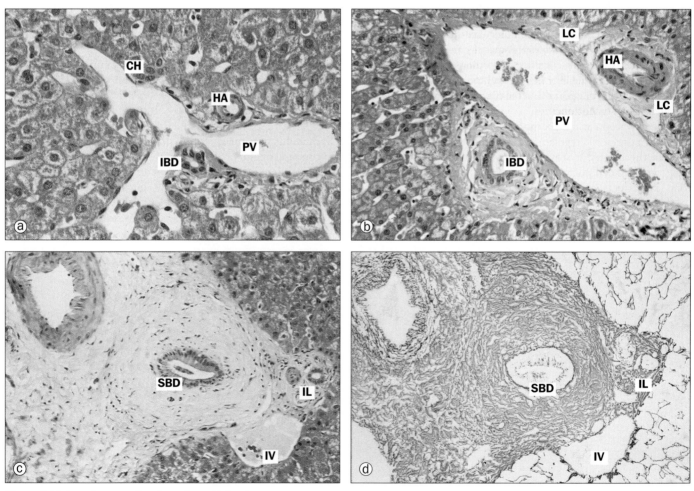

Figure 1.17 Portal tracts of various sizes. (a) Small portal tract with interlobular bile duct (IBD), a size matched arterial branch (HA) and a dividing portal venule (PV). A cholangiole or canal of Hering (CH) is shown. (b) Large interlobular, on the borderline of being a septal bile duct (IBD) with a low columnar epithelial lining. Hepatic arteriole (HA) and lymphatic channel (LC) are seen in the portal area. (c and d) Septal tract giving rise to an interlobular division to the right (IL) and an inlet portal venule (IV). Note the considerable amount of collagen normally surrounding the septal bile duct [SBD (d)].

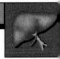

to 100μm to form larger septal (Fig. 1.17c) or segmental bile ducts that are lined by tall columnar cells with basally located nuclei. The portal tract fibrous tissue shows some condensation round these ducts, which through further anastomoses form the large hilar intrahepatic ducts. These are invested with intramural mucinous and extramural seromucinous glands. They anastomose further to give rise to the left and right hepatic ducts, which in turn join to form the common hepatic duct, itself joined by the cystic duct of the gallbladder to become the common bile duct (Fig. 1.18).

The common bile duct runs between the layers of the lesser omentum, lying anterior to the portal vein and to the right of the hepatic artery. It passes behind the first part of the duodenum in a groove on the back of the head of the pancreas, before entering the second part of the duodenum. The duct runs obliquely through the posteromedial duodenal wall, usually joining the main pancreatic duct to form a variable length common channel, the ampulla of Vater. In about 30% of individuals, the bile and pancreatic ducts open separately into the duodenum. The ampulla of Vater makes the duodenal mucous membrane bulge inwards to form an eminence, the duodenal papilla (Fig. 1.18).

During its passage through this collecting system, canalicular bile is modified by a process of absorption and secretion of water and electrolytes, and addition of seromucinous fluid by the peribiliary glands. There is evidence of immunoglobulin A (IgA) secretion by the bile duct epithelium which normally expresses HLA class I, γ-glutamyl transpeptidase (γ-GT), carcinoembryonic antigen (CEA), and epithelial membrane antigen (EMA). These represent phenotypic differences between bile duct epithelium and liver cells additional to their different cytokeratin profiles already mentioned.

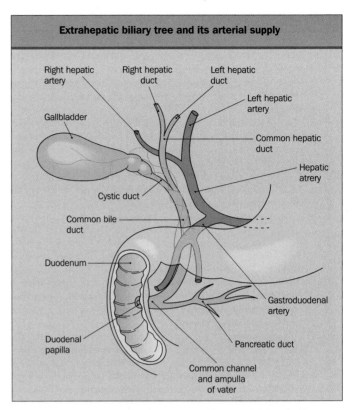

Figure 1.18 Extrahepatic biliary tree and its arterial supply. The gallbladder, cystic, duct and upper portion of the common hepatic and bile duct arterial supply is via the cystic artery and additional small branches that usually arise from the right hepatic artery, although there are several variations recorded. The rest of the common bile duct receives blood from the gastroduodenal artery. There are anastomoses between the two systems, but there may subsist a watershed zone which is important to recognize during the performance of an end-to-end biliary anastomosis at liver transplantation.

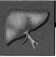

FURTHER READING

Bioulac-Sage P, Saric J, Balabaud C. Microscopic anatomy of the intrahepatic circulatory system. In: Okuda K, Benhamou J-P, eds. Portal hypertension. Clinical and physiological aspects. Tokyo: Springer-Verlag; 1991:13–26. *A comprehensive review of the intrahepatic vascular arrangements.*

Burt AD, Le Bail B, Balabaud C, Bioulac-Sage P. Morphologic investigation of sinusoidal cells. Semin Liver Dis. 1993;13:21–38. *A well documented account of the various cells encountered within the liver sinusoids and their recognised functions.*

Couinaud C. Le foie; études anatomiques et chirurgicales. Paris: Masson et Cie; 1957. *The original study on which the segmental division of the liver is based.*

De Pierre JW, Andersson G, Dallner G. Endoplasmic reticulum and Golgi complex. In: Arias I M, Jakoby WB, Popper H, Schachter D, Shafritz DA, eds. The liver: biology and pathobiology. New York: Raven Press; 1988:165–87. *A detailed review of the structure and function of the endoplasmic reticulum and Golgi complex.*

Elias H. A re-examination of the structure of the mammalian liver. I. Parenchymal architecture. Am J Anat. 1949;84:311–34. *Richly illustrated papers on the structure of the mammalian liver that remain the foundation of current knowledge.*

Elias H. A re-examination of the structure of the mammalian liver. II. The hepatic lobule and its relation to the vascular and biliary system. Am J Anat. 1949;85:379–456. *Richly illustrated papers on the structure of the mammalian liver that remain the foundation of current knowledge.*

Feldmann G. The cytoskeleton of the hepatocyte. Structure and functions. J Hepatol. 1989;8:380–386. *A well written review of the structure and function of the hepatocyte cytoskeleton.*

MacSween RNM, Scothorne RJ. Developmental anatomy and normal structure. In: MacSween RNM, Anthony PP, Scheuer PJ, Burt AD, Portmann BC, eds. Pathology of the liver, 3rd edn. Edinburgh: Churchill Livingstone, 1994:1–49. *A comprehensive and well illustrated account of the development and structure of the liver that has greatly assisted the compilation of this chapter.*

McCluskey RS, Reilley FD. Hepatic microvasculature: dynamic structures and its regulation. Semin Liver Dis. 1992;13:1–12. *Interesting considerations on the dynamic of the hepatic microcirculation.*

Nelson TM, Pollack R, Jonasson O, Abcarian H. Anatomic variants of the celiac, superior mesenteric and inferior mesenteric arteries and their clinical relevance. Clin Anat. 1988;1:75–91. *A summary of the major anatomical variants of the celiac axis and hepatic artery that are relevant to surgeons and radiologists.*

Rappaport M. The microcirculatory acinar concept of normal and pathological hepatic structure. Beitr Pathol. 1976;157:215–43. *The basic article on which the concept of the acinar and three-dimensional organisation of the liver is based.*

Rappaport M. Hepatic blood flow: morphological aspects and physiological regulations. Int Rev Physiol. 1980;21:1–63. *A dynamic demonstration of the hepatic blood flow in relation to the acinar organisation of the liver.*

Rojkind M. Extracellular matrix. In: Arias IM, Jakoby WB, Popper H, Schachter D, Shafritz DA, eds. The liver: biology and pathobiology. New York: Raven Press; 1988:707–16. *A broad review of the structure and function of the extracellular matrix.*

Schuppan D. Structure of the extracellular matrix in normal and fibrotic liver: collagens and glycoproteins. Semin Liver Dis. 1990;10:1–10. *An account of the structure and composition of the extracellular matrix in the normal and fibrotic liver.*

Van Eyken P, Sciot R, Callea F, Van der Steen K, Moerman P, Desmet V. The development of the intrahepatic bile ducts in man: a keratin-immunohistochemical study. Hepatology. 1988;8:1586–95. *A careful study describing the development of the intrahepatic biliary system in a series of human liver specimens throughout gestation.*

Winwood PJ, Arthur MJP. Kupffer cells: their activation and role in animal models of liver injury and human liver disease. Semin Liver Dis. 1993;13:50–59. *A good and clear description of the function of Kupffer cells.*

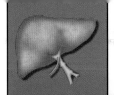

Section 1 Normal Structure and Function

Chapter 2

Cellular Biology of the Normal Liver

Guangsheng Fan and Clifford J Steer

INTRODUCTION

More than 50 years ago, EB Wilson believed that 'the key to every biological problem must finally be sought in the cell.' With the recent dramatic advances in technology and our understanding of cell function, cellular biology of the liver is beginning to take its rightful place as an application to clinical hepatology. In this chapter we present an overview of how hepatic cells are formed and

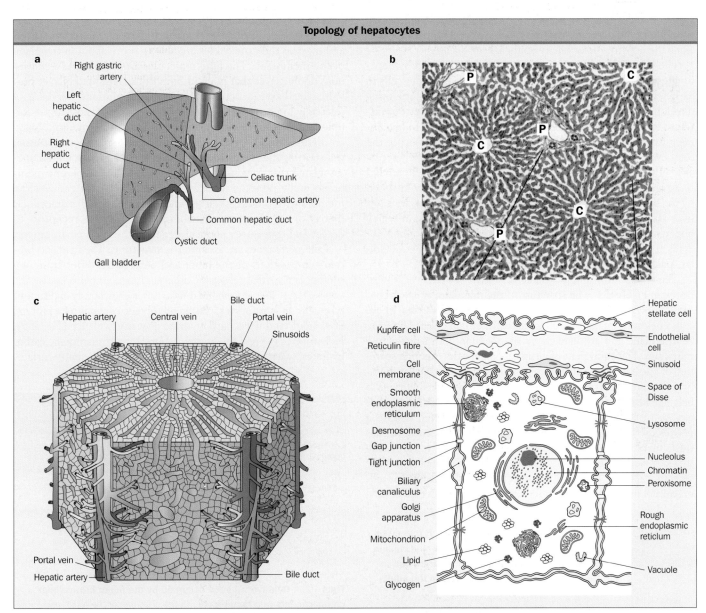

Figure 2.1 The topology of hepatocytes and liver lobules in a normal liver. (a) A cross section of an adult liver. (b) A magnified normal lobular section. The central veins (C) are surrounded by anastomosing cords of block-like hepatocytes. At the periphery of the lobule, typical portal areas (P) consist of branches of the portal vein, the hepatic artery, and the bile duct. (c) A schematic view of the relationship of the different liver cells to each other and to the sinusoids. The principal organelles and inclusions in the cytoplasm are shown. (d) Schematic view of a liver lobule.

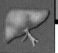

how they function and cooperate to form the amazing liver. In higher organisms, organ systems are like cellular cities in which groups of cells perform specialized functions and are linked by intricate systems of communication. Cells occupy a halfway point in the scale of biologic complexity (Fig. 2.1). A fetal liver has three main cellular compartments, which are:

- parenchymal cells (hepatocytes, bile duct cells);
- sinusoidal cells (endothelial and Kupffer cells); and
- perisinusoidal cells (Ito and hematopoietic cells).

In a human embryo, the hepatic diverticulum consists of a cranial and caudal portion. Hepatocytes develop from the cranial portions, while the caudal bud is the origin of extrahepatic bile duct cells and epithelial cells of the gallbladder. Generally, the proliferation of hepatic cells occurs by diffusion away from the thickening endoderm, but the formation of the extrahepatic ducts always proceeds from the caudal portion of the diverticulum. Studies in rat embryos suggest that the emerging hepatic tissue is composed of bipotential progenitor epithelial cells that are capable of differentiating either along the hepatocytic or biliary epithelial cell lineage.

The formation of intrahepatic bile ducts is initiated by hepatocytes. It has been suggested that the sinusoidal lining cells in early fetuses may be undifferentiated vascular stem cells. During development, these stem cells diverge, with one group committed to becoming an endothelial cell line and a second to becoming a Kupffer cell line. For mammals, the main function of the fetal liver is hematopoiesis, which begins soon after the appearance of the hepatic diverticulum. The hematopoietic cells are initially scattered throughout the liver, but are ultimately replaced by the developing and differentiating adult hepatic cells. An adult liver is occupied by hepatocytes and nonhepatocytes, in which hepatocytes constitute 78% of the tissue volume, nonhepatocytes account for 6.3% of the tissue volume, and the extracellular space for approximately 16% (Fig. 2.2).

The architecture and ultrastructure of the normal liver is illustrated in Figure 2.1. The structure of the muralium simplex consists of polygonal shaped parenchymal cells or hepatocytes. These cells enclose a chicken-wire-like network of bile canaliculi in the central plane and are flanked by sinusoids on both sides of the muralium. The equivalent of an apical pole for the exocrine secretion of bile by the hepatocyte corresponds to the canalicular membrane, which surrounds the parenchymal cell periphery in a belt-like fashion. This structural organization implies that the biliary secretory polarity of the hepatocyte is oriented toward a peripheral ring around the middle of the parenchymal cell. In contrast, metabolic uptake and secretion occur at, or towards, the surfaces facing the sinusoids, implying a bidirectional metabolic secretory activity. This complex secretory polarity requires a well-organized intracellular system for adequate and correct addressing

of secretory products to their respective destinations. Hepatocytes are large polyhedral cells of approximately 20–30μm diameter, which are arrayed in plates one or two cells thick along the hepatic sinusoids (see Fig. 2.1). As a metabolically highly active cell, the hepatocyte contains a vast array of organelles (Fig. 2.3). In human hepatocytes, approximately 30% of the cells are binucleate. While adult parenchymal cells display considerable heterogeneity in size, they all share at least one common constituent. The hepatocyte plasma membrane guarantees separation from but, at the same time, links the cell with its environment and matrix.

HEPATOCELLULAR PLASMA MEMBRANE

The plasma membrane encloses the cell, defines its boundaries, and maintains the essential differences between the cytosol and the extracellular environment. All biologic membranes have a common general structure; each is a very thin film of lipid and protein molecules, held together mainly by noncovalent interactions (Fig. 2.4). Cell membranes are dynamic, fluid structures, and most of their molecules are able to move about in the plane of the membrane. The lipid molecules are arranged as a continuous double layer that is about 5nm thick. This lipid bilayer provides the basic structure of the membrane and serves as a relatively impermeable barrier to the passage of most water-soluble molecules. Protein molecules 'dissolved' in the lipid bilayer mediate most of the other functions of the membrane, transporting specific molecules across it, or catalyzing membrane-associated reactions such as ATP synthesis. In the plasma membrane, some proteins serve as structural links that connect the membrane to the cytoskeleton and/or to either the extracellular matrix or an adjacent cell, while others serve as receptors to detect and transduce chemical signals in the cell's environment.

Cell membranes are asymmetric structures. The lipid and protein compositions of the inner and outer faces differ from one another in ways that reflect the different functions performed at the two surfaces. The protein–lipid ratio varies enormously in different type cells. In hepatocytes, plasma membrane contains 54% protein, 36% lipid, and 10% carbohydrate (by dry weight) (Fig. 2.5). Hepatocytes express the greatest abundance of membrane carbohydrates, where they occur almost exclusively on the outer surface.

Relative number and volume of different cell types in liver		
Cell type	Number (%)	Volume (%)
Hepatocytes	60	78
Nonhepatocytes	40	6.3
Endothelial cells	20	2.8
Kupffer cells	14	2.1
Ito cells	6	1.4
Extracellular space		15.7

Figure 2.2 Relative number and volume of different cell types in the adult liver.

Relative volumes occupied by the major intracellular compartments in a hepatocyte		
Intracellular compartment	Cell volume (%)	Approximate number per cell
Cytosol	54	1
Mitochondria	22	1700
Rough ER cisternae	9	1
Smooth ER cisternae plus Golgi cisternae	6	
Nucleus	6	1
Peroxisomes	1	400
Lysosomes	1	300
Endosomes	1	200

Figure 2.3 Relative volumes occupied by the major intracellular compartments in a hepatocyte. All the cisternae of the rough and smooth endoplasmic reticulum are thought to be joined to form a single large compartment. The Golgi apparatus, in contrast, is organized into a number of discrete sets of stacked cisternae in each cell, and the extent of interconnection between these sets has not been clearly established.

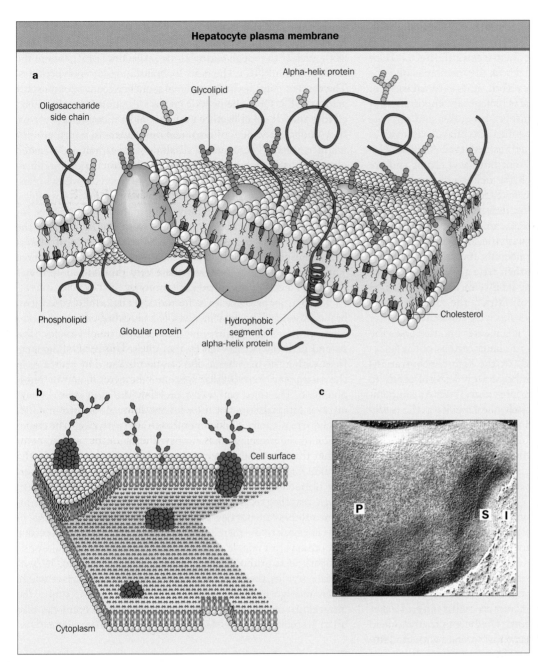

Hepatocyte plasma membrane

a

Oligosaccharide side chain

Glycolipid

Alpha-helix protein

Phospholipid

Globular protein

Hydrophobic segment of alpha-helix protein

Cholesterol

b

Cell surface

Cytoplasm

c

P   S I

Figure 2.4 The hepatocyte plasma membrane. (a) Schematic diagram of the membrane. The phospholipid molecules in the top layer, which faces the external medium, are shown as yellow spheres, each having two wiggly tails. The bottom layer, which faces the cytoplasm inside the cell, has a different phospholipid composition and is also shown in yellow. In some of these transmembrane proteins the polypeptide chain crosses the bilayer as a single α-helix (blue); in others the polypeptide chain crosses the bilayer multiple times, either as a series of α-helices or as a β-sheet in the form of multipass proteins. Other membrane-associated proteins do not span the bilayer but instead are attached to either side of the membrane. Rigid cholesterol molecules (red) tend to keep the tails of the phospholipids relatively fixed and orderly in the regions closest to the hydrophilic heads; the parts of the tails closer to the core of the membrane move about freely. Side chains of sugar molecules attached to proteins and lipids are shown in green. (b) The path followed by a fracture that splits a membrane into bilayers. (c) The membrane structure visible in a freeze-fracture preparation. P, membrane particles in bilayer; S, external membrane surface; I, ice crystals. [Part (a) from Bretscher MS. The molecules of the cell membrane. Scientific American. 1985;253:100–8. Parts (b) and (c) from Wolfe SL, ed. Molecular and cell biology, Belmont, CA: Wadsworth; 1993.]

Lipid, protein, and carbohydrate content in cellular membranes

Membrane	Dry mass (%)		
	Protein	Lipid	Carbohydrate
Plasma membrane	54	36	10
Nuclear envelope	66	32	2
Endoplasmic reticulum	62	27	10
Golgi complex	64	26	10
Mitochondrion outer membrane	55	45	trace
inner membrane	78	22	

Figure 2.5 Lipid, protein, and carbohydrate content in cellular membranes.

Membrane lipids

Lipid contribution to membranes is highly varied depending on the species and cell type. However, in most eukaryotic cells, there are three major classes of membrane lipid molecules: phospholipids, cholesterol, and glycolipids. Hydrophobic interactions between the fatty acyl chains of glycolipid and phospholipid molecules create a sheet that contains two layers of the amphipathic phospholipid molecules. The polar head groups face the surrounding water and the fatty acyl chains form a continuous hydrophobic interior. In such a lamellar structure, each layer of phospholipid is called a *leaflet*. In addition, the lipid compositions of the inner and outer leaflets are different. Most types of lipid molecules rarely flip-flop spontaneously from one monolayer to the other. The most complex of the glycolipids, gangliosides, contain oligosaccharides with one or more sialic acid residues, which give gangliosides a net negative charge. The glycolipids may serve as receptors for normal extracellular molecules that mediate cell-recognition

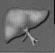

processes and protection of the membrane from the harsh conditions, and assist cells in binding to the extracellular matrix. Charged glycolipids may be important for their electrical effects. Their presence alters the electrical field across the membrane and the concentrations of ions, especially calcium, at its external surface.

The fluidity of a cell membrane is biologically important. For example, certain membrane transport processes and enzyme activities can be shown to cease when the bilayer viscosity is experimentally increased beyond a threshold level. All cell membranes contain a mixture of different fatty acyl chains and are fluid at the temperature at which the cell is grown and functions. Membrane cholesterol is a major determinant of bilayer fluidity. Cholesterol is too hydrophobic to form a sheet structure of its own, but it intercalates, or inserts, among phospholipids. Its polar hydroxyl group is in contact with the aqueous solution near the polar head groups of the phospholipids; the steroid ring interacts with and tends to immobilize their fatty acyl chains. The net effect of cholesterol on membrane fluidity varies, depending on the lipid composition. Cholesterol restricts the random movement of portions of the fatty acyl chains lying closest to the outer surfaces of the leaflets. However, it separates and disperses the tails of the fatty acyls and causes the inner regions of the bilayer to become slightly more fluid. At the high concentrations found in eukaryotic plasma membranes, cholesterol tends to restrict fluidity at growth temperatures near 37°C. At temperatures below the *phase transition*, cholesterol maintains the membrane in a fluid state by preventing the hydrocarbon fatty acyl chains of the membrane lipids from binding to each other. This offsets the drastic reduction in fluidity that would otherwise occur at low temperatures.

Membrane proteins

Whereas the lipid bilayer determines the basic structure of biologic membranes, proteins are responsible for most membrane functions, serving as specific receptors, enzymes, transport proteins, and so on. Most membranes contain 10–50 different major protein types with molecular masses ranging from 10kDa to more than 250kDa. Proteins that extend or are buried into the hydrophobic interior of the lipid bilayer are called *integral membrane proteins*, or *intrinsic proteins*. They contain amino acid residues with hydrophobic side chains that interact with the fatty acyl groups of the membrane phospholipids. These proteins can be removed only by the action of detergents, which displace the lipids bound to the hydrophobic side chains anchoring the membrane proteins. In contrast, *peripheral membrane proteins*, or *extrinsic proteins*, attach by noncovalently binding to other membrane components. Typically, they can be released from the membrane by solutions of high or low ionic strength or extreme pH.

To function correctly, membrane proteins must be properly oriented to the phospholipid bilayer. In contrast to membrane-associated proteins, only those that are transmembrane can function on both sides of the bilayer. The polypeptide chain of transmembrane proteins crosses the bilayer as a single α helix; in others, the polypeptide chain crosses the bilayer multiple times, either as a series of α helices or as a β sheet in the form of a closed barrel. Many membrane proteins are able to diffuse rapidly in the plane of the membrane including *rotational diffusion* (rotation about an axis perpendicular to the plane of the bilayer) and *lateral diffusion*. However, most membrane proteins do not tumble (*flip-flop*) across the bilayer.

Biogenesis and turnover

Most membrane proteins are synthesized on the membrane-bound ribosomes of the rough endoplasmic reticulum (RER), where the sequence of mRNA is the basis for translation into polypeptides. The nascent peptides utilize a signal sequence to initiate transport across the ER. Once the peptide chains are cotranslationally inserted into the ER, an obligatory event for most membrane proteins, they undergo a variety of chemical modifications, which are primarily covalent. These include disulfide bond formation, N-linked oligosaccharide maturation, O-linked oligosaccharide modification, fatty acid acylation and acetylation, addition of glycosyl-phosphatidylinositol (GPI) anchors, phosphorylation, proteolytic cleavage, and subunit assembly. The maturation pathway for plasma membrane proteins continues from the ER through the Golgi network to the cell surface. The concentration of plasma membrane proteins is affected by their biogenesis and degradation. The dynamic balance between these two processes determines the actual levels of the membrane proteins.

Three major pathways exist for the degradation of plasma membrane proteins. The first involves the shedding of intact membrane proteins along with phospholipids as small vesicles. The second pathway is triggered by the release of peptide fragments from within the membrane and can be mediated by proteases in the membrane, extracellular space, or the cytosol, and by phospholipase. The third pathway is probably the most common and involves internalization of the proteins through receptor-mediated endocytosis and/or bulky membrane internalization. The degradation of the proteins can be initiated either in the endosome or within the lysosome. After endosomal breakdown, the released peptide fragments either can be delivered to the lysosome for further degradation or released into the extracellular space through vesicle recycling to the cell surface. Therefore, many plasma membrane proteins are not degraded and simply undergo diacytosis, or recycling back to the membrane. In hepatocytes, receptor recycling is common after release of ligands in the more mature endosomal compartments. Although the ligand is frequently degraded by lysosomal enzymes, the receptor cycles back to the cell surface where it can undergo another round of endocytosis. As an example, the intracellular trafficking of an asialoglycoprotein receptor can take up to 10 minutes to recycle back to the plasma membrane.

Plasma membrane domains

The surface membrane of the hepatocyte is a complex structure. It has three specialized domains:
- the bile canalicular domain accounts for 13% of the cell surface, forms the microvilli, and functions in the secretion of bile;
- the intercellular domain makes up 50% and contains desmosomes, tight junctions for cell adhesion, and gap junctions for cell–cell communication; and
- the sinusoidal domain, which accounts for 37% of the membrane, also forms microvilli, and is the site of extensive interaction with the blood, such as secretion of plasma proteins.

The sinusoidal membrane domain represents a cellular frontier with remarkably active trafficking of molecules in and out of the cell. It is the site of numerous proteins involved in an array of processes including receptor-mediated endocytosis, channel formation, transporters, pinocytosis, as well as phagocytosis. With its highly specific domains, the hepatocellular plasma membrane reflects the polarity of the parenchymal cell.

CELL SURFACE AND INTERCELLULAR JUNCTIONS

Cell coat

In eukaryotic cells, the majority of plasma membrane proteins are not totally exposed on the cell surface. In fact, they are decorated and clothed by carbohydrates. These carbohydrates occur both as oligosaccharide chains covalently bound to membrane proteins and lipids, and as polysaccharide chains of *integral membrane* molecules. They are often described as a *cell coat* or *glycocalyx*. Proteoglycans, which consist of long polysaccharide chains linked covalently to a protein core, are found mainly outside of the cell. The oligosaccharide side chains of glycoproteins and glycolipids are enormously diverse in their arrangement of sugars. Although they usually contain fewer than 15 sugar residues, they are often branched, and the sugars can be bonded together by a variety of covalent linkages. Even three sugar residues can be assembled to form hundreds of different trisaccharides. In principle, both the diversity and the exposed position of these oligosaccharides on the cell surface make them especially well-suited to function in specific cell-recognition processes. The role of the cell coat is not merely to protect against mechanical and chemical damage, but also to keep foreign objects and other cells at a distance, preventing undesirable protein–protein interactions. Plasma membrane-bound lectins have been identified that recognize specific oligosaccharides on cell-surface glycolipids and glycoproteins, and mediate a variety of specific, transient, cell–cell adhesion events.

Hepatocyte surface

The hepatocyte is a polyhedral and multipolar cell (see Fig. 2.1). Most hepatocytes have two or three noncontiguous basal surfaces exposed to the perisinusoidal space of Disse. The lateral surface of the hepatocyte is typically divided by grooves of apical surface, which forms a segment of bile canaliculus. The apical and basal surfaces have irregular microvilli that amplify their areas three- and six-fold, respectively, over their hypothetical smooth counterparts. The basal surface is specialized for exchange of metabolites with the blood. This includes transport of small molecules across the basal membrane, secretion of plasma proteins via fusion of secretory vesicles with the basal membrane, and internalization of circulating macromolecules via clathrin-coated pits and vesicles. The lateral surface shares most of the functions of the sinusoidal front (basal surface) and additionally is specialized for cell attachments and cell–cell communication. The bile canaliculi are sealed off from the remainder of the intercellular space by junctional complexes placed at the boundaries between the lateral and apical surface of the hepatocytes. The junctional complexes contain tight junctions, adherens or intermediate junctions, and desmosomes like those of simple epithelia. Additional desmosomes and plaques of gap junctions can also be found distributed along the lateral surfaces of hepatocytes. The specialized functions of the bile canalicular (apical) membrane include transport of bile acids and products of detoxification across the membrane bilayer into bile, release/transport of lipids at the basal surface, and delivery of secretory immunoglobulin A to bile via fusion of transport vesicles with the apical membrane.

Cell polarity

Hepatocyte polarity is established at an early stage in the developing liver and the constituents of both the apical and basolateral domains appear at different rates. In contrast, in the regenerating liver, the hepatocyte retains its plasma membrane domains throughout the regenerative process, even during mitosis and cytokinesis when extensive rearrangements in microtubules and microfilaments occur. The membrane comprising the cleavage furrow of dividing hepatocytes is most often basolateral, which avoids potential problems that would arise from the joining of sinusoidal and bile canalicular lumina and the mixing of blood and bile. Moreover, it guarantees that bile canalicular domains are inherited by both daughter cells. Therefore, hepatocyte polarity is maintained with high fidelity during cell division. However, about 30% of hepatocytes appear to divide between basolateral and apical (bile canalicular) domains, which yields acinar arrangements of hepatocytes, like those that have been observed in both regenerating and developing livers. The new tight junctions form between the daughter cells on the basolateral side at the completion of cytokinesis, which prevents the joining of sinusoidal and bile canalicular lumina. In addition, hepatocyte surface polarity is also maintained in the face of the continued synthesis, delivery, removal, recycling, and degradation of the many protein components that make up each plasma membrane domain.

Cell junction

Many cells in tissues are linked to one another and to the extracellular matrix at specialized contact sites called *cell junctions*. As described above, the plasma membrane of hepatocytes is differentiated into sinusoidal, lateral, and bile canalicular domains. The lateral domain contains several junctional structures. In general, cell junctions fall into three functional classes: occluding, anchoring, and communicating junctions.

Tight junctions are occluding junctions that play a critical role in forming gasket-like seals as a permeability barrier. They maintain the concentration differences of small hydrophilic molecules across epithelial cell sheets and hepatocytes by sealing the plasma membranes of adjacent cells to create a continuous, impermeable, or semipermeable barrier to diffusion across the cell sheet; and by acting as barriers in the lipid bilayer to restrict the diffusion of membrane transport proteins between the apical and the basolateral domains of the plasma membrane in each cell. Desmosomes are specialized membrane structures that anchor intermediate filaments to the plasma membrane and link cells together. Eight major polypeptides have been identified in desmosomes. Four of the polypeptides are present on their cytoplasmic side, including desmoplakins I and II, plakoglobin, and band 6, a 76kDa polypeptide. Four of them are integral membrane proteins, including desmoglein, desmocolins I and II, and a 22kDa polypeptide. These integral proteins form the desmosomal adhesive structure. Desmoglein shares extensive sequence homology to the cadherin class of calcium-dependent cell adhesion molecules.

Gap junctions are communicating regions that play an important role in cell–cell communication. They consist of clusters of channel proteins that allow molecules smaller than 1kDa to pass directly from one cell to another. In liver, gap junctions occupy as much as 3% of the total membrane surface. Electron micrographs of stained, isolated gap junctions reveal a lattice of hexagonal particles with hollow cores as intercellular channels (Fig. 2.6). Each hexagonal particle consists of 12 *connexin* molecules: six formed in a hexagonal cylinder in one plasma membrane joined to six arranged in the same array in the adjacent cell membrane. The assemblage of the six connexin subunits is termed a *connexon* (Fig. 2.6b). The subunits make up a single cylinder and are radially symmetric around the central pore, and each is tilted

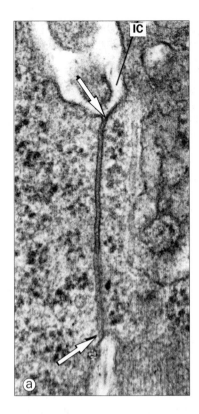

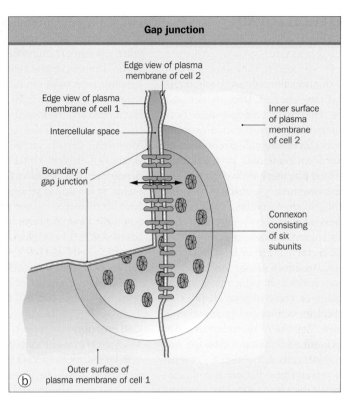

Figure 2.6 The gap junction.
(a) Electron micrograph showing the plasma membranes of two adjoining cells forming a gap junction. The unit membranes (arrows) approach one another narrowing the intercellular space to produce a 2nm-wide gap. IC, intercellular space. (b) Model of a gap junction showing the membranes of adjoining cells creating the 2nm gap and the structural components of the membrane that form channels or passageways between the two cells (double-headed arrow). The circular array of six subunits forms the basic connexon unit. (From Staehelin LA, Hull BE. Junctions between living cells. Sci Am. 1978;238:140–53.)

slightly relative to the plane of the membrane. They can interact in two different but related ways, by either opening or closing a channel. The cDNA encoding the subunit proteins of the hepatocyte gap junction channel have now been cloned and sequenced. At least two connexin proteins have been identified. Connexin 32 (Cx32) has a predicted molecular mass of about 32kDa, while connexin 26 (Cx26) is approximately 26kDa. It is well-established that gap junctions are involved in nutrient exchange, cell regulation, conduction of electrical impulses, development and differentiation, and synchronization and integration of cellular activities.

CYTOPLASMIC ORGANIZATION

Cytoskeleton

The cytoskeleton of the liver cell provides an important motor force for maintaining cell polarity, as well as for intracellular movement and transport of molecules. It also supports the organization of subcellular organelles that are located in functional positions within the differentiated hepatocyte. The cytoskeleton of the hepatocyte includes three basic filamentous components known as, microfilaments, microtubules, and intermediate filaments, together with cytoskeletal-associated proteins that play important roles in the dynamic movement and interaction of these filaments.

Intermediate filaments are the major components of the cytoskeleton. They are strong, rope-like polymers of fibrous polypeptides that resist stretch and play a structural or tension-bearing role in the cells (Fig. 2.7).

Intermediate filaments consist of five main types: cytokeratins, vimentin, desmin, lamins, neurofilaments, and glial filament acid protein. Liver cells *in vivo* only express the cytokeratins and lamins. However, vimentin can be expressed by hepatocytes in long-term tissue culture, and neurofilament proteins are found in injured hepatocytes and form Mallory bodies. Cytokeratins are het-

eropolymers that consist of two different coexpressed monomers with either an acidic or neutral-basic isoelectric pH. Hepatocytes express two cytokeratins: CK8, a basic protein with an isoelectric pH of 6.1 and molecular mass of 52.5kDa; and CK18, an acidic protein with an isoelectric pH of 5.7 and a molecular size of

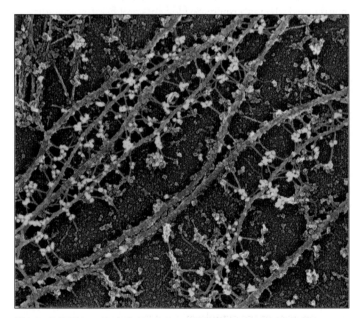

Figure 2.7 The cytoskeleton. Intermediate filaments interact with microtubules via numerous sidearms made of plectin. Electron micrograph of actin-depleted fibroblast cytoskeleton was digitally colorized to assist visualization of intermediate filaments (blue), microtubules (red), and plectin bridges (green) immunolabeled with 10nm colloidal gold (lime). (From Svitkina TM, Verhovsky AB, Borisy GG. Plectin sidearms mediate interaction of intermediate filaments with microtubules and other components of the microskeleton. J Cell Biol. 1996;135:991–1007.)

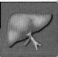

45kDa. Bile duct epithelium expresses not only these two cytokeratins but also CK19, an acidic protein with a molecular mass of 40kDa and an isoelectric pH of 5.2, and CK7, with an isoelectric pH of 6 and a molecular mass of 54kDa. The intermediate filaments of hepatocytes interact extensively with each other, the plasma membrane at the desmosomes, the membrane skeleton at the centrosomes, the nuclear lamina, mitochondria, microfilaments, and microtubules to form a supramolecular organizational state within the cell. In hepatocytes, cytokeratin filaments appear to maintain cell polarity, the adhesion plaques, the structure of the canaliculus, the localization of microfilaments at the canaliculus, endocytosis, and bile canalicular secretion of anions.

Microtubules within hepatocytes are found throughout the cytoplasm, including the perinuclear area, the centrosome, and along the plasma membrane. Morphometric analysis of electron micrographs of liver cells indicate that microtubules are more numerous in the vicinity of the Golgi area and close to the sinusoidal plasma membrane. Microtubules consist of polymerized dimers of α and β tubulins, which are in reversible equilibrium with free tubulin. They are polarized hollow cylindric structures with an outer diameter of 24nm and a 6nm thick wall. The cylindric nature of microtubules may confer rigidity, which contributes to cell shape and polarity. Side arms attached to microtubules exist between microtubules and intermediate filaments, actin filaments, and plasma membranes. The function of microtubules in the liver has been assessed using drugs that depolymerize microtubules. For instance, colchicine inhibits the secretion of plasma proteins by the liver without changing the rate of protein synthesis. These proteins include lipoprotein, albumin, retinol-binding protein, secretory component, fibrinogen, and other glycoproteins. Microtubules play a role in cellular organization through interaction with the Golgi apparatus and other cytoskeletal elements in the cytoplasmic matrix, including intermediate filaments and F-actin. In addition, they have been demonstrated to maintain the integrity of the canalicular plasma membrane during canalicular contraction. The integrity of the microtubular system is necessary for diacytosis, or retroendocytosis. Recent studies revealed that the loss of microtubules in the hepatocytes *in vivo* results in the retention of export proteins as the result of a block in the secretory apparatus such as Golgi complexes. Three motor proteins of cytoplasmic microtubules, which are associated with secretion and vesicle movement, have been identified primarily as kinesin, dynein, and dynamin. Kinesin, an ATPase active molecule, regulates gliding to the (−) end of microtubules by hydrolyzing ATP at both ends of the molecule. In contrast, cytoplasmic dynein promotes gliding toward the (+) end. Dynein also plays a role in retrograde organelle transport, including the endocytic pathway and Golgi apparatus organization. Kinesin and dynein may function as cross-bridges between microtubules and the membranes of organelles, and in this way provide the motor force for vesicle transport in hepatocytes.

Microfilaments, composed of F-actin, are associated with the plasma membrane and provide the physical basis for the mechanical properties of the cytoplasmic matrix and can be displayed by phalloidin-fluorescence-labeling (Fig. 2.8). F-actin has been shown by electron microscopy to be attached to isolated bile canalicular membrane together with intermediate filaments. However, by biochemical analysis most actin is associated with the lateral membrane fraction in liver. The F-actin filament is a double-helical strand comprising polymerized G-actin monomers. Actin polymers have two ends, referred to as barbed and pointed, based on the

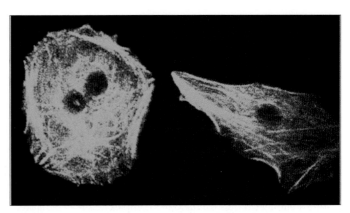

Figure 2.8 Actin filaments. Immunofluorescence of actin filaments in isolated primary hepatocytes with either one (right) or two (left) nuclei. Cultured primary hepatocytes were stained with antiactin FITC-labeled antibody (green). (Courtesy of X-H Zhang and J-G Aguilar).

polarity of myosin S-1 subunit decoration. Association of subunits at both ends of the actin filament is rapid, but subunit dissociation is slower. A large number of actin-binding proteins have been characterized and divided into five classes and nine major families. Examples of these are the profolins, which interact with monomeric actin; the cofilins and destrin, which depolymerize actin; the α-actinin family, which includes the fimbrins and human α-actinin, dystrophin, and spectrin; the myosin family; the caldesmon family; gelsolin and related proteins such as the villins; the tropomysins; neuronal synapsins; and a family of capping proteins. The dynamics of actin-binding proteins include the control of the cellular actin monomer pool, the sequestering, polymerization, and/or depolymerization of actin, the cross-linking of actin filaments, the binding of actin to cell membranes or other organelles, and the splicing of actin filaments. In addition, competing actin-binding proteins may provide a means of actin regulation. The roles of actin in the liver include facilitating bile canalicular contraction, participating in the control of tight junction permeability, and involvement in the integrity, composition, and characteristics of the cell matrix. Moreover, a large number of cellular functions are dependent on actin filaments, including receptor-mediated endocytosis and various transport processes.

Endoplasmic reticulum

Much of the cellular sorting and distribution system of proteins is through the endoplasmic reticulum (ER) and Golgi complexes. After synthesis and initial processing in the ER, proteins are transported to the Golgi complex where the majority are chemically modified before being sorted into vesicles and carried to their final destinations. The ER is a collection of membranous tubules, vesicles, and flattened sacs that extends throughout the cytoplasm of eukaryotic cells. It is the source of all membranes within the cell and the largest intracellular membrane compartment. Endoplasmic reticulum membranes are continuous and unbroken, and enclose a *lumen* or channel that is separate from the surrounding cytoplasm. The surface membrane of the *rough ER* is distinguished by the presence of ribosomes facing the surrounding cytoplasm. It is the site of synthesis, folding, assembly, and cotranslational membrane translocation of proteins. In contrast, the *smooth ER* has no ribosomes and functions in lipid biosynthesis, detoxification, and calcium regulation. Rough ER commonly extends into large, flattened

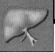
sacs called *cisternae*. Smooth ER membranes form primarily tubular sacs that are generally smaller in dimension than rough ER cisternae. At some points the smooth and rough ER membranes may connect, forming a continuous, inner channel enclosed by the two systems. In addition to the rough and smooth ER, there are at least four other morphologically distinct domains of the ER, including the nuclear envelope, transitional elements, crystalloid ER, and luminal ER bodies containing protein aggregates. Each of these domains perform distinct functions (Fig. 2.9).

Golgi complex

All newly synthesized proteins that are exported out of the ER system are funneled through the Golgi complex before being sorted to different final destinations within the cell. A Golgi complex consists of a localized stack of flattened, sac-like membranes. The ribosomes are characteristically absent from Golgi membranes as well as the spaces between and immediately surrounding the Golgi sacs. An entire Golgi complex often appears to be cup-shaped in cross-section, giving the structure convex and concave faces. The individual sacs of a Golgi complex, called *cisternae*, as in the ER, are typically dilated or swollen at their margins. Dispersed around the Golgi cisternae are numerous vesicles of varying sizes. Some of these bud from or fuse with the edges of the cisternae. Golgi complexes are usually closely associated with the rough ER, separated only by a layer of small, protein-filled vesicles. Some of these vesicles arise as buds from the rough ER and others join with the face

ER and Golgi compartments	
Compartment	**Function**
ER	
RER	Protein synthesis and translocation Protein folding and assembly Lipid synthesis
SER	Lipid synthesis Detoxification Ca²⁺ storage and release
Nuclear envelope	Compartmentalization of nuclei Nucleocytoplasmic transport Attachment to lamins
Transitional elements	Membrane export out of the ER
Crystalloid ER	Storage of specific membrane proteins
Luminal ER bodies	Storage of luminal protein aggregates
Golgi	
CGN	Receives material from ER
Golgi stacks	Processing of N-linked and O-linked glycoproteins Phosphorylation of glycoproteins Elongation of GAGs and glycolipids Addition of lipid to secretory lipoproteins
TGN	Terminal glycosylation Tyrosine sulfation Proteolytic cleavages Sorting to lysosomes and plasma membrane Concentration of content

Figure 2.9 Endoplasmic reticulum and Golgi compartments. CGN, *cis*-Golgi network; TGN, *trans*-Golgi network; RER, rough endoplasmic reticulum; SER, smooth endoplasmic reticulum; GAGs, glycosaminoglycan side chains.

of the nearest Golgi sac. At least some of these structures are considered to be *transition vesicles* transporting proteins from the ER to the Golgi complex. The side of the Golgi complex facing the ER is known as the *cis* or *forming* face. The opposite *trans* or *maturing* face of the Golgi complex typically contains larger vesicle structures. Sacs in the region between the *cis* and *trans* faces form the medial segment of the Golgi complex. *Shuttle vesicles* are believed to move proteins and glycoproteins between the Golgi sacs.

The Golgi complex has three major functions within cells:
- the receipt and sorting of membrane and soluble components arriving from the ER;
- N- and O-linked glycosylation and processing of glycoproteins and glycolipids; and
- sorting of membrane and soluble components that exit the Golgi to different destinations within the cell.

Each of these functions is predominantly associated with specific morphologic domains or subcompartments of the Golgi complex (see Fig. 2.9).

Lysosomes

All of the proteins that pass through the Golgi apparatus, except those that are retained there as permanent residents, are sorted in the *trans*-Golgi network according to their final destination. The sorting establishes a link for some of the proteins to lysosomes, a ubiquitous cytoplasmic organelle interconnected with other subcellular compartments through selective membrane budding and fusion processes. Lysosomes are membrane-bound sacs containing a combination of hydrolytic enzymes (>50) capable of breaking down most biologic substances. In general, the hydrolytic reactions catalyzed by lysosomal enzymes occur at pH 4.5–5, which is a typical environment for primary lysosomes. The boundary membranes of lysosomes contain characteristic proteins, among them a H⁺-ATPase active transport pump that continually moves H⁺ from the surrounding cytoplasm into the lysosomal interior, thereby maintaining the acidic pH characteristic of these organelles. Newly synthesized lysosomal proteins are transferred into the lumen of the ER, transported through the Golgi apparatus, and then carried from the *trans*-Golgi network to the lysosomal compartment by vesicular trafficking.

Lysosomal hydrolases contain N-linked oligosaccharides that are covalently modified in the *cis*-Golgi network so that their mannose residues are phosphorylated. These mannose 6-phosphate (M6P) groups are recognized by the M6P receptor in the *trans*-Golgi network that segregates the hydrolases and helps to package them into budding transport vesicles, en route to late endosomes as they transform into lysosomes. These transport vesicles act as shuttles that move the M6P receptor to and from the *trans*-Golgi network and the endosomal compartment. The low pH in the late endosome dissociates lysosomal hydrolases from the M6P receptor, making the transport of the hydrolases unidirectional.

Exocytosis and endocytosis

Exocytosis provides the route by which proteins that are synthesized within the cell are exported to the cell's exterior. Some of the final steps of the pathway are similar to those exhibited by endocytosis, a route of entry for selected materials from outside the cell. However, endocytosis is more than a simple reversal of exocytosis and utilizes receptors and other elements that are not typically associated with exocytosis.

In the exocytotic pathway the secreting proteins take a route from ER to *cis*-Golgi, to *medial*-Golgi, from *medial*- to *trans*-Golgi, and finally from the *trans*-Golgi network to the cell surface. This transport is mediated by a novel class of coated vesicles. Unlike the coated vesicles that are involved in endocytosis, these transporting vesicles do not contain clathrin. However, the protein components involved in the formation of these novel coat structures share extensive similarities to those of clathrin coats in both polypeptide composition and even primary amino acid sequence. Liver cells can secrete more than one type of protein in a secretory vesicle. For example, two commonly secreted but unrelated proteins, albumin and transferrin, have been found to be packaged in the same secretory vesicles at the Golgi complex and released together to the extracellular medium.

Endocytosis is defined as the process by which cells bind and internalize macromolecules from the environment. Cells can take up materials from the surrounding medium through three distinct but closely related pathways: pinocytosis, phagocytosis, and receptor-mediated endocytosis (RME). Pinocytosis is a constitutive type of process described as the nonselective uptake of extracel-

lular fluid by small smooth-surfaced invaginations in the plasma membrane. Phagocytosis is the ingestion of particles and, not infrequently, internalization of expansive regions of the cell surface. In contrast, RME is the process by which cells specifically bind and internalize a variety of macromolecules, or ligands.

Of the three endocytotic pathways, RME has been studied in greatest detail in liver cells. It proceeds in several steps (Fig. 2.10). After binding to specific receptors that are randomly distributed on the hepatocyte sinusoidal plasma membrane, the ligand–receptor complexes are concentrated in distinctive regions of the membrane called *coated pits*. They are characterized by a dense material or bristle coat that covers the cytoplasmic surface. The major building block of the coat material is the triskelion, a three-legged structure composed of three clathrin molecules. Invagination of the coated pits proceeds rapidly until they pinch free from the plasma membrane and sink into the underlying cytoplasm as a coated vesicle. As the vesicle forms, the membrane quickly loses its clathrin coat and becomes an endosome. At this stage, some ligand–receptor complexes may return to the surface membrane by the process of retroendocytosis, or diacytosis, where the endo-

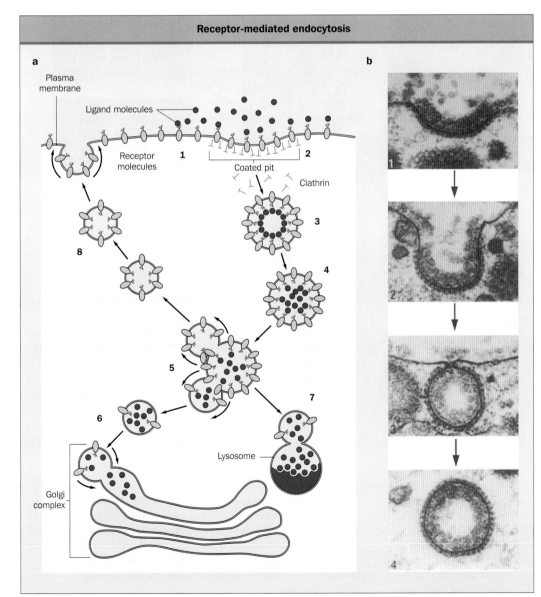

Receptor-mediated endocytosis

Figure 2.10 Pathways in receptor-mediated endocytosis. (a) After ligands bind to the specific receptors (1), the ligand/receptor complexes are concentrated in coated pits (2). The pits invaginate and sink into the underlying cytoplasm as endocytotic vesicles (3). During vesicle movement and fusion, the ligands within the vesicles are sorted and, in many cases, released from their receptors (4 and 5). The sorted molecules may proceed to the Golgi complex (6) or to lysosomes (7). After release from their ligand, some receptors are recycled to the plasma membrane (8); others are degraded in the vesicles that fuse with lysosomes. (b) Electron micrographs showing the transition of a coated pit to a coated vesicle (steps 1–4). Binding of lipoprotein ligands at the surface membrane is followed by invagination of the coated pit region and formation of a coated vesicle, with its distinctive fuzzy outer covering. [Part (a) from Wolfe SL, ed. Molecular and cell biology. Belmont, CA: Wadsworth; 1993. Part (b) from Alberts et al., eds. Molecular biology of the cell, 3rd edition. New York: Garland; 1994.]

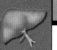

cytotic process begins again. The endosomal vesicles may be spheric or extend into elongated and variously branched tubules. As they travel along microtubules deeper into the cytoplasm, vesicles often fuse into larger structures.

During vesicle movement and fusion, the ligands within the interior space are released from their receptors and begin to be sorted into separate compartments. Hydrogen ions pumped into the intravesicular space induce ligand–receptor dissociation. A small fraction of internalized ligand is transported directly to the bile canalicular membrane. The majority of ligands remain within the acidified vesicle interior. Although the basis for sorting is presently unknown, it presumably involves an interaction between recognition sites on the endocytotic vesicles. The sorted molecules may proceed to the Golgi complex as smaller vesicles that pinch off from the endocytic vesicle.

Molecules that are sorted into vesicles that travel to the Golgi complex may remain there or may be distributed further to the ER or perinuclear space. They may also be resorted and secondarily routed in vesicles to the plasma membrane or to lysosomes. Fusion of vesicles with lysosomes exposes their contents to degradation by the lysosomal enzymes. Most hepatocyte receptors, devoid of bound ligand, return to the plasma membrane attached to small vesicles, and are reintroduced by membrane fusion. Not all receptors recycle, however; some undergo lysosomal degradation together with their associated ligands.

In most cells coated pits occupy approximately 2% of the surface membrane area. It has been estimated that about 2500 clathrin-coated vesicles invaginate from the plasma membrane of a cultured fibroblast every minute. In liver, the coated pit regions are particularly abundant along the hepatocyte sinusoidal membrane base of the microvilli. The technique of freeze-etching has provided a unique electron microscopic view of coated membrane dynamics at the cell surface (Fig. 2.11). It is now well-established that the coat structure of both coated

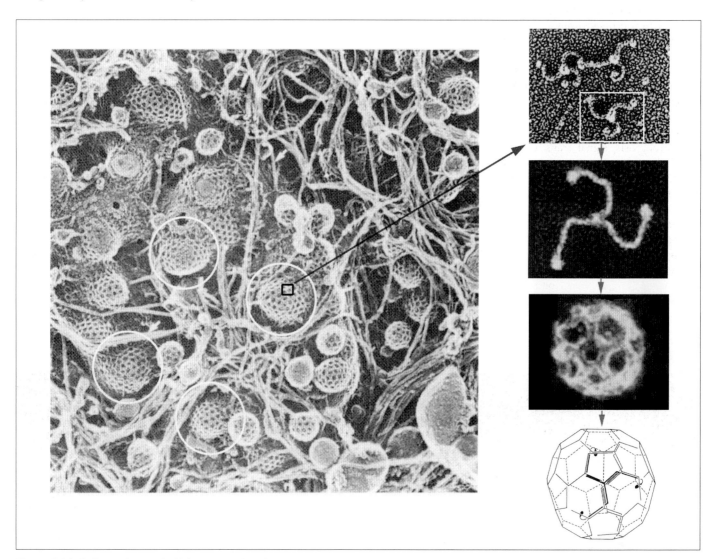

Figure 2.11 Cell membrane. (Left) Schematic view of a coated membrane region from within the cell. Clathrin basketworks (encircled) form coated membranes, pits and vesicles. Smooth-surfaced membranes and intermediate filaments are particularly numerous. (Right) Electron micrographs of clathrin triskelions (×230,000), a clathrin shell reformed from triskelions and a schematic representation of the clathrin coat lattice. Each structure is composed of 12 pentagons and a variable number of hexagons forming an outer cage of clathrin, an inner layer of clathrin terminal domains and an innermost shell consisting of unrelated proteins that interact directly with receptors in the coated regions. (From Steer CJ. Receptor-mediated endocytosis: mechanisms, biologic function, and molecular properties. In: Zakim D, Boyer TD, eds. Hepatology: a textbook of liver disease, 3rd edn. Philadelphia: WB Saunders; 1996:149–214.)

pits and coated vesicles consists of a highly ordered array of specific macromolecules organized into polygonal lattices consisting primarily of a single protein, clathrin. Clathrin subunits associate into three-legged structures called *triskelions* (Fig. 2.11). Each leg is bent to a shallow angle at a position roughly halfway along its length. This remarkable structure consists of three molecules of clathrin heavy chain (180kDa) and three molecules of clathrin light chain (33–36kDa). The three light chains overlap with the three heavy chains to form a triskelion with its prominent vertex and terminal domains at the end of each clathrin molecule. Triskelions assemble in an overlapping network to form the lattice lining a coated pit. The structure and assembly of clathrin triskelions is illustrated in and consists of a geometric array of 12 pentagons and a variable number of hexagons depending on the size of the coat.

Caveolae or plasmalemmal vesicles are a characteristic feature of the plasma membrane of many mammalian cell types and especially fibroblasts, endothelial cells, and smooth muscle cells (Fig. 2.12). Morphologically, caveolae are 50–60nm invaginations of the plasma membrane with a characteristic flask shape. Unlike clathrin-coated pits, caveolae exhibit a characteristic spiral coat on the cytoplasmic side of the caveolae, consisting in part of the integral membrane protein caveolin. A number of molecules have now been localized to caveolae including GPI-anchored proteins, the β-adrenergic receptor, as well as tyrosine kinase and substrates. Caveolae exhibit a number of different functions including potocytosis, signal transduction, calcium regulation, and nonclathrin-dependent endocytosis and transcytosis. Caveolin is a unique protein of 178 amino acids and displays little sequence homology to other proteins.

Mitochondria

Mitochondria are respiratory organelles that constitute about 20% of the cytoplasmic volume of hepatocytes. Their primary function is to conserve the energy from the oxidation of substrates by oxygen as the high-energy phosphate anhydride bonds of ATP. They contain the enzymes of the tricarboxylic acid cycle, fatty acid oxidation, and oxidative phosphorylation. Other functions in liver cells include parts of the urea cycle, gluconeogenesis, fatty acid

synthesis, and regulation of intracellular calcium concentrations. Normal human hepatocytes contain numerous mitochondria throughout the cytoplasm (Fig. 2.13). All mitochondria contain two very different membranes: the outer membrane, which defines the smooth surface perimeter of the mitochondrion; and the inner membrane, which is highly folded. The folds, called cristae, greatly increase the area of the inner membrane. These membrane structures define two submitochondrial compartments: the intermembrane space between the two membranes, and the matrix or central compartment (Fig. 2.13).

Liver mitochondria vary in size and shape, depending on their location in relation to the blood supply. The location of mitochondria in a cell is often controlled so they are positioned near major sites of ATP utilization. This is accomplished by transport of mitochondria along microtubules. The mitochondrial matrix is a concentrated protein solution of enzymes of the tricarboxylic acid cycle, fatty acid oxidation, and urea synthesis. The matrix, however, may contain a variety of discrete structures, including granules of various sizes, fibrils, and crystals. The most common large granule is the so-called *intramitochondrial granule*, a dense, spheric particle that may store calcium and other ions. In contrast, the smaller granules contain the *mitochondrial ribosomes*. Interestingly, mitochondria contain their own DNA, which is embedded within the matrix and codes for a number of protein constituents. The mitochondrion may also be the key organelle in the regulation of programmed cell death, or apoptosis.

Peroxisomes

By electron microscopy, peroxisomes appear as roughly spheric structures that are somewhat smaller than mitochondria. Peroxisomes are enclosed by a single membrane; the material inside the membrane, called the *matrix*, contains a *core* that exhibits a regular lattice or crystalline structure. They are particularly abundant in hepatocytes and provide many important links between the metabolism of carbohydrates, lipids, proteins, fats, and nucleic acids. Many of the biochemical reactions of peroxisomes are oxidative and function in catabolic pathways; however, some are anabolic reactions in which the end-products serve as building blocks for anabolic reactions elsewhere in the cell.

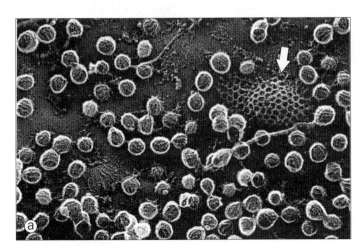

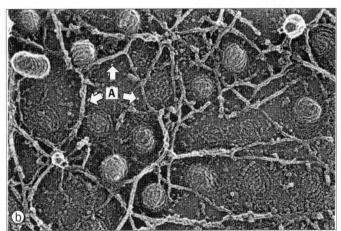

Figure 2.12 Freeze-etch images of caveolae. They are smaller and are usually more round than clathrin-coated pits [(a), arrow]. Caveolae are coated with ridges of material on their surface that resemble fingerprints. Typically, they occur in clusters and often in actin filament (A)-rich regions of the cell (b). ×130,000 (a); ×177,000 (b). (From Steer CJ. Receptor-mediated endocytosis: mechanisms, biologic function, and molecular properties. In: Zakim D, Boyer TD, eds. Hepatology: a textbook of liver disease, 3rd edition. Philadelphia: WB Saunders; 1996:149–214.)

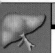

Mitochondrial distribution and structure

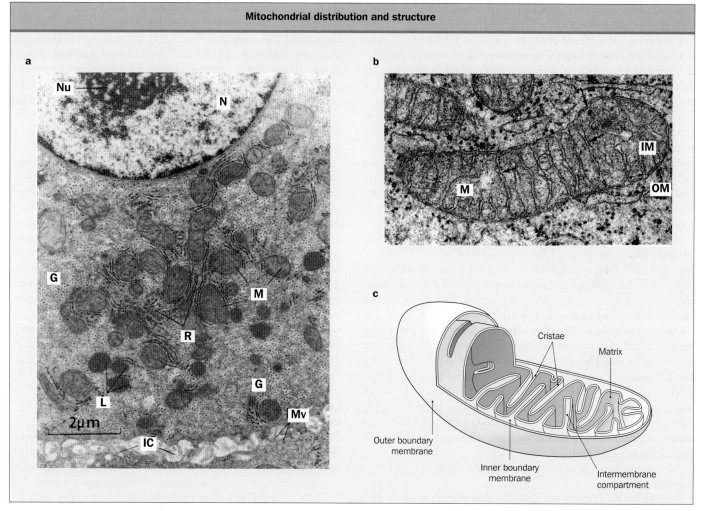

Figure 2.13 Mitochondrial distribution and structure. (a) Electron microscopic view of mitochondrial distribution in a normal human liver cell. N, nucleus; Nu, nucleolus; M, mitochondria; R, rough endoplasmic reticulum; G, glycogen granules; Mv, microvilli in intracellular space; L, lysosomes; IC, intercellular space. (b) A magnified view of a mitochondrion with (c) a schematic diagram of its structure. [Part (a) from Sherlock S, Dooley J, eds. Diseases of the liver and biliary system, 10th edn. London: Blackwell Science; 1997:10–1. Parts (b) and (c) from Wolfe SL, ed. Molecular and cell biology. Belmont, CA: Wadsworth; 1993.]

Failure to form peroxisomes during gestation causes death in early infancy and supports the notion that peroxisomal function is essential to human life.

THE NUCLEUS AND ITS MOLECULAR CONSTITUENTS

Morphology of the nucleus

Hepatocytes have large, active nuclei, with prominent nucleoli where ribosomal precursors are processed. The nucleus is delimited by a nuclear envelope formed by two concentric membranes. These membranes are punctured at intervals by nuclear pores, which actively transport selected molecules to and from the cytosol. The envelope is directly connected to the extensive membranes of the ER, and it is supported by two networks of intermediate filaments. In one, the nuclear lamina forms a thin shell just inside the nucleus underlying the inner membrane, while the other, less regularly organized, surrounds the outer nuclear membrane. The nucleus contains the nucleolus, a fibrous matrix, and DNA–protein complex (Fig. 2.13a). Both the ribonu-

clear protein (RNP) network and the perinucleolar chromatin radiate from the nucleolus, which is the largest intranuclear structure. The chromacenters are widely distributed in the nucleoplasm and the perichromatin granules are often found associated with the chromocenters. A layer of dense chromatin is often found in close proximity to the nuclear envelope.

Function of the nucleus

The nucleus is the ultimate control center for cell activities. Within the chromatin, the information required to synthesize cellular proteins is written into the DNA. Each DNA segment encoded for a specific protein molecule constitutes a gene. In a process called *transcription*, the information from a gene is copied into a mRNA molecule which, after some processing, moves across the nuclear pore complex into the cytoplasm where it becomes part of a ribosome. The DNA of the human genome contains the codes for many thousands of different proteins. In addition, DNA stores the information for making additional RNA types that carry out accessory roles in protein synthesis and other nucleocytoplasmic functions. For example, ribosomal RNAs

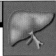

(rRNAs) are encoded in DNA regions within the nucleolus and become important participants of the mature ribosome. In addition, transfer RNA (tRNA) binds to amino acids during protein synthesis and provides a necessary link between the nucleic acid code and the amino acid sequence of proteins during protein *translation*. Finally, other RNAs are involved in the processing of mRNA, rRNA, and tRNA molecules.

A second major function of the nucleus involves duplication of the chromatin as a part of cell replication. Just before cell division all the components of chromatin, including both DNA and chromosomal proteins, are precisely duplicated and transmitted to the two identical daughter cells. During cell division the two copies of each duplicated chromosome are separated and exactly divided so that the two cells resulting from the division each receive a complete set of genes.

Nuclear envelope

The nuclear envelope consists of three primary structure elements: the *outer* and *inner membranes*, and the *pore complexes*. The outer membrane, which faces the cytoplasm, is covered with ribosomes on its cytoplasmic side. At scattered points, it is continuous with the ER. The inner membrane, which faces the nucleoplasm, has no ribosomes. The outer and inner nuclear membranes enclose a narrow space about 40nm wide, the *perinuclear compartment*. The perinuclear compartment encircles the nucleus and, through the connections made by the outer nuclear membrane with the ER, is continuous with the space enclosed in the ER cisternae. Proteins synthesized by the ribosomes on the outer nuclear membrane can enter the perinuclear compartment and eventually make their way to the ER cisternae and other destinations in the cellular-secretion pathways.

Nuclear pore complex

The nuclear envelope of a typical mammalian cell contains 3000–4000 pore complexes. However, the number of pore complexes varies with the transcriptional activity of the nucleus. The nuclear pore complex is a large, elaborate structure that has an estimated molecular mass of about 125MDa and is thought to be composed of more than 100 different proteins, arranged with a striking octagonal symmetry. Models of the pore complex have been based on negatively stained electron micrographic images (Fig. 2.14a). The nuclear pore complex is often described as having three parallel rings inserted into and oriented along the same plane of the envelope such that the outer rings face either the cytoplasm or nucleoplasm (Fig. 2.14b). In negatively stained samples a large central plug or granule is often observed between the cytoplasmic and nucleoplasmic rings that associates with a middle ring of spokes. The surface of the cytoplasmic ring is decorated with eight 22nm granules that are thought to be ribosomes, ribosomal precursors, or circular polysomes. The channels in the outer ring appear to control diffusion. The diameter of the opening in the nuclear envelope is roughly 72–94nm, while the diameter of the pore complex measured along the axis of the envelope is 120–150nm, depending upon whether the distances contributed by the radial arms are included. The depth of the pore complex is approximately 70nm. Thus, the pore complex is an extremely large macromolecular assembly.

Nucleocytoplasmic transport

Bidirectional traffic occurs continuously between the cytosol and the nucleus. The many proteins that function in the nucleus, including histones, DNA and RNA polymerases, gene regulatory proteins, and RNA-processing proteins, are selectively imported

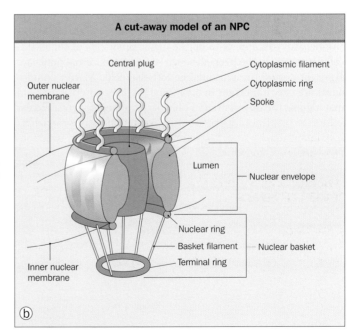

Figure 2.14 Nuclear pore complex (NPC). (a) An oblique view of a three-dimensional map of the nuclear pore complex calculated from electron micrograph images (shown in the background). The nuclear pore is highly symmetric. The arrangement of the subunits within the membrane pore creates a large central channel thought to be involved in active nuclear transport. Eight peripheral channels are also created, which could serve for the diffusion of small ions and proteins. (b) A cut-away model identifying the major structural components of a nuclear pore complex (NPC). [(a) From Hinshaw JE, Carragher BO, Milligan RA. Architecture and design of the nuclear pore complex. Cell. 1992;69:1133–41. (b) From Ohno M, Fornerod M, Mattaj IW. Nucleocytoplasmic transport: the last 200 nanometers. Cell. 1998:92:327–36.]

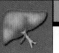

into the nuclear compartment from the cytosol where they are made. At the same time, tRNAs and mRNAs are synthesized in the nuclear compartment and then exported to the cytosol. Both the export and import processes are selective. Messenger RNAs, for example, are exported only after they have been properly modified by RNA-processing reactions in the nucleus. In some cases, the transport process is complex. For instance, ribosomal proteins are synthesized in the cytosol, imported into the nucleus where they assemble ribosomal RNA into particles, and then exported again to the cytosol as part of a ribosomal subunit. Each of these steps involves selective transport across the nuclear envelope.

Macromolecules are actively transported into and out of the nucleus through nuclear pores and appear to require energy supplied by specific ATPase/GTPase enzymes. Two mechanisms have been considered for the uptake of large nuclear proteins. In the first, referred to as *retention*, large molecules diffuse slowly through the nuclear pore complex and subsequently bind to specific intranuclear sites. In the second mechanism, *signal-mediated* vectorial transport increases the rate of movement across the nuclear membrane. The signals are short amino acid sequences and recognized by receptors in the pore complex. After recognition and binding, the proteins are transported through the pores into the nucleus. The nuclear envelope is freely permeable to small molecules ($<5kDa$), which diffuse rapidly across the pore complex.

EXTRACELLULAR MATRIX

Functions of the extracellular matrix

Animals contain many types of extracellular matrices, each specialized for a particular function. Cells bind to extracellular matrices as a means of anchoring themselves, to derive traction for migration, and to receive signals from the matrix and matrix-bound growth factors. The adult liver has been shown to contain many of the known extracellular matrix components. Lipocytes and hepatocytes appear to be the major producers of the extracellular matrix in the liver, although some matrix components are also synthesized by sinusoidal endothelial cells. Matrix components are very important in organizing the liver parenchyma and maintaining the differentiated phenotype of hepatocytes. Excess

deposition of connective tissue in the liver is associated with structural alterations in the liver, with changes in hemodynamic properties and ultimately in impairment of liver function.

Cell–matrix interactions

Cell phenotype appears to be regulated by specific cell–matrix interactions that are modulated by the molecular organization of the extracellular matrix and by the type and availability of distinct matrix receptors on the cell surface. The primary class of these receptors is a family of transmembrane proteins known as *integrins*. The integrin receptors bind to extracellular matrix proteins at specialized cell attachment sites that often have the tripeptide sequence Arg-Gly-Asp as the target sequence for binding. They mediate attachment of the extracellular matrix to the intracellular cytoskeleton network, thereby promoting changes in cell shape, spreading, and migration. Nonintegrin surface receptors have also been identified in hepatocytes that mediate cell attachment by different mechanisms. Cell–matrix interactions in the liver play important roles in maintaining hepatocyte morphology and proliferation. For example, when plated on collagen, hepatocytes can undergo four-fold higher levels of DNA synthesis than when they are grown on basement membrane gels. Moreover, the level of expression of liver-specific gene products, such as albumin, is also significantly influenced by the type of extracellular matrix used for hepatocyte culture. Cell–cell and cell–matrix interactions in the liver appear to determine the level of synthesis and deposition of extracellular matrix components by different cells, as well as to regulate matrix remodeling by the production of specific enzymes and inhibitors.

Components of extracellular matrix

All extracellular matrices, including the connective tissues and basement membrane structures, are composed of molecules that fall into three distinct classes: collagens, noncollagenous glycoproteins, and proteoglycans. These components, particularly those in the latter two classes, form the *ground substance* which can be visualized in the extracellular space by electron microscopy. In liver, the extracellular matrix is composed of five distinct types of collagen (types I, III, IV, V, VI) (Fig. 2.15), seven classes of noncollagenous proteins (fibronectin, laminin, entactin/nidogen, tenascin, thrombospondin, SPARC, undulin), and an undetermined number of

Extracellular matrix proteins in normal liver					
Collagen type	Associated anchorage protein	Associated proteoglycans	Cell-surface receptor	Source	Localization
I	Fibronectin	Chondroitin sulfate	Integrin	Fibroblasts	Vascular space, Glisson's capsule, space of Disse
III	Fibronectin	Heparan sulfate Heparin	Integrin	Hepatocytes, fibroblasts	Vascular space, Glisson's capsule, space of Disse
IV	Laminin	Heparan sulfate	Laminin	Epithelial cells, hepatocytes	Vascular, lymphatic, canalicular structure, and sinusoids
V	Fibronectin	Heparan sulfate Heparin	Integrin	Fibroblasts	Periportal tissue, basal lamina of bile ducts
VI	Fibronectin	Heparan sulfate	Integrin	Fibroblasts	Periportal spaces, space of Disse

Figure 2.15 Extracellular matrix proteins in normal liver.

proteoglycans and glycosaminoglycans, such as membrane-associated syndecan, thrombomodulin, and betaglycan; and the extracellular matrix-associated versican, biglycan, decorin, fibromodulin, and perlecan. The extracellular matrices are highly structured. The distribution and organization of the extracellular matrix of the liver is unique and during development is produced along the migration path of the hepatocytes. The absence of a continuous basement membrane between the hepatocytes and liver endothelial cells is another unique feature of the liver.

SIGNAL TRANSDUCTIONS

Each cell of the human body is programmed during development to respond to a specific set of signals that act in various combinations to regulate its behavior as well as its lifespan and rate of replication. Most of these signals are paracrine, in which local mediators are rapidly taken up, destroyed, or immobilized, so that they act only on neighboring cells. Centralized control is, in general, exerted by endocrine signaling, in which secreted hormones are carried in the blood to target cells throughout the body. In synaptic signaling, neurotransmitters are secreted by

nerve cells which act locally on the postsynaptic cells in contact with their axons.

The liver plays a critical role in the adaptive response to systemic changes such as inflammation and alteration of energy requirements. Hepatocytes are particularly sensitive to signals generated in these environments. Some small hydrophobic signaling molecules, including the steroid and thyroid hormones and the retinoids, diffuse across the plasma membrane of hepatic cells and activate intracellular receptor proteins, which directly regulate the transcription of specific genes. Some dissolved gases such as nitric oxide act as local mediators by diffusing across the plasma membrane of the target cell and activating an intracellular enzyme, usually guanylyl cyclase, which produces cyclic GMP in the target cell. But most extracellular signaling molecules are hydrophilic and are able to activate receptor proteins only on the surface of the target cell (Fig. 2.16). These receptors act as signal transducers, converting the extracellular binding event into intracellular signals that alter the behavior of the target cell. Plasma membrane receptors exhibit a variety of topologies and, of course, are responsive to many different ligands (Fig. 2.17). In general, there are three main families of cell-surface receptors, each of which transduces extracellular signals in a different way. Ion-channel-linked receptors open or close briefly in response to their respective stimuli. G-protein-linked receptors indirectly activate or inactivate plasma-membrane-bound enzymes or ion channels via trimeric GTP-binding proteins (G-proteins). Enzyme-linked receptors act either directly as or indirectly through enzymes that are usually protein kinases. In general, kinases regulate the phosphorylation state of specific proteins in the target cell. Through cascades of highly regulated protein phosphorylations, elaborate sets of interacting proteins relay most signals from the cell surface to the nucleus, thereby altering the cell's pattern of gene expression and, as a consequence, its behavior.

Transforming growth factor (TGF)-β signaling is one of the better understood examples in this class of signal transduction pathways (Fig. 2.18). The isoforms of TGF-β exist as homodimers that are excreted from hepatocytes and liver nonparenchymal cells as latent molecules (pro-TGF-βs). The pro-TGF-β undergoes plasmin-mediated activation when bound to the mannose 6-phosphate receptor. There are three types of TGF-β receptor. Type I and II

Cell surface receptors in normal liver		
Ligand	Binding sites/cell	Cell type
ASGP	150–250,000	Hepatocyte
LDL	20–50,000	Hepatocyte
Transferrin	31,000	Hepatocyte
Insulin	16,000	Hepatocyte
EGF	300,000	Hepatocyte
M6P (CI)	19,000	Hepatocyte
IgA	200,000	Hepatocyte
Fucose		Kupffer cell
		Endothelial cell
GlcNAc (Avian)	33,000	Hepatocyte
Mannose	50–150,000	Kupffer cell
		Endothelial cell

Figure 2.16 Cell surface receptors in normal liver. CI, cation-independent; ASGP, asialoglycoprotein; LDL, low-density lipoprotein; EGF, epidermal growth factor; GlcNAc, N-acetylglucosamine; M6P, mannose 6-phosphate.

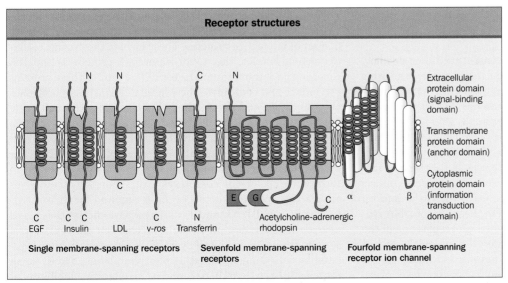

Figure 2.17 Topology of different receptor structures in the membrane. E, effector protein; G, G protein; C, C-terminus; N, N-terminus; EGF, epidermal growth factor; v-ros, viral ros receptor; LDL, low-density lipoproteins. (From Hesch RD. Classification of cell receptors. Curr Topics Pathol. 1991;83:13–51.)

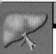

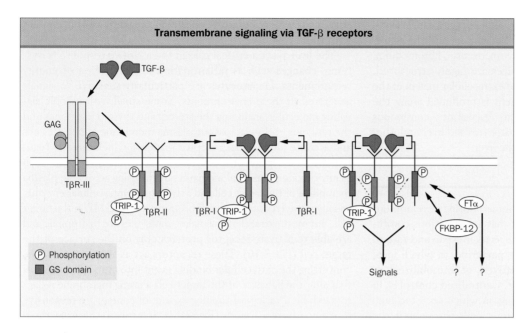

Transmembrane signaling via TGF-β receptors

Ⓟ Phosphorylation

▮ GS domain

Figure 2.18 Transmembrane signaling via TGF-β receptors. Accessory receptors, such as homo-oligomeric TGF-β receptor (TβR)III, may present TGF-β to homo-oligomeric TβR-II, which is a constitutively active serine/threonine kinase. The TGF-β–TβR-II complex recruits TβR-I into the complex, after which TβR-I is phosphorylated by TβR-II and activated. In such a state, TβR-I propagates signals to downstream components. The functional significance in TGF-β signaling of TβR-II interaction with TRIP-1, and TβR-I interaction with FKBP-12 and farnesyl protein transferase α (FTα) remains to be determined. GAG, glycosaminoglycan side chains. (From ten Dijke et al. Signaling via hetero-oligomeric complexes of type I and type II serine/threonine kinase receptors. Curr Opin Cell Biol. 1996;8:139–45.)

receptors form heterodimers that transmit the TGF-β signal into the hepatocyte. The type III receptor does not transduce an intracellular signal, but serves as a repository for TGF-β on the plasma membrane. The type II receptor binds ligand with high affinity, resulting in the recruitment of a type I receptor to form a receptor-ligand complex. Upon dimerization, the type II receptor phosphorylates the type I receptor in a cluster of glycine and serine residues near the membrane, known as the GS domain. Phosphorylation of the GS domain stimulates intracellular responses to the bound ligand. Therefore, the type I receptor is considered to be the primary transducer of the signal, whereas the type II receptor functions as the primary ligand-binding component. Studies have revealed that the TGF-β-signaling cascade is mediated by a family of serine/threonine receptor kinases. However, multiple independent, intracellular signal transduction pathways exist that mediate pleiotropic genomic responses to TGF-β. For example, it has recently been shown that the Smads (Sma and Mad), are major intracellular players of the TGF-β signal transduction pathway. Smads are activated near the membrane through receptor signaling and are subsequently translocated into the nucleus to activate transcription by associating with DNA-binding proteins.

Regulation of the cell cycle

Cells reproduce by duplicating their contents and then dividing. This *cell division cycle* is the fundamental means by which all living things are propagated. Within the liver, the normal state of hepatocytes is a quiescent or nonproliferative one, but they exhibit a tremendous capacity to replicate. For example, after loss of hepatic tissue, hepatocytes, which may have been quiescent for years, dramatically enter into the cell cycle and proliferate until the liver mass is completely restored. Then, just as acutely, they become quiescent again. A typical cell division cycle in somatic cells consists of four major phases (Fig. 2.19). The *G1 phase* is the interval between the completion of mitosis and the beginning of DNA synthesis; *S phase* (synthesis phase) is the period of replication of the nuclear DNA; the *G2 phase* is the interval between the end of DNA synthesis and the beginning of mitosis; and finally, the *M phase* is the period of mitosis in which nuclear division takes place.

In mitosis, the nuclear envelope breaks down, the contents of the nucleus condense into visible chromosomes, and the cell's microtubules reorganize to form the *mitotic spindle* that will eventually separate the chromosomes. As mitosis proceeds, the cell seems to pause briefly in a state called *metaphase*, in which the chromosomes, already duplicated, are aligned on the mitotic spindle, poised for segregation. The separation of the duplicated chromosomes marks the beginning of *anaphase*, during which the chromosomes move to the poles of the spindle, where they decondense and reform intact nuclei. The cell is then pinched in two by a process called *cytokinesis*, which marks the end of M phase. In most cells the M phase takes only about an hour, which represents only a small fraction of the total cell cycle division time. The much longer period that elapses between one M phase and the next is known as *interphase*, and represents the time required to grow before the next division. Cells which have not yet committed themselves to DNA replication can pause in their progress. They enter a specialized resting state, called *G0*, where they can remain for days, weeks, or years before resuming proliferation.

The sequence of the cell cycle events is governed by a control system that delicately balances the expression and activity of a set of interacting proteins. These include the cyclins, cyclin-dependent kinases, the tumor-suppressor proteins retinoblastoma and p53, transcription factor E2F, and p21. These proteins can induce and coordinate the essential downstream processes that duplicate and divide the cell's contents. The cell cycle control system is primarily based on the regulation of certain protein kinases. Cyclins and cyclin-dependent kinases (cdks) are essential for cell-cycle regulation in eukaryotes (Fig. 2.20). The cyclins (regulatory subunits) bind to cdks (catalytic subunits) to form active cyclin–cdk complexes. Cdk subunits by themselves are inactive and binding to a cyclin is required for their activity. Cyclins A, B1, D, and E undergo periodic synthesis and degradation, thereby providing a mechanism to regulate cdk activity throughout the cell cycle. Cdk activity is further regulated by activating or inhibiting phosphorylation, and by small proteins (p15, p18, p19, p21, and p27), which are inhibitors of

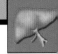

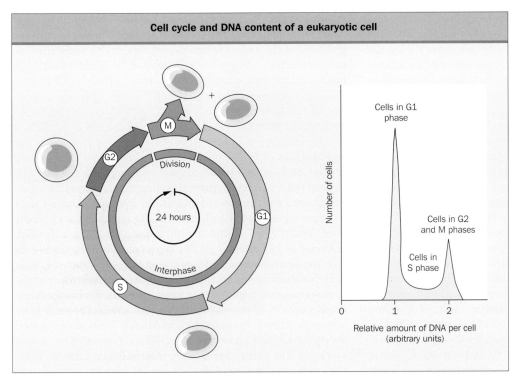

Cell cycle and DNA content of a eukaryotic cell

Fig. 2.19 Cell cycle and DNA content of a eukaryotic cell. (Left) The four successive phases of the cell cycle in which the cell grows continuously during interphase and divides during M phase. DNA replication is confined to the part of interphase known as S phase. G1 phase is the gap between M phase and S phase; G2 exists between S phase and M phase. (Right) Analysis of DNA content during the cell cycle. In this example, there are greater numbers of cells in G1 than in G2+M, implying that G1 is longer than G2+M. The cells in the G1 phase have an unreplicated complement of DNA (one arbitrary unit); the G2 and M phase cells have a fully replicated complement of DNA (two arbitrary units), and the S phase cells have an intermediate amount of DNA. (From Alberts et al. Molecular biology of the cell, 3rd edition. New York: Garland; 1994.)

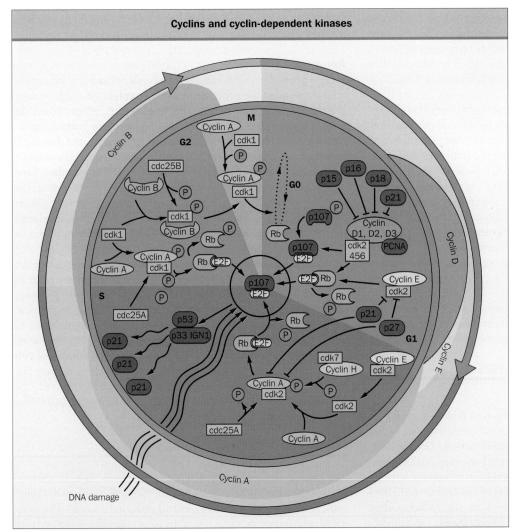

Cyclins and cyclin-dependent kinases

Figure 2.20 Cyclins and cyclin-dependent kinases (cdks). Modulation of cyclins A, B1, D and E provides a mechanism to regulate cdk activity throughout the cell cycle. Cdk activity is further regulated by activating or inhibitory phosphorylation, and by a variety of small proteins which bind to cyclins, cdks, or their complexes and inhibit cdk activity. The active cyclin–cdk complexes drive cells through the various cell cycle phases, or checkpoints, by phosphorylating the unique set of proteins substrates that are essential to achieve phase transition. Nine different cyclins have been identified and are designated A through I. The cyclin–cdk complexes induce phosphorylation of the retinoblastoma family of proteins. [From PharMingen cell cycle regulation. Applied Reagents and Technologies (brochure, p.2.)]

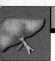

cdk activity, that bind to cyclins, cdks, or cyclin–cdk complexes. Active cyclin–cdk complexes drive cells through particular cell cycle phases, called checkpoints, by phosphorylating the unique sets of protein substrates that are essential to achieve transition to the next phase. In yeast, there appear to be three major checkpoints that regulate progression through the cell cycle. One is at late G1, just before S phase, where a commitment to enter into the cell cycle is made; the second is at late G2, just before M phase, where successful progression through the cell cycle is monitored; and the third regulates exit from mitosis by monitoring the completion of spindle assembly.

When hepatocytes are stimulated to replicate, an early response is the transcription and translation of G1 cyclins. These G1 cyclins bind to appropriate kinases to form the activated cyclin–cdk complexes that subsequently phosphorylate a set of specific downstream targets. The potential downstream targets of the G1 specific cyclin–cdk complexes include p53, retinoblastoma, and p107 (a retinoblastoma-family protein). Retinoblastoma is a nuclear tumor suppressor phosphoprotein that is hypophosphorylated throughout most of G1 and becomes progressively phosphorylated in the late G1, S, G2, and M phases of the cell cycle. It regulates through modification of gene expression, achieved by sequestration, active repression, or stimulation of a series of transcription factors by the hypophosphorylated form of retinoblastoma that is present in G1 phase. Phosphorylation of retinoblastoma via interaction with various cdks and cyclins in mid-to-late G1 phase, results in release of E2F and other transcriptional factors, which then activates S-phase and DNA replication. It undergoes additional phosphorylation as cells progress through S and into G2/M phase. Most of the phosphate groups are removed as the cell re-enters into G0/G1 phase.

In general, a common feature of the retinoblastoma-family proteins, p53 and p33^{ING1} is their ability to inhibit cell proliferation. For example, in hepatocytes, TGF-β inhibits cellular proliferation largely through its ability to downregulate the activity of the cyclin-dependent kinases cdk2 and cdk4; TGF-β decreases the transcription of cdk4 and downregulates cdk2 activity by inactivating cyclin E–cdk2 complexes. These events lead to accumulation of hypophosphorylated retinoblastoma and prevent activation of E2F transcriptional factor. P33^{ING1} facilitates the activity of p53 and leads to increased expression of p21, a major target of p53 transcription regulation. In addition, the proto-oncogene c-Myc is a positive regulator of cyclin-cdk complexes. c-Myc can enhance cdk activity via functional inactivation of the cdk inhibitors as well as by inducing the cdk-activating phosphatase cdc25. All these particular proteins exert control through their kinase activities, which are abruptly switched on or off at particular points in the cycle.

REGENERATION AND APOPTOSIS

Liver regeneration

Regeneration is the capability of an organ to replace tissue mass after partial removal or injury. The normal adult liver is a quiescent organ exhibiting minimal replicative activity and, in fact, mitosis is observed only in approximately 1 in every 20,000 hepatocytes. After partial hepatectomy (PH) the remaining hepatocytes can proliferate to restore the mass of the organ within days to weeks. In the rat, peak DNA synthesis occurs 24 hours after PH, when approximately 35% of hepatocytes are actively

involved in cell replication. Mitosis follows DNA synthesis 6–8 hours later, and during the course of regrowth most hepatocytes will have replicated at least once or twice. The replication of nonhepatocyte cells generally is delayed by approximately 24 hours, but exhibits a similar synchronous pattern of DNA synthesis and mitosis as observed in hepatocytes. Once the original size of the liver is attained, hepatocytes revert to their non-replicative, quiescent state. Liver regeneration is actually a process of compensatory growth of the remnant liver and is not regeneration of the removed tissue. During the regenerative process, there is an increase in mass resulting from cell proliferation of the remaining hepatocytes. In general, progenitor, or so-called stem cells do not participate in liver regeneration after PH, but are activated and differentiate into hepatocytes only after certain types of toxic injury. In addition, the proliferative response of hepatocytes to PH begins almost immediately. In fact, the immediate-early genes that are rapidly induced as liver cells exit from their normally quiescent state include many of the proto-oncogenes implicated in cancer growth. Their expression is independent of protein synthesis and appears to result from mitogenic stimuli. In contrast, delayed-early genes are expressed during the G0–G1 phase transition and are dependent on protein synthesis. The entire regenerative process is a cascade of events that moves cells from G0 through G1 and DNA synthesis, through G2 to M phase and cell division, and is tightly regulated by both extrahepatic and intrahepatic signals. When the optimal ratio between functional hepatic mass and body mass is reached, the cells return to their resting G0 state.

Apoptosis

Liver regeneration after PH also involves a remodeling process in which apoptosis, or programmed cell death, plays an important role in reconstruction of the infrastructure of hepatic tissue. In a sense, it fine tunes the regenerative process. In general, apoptosis is a form of cell death that permits the removal of damaged, senescent, or unneeded cells in multicellular organisms, without damage to the cellular microenviroment. Recent studies have shown that genes involved in apoptosis are actively expressed in the regenerating liver. They include the inducing genes c-*fos*, c-*jun*, c-*myc*, p53, *Bax*, *Bad*, *Bak*, and TGF-β; the apoptosis inhibitory genes, *Bcl*-2, *Bcl*-X$_L$, TRPM-2/clusterin; and the retinoblastoma gene. Ironically, some of these genes are also involved in cell proliferation, through regulation of the cell cycle; TGF-β can induce hepatocytes to undergo apoptosis both *in vitro* and *in vivo*. In fact, this multifunctional cytokine has been identified as a key factor in terminating the regenerative process, presumably regulated by the optimal ratio of functional liver to body mass. However, liver regeneration after PH is a complicated process, and probably involves an orchestrated balance of cell replication, apoptosis, and remodeling by a number of molecular players. When the surviving hepatocytes are also injured, the process may be even more complicated and involve additional factors, including stem-cell proliferation.

NONPARENCHYMAL CELLS

The hepatic sinusoidal cells play a critical role in the maintenance of liver function and are composed of four cell types: endothelial cells, Kupffer cells, fat-storing (or Ito) cells, and pit cells. The sinusoidal cells represent about 6% of the total liver volume but account

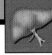

for 35–40% of the total number of liver cells. The endothelial and Kupffer cells are in close contact with the bloodstream, whereas parenchymal cells are in contact with the plasma only via the space of Disse (Fig. 2.21). The fenestrated endothelial cells form a physical barrier, which enables direct contact of parenchymal cells with most plasma proteins in the space of Disse, but prevents direct interaction of parenchymal cells with blood cells, large chylomicrons, viruses, and bacteria. Kupffer cells, which constitute the majority of the fixed tissue macrophages of the reticuloendothelial system, are anchored to the endothelial cells by long cytoplasmic processes. Within the liver acinus, Kupffer cells are located preferentially in the periportal region. They are highly phagocytic cells, which enables them to phagocytose particulate matter such as bacteria. Both endothelial and Kupffer cells contain several specific receptors on their cell membrane which significantly increases the endocytic capacity of the liver. The fat-storing cells serve as specialized pericytes extraluminally. The pit cells are immunoreactive cells attached to the luminal surface of the sinusoid.

Kupffer cells

Kupffer cells constitute 80–90% of the total population of fixed macrophages in the body. These cells are components of the wall of hepatic sinusoids and play a significant role in the removal of particulates and cells as well as toxic, ineffective, and foreign substances from the portal blood, particularly those of intestinal origin. Kupffer cells also are the source of a variety of beneficial vasoactive toxic mediators, which are thought to be involved in host defense mechanisms as well as in some disease processes in the liver. Kupffer cells appear to be derived from monocytes or stem cells in the bone marrow and possess a typical morphology. Their cell body shows microvilli, lamellapodia, and occasional filopodia. The cell coat consists of a 50–70nm thick fuzzy outer layer and a thin layer close to the plasma membrane. Kupffer cells have several specific structures related to pinocytosis, including bristle-coated micropinocytic vesicles, fuzzy-coated vacuoles, and worm-like structures. In addition, the abundance of lysosomes

and their variety of enzymes reflect the prominent role of these cells in the degradation of particles and substances taken up from the bloodstream. Both the number and activity of Kupffer cells may vary due to the immunologic and pathophysiologic conditions of the liver. The mean turn over rate of the total Kupffer cell population varies from 21 days to 14 months.

Endothelial cells

The endothelial cells account for 20% of total liver cells, but for only 3.3% of the protein content of the liver. They possess slender extended processes containing pores (fenestrae) that are arranged in so-called sieve plates. These fenestrae constitute only 6–8% of the surface area of the endothelial lining, so that the endothelium is thought to act as a selective barrier between the blood and the parenchyma. The size of fenestrae is dynamic and can be modified by both physical and chemical forces, which are actively controlled by the actin-containing components of the cytoskeleton, particularly microtubules. The surface of the sinusoidal endothelial cells are relatively smooth compared with those of Kupffer cells, and generally are lacking in filopodia or lamellopodia. They possess numerous bristle-coated membrane invaginations and vesicles and many other lysosome-like vacuoles, which correlates with the high degree of endocytotic activity present in these cells. Unlike cells of the vascular endothelium, liver endothelial cells lack an underlying basement membrane so that solutes and small particles have access to the perisinusoidal space. However, scattered connective tissue elements and extracellular matrix material are associated with the abluminal surfaces of the endothelial cells. The endothelial cells can secret a wide variety of proteins, such as interleukins, interferon, and TNF-α. Thus, along with Kupffer cells, the endothelium participates in host defense mechanisms in the liver.

Fat-storing (Ito) cells

Fat-storing, or Ito, cells are located in the space of Disse, under the endothelial lining, in close contact with liver parenchymal cells. They are derived from mesenchymal cells in the subendothelial space of the embryonic liver. In normal liver, these cells represent 5–8% of all liver cells. They are phenotypically long-lived cells with a low level of proliferative activity. The nucleated portion of the cell is often located in a recess between two parenchymal cells, and their cytoplasmic processes run in the space of Disse parallel to the endothelial lining. These extrusions cover several sinusoids, not only allowing their contact with a significant portion of the liver blood supply, but also allowing an intimate cell–cell contact with numerous other liver cells. These cytoplasmic extensions show numerous filaments and microtubules. The cytoplasm contains characteristic vitamin A-rich lipid droplets whose number and diameters seem to vary between species and under different physiologic conditions. In certain liver diseases, fat-storing cells develop a very different phenotype, in which they proliferate actively, alter their morphology, and acquire features of myofibroblasts with an accompanying loss of lipid droplets. These activated fat-storing cells play a major role in development of fibrosis.

In general, fat-storing cells which undergo activation exert the following functions:
- uptake, storage, and release of retinoids;
- synthesis and secretion of extracellular matrix proteins (collagens I, III, IV, V, and VI; laminin; tenascin; undulin; hyaluronic acid; and proteoglycans);

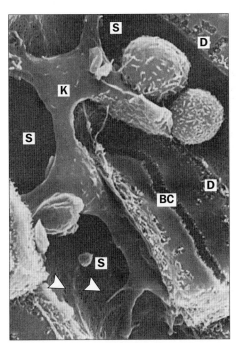

Figure 2.21 Scanning electron micrograph of a guinea pig liver. The centrally located hemibile canaliculus (BC) is between liver cells and the fenestrae are within the endothelial cells (arrowheads). A large Kupffer cell (K) reaches into two sinusoids (S) through a lacuna in the hepatic plates. D, space of Disse. ×6500. (From Jones AL. Anatomy of the normal liver. Zakem and Boyer, eds. 1996;3–32.)

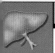

- synthesis and secretion of inflammatory and fibrogenic cytokines; and
- synthesis of additional and dilated rough ER and a prominent Golgi apparatus.

In addition, they often become surrounded by abundant interstitial collagen bundles.

Pit cells

In normal liver, most pit cells are located within the sinusoidal lumen and are adherent to the sinusoidal wall or anchored with villous extensions (pseudopods). Under physiologic conditions, pit cells are short-lived and continuously replaced by cells originating from extrahepatic sources. They were originally called large granular lymphocytes. In human liver they are present at very low frequencies in contrast to rat liver. The human pit cells have pronounced polarity, abundant cytoplasm containing dense granules, a conspicuous cytocenter, and locomotory shape with hyaloplasmic pseudopods and a uropod. The number of typical granules is significantly smaller than in the rat hepatocyte, however, and rod-cored vesicles are extremely rare. Another characteristic for human pit cells is the 'parallel tubular arrays', in which the tubular structures frequently associate with dense granules. They are thought to function in the liver:

- against cancer because of their strong cytotoxic activity against various tumor cell lines *in vitro*;
- in antiviral activity similar to that of natural killer cells; and
- in control of growth and differentiation of liver cells.

FURTHER READING

Bouwens L, De Bleser P, Vanderkerken K, Geerts B. Wisse E. Liver cell heterogeneity: functions of non-parenchymal cells. Enzyme. 1992;46:155–68. *Sinusoidal cells represent a functional unit at the border between hepatocytes and the blood, and their own heterogeneity provides the basis for a complex and important cellular cooperation.*

Crawford JM. Role of vesicle-mediated trasnport pathways in hepatocellular bile secretion. Semin. Liver Dis. 1996;16:169–89. *An excellent review of the plasma-to-bile trafficking of bile salts, phospholipids, cholesterol and proteins with emphasis on vesicle-mediated pathways.*

Darlington GJ. Molecular mechanisms of liver development and differentiation. Curr. Opin. Cell Biol. 1999;11:678–82. *A review of liver differentiation through the developing embryo, cell and tissue culture, knockout mice and cell transplantation.*

Diehl AM. Roles of CCAAT/enhancer-binding protein in regulation of liver regenerative growth. J. Biol. Chem. 1998;273:30843–6. *A review supporting the notion that members of the CCAAT/enhancer-binding proteins (C/EBP) family of transcription factors actively participate in many aspects of the regenerative response to liver injury.*

Friedman SL. Cytokines and fibrogenesis. Semin. Liver Dis. 1999;19:129–40. *Cytokines are critical effectors of stellate cell activation for a number of functions, including proliferation, contractility, chemotaxis, and fibrogenesis.*

Graf J, Haussinger D. Ion transport in hepatocytes: mechanisms and correlations to cell volume, hormone actions and metabolism. J. Hepatol. 1996;24 Suppl 1:53–77. *Transduction of a hormonal signal primarily involves alteration of membrane ion transport followed by a change in cell volume, which appears to assist in executing the stimulus on cell function.*

Gressner AM. The cell biology of liver fibrogenesis - an imbalance of proliferation, growth arrest and apoptosis of myofibroblasts. Cell Tissue Res. 1998;292:447–52. *Fibrosis following liver damage and factors influencing this process are discussed with special reference to hepatic stellate cells and their transformation to myofibroblasts.*

Hayashi Y, Wang W, Ninomiya T, Nagano H, Ohta K, Itoh H. Liver enriched transcription factors and differentiation of hepatocellular carcinoma. Mol. Pathol. 1999;52:19–24. *A review of transcription factors which are key elements in normal hepatocyte function and their potential role in the development of hepatocellular carcinoma.*

Lemasters JJ. V. Necrapoptosis and the mitochondrial permeability transition: shared pathways to necrosis and apoptosis. Am. J. Physiol. 1999;276:G1–6. *An important and timely commentary on cell death that involves characteristics of both necrosis and apoptosis.*

Makita T. Molecular organization of hepatocyte peroxisomes. Int. Rev. Cytol. 1995;160:303–52. *An exhaustive review of the biochemical, functional and structural characteristics of hepatocyte peroxisomes, providing some interesting surprises.*

Mannella CA, Buttle K, Rath BK, Marko M. Electron microscopic tomography of rat-liver mitochondria and their interaction with the endoplasmic reticulum. Biofactors. 1998;8:225–8. *Three-dimensional analysis suggests that the conventional model of the mitochondrion is incorrect, and that there is a complex tubular connection of inner membranes (cristae) to each other and the outside.*

Meier PJ. Molecular mechanisms of hepatic bile salt transport from sinusoidal blood into bile. Am. J. Physiol. 1995;269:G801–12. *An excellent review of the increasingly complex mechanisms involved in the Na⁺-dependent and -independent transport of bile acids across the hepatocyte membrane.*

Mitaka T, Mizuguchi T, Sato F, Mochizuki C, Mochizuki Y. Growth and maturation of small hepatocytes. J. Gastroentol. Hepatol. 1998;13:S70–7. *The data suggest that the so-called 'small hepatocytes' may, in fact, be committed progenitor cells that will further differentiate into mature hepatocytes.*

Morré DJ. Cell-free analysis of Golgi apparatus membrane traffic in rat liver. Histochem. Cell Biol. 1998;109:487–504. *Review of cell-free systems developed to study the complex mechanisms involved in vesicular trafficking along the endoplasmic reticulum/Golgi system/plasma membrane pathways.*

Nakielny S, Dreyfuss G. Transport of proteins and RNAs in and out of the nucleus. Cell. 1999;99:677–90. *A detailed review discussing all the major areas of nuclear import and export from cargos and transporters to routes, direction, translocation mechanisms and regulation.*

Piek E, Heldin C-H, Ten Dijke P. Specificity, diversity, and regulation in TGF-β superfamily signaling. FASEB J. 1999;13:2105–24. *An outstanding review of the molecular mechanisms of signaling specificity and regulation by the different superfamily members and how a single one can elicit a broad spectrum of biological responses.*

Sokol RJ, Treem WR. Mitochondria and childhood liver diseases. J. Pediatr. Gastroenterol. Nutr. 1999;28:4–16. *The newly recognized primary and secondary mitochondrial hepatopathies should be considered in the differential diagnosis of childhood acute and chronic liver diseases.*

Steer CJ. Receptor-mediated endocytosis: mechanisms, biologic function, and molecular properties. In Zakim D and Boyer TD (Eds): Hepatology: A Textbook of Liver Disease. 3rd ed., Philadelphia, W. B. Saunders, 1996, pp. 149–214. *A comprehensive review of hepatocyte receptors, ligand internalization and both the caveolar and clathrin-coated pit pathways of endocytosis, with an extensive reference list.*

Taub R, Greenbaum LE, Peng Y. Transcriptional regulatory signals define cytokine-dependent and -independent pathways in liver regeneration. Semin. Liver Dis. 1999;19:117–27. *A comprehensive review of transcriptional regulatory pathways which are critical for the normal regeneration of the liver after injury.*

Treem WR, Sokol RJ. Disorders of the mitochondria. Semin. Liver Dis. 1998;18:237–53. *An excellent and convincing review that inherited and acquired mitochondrial dysfunction are responsible for a number of diseases affecting the liver.*

Trembley JH, Kren BT, Steer CJ. Cyclins and gap junctions. In Strain A and Diehl AM (Eds): Liver Growth and Repair, London, Chapman & Hall Ltd.,1998, pp. 311–65. *A comprehensive chapter reviewing both the cell cycle and gap junctions in hepatocyte function with an excellent, inclusive reference list.*

Wisse E, Luo D, Vermijlen D, Kannellopoulou C, De Zanger R, Braet F. On the function of pit cells, the liver-specific natural killer cells. Semin. Liver Dis. 1997;17:265–86. *They probably originate in bone marrow as lymphoid cells, and migrate to the liver where they act as natural killer cells against a growing list of intruders.*

Zaret K. Early liver differentiation: genetic potentiation and multilevel growth control. Curr. Opin. Genet. Dev. 1998;8:526–31. *A comprehensive review of the regulatory transcription factors and cell signalling molecules that control the development of the mature liver.*

Zegers MMP, Hoekstra D. Mechanisms and functional features of polarized membrane traffic in epithelial and hepatic cells. Biochem. J. 1998;336:257–69. *The hepatocyte, with its distinct membrane domains, provides an excellent system to elucidate mechanisms of sorting and intracellular trafficking of both lipids and proteins in polarized cells.*

Zucker SD, Goessling W, Gollan JL. Intracellular transport of small hydrophobic compounds by the hepatocyte. Semin. Liver Dis. 1996;16:159–67. *This review summarizes recent developments in the field of intracellular transport, with particular reference to the metabolism of small hydrophobic and amphipathic molecular species, such as bilirubin, bile salts and fatty acids.*

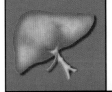

Section 1 Normal Structure and Function

Chapter 3

Function of the Normal Liver

Richard H Moseley

INTRODUCTION

The liver is composed of parenchymal cells, hepatocytes, and nonparenchymal cells. This latter cell population includes the sinusoidal endothelial cells, the Kupffer cells (the hepatic macrophages), the hepatic stellate cells (also termed the fat-storing, Ito, perisinusoidal cells or lipocytes), the bile duct epithelial cells, and the pit cells (a nonparenchymal cell type with natural killer cell activity). Each cell type contributes to the overall function of the liver, which in broad terms can be defined as the regulation of the concentration of solutes in blood that affect the function of other organs, such as the brain, heart, muscle, and kidneys. This regulation is achieved by the uptake, metabolism, biotransformation, storage, and secretion of endogenous and exogenous solutes and by *de novo* synthesis and secretion. The function of the hepatocytes in this regulatory process is the focus of this chapter.

MORPHOLOGIC CONSIDERATIONS

Hepatocytes are arranged in single-cell thick plates extending from the portal tract to the terminal hepatic venule (Fig. 3.1). Adjacent plates of hepatocytes are separated by the hepatic sinusoids, lined by endothelial cells with several characteristic ultrastructural features. Slender processes extending from the cell body contain pores (fenestrae), which are arranged in sieve plates. The fenestrae are dynamic structures under the regulation of an actin cytoskeleton. Unlike other endothelia, sinusoidal endothelial cells lack an underlying basement membrane, allowing direct exchange between plasma and the perisinusoidal space of Disse. This feature facilitates the transfer of protein-bound solutes, such as drugs, bilirubin, and bile acids, from sinusoidal blood to the hepatocyte, and promotes the excretion of, for example, lipoproteins and other proteins from the hepatocyte to the sinusoid. In cirrhosis, a continuous basement

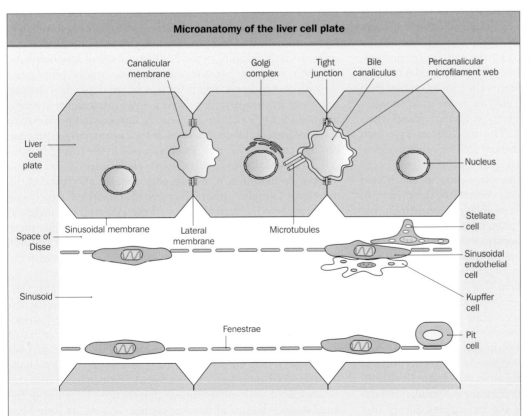

Microanatomy of the liver cell plate

Canalicular membrane · Golgi complex · Tight junction · Bile canaliculus · Pericanalicular microfilament web · Liver cell plate · Nucleus · Sinusoidal membrane · Lateral membrane · Microtubules · Stellate cell · Space of Disse · Sinusoidal endothelial cell · Sinusoid · Kupffer cell · Fenestrae · Pit cell

Figure 3.1 Microanatomy of the liver cell plate. The relationship of the four nonparenchymal cells to the hepatocytes is shown on the right. Kupffer cells and pit cells lie within the sinusoidal lumen. Endothelial cells separate the sinusoidal lumen from the space of Disse. Stellate cells (lipocytes) lie within the space of Disse. Intracellular organelles and features that play a role in bile secretion are shown within the hepatocytes.

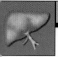

membrane accumulates between hepatocytes and endothelial cells, obliterating the fenestrae and impairing solute transfer in both directions. Defenestration also occurs early in liver cancer and in chronic alcohol abuse, contributing to the hyperlipoproteinemia associated with alcoholism.

Hepatocyte membranes

Neighboring hepatocytes are joined by junctional complexes that serve to demarcate the canalicular space from the basolateral, or sinusoidal, domain. Differences in the structure and function of the sinusoidal and canalicular membrane define the hepatocyte as a polarized cell. A lipid composition of a higher cholesterol–phospholipid and a lower phospholipid–sphingomyelin molar ratio in the canalicular than in the sinusoidal domain confers a relative resistance to the detergent actions of bile acids on the canalicular membrane. Morphologically similar to other transporting epithelia, the surface area of the sinusoidal and canalicular membranes is increased by microvilli. Major alterations in canalicular microvilli occur in intrahepatic and extrahepatic forms of cholestasis, including a reduction in the number of microvilli and the development of giant microvilli secondary to edema and bleb formation, which occlude the canalicular lumina to some degree. These findings suggest that canalicular microvilli, like their morphologic counterparts in the enterocyte, play a role in solute transport.

The sinusoidal membrane is primarily involved in the bidirectional exchange of solutes, and has uptake mechanisms for amino acids, glucose, and organic anions such as bile acids, fatty acids, and bilirubin; receptor-mediated endocytotic processes; Na^+,K^+-ATPase and glucagon-stimulatable adenylate cyclase activity; and export processes for albumin, lipoproteins, and clotting factors. The predominant function at the canalicular membrane surface is secretion, although limited reabsorptive capacity has been demonstrated. Certain membrane enzymes are selectively localized to the canalicular domain, including alkaline phosphatase, leucine aminopeptidase, and γ-glutamyl transpeptidase. Increased protein synthesis rather than impaired biliary secretion of the enzyme is the major mechanism underlying the elevation in hepatic alkaline phosphatase activity observed in cholestasis. The mechanism by which increased hepatic alkaline phosphatase activity leads to elevations in serum activity is less clear. Alkaline phosphatase contained within the bile canalicular membrane may be solubilized by bile acids that accumulate during cholestasis; these, in turn, would alter the tight junction permeability. Alternatively, the distribution of hepatic alkaline phosphatase activity may be altered, again by the high intrahepatic concentrations of bile acids in patients with cholestasis, so that it is found in all domains of the hepatocyte plasma membrane and enters serum directly from the plasma membrane.

From adjacent canaliculi, bile enters small terminal bile ductules, the canals of Hering, which consist of fusiform cells in close association with neighboring hepatocytes. These short channels traverse the limiting plate to form successively larger ductules and intralobular bile ducts, composed of cuboidal epithelial cells. Interlobular bile ducts, ranging in size from 30–40μm, convey bile to the extrahepatic bile duct, the gallbladder, and the duodenum. Cholangiocytes along the intrahepatic biliary tree are morphologically and functionally heterogeneous; regulated transport of water and electrolytes primarily occurs in the medium and large interlobular bile ducts.

Hepatocyte membrane junctions

The junctional complexes that join adjacent hepatocytes consist of several discrete structures. The tight junctions (i.e. zonulae occludens) function as a barrier to unrestricted movement of solutes from the space of Disse to the canalicular lumen. The tight junction, seen with freeze-fracture electron microscopy, is a network of anastomosing intramembrane strands or fibrils in the outwardly facing cytoplasmic leaflet (Fig. 3.2a). This barrier for entry into bile acts as if it is associated with a net negative charge, since the paracellular movement of negatively charged solutes from blood to bile is impaired. Likewise, negatively charged species, such as conjugated bile acids, secreted across the canalicular membrane may be retained in the canalicular lumen by this selective permeability barrier. Tight junction permeability, altered in intrahepatic and extrahepatic cholestasis, is determined by at least three tight junction-specific proteins. Rows of the transmembrane protein, occludin, act as the intercellular seal. Occludin is linked on its cytoplasmic surface zonula occludens to ZO1 and ZO2 (Fig. 3.2b). Both of these proteins are members of the membrane-associated guanylate kinase family of proteins involved in signal transduction pathways. Adjacent to the tight junction is the adherens junction or zonula adherens (Fig. 3.2b). The adhesion molecules, the cadherins, form zipper-like connections between hepatocytes. The cytoplasmic domains of cadherins interact with catenins, which are cytoplasmic proteins linked to the actin cytoskeleton. Cadherins have a critical role in the malignant behavior of some forms of cancer.

Located distal to the tight junction is the nexus or gap junction. One of the proposed functions for gap junctions is mediation of intercellular communication under physiologic conditions. Individual gap junction proteins, termed connexins, form hexameric channels that allow the exchange of ions and small molecules, such as calcium, cyclic AMP, and inositol trisphosphate, between adjacent hepatocytes. Calcium waves propagated through this pathway may activate calcium-dependent cellular responses, such as glycogenolysis. Loss of intracellular communication via gap junctions may lead to unregulated proliferation and liver tumors. Downregulation of the hepatocyte gap junction protein, connexin 32, may also play a role in the loss of hepatocellular function seen in extrahepatic cholestasis.

Spot desmosomes, or macula adherens, are also found in the junctional complex, where they are also involved in cell–cell adhesion. Intermediate filaments of the cytoskeleton anchor at these structures (Fig. 3.3). Composed of desmogleins, these structures serve a bridging function, maintaining contact between hepatocytes during pathologic situations that interfere with the function of gap junctions.

Actin-containing microfilaments are numerous in the pericanalicular cytoplasm, where they insert into the canalicular microvilli and into the junctional complex to form a pericanalicular web (Fig. 3.3). Coordinated and periodic contractions of canaliculi, responsive to intracellular calcium and bile acids, have been observed *in vitro* and *in vivo*. The 17α-alkylated anabolic steroid, norethandrolone, causes a form of drug-induced cholestasis associated with microfilament dysfunction. Increases in the number and density of hepatocyte microfilaments have been observed in other cholestatic disorders.

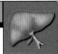

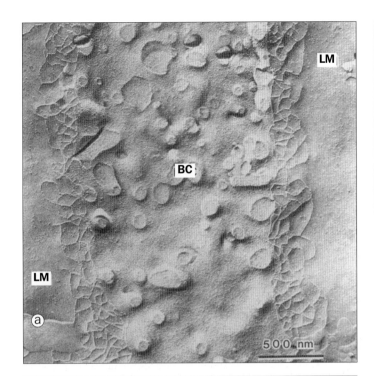

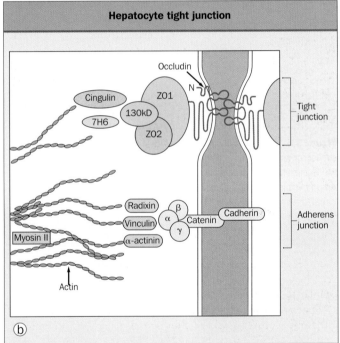

Figure 3.2 Hepatocyte tight junction. (a) Freeze fracture replica of hepatocyte tight junction. The grid-like tight junction elements act as a barrier between the bile canaliculus (BC) and the intracellular space lined by the lateral membrane (LM) (From Boyer JL. Hepatology. 1983;3:615.) (b) Schematic diagram of hepatocyte tight junction. An intercellular seal is formed by contact between pairs of the transmembrane protein, occludin, which are bound on the cytoplasmic surface to ZO1 and ZO2. Junctional proteins without known functions include cingulin and 7H6. The adherens junction is formed by the association of cadherins, which interact with α-, β-, and γ-catenin, cytoplasmic proteins that are linked to the actin cytoskeleton. (Adapted from Anderson JM, van Itallie CM. Am J Physiol. 1995;269:G468.)

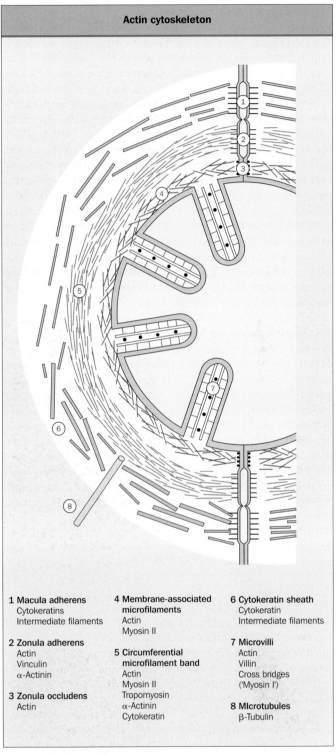

Actin cytoskeleton

1 **Macula adherens**
Cytokeratins
Intermediate filaments

2 **Zonula adherens**
Actin
Vinculin
α-Actinin

3 **Zonula occludens**
Actin

4 **Membrane-associated microfilaments**
Actin
Myosin II

5 **Circumferential microfilament band**
Actin
Myosin II
Tropomyosin
α-Actinin
Cytokeratin

6 **Cytokeratin sheath**
Cytokeratin
Intermediate filaments

7 **Microvilli**
Actin
Villin
Cross bridges
('Myosin I')

8 **MIcrotubules**
β-Tubulin

Figure 3.3 Actin cytoskeleton of the bile canaliculus. Three distinct zones of microfilaments are present: the microvillous core, a membrane-associated zone, and a circumferential pericanalicular microfilament band. The contraction control proteins of muscle, α-actinin and tropomyosin, and myosin II are present in this microfilament band. Intermediate filaments are present in a cytokeratin sheath that associates with the macula adherens and defines the outer limits of the bile canaliculus. (From Tsukada N, Ackerley CA, Phillips MJ. Hepatology. 1995;21:1111.)

Hepatocyte intracellular organelles

A variety of vesicular transport processes in cells is dependent on the integrity of microtubules. Vesicular transport is an energy-dependent process mediated partially by the microtubule-associated motor ATPases, dynamin, kinensin, and dynein, which are all present in abundance in hepatocytes. The role of microtubules in normal bile formation, in particular, appears to be primarily that of delivery of transport proteins to the canalicular membrane from intracellular compartments more proximal than subapical endosomes. The Golgi apparatus is preferentially located at the canalicular pole of the hepatocyte. Besides its role in protein synthesis, intact Golgi function is critical in the intracellular processes involved in bile formation. Dynamins, a family of 100kDa GTPases that associate with the Golgi apparatus to facilitate the formation of endocytic vesicles and promote intracellular vesicular traffic, also play a role in bile secretion. Bile acids interact with another intracellular organelle, the smooth endoplasmic reticulum (ER). Permeabilization of this intracellular compartment may play a role in the inhibition of bile secretion seen with the hydrophobic bile acids.

The hepatic acinus – a functional unit

A unique feature of hepatic architecture is the organization of hepatocytes within a hepatic acinus that is arbitrarily divided into three functional zones (Fig. 3.4). Zone 1 hepatocytes abut the portal tract and are exposed to sinusoidal blood containing the highest concentration of solutes and oxygen. In contrast, zone 3 hepatocytes, present in the pericentral region around the terminal hepatic venule, are exposed to a relatively oxygen-poor environment. As a result, ischemic hepatitis preferentially causes centrizonal hepatocyte necrosis. In addition, zone 3 hepatocytes actively participate in drug metabolism and disposition. Consequently, most drugs in clinical use, if hepatotoxic, induce zone 3 necrosis.

BILE FORMATION

Bile is composed primarily of water, inorganic electrolytes, and organic solutes such as bile acids, phospholipids, cholesterol, and bile pigments (Fig. 3.5). The volume of hepatic bile excreted is between 500 and 600mL/day. The relative proportions of the major organic solutes of bile are illustrated in Fig. 3.6. Bile acids are the major organic solutes in bile and are derived from two sources. Primary bile acids (i.e. cholic and chenodeoxycholic acid in

Composition of hepatic bile	
Component	**Concentration (mmol/L)**
Electrolytes	
Na+	141–165
K+	2.7–6.7
Cl–	77–117
HCO₃–	12–55
Ca²+	2.5–6.4
Mg²+	1.5–3.0
Organic anions	
Bile acids	3–45
Bilirubin	1–2
Lipids	
Lecithin	140–810 (mg/dL)
Cholesterol	97–320 (mg/dL)
Proteins	2–20 (mg/mL)
	0.02–0.2 (g/L)
Peptides and amino acids	
Glutathione	3–5
Glutamate	0.8–2.5
Aspartate	0.4–1.1
Glycine	0.6–2.6

Figure 3.5 Composition of hepatic bile. Values obtained from measurements of human, rat and rabbit bile. (Derived from Boyer JL. Mechanisms of bile secretion and hepatic transport. In: Andreoli et al., eds. Physiology of membrane disorders. New York: Plenum; 1986:609.)

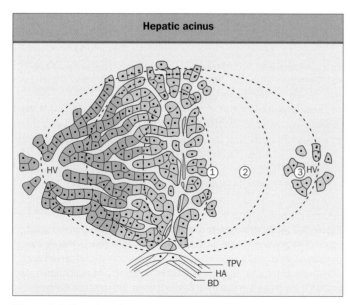

Figure 3.4 Hepatic acinus. The acinar axis is formed by the terminal branch of the portal vein (TPV), hepatic artery (HA), and bile ductule (BD). Blood enters the sinusoids in zone 1 and flows sequentially through zone 2 and zone 3, where it exits the acinus through the terminal branch of the hepatic vein (HV). (From Traber PG, Chianale J, Gumucio JJ. Gastroenterology. 1988;95:1131.)

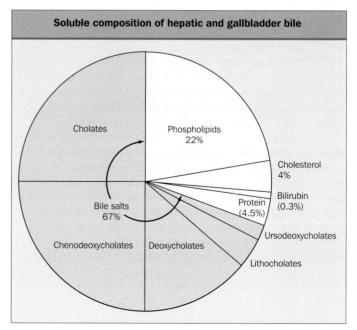

Figure 3.6 Typical solute composition in percentage by weight of hepatic and gallbladder bile in healthy humans.

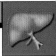

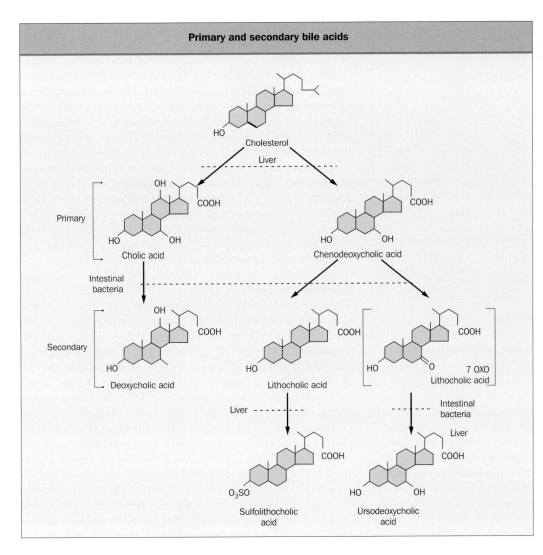

Primary and secondary bile acids

Cholesterol

Liver

Primary

Cholic acid

Chenodeoxycholic acid

Intestinal bacteria

Secondary

Deoxycholic acid

Lithocholic acid

7 OXO Lithocholic acid

Liver

Intestinal bacteria

Liver

Sulfolithocholic acid

Ursodeoxycholic acid

Figure 3.7 Major primary and secondary bile acids and their sites of synthesis and metabolism.

humans) are synthesized from cholesterol in the liver. Microsomal 7α-hydroxylase is the rate-limiting enzyme in bile acid synthesis. The secondary bile acids (i.e. deoxycholic, lithocholic, and ursodeoxycholic acid in humans) are produced from primary bile acids by bacterial enzymes in the intestine (Fig. 3.7). Bile acids consist of two components that determine their physiologic and physicochemical properties: a steroid nucleus with its hydroxyl substituents, and an aliphatic side chain. All of the major mammalian primary bile acids contain a 3- and a 7-hydroxyl substituent, which greatly increase water solubility or hydrophilicity.

The terminal carboxylic acid group of the side chain is modified after the synthesis of the primary bile acids and during the hepatic phase of the enterohepatic cycling of the secondary bile acids by enzymatic conjugation to taurine or glycine. Conjugation decreases the ability of bile acids to traverse cell membranes by passive diffusion in their transit down the biliary tract and small intestine. Glycine and taurine conjugates of bile acids also demonstrate selective resistance to hydrolysis by pancreatic enzymes during small intestinal transit. The net effect of conjugation is to permit bile acids to accumulate at an intralumenal concentration in the small intestine high enough to facilitate fat digestion and absorption.

The presence of hydrophilic (i.e. hydroxyl substituents and the amide linkage on the aliphatic side chain) and lipid-soluble or hydrophobic (i.e. the steroid nucleus) regions allows conjugated bile salts to act as amphiphilic molecules that form micelles or

polymolecular aggregates above a critical micellar concentration. Bile salt micelles can solubilize other biologically important amphiphilic solutes, such as cholesterol and phospholipids, to form mixed micelles. This detergent-like property of bile acids is important in stabilizing the physical state of bile and in promoting fat digestion and absorption.

The dihydroxy bile acid ursodeoxycholic acid (UDCA) is used in the treatment of chronic cholestatic disorders, such as primary biliary cirrhosis. Under normal conditions, UDCA represents less than 3% of the bile acid pool; it is more hydrophilic than the other major dihydroxy bile acids chenodeoxycholic acid and deoxycholic acid. The mechanism of action of UDCA is not clear, but it stimulates the biliary secretion and inhibits the intestinal reabsorption of endogenous bile acids, becoming the predominant bile acid in serum and in bile after long-term administration. It may, therefore, protect against bile duct and hepatocyte injury from hydrophobic bile acids, such as chenodeoxycholic acid, deoxycholic acid, and lithocholic acid, and other potential hepatotoxins.

As shown in Fig. 3.5, the predominant biliary cation is Na⁺, and the concentrations of inorganic electrolytes in bile are similar to their plasma concentrations. The inorganic electrolytes are largely responsible for the osmotic activity of bile, because the osmotic activity of most of the organic solutes, such as bile acids, is lost by aggregation into mixed micelles.

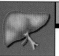

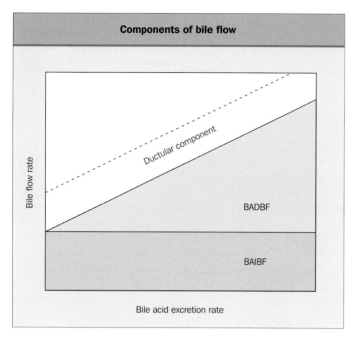

Figure 3.8 Components of bile flow. BADBF, bile acid-dependent bile flow; BAIBF, bile acid-independent bile flow.

In contrast to the passive, hydrostatic forces that govern glomerular filtration by the kidney, bile formation by hepatocytes is an osmotic process that involves the active secretion of osmotically active inorganic and organic solutes into the canalicular lumen, followed by passive water movement. In this important respect, hepatic bile secretion can be characterized by the same processes found in more conventional secretory epithelia.

Canalicular bile formation is classically measured using metabolically inert solutes, such as erythritol and mannitol, which are assumed to enter bile passively only at the level of the canaliculus and not to undergo modification by biliary ductular cells. Using

these markers, canalicular bile formation has been traditionally divided into two components (Fig. 3.8): bile acid-dependent bile flow (BADBF), which is defined as the slope of the line relating canalicular bile flow to bile salt excretion; and bile acid-independent bile flow (BAIBF), which is attributed to the active secretion of inorganic electrolytes and other solutes and defined as the extrapolated y-intercept of this line. Although these two components are typically discussed separately, BAIBF and BADBF should be viewed as interrelated components of bile flow.

There are two hypotheses to explain the apparent linear relation between bile acid secretion rates and bile flow. Because bile acids are in a micellar form in bile, the bile acids or, more accurately, their accompanying counterions (Na^+ predominantly), may provide an osmotic driving force for water and electrolyte movement. Another way in which bile acids may affect bile flow is by increasing the secretion of other solutes into bile.

Bile acid transport

The sinusoidal uptake of conjugated bile acids, such as taurocholate, is primarily mediated by a secondary active transport process, which is driven by the inwardly directed Na^+ gradient maintained by Na^+,K^+-ATPase activity. The negative electrical potential difference (PD) across the membrane maintained by Na^+,K^+-ATPase activity is also an important driving force, because Na^+–taurocholate cotransport is electrogenic (i.e. associated with the net entry of positive charge). This bile salt transporter has been cloned from both rat and human liver and termed the Na^+-taurocholate cotransporting polypeptide, ntcp and NTCP, respectively. Expression and function of ntcp is downregulated in several models of experimental cholestasis, including a model of sepsis-associated cholestasis. Findings in patients with extrahepatic biliary atresia suggest similar regulation of NTCP. The molecular mechanism for the downregulation of sinusoidal bile acid uptake is beginning to be defined (Fig. 3.9).

The uptake of unconjugated bile acids at the sinusoidal membrane, in contrast, is a Na^+-independent process mediated, in

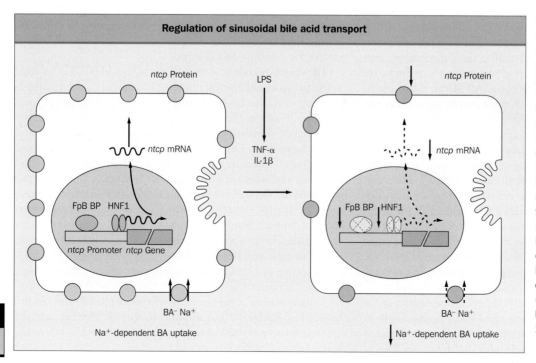

Regulation of sinusoidal bile acid transport

Figure 3.9 Regulation of sinusoidal bile acid transport. Sodium-dependent sinusoidal bile acid (BA^-) uptake in the rat is mediated by the protein ntcp. Under normal conditions, *ntcp* gene expression is regulated by the binding of the transcription factors hepatocyte nuclear factor 1 (HNF1) and footprint B binding protein (FpB BP) to the *ntcp* promoter. Endotoxin (LPS) and cytokines released in response to LPS, tumor necrosis factor (TNF)-α and interleukin (IL)1β, reduce levels of HNF1 and FpB BP in the nucleus, leading to decreased *ntcp* mRNA expression. In turn, ntcp protein and Na^+-dependent BA uptake are reduced. (From Trauner M, Arrese M, Lee H, Boyer JL, Karpen SJ. J Clin Invest. 1998;101:2099.)

part, by the organic anion transporting polypeptide, oatp1. The Na^+-independent uptake of bile salts exhibits a broad substrate specificity that includes electroneutral steroids, such as ouabain and progesterone; cyclic oligopeptides, such as phalloidin, somatostatin analogs, and cyclosporine; and a wide variety of xenobiotics. Hepatic uptake of amatoxins, the toxic product in toadstools of the genus *Amanita* and the cause of most accidental mushroom poisonings, is also mediated by this multispecific organic anion transport process.

Serum bile acids are frequently elevated in patients with cirrhosis. It is unclear whether this is the result of hemodynamic alterations, shunts, and the reduced liver cell mass observed in cirrhosis, as proposed in the intact cell hypothesis; or a result of dysfunction at the level of the individual hepatocyte, as proposed in the sick cell hypothesis.

The mechanism for intracellular transport of bile acids from the sinusoidal to the canalicular pole of hepatocytes is not as well understood. Intracellular binding of bile acids has been proposed as a mechanism for hepatic transport and a protective mechanism against potential toxic effects of free bile acids. Two unrelated families of cytosolic proteins with high affinities for bile acids have been identified: ligandins and Y′ proteins. The Y′ bile acid binders belong to the monomeric reductase gene family that also bind derivatives of polycyclic aromatic hydrocarbon carcinogens. These cytosolic proteins may be involved in the intracellular transport of bile acids and carcinogens to the canalicular membrane or to intracellular organelles by diffusion. Extrahepatic cholestasis downregulates these bile acid binders at a post-transcriptional level. Bile acids are also transported into smooth endoplasmic reticulum by a Na^+-independent, electrogenic process, which is mediated by microsomal epoxide hydrolase.

On the basis of morphometric studies of ER, Golgi apparatus, and pericanalicular cytoplasm after bile acid-induced choleresis, a vectorial vesicular transport of bile acids across the hepatocyte

was proposed. Despite these observations, morphologic evidence of exocytosis of bile acid-loaded vesicles at the canalicular membrane has not been reported. Instead, the dependence of bile salt secretion on intact microtubule function appears to be an indirect consequence of microtubule-dependent delivery of bile salt transporters to the canalicular membrane.

Canalicular excretion represents the rate-limiting step in the hepatic transport of bile acids. Canalicular secretion of anionic bile acids was believed to occur by passive facilitated diffusion down an energetically favorable electrochemical gradient. However, the magnitude of the membrane potential is too small to account for the bile salt concentration gradient that exists across the canalicular membrane, and alternative mechanisms have been identified for carrier-mediated bile acid secretion at this membrane domain. A member of the P-glycoprotein family encoded by the *spgp* gene is an ATP-dependent canalicular bile acid transporter. A defect in this canalicular bile acid transporter is responsible for a form of progressive familial intrahepatic cholestasis, PFIC type 2. The vectorial movement of bile acids from sinusoidal blood to canalicular bile is schematically depicted in Fig. 3.10.

Electrolyte transport

In contrast to the information regarding BADBF, less is known about the hepatocellular mechanisms that underlie BAIBF. Inhibition of Na^+,K^+-ATPase activity does not appear to have a significant effect on BAIBF, and indirect evidence points to a primary role for bicarbonate (HCO_3^-) transport. In other epithelia, such as the pancreas, HCO_3^- transport has been attributed to Na^+–H^+ exchange (i.e. antiport) activity. With the identification and characterization of sinusoidal Na^+–H^+ exchange and canalicular Cl–HCO_3^- exchange, a model was proposed (Fig. 3.11) in which these two transport processes are functionally coupled by way of cytosolic carbonic anhydrase to generate net biliary bicar-

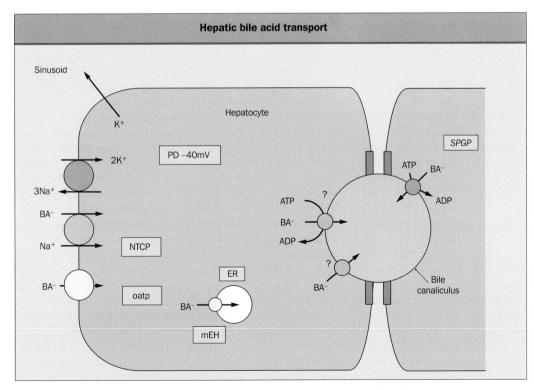

Figure 3.10 Hepatic bile acid transport. The sinusoidal uptake of conjugated bile acids (BA^-), such as taurocholate, is primarily mediated by the Na^+–taurocholate cotransporting polypeptide NTCP. The uptake of unconjugated bile acids at the sinusoidal membrane, in contrast, is a Na^+-independent process that is mediated, in part, by the organic anion transporting polypeptide oatp. Intracellular transport of bile acids involves binding to ligandins and Y′ proteins and uptake into smooth endoplasmic reticulum by a Na^+-independent, electrogenic process, mediated by microsomal epoxide hydrolase (mEH). A member of the P-glycoprotein family encoded by the *SPGP* gene mediates ATP-dependent bile acid excretion at the canalicular membrane.

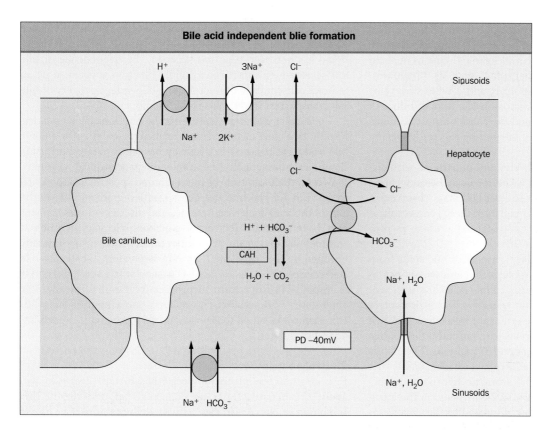

Bile acid independent blie formation

H⁺ 3Na⁺ Cl⁻

Sinusoids

Na⁺ 2K⁺

Hepatocyte

Cl⁻

Cl⁻

Bile canilculus

H⁺ + HCO₃⁻

CAH

HCO₃⁻

H₂O + CO₂

Na⁺, H₂O

PD –40mV

Na⁺ HCO₃⁻

Na⁺, H₂O

Sinusoids

Figure 3.11 Bile acid-independent bile formation. Sinusoidal Na⁺-H⁺ exchange and canalicular Cl—HCO₃ exchange are functionally coupled by means of cytosolic carbonic anhydrase (CAH) to generate net biliary bicarbonate secretion. A sinusoidal Na⁺-HCO₃ symport in conjunction with canalicular Cl—HCO₃ exchange may also play a role in biliary HCO₃ secretion (Adapted from Moseley RH, Meier PJ, Aronson PS, et al. Am J Physiol. 1986;250:G42).

bonate secretion. A sinusoidal Na^+-HCO_3^- symport in conjunction with canalicular Cl–HCO_3^- exchange may also play a role in biliary bicarbonate secretion. Support for this model comes primarily from studies examining the effects of certain cholestatic and choleretic agents on membrane transport. Ethinyl estradiol, which causes a diminution in BAIBF, inhibits Na^+-H^+ exchange activity; UDCA, which results in a HCO_3^-–rich choleresis, stimulates Na^+-H^+ exchange activity. Amiloride and acetazolamide, inhibitors of Na^+–H^+ exchange and carbonic anhydrase activity, respectively, produce a concentration-dependent inhibition of UDCA-stimulated bile flow and biliary HCO_3^- output.

Inorganic electrolytes may not provide a sufficient driving force for BAIBF, however, because their biliary secretion depends primarily on passive diffusion and solvent drag. This has led to the alternative suggestion that nonbile salt organic anions may provide a major driving force for canalicular BAIBF. The tripeptide glutathione (γ-L-glutamyl-L-cysteinylglycine; GSH) may fulfill this role. It is present in bile in high concentrations (see Fig. 3.5) and, as a result of intrabiliary catabolism of GSH by γ-glutamyl transpeptidase located on the lumenal membranes of bile ductule cells and the bile canalicular membrane, the concentration of this solute in the canalicular lumen may be substantially higher than that measured in excreted bile. At concentrations that exceed free (i.e. nonmicelle associated) bile acids and bile pigments, GSH may generate a potent osmotic driving force for canalicular bile formation. Because biliary secretion of GSH is a carrier-mediated process, the requirement that the solute providing the driving force for BAIBF not be governed by passive diffusion or solvent drag is met. Additional indirect evidence supports a role for GSH in BAIBF, including the strong correlation of GSH excretion with drug-induced changes in BAIBF and with ontogenic changes in bile formation. However, other unidentified solutes, in addition to GSH, may also contribute to BAIBF.

Bilirubin metabolism and transport

For a full discussion of bilirubin metabolism and transport, see Chapter 5.

Bilirubin is generated by the breakdown of heme. Approximately 80% of bilirubin is derived from heme released by senescent erythrocytes, while the remainder comes from the heme moieties of other hemoproteins, such as myoglobin and tissue cytochromes. The microsomal enzyme, heme oxygenase, converts heme to biliverdin, which is then converted to bilirubin by biliverdin reductase. The unconjugated bilirubin produced by these enzymatic reactions is transported in the plasma tightly bound to albumin. Competition for albumin binding by certain drugs displaces unconjugated bilirubin and, in the neonate, may result in the diffusion of bilirubin across the blood–brain barrier and bilirubin encephalopathy, or kernicterus.

Bilirubin uptake and secretion is mediated by transport processes distinct from those identified for bile acid transport (Fig. 3.12). Sinusoidal uptake of bilirubin and other non-bile acid organic anions is a Na^+-independent process mediated, in large part, by oatp1. Glutathione efflux from the hepatocyte appears to provide the driving force for uptake via oatp1. Within the hepatocyte, bilirubin and other organic anions bind to cytosolic glutathione S-transferases or ligandins. Conjugation of bilirubin to its monoglucuronides and diglucuronides, catalyzed by bilirubin-UDP-glucuronosyl-transferase (UDP-GT), is required for canalicular secretion. Canalicular secretion, in turn, involves a homolog of the multidrug resistance protein, MRP2. A point mutation in MRP2 is the molecular basis for the Dubin–Johnson syndrome, an autosomal-recessive disorder characterized by a conjugated hyperbilirubinemia. Sepsis-associated cholestatic jaundice may be, in part, the result of downregulation of this rate-limiting step in overall hepatic bilirubin transport.

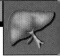

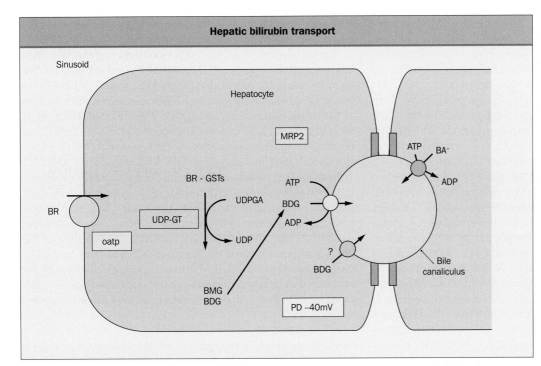

Hepatic bilirubin transport

Figure 3.12 Hepatic bilirubin transport. Unconjugated bilirubin (BR), disassociated from albumin, is taken up at the sinusoidal membrane by a Na^+-independent process, mediated by organic anion transporting polypeptide (oatp). Within the hepatocyte, bilirubin and other organic anions bind to cytosolic glutathione S-transferases or ligandins. Conjugation of bilirubin to its monoglucuronides and diglucuronides (BMG and BDG), catalyzed by bilirubin-UDP-glucuronosyl-transferase (UDP-GT), is required for canalicular secretion. Canalicular secretion involves a homolog of the multidrug resistance protein, MRP2.

Pathophysiologically, jaundice is classified as either the result of an unconjugated or conjugated hyperbilirubinemia. Unconjugated hyperbilirubinemia results from either increased bilirubin production, impaired hepatic uptake, or impaired conjugation. Increased red blood cell destruction in disorders associated with ineffective erythropoiesis and in hemolytic disorders results in increased bilirubin production and a mild unconjugated hyperbilirubinemia. Reductions in hepatic bloodflow due to congestive heart failure or portosytemic shunting impair the delivery of bilirubin to hepatocytes, resulting in a mild unconjugated hyperbilirubinemia. Impaired hepatic uptake at the sinusoidal membrane occurs in Gilbert's syndrome and following the administration of certain drugs, such as rifampin (rifampicin). Reduced activity of UDP-GT leads to impaired bilirubin conjugation and is observed in the neonate and in patients with Gilbert's and Crigler–Najjar type I and II syndromes. Activity of UDP-GT can be induced by phenobarbital, effectively reducing the jaundice in Crigler–Najjar type II syndrome.

Hepatic bilirubin uptake and conjugating activity are preserved in most forms of liver disease. Accordingly, conjugated hyperbilirubinemias can occur in a wide spectrum of hepatic diseases, including disorders associated with acute and chronic hepatocellular and cholestatic injury and extrahepatic biliary obstruction.

Ductular events

Experimental approaches, such as the isolation of intact segments from small interlobular bile ducts, the site of injury in the vanishing bile duct syndromes, have led to a better understanding of the biology and pathology of the biliary epithelium; the biliary tract is no longer considered merely a conduit for bile. The mechanism for the HCO_3^--rich fluid secretion by bile duct epithelial cells has been examined at both a cellular and molecular level. As shown in Fig. 3.13, the binding of the hormone secretin, and possibly of other agonists, to receptors localized to the basolateral domain of the bile duct epithelial cell leads to an increased intracellular level of the second messenger cAMP.

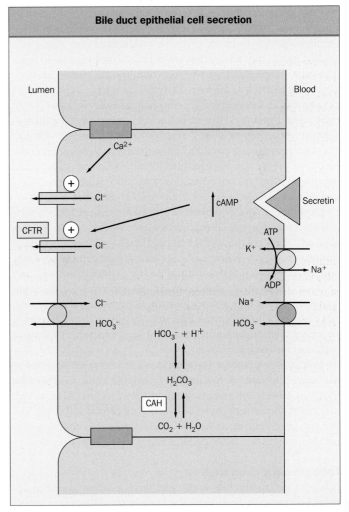

Bile duct epithelial cell secretion

Figure 3.13 Bile duct epithelial cell secretion. See text for details. CFTR, cystic fibrosis transmembrane conductance regulator; CAH, carbonic anhydrase; cAMP, adenosine 3′,5′-cyclic monophosphate.

Chloride exits from the apical membrane through cAMP-responsive cystic fibrosis transmembrane conductance regulator (CFTR)-associated Cl^- channels. The resulting cell depolarization facilitates the uptake of HCO_3^- at the basolateral membrane, mediated by a Na^+–HCO_3^- symport (or a Na^+–Cl^-–HCO_3^- cotransporter). Intracellular HCO_3^-, increased by either this mechanism or by enhanced carbonic anhydrase activity, then enters the bile duct lumen by means of apical Cl^-–HCO_3^- exchange. The mechanism for the HCO_3^--rich secretin-induced choleresis may involve cAMP-dependent insertion of vesicles containing CFTR or Cl^-–HCO_3^- exchange into the apical membrane of the bile duct epithelial cell, a process that is inhibited by somatostatin. In addition to the cAMP-regulated CFTR, bile duct epithelial cells also possess a calcium-dependent Cl^- channel. Because the biliary epithelium appears to be less susceptible to injury than other secretory epithelia in cystic fibrosis, this Cl^- channel may play a more dominant role in biliary secretion. A clinical correlation of the secretory activity of the biliary epithelium can be found in the increased response to secretin and increased bile flow observed in patients with chronic liver diseases associated with ductular proliferation.

Gallbladder function

The physiologic functions of the gallbladder include concentration and storage of bile during interdigestive periods; evacuation by smooth muscle contraction in response to cholecystokinin (CCK); moderation of hydrostatic pressure within the biliary tract; bile acidification; and absorption of organic components of bile. Although not essential for bile secretion, the gallbladder concentrates bile as much as 10-fold. This process is largely the result of electroneutral Na^+-coupled Cl^- transport and passive water movement. The exact mechanism is unclear; experimental evidence supports either coupled NaCl entry or a Na^+–H^+ and Cl^-–HCO_3^- exchange operating in parallel. The net result of this concentrative process is the formation of gallbladder bile, isotonic to plasma and composed of higher concentrations of Na^+, bile salts, K^+, and Ca^{2+} and lower concentrations of Cl^- and HCO_3^- than hepatic bile.

Despite the considerable concentration gradient for bile salts and bile pigments, the absorption of highly ionized organic solutes such as taurocholate, sulfobromophthalein, and iodipamide is minimal. In acute cholecystitis, increased permeability to water and to highly ionized solutes has been demonstrated, and enhanced absorption of iodipamide may account for the non-visualization of the gallbladder that occurs in this setting. Accelerated absorption of bile salts resulting from bacterial deconjugation or gallbladder mucosal injury may be a factor in gallstone formation.

Mucus is released by the exocytosis of secretory granules in the apical portion of gallbladder epithelial cells. Gallbladder mucin synthesis and release are markedly accelerated in animal models of cholesterol cholelithiasis before crystal and stone formation. Formation of an insoluble mucin–bilirubin complex may provide a nidus for cholesterol monohydrate nucleation.

Enterohepatic circulation

It is best to consider bile acid secretion as a cyclic flow of molecules anatomically limited to the hepatocyte, biliary tree, small intestine, enterocyte, and portal blood, known as the *enterohepatic circulation* (Fig. 3.14). Intestinal conservation of bile acids is approximately 90% efficient, reflecting the additive effects of both passive and active reabsorptive processes. The bile acid pool cycles 5–15 times daily through this pathway.

Passive absorption of bile acids occurs throughout the small intestine and depends on intestinal pH and bile acid structure. The most hydrophobic bile acids (i.e. glycine-conjugated dihydroxy bile acids) are passively absorbed in the more acidic environment of the duodenum, where the fraction in protonated (uncharged) form is greatest. Bile acids are transported across the ileal brush border membrane by a Na^+-dependent transporter, referred to as the apical sodium-dependent bile acid transporter (ASBT). Trihydroxy (i.e. cholic acid) bile acids are favored over dihydroxy (i.e. chenodeoxycholic acid) bile acids, and conjugated over unconjugated species. Similar to NTCP, ASBT is not fully operative at birth, and the inability to conserve bile salts may contribute to the diminished bile salt pool size and 'physiologic steatorrhea' of the immediate postnatal period. Mutations in ABST have been associated with idiopathic bile acid diarrhea, a chronic diarrheal illness characterized by bile acid malabsorption, lack of association with other forms of ileal dysfunction, and a response to cholestyramine.

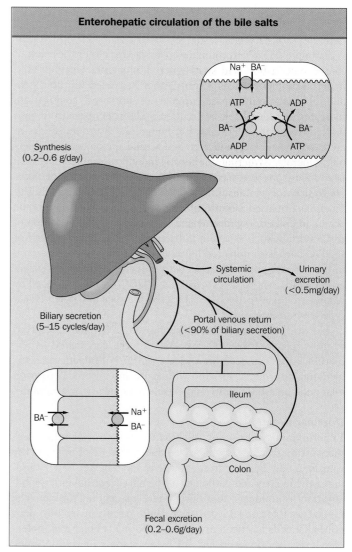

Figure 3.14 Enterohepatic circulation of bile salts and typical kinetic values for healthy humans. Insets depict bile acid transport at the level of the hepatocyte and the enterocyte. BA, bile acid.

Intracellular transport of bile acids in enterocytes is mediated by several cytosolic and microsomal proteins. The best characterized of these proteins is the ileal lipid-binding protein, a member of the fatty acid-binding protein family. At the basolateral membrane of the ileum, bile acids leave the enterocyte by a Na^+-independent anion exchange process, recently attributed to a member of the organic anion transporting polypeptide family, oatp3. Absorption of bile acids occurs solely into portal blood.

The small fraction of bile acids that escapes active or passive absorption in the small intestine undergoes bacterial modification in the colon. The secondary bile acids formed are also reabsorbed to various degrees, depending on their physicochemical properties, their interaction with lumenal constituents, and the permeability characteristics of the colon. Lithocholate and deoxycholate, formed from the 7-dehydroxylation of chenodeoxycholate and cholate, respectively, are the major fecal bile acids in humans.

Continuous bile acid synthesis from cholesterol is required to maintain the bile acid pool in the enterohepatic circulation. The maximal rate of synthesis is on the order of 4–6g/day. The importance of bile acid synthesis in health is evident if the effects of a cessation in synthesis are considered. Fecal loss would not be repleted, cholesterol would not be excreted, bile acid-dependent bile formation would stop, and fat-soluble substances would not be absorbed. Cerebrotendinous xanthomatosis is a rare inherited defect in bile acid synthesis characterized by progressive neurologic disturbances, premature atherosclerosis, cataracts, and tendinous xanthomas. Low plasma cholesterol but elevated plasma cholestanol levels are the result of mitochondrial 26-hydroxylase deficiency, an enzyme involved in cholesterol side-chain oxidation. Bile acid synthesis is decreased in this disorder, preferentially affecting chenodeoxycholate levels. The loss of bile acid feedback inhibition of cholesterol synthesis leads to the formation of cholestanol, which accumulates in myelin. Hydroxylation of cholesterol to form bile alcohols, which are then conjugated to glucuronides and excreted in bile and urine,

accounts for the low cholesterol levels. Treatment with chenodeoxycholate suppresses the biochemical abnormalities and may improve neurologic symptoms.

CENTRAL METABOLIC MECHANISMS

Apart from its unique role in biliary metabolism, the liver is central to the metabolism of lipids, carbohydrates and proteins, as well as being closely involved in drug metabolism. Some of these metabolic pathways are summarized in Fig. 3.15.

CHOLESTEROL AND LIPOPROTEIN METABOLISM

The liver plays a pivotal role in normal cholesterol and lipoprotein metabolism. Cholesterol homeostasis is maintained by pathways that either increase or decrease hepatic cholesterol. Pathways that increase hepatic cholesterol include uptake from lipoproteins [chylomicrons and low-density lipoprotein (LDL)] and *de novo* synthesis of cholesterol, regulated by the enzyme, 3-hydroxy-3-methylglutaryl (HMG)-coenzyme A (CoA) reductase. Cholesterol present in the liver exists either as cholesterol esters, a storage form, or free cholesterol. Concentrations of these two forms of cholesterol are governed by acyl-CoA:cholesterol acyltransferase (ACAT), which esterifies free cholesterol, and cholesterol ester hydrolase (CEH), which hydrolyzes cholesterol esters. The two major pathways that decrease hepatic cholesterol are synthesis of bile acids from free cholesterol and biliary excretion of free cholesterol.

The pathways responsible for cholesterol homeostasis are tightly regulated. Cholesterol inhibits HMG-CoA reductase and bile acids decrease bile acid biosynthesis from cholesterol by inhibition of cholesterol 7α-hydroxylase.

The major lipoprotein secreted by the liver is very-low-density lipoprotein (VLDL). The amounts of free fatty acids taken up by the liver and diet are the principal regulatory factors in the

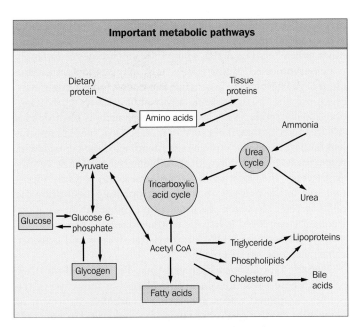

Figure 3.15 Important metabolic pathways of proteins, carbohydrates and lipids in the liver.

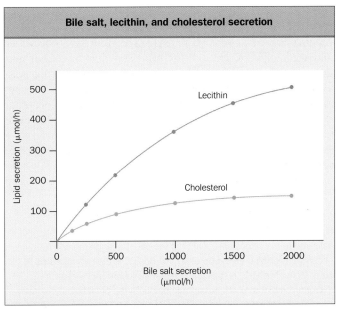

Figure 3.16 Influence of bile salt excretion rates on lecithin and cholesterol secretion rates.

rate of production, composition, and rate of secretion of VLDL.

Biliary bile acids promote endogenous lipid secretion and stabilize the physicochemical state of bile. Biliary output of nonesterified cholesterol and phosphatidylcholine (PC) (i.e. lecithin), the two major lipids in bile, is curvilinearly related to bile acid output. Lecithin secretion exceeds cholesterol secretion (Fig. 3.16). Bile salts appear to promote biliary secretion of phospholipids following their secretion into bile by preferential partitioning into microdomains of the outer leaflet of the canalicular membrane that are also enriched with biliary-type PCs. These bile salts in the canalicular lumen induce vesiculation of the canalicular membrane. The inner or cytoplasmic leaflet of the canalicular membrane is resupplied with biliary-type PCs derived from smooth ER membranes by PC transfer protein (TP) and sterol carrier protein 2. Translocation of phospholipid from the inner to the outer leaflet of the canalicular membrane bilayer is mediated by the product of the *mdr2* gene, the mouse homolog of human *MDR3*.

The pathway for phospholipid secretion proposed in Fig. 3.17 appears to be specific for PCs; although the mechanism is unclear, a largely separate secretory pathway exists for cholesterol secretion. However, the initiating event in the pathogenesis of cholesterol cholelithiasis may involve disruption of the coupling of biliary cholesterol excretion to simultaneous secretion of phospholipid and bile acids.

Liver disease causes significant lipid abnormalites. Chronic cholestasis, as found in primary biliary cirrhosis, results in hypercholesterolemia, mainly due to unesterified cholesterol, and xanthelasma, in the presence of moderate hyperlipidemia, and eventually xanthoma, in the presence of severe hyperlipidemia. Much of the elevated serum cholesterol in these patients is associated with a novel LDL, lipoprotein-X, and accelerated atherosclerosis does not occur. Lipoprotein-X particles most likely represent biliary vesicles that are regurgitated into the plasma of cholestatic subjects. In patients with acute hepatitis, hypertriglyceridemia and a moderate increase in total cholesterol, with a markedly decreased fraction as cholesterol ester, are observed. In chronic liver disease, similar lipid abnormalities are observed, although not as pronounced.

DRUG METABOLISM

The liver plays a major role in drug metabolism or biotransformation. Products of hepatic biotransformation destined for urinary elimination are transported back into sinusoidal blood. Organic lipophilic drugs undergo biliary excretion, because these substances are poorly filtered at the glomerulus and minimally secreted by the renal tubule. Hepatic uptake of many drugs is mediated by the same transport processes that are involved in hepatic bile formation discussed above. In addition, the hepatic uptake of organic cations, a class of substances that accounts for about 70% of drugs used in clinical practice, is mediated by a membrane potential-dependent carrier on the sinusoidal membrane, termed OCT1 (Fig. 3.18). Once drugs are taken up by the liver, they are processed or metabolized by several families of enzymes located in the endoplasmic reticulum, the cytosol, and, to a lesser extent, other organelles (Fig. 3.19). The p450 cytochromes are a family of hemoproteins situated predominantly in the endoplasmic reticulum of the hepatocyte in a membrane-bound form. Drug metabolism by the p450 system, although typically detoxifying, occasionally produces toxic intermediates such as electrophiles and free radicals that, if not further metabolized, can lead to covalent binding to cellular proteins and membrane lipid peroxidation, respectively. Conjugation with glutathione is mediated by cytosolic enzymes, the glutathione S-transferases, and plays an important role in the detoxification of electrophiles produced by the p450 system. However, glucuronidation and sulfation are more frequently employed in hepatic biotransformation and are mediated by microsomal UDP-glururonyl transferases and cytosolic sulfotransferases, respectively.

Hepatic biotransformation can thus, be classified into two phases. Phase I reactions involve oxidation or reduction of the parent compound, often generating a carboxyl, hydroxyl, or epoxide group that can subsequently be conjugated in a phase II reaction with, for example, glucuronic acid, glutathione, sulfate, or acetate. However, many drugs do not undergo sequen-

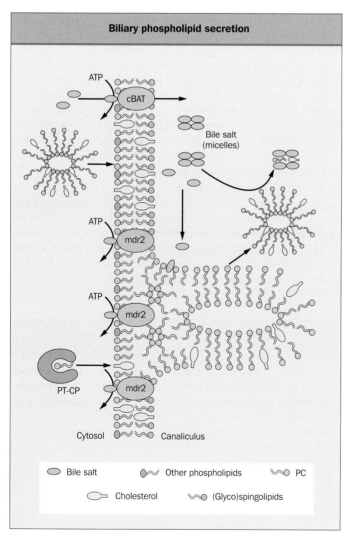

Biliary phospholipid secretion

ATP

cBAT

Bile salt
(micelles)

ATP

mdr2

ATP

mdr2

PT-CP

mdr2

Cytosol   Canaliculus

◯ Bile salt   ◯〜 Other phospholipids   〜◯ PC

◻ Cholesterol   〜◯ (Glyco)spingolipids

Figure 3.17 Biliary phospholipid secretion. Phosphatidylcholine (PC) is delivered to the cytoplasmic leaflet of the canalicular membrane by phosphatidylcholine transfer protein (PC-TP). PC is then translocated to the outer leaflet by mdr2, resulting in a relative phospholipid excess in microdomains of the canalicular membrane. In the presence of bile salts, secreted into the lumen by the canalicular bile acid transporter (cBAT), SPGP, these microdomains are destabilized and vesicular structures develop that pinch off to yield biliary lipid vesicles.

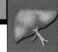

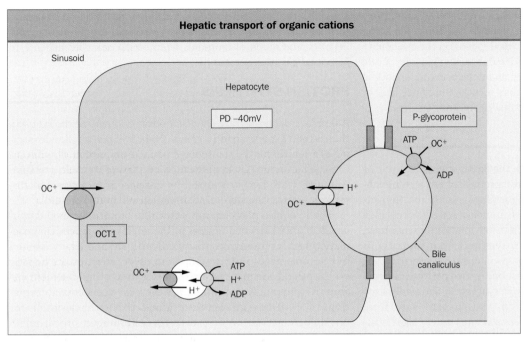

Hepatic transport of organic cations

Sinusoid

Hepatocyte

PD –40mV

P-glycoprotein

ATP   OC⁺

ADP

OC^+

H^+

OC^+

OCT1

OC^+ ATP
H^+
H^+ ADP

Bile
canaliculus

Figure 3.18 Hepatic transport of organic cations. The uptake of organic cations (OC⁺) is mediated by a membrane potential-dependent carrier on the sinusoidal membrane, termed OCT1. Organic cations may then be sequestered into acidified intracellular organelles by a H⁺-ATPase-dependent organic cation–H⁺ exchanger. In addition to P-glycoprotein-mediated organic cation efflux, biliary secretion of small-molecular-weight organic cationic drugs may be mediated by an organic cation–H⁺ exchanger.

Key enzyme families in hepatic drug metabolism

Enzyme family	Cofactors	Intracellular site
Cytochromes P450	NADPH, O2	Endoplasmic reticulum
Glucuronyltransferases	UDP-glucuronic acid	Endoplasmic reticulum
Sulfotransferases	Sulfate (PAPS)	Cytosol
Glutathione S-transferases	Reduced glutathione (GSH)	Cytosol and endoplasmic reticulum

Figure 3.19 Key enzyme families in hepatic drug metabolism. PAPS, 3′-phosphoadenosine-5′-phosphosulfate.

tial phase I and II reactions. The effect of phase I reactions is increased polarity, or water solubility, and, therefore, enhanced excretory potential. Phase II reactions further increase the water solubility of a compound. Although the products of phase II reactions tend to be less toxic and less active than the parent compound, phase I reactions may produce toxic intermediates. Exposure to specific substrates of an hepatic drug-metabolizing enzyme may induce the activity of that enzyme. Such induction may be clinically relevant if the enzyme induced produces a toxic intermediate. One of the best examples of such a phenomenon is acetaminophen (paracetamol) hepatotoxicity. Although metabolized largely by sulfation and glucuronidation (phase II reactions), a small percentage of the drug is oxidized by cytochrome p450 to a reactive metabolite. Chronic alcohol exposure induces this form of cytochrome p450, providing an explanation for the enhanced susceptibility of chronic alcoholics to acetaminophen hepatotoxicity.

A specific example of a biliary excretory mechanism for drugs is the multidrug transport protein, known as P-glycoprotein or 9170, encoded by the *MDR1* gene. Originally described in tumor-derived tissue culture systems resistant to cytotoxic hydrophobic agents, such as vinblastine, vincristine, and daunomycin, this ATP-dependent drug efflux system is located on the canalicular membrane and the apical surface of biliary epithelial cells lining small biliary ductules. This selective localization suggests that this membrane transport protein may serve as a pathway for the detoxification of physiologic metabolites and chemotherapeutic agents. In addition to P-glycoprotein-mediated drug efflux, biliary secretion

of small-molecular-weight organic cationic drugs may be mediated by an organic cation–H⁺ exchanger, a process that shares similarities with renal drug transport (see Fig. 3.18).

CARBOHYDRATE METABOLISM

Carbohydrate metabolism by the liver appears to be compartmentalized. In the fed state, the liver is involved in glycogen synthesis from glucose and glycolysis, metabolic processes that are preferentially located in perivenular hepatocytes. In the postabsorptive or fasted state, there is a shift from glucose uptake to glucose production mediated by glycogenolysis and gluconeogenesis predominantly in periportal hepatocytes.

Glucose is not the only ingested carbohydrate that is metabolized by the liver. Fructose is metabolized by the liver via a unique pathway and the metabolism of galactose depends on a conversion to glucose that occurs almost exclusively in the liver. Portosystemic shunting in cirrhosis results in impaired galactose elimination capacity, a finding that may have prognostic importance.

FATTY ACID METABOLISM

Fatty acids continuously cycle between the liver and adipose tissue. During the fed state, hepatocytes synthesize fatty acids that are then incorporated into lipoproteins to be delivered to adipocytes. During fasting, fatty acids derived from triglycerides stored in adipocytes are delivered to the liver where they undergo oxidation to ketone bodies in mitochondria and, in the case of very long chain fatty acids, in peroxisomes. In cirrhosis, fatty acids are preferentially used as a energy source, even in the nonfasted state. Mitochondrial oxidation of fatty acids depends on the availability of the amino acid carnitine. Carnitine deficiency may play a role in valproate-induced hepatotoxicity, and defects in mitochondrial fatty acid oxidation underlie disorders such as acute fatty liver of pregnancy, Reye's syndrome, and Jamaica vomiting sickness.

AMMONIA METABOLISM

Urea synthesis in the liver, through the Krebs–Henseleit cycle, is required for the disposal of the toxic product of nitrogen metabolism, ammonia. Glutamine synthesis plays a minor role in overall ammonia metabolism. Removal of ammonia from the circulation is compartmentalized in the liver. Carbamoylphosphate synthetase, the key regulatory enzyme in urea synthesis from ammonia, is expressed in all but the last one or two hepatocytes surrounding the terminal hepatic venule. The last one or two perivenous hepatocytes, in contrast, express glutamine synthetase, and avidly scavenge any remaining ammonia from the circulation to form glutamine, which is subsequently released into the terminal hepatic venule and the systemic circulation (Fig. 3.20). Elevated serum ammonia levels are often observed in both acute and chronic forms of liver disease. The striking elevations seen in fulminant hepatic failure are the result of impaired conversion of ammonia to urea in the setting of severe hepatocellular necrosis, whereas the hyperammonemia present in patients with cirrhosis and portal hypertension reflects loss of glutamine synthetic capacity by the perivenous scavenger cells in the liver as well as portosystemic shunting of ammonia derived from colonic bacteria. Additional factors that influence the level of serum ammonia in patients with cirrhosis include intestinal production of ammonia by bacterial deamination of blood or dietary protein, renal production of ammonia by glutaminase in response to metabolic alkalosis or hypokalemia, intestinal production of ammonia from urea by urease-forming bacteria in the setting of diminished renal function, and hepatic production of ammonia from amino acids in response to increased glucagon secretion.

PROTEIN SYNTHESIS

Albumin is the single most abundant serum protein and the liver synthesizes and exports up to 12 grams of albumin per day. Besides serving as a vehicle for the transport of many drugs, serum albumin is a critical factor in the maintenance of plasma oncotic pressure. Albumin synthesis is regulated by changes in nutritional status, osmotic pressure, systemic inflammation and corticosteroids.

The liver also plays an important role in normal blood coagulation. Normal serum activities of the vitamin K-dependent coagulation-factor proenzymes (factors II, VII, IX, and X), as assessed by the one-stage prothrombin time, depend on intact hepatic synthesis and adequate intestinal absorption of lipid-soluble vitamin K. Vitamin K is required for the post-translational formation of γ-carboxyglutamyl residues that are essential for physiologic activation of the factors. Prolonged prothrombin times can be observed in both hepatocellular disorders that impair hepatic synthetic function, such as hepatitis and cirrhosis, and in cholestatic syndromes that interfere with lipid absorption. Hepatocellular injury can be differentiated from cholestatic causes of prothrombin time prolongation by the parenteral administration of vitamin K; intact hepatic function is established by an improvement in prothrombin time greater than 30% within 24 hours of administration.

The liver is also a major site for the synthesis of antithrombin III, protein C, and protein S. Despite reductions in these plasma inhibitors of hemostasis in chronic liver disease, thrombosis is a rare complication, presumably because of a disproportionate deficiency in procoagulants in most patients.

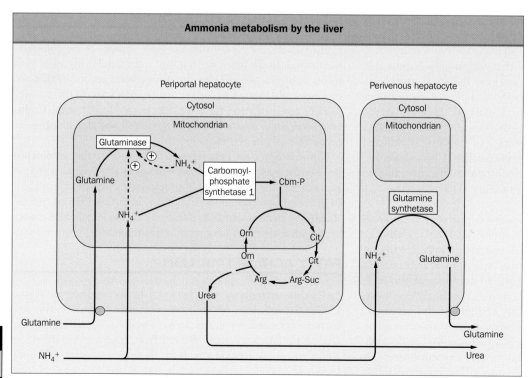

Ammonia metabolism by the liver

Figure 3.20 Ammonia metabolism by the liver. Ammonia is removed from the circulation by periportal hepatocytes expressing glutaminase and carbamoyl phosphate synthetase. Periportal glutaminase is activated by ammonia. Ammonia that is not taken up by periportal hepatocytes is scavenged by perivenous hepatocytes that selectively express glutamine synthetase. (From Haussinger D. Biochem J. 1990;267:285.)

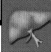

CELL VOLUME REGULATION

Hepatocyte function is regulated by its hydration state, a dynamic parameter that is altered by hormones, oxidative stress and substrates, such as amino acids and bile salts (Fig. 3.21). Changes in hepatocyte volume occur despite the activation of specific transport processes in hepatocytes that are responsible for regulatory volume increase, namely Na^+–H^+ and Cl^-–HCO_3^- exchange, and regulatory volume decrease, namely K^+ and Cl^- channels. Increases in cell volume despite these counter-regulatory processes stimulate protein and glycogen synthesis and bile formation. In contrast, a catabolic state is triggered by cell shrinkage. Disrupted cellular osmoregulation has been associated with many disease states and their complications. Defective hepatocellular volume regulation may play a role in portal hypertension, chronic viral hepatitis, and hepatocarcinogenesis.

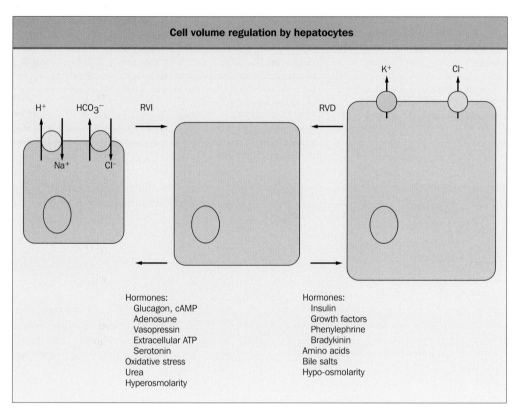

Figure 3.21 Cell volume regulation by hepatocytes. Osmotic water shifts out of and into hepatocytes in response to the listed effectors and results in activation of regulatory volume increase (RVI), due to Na^+:H^+ exchange and Cl^-–HCO_3^- exchange, and regulatory volume decrease (RVD), due to K^+ and Cl^- channels, respectively.

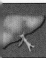

FURTHER READING

Anderson JM, van Itallie CM. Tight junctions and the molecular basis for regulation of paracellular permeability. Am J Physiol. 1995; 269:G467–75. *This review focuses on insights provided by the identification of several tight junction proteins and evidence supporting a role for the perijunctional actin cytoskeleton in regulating paracellular permeability.*

Moseley RH. Bile secretion. In: Yamada T, ed. Textbook of gastroenterology, 2nd edition. Philadelphia: JB Lippincott Company; 1995:383–404. *Comprehensive review of the mechanisms of bile formation and cholestasis.*

Moseley RH. Bile secretion and cholestasis. In: Kaplowitz N, ed. Liver and biliary diseases, 2nd edition. Baltimore: Williams & Wilkins; 1996: 185–204. *Broad overview of the mechanisms of bile formation and cholestasis.*

Muller M, Jansen PLM. Molecular aspects of hepatobiliary transport. Am J Physiol. 1997;272:G1285–G1303. *Review of recent advances in the functional and molecular characterization of transport proteins in the liver.*

Oude Elferink RPJ, Meijer DKF, Kuipers F, Jansen PLM, Groen AK, Groothuis GMM. Hepatobiliary secretion of organic compounds: molecular mechanisms of membrane transport. Biochim Biophys Acta. 1995;1241:215–68. *One of the main functions of the liver, the formation of bile, involves transport of compounds, such as bile acids, phospholipids, cholesterol, and other organic anions and cations. This review discusses the specific mechanisms involved in the transport of these compounds.*

Oude Elferink RPJ, Tytgat GNJ, Groen AK. The role of mdr2 P-glycoprotein in hepatobiliary lipid transport. FASEB J. 1997;11:19–28. *Fascinating review of the physiologic role of this canalicular ATP-binding cassette transporter and its likely role in human liver disease.*

Roberts SK, Ludwig J, LaRusso NF. The pathobiology of biliary epithelia. Gastroenterology. 1997; 112:269–79. *Review of the advances made in understanding the mechanisms of bile formation by the bile duct epithelial cells, or cholangiocytes, and the role of these cells as targets in a variety of hepatobiliary diseases.*

Trauner M, Meier PJ, Boyer JL. Molecular pathogenesis of cholestasis. N Engl J Med. 1998;339:1217–27. *Summary of the molecular defects in hepatic membrane transporters that are associated with various forms of cholestatic liver disease.*

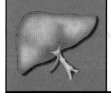

Section 2 Clinical Manifestations of Liver Disease

Chapter 4

Clinical Evaluation of the Patient with Liver Disease

Peter D Howdle

INTRODUCTION

Patients who have liver disease present in a variety of ways with a multiplicity of symptoms and signs of varying severity. At one end of the spectrum is the patient who is found incidentally to have an abnormal liver function test but no clinical features of liver disease; at the other end is the patient who has obvious symptoms and signs of acute or chronic hepatocellular failure. Some of these symptoms and signs are quite specific for liver disease; others are suggestive but may also reflect disease or dysfunction in another system. Consequently, the physician has to maintain a high standard of clinical expertise and a low diagnostic threshold for liver disease in order to evaluate patients properly.

THE HISTORY

Good clinical practice always entails obtaining a comprehensive history about the patient's illness. The presenting symptoms can be very varied in patients who have liver disease, as reviewed below. The astute physician should remember to obtain details of all aspects of the history both present and past, including reviewing the presence of symptoms in all body systems

SYMPTOMS OF LIVER DISEASE

General ill health
In patients who have liver disease, the level of consciousness and higher mental functions may be disturbed to such an extent that it is impossible to obtain a full or satisfactory history. Usually this is caused by the presence of encephalopathy (see below).

Weakness, increased fatiguability, and general malaise are common but nonspecific symptoms of both acute and chronic liver disease, occurring in up to 60% of individuals. These symptoms tend to improve rapidly when specific treatment is given for the liver disease (particularly following successful liver transplantation). It is not uncommon, however, for such symptoms to persist following acute hepatitis. There is no effective treatment for the weakness and malaise, and their pathogenesis is unknown.

Gastrointestinal symptoms
Gastrointestinal symptoms are common in liver disease, although they are very nonspecific. Anorexia, particularly in jaundiced patients, frequently occurs in acute hepatitis of any cause. Long-term anorexia inevitably leads to weight loss; in patients who have end-stage chronic liver disease, the muscle wasting and loss of adipose tissue is often striking. There is often a remarkable contrast between the thin, wasted chest and the distended abdomen in patients with end-stage disease who have developed ascites.

Nausea and vomiting are common at some stage in most cases of liver disease. Nausea is noteworthy in the prodromal phase of acute hepatitis; vomiting is particularly associated with obstructive biliary disease. Following paracetamol overdose, there is frequently nausea and vomiting. It should be remembered that excess alcohol often causes these symptoms, particularly in the morning.

Hematemesis is frequent in patients who have liver disease. It should not be assumed that the blood always comes from esophageal varices. In acute liver failure patients often develop gastritis, and 20% of patients who have varices and chronic liver disease bleed from nonvariceal lesions such as peptic ulcers or gastric erosions.

Abdominal pain is also common in hepatobiliary disease. It can be present anywhere across the upper abdomen, but is frequently localized to the right upper quadrant. The pain may result from rapid or gross enlargement of the liver. There may be associated tenderness in acute hepatitis, hepatic abscess or hepatic malignancy. Peritoneal pain is present if the capsule and/or parietal peritoneum is involved. Severe pain associated with jaundice and fever suggests biliary disease and/or cholangitis. On occasions an enlarged spleen is painful.

Abdominal discomfort, as opposed to pain, may be described by patients who have an enlarged liver or spleen, but it is frequently caused by distension with ascites. Patients who have gross ascites often complain of the development of an umbilical hernia, difficulty in mobilization, and dyspnea (Fig. 4.1). There is an increased risk of spontaneous bacterial peritonitis and this

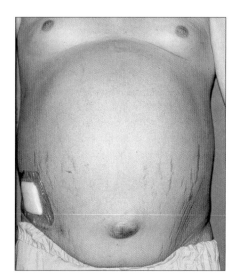

Figure 4.1 Ascites in a patient with chronic liver disease. There are dilated abdominal wall veins, striae, and an everted umbilicus.

should always be borne in mind, particularly when a patient who has ascites suddenly deteriorates. The sudden development of ascites raises the possibility of Budd–Chiari syndrome.

There is commonly a change in bowel function or stool appearance in liver disease. Mild diarrhea with soft stools is frequent. Stools suggestive of steatorrhea are less common, but if present suggest biliary obstruction or cholestasis. Severe diarrhea should prompt the search for a cause other than liver disease, although associated conditions such as ulcerative colitis should be considered. Those who drink alcohol excessively also develop diarrhea. Melena is obviously an important symptom and in patients who have chronic liver disease may herald the development of encephalopathy. Constipation, although not a consequence of liver disease, may also precipitate encephalopathy.

Jaundice and associated symptoms

Jaundice is the most striking symptom of hepatobiliary disease and is well recognized as such by lay people. It is often first brought to the attention of patients by friends, relatives, or a primary care physician. It is first obvious when the serum bilirubin level exceeds approximately 45μmol/L (2.6mg/dL) and is most easily observed in the sclerae. In hepatobiliary disease, the serum bilirubin is usually much higher than this, however, and this points to a major hepatocellular pathology or to extrahepatic cholestasis. Other symptoms may help to differentiate the cause of jaundice. Prodromal symptoms of nausea, anorexia, and malaise may suggest acute hepatitis. Cholestatic or biliary disease is often associated with dark urine and pale stools. Symptoms of infection or severe pain also suggest biliary problems such as cholangitis or cholelithiasis. In hepatocellular damage there are generalized symptoms and the patient feels ill, whereas with a slowly developing cholestatic lesion the patient often feels well in general, although he or she may be quite deeply jaundiced. Progressive pruritis (prior to jaundice) suggests developing cholestatic liver disease. Pruritis can be one of the most severe symptoms of liver disease and may become disabling. The patient almost always complains that it is worse at night.

Circulatory, cardiorespiratory, and hematologic symptoms

There is a variety of symptoms that can be classified as cardiovascular/respiratory. Fluid retention, reflected by the development of ascites, can also lead to symptoms of ankle swelling and dyspnea. Such symptoms are common in the patient who has chronic liver disease and they can be expected at some stage in almost all patients. Dyspnea has a number of causes in liver disease apart from fluid retention (see below). Oliguria and nocturia occur as fluid retention develops and liver disease increases in severity.

Spontaneous (or easily induced) bleeding is commonly seen in patients who have liver disease and are developing either acute or chronic liver failure. Such symptoms are attributable to the defective hepatic synthesis of coagulation factors and the thrombocytopenia that occur in such conditions. In severe acute liver failure, as seen in paracetamol overdose, patients may develop an almost uncontrollable bleeding tendency (Fig. 4.2).

Nervous system

The most striking neurologic symptoms occurring in liver disease are those associated with encephalopathy. This occurs to some degree in up to 80% of patients who have chronic liver disease; in such patients, it is often chronic and variable in extent. In severe acute liver failure, encephalopathy develops rapidly with

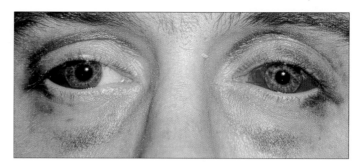

Figure 4.2 Subconjunctival hemorrhage, periorbital bruising, and jaundice in a patient who has acute liver failure.

the increasing severity of the liver failure. It is a complex neuropsychiatric syndrome; patients develop such symptoms as sleep disturbance, altered personality, deterioration of higher mental functions, increasing drowsiness and confusion, and eventually coma. More specific symptoms may occur if particular areas of the central nervous system are affected by pathologic change, for example demyelination of the cord leading to a paraplegic gait.

Specific diseases can lead to characteristic neurologic symptoms, for example abnormal movements in Wilson's disease or nightblindness in vitamin A deficiency.

Endocrine system

In men who have chronic liver disease, there is decreased libido, together with frequent impotence and sterility. Women also have infertility and oligomenorrhea. These symptoms are more severe in patients who have alcoholic liver disease. Males may complain of painful or embarrassing gynecomastia (see Fig. 4.11).

Systematic review

When evaluating a patient who has liver disease, as in all comprehensive histories, a general systematic review is important. As seen above, symptoms referable to any body system can occur that may indicate liver disease.

Wider history
Past medical history

Past medical history is of great importance. Previous jaundice is always important, suggesting hepatitis, gallstones, or even congenital biliary disease. Previous surgery, other medical conditions, psychologic or psychiatric treatment, and administration of blood products are important features.

Family history

A positive family history helps to establish the cause of liver disease in some patients, for example genetic hemochromatosis. In some families, an infective cause such as hepatitis B virus may also be likely.

Drug history

Many drugs can cause hepatic dysfunction and disease; therefore, a careful drug history is important, even from the distant past. For example, hepatic dysfunction can occur after patients have been taking amiodarone or methotrexate for some months. Routine monitoring of liver function is recommended and full assessment may require liver biopsy. Drug-induced liver disease is discussed in detail in Chapter 29.

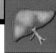

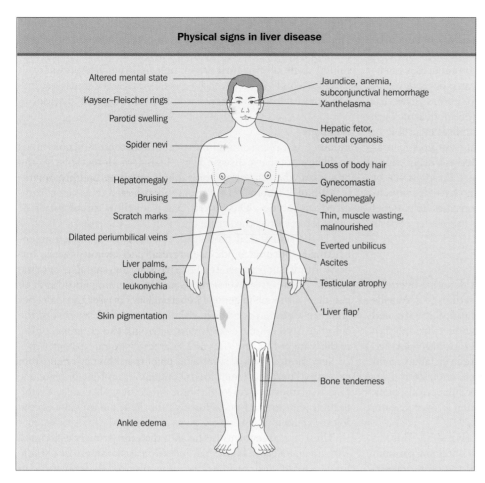

Physical signs in liver disease

- Altered mental state
- Kayser–Fleischer rings
- Parotid swelling
- Spider nevi
- Hepatomegaly
- Bruising
- Scratch marks
- Dilated periumbilical veins
- Liver palms, clubbing, leukonychia
- Skin pigmentation
- Ankle edema

- Jaundice, anemia, subconjunctival hemorrhage
- Xanthelasma
- Hepatic fetor, central cyanosis
- Loss of body hair
- Gynecomastia
- Splenomegaly
- Thin, muscle wasting, malnourished
- Everted unbilicus
- Ascites
- Testicular atrophy
- 'Liver flap'
- Bone tenderness

Figure 4.3 Physical signs in liver disease.

Social history

Intravenous drug abuse, alcohol consumption, sexual orientation and practice, foreign travel, and type of work (now and previously), including exposure to industrial chemicals and toxins, must all be enquired about when seeking a cause of liver disease in a newly presenting patient.

THE PHYSICAL EXAMINATION

Evaluation of any patient always includes a comprehensive history and a complementary examination for the presence or absence of relevant physical signs. Physical signs in liver disease vary in their significance. Some can be quite specific for a particular condition [e.g. Kayser–Fleischer (K–F) rings in Wilson's disease] or for a complication and, therefore, prognosis of liver disease (e.g. liver flap in hepatic encephalopathy). Others are really quite nonspecific (e.g. clubbing, spider nevi) but do suggest that liver disease is the underlying pathology.

In order to elucidate properly and reliably the physical signs in liver disease, the young physician must practise regularly; some of the signs are genuinely difficult to elicit and there is considerable inter- and intraobserver variation.

Physical examination can give information about the nature, complications, and prognosis of the liver disorder.

SIGNS OF LIVER DISEASE

The physical signs found in liver disease are summarized in Figure 4.3.

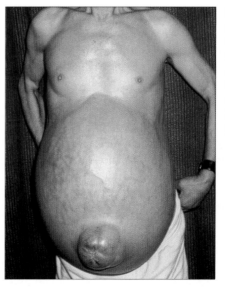

Figure 4.4 Gross ascites in a patient who has chronic liver disease. There is an umbilical hernia, dilated abdominal wall veins and a pigmented skin. Marked muscle wasting is evident.

General examination

It is important to note the general bodybuild of the patient. Muscle wasting, loss of fat deposits, and thinning of the skin are all signs of malnutrition, which occurs as chronic liver disease progresses. The onset of fluid retention can mask some of these signs. There is often a remarkable contrast between a thin wasted chest and an abdomen distended by ascites (Fig. 4.4).

Patients who have acute liver disease usually look well nourished. Obesity is a common cause of abnormal liver function tests.

Fever and infection

Patients who have liver disease have an increased risk of infection. Up to 50% of patients present with, or acquire in hospital, a bacterial infection. Urinary tract infections are common, as is pneumonia, particularly in alcoholics. Septicemia can quickly develop, leading to shock. In patients who have severe chronic liver disease there is a high mortality from infections (38%). In acute liver failure fungal infections are an important complicating problem. If the patient who has liver disease deteriorates for no apparent reason, underlying infection should be suspected as a major cause.

Nevertheless, fever does not always reflect the presence of infection. Approximately 30% of patients who have decompensated cirrhosis have a continuous low-grade fever, as do patients who have alcoholic hepatitis. In 50% of these the fever persists for more than 2 weeks.

Facial signs

There are no particular facial characteristics denoting liver disease, but there are rare instances of specific features (e.g. Alagille syndrome: widely set eyes, prominent forehead, flat nose, and small chin associated with congenital hepatic duct hypoplasia). Other facial signs include subconjunctival hemorrhage (see Fig. 4.2), which is commonly seen in severe acute liver failure, xanthelasma around the eyes, suggesting chronic cholestatic liver disease (e.g. primary biliary cirrhosis), and conjunctival pallor. The last may suggest anemia, which is common in liver disease, but so is central cyanosis.

A specific sign in the eye is the K–F ring (Fig. 4.5). This is a ring resulting from the deposition of copper-containing pigment in Descemet's membrane at the periphery of the posterior surface of the cornea. The K–F ring is usually greenish brown in color; although visible to the naked eye, it is best seen by an ophthalmologist using a slit lamp. It is present in more than 90% of all patients who have Wilson's disease with neurologic signs, and in the majority of those with hepatic involvement. It may be absent (or very difficult to visualize) in approximately 50% of adolescents or in fulminant cases of Wilson's disease. A similar ring may rarely be found in chronic cholestasis or cirrhosis.

Observation of the face may reveal bilateral parotid swelling, usually associated with alcoholic cirrhosis and the accompanying malnutrition. This sign must be distinguished from the pseudo-Cushing's syndrome induced by alcohol abuse.

Fetor

Hepatic fetor complicates severe hepatocellular disease. It is described as a sweet, slightly fecal smell of the breath that is presumed to be of intestinal origin, being particularly prevalent in patients who have an extensive portal collateral circulation. It is a frequent finding in patients who have chronic liver disease.

Skin signs

Jaundice is a physical sign most often regarded as synonymous with hepatobiliary disease (Fig. 4.6). It is detectable by the physician when the serum bilirubin level exceeds approximately 45μmol/L (2.6mg/dL). Patients are referred to as being 'jaundiced' or 'icteric'. The earliest sign is a yellow discoloration of the sclerae, but as the serum bilirubin rises the jaundice is obvious in the skin and, if prolonged, the skin can develop a greenish tinge. Bilirubin binds preferentially to elastic tissues, but body fluids such as ascites, sweat, or urine can also become yellow. There are several mechanisms affecting the depth of jaundice, although in general hepatobiliary diseases cause deeper jaundice than that occurring with hemolysis. The severity of the jaundice does not necessarily correlate with the prognosis of the underlying pathology.

Very rarely, a yellow pigmentation of the skin may result from excessive consumption of foods containing carotene or lycopene (e.g. tomatoes and carrots). Some drugs may also cause discoloration (e.g. mepacrine). However, in these circumstances, the sclerae remain white.

There are other signs in the skin that are strongly associated with liver disease. Hyperpigmentation is common in chronic liver disease and results from the increased deposition of melanin. It is seen particularly in primary biliary cirrhosis and hemochromatosis (bronze diabetes). Local areas of hyperpigmentation occur at sites of irritation, trauma, or in more exposed areas. In addition, patients with marked hyperbilirubinemia can have general hyperpigmentation. Vitiligo is much more obvious in pigmented patients and is associated with autoimmune diseases (e.g. primary biliary cirrhosis and chronic hepatitis). Pruritis is a frequent symptom of cholestatic conditions. Scratch marks on the skin are commonly observed. These are in accessible areas and so the center of the back is usually spared. The nails in such patients are highly polished; this is a striking phenomenon on examination.

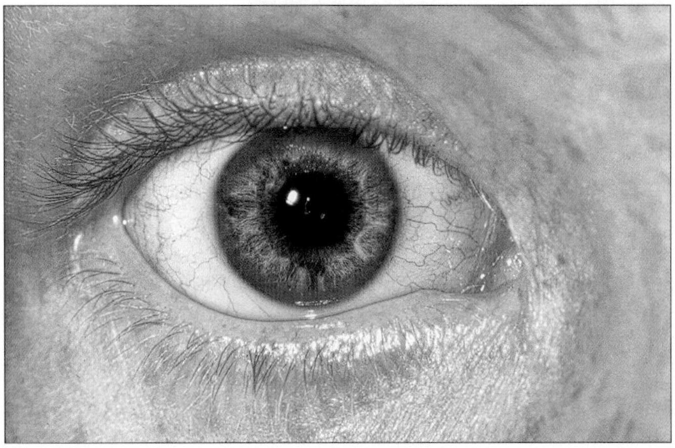

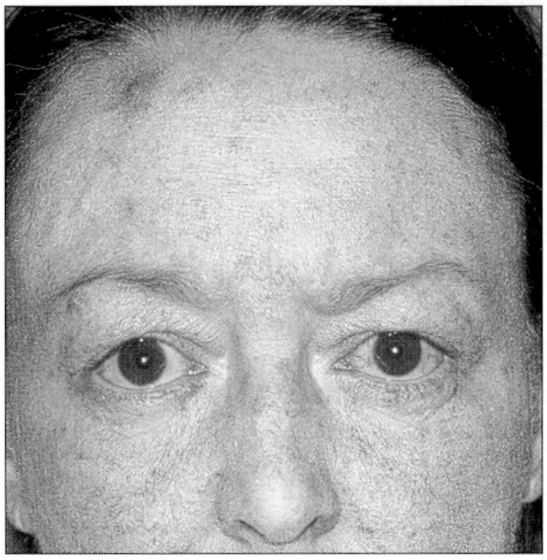

Figure 4.6 Jaundice in a patient with alcoholic liver disease. There is also a spider nevus and paper money skin.

Figure 4.5 A K–F ring in a patient with Wilson's disease.

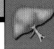

Lichen planus is associated with primary biliary cirrhosis and also with chronic liver disease due to HCV. The increased plasma lipids in chronic cholestatic conditions lead to xanthelasma around the eyes and xanthomata over pressure areas such as buttocks, knees, and elbows.

Excessive bruising and purpura occur in patients where the coagulation factors and platelet count are disturbed. Often sites of venepuncture show excessive extravasation of blood. Needle marks from intravenous drug abuse should be noted since they may suggest the cause of viral hepatitis. Tattoos similarly should be noted. Leukocytoclastic vasculitis, a necrotic rash with transient erythema multiforme, may be an early manifestation of both hepatitis B and C infection.

Vascular 'spiders' are commonly seen in association with chronic liver disease. There are several synonyms: spider telangiectasia, spider nevi, arterial spiders, and spider angioma. The lesion consists of a central arteriole with numerous small radiating vessels resembling a spider's legs, hence the various names for this lesion (Fig. 4.7). Pressure on the central prominence causes blanching of the whole lesion. Occasionally such lesions can be seen or felt to pulsate. The spiders can vary in size from 1mm to 1–2cm in diameter (Fig. 4.8). They are found in the drainage area of the superior vena cava and are commonly found in the neck, face, arms, and hands. Approximately 2–3% of normal individuals have two or three spiders, but any more than that, especially if they are developing or enlarging, suggests parenchymal liver disease. Spiders can occur briefly in acute hepatitis, but they usually reflect cirrhosis. They can develop during pregnancy but fade after delivery. There are two other lesions associated with spiders. White spots occur on the arms and buttocks on exposure to cold; these indicate the position of a spider's central arteriole. There

may also be numerous, random small vessels in the area of the spiders. These resemble the pattern on the paper used for US dollar bills, hence the skin is called 'paper money skin' (see Fig. 4.6).

The skin may occasionally reveal several relatively specific signs. The CREST syndrome (Calcinosis Raynaud's phenomenon Esophageal dysfunction Sclerodactyly and Telangiectasis) suggests primary biliary cirrhosis; hereditary hemorrhagic telangiectasia may cause cirrhosis and hepatic vascular ectasia; striae and a facial rash occur with autoimmune chronic hepatitis; and porphyria cutanea tarda is strongly associated with HCV infection, with up to 80% of porphyria patients being HCV positive.

Examination of the limbs

Examination of the limbs in patients who have liver disease may reveal proximal myopathy associated with alcohol abuse or a deficiency of either vitamin D or E. Bone tenderness is related to the osteopenia of chronic liver disease and arthritides are associated with primary biliary cirrhosis or hemachromatosis.

Hand and nail signs

Examination of the hands can reveal several signs in patients who have liver disease. None of these signs, however, are specific to liver disease. The hands may be warm and the palms bright red. This palmar erythema is a mottled red discoloration affecting the thenar and hypothenar eminences, and the pulps and bases of the fingers (Fig. 4.9). The feet may be similarly affected. This appearance is associated with acute and chronic liver disease but can also occur in rheumatoid arthritis, thyrotoxicosis, fever, and pregnancy.

Dupuytren's contracture has been traditionally associated with alcoholic cirrhosis. In this condition, there is a thickening and shortening of the palmar fascia causing flexion deformities of the fingers. The abnormality is now known to have a multifactorial origin but to be strongly associated with cigarette smoking and alcohol consumption rather than primary liver disease. It affects approximately 10% of men over 65 years of age and consequently will be commonly seen in older males who drink regularly, whether or not liver disease is present.

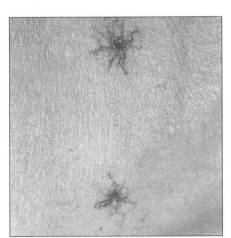

Figure 4.7 Spider nevi on the neck.

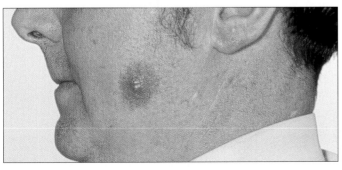

Figure 4.8 A large spider nevus on the cheek.

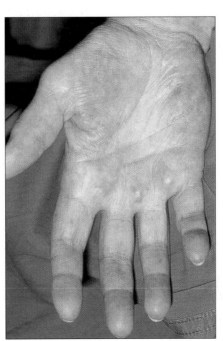

Figure 4.9 Palmar erythema in a patient who has chronic liver disease.

Reference has already been made to the highly polished nails associated with pruritis. The nails can also appear white (leukonychia). This occurs because of the opacity of the nail bed and is seen in up to 80% of patients who have chronic liver disease. The distal border may retain a 1–2mm pink edge, but the lunulae are often obscured by the white nail bed (see Fig. 4.10). An alternative appearance is one of transverse white lines, parallel to the lunula (Muehrcke's lines). Both these forms of leukonychia are said to be related to a low serum albumin, such as occurs in chronic liver disease. Other conditions in which leukonychia is found include nephrotic syndrome, diabetes mellitus, pulmonary tuberculosis, rheumatoid arthritis, and multiple sclerosis. Blue discoloration of the lunulae has been described in Wilson's disease and argyria.

Finger clubbing occurs in chronic liver disease and even regresses after hepatic transplantation. It is most commonly seen in the setting of hypoxemia associated with the hepato-pulmonary syndrome; in these conditions, hypertrophic osteo-arthropathy with periostitis may also occur. This is seen radiologically in up to 40% of patients who have chronic liver disease.

Cardiovascular examination

Patients in the early stages of liver disease have a normal cardiovascular system on clinical examination. Alcohol has an effect on blood pressure and this may contribute towards hypertension in some cases. Patients who have advanced hemochromatosis and alcohol abuse can develop cardiomyopathies, with the consequent heart failure.

As patients who have chronic liver disease slowly deteriorate, cardiovascular changes develop. Similar hemodynamic effects occur rapidly if the patient has acute liver failure. In these conditions, a hyperdynamic circulation develops. The patient has warm peripheries, a bounding pulse, a tachycardia at rest, and systemic hypotension. There is an evident precordial impulse and an ejection flow murmur.

If the disease progresses, the blood pressure falls further. This has serious effects on already compromised renal, hepatic, and cerebral bloodflows.

These circulatory changes are a result of an increased cardiac output and reduced peripheral vascular resistance. The cause is thought to be the release of a variety of vasodilators, often acting via the induction of nitric oxide synthase. When a patient presents with such circulatory signs, their increasing severity reflects either significant deterioration of the underlying liver disease or the development of serious complications.

Pulmonary hypertension rarely produces symptoms but can occur in 2% of those patients who have portal hypertension. It can contribute to the signs of right heart failure and low cardiac output that may be found in severely affected patients.

Respiratory examination

There is a wide variety of pulmonary pathologies that can affect patients who have liver disease and these produce abnormal physical signs. Cyanosis occurs in up to 30% of patients who have chronic liver disease. Reduced chest expansion, evidence of pleural effusions, dyspnea, orthopnea, and signs of intrapulmonary fluid, infection, or pulmonary fibrosis can all be found in patients who have acute or chronic liver disease.

Many of these symptoms and signs can be caused by the hepatopulmonary syndrome. In this condition there is evidence of intrapulmonary arteriovenous (A–V) shunts, vasodilatation leading to ventilation–perfusion mismatching, and capillary wall thickening leading to diffusion defects.

Pleural effusions occur in approximately 6% of cirrhotic patients but are more common in decompensated cirrhosis, usually occurring on the right and in association with ascites. However, they can occur bilaterally and in the absence of ascites or can still be present when ascites has responded to diuretic treatment. A right-sided effusion is the norm in the postoperative phase following liver transplantation.

More specific associations between the lung and liver are seen in autoimmune conditions such as fibrosing alveolitis and Sjögren's syndrome. In α_1-antitrypsin deficiency emphysema may be present and in cystic fibrosis chronic suppurative lung disease is usual.

Abdominal examination
Observation

Observation of the abdomen may reveal wasting caused by severe malnutrition or cachexia caused by malignancy. Alternatively, distension, especially in the flanks, may be present, suggestive of

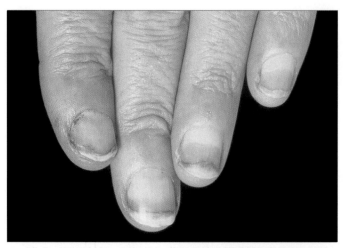

Figure 4.10 Leukonychia of the proximal nail bed in a patient who has alcoholic liver disease.

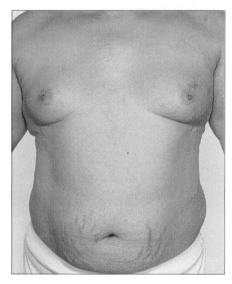

Figure 4.11 Gynecomastia in a patient who has chronic liver disease. Striae are seen on the arms and abdominal wall.

ascites. Normal abdominal wall movement may be restricted by intra-abdominal pathology, causing tenderness and pain.

The abdominal skin may show petechiae, scratch marks or striae, all of which are related to possible liver disease (Figs 4.1 & 4.11).

Dilated abdominal wall veins are a notable finding in liver disease (see Figs 4.1 & 4.4). Prominent superficial veins occur around the umbilicus if the portal venous bloodflow is obstructed beyond the origin of the umbilical veins from the left branch of the portal vein, as occurs in intrahepatic pathology. Such portal hypertension allows the umbilical and para-umbilical veins to open up and produce dilated veins on the abdomen and the umbilicus. Blood in these veins flows away from the umbilicus. The appearance is classically called 'caput medusae' since the serpiginous veins are supposed to resemble snakes on the head of the mythologic gorgon Medusa. Such an appearance is rarely seen in practice, although the commonly seen dilated veins that flow away from the umbilicus are usually loosely termed 'a caput medusae'. Dilated veins resulting from an obstructed inferior vena cava are usually contrasted with para-umbilical veins. In inferior vena caval obstruction, the distended veins are more commonly seen in the sides of the abdomen and the flow is upwards from legs to chest.

Palpation

Palpation of the abdomen may reveal general features such as abnormal masses or areas of tenderness. These may be associated with hepatobiliary problems, for example intra-abdominal malignancy or biliary infection. More specifically, the clinician needs to palpate the liver and spleen. The shape and size, the contour, and the consistency of the liver are all important features. Normally the liver may just be palpable. A Riedel's lobe or downward displacement by pulmonary disease may suggest that the liver is enlarged. Hepatomegaly usually, however, supports a diagnosis of liver disease. The development of cirrhosis often leads to shrinkage of a previously enlarged liver, perhaps with compensatory hypertrophy of the left lobe. The cirrhotic liver becomes irregular. An enlarged, hard, irregular liver suggests malignancy. Hepatomegaly can be caused by conditions other than those leading to cirrhosis (Fig. 4.12).

Splenomegaly is an important physical sign in liver disease (Fig. 4.13). The spleen is normally impalpable, although in one study it was felt in 3% of 2200 healthy college students. It enlarges mainly as a result of portal hypertension and hyperplasia of the reticuloendothelial component and can consequently be felt in chronic or acute liver disease. In the presence of chronic liver disease, splenomegaly is the most important sign of portal hypertension. In the presence of splenomegaly, the peripheral blood may show features of hypersplenism. The splenic size is most easily assessed by ultrasound examination.

Palpation of the kidneys is usually unhelpful in liver disease, although 70% of patients who have adult renal polycystic disease may develop liver cysts.

Percussion

Percussion of the abdomen is useful in assessing the size of the liver, especially when it is small, and in detecting the presence of ascites (see Figs 4.1 & 4.4). The cardinal sign of ascites is 'shifting dullness' present on both sides of the abdomen. At least 2L of fluid must be present before it can be detected in this way. A fluid thrill requires marked ascites before it is detected. An everted umbilicus is frequently associated with gross ascites (see Figs 4.1 & 4.4).

Auscultation

Auscultation of the abdomen in relation to liver disease may reveal three types of sound.

- Arterial bruits heard over the liver suggest the presence of a vascular hepatocellular carcinoma or other malignancy, an A–V malformation, very rarely tortuous arteries in a cirrhotic liver, or severe alcoholic hepatitis.
- Venous hums are occasionally heard in portal hypertension and reflect turbulent flow in collateral veins. A venous hum at the umbilicus in association with dilated abdominal wall veins and occasionally a venous thrill is termed the Cruveilhier–Baumgarten syndrome. This rare and unusual association may result from a congenitally patent umbilical vein or portal hypertension in well-compensated cirrhosis.
- Friction rubs over the liver suggest inflammation or infiltration. They may be caused by tumor or abscess invading the peritoneum or by hepatic infarction. A transient rub is often heard over the site of a liver biopsy. The Fitz–Hugh–Curtis syndrome refers to a rub from a perihepatitis, often caused by

Common causes of hepatomegaly	
Causes	Examples
Chronic liver disease	Multiple causes often leading to cirrhosis
Inflammation	Viral, bacterial (including abscess), parasitic
Venous congestion	Cardiac, venous occlusion (e.g. hepatic vein)
Tumors	Primary hepatobiliary, secondary carcinoma, hematologic malignancies
Biliary disease	Extrahepatic obstruction, congenital cystic disease
Metabolic	Fatty liver, amyloidosis, storage diseases

Figure 4.12 Common causes of hepatomegaly. The differential diagnosis of hepatomegaly

Common causes of splenomegaly	
Causes	Examples
Venous congestion	Liver disease, hepatic/portal vein occlusion
Infection	Viral, bacterial, parasitic
Inflammation	Rheumatoid arthritis, sarcoidosis, systemic lupus erythmatosus
Hematologic disturbances	Chronic hemolysis, hemoglobinopathies, myeloproliferative disease, leukemia, lymphoma
Miscellaneous	Storage diseases, amyloidosis

Figure 4.13 Common causes of splenomegaly. The various etiologies of splenomegaly.

chlamydial infection.

Examination for endocrine abnormalities

Endocrine changes may occur in the presence of chronic liver disease and are more common when there is an alcoholic cause. In patients who have cirrhosis, hypogonadism is common, which in men produces feminization leading to testicular atrophy, a female body habitus and distribution of body hair, and gynecomastia (see Fig. 4.11). The last particularly occurs in alcoholics but is also seen in patients taking spironolactone. This combination of factors may frequently be present in patients who have liver disease. Gonadal atrophy in women produces very few clinically detectable physical signs, although the premenopausal patient loses female characteristics such as breast and pelvic fatty tissue.

It is important to recognize that alcohol abuse can produce features of pseudo-Cushing's syndrome and that some of the above features in men with hemachromatosis can occur before evidence of chronic liver disease.

Neurologic examination

Neurologic abnormalities caused by underlying liver disease are rare, apart from hepatic encephalopathy. The neurologic examination is usually, therefore, unremarkable. Specific associations should be borne in mind, for example the neurologic features of Wilson's disease, the effects of vitamin A and E deficiency, and the neurologic consequences of viral hepatitis or alcohol abuse.

The most common neurologic syndrome is encephalopathy. This is a reversible neuropsychiatric condition that can complicate liver disease. The clinical course of hepatic encephalopathy fluctuates and patients can deteriorate very rapidly in some situations (e.g. acute liver failure). The clinical features vary from subtle signs with mild cognitive impairment to coma. A clinical grading system from 1 to 4 is useful (Fig. 4.14), particularly when frequent observations need to be made to follow the development of the condition or the effect of treatment. Early changes may be monitored by serial use of a number connection test where the time taken by a patient to join together sequential but randomly spaced numbers is recorded. The time taken increases with the development of encephalopathy.

One of the most characteristic signs of encephalopathy is that of a flapping tremor ('asterixis' or 'liver flap'). This is demonstrated best with the arms outstretched, the wrists dorsiflexed, and the fingers separated. The flapping tremor consists of brief, rapid flexion and extension movements of the fingers or wrists. If it is severe, a similar tremor may be seen in the arms, head, and feet. The tremor is seen best on sustained posture and disappears if coma develops. The 'liver flap' is not specific for liver disease and can occur in renal failure, respiratory failure, metabolic disturbances, and drug intoxication.

When neurologic deterioration of this nature occurs, the clinician should evaluate the patient carefully because intracranial lesions such as infection, hemorrhage, or tumor can produce a similar clinical picture, as can metabolic and drug-induced pathology. In patients who have chronic liver disease and consequent hemostatic disturbances, even minor head injury can lead to significant intracranial bleeding. Hepatic encephalopathy can progress rapidly to coma in acute liver failure and is a severe prognostic sign. In patients who have chronic liver disease, it is often precipitated by a number of factors, particularly if there is significant portal–systemic shunting (Fig. 4.15).

More focal neurologic signs may rarely be present in chronic hepatic encephalopathy as a result of irreversible neurologic degeneration in the cerebral cortex, the basal ganglia, the cerebellum, or the spinal cord.

INVESTIGATIONS IN LIVER DISEASE

After the clinical evaluation of a patient who has liver disease, the physician assesses the history and examination and decides on the need for special investigations. Those specific to particular diseases will be described in the relevant chapters, but the vast majority of patients will have 'liver function tests' measured, a large proportion will undergo some form of radiologic investigation, and a majority will require a liver biopsy. The various investigations and their role are described below in the context of the evaluation of the patient who has liver disease.

Liver function tests

The liver function tests (LFTs) consist of a number of relatively

Clinical grading of hepatic encephalopathy		
Clinical grade	Clinical signs	Flapping tremor
Grade 1 (prodrome)	Alert, euphoric, occasionally depression. Poor concentration, slow mentation and affect, reversed sleep rhythm	Infrequent at this stage
Grade 2 (impending coma)	Drowsiness, lethargic, inappropriate behavior, disorientation	Easily elicited
Grade 3 (early coma)	Stuporose but easily rousable, marked confusion, incoherent speech	Usually present
Grade 4 (deep coma)	Coma, unresponsive but may respond to painful stimulus	Usually absent

Figure 4.14 Clinical grading of hepatic encephalopathy. The spectrum of encephalopathy is divided into four clinical grades.

Hepatic encephalopathy: precipitating factors in chronic liver disease	
Causes	Examples
Gut factors	Constipation, high protein intake, upper gastrointestinal bleeding
Electrolyte/water imbalances	Vomiting, diarrhea, diuretic treatment, renal failure, paracentesis
Infection	Chest, urinary, spontaneous bacterial peritonitis
Drugs	Hypnotic/sedative drugs, alcohol
Severe factors affecting major metabolic functions	Hypoxia, hypotension, hypoglycemia

Figure 4.15 Hepatic encephalopathy: precipitating factors in chronic liver disease. A number of clinical conditions not involving the liver can worsen hepatic encephalopathy.

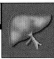

simple assays of various serum constituents that give an indication of the metabolic activity and cellular integrity of the liver; an abnormality in these tests, therefore, probably indicates the presence of liver disease and its severity and is thus reflecting injury rather than purely function. The individual tests all have low sensitivities and specificities; isolated abnormalities found in any patient, particularly if found as a result of a screening program or simply because of the availability of autoanalysers, must be interpreted with caution, taking into account the overall clinical situation of the patient. Nevertheless, part of the evaluation of a patient with liver disease almost always includes LFTs. Certainly, if there is any clinical suspicion of hepatobiliary disease, the results of these tests, taken as a group, are useful in the evaluation of the patient.

The most commonly used tests are listed in Figure 4.16, with their normal ranges and an indication of their most useful roles.

Total bilirubin

Elevated serum bilirubin levels reflect increased production, reduced hepatic uptake and/or conjugation, or decreased biliary excretion. In acute liver disease, the serum bilirubin reflects severity of the disease but is of little prognostic value because it usually resolves completely. In chronic liver disease, a gradual increase (for no obvious cause) reflects serious disease progression.

Aminotransferase enzymes

Two intracellular enzymes, alanine aminotransferase (ALT) and asparate aminotransferase (AST), are present in a number of tissues including hepatocytes. They are released when cells are damaged. Of the two, ALT is slightly more specific to liver damage. Very high levels are seen in acute hepatic injury, modest increases in many types of liver disease, and mild increases in some situations (e.g. obesity) when liver histology can be shown to be virtually normal. In alcoholic liver disease, the AST activity is generally more than two times greater than the ALT activity and is often useful in making this diagnosis.

Alkaline phosphatase

Alkaline phosphatase is present in many tissues, notably the hepatobiliary system, bone, and intestine. Up to 20% of activity in normal individuals is of intestinal origin. Isoenzyme estimations can indicate the source of the alkaline phosphatase,

whether it is principally hepatobiliary or bony in origin. Isoenzymes are rarely estimated routinely since other assays help in this differentiation (see below).

A raised alkaline phosphatase level is seen in a variety of liver diseases, but the highest levels are in cholestatic conditions or biliary obstruction, and in hepatic infiltrations.

5-Nucleotidase is a form of alkaline phosphatase that is elevated in liver disease and its presence helps to confirm the hepatobiliary origin of a raised alkaline phosphatase. This is also the case for the enzyme gammaglutamyl transpeptidase (γ-GT), the levels of which reflect the level of alkaline phosphatase, bile being rich in γ-GT. The highest levels of γ-GT are found in intrahepatic biliary obstruction. However, it is an enzyme that is easily induced, particularly by alcohol. Therefore, while it is a sensitive test of hepatobiliary dysfunction, it is not specific and in isolation certainly is not a useful measurement.

Synthetic function

Serum albumin and the prothrombin time are commonly used as estimates of hepatic synthetic function. Assuming there is no excess loss from the intestine or kidney, and the patient is not in a catabolic state, then the serum albumin is a reasonable indication of synthetic function. A low serum albumin reflects chronic liver disease and is a sign of a poor prognosis (see Fig. 4.26).

The liver also synthesizes the majority of the clotting factors, the function of which can be assessed by estimating the prothrombin time. All these factors (I, II, V, VII, IX, X) are dependent upon vitamin K (except factor V). Hence, if the prothrombin time remains prolonged after attempts at correction with vitamin K, the prolongation indicates the severity of liver disease and is a sign of a poor outcome, most notably in acute liver failure (see Fig. 4.28).

Full blood count and blood film

Although not strictly regarded as part of the LFTs, the blood count and blood film provide useful indications of liver disease. The erythrocytes are usually normocytic. In patients with cirrhosis, the erythrocytes are usually macrocytic. Chronic blood loss can induce hypochromia. The erythrocytes may show a variety of shapes so that the film shows macrocytosis, target cells, spur cells and acanthocytes. Hemoglobin is often moderately reduced, which can result from reduced red cell survival, partial marrow suppression, and an element of hemolysis. The white cells may show a neutrophil leukocytosis in the presence of infections but also a leukopenia when splenomegaly is present. Similarly, the platelet count may be reduced through hypersplenism, although a deficiency of thrombopoetin may also play a part.

RADIOLOGY

In modern hepatologic practice, the evaluation of a patient almost always involves the use of radiology. The role of specialized radiologic investigations will be described in the relevant chapters on specific conditions. However, it is useful to consider their routine use in the initial assessment of hepatobiliary disease.

Plain radiography

A plain radiograph of the abdomen is generally not helpful. However, diffuse hepatic calcification suggests hepato-biliary tuberculosis and air in the biliary tree may indicate either previ-

Commonly measured tests of 'liver function'		
Test	**Normal range**	**Role**
Total bilirubin	3–17μmol/L 0.2–1.0mg/dL	Diagnosis of jaundice, severity of liver disease
Aminotransferase: Alanine (ALT) Aspartate (AST)	5–35IU/L 5–40IU/L	Diagnosis of hepatocellular damage Follow progression of disease
Alkaline phosphatase	35–130IU/L	Diagnosis of cholestasis, biliary obstruction, hepatic infiltration
Serum albumin	35–50g/L 3.5–5.0g/dL	Severity of chronic liver disease
Prothrombin time	12–15s	Assess severity of hepatic synthetic function

Figure 4.16 Commonly measured tests of 'liver function'. Tests used in the preliminary assessment of liver function.

ous instrumentation or anaerobic infection. The presence of pancreatic calcification indicates chronic pancreatitis.

Abdominal ultrasound

Ultrasound is the most frequently used radiologic investigation and is regarded as a screening test for hepatobiliary abnormalities.

Ultrasound is freely available, easy to perform, and relatively inexpensive. It depends upon an experienced operator for the correct interpretation of findings, but sensitivities and specificities of over 90% are reported for the diagnosis of gallbladder stones and for hepatocellular carcinomas over 2cm in diameter.

Ultrasound imaging is used to examine the biliary system, the liver size and texture, the vascular supply of the liver, and the size of the spleen. Useful information from all these areas can be obtained. It is an ideal screening test for cholestasis because the gallbladder and bile ducts are clearly seen and biliary dilatation can be easily diagnosed (Fig. 4.17).

Focal hepatic lesions more than 1cm in diameter are seen, including cysts, abscesses, and tumors of all types. Diffuse liver

abnormalities suggesting 'fatty' infiltration, an irregular outline, or 'coarse' texture all suggest diffuse, probably chronic liver disease. Doppler ultrasound is extremely useful in assessing the portal and hepatic venous systems in patients who have ascites, splenomegaly, or peripheral edema. Examination of the hepatic artery is particularly useful after liver transplantation.

Ultrasound can also be used to target a guided liver biopsy to a focal lesion.

Computed tomography

Computed tomography (CT) is an extremely useful technique for demonstrating the abdominal anatomy (Fig. 4.18). It is used to image the liver and surrounding organs and is more accurate than ultrasound but is less convenient and more expensive.

Focal hepatic lesions (over 1cm in diameter) are visualized well, as is the diffuse abnormal texture of the liver with chronic disease. Intravenous contrast can be used with CT to enhance the findings and in this way the vascular supply to the liver or tumors can be demonstrated. CT arterio-portography (CTAP) and helical (spiral) CT are particularly useful for demonstrating small focal liver lesions. CT-guided biopsies are used by some investigators.

Magnetic resonance imaging

Magnetic resonance imaging (MRI) is the most sophisticated of the three imaging techniques in common use. It is the most expensive and least freely available. It is excellent for demonstrating the anatomy of the abdomen, including the liver and its vessels and ducts. It is usually used as a second-line investigation when CT findings are unclear or when further delineation of focal hepatic lesions is needed, such as when assessing the suitability of a tumor for resection.

A relatively recent development in noninvasive imaging is magnetic resonance cholangiopancreatography (MRCP). MRCP produces high quality images without the injection of contrast agents (Fig. 4.19), and the sensitivity in defining biliary stones or strictures is similar to that of endoscopic retrograde cholangiopancreatography (ERCP; see below). Its major limitation is that there are no therapeutic options. However, if ERCP has failed or there has been a previous surgical anastomosis preventing

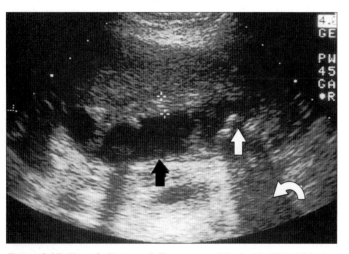

Figure 4.17 Use of ultrasound. The common bile duct is dilated (black arrow) and in the duct there are three gallstones (centred on straight white arrow) that cast an 'acoustic shadow' (curved white arrow). (Courtesy of Dr MB Sheridan.)

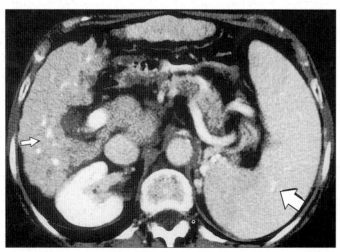

Figure 4.18 Use of CT. The liver is small and irregular (small arrow) and the spleen is grossly enlarged (large arrow). (Courtesy of Dr MB Sheridan.)

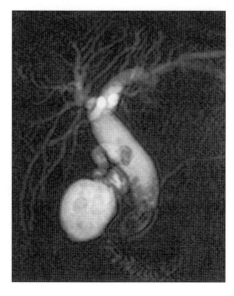

Figure 4.19 An MRCP image of stones in the common bile duct and gall bladder. (Courtesy of Dr. A. Chalmers.)

ERCP, then MRCP provides very useful diagnostic information.

Endoscopic retrograde cholangiopancreatography

ERCP has greatly increased our ability to evaluate correctly the patient suspected of biliary or pancreatic disease. As a result it is frequently used in patients who have jaundice. It is an invasive test and, therefore, complications are possible. It will usually have been preceded by ultrasound and possibly CT to image the common bile duct and pancreatic head. Indications include diagnosis and management of cholelithiasis (Fig. 4.20), biliary tract abnormalities, pancreatic disease, and postbiliary surgery problems.

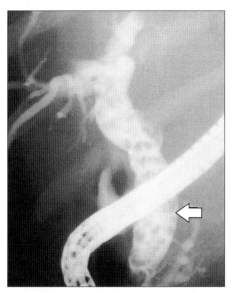

Figure 4.20 Use of endoscopic retrogradecholangiopancreatography. The common bile duct is dilated and full of stones (arrow). (Courtesy of Dr MB Sheridan.)

Management in these situations includes sphincterotomy and removal of stones, sampling of stricture or tumors, and positioning of stents for drainage. In patients who have received liver transplant, ERCP is particularly useful in examining the biliary system.

However, ERCP is an invasive procedure. The complication rate is 2–3% and mortality rate is 0.1–0.2%. The common complications seen include pancreatitis, cholangitis, hemorrhage, and perforation and their incidence is directly related to the skill of the endoscopist. Usually, an experienced endoscopist will obtain a successful examination in 80–90% of patients. In patients for whom ERCP fails or is impossible for anatomic reasons, and for whom visualization of the biliary system is required, then MRCP and/or percutaneous transhepatic cholangiography (PTC) will be required.

Radiology and the diagnosis of jaundice

One of the most frequent clinical problems is the diagnosis of jaundice. After clinical evaluation and LFTs, the physician employs radiologic techniques. A scheme of investigation is outline in Figure 4.21. The value of the radiologic techniques described in diagnosing jaundice is summarized in Figure 4.22.

BIOPSY OF THE LIVER

Biopsy of the liver is an important part of the evaluation of a patient who has liver disease and often follows from the clinical assessment and initial investigation. Although many other advances have been made that facilitate diagnosis (e.g. improved imaging techniques, virologic markers, immunologic assessments), there is still a need for histologic examination of a liver specimen in order to obtain a definitive diagnosis in many cases. Most liver lesions are fortunately diffuse and, therefore, a small biopsy, usually obtained percutaneously with a biopsy needle, is sufficiently representative for the pathologist to make an accurate diagnosis. Biopsy of the liver is now extremely important in the management of liver transplant recipients.

The situations in which a liver biopsy would be useful in diagnosis are given in Figure 4.23. In acute hepatitis, liver biopsy is only occasionally helpful and is not normally performed. In cases where clinical evaluation indicates end-stage liver disease and

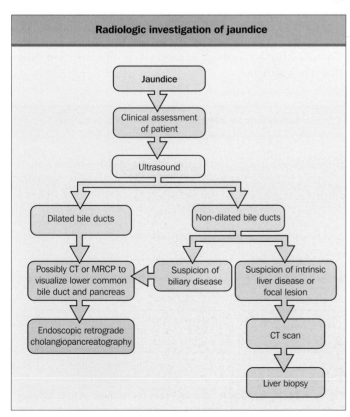

Figure 4.21 Radiologic investigation of jaundice.

Imaging techniques in the diagnosis of jaundice			
Technique	Sensitivity (%)	Specificity (%)	Specific features
Ultrasound	55–91	82–95	Noninvasive, easy to perform, cheap Bowel gas/obesity interfere with images Operator dependent
CT	63–96	93–100	Noninvasive, more specific and objective than ultrasound Not portable, more expensive
ERCP	89–98	89–100	Direct images of biliary system Therapeutic possibilities Occasionally anatomically impossible to perform 3% morbidity, 0.2% mortality

Figure 4.22 Imaging techniques in the diagnosis of jaundice. The different imaging techniques used to evaluate patients with liver disease have differing specificities and sensitivity.

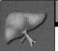

where there is a known etiology, most hepatologists would not require a liver biopsy.

The specific findings in various liver diseases are described in other chapters. However, there are some important common guidelines that will be described here as an introduction.

Patient selection and preparation

Many patients are admitted to hospital for liver biopsy and observed for 24 hours following the procedure. A substantial number of selected patients are managed as day cases. Such patients should not be jaundiced or have complications of liver disease such as ascites or encephalopathy. The usual indication for outpatient biopsy would be assessment of chronic hepatitis or alcoholic liver disease.

Knowledge of the patient's blood group (with facilities for transfusion), prothrombin time, and platelet count is essential. It should be remembered that in some patients, for example with uremia or myeloproliferative disorders, the bleeding time or activated partial thromboplastin time may be prolonged. Liver biopsy is generally regarded as being safe if the prothrombin time is prolonged by no more than 3 seconds and the platelet count is greater than 80,000 (80×10^9 cells/L). Nowadays, many patients will have the liver biopsy using ultrasound guidance.

Technique

Tissue is obtained in amounts adequate to provide a satisfactory diagnosis in 75–95% of patients using the needle techniques described here.

The usual technique is a percutaneous, intercostal approach with local anesthesia to the superficial tissues. Using a Menghini needle is probably the safest and quickest technique as it obtains a specimen via suction and takes '1 second'. In the presence of fibrosis or cirrhosis, a 'Trucut' needle provides a better sample with less fragmentation, but there is the slight risk of more complications.

A biopsy can be obtained under radiologic guidance, usually ultrasound. The needle can be targeted to a particular area of interest. Usually an automatic biopsy gun is used that incorporates a Trucut-type biopsy needle. This last technique is also used in patients who are at increased risk of bleeding; the biopsy site can then be 'plugged' with gel foam injected through the outer cannula of the Trucut needle.

In patients who have a coagulopathy or for whom a percutaneous method would be dangerous or not possible, a transvenous biopsy can be obtained. This is obtained using a modified Trucut needle that is passed intravenously into a hepatic vein via the jugular (or, rarely, the femoral) vein.

In some centers, laparoscopic liver biopsy is used, and this may be the best approach in specific cases. Open-liver biopsy at laparotomy is occasionally necessary and is often found to be useful in retrospect when obtained in patients who have liver disease who require abdominal surgery for a coincidental reason.

There are various absolute or relative contraindications to 'blind' percutaneous liver biopsy, including:
- bleeding diathesis,
- dilated intrahepatic biliary system,
- cystic lesions (parasitic or biliary),
- vascular tumours,
- amyloidosis,
- myeloproliferative disorders,
- gross ascites,
- severe emphysema.

Indications for the different techniques are given in Figure 4.24.

Follow-up and complications

After liver biopsy, by whichever technique, the patient should be carefully monitored because there may be complications (Fig. 4.25).

The mortality rate following liver biopsy is reported to be 0.01% and complications occur in 0.1–1.0% of cases. Complicating hemorrhage is most likely to occur 3–4 hours after the procedure.

Indications for liver biopsy

Chronic hepatitis

Drug-induced hepatitis

Acute hepatitis (occasionally)

Suspected cirrhosis

Suspected liver disease in an alcoholic

Intrahepatic cholestasis

Infective conditions (including pyrexia of unknown origin)

Storage diseases

Space-occupying lesions

Unexplained hepatomegaly

Unexplained raised liver enzymes

Follow-up after liver transplant

Figure 4.23 Indications for liver biopsy. A liver biopsy is an important diagnostic test for the evaluation of several clinical disorders.

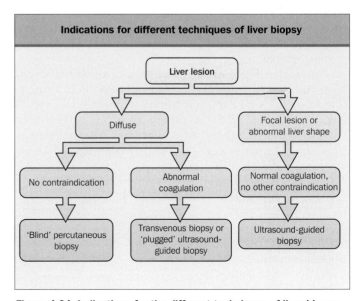

Figure 4.24 Indications for the different techniques of liver biopsy. Liver biopsy may be 'blind', targeted, or performed endovascularly, depending upon the indication and degree of coagulopathy.

Complications of liver biopsy	
Complication	**Extent**
Pain	Locally, including perihepatitis; radiating to epigastrium/shoulder
Vagal shock	—
Hemorrhage	Intraperitoneal, intrahepatic, hemobilia
Perforation	Gallbladder: biliary peritonitis Diaphragm: pneumothorax Intrahepatic vessels: A–V fistula Other organs: rarely significant
Transient bacteremia	—
Tumor dissemination (rare)	—

Figure 4.25 Complications of liver biopsy. Liver biopsy is generally safe, but complications do occur in 0.1–1% of procdures.

If an inpatient, the patient is kept in bed for 24 hours' observation. During the first 2 hours the pulse and blood pressure are monitored frequently, and hourly thereafter . Adequate analgesia should be given, if required, after careful assessment for complications. If an outpatient, the biopsy should be obtained in the early morning and the patient observed in hospital until the evening. Thereafter they should be within easy reach of the hospital and not be alone overnight.

DIAGNOSIS AND PROGNOSIS

The evaluation of the patient who has liver disease in order to arrive at a definitive diagnosis and management plan requires careful clinical assessment and the use of various investigations. The analysis of the information obtained also allows an assessment of the severity of the disease and the prognosis for the patient.

Grading the overall severity of liver disease is now more important than it used to be because of the routine use of liver transplantation in the management of patients. An estimate of prognosis is essential if the timing of transplantation is to be optimal.

Various classifications have been used to assess the severity of disease. In patients who have chronic liver disease, Child's grading with Pugh's modification is frequently used. In fact, the Child–Pugh score is the basis of the standardized criteria needed to list patients for liver transplantation in the USA. Each feature is scored from 1 to 3 points and the total score equated with a Child's grade (from A to C) (Fig. 4.26). The Child's grade has been equated with survival (Fig. 4.27), C being the most severe with an overall mortality of 88% (see Fig. 4.26).

There are some important clinical points that have a bearing on survival in individual patients who have chronic liver disease when they are assessed. Serious factors include:
• persistent jaundice,
• intractable ascites,
• spontaneous bacterial peritonitis,
• progressive encephalopathy,
• persistent hypotension,

Child's grading of disease severity in chronic liver disease with Pugh's modifications			
Criteria assessed	**Points scored for increasing abnormality**		
	1	**2**	**3**
Encephalopathy (grade)	None	1–2	3–4
Ascites	Absent	Slight	Moderate
Serum bilirubin [μmol/L (mg/dL)]	<35 (<2)	35–50 (2–3)	>50 (>3)
In primary biliary cirrhosis	<70 (<4)	70–170 (4–10)	>170 (>10)
Serum albumin [g/L (g/dL)]	>35 (3.5)	35–28 (3.5–2.8)	<28 (<2.8)
Prothrombin time [prolongation (s)]	1–4	4–10	>10
Total score	5–6	7–9	10–15
Child's grade equivalent	A	B	C
Overall mortality in Pugh's series (%)	29	38	88

Figure 4.26 Child's grading of disease severity in chronic liver disease with Pugh's 1973 modifications. The Child–Pugh score is universally used to quantify the severity of liver disease. (Modified from Pugh et al. Br J Surg, 1973).

Percentage survival in chronic liver disease			
Child's grade	**At 1 year**	**At 5 years**	**At 10 years**
A	84	44	27
B	62	20	10
C	42	21	0

Figure 4.27 Survival in chronic liver disease. The risk of death in patients with chronic liver disease correlates well with the Child's grade. (Data extracted from Christensen et al. Hepatology, 1984).

• low serum albumin,
• persistent hyponatremia,
• prolonged prothrombin time.

In those patients who have acute liver disease who develop acute liver failure, transplantation may be the only successful treatment. Prognosis can be predicted in order to assess the chances of successful recovery without transplantation and to decide the timing of transplantation. The prognostic criteria in acute hepatic failure are summarized in Figure 4.28. If a patient who has acute hepatic failure fulfills these criteria, one would predict that there is only an approximate 10% chance of spontaneous recovery. Acute hepatic transplantation is, therefore, a serious option to be considered, bearing in mind the approximate 50% chance of recovery following the procedure in such a situation.

Apart from these predictive assessments, there are very few useful mathematical models that have proven beneficial in the management of individual patients.

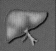

Prognostic criteria for assessing acute liver failure	
Cause of liver damage	Criteria indicating <10% chance of spontaneous recovery
Paracetamol overdose	pH <7.30 at 24 hours or more (irrespective of grade of encephalopathy) or: Serum creatinine >300µmol/L (>3.5mg/dL), prothrombin time >100s, and encephalopathy grade 3 or 4
Nonparacetamol causes	Prothrombin time >100s (irrespective of grade of encephalopathy) or: three of the following five criteria: Age <10 years or >40 years Duration of jaundice to encephalopathy >7 days Etiology: drugs, non-A, non-B hepatitis, indeterminate Prothrombin time >50s Serum bilirubin >300µmol/L (>17mg/dL)

Figure 4.28 Prognostic criteria for assessing acute hepatic failure. These criteria allow the prediciton of prognosis for patients with acute liver failure within a short time following their presentation. Patients fulfilling these criteria have an approximately 10% chance of spontaneous recovery.

In clinical practice, the experienced physician uses his or her skills to elicit many of the features described in this chapter. Clinical diagnoses are dependent upon a process of pattern recognition and the astute clinician integrates all the information obtained in evaluating the patient. It is perhaps useful to remember that the liver is affected by a variety of etiologies but often reacts in a similar, diffuse pathologic fashion. As a result, a number of clinical effects can be reliably predicted (Figs 4.29 & 4.30).

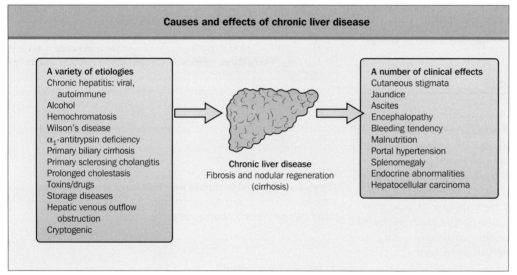

Causes and effects of chronic liver disease

A variety of etiologies
Chronic hepatitis: viral, autoimmune
Alcohol
Hemochromatosis
Wilson's disease
α_1-antitrypsin deficiency
Primary biliary cirrhosis
Primary sclerosing cholangitis
Prolonged cholestasis
Toxins/drugs
Storage diseases
Hepatic venous outflow obstruction
Cryptogenic

Chronic liver disease
Fibrosis and nodular regeneration (cirrhosis)

A number of clinical effects
Cutaneous stigmata
Jaundice
Ascites
Encephalopathy
Bleeding tendency
Malnutrition
Portal hypertension
Splenomegaly
Endocrine abnormalities
Hepatocellular carcinoma

Figure 4.29 Causes and effects of chronic liver disease. This figure shows the common clinical manifestations of liver disease together with the common etiologies of cirrhosis.

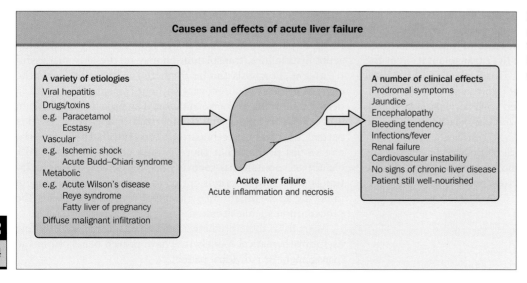

Causes and effects of acute liver failure

A variety of etiologies
Viral hepatitis
Drugs/toxins
e.g. Paracetamol
Ecstasy
Vascular
e.g. Ischemic shock
Acute Budd–Chiari syndrome
Metabolic
e.g. Acute Wilson's disease
Reye syndrome
Fatty liver of pregnancy
Diffuse malignant infiltration

Acute liver failure
Acute inflammation and necrosis

A number of clinical effects
Prodromal symptoms
Jaundice
Encephalopathy
Bleeding tendency
Infections/fever
Renal failure
Cardiovascular instability
No signs of chronic liver disease
Patient still well-nourished

Figure 4.30 Causes and effects of acute liver failure. This figure shows the common clinical manifestations of liver failure together with the common etiologies of acute liver injury.

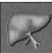

FURTHER READING

Bean WB. Vascular spiders and related lesions of the skin. Oxford: Blackwell; 1958. *An interesting historic record of skin lesions in a variety of conditions. Of especial note are the extensive descriptions of vascular spiders and palmer erythema, particularly in liver disease. Professor Bean obviously made many careful observations.*

Christensen E, Schlichting P, Fauerholdt L, et al. Prognostic value of Child–Turcotte criteria in medically treated cirrhosis. Hepatology. 1984;4:430–5. *A good attempt at predicting outcome in chronic liver disease using routine clinical information.*

Hislop WS, Bouchier IAD, Allan JG, et al. Alcoholic liver disease in Scotland and North Eastern England: presenting features in 510 patients. Q J Med. 1983;52:232–43. *Comprehensive clinical review of 510 patients with alcoholic liver disease. Good description of clinical features and laboratory data.*

Lange PA, Stoller JK. The hepatopulmonary syndrome. Ann Intern Med. 1995;122:521–9. *A comprehensive review with extensive bibliography. A good definition of the clinical features as well as the mechanisms and treatment.*

Menghini G. One-second needle biopsy of the liver. Gastroenterology. 1958;35:190–9. *The first description by Menghini of his technique for a 1-second liver biopsy. He records experience of 2000 biopsies with almost 100% success.*

Menghini G. One-second biopsy of the liver – problems of its clinical application. N Engl J Med. 1970;283:582–5. *A review of some problems of the Menghini technique for the inexperienced. By 1970 the technique was in common clinical use and the mortality was only 10% of that of other techniques of liver biopsy.*

O'Grady J, Alexander GJM, Hayllar KM, Williams R. Early indicators of prognosis in fulminant hepatic failure. Gastroenterology. 1989;97:439–45. *A seminal paper using two groups of patients (a learning and a validation set) to establish criteria for predicting outcome in acute liver disease.*

Pugh RNH, Murray-Lyon IM, Dawson JL, Pietroni MC, Williams R. Transection of the oesophagus for bleeding oesophageal varices. Br J Surg. 1973;60:646–9. *A modification and refinement of Child's grading system which produced a good predictor of survival in patients who have chronic liver disease undergoing esophageal transection and variceal ligation for bleeding varices.*

Riley SA, Ellis WR, Irving HC, et al. Percutaneous liver biopsy with plugging of needle track: a safe method for use in patients with impaired coagulation. Lancet. 1984;ii:436. *First description of plugged liver biopsy in routine use for patients with a coagulation disorder. Adequate biopsies were obtained in 19 out of 20 patients and there was one death.*

Runyon BA. Spontaneous bacterial peritonitis: an explosion of information. Hepatology. 1988;8:171–5. *Useful review of spontaneous bacterial peritonitis and its presentation, diagnosis, and treatment. The importance of making the diagnosis and its influence on prognosis is stressed.*

Saunders JB, Walters JRF, Davies P, Paton A. A 20-year prospective study of cirrhosis. Br Med J. 1981;282:263–6. *A useful description of the causes and prognosis of cirrhosis in an English health district during the 1960s and 1970s. Alcoholic cirrhosis was seen to increase rapidly in prevalence.*

Scheuer PJ, Lefkowitch JH. Liver biopsy interpretation, 5th edn. London: Saunders; 1994. *An excellent guide for physicians and pathologists about the correct interpretation of liver histology.*

Sherlock S. Aspiration liver biopsy. Technique and diagnostic application. Lancet. 1945;2:397–401. *Early results of aspiration liver biopsy. A series of 264 biopsies in 222 patients is presented. The risks, contraindications, and difficulties are discussed. This is a seminal paper in hepatology as liver biopsy was being introduced into routine clinical practice.*

Sherlock S, Summerskill WHJ, White LP, Phear EA. Portal-systemic encephalopathy. Neurological complications of liver disease. Lancet. 1954;ii:453–7. *Eighteen patients are described with chronic liver disease and the now 'classical' features of encephalopathy. These changes were related to portal–systemic shunting of nitrogenous substances to the brain. A good description of this common clinical problem in hepatology.*

Sherman KE. Alanine aminotransferase in clinical practice: a review. Arch Intern Med. 1991;151:260–5. *A practical review of the advantages and limitations of ALT measurement in clinical practice and its role in the diagnosis of liver disease.*

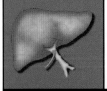

Section 2 Clinical Manifestations of Liver Disease

Chapter 5

Jaundice

Steven D Lidofsky

INTRODUCTION

Jaundice, which gives rise to a yellow appearance of the skin, occurs as a consequence of bilirubin deposition into subcutaneous tissues. In darker skinned individuals (or early in the course of jaundice), this yellow discoloration may be confined to the sclerae and mucous membranes. Jaundice is classically associated with liver and biliary tract disease, but extrahepatic causes of jaundice are well-recognized. In the past, distinction was made between 'medical' and 'surgical' jaundice (referring to the absence versus presence of biliary tract obstruction, respectively). However, this distinction has been rendered artificial because transplant surgeons now correct certain causes of 'medical' jaundice, and interventional gastroenterologists and radiologists now correct certain causes of 'surgical' jaundice.

The etiology of jaundice can be identified in the vast majority of cases. Indeed, with a simple history, physical examination, and routine biochemical screening tests, the presence versus absence of biliary tract obstruction can be correctly distinguished 75% of the time. Additional tests are often necessary to make a precise diagnosis, however. The diversity of currently available laboratory and imaging techniques requires judicious selection in order to minimize cost and patient discomfort.

This chapter covers five principal areas. It begins with a discussion of bilirubin formation and metabolism, especially as it relates to the pathophysiology of jaundice. It then presents a rational clinical classification of the causes of jaundice. Some of the causes described are delineated with brevity, as they are discussed in greater detail in other chapters in this book. This section is followed by clinical clues to various types of jaundice. With this as a background, the chapter moves toward a presentation of the strengths and weaknesses of different diagnostic modalities. The chapter concludes with a general approach to the management of the jaundiced patient, building upon the conceptual framework already established.

PATHOPHYSIOLOGY

Overview

Jaundice ultimately occurs in response to an elevated bilirubin concentration. Serum bilirubin concentration is generally less than 1–1.5mg/dL (17–25µmol/L), and jaundice is not usually detectable until bilirubin concentration exceeds 3mg/dL (50µmol/L). The level of bilirubin elevation is a critical determinant of overall prognosis in several diseases of the liver. This includes acute liver failure, alcoholic hepatitis, and cholestatic liver diseases such as primary biliary cirrhosis and sclerosing cholangitis. An understanding of the origins of an elevated bilirubin concentration is particularly germane to the management of these clinical entities, as is elucidating the cause of jaundice in patients who do not have a defined illness.

Bilirubin formation

Bilirubin is a potentially toxic compound that is an end-product of heme degradation. It has the chemical structure of a tetrapyrrole, which renders it highly water-insoluble due to internal hydrogen bonding. As such, the elimination of bilirubin from the circulation requires chemical conversion in the liver to water soluble conjugates that are normally excreted into bile. This multistep process is schematically illustrated in Figure 5.1. An abnormality at any of these steps can lead to hyperbilirubinemia and jaundice.

Daily bilirubin production is considerable. In healthy adults, this averages 4mg/kg (i.e. nearly 0.5mmol in a 70kg individual) each 24 hours. Bilirubin arises from heme breakdown from both red cells and extrahematopoietic tissues (see Fig. 5.1). Most (70–80%) is derived from hemoglobin degradation from senescent erythrocytes, and a small proportion comes from premature destruction of developing erythrocytes in the bone marrow (ineffective erythropoiesis). The liver represents the dominant source of the remaining 20–30% of bilirubin formed. The principal intracellular sources for this are heme-containing enzymes such as catalase and cytochrome oxidases. Other heme-containing proteins are present in extrahepatic tissues (e.g. myoglobin). However, the overall contribution of such proteins to bilirubin production is minimal due to their low mass or slow degradation rate.

Heme is converted to bilirubin via a two-step process (Fig. 5.2). First, heme is converted to biliverdin by the microsomal enzyme heme oxygenase. Second, biliverdin is converted to bilirubin by the cytosolic enzyme biliverdin reductase. Degradation of heme derived from erythrocyte hemoglobin primarily takes place in macrophages in the spleen, liver, and bone marrow. By contrast, hepatocytes produce bilirubin from heme derived from free hemoglobin, haptoglobin-bound hemoglobin, and methemealbumin.

Bilirubin metabolism

Bilirubin metabolism is a complex process in which several inherited disorders and associated gene products have been identified. This is illustrated in Fig. 5.1. Bilirubin circulates in plasma tightly bound to albumin. Extraction of bilirubin from plasma occurs in the liver, where bilirubin is metabolized and transported into bile through the actions of hepatocytes.

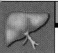

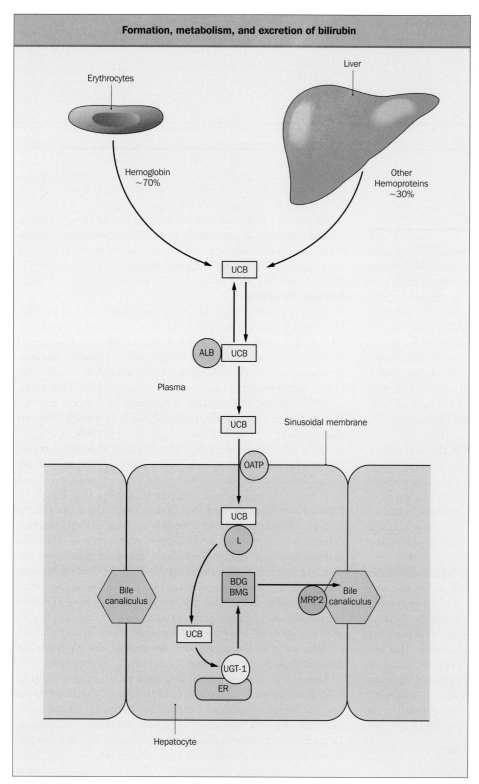

Formation, metabolism, and excretion of bilirubin

Figure 5.1 Formation, metabolism and excretion of bilirubin. Unconjugated bilirubin (UCB), formed from breakdown of hemoglobin from erythrocytes and heme-containing proteins from other tissues (principally liver), circulates in plasma bound to albumin (ALB). It is taken up by the hepatocyte (possibly via the transport protein OATP), diffuses through the cytosol bound to ligandins (L), and undergoes conjugation in the endoplasmic reticulum (ER) by bilirubin glucuronyltransferase (UGT-1). Mono- and diglucuronidated bilirubins (BMG, BDG) are exported into the bile canaliculus via the transport protein MRP2.

Bilirubin uptake occurs at the sinusoidal (basolateral) membrane of hepatocytes. The mechanism appears to be carrier-mediated. This process is competitively inhibited by certain organic anions such as bromosulfophthalein (BSP) and indocyanine green. In addition, the drug rifampin (rifampicin) may lead to hyperbilirubinemia by a similar process.

A candidate gene product, organic anion transporting polypeptide (OATP), has been implicated in sinusoidal biliru-bin uptake, but its role remains to be determined. Once sinu-soidal uptake has occurred, bilirubin is directed to the endo-plasmic reticulum by several cytosolic binding proteins, which serve to facilitate diffusion of this hydrophobic molecule. These cytosolic proteins include the ligandins and fatty acid binding protein. Bilirubin conjugation occurs in the endoplasmic retic-ulum. There it is principally converted to water-soluble monoglucuronides and diglucuronides via conjugation with uri-

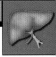

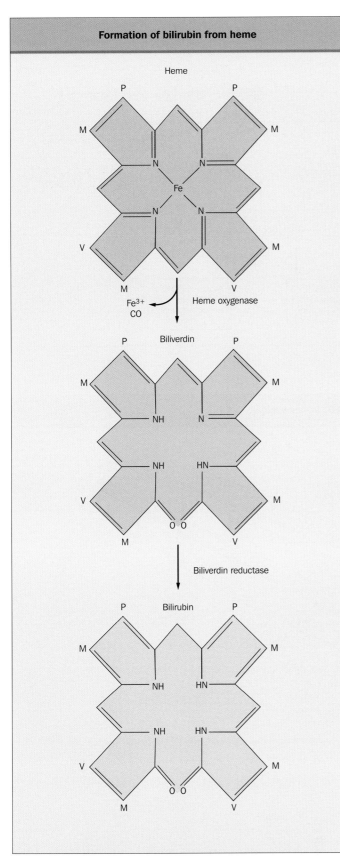

Figure 5.2 Formation of bilirubin from heme. Shown here are the chemical reactions that are catalyzed by heme oxygenase and biliverdin reductase, in which heme is sequentially converted to biliverdin and then to bilirubin. In the chemical structure shown, side groups are abbreviated as follows: methyl (M), propionyl (P), and vinyl (V).

dine diphosphate (UDP)-glucuronic acid. This is accomplished by the enzyme bilirubin UDP-glucuronosyl transferase (bilirubin UGT-1), the *HUG-Br1* gene product. Conjugation serves to convert hydrophobic bilirubin into a water-soluble form that can be readily excreted into bile.

Three inherited disorders of bilirubin metabolism are associated with defects in bilirubin UGT-1 activity (Fig. 5.3). In Gilbert's syndrome, bilirubin UGT-1 activity is decreased in response to an apparent decrease in *HUG-Br1* gene transcription. Mutations in the promoter region of the *HUG-Br1* gene have been reported in patients with Gilbert's syndrome and have been thought to contribute to this decrease in transcription. In the Crigler–Najjar syndromes, bilirubin UGT-1 activity is either reduced due to absence of the *HUG-Br1* gene product (type I Crigler–Najjar syndrome) or to mutations in the coding region of the *HUG-Br1* gene (type II Crigler–Najjar syndrome). Developmental delay of *HUG-Br1* expression appears to be the cause of physiologic jaundice of the newborn, a condition that resolves spontaneously.

Once conjugated, bilirubin is directed toward the canalicular (apical) membrane of hepatocytes, where it is transported into the bile canaliculus by an ATP-dependent export pump. The responsible protein has been identified through molecular cloning techniques as the multidrug resistance-associated protein MRP2 (also known as cMOAT), a member of the ATP-binding cassette protein superfamily. MRP2 appears to function as a multispecific transporter of a variety of organic anions (including BSP, but not hydrophilic bile acids). Of interest, MRP deficiency has been identified as the cause of Dubin–Johnson syndrome, another inherited hyperbilirubinemic disorder.

Bilirubin excretion
Virtually all bilirubin in human bile is conjugated. Approximately 80% is in the form of bilirubin diglucuronides. Nearly all the rest is in the form of bilirubin monoglucuronides, and only trace amounts are unconjugated. Bilirubin is propelled with biliary contents into the duodenum, where it is ultimately eliminated in the stool. Clearly, obstruction of the biliary tree at any level, from the canals of Hering to the ampulla of Vater, can lead to jaundice (Fig. 5.4).

Resorption of conjugated bilirubin by the gallbladder and gut is minimal. However, bilirubin breakdown products can be reabsorbed by the gut. In particular, conjugated bilirubin can be hydrolyzed by bacterial β-glucuronidase in the terminal ileum and colon. The resulting unconjugated bilirubin is converted in the intestinal lumen to tetrapyrroles called urobilinogens. Up to 20% of these colorless compounds are resorbed by the gut and ultimately excreted in bile and urine.

CAUSES

Overview
Jaundice can result from either an increase in bilirubin production or a decrease in hepatobiliary elimination of bilirubin (Fig. 5.5). In practice, the latter entity can be subdivided into three broad categories:
- isolated disorders of bilirubin metabolism;
- liver disease; and
- obstruction of the bile ducts.

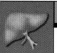
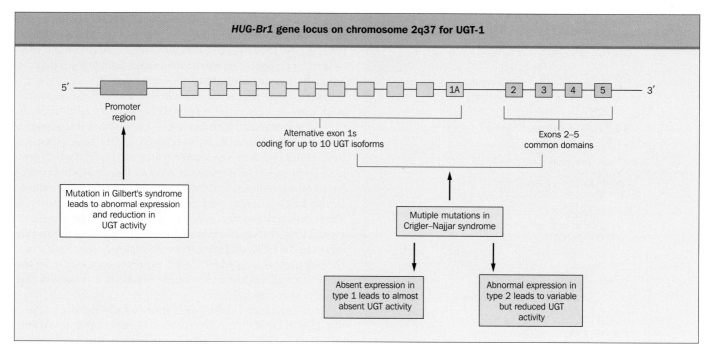

Figure 5.3 *HUG-Br1* gene locus on chromosome 2q37 for UGT-1.

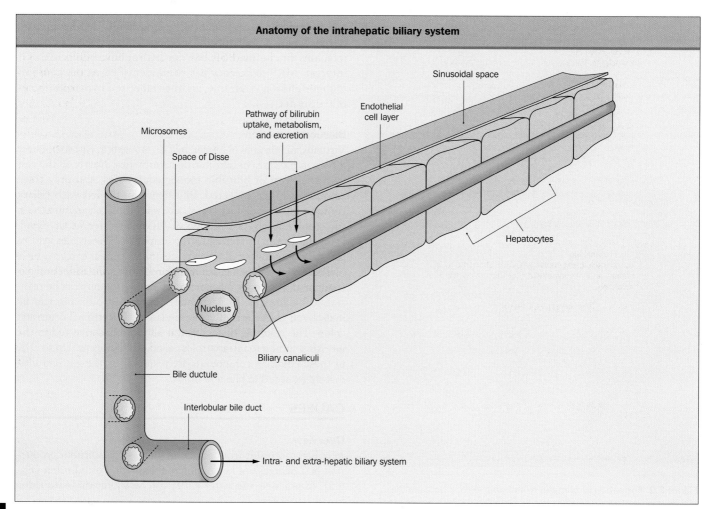

Figure 5.4 Anatomy of the intrahepatic biliary system.

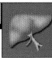

Differential diagnosis of Jaundice

Isolated disorders of bilirubin production or metabolism

Unconjugated hyperbilirubinemia
  Increased bilirubin production
  e.g. Hemolysis, ineffective erythropoiesis, massive
    blood transfusion, resorption of hematomas

Decreased hepatocellular uptake of bilirubin
e.g. Rifampin (rifampicin)

Decreased bilirubin conjugation
e.g. Gilbert's syndrome,
  Crigler–Najjar syndrome types I and II,
  physiologic jaundice of the newborn

Conjugated hyperbilirubinemia
  Impaired canalicular excretion of bilirubin
  e.g. Dubin–Johnson syndrome, Rotor's syndrome

Liver disease

Hepatocellular injury
  Acute or subacute hepatocellular injury
  e.g. Viral hepatitis, hepatotoxins (e.g. ethanol), drugs [e.g.
    acetaminophen (paracetomol), many others], ischemia,
    metabolic disorders (e.g. Wilson's disease, Reye's
    syndrome), pregnancy-related (e.g. acute fatty liver of
    pregnancy, pre-eclampsia), autoimmune hepatitis

Chronic hepatocellular injury
  e.g. Viral hepatitis, hepatotoxins (e.g. ethanol), autoimmune
    hepatitis, metabolic (Wilson's disease, hemochromatosis,
    α_1-antirypsin deficiency)

Intrahepatic cholestasis
  Diffuse infiltrative disorders
  e.g. Granulatomous disease, amyloidosis, malignancy

Inflammation of intrahepatic bile ductules and/or portal tracts
e.g. Primary biliary cirrhosis, graft versus host disease, drugs

Miscellaneous conditions
e.g. Benign recurrent intrahepatic cholestasis, intrahepatic
  cholestasis of pregnancy, drugs (many, e.g. estrogens, anabolic
  steroids), total parenteral nutrition, sepsis, atypical presentations
  of viral or alchoholic hepatitis, postoperative cholestasis

Obstruction of the bile ducts

Choledocholithiasis
  Cholesterol gallstones
  Pigment (black or brown) gallstones

Diseases of the bile ducts
  Inflammation/infection
  e.g. Primary sclerosing cholangitis, AIDS cholangiopathy,
    hepatic arterial chemotherapy or trauma, postsurgical
    strictures

Neoplasms (e.g. cholangiocarcinoma)

Extrinsic compression of the biliary tree
  Neoplasms
  e.g. Pancreatic carcinoma, hepatocellular carcinoma,
    metastatic lymphadenopathy

Pancreatitis

Vascular enlargement (e.g. aneurysm, cavernous transformation
  of portal vein)

Figure 5.5 Differential diagnosis of jaundice.

Disorders associated with increased bilirubin production
Several processes can lead to increased bilirubin production. These include hemolysis, ineffective erythropoiesis, or resorption of a hematoma. For these reasons, jaundice may complicate the

clinical course of patients with hemolytic anemias, either hereditary or acquired. Megaloblastic anemia from either folate or vitamin B12 deficiency, iron deficiency anemia, sideroblastic anemia, and polycythemia vera may also increase bilirubin production. With these disorders, bilirubin concentration does not generally exceed 4–5mg/dL (68–85μmol/L).

Massive transfusion can lead to jaundice because the foreshortened life span of transfused erythrocytes leads to excessive bilirubin production. This, in conjunction with resorption of hematomas, is a significant factor in the development of hyperbilirubinemia that follows major trauma. Each of these disorders involves excessive delivery of unconjugated bilirubin to the liver without intrinsic organ dysfunction. Characteristically, these disorders produce an unconjugated hyperbilirubinemia.

Isolated disorders of bilirubin metabolism
Each of the following inherited conditions is characterized by a disorder at a specific step of bilirubin metabolism (see Fig. 5.1) without generalized hepatocellular dysfunction. In some of these disorders, the mutated gene has been identified. These disorders can be divided into unconjugated hyperbilirubinemias and conjugated hyperbilirubinemias (Fig. 5.6; also see Figs. 5.1 & 5.5).

Gilbert's syndrome
The most common of the inherited hyperbilirubinemias is Gilbert's syndrome. Gilbert's syndrome is present in up to 10% of Caucasian individuals. As discussed above, Gilbert's syndrome is thought to be attributable to decreased bilirubin glucuronidation. Thus, it is characterized by unconjugated hyperbilirubinemia. Gilbert's syndrome is entirely benign and rarely produces clinical jaundice. Because fasting is associated with downregulation of bilirubin UGT-1 activity, serum bilirubin may rise twofold to threefold in this condition. This is the basis of the diagnostic 'caloric test' for Gilbert's syndrome, which involves a prolonged fast. The test, however, has low sensitivity. In general, bilirubin remains below 4mg/dL (68μmol/L). Patients with Gilbert's syndrome are commonly identified during or after adolescence, when isolated hyperbilirubinemia is detected incidentally during routine multiphasic biochemical screening, or during an intercurrent illness whose symptoms of nausea, vomiting and fasting may thus provoke an unconjugated hyperbilirubinemia.

Crigler–Najjar syndromes
More profound defects in bilirubin conjugation are encountered in Crigler–Najjar syndrome. In type I Crigler–Najjar syndrome, unconjugated bilirubin levels often exceed 20mg/dL (340μmol/L), and the majority of patients die of kernicterus in the neonatal period. Liver transplantation can be lifesaving. Patients with type II Crigler–Najjar syndrome have serum bilirubin levels between those of Gilbert's syndrome and those of type I Crigler–Najjar syndrome (see Fig. 5.6). In contrast to type I Crigler–Najjar patients, patients with type II Crigler–Najjar syndrome experience a fall in serum bilirubin concentration to levels of 2–5mg/dL (34–85μmol/L) with phenobarbital (phenobarbitone), which increases bilirubin UGT-1 activity. These patients generally survive to adulthood without neurologic impairment.

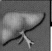

Clinical Manifestations of Liver Disease

Inherited disorders of hepatic bilirubin metabolism and transport					
	Gilbert's syndrome	Type I Crigler–Najjar syndrome	Type II Grigle–Najjar syndrome	Dubin–Johnson syndrome	Rotor's syndrome
Incidence	<10% of population	Extremely rare	Uncommon	Uncommon	Rare
Genetic defect	Mutations in promotor region of HUG-Br1	Absent HUG-Br1 expression	Mutations in coding region of HUG-Br1	Absent expression of MRP2	Unknown
Inheritence	Autosomal recessive	Autosomal recessive	Autosomal recessive	Autosomal recessive	Autosomal recessive
Mechanism	Decreased bilirubin conjugation	Absent bilirubin conjugation	Markedly decreased bilirubin conjugation	Impaired canalicular excretion of conjugated bilirubin via multispecific anion transporter	Unknown
Serum bilirubin concentration (mg/dL) (μmol/L)	<3–4 (51–68), virtually all unconjugated	Usually >20 (340), unconjugated	Usually <20 (340), virtually all unconjugated	Usually <7 (120), about 50% conjugated	Usually <7 (120), about 50% conjugated
Other laboratory abnormalities	Bilirubin decreases with phenobarbital	No change in bilirubin with phenobarbital	Bilirubin decreases with phenobarbital	Normal total urinary coproporphyrin (>80% type I)	Elevated total urinary coproporphyrin (<80% type I)
Liver histology	Normal	Normal	Normal	Dark pigment, predominantly centrilobular	Normal
Prognosis	Good	Poor, death in infancy from kernicterus unless specific therapy employed	Good	Good	Good
Treatment	None required	Phototherapy initially, liver transplantation necessary for long-term survival	Phenobarbital for marked hyperbilirubinemia	None available; avoid estrogens (worsens hyperbilirubinemia)	None

Figure 5.6 Inherited disorders of hepatic bilirubin metabolism and transport.

Dubin–Johnson and Rotor's syndromes

Two inherited disorders are associated with conjugated hyperbilirubinemia. Each appears to result from a selective decrease in bilirubin secretion into the bile canaliculus. Patients with Dubin–Johnson syndrome, which has been linked to the MRP2 gene (see discussion above), also exhibit impaired canalicular transport of other organic anions such as BSP. The molecular basis of Rotor's syndrome is currently unknown. Both Dubin–Johnson syndrome and Rotor's syndrome are not associated with impaired hepatic function.

Liver disease

Jaundice is a classic feature of hepatic dysfunction. In distinction to isolated disorders of bilirubin metabolism, icteric liver disease is characterized by an increase in serum bilirubin concentration in association with abnormalities in other standard liver function tests. The extensive differential diagnosis of icteric liver disease is briefly outlined here. Two broad categories of liver disease can be defined: those in which hepatocellular injury is the predominant mechanism; and those in which cholestasis predominates. The latter types of diseases are the most problematic from a diagnostic standpoint, because they are often difficult to distinguish clinically from obstruction of the bile ducts. The following discussion is arbitrarily organized according to the above classification. Clearly, however, there are instances in which hepatocellular injury and cholestasis contribute similarly to the development of jaundice.

Acute hepatocellular injury

A variety of disorders can produce acute or subacute hepatocellular injury, including viral hepatitis, exposure to hepatotoxins, hepatic ischemia, and certain metabolic derangements. In these situations there is usually evidence of severe disruption to hepatocytes with widespread necrosis and often associated inflammatory cell infiltration. This severe damage leads to metabolic dysfunction and destruction of excretory mechanisms, resulting in jaundice.

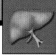

Five major hepatotropic viruses have been isolated. Hepatitis A and E viruses are transmitted enterally. Each typically produces a self-limited illness that does not progress to chronic liver disease. By contrast, hepatitis B, C, and D viruses are transmitted parenterally, and illness produced by these agents may be prolonged and progress to chronic disease. Major risk factors for hepatitis B, C, and D include intravenous drug use, exposure to blood products, and sexual exposure. The diagnosis of each these disorders is aided by serologic testing (see Chapters 11, 12 & 13).

Toxins and drugs can produce hepatocellular injury, either in a dose-dependent fashion, or idiosyncratically. The most common agent to produce acute dose-dependent hepatocellular injury is acetaminophen (paracetamol). A wide variety of drugs produce idiosyncratic hepatocellular injury and jaundice. These include isoniazid, and disulfiram, and nonsteroidal anti-inflammatory drugs (see Chapter 29). In a patient with ethanol dependency, alcoholic hepatitis should be always be a diagnostic consideration when there is jaundice and biochemical evidence of hepatocellular injury. Of note, alcoholic hepatitis can also have an atypical cholestatic presentation that can create diagnostic confusion (see Chapter 19).

Several forms of hepatic ischemia produce hepatocellular injury and jaundice. These include hypotension, hypoxia, or occlusive vascular disorders. Thrombosis of the hepatic vein (Budd–Chiari syndrome) should be suspected in patients with hypercoaguable states and, in particular, myeloproliferative disorders. Hepatic veno-occlusive disease should be suspected in a patient receiving cytotoxic agents in the setting of bone marrow transplantation (see Chapter 27).

Jaundice is a recognized complication of Wilson's disease, an inherited disorder of copper excretion into bile with copper overload and hepatocellular injury. Patients with Wilson's disease can also develop a Coombs negative hemolytic anemia, which contributes to the disproportionate hyperbilirubinemia that is often present (see Chapter 21). Several mitochondriopathies are associated with impaired fatty acid metabolism and hepatocellular injury from fatty acid overload. These include Reye's syndrome, which classically follows a viral illness in children, valproic acid toxicity, and fatty liver of pregnancy.

Chronic hepatocellular injury

Jaundice is a good indicator of significant hepatic dysfunction in the setting of liver diseases produced by chronic hepatocellular injury. In such situations there is a variety of pathogenetic mechanisms that cause liver damage. In general there is diffuse hepatocyte necrosis of varying severity, portal tract inflammation, and the development of fibrosis and subsequently cirrhosis. The hepatocytes are therefore severely affected at a functional level and biliary excretion is also substantially affected at both the cannicular and more distal levels due to the grossly deranged architecture. Although the broad categories of chronic hepatocellular injury are similar to those of acute injury, there are differences in the specific details. For example, causes of chronic viral hepatitis are largely limited to hepatitis B, C, and D viruses. The major hepatotoxin-associated chronic hepatocellular disease is alcoholic cirrhosis, whereas drug toxicity is a much less common cause of chronic as opposed to acute hepatocellular injury. The possibility of industrial exposure to toxic compounds such as vinyl chloride should be a diagnostic consideration in jaundiced patients with an appropriate background; carbon tetrachloride, a classic

industrial hepatotoxin, is no longer used in the USA.

Two metal storage diseases merit consideration. Wilson's disease clearly produces chronic hepatocellular injury (see Chapter 21). However, the most common metal storage disease worldwide is the iron overload disorder genetic hemochromatosis, with an estimated prevalence of 0.05% in Caucasian populations. Hepatocytes are a major target of iron-mediated injury in hemochromatosis, but jaundice does not generally occur until end-stage liver disease develops (see Chapter 20). Miscellaneous causes of chronic hepatocellular injury include autoimmune hepatitis and α_1-antitrypsin deficiency.

Cholestasis

Cholestasis is a term referring to the interruption of bile flow or bile formation. It can therefore occur anywhere from the sinusoidal membrane of the hepatocyte to the exit of the common bile duct into the duodenum. Thus cholestasis can be classified as intra- or extrahepatic, and there are many causes of each. This classification is adhered to here with a discussion of hepatic disorders that cause intrahepatic cholestasis and of obstruction of the bile ducts that causes extrahepatic cholestasis.

Functionally, if bile flow is interrupted, at whatever level, there will be decreased hepatic secretion of water and organic anions (including bile acids and bilirubin). The place of bilirubin is important here in a discussion of the causation of jaundice. Normal bile flow is obviously necessary for bilirubin excretion, but it should be noted that many of the pathologic processes affecting overall bile production also affect bilirubin metabolism (see Figs 5.1 & 5.4). Morphologically, bile will accumulate in the liver and biliary system and evidence of this is seen on liver biopsy.

Clinically, there will be features resulting from the decreased secretion and retention of bile, such as jaundice, pruritus, and evidence of malabsorption (Fig. 5.7).

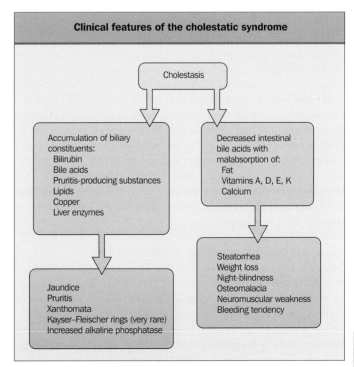

Figure 5.7 Clinical features of the cholestatic syndrome.

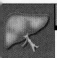

As indicated, in the diagnosis of jaundice, one of the most difficult differentials is between intra- and extrahepatic cholestasis.

Hepatic disorders with prominent cholestasis (intrahepatic cholestasis)

Overview
The following diseases are characterized by biochemical abnormalities that mimic obstruction of the bile ducts. These disorders have the greatest potential to generate diagnostic confusion. Such disorders can be categorized histologically according to those that infiltrate the liver, those that mainly involve injury to intrahepatic bile ductules or portal triads, and those in which major histologic changes are not evident.

Infiltrative diseases
A variety of infiltrative liver diseases is often associated with striking cholestasis and jaundice. Infiltrative diseases of the liver can be conveniently divided into granulomatous diseases, amyloidosis, and neoplastic replacement of hepatic parenchyma. The latter should be suspected if there is a known underlying malignancy. These disorders are likely to produce cholestasis by compression or obliteration of small bile ductules. Granulomatous diseases of the liver include:

- infections, such as tuberculosis, *Mycobacterium avium-intracellulare* (particularly in the immunocompromised host), leprosy, brucellosis, Q fever, syphilis, fungal diseases, parasitic diseases, and mononucleosis;
- toxins, such as beryllium, quinidine, allopurinol, and sulfonamides; and
- systemic disorders, including sarcoidosis, lymphoma (in particular, Hodgkin's disease), and Wegener's granulomatosis.

Tuberculosis and sarcoidosis are the most common forms of granulomatous liver diseases to produce jaundice. Although amyloidosis is in the differential diagnosis of infiltrative liver diseases, jaundice is extremely uncommon in that setting.

Disorders involving bile ductules
Inflammation and loss of small intrahepatic bile ductules are characteristic of primary biliary cirrhosis. When jaundice occurs, the disease is generally advanced. In particular, the presence of a serum bilirubin concentration of greater than 10mg/dL (170μmol/L) carries an extremely poor prognosis. A distinct form of bile ductular injury occurs with hepatic involvement in graft versus host disease, encountered in organ transplant recipients. Certain drugs can produce inflammation of the portal tracts with resultant cholestasis. These include chlorpromazine, erythromycin (particularly the estolate salt), chlorpropamide, and methimazole. Cholestasis generally resolves within several months after drug discontinuation.

Cholestasis with minimal histologic abnormalities
Jaundice may accompany conditions characterized by minimal hepatocellular injury or histologic abnormalities. The mechanism of cholestasis in these conditions is not well understood at present and may be multifactorial. In benign recurrent cholestasis, an autosomal recessive disorder that has been mapped to the same gene that is mutant in progressive familial intrahepatic cholestasis type I (Byler's disease), there is a defect of canalicular secretion of several classes of organic anions, including bile acids, into bile.

Sex hormones can produce a histologically bland intrahepatic cholestasis. Estrogens reduce bile formation through several mechanisms. These include:

- inhibition of the hepatocellular plasma membrane sodium pump, an important modulator of solute transport from blood to bile;
- impaired acidification of intracellular organelles, which may disrupt the targeting of organic anion transporters to their proper membrane domain; and
- decreased membrane fluidity, which may perturb the function of such transporters.

Each of these mechanisms may contribute to jaundice resulting from the use of oral contraceptives. Anabolic steroids can produce a syndrome that is clinically indistinguishable from that of estrogen-induced cholestasis. Of interest, the anabolic steroids methyltestosterone and norethandrolone may impair the integrity of hepatocellular microfilaments and thus increase back diffusion of biliary solutes through tight junctions into serum.

The features of cholestasis associated with total parenteral nutrition (TPN) can resemble those of cholestasis associated with estrogens and anabolic steroids. However steatohepatitis can also be seen with TPN. It has been proposed that TPN-induced cholestasis is also related to an altered enterohepatic circulation as well as diminished neuroendocrine stimulation of bile flow.

Cholestasis and jaundice may also develop during bacterial infections. At least two mechanisms have been proposed, each related to cytokines released during infection. First, tumor necrosis factor-α causes decreased expression of several hepatocellular organic anion transporters (including MRP2 – see above) and decreased bile flow. Second, interleukin-6 inhibits hepatocellular bile acid transport by reducing sodium pump activity. Sepsis-related cholestasis in the critically ill patient may be extremely difficult to distinguish from obstruction of the bile ducts. Helpful diagnostic clues are discussed below.

Atypical presentations of cholestasis
Viral hepatitis may rarely produce profound cholestasis with marked pruritus. Unless there are risk factors for viral hepatitis, no features reliably distinguish this disorder from those of other cholestatic syndromes or biliary tract obstruction. A high level of suspicion and appropriate serologies will aid in establishing the diagnosis. Similarly, alcoholic hepatitis can uncommonly have a cholestatic presentation. This is one setting in which urgent liver biopsy may be required to make the diagnosis.

Jaundice in pregnancy
Several cholestatic disorders associated with pregnancy merit discussion. Each of these characteristically occurs in the third trimester. Intrahepatic cholestasis of pregnancy typically presents with pruritus. Infrequently, it is associated with jaundice. It generally resolves within 2 weeks of delivery, and tends to recur with subsequent pregnancies. Two far more serious syndromes are acute fatty liver of pregnancy and pre-eclampsia. The former histologically resembles Reye's syndrome with microvesicular steatosis in hepatocytes. The latter is a microvascular disorder of the third trimester that is heralded by hypertension and proteinuria. Each requires prompt delivery (see Chapter 28).

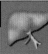

Jaundice in the postoperative patient

Postoperative jaundice is often multifactorial. Possible factors include inhalational anesthetic agents, other potentially hepatotoxic drugs, hepatic ischemia, blood transfusions, TPN, and sepsis. These can be distinguished from benign postoperative cholestasis, a self-limited (less than 1–2 weeks) syndrome characterized by transient hyperbilirubinemia without biochemical evidence of hepatocellular injury (see Chapter 31).

The liver transplant recipient represents a special case, in which the differential diagnosis of jaundice may not only include the disorders common to all postoperative patients, but those that relate to transplantation in particular. Specific diagnostic considerations include graft dysfunction due to ischemia-reperfusion injury or vascular occlusion, graft rejection, obstruction of the bile ducts, bile leak, viral hepatitis (e.g. cytomegalovirus, recurrent hepatitis B or C), immunosuppressive drug toxicity (e.g. azathioprine), and lymphoproliferative disorders.

Obstruction of the bile ducts

Obstructive disorders of the biliary tree include occlusion of the bile duct lumen by gallstones, intrinsic disorders of the bile ducts, and extrinsic compression.

Choledocholithiasis

The most common cause of biliary obstruction is choledocholithiasis. Two types of gallstones are associated with this problem: cholesterol gallstones and pigment gallstones. Cholesterol gallstones typically originate in the gallbladder, migrate into the common bile duct, and either impact at the ampulla of Vater or produce partial obstruction in a ball-valve fashion. Calcium bilirubinate (black pigment) gallstones characteristically develop in patients with unconjugated hyperbilirubinemia. Black pigment stones, like cholesterol stones, can form in the gallbladder, but they may also form *in situ* at any level of the biliary tree including the common bile duct. A distinct type of bilirubinate stone, so-called brown pigment gallstones, also forms *in situ* within the biliary tree. Obstruction of the bile ducts by these stones leads to repeated bouts of cholangitis (recurrent pyogenic cholangitis) in patients from certain regions in Asia, in association with biliary parasitic infestations, and in patients with prior biliary tract surgery.

Diseases of the bile ducts

Intrinsic disorders of the bile ducts may be inflammatory, infectious, or neoplastic. Primary sclerosing cholangitis, an inflammatory disorder of the bile ducts, characterized by focal and segmental strictures, is extensively discussed elsewhere in this book (see Chapter 18). A similar picture of focal narrowing and localized obstruction of the bile ducts is seen in patients infected with human immunodeficiency virus (so-called AIDS cholangiopathy), but jaundice is distinctly unusual in this setting. Biliary strictures may also follow hepatic arterial infusion of certain chemotherapeutic agents or result from surgical injury to the bile duct or hepatic artery. Neoplasms of the biliary tree, including cholangiocarcinoma, are discussed elsewhere in this book (see Chapter 26).

Extrinsic compression of the bile ducts

Extrinsic compression of the biliary tree may result from neoplastic involvement or inflammation of surrounding viscera.

Rarely, marked enlargement of surrounding vessels (e.g. arterial aneurysms, cavernous transformation of the portal vein) can compress the bile ducts as well.

Painless jaundice is a classic sign of carcinoma of the head of the pancreas. Occasionally, hepatocellular carcinoma or periportal lymph nodes enlarged by any metastatic tumor or lymphoma obstruct the extrahepatic bile ducts (Fig. 5.8). Pancreatitis may also produce extrinsic biliary compression, as a result of edema, pseudocyst formation, or fibrosis.

CLINICAL FEATURES

Overview

In a jaundiced individual, associated clinical features can be very helpful in distinguishing isolated disorders of hyperbilirubinemia from intrinsic liver disease or from biliary tract obstruction. Important clues can be obtained from the history and physical examination. These, in conjunction with standard biochemical tests, will substantially improve the efficiency of subsequent diagnostic studies.

It should be remembered that jaundice is one of the features of cholestasis, but that other effects of cholestasis are encountered in such patients. Some of these features can be present without jaundice (see Fig. 5.7).

History

The absence of any symptoms other than jaundice is consistent with hemolysis or an isolated disorder of bilirubin metabolism, but it does not exclude liver disease or biliary tract obstruction. Clues to the presence of liver disease versus biliary tract obstruction are featured in Fig. 5.9.

Symptoms compatible with a viral prodrome, such as anorexia, malaise, and myalgias, make viral hepatitis a strong possibility, as does a history of known infectious exposure, intravenous drug use, or receipt of blood products. The presence of arthralgias and rash heightens the suspicion for autoimmune hepatitis. Symptoms of pruritus are encountered with several disorders of intrahepatic cholestasis, such as primary biliary cirrhosis. Important clues to chronic liver disease include a history of fluid retention or confusion. A history of rapid fluid retention and jaundice raises the concern of Budd–Chiari syndrome or venoocclusive disease. A careful history may suggest that environmental hepatotoxins, ethanol, or medications underlie hepatic dysfunction that is responsible for jaundice. Finally, a family

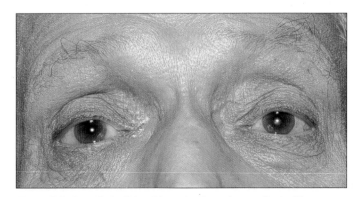

Figure 5.8 Jaundice of the skin and sclerae in a patient with malignant nodes at the porta hepatis.

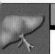

Features that differentiate biliary tract obstruction from cholestatic liver disease in the diagnosis of jaundice		
	Favors biliary obstruction	**Favors liver disease**
History	Abdominal pain	Malaise, myalgias, arthralgias, suggestive of viral syndrome
	Fever, rigors	Known infectious exposure
	Prior biliary surgery	Receipt of blood products, intravenous or nasal use
	Older age	of illicit drugs
		Exposure to known hepatotoxin
		Family history of liver disease
Physical examination	Fever	Ascites
	Abdominal tenderness	Signs of chronic liver disease (e.g. prominent abdominal veins, gynecomastia, spider angiomata, asterixis, encephalopathy)
	Palpable abdominal mass	
	Surgical scar	
		Signs of specific liver disease (e.g. Kayser–Fleischer rings, xanthelasmas)
Routine laboratory studies	Predominant elevation of alkaline phosphatase	Predominant elevation of serum transaminases
	Prothrombin time that is normal or normalizes with vitamin K administration	Prolonged prothrombin time that does not correct with vitamin K administration
	Elevated serum lipase	Decreased albumin concentration

Figure 5.9 Features that differentiate biliary tract obstruction from cholestatic liver disease in the diagnosis of jaundice.

history of liver disease suggests the possibility of a hereditary liver disease, such as hemochromatosis, Wilson's disease, or α_1-antitrypsin deficiency.

There are several historic clues to the presence of biliary tract obstruction. A history of fever, especially when accompanied by rigors, or abdominal pain, particularly in the right upper quadrant, is suggestive of cholangitis due to obstructive diseases (particularly choledocholithiasis). A history of prior biliary surgery also increases the likelihood that biliary tract obstruction is present. Although weight loss is often a nonspecific symptom, it is suggestive of malignancy in an older individual with jaundice. Obstructive jaundice from gallstone disease is also more common in the elderly.

Physical examination

Like the history, physical examination can offer important clues that distinguish liver disease from biliary tract obstruction. Several signs suggest that liver disease is the cause of jaundice. These include evidence of portal hypertension (i.e. ascites, splenomegaly, or prominent abdominal veins) or other characteristic features, such as spider angiomata, gynecomastia, and asterixis. Certain physical findings may suggest particular liver diseases. Examples of such classic signs include hyperpigmentation in hemochromatosis, xanthomas in primary biliary cirrhosis (see Figs 5.10 & 5.11), and Kayser–Fleischer rings in Wilson's disease. By contrast, certain findings suggest biliary tract obstruction. For example, high fever or abdominal tenderness (particularly right upper quadrant) suggests cholangitis. A palpable abdominal mass or palpable gallbladder suggests a neoplastic cause of obstructive jaundice. Finally, an abdominal scar in the midline or right upper quadrant may be the only clinical clue to prior biliary surgery.

A caveat

All clues in the history and physical must be interpreted with caution, because fever and abdominal pain accompany diseases other than biliary obstruction, and patients with prior biliary surgery may fortuitously develop viral hepatitis. Conversely, anorexia and malaise are not exclusively symptoms of viral hepatitis, and patients with parenchymal liver disease can certainly develop gallstones. Nonetheless, when these clues are evaluated with physical findings and routine laboratory tests, jaundice is correctly characterized as obstructive or nonobstructive in most cases.

DIAGNOSIS AND EVALUATION

Overview

A general algorithm for evaluating the patient with jaundice is presented in Fig. 5.12. The sequential approach involves: a careful patient history, physical examination, and screening laboratory studies; formulation of a working differential diagnosis; selection of further specialized tests to narrow the diagnostic possibilities; and development of a strategy for treatment or further testing if unexpected diagnostic possibilities are suggested.

Screening laboratory studies

Essential laboratory studies include serum total bilirubin, alkaline phosphatase, transaminases [asparate aminotransferase (AST) and alanine aminotransferase (ALT)], and prothrombin time. Serum alkaline phosphatase activity reflects the presence of a number of related enzymes of different tissue origins. In liver, alkaline phosphatase is associated with the apical domain of the plasma membrane of hepatocytes and bile duct

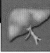

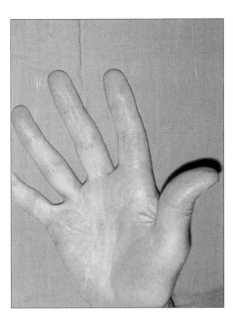

Figure 5.10 Xanthomata (fatty deposits) in the skin creases and palm of a patient with primary biliary cirrhosis.

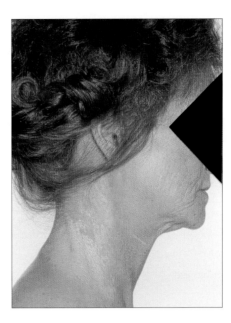

Figure 5.11 Extensive xanthoma in the neck of a pigmented patient with primary biliary cirrhosis.

epithelial cells. Under physiologic conditions, this protein is enzymatically cleaved and released into bile, but small amounts are released into serum as well. Biliary obstruction or intra-hepatic cholestasis increase serum alkaline phosphatase activity by increasing its synthesis and release into serum. However, increased serum alkaline phosphatase activity may reflect release of alkaline phosphatase isoenzymes from extrahepatic tissues. Hence, other more specific markers, such as the serum activities of the canalicular enzymes γ-glutamyl transpeptidase, leucine aminopeptidase, or 5′-nucleotidase are useful to confirm the hepatic origin of alkaline phosphatase. In a jaundiced patient, a predominant increase in (hepatic) alkaline phosphatase activity relative to those of serum transaminases suggests the possibility of biliary tract obstruction. It should be noted that intrahepatic cholestatic disorders can produce an identical biochemical picture. By contrast, in hemolysis or an isolated disorder of bilirubin metabolism, alkaline phosphatase is normal.

Measurements of transaminases, in particular, AST and ALT, are useful in the evaluation of jaundice. Serum AST reflects a mixture of isozymes released from both the cytosol and mitochondria of hepatocytes as well as AST released from other tissues. Alanine aminotransferase is a cytosolic enzyme found predominantly in hepatocytes. Each of these enzymes ordinarily circulates in low concentrations in serum. However, liver cell damage, due to ischemia, viral infection, or toxins, significantly increases serum transaminase activity. Thus, predominant elevation of serum transaminase activity in comparison with alkaline phosphatase activity suggests that jaundice is due to intrinsic hepatocellular disease. By contrast, in hemolysis or an isolated disorder of bilirubin metabolism, transaminases are normal.

Of note, a serum activity of AST that exceeds that of ALT by at least a factor of 2, but is less than 10 times the upper limit of normal, represents a clue to the diagnosis of alcoholic liver disease. However, acute Wilson's disease may present with similar biochemical abnormalities. There are exceptions to the above generalizations. For example, transient biliary obstruction from choledocholithiasis is occasionally associated with a brief but

dramatic elevation (exceeding 10 to 20 times normal) of serum transaminase activity.

The prothrombin time is a measure of the plasma activities of the coagulation factors I, II, V, VII, and X, each of which is synthesized in the liver. Prolongation of the prothrombin time can result from impaired hepatic synthesis of these proteins but may also reflect deficiency of vitamin K, which is essential for post-translational γ-carboxylation of lysine residues of factors II, VII, IX, and X. Vitamin K absorption requires an intact enterohepatic circulation (hence an unobstructed biliary tree) of bile acids. Thus, parenteral administration of vitamin K will generally normalize a prolonged prothrombin time in patients with obstructive jaundice but not in patients with liver disease. In hemolysis or an isolated disorder of bilirubin metabolism, the prothrombin time is (generally) normal.

In most cases, the measurement of the total bilirubin concentration is sufficient to aid in the diagnosis of jaundice, especially when it is interpreted in conjunction with the alkaline phosphatase and transaminases. In patients with liver disease or biliary tract obstruction, there are either signs or symptoms of hepatobiliary disease or more than one of the above laboratory tests is abnormal. By contrast, patients with hemolysis or isolated disorders of bilirubin metabolism have no signs or symptoms of hepatobiliary disease, and the only abnormality in screening laboratory studies is hyperbilirubinemia.

Although some laboratories provide colorimetric estimates of conjugated and unconjugated bilirubin, these are not usually necessary in practice (with the exception of neonatal jaundice, in which unconjugated hyperbilirubinemia has therapeutic implications). In general, such tests may have greatest utility in distinguishing unconjugated hyperbilirubinemias (e.g. hemolysis, and Gilbert's Criggler–Najjar syndromes), from isolated conjugated hyperbilirubinemias (e.g. Rotor's and Dubin–Johnson syndromes). These are uncommon issues. Moreover, accurate distinction between these conditions usually requires more sophisticated chromatographic tools that are available only in specialized centers. Thus, reliance on the relative concentrations of unconjugated versus conjugated bilirubin is not helpful in most cases.

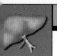

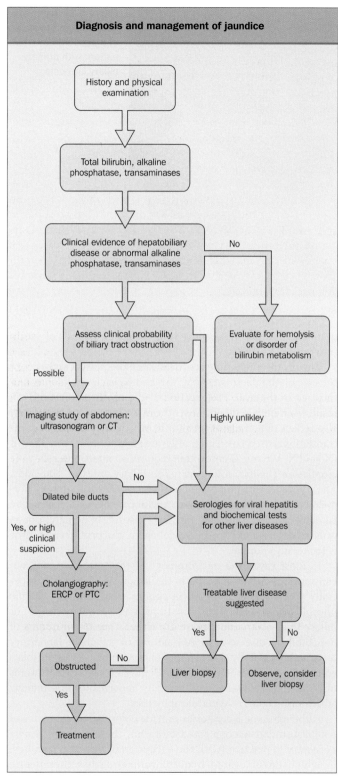

Figure 5.12 Diagnosis and management of the jaundiced patient.

phosphatase and transaminases is unlikely to have liver disease or biliary obstruction. Further testing for specific disorders, such as hemolysis or isolated defects in bilirubin metabolism, is warranted (see Fig. 5.12).

If classic features of liver disease are present on the basis of history and physical examination, and screening laboratory studies, and biliary tract obstruction is not suspected, then a further evaluation for causes of liver disease should ensue. On the other hand, if the history, physical examination, and laboratory studies suggest that biliary tract obstruction is possible, an imaging study is appropriate to confirm either the presence or absence of biliary tract obstruction. Selection of an imaging study depends on the likelihood of obstruction, diagnostic accuracy, cost, complication rate, and availability, especially if simultaneous therapeutic intervention is anticipated.

Imaging studies (see Chapter 4 also)
Abdominal ultrasonography

Abdominal ultrasonography is an accepted tool in the evaluation of hepatobiliary disease, because it determines the caliber of the extrahepatic biliary tree, and it reveals intra- or extrahepatic mass lesions. The sensitivity of abdominal ultrasonography for the detection of biliary obstruction in jaundiced patients ranges from 55 to 91%, and the specificity from 82 to 95% (Fig. 5.13). Ultrasonography can also demonstrate cholelithiasis (although common duct stones may not be well seen) and space occupying lesions in the liver greater than 1cm in diameter. Ultrasonography has three major advantages. First, it is noninvasive. Second, it is portable (this may be invaluable in the evaluation of the critically ill patient). Third, it is relatively inexpensive. However, there are several potential disadvantages with ultrasound. For example, studies may be difficult to interpret in obese patients or patients with overlying bowel gas. Also, dilatation of the common bile duct, which usually indicates biliary tract obstruction, is common in patients who have undergone previous cholecystectomy. A final caveat is that in patients with cirrhosis and other conditions associated with poorly compliant hepatic parenchyma such as primary sclerosing cholangitis, intrahepatic ducts may not dilate with obstruction.

Computed tomography of the abdomen

Computed tomography (CT) of the abdomen with intravenous contrast is an excellent alternative to ultrasound in evaluating the possibility of biliary tract obstruction in jaundiced patients. Abdominal CT has a diagnostic accuracy comparable to that of ultrasound in the diagnosis of biliary obstruction, with a sensitivity and specificity of 63–96% and 93–100%, respectively (see Fig. 5.13). A technical refinement, spiral (helical) CT may improve the diagnostic accuracy of this method. Abdominal CT has several advantages over ultrasound. First, it detects space occupying lesions as small as 5mm. Second, it is not operator-dependent as in ultrasonography. Third, it provides technically superior images in obese individuals and in patients in whom the biliary tree is obscured by bowel gas. The caveats that apply to the accuracy of ultrasonography for the diagnosis of biliary obstruction also apply to abdominal CT. In particular, CT it is not as accurate as ultrasonography in detecting cholelithiasis because it only images calcified stones. Other considerations in the utilization of abdominal CT in patients with jaundice are its lack of portability, requirement for use of intravenous contrast, and expense.

Decision analysis

In aggregate, history, physical examination, and screening laboratory provide a good estimate of the likelihood that obstructive jaundice is present or absent. For example, an asymptomatic hyperbilirubinemic patient who has an unremarkable physical examination and normal serum alkaline

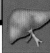

Endoscopic retrograde cholangiopancreatography

Endoscopic retrograde cholangiopancreatography (ERCP) permits direct visualization of the biliary tree as well as the pancreatic ducts. In contrast to abdominal ultrasonography and CT, ERCP is more invasive. The procedure involves passage of an endoscope into the duodenum, introduction of a catheter into the ampulla of Vater, and injection of contrast medium into the common bile duct and/or pancreatic duct. Importantly, conscious sedation is necessary.

The technique of ERCP is highly accurate in the diagnosis of biliary obstruction, with a sensitivity of 89–98% and specificity of 89–100% (see Fig. 5.13). It offers the possible implementation of other diagnostic maneuvers in addition to simple visualization and radiography. For example, it permits biopsies and brushings for cytology of periampullary lesions. Moreover, if a focal cause for biliary obstruction is identified (e.g. choledocholithiasis, biliary stricture), maneuvers to relieve obstruction (e.g. sphincterotomy, stone extraction, dilatation, stent placement) can be performed during the same session. It should be noted that acquisition of biopsy material and therapeutic intervention via ERCP are largely limited to lesions that are distal to the bifurcation of the right and left hepatic bile ducts.

The technical success rate of ERCP is higher than 90%; the rate limiting step is cannulation of the ampulla of Vater. This may be a particularly important consideration in patients with prior abdominal surgery and altered anatomy (e.g. choledochojejunostomy, gastrojejunostomy). As an invasive procedure, ERCP should be employed thoughtfully. The morbidity and mortality associated with ERCP from untoward events such as respiratory depression, aspiration, bleeding, perforation, cholangitis, and pancreatitis, are 3% and 0.2%, respectively. These rates are increased when interventional procedures are concomitantly employed. A final consideration is cost, as ERCP is more expensive than noninvasive imaging procedures.

Percutaneous transhepatic cholangiography

Percutaneous transhepatic cholangiography (PTC) is a procedure that complements ERCP. It requires the passage of a needle through the skin and subcutaneous tissues into the hepatic parenchyma and advancement into a peripheral bile duct. When bile is aspirated, a catheter is introduced through the needle, and radio-opaque contrast medium is injected. It has an accuracy comparable to that of ERCP in the diagnosis of biliary tract obstruction in the setting of jaundice, with a sensitivity and specificity of approximately 98–100% and 89–100%, respectively (see Fig. 5.13). Like in ERCP, interventional procedures, such as balloon dilatation and stent placement to relieve amenable focal obstructions of the biliary tree, can be performed at the time of PTC.

Percutaneous transhepatic cholangiography is potentially technically advantageous under conditions in which the level of biliary obstruction is proximal to the common hepatic duct or in which altered anatomy precludes ERCP (see above). It may be technically difficult in the absence of dilatation of the intrahepatic bile ducts; under these conditions, multiple passes are frequently required, and cannulation of the biliary tree may be unsuccessful

Imaging studies for the evaluation of jaundice					
Test	Sensitivity (%)	Specificity (%)	Morbidity (%)	Mortality (%)	Comments

Abdominal ultrasonogram	55–91	82–95	–	–	Advantages:
					  Noninvasive, portable, less expensive
					
					Disadvantages:
					  Bowel gas may obscure common bile duct; interpretation difficult in obese individuals and in those with ileus

Abdominal CT	63–96	93–100	–	–	Advantages:
					  Noninvasive, not operator- dependent, interpretation less affected by obesity or ileus
					
					Disadvantages:
					  Not portable, intravenous contrast required (potential for nephrotoxicity)

ERCP	89–98	89–100	3	0.2	Advantages:
					  Provides direct imaging of bile ducts, permits direct visualization of periampullary mucosa, potential for simultaneous tissue acquisition or therapeutic intervention, especially useful for lesions distal to bifurcation of hepatic ducts
					
					Disadvantages:
					  Cannot be performed if altered anatomy precludes endoscopic access to ampulla (e.g. gastro- or choledochojejunostomy)

PTC	98–100	89–100	3	0.2	Advantages:
					  Provides direct imaging of bile ducts, poptential for simultaneous tissue aquisition or therapeutic intervention, especially useful for lesions proximal to common hepatic duct
					
					Disadvantages:
					  More difficult with non dilated intrahepatic bile ducts

Figure 5.13 Imaging studies for the evaluation of jaundice.

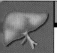
in up to 25% of attempts. The morbidity and mortality of PTC from bleeding, perforation, and cholangitis are 3% and 0.2%, respectively. Like ERCP, it is more expensive than abdominal ultrasonography or CT.

Other imaging studies

Magnetic resonance cholangiography (MRC) is a technical refinement of standard magnetic resonance imaging that permits rapid clear-cut delineation of the biliary tree without the requirement for intravenous contrast. Emerging evidence suggests that its accuracy for detecting biliary tract obstruction approaches that of ERCP. Although promising as an imaging modality, MRC is expensive, making it uncertain whether it will supplant abdominal ultrasonography or CT as an initial imaging test. Moreover, at the time of this writing, it is not clear whether MRC should be performed before ERCP or PTC if ultrasonography or CT are inconclusive.

Nuclear scintigraphy of the biliary tree, while helpful in the diagnosis of cholecystitis, is not sufficiently sensitive to justify its use in the diagnostic evaluation of jaundice. Furthermore, hepatic uptake of radiolabeled derivatives of iminodiacetic acid [e.g. 2,6-dimethyl iminodiacetic acid (HIDA)] is quite limited when the serum bilirubin exceeds 7–10mg/dL (119–170μmol/L).

Suggested strategies for imaging

The order of imaging studies will depend largely on the clinical likelihood of obstructive jaundice (see Fig. 5.12). Clinical decision analysis has compared several diagnostic strategies by mathematical modeling. For example, if the probability of biliary obstruction is 20%, the positive and negative predictive values of a strategy that employs ultrasonography as the initial test would be 96 and 98%, respectively. This compares quite favorably with a strategy that employs ERCP as the initial test. On the other hand, if the probability of biliary obstruction is 60%, a strategy that employs ultrasonography as the first test would yield a positive predictive value of 99%. However, the negative predictive value would fall to 89%. By contrast, when ERCP is the initial diagnostic procedure, the predictive value of a positive test would be 99% and that of a negative test would be 95%.

Stated differently, among patients in whom the probability of biliary obstruction is felt to be low (but not zero), information regarding the hepatic parenchyma may be just as important as excluding the possibility of biliary obstruction. Therefore, in such patients an abdominal ultrasonogram or CT are appropriate as initial imaging studies. If no evidence of biliary obstruction is found, the patient can be followed and should undergo further evaluation for hepatic parenchymal disease as appropriate (see Fig. 5.12). On the other hand, if dilated bile ducts are visualized, then direct imaging of the biliary tree should be performed.

If biliary obstruction is felt to be likely on clinical and biochemical grounds, ERCP (or PTC) could be considered as the initial study, since the absence of dilated ducts on abdominal ultrasound or CT would not rule out biliary obstruction. If ERCP or PTC do not show biliary obstruction, then abdominal ultrasonography or abdominal CT should be performed (if this has not been done) to image the hepatic parenchyma, and further studies, as outlined below, should be obtained.

The decision to employ ERCP versus PTC will be influenced by a variety of factors (see above and Fig. 5.13). These include the availability of each procedure at a particular facility, the presence or absence of dilated bile ducts, the suspected level of biliary obstruction, and the importance of accurately localizing the obstructing lesion (proximal with PTC, or distal with ERCP) in order to facilitate a plan of therapy. Under most circumstances, ERCP should be the procedure of choice, since it is comparable to PTC in availability, accuracy, technical success rate, and frequency of complications, and offers a broader range of interventional options than PTC.

Further studies
Serologic testing

When imaging studies do not suggest biliary obstruction, evaluation for underlying liver disease is indicated in jaundiced patients with biochemical evidence of hepatocellular dysfunction or cholestasis (see Fig. 5.12). If there is evidence of hepatocellular injury, appropriate screening laboratory studies would include viral serologies (including those for hepatitis B and C viruses; if acute then hepatitis A virus as well), serum levels of iron, transferrin, and ferritin (for hemochromatosis), ceruloplasmin (for Wilson's disease, especially in patients younger than 40 years of age), autoantibodies (for autoimmune hepatitis), and α_1-antitrypsin (for α_1-antitrypsin deficiency). If there is biochemical evidence of predominantly cholestasis, antimitochondrial antibodies (for primary biliary cirrhosis) should be measured. Confirmation of these diagnoses as well as elucidation of diagnoses not revealed by serologic analysis may be made by liver biopsy.

Liver biopsy

Liver biopsy provides precise information regarding details of hepatic lobular architecture. It has greatest utility in two types of patient. These are patients in whom a treatable cause of liver disease is suspected by serologic evaluation or patients with persistent jaundice that remains undiagnosed. With special histologic stains and/or quantitation of copper or iron content as appropriate, liver biopsy permits the accurate diagnosis of a number of liver diseases. These include viral hepatitis, alcoholic hepatitis, Wilson's disease, hemochromatosis, α_1-antitrypsin deficiency, fatty liver of pregnancy, primary biliary cirrhosis, granulomatous hepatitis, and neoplasms. Occasionally, liver biopsy provides clues to otherwise unsuspected biliary tract obstruction (Figs 5.14 & 5.15). The absence of these findings does not exclude biliary tract obstruction, however.

Despite its potential advantages, liver biopsy carries a small risk of complications. These include bleeding and perforation, with a morbidity of less than 0.5% and mortality of 0.1%. For these reasons, liver biopsy should be employed only after a careful evaluation of the jaundice has been performed.

MANAGEMENT

Biliary obstruction

In the patient with obstruction of the bile ducts, the goal of therapy is mechanical relief of obstruction. There are three alternative approaches: endoscopic, radiologic, and surgical. Both interventional endoscopic or radiologic approaches permit sphincterotomy, balloon dilatation of focal strictures, and placement of drains or stents. These techniques are less invasive than surgery, but they may not permit definitive treatment under specialized circumstances. The therapeutic strategy chosen will depend, in

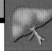

Abnormalities seen on liver biopsy that are associated with obstructive jaundice
Findings seen with either extra- or intrahepatic cholestasis
Bile plugs in canalicular spaces Bile staining of hepatocytes or Kupffer cells
Findings suggestive of biliary obstruction
Feathery degeneration of hepatocytes Portal tract 'edema' Proliferation of bile ductules Periductular fibrosis
Findings 'diagnostic' of biliary obstruction
Bile infarct Bile lake Neutrophils in the wall or lumen of interlobular bile (cholangitis) Bile plugs in interlobular ducts

Figure 5.14 Abnormalities seen on liver biopsy that are associated with obstructive jaundice.

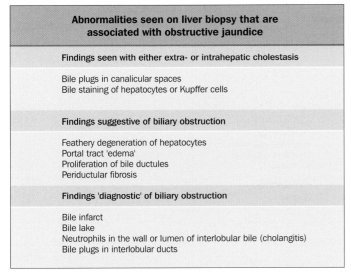

Figure 5.15 Histologic section showing biliary cirrhosis and a bile lake (arrow) in a patient with prolonged extrahepatic biliary obstruction.

part, on the location and likely etiology of the obstructing lesion. For example, focal intrahepatic strictures may be best treated by an interventional radiologic approach. By contrast, lesions distal to the bifurcation of the hepatic ducts may be more suitably managed endoscopically. Mass lesions may require surgery.

Cholestatic liver disease

In cholestatic liver disease, the optimal treatment is directed toward the underlying etiology. Such treatments might include cessation of ethanol, discontinuation of a drug, antiviral agents, phlebotomy for hemochromatosis, corticosteroids for autoimmune hepatitis, ursodiol (ursodeoxycholic acid) for primary biliary cirrhosis, or penicillamine for Wilson's disease. In irreversible liver disease, liver transplantation is a clear-cut option.

In adults, therapy for hyperbilirubinemia *per se* is not usually required. In particular, the neurotoxicity of bilirubin is confined to disorders characterized by extreme elevations of unconjugated bilirubin such as type I Crigler–Najjar syndrome. In these special cases, clearance of bilirubin can be achieved by phototherapy. With this technique, exposure to blue or green light produces photo-isomerization of bilirubin to more water-soluble enantiomers that do not require conjugation for excretion into bile.

Management of other cholestatic features
Pruritus
Pruritus is a complication of cholestasis that is worthy of discussion. It should be emphasized that it develops independently of jaundice. Not all jaundiced individuals have pruritus, and not all patients with pruritus and cholestasis are jaundiced. Regardless of the mechanism, pruritus can be devastating to the quality of life of patients with cholestasis.

Although it has been assumed that the pruritogen is excreted in bile and undergoes an enterohepatic circulation, its chemical structure remains unknown. Indirect evidence suggests that it may be chemically related to bile acids, since bile acid-binding resins such as cholestyramine have been of some benefit. Other lines of evidence suggest that endogenous opiate-like compounds may be involved. First, opiates are excreted in bile, and endogenous opiomimetic activity is elevated in animal models of cholestasis. Second, opiate receptor antagonists such as naloxone and naltrexone have shown promise in eliminating pruritus in preliminary trials.

The choleretic bile acid ursodiol improves biochemical indices and slows disease progression in primary biliary cirrhosis, but it has variable efficacy with respect to pruritus. Ursodiol appears to improve biochemical markers in TPN-induced cholestasis as well as pruritus in intrahepatic cholestasis of pregnancy. However, it does not appear to be of benefit in primary sclerosing cholangitis. Ursodiol has not been extensively studied in other cholestatic disorders. Phenobarbital, an inducer of xenobiotic metabolism, may relieve pruritus in individual patients, but its utility has not been supported in controlled trials. Rifampin, another inducer of xenobiotic metabolism, has been shown in some, but not all studies, to reduce pruritus in primary biliary cirrhosis and pediatric cholestatic disorders. In addition to these specific therapies, simple measures have been recommended, such as less frequent bathing, wearing of light clothing, and frequent cutting of fingernails. The use of skin emollients and mild fragrance-free soaps has been recommended as well. Each of these approaches is summarized in Fig. 5.16.

Effects of malabsorption
Malabsorption has important effects in chronic cholestasis. If steatorrhoea is present, a low fat diet may help the resulting diarrhea, and medium chain triglycerides, as a dietary supplement that does not require bile acids for absorption, may improve nutrition. Fat soluble vitamins A, D, E, and K should be given, together with calcium supplements.

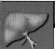

Medical therapy for cholestasis-associated pruritus			
Drug	**Regimen**	**Efficacy**	**Adverse effects**
Antihistamines, eg: Diphenhydramine Hydroxyzine	25–50mg q6h 25mg q8h	Rarely provides significant relief apart from sedation	Drowsiness
Cholestyramine	4–6g 30 minutes before meals (may take double dose at breakfast and skip evening dose)	Beneficial in most patients	Constipation, fat malabsorption, decreased absorption of other medications
Ursodiol (ursodeoxycholic acid)	10–15mg/kg per day	Beneficial in primary biliary cirrhosis, possibly in intrahepatic cholestasis of pregnancy	No major toxicity reported
Rifampin (rifampicin)	300mg q12h	Beneficial in most but not all controlled trials to date	Inducer of hepatic enzymes involved in drug metabolism, potential hepatotoxicity, red–orange discoloration of secretions
Naltrexone	50mg/day	Beneficial in primary biliary cirrhosis, no extensive study in other disorders	Opiate withdrawal symptoms, generally transient

Figure 5.16 Medical therapy for cholestatis-associated prurititus.

PRACTICE POINTS

Illustrative case

A 30-year-old woman had a 10-year history of recurrent attacks of abdominal pain and facial swelling. She had had three successful pregnancies with no problems. She was overweight but there were no other abnormal physical signs. Investigation revealed C1 esterase inhibitor deficiency. In view of the increasing frequency of her symptoms, she was treated with stanozolol 2.5–5.0mg/day and her attacks of abdominal pain and facial swelling were reduced.

One year later she had a severe attack of abdominal pain and jaundice. The stanozolol was stopped and the jaundice cleared over 1 week. Abdominal ultrasound was performed, which showed multiple stones in the gallbladder and a dilated common bile duct, but no stone was detected in the duct. Subsequent ERCP showed that the duct was clear. The stanozolol was restarted after a further attack of facial swelling.

Interpretation

Stanozolol is a C-17 alkyl substituted anabolic steroid which is useful in preventing attacks of oedema in patients with C1

esterase inhibitor deficiency. Patients taking this drug have to be carefully monitored due to the possibility of developing cholestatic jaundice. The steroid is believed to effect bile acid transport across the sinusoidal membrane of the hepatocyte, but also the excretion of conjugated bilirubin into the cannaliculi. Damage is also caused to the pericannalicular microfilamantous network, thus impairing canalicular contractions and contributing to the cholestasis due to reduced bile flow. These changes resolve when the drug is stopped.

In this case, however, the severe attack of abdominal pain associated with jaundice was due to a gallstone in the common bile duct, which the patient was presumed to have passed spontaneously. The pain was not due to the C1 esterase inhibitor deficiency on this occasion, nor was the jaundice due to the stanozolol. The jaundice cleared rapidly, which is consistent with passage of a gallstone. The patient had several risk factors for cholethiasis but, interestingly, had not had any evidence of cholestasis of pregnancy, which might have indicated stanozolol could have caused jaundice.

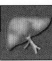

FURTHER READING

Berk PD, Noyer C. Bilirubin metabolism and the hereditary hyperbilirubinemias. Semin Liver Dis. 1994;14:321–94. *A detailed and comprehensive review of hereditary hyperbilirubinemias.*

Bosma PJ, Chowdhury JR, Bakker C, et al. The genetic basis of the reduced expression of bilirubin UDP-glucuronosyltransferase 1 in Gilbert's syndrome. N Engl J Med. 1995;333:1171–5. *A useful paper describing the genetic abnormality in the 5′-promoter region for the UGT gene in Gilbert's syndrome.*

Malchow-Møller A, Gronvall S, Hilden J, et al. Ultrasound examination in jaundiced patients. Is computer-assisted preclassification helpful? J Hepatol. 1991;12:321–6. *Ultrasound needs to be combined with clinical information in order to make an accurate diagnosis of jaundice.*

Matzen P, Malchow-Møller A, Brun B, et al. Ultrasonography, computed tomography, and cholescintigraphy in suspected obstructive jaundice: a prospective comparative study. Gastroenterology. 1983;84:1492–7. *An early paper demonstrating the superiority of ultrasound in the diagnosis of obstructive jaundice.*

O'Connor KW, Snodgrass PJ, Swonder JE, et al. A blinded prospective study comparing four current non-invasive approaches in the differential diagnosis of medical versus surgical jaundice. Gastroenterology. 1983;84:1498–504. *Paper indicating that careful clinical assessment is an accurate means of detecting extrahepatic biliary obstruction. This can be reliably confirmed by the imaging techniques used.*

Pasanen PA, Partanen KP, Pikkarainen PH, Alhava EM, Janatuinen EK, Pirinen AE. A comparison of ultrasound, computed tomography and endoscopic retrograde cholangiopancreatography in the differential diagnosis of benign and malignant jaundice and cholestasis. Eur J Surg. 1993;159:23–9. *A study which shows that the three imaging methods are complementary in the diagnosis of obstructive jaundice.*

Richter JM, Silverstein MD, Schapiro R. Suspected obstructive jaundice: a decision analysis of diagnostic strategies. Ann Intern Med. 1983;99:46–51. *An early attempt at decision analysis of a diagnostic strategy for the diagnosis of obstructive jaundice. Ten diagnostic strategies were evaluated.*

Rubin R, Kowalski TE, Khandewali M, Malet PF. Ursodiol for hepatobiliary disorders. Ann Intern Med. 1994;121:207–18. *A useful review of the use of ursodiol (ursodeoxycholic acid) in the treatment of cholestasis. The rationale for its use is discussed.*

Soto JA, Barish M, Yucel EK, Siegenberg D, Ferrucci JT, Chuttani R. Magnetic resonance cholangiography: comparison with endoscopic retrograde cholangiography. Gastroenterology. 1996;110:589–97. *A paper showing that MRC is highly sensitive and specific in detecting abnormalities of the biliary tract.*

Te Boekhorst T, Urlus M, Doesburg W, Yap SH, Goris RJ. Etiologic factors of jaundice in severely ill patients. J Hepatol. 1988;7:111–7. *A retrospective study elucidating the multiple factors contributing to jaundice in severely ill patients.*

Trauner M, Meier PJ, Boyer JL. Molecular pathogenesis of cholestasis. N Engl J Med. 1998;339:1217–27. *An excellent up-to-date review of the modern understanding of the molecular basis of cholestasis.*

Van der Veere CN, Sinaasappel M, McDonagh AF, et al. Current therapy for Crigler–Najjar syndrome type I: report of a world registry. Hepatology. 1996;24:311–15. *A review of an important database of cases of Crigler–Najjar type 1. It is concluded that the only effective therapy is hepatic transplantation, which should be performed early enough to prevent permanent brain damage.*

Wolfhagen FH, Sternieri E, Hop WC, Vitale G, Bertolotti M, Van Buuren HR. Oral naltrexone treatment for cholestatic pruritus: a double-blind, placebo-controlled study. Gastroenterology. 1997;113:1264–9. *A double-blind trial showing that naltrexone is useful in cholestatic patients with refractory pruritus.*

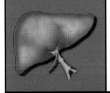

Section 2 Clinical Manifestations of Liver Disease

Chapter 6

Gastrointestinal Hemorrhage and Portal Hypertension

John R Lake and Peter D Howdle

INTRODUCTION

Gastrointestinal bleeding driven by portal hypertension represents a common and potentially life-threatening complication of chronic liver disease. Virtually any lesion in the upper gastrointestinal tract, including peptic ulcer disease, Mallory–Weiss tear, gastritis, and oesophagitis, is more likely to bleed in the presence of portal hypertension and may bleed briskly. The most common and most serious site of bleeding is from gastroesophageal varices. Varices occur as a result of the development of a collateral bloodflow around the liver in response to impaired portal bloodflow. The most common cause of this is cirrhosis of the liver. However, presinusoidal causes such as portal vein thrombosis or schistosomiasis can lead to a similar presentation in the absence of cirrhosis. The management of patients with variceal hemorrhage has changed quite markedly in recent years. While endoscopic sclerotherapy has been used successfully in the management of esophageal varices for more than two decades, more recently variceal band ligation has lessened the morbidity associated with endoscopic therapy, in particular the incidence of esophageal strictures and ulcers, and has substantially improved its results.

The fashioning of a surgical shunt to manage refractory variceal hemorrhage has become much less common and is now rare in the Western world. By contrast, the use of a transjugular intrahepatic portosystemic shunt (TIPS) has emerged as the most important therapeutic option for recurrent or refractory variceal hemorrhage. It is particularly useful in patients awaiting liver transplantation, as it does not alter the extrahepatic vascular anatomy. Finally, pharmacologic therapy for the prevention and treatment of portal hypertensive bleeding has also markedly improved, with β blockers emerging as a very effective method for preventing recurrent bleeding. The continuous infusion of somatostatin and its analogs has been shown to control the rate of bleeding with relatively few side effects.

PORTAL VENOUS ANATOMY

The portal venous system drains blood from the gastrointestinal tract within the abdomen and from the pancreas, gallbladder, and spleen (Fig. 6.1). The portal bloodflow is approximately 1 litre per minute, the mean pressure is about 7mmHg, and 70% of the hepatic oxygen is supplied by the portal system.

Changes with portal hypertension

If the portal venous flow becomes obstructed, there is a rise in

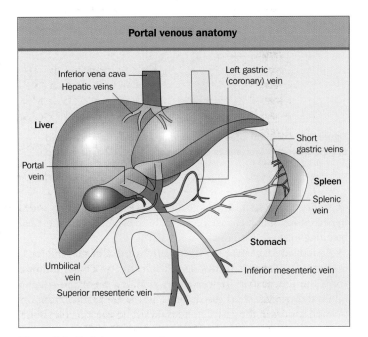

Figure 6.1 Portal venous anatomy.

portal pressure and a collateral circulation develops, diverting the portal flow into systemic veins (Fig. 6.2). Thus, while in normal circumstances 100% of portal blood flows through the liver, in cirrhosis with a severe intrahepatic block to portal venous flow, only approximately 10% of the bloodflow reaches the hepatic veins, and the rest circumvents the liver via the collateral circulation.

Many of these collateral systems are clinically benign, but the most important and dangerous are gastroesophageal collaterals, so-called varices. Apart from gastroesophageal varices, similar collaterals develop between the inferior mesenteric vein and the hemorrhoidal veins, and the umbilical veins and the cutaneous veins of the abdominal wall. Similarly, blood from the portal system drains in a retrograde fashion via the left renal vein, the gonadal veins and many retroperitoneal veins into the azygos systems and the vena cavae. Collaterals also develop at the sites of previous surgery or inflammation and frequently around an ileostomy or colostomy stoma.

Longstanding portal hypertension is not only the cause of discrete collaterals with resulting dilated and tortuous varices, but also causes mucosal changes due to abnormalities in the microcirculation. Thus portal gastropathy is well recognized with vascular ectasia of the gastric mucosa. Similar changes have been

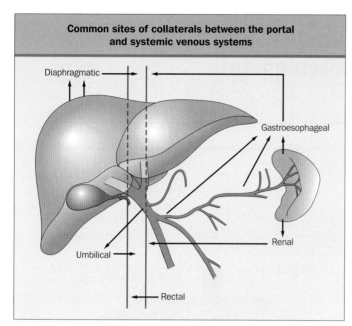

Figure 6.2 **Common sites of collaterals between the portal and systemic venous systems in the presence of portal hypertension.**

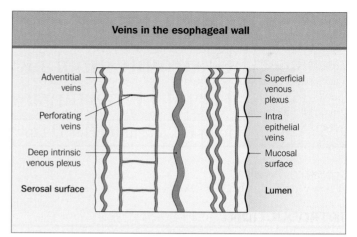

Figure 6.3 **Veins in the esophageal wall.**

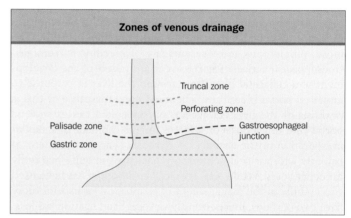

Figure 6.4 **Zones of venous drainage at the gastroesophageal junction.**

described in the small and large intestines of patients with portal hypertension. Such changes contribute to occult gastrointestinal bleeding in these patients.

As indicated, gastroesophageal varices are clinically the most important collaterals to develop. There are two main inflows: from the left gastric (or coronary) vein and from the splenic hilum through the short gastric veins. Interestingly, the finding of isolated varices in the gastric fundus raises the question of a block in the splenic vein with the formation of collaterals only via the short gastric vessels. Esophageal varices are fed principally due to reversed flow in the left gastric vein.

Formation of esophageal varices

Normally there are four layers of veins in the lower esophagus (Fig. 6.3). The veins within the epithelium form 'cherry red spots' under conditions of portal hypertension, which predict hemorrhage. Typical large varices occur when portal hypertension causes dilatation and tortuosity of the deep intrinsic veins in this region where portal and systemic circulations connect. The causes of rupture of esophageal varices resulting in a major hemorrhage are complex. The venous system in the gastroesophageal region has been classified into zones (Fig. 6.4). The palisade zone is believed to be the watershed between the portal and systemic systems. Turbulent flow in the veins of the perforating zone is one explanation of why rupture of varices in this region is frequent.

CAUSES OF PORTAL HYPERTENSION

Hemodynamics of portal hypertension

The pressure gradient within the portal venous system is a product of portal bloodflow and vascular resistance: pressure = flow × resistance. It is important to remember that flow includes that within the portal venous system as a whole, including the collaterals that develop. Likewise, the resistance includes that in the portal vein, the hepatic vascular bed, and the collaterals. The main factor influencing resistance is the radius of the vessels. It is obvious that portal pressure increases if either portal bloodflow or vascular resistance, or both, increase. Attempts to lower portal pressure have therefore been aimed at reducing flow or resistance, or both.

Increased vascular resistance

It has become apparent that the major factor in increased portal pressure is increased resistance. This is mainly as a result of morphologic changes in the liver related to fibrosis, scarring and regenerative nodules. In hepatic fibrosis there is disturbance of the microcirculation of the liver related to the deposition of collagen in the hepatic sinusoids. Pathologic studies have also shown that thrombosis in small vessels contributes to the increased vascular resistance.

Recent evidence suggests there is also a reversible element to increased vascular resistance. For example, hepatic stellate cells under appropriate conditions can take on the morphology of myofibroblasts and possess a contractile function. Endothelin-1 acts as a stimulator of contraction and high blood levels have been found in cirrhotic patients. Nitric oxide and prostacyclin are important vasodilators and disturbances of their metabolism

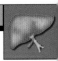

probably have effects on vascular resistance. It has long been observed that patients with alcoholic liver disease who are able to abstain from alcohol can experience a fall in portal hypertension. This change occurs over several weeks, and thus a good candidate for the change would be altered myofibroblast morphology or contractility in response to normalization of metabolic function. In the future it may be possible to exploit these observations in order to develop better pharmacologic treatment for portal hypertension.

Increased bloodflow

There is no doubt that increased portal flow is observed in cases with advanced portal hypertension. This increased flow is a result of arteriolar vasodilatation of the splanchnic organs so that the portal system becomes hyperdynamic. This is part of a systemic effect with a generally hyperdynamic circulation, as evidenced by an increased cardiac index and a reduced systemic blood pressure and arterial resistance.

As regards the portal system, it is still unclear whether the hyperdynamic circulation is a result of the need to increase flow as the resistance increases in the liver and collaterals develop increasing venous space, or whether the increased flow is a primary event. In either case, the increased portal venous flow will contribute towards portal hypertension.

It must be noted that these factors of increased resistance and flow that cause increased portal pressure apply to the total portal system, including collaterals. Thus, despite a hyperdynamic circulation, actual flow through the liver is severely reduced.

CLASSIFICATION OF PORTAL HYPERTENSION

The causes of portal hypertension are usually classified into prehepatic, intrahepatic, and posthepatic. Prehepatic causes are those affecting the venous system before it enters the liver, an obvious cause would be thrombosis of the portal vein. Intrahepatic causes form the main group, with cirrhosis accounting for the vast majority of cases. Posthepatic causes encompass those affecting the hepatic veins and venous drainage to the heart. These are discussed in Chapter 27.

The classification is modified, however, by consideration of the intrahepatic anatomy of the venous connections. The portal vein divides and branches throughout the liver, eventually forming portal venules at the lobular level. These connect to the central veins via the hepatic sinusoids. The pressure in the portal venules is the same as that in the portal system, whereas the pressure in the hepatic veins is the same as that in the systemic venous circulation (vena cavae). There is a normal gradient of approximately 3mmHg across the liver from portal (7mmHg) to hepatic (4mmHg) venous systems. This pressure gradient falls across the sinusoids (Fig. 6.5). The pressures can be measured by a catheter in the inferior vena cava for the systemic venous pressure, and by wedging the catheter into a small hepatic vein such that flow is blocked and measuring the pressure, which reflects that in the portal venule and thus the portal system [the wedged hepatic venous pressure (WHVP)].

In cases of portal hypertension a high WHVP suggests an intrahepatic block at the level of the sinusoids (flow being obstructed between a portal venule and central vein, with a resulting high pressure in the venule), whereas a normal WHVP reflects normal pressure in the portal venule and thus a presinusoidal cause of portal hypertension, such as disease around the portal tracts or outside the liver (see Fig. 6.5). Thus, portal hypertension can be classified as presinusoidal (both prehepatic and intrahepatic), sinusoidal (intrahepatic), and post-sinusoidal (intrahepatic and posthepatic) (Fig. 6.6).

The relevance to clinical practice is that in presinusoidal portal hypertension (both pre- and intrahepatic) the liver function is well preserved and liver failure is infrequent following variceal hemorrhage, as is the precipitation of hepatic encephalopathy. Nevertheless, many hepatic causes of portal hypertension produce pathologic changes that cause a block at both the pre-sinusoidal and sinusoidal levels and often, therefore, the distinction is academic. There are clear therapeutic implications for differentiating hepatic venous outflow obstruction (posthepatic) from other causes of portal hypertension (see Chapter 27).

The causes of portal hypertension are summarized in Figs 6.6 & 6.7.

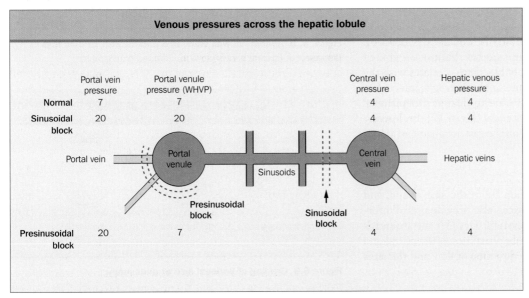

Venous pressures across the hepatic lobule

	Portal vein pressure	Portal venule pressure (WHVP)		Central vein pressure	Hepatic venous pressure
Normal	7	7		4	4
Sinusoidal block	20	20		4	4
Presinusoidal block	20	7		4	4

Figure 6.5 Venous pressures across the hepatic lobule in the normal liver, and in the presence of either a sinusoidal or presinusoidal block. Wedged hepatic venous pressure (WHVP) reflects portal venule pressure by allowing the pressures in the portal venule and central vein to equalize.

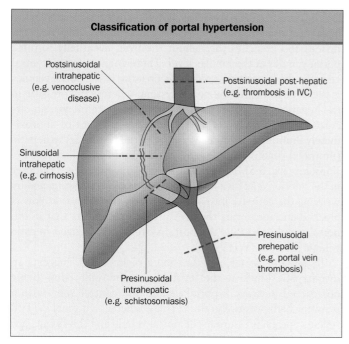

Classification of portal hypertension

Postsinusoidal intrahepatic (e.g. venocclusive disease)

Postsinusoidal post-hepatic (e.g. thrombosis in IVC)

Sinusoidal intrahepatic (e.g. cirrhosis)

Presinusoidal prehepatic (e.g. portal vein thrombosis)

Presinusoidal intrahepatic (e.g. schistosomiasis)

Figure 6.6 Classification of portal hypertension. IVC, inferior vena cava.

Causes of portal hypertension	
Prehepatic	Splenic vein thrombosis Portal vein thrombosis Congenital anomaly of the portal vein Extrinsic compression of the portal vein
Intrahepatic presinusoidal	Schistosomiasis Congenital hepatic fibrosis Early primary biliary cirrhosis Sarcoidosis Idiopathic, noncirrhotic portal hypertension Toxins (e.g. arsenic, copper, vinyl chloride, methotrexate, azathioprine)
sinusoidal	Cirrhosis Acute alcoholic hepatitis Hypervitaminosis A Non-cirrhotic nodule formation
post-sinusoidal	Veno-occlusive disease Alcoholic hyaline sclerosis
Posthepatic	Budd–Chiari syndrome Thrombosis of the IVC Congenital web in the IVC Constrictive pericarditis

Figure 6.7 Causes of portal hypertension. IVC, inferior vena cava.

CLINICAL PRESENTATION OF PORTAL HYPERTENSION

Hematemesis is the most common presenting feature of portal hypertension. However, other features in the patient's history should be sought, including etiologic factors for chronic liver disease and for extrahepatic portal vein block, such as previous abdominal inflammation or a predisposition to thrombosis.

Examination should include a search for other complications of liver disease (e.g. ascites and encephalopathy), as well as signs that indicate liver disease and portal hypertension (see Chapter 4). Abdominal wall veins, splenomegaly, and hepatic size should be assessed (Fig. 6.8).

DIAGNOSIS OF PORTAL HYPERTENSION

Endoscopy

Gastric and esophageal varices are best viewed using endoscopy. This has replaced the use of barium studies. Varices are graded 1–3 (see Fig. 6.9). The probability of bleeding correlates with the size of the varices. Varices look white or bluish in appearance, but the presence of 'cherry red spots' due to dilated subepithelial veins is an indicator of bleeding potential (Fig. 6.10). Endoscopy may also show the mosaic pattern on the gastric mucosa of portal gastropathy (Fig. 6.11).

Ultrasound

Ultrasound can provide information about the size, shape, and any echogenic areas of the liver. It can also provide useful information about the portal venous system. Doppler ultrasound is extremely accurate at diagnosing abnormalities in the portal and hepatic vasculature, including the direction of flow and the sites of blockage (Fig. 6.12).

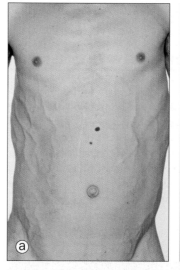
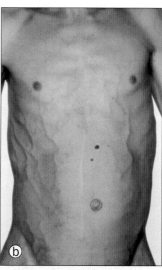

Figure 6. 8 Abdominal wall veins in a patient with chronic liver disease. (a) Routine photograph, (b) infra-red photograph.

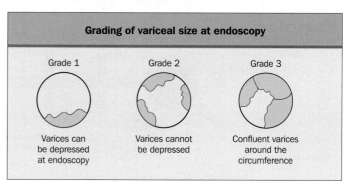

Grading of variceal size at endoscopy

Grade 1 — Varices can be depressed at endoscopy

Grade 2 — Varices cannot be depressed

Grade 3 — Confluent varices around the circumference

Figure 6.9 Grading of variceal size at endoscopy.

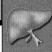

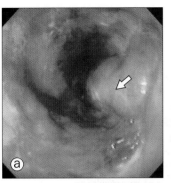
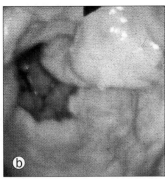

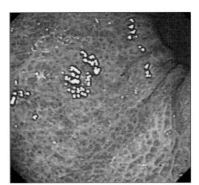

Figure 6.11 Mosaic appearance of portal gastropathy.

Figure 6.10 Endoscopic appearance of esophageal varices. (a) Grade 1 varix (arrow); (b) grade 2 varices. (By kind permission of Dr. K J A Miloszewski.)

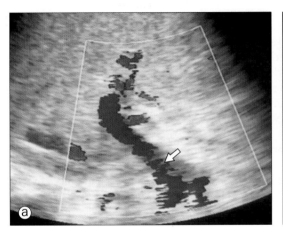
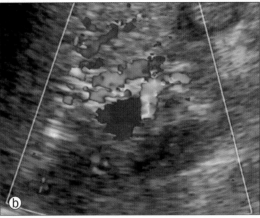

Figure 6.12 Color flow Doppler ultrasounds of a cirrhotic liver.
(a) With reversed flow in the portal vein (arrow). (b) With cavernous transformation at the porta hepatis and variceal flow in all directions. (By kind permission of J. Bates.)

Computed tomography scan and magnetic resonance imaging

Computed tomography scan with contrast establishes portal vein patency and CT arterial portography shows collaterals and arteriovenous shunts. Magnetic resonance imaging gives excellent views of the vasculature and magnetic resonance angiography is more reliable than Doppler ultrasound (Fig. 6.13).

Venography

Venography is the 'gold standard' for demonstrating the portal venous system. Due to the accuracy of the various scanning procedures, however, it is rarely needed. Pure venography via percutaneous splenic puncture is rare. If direct views of the vasculature are needed as a prelude to surgery or transplantation, visceral angiography is usually undertaken. The venous phase of a celiac angiogram gives good pictures of the portal and splenic veins (Fig. 6.14).

The above techniques are used to diagnose the presence of varices and hence portal hypertension. They also provide diagnostic data about the cause of the portal hypertension as regards prehepatic or posthepatic venous problems. A strong indication is also obtained about the state of the liver parenchyma. Other

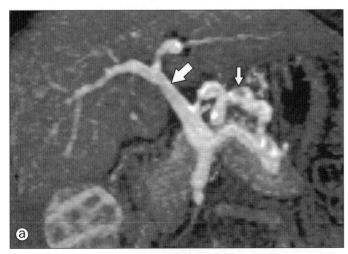
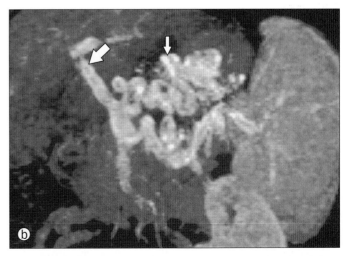

Figure 6.13 Magnetic resonance images of a cirrhotic liver showing an attenuated portal vein within the liver. (large arrow), left gastric varices (small arrow) and splenomegaly [on figure (b)]. (By kind permission of Dr A. Guthrie.)

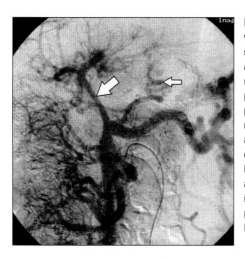

Figure 6.14 The venous phase of a superior mesenteric angiogram. There is recanalization of a previously thrombosed portal vein, which remains narrow (large arrow). Varices have developed from the left gastric vein (small arrow) and the spleen is enlarged. (By kind permission of Dr I. Robertson.)

diagnostic tests will often be necessary, however, including liver biopsy, to diagnose the specific cause of portal hypertension.

MANAGEMENT OF GASTROINTESTINAL HEMORRHAGE

Initial management

Gastrointestinal hemorrhage is not only the commonest presenting feature of portal hypertension, but also the most life-threatening. Although bleeding can be from any of the causes of upper gastrointestinal hemorrhage, esophageal varices are the most likely and most serious. It should go without saying that the initial management of major gastrointestinal hemorrhage is volume resuscitation. This usually requires blood transfusion and clotting factors, and platelets may be necessary. Too often, the initial management is focused on preparing the patient for endoscopy. Endoscopy should only be performed once the patient is adequately resuscitated. However, it is equally important not to 'over-resuscitate' the patient. Portal pressure correlates directly with central venous pressure; over-resuscitation may therefore increase the risk of rebleeding. Thus, monitoring central venous pressure is important in the management of these patients. Once the patient is adequately resuscitated, endoscopy should be performed. The purpose of early endoscopy is two-fold. First, it enables diagnosis; up to 50% of the patients with cirrhosis and gastrointestinal hemorrhage will be bleeding from sites other than gastroesophageal varices. Second, if the patient is bleeding from varices, endoscopic therapy is generally effective as is discussed below.

While these efforts are ongoing, it is also important to anticipate the standard complications that can occur as a result of variceal hemorrhage. These include the development of hepatic encephalopathy, infections such as spontaneous bacterial peritonitis (SBP) and fluid retention (i.e. ascites and pleural effusions). To prevent the development, or lessen the severity of encephalopathy, cathartics such as lactulose should be administered to clean out the blood from the gastrointestinal tract. Encephalopathy may also impair the ability of the patient to protect their airway and intubation before endoscopy may be indicated. Sedation should be avoided if possible, but may be necessary in the presence of alcohol withdrawal symptoms. The risk of infection developing during the course of variceal hemorrhage is substantial enough to recommend prophylaxis with a 3rd generation cephalosporin. Some also give oral antibiotics (e.g. norfloxacillin, ciprofloxacillin or trimethoprim-sulfa) to decrease the risk of bacterial translocation from the

gastrointestinal tract. This type of therapy has been shown to lower the rate of subsequent infections such as SBP. Infusion of large amounts of crystalloid often leads to ascites or pleural effusions. It again emphasizes the need to avoid over-resuscitation and diuretics should be considered early. For patients who develop marked ascites, large volume paracentesis has been shown actually to decrease the risk of variceal hemorrhage.

Acid suppressant drugs are often given to prevent stress-induced ulcers, although their effect on gastrointestinal hemorrhage itself is unproven.

Diagnosis of acute gastrointestinal hemorrhage

As indicated above, diagnostic endoscopy is performed as soon as possible, usually within 6 hours of admission. The diagnosis of bleeding varices is made if there is a venous spurt or ooze, or adherent clot on a varix (Fig. 6.15). If active bleeding is present, it is usually seen just above the gastroesophageal junction. In the absence of these signs, variceal bleeding is surmised to have occurred if there are varices and no other lesions in the stomach or duodenum. Bleeding from gastric varices (10% of cases) is often difficult to diagnose since the stomach may contain much fresh blood which obscures the varices.

Specific therapy for bleeding gastroesophageal varices

Endoscopic therapy is the treatment of choice for the control of acute variceal hemorrhage. However, there is a number of techniques that have been used:
* vaso-active drugs;
* esophageal tamponade;
* endoscopic sclerotherapy;
* endoscopic banding;
* TIPS;
* shunt surgery;
* esophageal transection; and
* liver transplantation.

Some of these are useful in combination with endoscopic therapy or while awaiting further treatment.

Vasoactive drugs

Vasopressin is a powerful vasoconstrictor; it reduces bloodflow to splanchnic organs and therefore portal bloodflow and portal pressure. Despite several clinical trials, its efficacy is still not proven. There is some evidence that it reduces variceal bleeding but not

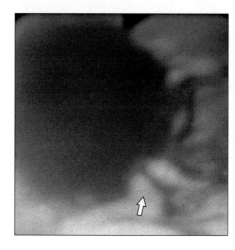

Figure 6.15 Blood oozing from a varix (arrow) at the lower end of the esophagus.

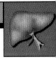

mortality. The main problem is the complication rate, which varies between 32 and 64%. This is due to its vasoconstrictor effect on the systemic circulation, leading to myocardial ischemia, arrhythmias, mesenteric ischemia, limb ischemia, heart failure and cerebrovascular accidents.

Nitroglycerine is principally a venous dilator and has been used in combination with vasopressin. It reduces the transfusion requirements and side effects compared with vasopressin alone, but mortality is unchanged.

Glypressin is a synthetic analog of vasopressin with a longer period of action. It is more effective than vasopressin and has less side effects.

Somatostatin causes splanchnic vasoconstriction and thus reduces portal flow and pressure. It does not have the systemic effects of vasopressin. It has been shown to be effective in clinical trials and is virtually free of side effects. Its role may be particularly useful once acute bleeding has been controlled by tamponade or endoscopic therapy.

Octreotide is a synthetic peptide of somatostatin with a longer half-life. It is as safe and effective as somatostatin in controlling acute variceal hemorrhage.

Esophageal tamponade

Balloon tamponade is aimed at obtaining temporary hemostasis by direct compression of varices. Its use has declined dramatically with the introduction of vasoactive drugs and endoscopic therapy. It is now only used to gain temporary control of bleeding when other measures have not been successful and while awaiting more definitive treatment such as TIPS. Balloon tamponade should not be used unless experienced medical and nursing staff are available.

The Sengstaken–Blakemore tube has two balloons, one which compresses the esophageal varices and the other which fixes the tube in the stomach and produces some compression at the cardia (Fig. 6.16). The Linton–Nachlas tube has one balloon in the stomach, which when distended compresses gastric varices and prevents bloodflow into the esophageal venous plexuses at the cardia.

In experienced hands balloon tamponade can be very effective in controlling variceal hemorrhage, with control rates of 40–90%. However, this control is only temporary and 50% of cases rebleed within 24 hours of balloon deflation. The main complications are aspiration and airway obstruction. Hence the need for experienced clinical care.

Endoscopic therapy: sclerotherapy and banding

Endoscopic therapy is the 'gold standard' for the treatment of acute variceal hemorrhage. There are currently two forms of endoscopic therapy that are used in this setting: sclerotherapy and band ligation. Sclerotherapy is now the time-honored therapy and is still probably most commonly used in this setting (Fig. 6.17). This will control bleeding in 80–90% of cases. Whether the injection of a sclerosing material is directly into or alongside a varix probably makes little difference. The most common complications include the development of esophageal ulcers and strictures, which occur in up to 18% of cases (Fig. 6.18). The most serious complication is esophageal perforation (0.5% procedures) (Fig. 6.19). Other complications include fever, chest pain and mediastinitis and the development of pleural effusions in up to 50% of cases.

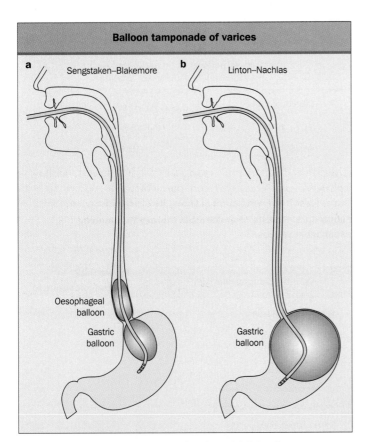

Balloon tamponade of varices

a Sengstaken–Blakemore

b Linton–Nachlas

Oesophageal balloon

Gastric balloon

Gastric balloon

Figure 6.16 Balloon tamponade of varices. (a) Using the Sengstaken–Blakemore tube; (b) using the Linton–Nachlas tube.

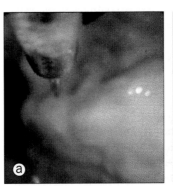
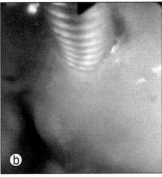

Figure 6.17 Injection sclerotherapy of an esophageal varix. (a) Needle entering varix; (b) swelling due to injection of sclerosant.

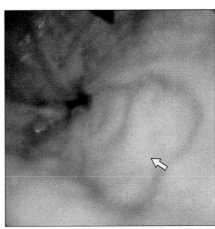

Figure 6.18 Healed sclerotherapy ulcer (arrow).

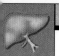

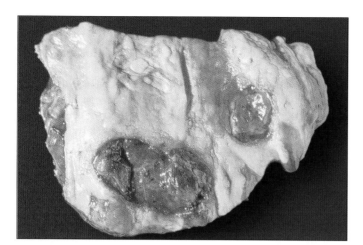

Figure 6.19 Surgical specimen from a patient with perforated sclerotherapy ulcers. (By kind permission of Dr. K J A Miloszewski.)

Clinical trials show that sclerotherapy is superior to tamponade or vasopressin and nitroglycerin, and comparable to somatostatin for the control of acute bleeding. In experienced hands it is the first-choice treatment.

Band ligation represents a relatively new approach to the management of variceal bleeding. It is similar to hemorrhoidal ligation in that the varix is 'sucked' up into the ligator and a rubber band is then placed around the varix (Fig. 6.20). It has been used for both the acute and chronic control of variceal bleeding. Studies have compared these two modalities for the control and prevention of variceal bleeding. As shown in Fig. 6.21, these two therapies are comparable in their ability to control variceal bleeding. The complication rate with banding, however, is less than that with sclerotherapy.

Multiple band delivery devices are now in common use and, as gastroenterologists become more experienced with their use, band ligation will probably supplant sclerotherapy in the management of variceal bleeding.

Transjugular intrahepatic portosystemic shunts (TIPS)

Portosystemic shunting has been a mainstay for the treatment of refractory variceal hemorrhage where other methods have failed. Hitherto, these shunts were created surgically. The first intrahepatic portosystemic shunt in a human was created by Colapinto and colleagues in 1982. The technique failed due to almost universal

occlusion related to the elasticity of the liver tissue. Transjugular intrahepatic portosystemic shunts emerged as a viable technique when Palmaz first deployed an expandable metal stent in a human in 1989. While some groups still use the Palmaz-type stent, many currently use a slightly modified technique involving a similar stent called the 'Wallstent'.

In the acute situation, TIPS is considered when endoscopic therapy and vasoactive drugs have failed to control the bleeding. Balloon tamponade may be an interim measure. The full evaluation of patients before TIPS includes a Doppler ultrasound to assess patency of the portal veins, endoscopy to confirm gastroesophageal varices as a source of hemorrhage, and a routine physical examination to exclude other active medical problems. Coagulopathy or thrombocytopenia are corrected if indicated. There are several contraindications to the procedure, listed in Fig. 6.22.

The TIPS procedure itself is performed in a fluoroscopy suite with the patient under conscious sedation. A puncture is made into the right internal jugular vein and an angiographic catheter is advanced into a large hepatic vein (usually the right or middle hepatic vein). A Colapinto needle is then advanced into the hepatic parenchyma. The needle is placed under suction and, when blood is aspirated, a contrast injection is performed to confirm the presence of the needle in the portal vein (generally, the right portal vein). After position has been secured in the portal vein, a balloon catheter replaces the Colapinto needle and the parenchymal tract is created and dilated. Finally, the Wallstent, which comes collapsed onto a 7-Fr delivery catheter, is advanced across the tract and is deployed by pulling back the 'rolling' membrane. Repeat angiographic images are obtained (Fig. 6.23). If a further decrease in portal pressure is needed, the diameter of the Wallstent can be increased using angiographic balloons.

Efficacy of band ligation compared with sclerotherapy in 4 different studies	
Efficacy of ligation	Efficacy of sclerotherapy
12/14 (86%)	10/13 (77%)
8/9 (89%)	8/9 (89%)
17/18 (94%)	12/15 (80%)
12/12 (100%)	8/10 (80%)

Figure 6.21 Results of endoscopic therapy for bleeding esophageal varices.

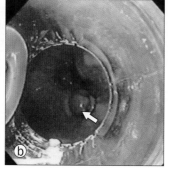

Figure 6.20 Banding of esophageal varix. (a) varix aspirated into banding device (arrow); (b) varix with band in place (arrow). (By kind permission of Dr. C Millsom.)

Contraindications to TIPS
Polycystic liver disease
Hepatic neoplasm
Hepatic abscess
Bacterial cholangitis
Occluded portal vein
Anomalous vena caval anatomy
Severe coagulopathy
Severe hepatic encephalopathy

Figure 6.22 Contraindications to TIPS.

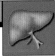

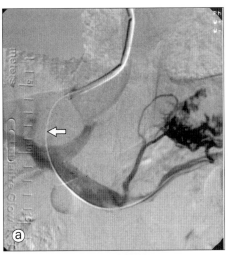

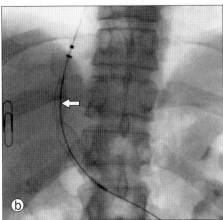

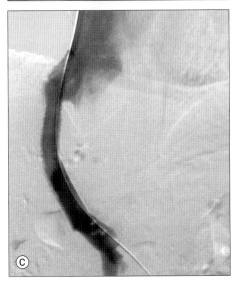

Figure 6.23 The TIPS procedure. (a) A catheter is in place from hepatic vein, through hepatic parenchyma (arrow) into portal vein (outlined with contrast); (b) unexpanded stent in place (arrow) between hepatic vein and portal vein; (c) expanded stent filled with contrast showing shunt between portal vein and hepatic vein.

The indications for TIPS, both for the management of acute variceal hemorrhage and for other complications of portal hypertension, are shown in Fig. 6.24.

As indicated, TIPS has been used most frequently for the treatment of bleeding esophageal and gastric varices, which are deemed refractory to endoscopic therapy. With the exception of several small randomized trials, all reported results to date have been uncontrolled. The initial experience reported from a variety of centers has clearly demonstrated TIPS to be an effective technique in reducing portal hypertension and controlling variceal hemorrhage (Fig. 6.25). Of the first 250 patients undergoing TIPS at University of California at San Francisco (UCSF), shunts were successfully placed in 97% of these patients. All eight cases in whom a shunt could not be successfully placed had portal vein thrombosis. In the 75 patients for whom the indication was acute variceal hemorrhage, TIPS led to cessation of hemorrhage in 70. Recurrence of variceal bleeding following TIPS was seen in 10% of patients. All had either shunt stenosis or occlusion. Almost all of these patients with recurrent bleeding were treated successfully with dilatation and re-stenting of the TIPS, or placement of a second shunt.

Transjugular intrahepatic portosystemic shunting appears to be especially useful in liver transplant candidates, in whom one would want to avoid surgery in the right upper quadrant. The stent is completely contained within the liver and, as such, is removed at the time of hepatectomy. In addition to controlling variceal hemorrhage, TIPS has other positive byproducts. For example, it usually improves ascites control and possibly nutritional status in patients awaiting transplant. It has been the prevailing opinion of many transplant surgeons that the presence of a TIPS decreases intraoperative bleeding and possibly the duration of surgery. However, a recent study from the NIDDK Liver Transplantation Database was unable to confirm that TIPS leads to such benefits.

Indications to TIPS
Control* and prevention of portal hypertensive bleeding
Control of refractory ascites
Management of hepatorenal syndrome
Treatment of refractory hepatic hydrothorax
Management of Budd–Chiari syndrome
Portal decompression before liver transplantation

Figure 6.24 Indications for TIPS. (* As indicated in the acute situation for refractory variceal hemorrhage.)

Which clinical end-point should be used to determine when the shunt diameter is sufficient to control and prevent future variceal hemorrhage is unclear. Some investigators have used a net portal pressure (i.e. portal pressure minus central venous pressure) of <13mmHg as the end-point. Others have used the absence of angiographic evidence of variceal flow. On occasion, one fails to see an adequate drop in portal pressure in spite of maximal deployment of the stent. In this situation, some investigators have advocated the use of 'parallel' shunts. This, however, may increase the risk of post-TIPS encephalopathy.

Results of TIPS for acute variceal haemorrhage			
Number of patients	Immediate success (%)	Short-term success (%)	Complications (%)
100	96	94	9
59	93	81	14
45	100	93	0
100	93	93	15

Figure 6.25 Results of TIPS for acute variceal hemorrhage in four reported series.

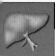

While the results at many centers are encouraging, the true role of TIPS in the chronic control of variceal hemorrhage remains to be defined by randomized, controlled trials. It must be remembered that TIPS is technically demanding of the interventional radiologist and may be associated with a variety of complications. It should only be undertaken at centers with special expertise.

Complications of transjugular intrahepatic portosystemic shunting

A variety of complications, directly related to the TIPS procedure, may be seen. These may be minor, such as a hematoma at the site of the right internal jugular puncture, or major in nature, such as intra-abdominal hemorrhage due to puncture of the liver capsule or hemobilia, each of which was seen once in the first 100 patients treated at UCSF.

The most notable complication of TIPS is hepatic encephalopathy. At UCSF, 24% of patients who did not have coexisting multiorgan system failure experienced new or worsened hepatic encephalopathy after TIPS. This was most commonly seen during the first month after TIPS and was controlled with lactulose therapy in the majority of cases. Factors associated with an increased risk of developing post-TIPS encephalopathy included age, an etiology of liver disease other than alcohol, female gender, and hypoalbuminemia. Of note, only 10% of those patients with a prior history of encephalopathy and who were continued on lactulose experienced worsening of encephalopathy. Hepatic encephalopathy was not confined to Child's class C patients. Other groups have similarly demonstrated an incidence of encephalopathy in the range of 10–25%. This is similar to the incidence of hepatic encephalopathy seen following small diameter H-graft portacaval shunts or distal splenorenal shunts.

As mentioned above, the most common cause of recurrent gastrointestinal bleeding following TIPS is shunt dysfunction. The lumen of the stent can become narrowed by either thrombosis or neointimal hyperplasia. This progresses to stent occlusion in approximately 10–15% patients, although some series have shown rates of occlusion up to 40%. This complication occurs at any time from day 1 to many months after the placement of the stent. Early (<14 days after the procedure) occlusions are generally the result of shunt thrombosis, while later occlusions are the result of neointimal hyperplasia. Most often, occlusion presents with recurrent variceal bleeding or worsening ascites. However, some cases may be identified by screening ultrasound examinations in the absence of symptoms. In almost all cases, the TIPS can be revised radiologically.

Thromboses may have other secondary effects. Clots may extend into the portal vein and produce portal vein thrombosis. In addition, clots may move to the lung. However, the occurrence of clinically significant pulmonary embolism during and after TIPS is surprisingly uncommon.

Acute increases in central venous pressure, pulmonary wedge pressure, and cardiac output were recognized sequelae of surgical shunting and occur following TIPS as well. The mechanism of these hemodynamic changes is unclear. Redistribution of blood volume from the portal to the systemic venous systems, reduction in the rate of ascites formation, shunting of vasoactive substances, and iatrogenic volume expansion may all contribute. Increased central vascular volume following TIPS has been associated with acute pulmonary edema and cardiac dysfunction. Patients with pulmonary hypertension or baseline cardiac dysfunction may be at particular risk of developing significant hemodynamic problems following TIPS.

It is not unusual for patients undergoing TIPS to receive between 300–400mL of radiographic contrast. Transient rises in serum creatinine are commonly observed following TIPS. However, the incidence of clinically significant contrast-induced acute renal failure is quite low (2–3%). Patients with functional renal dysfunction and chronic renal disease are at particular risk.

Increases in serum bilirubin concentration, transaminase activity, prothrombin time, and blood ammonia concentration occur in 10–20% of patients after TIPS. The pathogenesis of these early, transient abnormalities is unclear, but may include parenchymal trauma, transient hepatic decompensation, low-grade disseminated intravascular coagulation, and hemolysis. Fever of 38°C or greater within 24 hours after TIPS has been reported in up to 10% of patients. In most cases, blood cultures are negative.

Conclusions regarding transjugular intrahepatic portosystemic shunting

The TIPS clearly has had a major impact on the treatment of complications of portal hypertension in the cirrhotic patient. While the shunt is placed under local anesthesia in a nonoperative fashion, it must be remembered that it does function as a highly effective side-to-side shunt with the attendant complications including hepatic encephalopathy as well as acute liver failure.

Early reports of clinical and hemodynamic results after TIPS have clearly demonstrated it to be an effective bridge to liver transplantation. Nonetheless, transplant candidates who experience their initial episode of variceal hemorrhage should be managed with sclerotherapy or variceal banding. However, if bleeding recurs during a course of treatment or cannot be controlled, TIPS has proved invaluable in stabilizing patients before liver transplantation. Refractory variceal bleeding in Child's class C patients, in whom the perioperative mortality associated with surgical shunts is high, also seems to be a reasonable indication for TIPS.

In spite of increasing use of TIPS, it will be important to continue studying its indications and its complications so that it can be optimally utilized in the treatment of patients with portal hypertension and gastrointestinal hemorrhage.

Emergency surgery: shunt surgery and esophageal transection

Emergency surgery to control acute variceal hemorrhage is now only used as a last resort. Patients with uncontrolled variceal hemorrhage should be managed in centers with special expertise where all other modalities of treatment are available. Emergency surgery is indicated where hemorrhage is uncontrolled or recurrent and massive. It causes least risk in patients with Child's classes A and B. Once decided upon, it should not be delayed. Portacaval shunt surgery or staple transection of the esophagus are highly effective emergency means to stop bleeding.

Surgery has a high mortality in high risk patients and following shunts there is up to a 40% occurrence of encephalopathy, which becomes chronic. Because of this latter problem, small diameter interposition graft shunts have been developed. In this technique a vein graft or an artificial material is used to join the portal vein to the inferior vena cava. The perceived advantage of this H-graft shunt is that one can control the diameter of the shunt and thus minimize the diversion of portal bloodflow. This minimizes the incidence of post-shunt encephalopathy and ascites. The H-graft can also be used to join the mesenteric vein to the inferior vena cava leading to similar degrees of portal decompression.

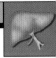

Rightly or wrongly, TIPS has largely replaced surgical shunts in the management of refractory variceal bleeding. Nonetheless, it is important to realize that surgical shunts have been highly effective at controlling variceal bleeding. The major concerns regarding surgical shunts, and where TIPS is perceived to have an advantage, include the requirement for a general anesthetic, and the presence of an incision with the attendant problem of post-operative ascitic leaks from the wound and the worsening of ascites. However it is important to remember that they have a track record of excellent long-term patency. In low-risk patients, it remains unknown as to whether TIPS or surgical shunts will represent the optimal therapy for refractory variceal bleeding.

Liver transplantation

This should always be considered in patients with chronic liver disease. In poor risk patients long-term survival may well be better after transplantation than after shunt surgery for the management of refractory variceal hemorrhage. There are no clinical trials on this point. Care should always be taken with TIPS or surgery in order not to make subsequent transplantation more difficult.

Treatment of acute bleeding for gastric varices

Bleeding from gastric varices can be more difficult to control than that from esophageal varices. In the presence of isolated fundal varices one should always consider the possibility of splenic vein thrombosis.

Gastric varices (usually in the fundus of the stomach) are often large and under relatively low pressure (Fig. 6.26). Control of bleeding may require balloon tamponade with a Linton–Nachlas tube. There are very few clinical trials of sclerotherapy in this situation, but some endoscopists have had remarkable success with bucrylate, cyanoacrylate, or thrombin injections. Recent results with banding are promising and this may be better than sclerotherapy. A large diameter TIPS may be necessary or definitive shunt surgery.

Prevention of rebleeding from varices

Patients with chronic liver disease who survive their first variceal hemorrhage have up to a 70% risk of rebleeding. Of those that do rebleed, there is a 20–35% mortality. Thus, effective preventive treatment is mandatory in patients surviving an episode of acute variceal hemorrhage. Treatment options include endoscopic therapy, pharmacologic therapy, and surgery.

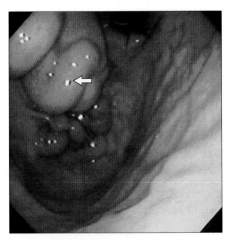

Figure 6.26 Gastric fundal varix (arrow).

Endoscopic therapy

There is good evidence that endoscopic sclerotherapy continued on a weekly basis in order to eradicate varices significantly reduces rebleeding and overall mortality. In fact, rebleeding is uncommon after achieving eradication. Complications do occur, particularly ulceration and stricture. Regular review is necessary since although in one-third the varices never recur, new varices do occur and 30% of patients rebleed.

Band ligation has also been used for the prevention of rebleeding and has been shown to be better with fewer side effects than sclerotherapy. Eradication of the varices can also be achieved in fewer endoscopy sessions. However, it now appears that more varices recur following banding than sclerotherapy. Hence banded patients require more frequent follow-up.

Pharmacologic therapy

Portal pressure can be reduced in patients with cirrhosis by the use of nonselective β blockers such as propanolol, nadolol, and timolol. This is because the β blockers cause splanchnic vasoconstriction and thus reduce the portal–collateral bloodflow. They also reduce heart rate and cardiac output, which has an effect on portal bloodflow. Although the individual patient response to β blockers varies, the dose is usually increased to produce a 25% decrease in heart rate. Clinical trials show that with this treatment there is a highly significant reduction in rebleeding from varices and also an improvement in mortality.

Comparative studies show that endoscopic sclerotherapy is slightly more effective than β blockers in preventing recurrent variceal hemorrhage. However, recent studies using a combination of a β blocker and a nitrate suggest this may be as good as sclerotherapy. Such a combination requires comparison with band ligation.

There is some evidence to support endoscopic therapy and β blockade combined; it would be logical to continue β blockers long term in such patients in an attempt to reduce the rebleeding rate as low as possible.

Elective surgery

In the acute situation surgery is effective in controlling bleeding and portal hypertension but the patients are often at high risk and complications are frequent.

Following elective shunt surgery for the prevention of rebleeding, there is a significant reduction in the rebleeding rate. Survival, however, is not significantly prolonged. Encephalopathy is more common following shunt surgery. Such results are representative of many operations over many years in different centers, and refer principally to portacaval shunts. Distal shunts have been shown to be as effective in preventing rebleeding, with slightly less encephalopathy and mortality, but require very experienced surgeons.

Transjugular intrahepatic portosystemic shunting

As referred to above, TIPS is effective at controlling acute bleeding and preliminary clinical trials suggest that it is effective in preventing rebleeding. However, the place of TIPS in long-term management has still to be clearly defined.

Prevention of the first variceal bleeding episode

Although the vast majority of patients with chronic liver disease and portal hypertension develop gastroesophageal varices, not

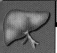
all suffer from variceal hemorrhage. Observations over many years suggest that approximately one-third will bleed, but that the mortality associated with that first bleed is 50%. Although these observations are made in the main on selected groups of patients at specialist centers, nevertheless there is a high morbidity and mortality from gastrointestinal variceal hemorrhage secondary to portal hypertension. It would seem logical to try to prevent the first bleed in such patients.

Prophylactic shunt surgery has been tried and does prevent variceal bleeding, but the complications and mortality rates mitigate against such prophylaxis.

Similarly, prophylactic endoscopic sclerotherapy is controversial and cannot be recommended. However, as techniques develop and are combined with pharmacologic therapy, the management of these patients may change.

A consensus view of several trials of β blockers in this situation is that such treatment is safe and beneficial in patients with chronic liver disease who have varices and who have not bled. This treatment is currently recommended for patients with moderate or large varices, since most studies were conducted in such patients.

CONCLUSION

Gastrointestinal hemorrhage in the presence of portal hypertension is a major medical emergency. Portal hypertension results from restriction of flow from the portal venous system into the system venous system via the liver. The commonest cause is chronic liver disease. A number of collateral circulations develop, the most important clinically being the development of gastroesophageal varices.

The treatment of bleeding esophageal varices has progressed in recent years, with endoscopic therapy and pharmacologic agents being the principal means of management in the acute situation. Transjugular intrahepatic portosystemic shunting is finding its place in the management of refractory or recurrent hemorrhage and is replacing some of the shunt surgery of the past.

A number of caveats should be noted.
- Several treatments have not undergone rigorous clinical trials.
- Trials should be interpreted carefully, since patients with liver disease vary widely and comparable groups are difficult to obtain.
- It is usually possible to stop acute variceal hemorrhage by one means or another, and deaths from bleeding should not occur.
- Shunting procedures (including TIPS) are often complicated by encephalopathy.
- Although there are effective treatments to stop bleeding, these do not prolong survival.
- Hepatic transplantation is often the best treatment and this should be considered in the patient with chronic liver disease sooner rather than later.

PRACTICE POINT

Illustrative case

A 63-year-old male was admitted with hematemesis. On arrival his clinical condition was stable, but while in the emergency room he had a further hematemesis of approximately 1 liter fresh blood. He became tachycardic and hypotensive. He was resuscitated with intravenous colloid and that same evening endoscopy was performed. This revealed esophageal varices with fresh blood oozing rapidly. The stomach was full of fresh blood and it was not possible to visualize the whole of the mucosa. The duodenal mucosa looked normal. Endoscopic sclerotherapy was performed with injections into three varices. The bleeding was controlled.

From his past history it emerged that 3 years previously he had had a hepatic abscess following an episode of diverticulitis with perforation. This had been treated medically at that time with a satisfactory outcome. The hepatic abscess had resolved on scanning. A biopsy had shown normal hepatic architecture. Following the upper gastrointestinal hemorrhage, an ultrasound showed thrombosis of the portal vein at the porta hepatis. There was mild splenic enlargement and splenic, as well as gastroesophageal varices.

A further endoscopy was performed 1 week later with banding of the esophageal varices. Two further weekly sessions of banding were performed, but before the next session he was readmitted with a further hematemesis from bleeding varices.

This was controlled with sclerotherapy and octreotide infusion for 24 hours. He continued with weekly banding and only after two further sessions did the varices begin to regress.

Magnetic resonance imaging confirmed the portal vein thrombosis at the porta hepatis with the formation of collaterals, allowing some portal venous blood to bypass the thrombosed vein. The varices at the gastroesophageal junction and around the spleen were confirmed. A repeat liver biopsy confirmed normal histologic appearances.

Interpretation

This patient had portal hypertension as a consequence of portal vein thrombosis. It was assumed that this had occurred as a result of the previous intra-abdominal sepsis. It was important to document normal hepatic histology. This accounted for the fact that he never developed encephalopathy following any of the episodes of variceal hemorrhage.

The initial difficulty in producing satisfactory resolution of the varices led to consideration of a TIPS or shunt surgery in order to relieve the portal hypertension; TIPS would have been technically possible in this case, since the portal vein thrombosis was at the porta hepatis. However, resolution of the varices with banding, and the good prognosis as a consequence of the normal hepatic function, led to the conclusion that no further intervention would be necessary.

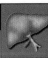

FURTHER READING

Bornmann PC, Krige JE, Terblanche J. Management of oesophageal varices. Lancet. 1994;343:1079–84. *A useful and comprehensive summary of the range of management options for the control of variceal bleeding.*

Bradley SE, Ingelfinger FJ, Bradley GP, Curry JJ. The estimation of hepatic blood flow in man. J Clin Invest. 1945;24:890–97. *An important historic paper demonstrating that it is possible to measure reliably hepatic bloodflow in humans.*

Burroughs AK, Jenkins WJ, Sherlock S, et al. Controlled trial of propranolol for the prevention of recurrent variceal haemorrhage in patients with cirrhosis. N Engl J Med. 1983;309:1539–42. *A controlled trial showing that propranolol was not efficacious in preventing rebleeding from esophageal varices. This contrasts with the results of the trial of Lebrec et al. and points up the difficulties of clinical trials in liver disease because of the great variability between patients.*

Burroughs AK, McCormick A, Hughes MD, Sprengers D, D'Heygere F, McIntyre N. Randomised, double-blind, placebo-controlled trial of somatostatin for variceal bleeding. Gastroenterology. 1990; 99:1388–95. *Somatostatin was shown to be safe and more effective than placebo in controlling variceal bleeding. There was a 41% reduction in the hazard of failure.*

Conn HO. Transjugular intrahepatic portal-systemic shunts: the state of the art. Hepatology. 1993;17:148–58. *A comprehensive review article, now of historical importance, about the development and use of TIPS. In 1993 Conn felt that TIPS was a major breakthrough that would find its role after careful clinical assessment.*

D'Amico G, Pagliaro L, Bosch J. The treatment of portal hypertension: a meta-analytic review. Hepatology. 1995;22:332–54. *An important review article that summarizes the treatment options and makes useful recommendations about the management of variceal hemorrhage.*

Gimson AES, Ramage JK, Panos MZ, et al. Randomised trial of variceal banding ligation versus injection sclerotherapy for bleeding oesophageal varices. Lancet. 1993;342:391–4. *An important trial soon after banding was introduced routinely. This showed that banding ligation was safe and effective and obliterated varices with a lower rebleeding rate than injection sclerotherapy.*

Gimson AES, Westaby D, Hegarty J, Watson A, Williams R. A randomized trial of vasopressin and vasopressin plus nitroglycerin in the control of acute variceal hemorrhage. Hepatology. 1986;6:410–413. *An important study showing that the addition of nitroglycerin to a vasopressin infusion resulted in a lower rate of complications and was more effective in controlling variceal hemorrhage.*

Graham DY, Smith LJ. The course of patients after variceal hemorrhage. Gastroenterology. 1981;80:800–809. *An analysis of the prognosis of patients with chronic liver disease and variceal hemorrhage. The mortality was high and at that time had not significantly changed over four decades.*

La Berge JM, Ring EJ, Gordon RL, et al. Creation of transjugular intrahepatic portosystemic shunts with the Wallstent endoprosthesis: results in 100 patients. Radiology. 1993;187:413–20. *An early report of the clinical use of TIPS. It was an effective and reliable means of lowering portal pressure and controlling variceal bleeding.*

Laire L, Cook D. Endoscopic ligation compared with sclerotherapy for treatment of esophageal variceal bleeding. Ann Intern Med. 1995;123:280–87. *An important meta-analysis of the results of ligation banding versus injection sclerotherapy for the management of esophageal hemorrhage. Seven randomized trials were selected for review. Ligation banding was considered the treatment of choice due to its lower rebleeding rate, lower mortality, fewer complications, and more rapid resolution of varices.*

Lebrec D, Poynard T, Hillon P, Benhamou JP. Propranolol for prevention of recurrent gastrointestinal bleeding in patients with cirrhosis. N Engl J Med. 1981;305:1371–4. *The first controlled study of β blockers, which showed propranolol was effective in preventing recurrent gastrointestinal bleeding in patients with cirrhosis.*

Palmaz JC, Sibbitt RR, Reuter SR, Garcia F, Tio FO. Expandable intrahepatic portacaval shunt stents: early experience in the dog. Am J Roentgenol. 1985;145: 821–5. *The original description of the use of an expandable stent in dogs to keep a shunt patent. Eight out of 12 shunts remained functioning for as long as 9 months after placement.*

Rossle M, Haag K, Ochs A, Sellinger M, et al. The transjugular intrahepatic portosystemic stent-shunt procedure for variceal bleeding. N Engl J Med. 1994;330:165–71. *An early report of 100 patients who underwent TIPS. In this specialized unit the results showed that the procedure was safe and effective treatment for variceal hemorrhage in patients with portal hypertension due to cirrhosis.*

Shiffman ML, Jeffers L, Hoofnagle JH, Tralka TS. The role of transjugular intrahepatic portosystemic shunt for treatment of portal hypertension and its complications: a conference sponsored by the National Digestive Diseases Advisory Board. Hepatology. 1995;22:1591–7. *A useful summary of the use of TIPS in 1995. The role needed to be defined more clearly, which is still the case.*

Vianna A, Hayes PC, Moscoso G, et al. Normal venous circulation of the gastro-oesophageal junction. Gastroenterology. 1987;93:876–9. *An important study outlining the normal venous drainage of the lower esophagus using radiologic and histologic techniques.*

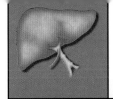

Section 2 Clinical Manifestations of Liver Disease

Chapter 7

Ascites and Spontaneous Bacterial Peritonitis

Vicente Arroyo, Ramón Bataller and Pere Ginès

INTRODUCTION

The natural course of patients who have cirrhosis is frequently complicated by ascites, which consists of the excessive accumulation of fluid in the peritoneal cavity. Ascites is one of the earliest and most common complications in patients who have cirrhosis and is associated with a poor prognosis. A typical circulatory dysfunction characterized by arterial vasodilatation, high cardiac output, and stimulation of vasoactive systems (renin–angiotensin–aldosterone system, sympathetic nervous system, and antidiuretic hormone) is commonly present in these patients. The development of ascites is closely related to renal disturbances of functional origin (sodium retention, impaired capacity to excrete free water and renal vasoconstriction). Patients who have advanced cirrhosis and ascites are liable to develop a form of renal failure called hepatorenal syndrome (HRS), which is the condition with the worst prognosis in cirrhosis. Finally, the development of ascites is associated with a high risk of bacterial infections, the most typical being spontaneous bacterial peritonitis (SBP). In the current chapter the pathophysiology, clinical features, and management of these conditions will be discussed.

ASCITES

Pathogenesis

The formation of ascites in cirrhosis is a consequence of a combination of abnormalities in renal function that cause sodium and water retention, with the subsequent expansion of extracellular fluid volume. This causes circulatory changes in the portal and splanchnic vascular beds and leads to the accumulation of fluid in the peritoneal cavity by increasing lymph formation. Sodium retention is the earliest and most common renal abnormality observed in patients who have cirrhosis. The pathogenesis of sodium retention and ascites formation in cirrhosis is currently explained by the arterial vasodilatation theory. According to this hypothesis, sodium retention is the consequence of a homeostatic response triggered by an underfilling of the arterial circulation, secondary to arterial vasodilatation in the splanchnic vascular bed.

The systemic circulation is also frequently disturbed in cirrhotic patients who have ascites. Plasma volume and cardiac output are increased while arterial pressure and systemic vascular resistance are reduced, leading to a hyperdynamic circulatory syndrome. Finally, many if not all vasoconstrictor and antinatriuretic systems may be activated in patients who have cirrhosis and ascites. Values of parameters used to estimate the activity of these systems, such as plasma renin activity (PRA) and plasma norepinephrine (noradrenaline), antidiuretic hormone and endothelin concentrations, are, in cirrhotic patients, among the highest reported in several pathologic conditions.

Functional renal abnormalities

Sodium retention is the most frequent abnormality of renal function in patients who have cirrhosis and ascites, and plays a key role in the pathophysiology of ascites and edema formation. As in other sodium-retaining disorders, the sodium retained by cirrhotic patients depends on the balance between sodium intake and the sodium excreted in the urine. As long as the amount of sodium excreted is lower than that ingested, patients accumulate ascites and/or show edema. This sodium retention has an important role in ascites formation, as indicated by the fact that ascites diminishes and can even disappear just by reducing the dietary sodium content or by increasing urinary sodium excretion with the administration of diuretics. Conversely, a high sodium diet or diuretic withdrawal may lead to the reaccumulation of ascites. Chronologically, sodium retention is the earliest alteration of kidney function observed in patients who have cirrhosis and usually precedes ascites formation, further emphasizing the important role of this abnormality of renal function in the pathogenesis of ascites in cirrhosis. The severity of sodium retention varies considerably from patient to patient. Some patients have relatively high urinary sodium excretion, whereas in other patients urinary sodium is very low. The response to diuretics is usually better in the former than in the latter patients.

In most instances, sodium retention in cirrhosis is due to increased tubular reabsorption of sodium, because it occurs in the presence of a normal or only slightly reduced glomerular filtration rate (GFR). In patients who have renal failure sodium retention is usually more marked than in patients without renal failure due to a reduction in filtered sodium load and a possibly greater increase in tubular sodium reabsorption. Patients who have cirrhosis in the preascitic stage (without past history of ascites or edema) do not exhibit overt sodium retention, but may have subtle abnormalities in renal sodium handling. In particular, they may be unable to handle an increased sodium load. In this stage of the disease, sodium retention and the resulting expansion in blood volume may represent a homeostatic circulatory mechanism to compensate for the increased capacity of the arterial circulation, especially in the splanchnic area.

Impairment in renal water excretion occurs frequently in cirrhotic patients who have ascites. The clinical consequences of this abnormality are an increased total body water and, in severe cases, dilutional hyponatremia. In healthy subjects, total body water is

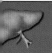
maintained within narrow limits despite daily variations in water intake in such a way that any increase in water intake is rapidly followed by an increase in water excretion, thus preventing the dilution of body fluids and hyponatremia. Conversely, a decrease in water intake is associated with a decrease in water excretion to prevent dehydration and hypernatremia. Cirrhotic patients without ascites (and without sodium retention) usually have renal water handling similar to healthy subjects and normal total body water, plasma osmolality, and serum sodium concentration, and do not develop hyponatremia, even in conditions of excessive water intake. By contrast, an impairment in the renal capacity to excrete water is very common in patients who have ascites.

Up to 75% of hospitalized cirrhotic patients who have ascites have impaired renal water handling. The intensity of this disorder varies markedly from patient to patient. Thus, in some patients, water retention is moderate and can only be detected by measuring water excretion after a water load. These patients are usually able to eliminate water normally and maintain a normal serum sodium concentration as long as their water intake is kept within normal limits, but hyponatremia may develop when water intake is increased. Therefore, a normal serum sodium concentration in a cirrhotic patient who has ascites is not synonymous with a normal renal capacity to excrete solute-free water. In other patients, the severity of the disorder is such that they retain most of the water taken in the diet, causing hyponatremia and hypo-osmolarity. Therefore, hyponatremia in cirrhotic patients who have ascites is almost always dilutional in origin as it occurs in the setting of an increased total body water. The prevalence of spontaneous hyponatremia [serum sodium <130mmol/L (130mEq/L)] in hospitalized cirrhotic patients who have ascites is of approximately 30%. Most patients, hyponatremia is asymptomatic, but in some patients it may be associated with clinical symptoms similar to those found in dilutional hyponatremia of other etiologies, including anorexia, headache, difficulty in mental concentration, lethargy, nausea, vomiting, and, occasionally, seizures. The impairment in water excretion in patients who have cirrhosis is usually a late event in the natural history of the disease and follows sodium retention.

Renal vasoconstriction is also a common finding in patients who have cirrhosis and ascites. This renal abnormality leads to reductions in renal bloodflow and GFR. As with sodium and water retention, the degree of renal vasoconstriction is very variable among patients who have ascites. Renal bloodflow and GFR are normal in some cases, whereas they may be extremely reduced in others. This latter condition is known as hepatorenal syndrome (HRS).

Portal hypertension
Portal hypertension induces profound changes in the splanchnic circulation. Classically, portal hypertension was considered to be due solely to an increased resistance to portal venous flow. However, studies in animals with portal hypertension indicate that an increased portal venous inflow secondary to a generalized splanchnic arteriolar vasodilatation also plays an important role in the increased pressure in the portal circulation. This high portal venous inflow may explain why portal pressure remains increased in these animals despite the development of a marked collateral circulation. This arteriolar vasodilatation is also responsible for marked changes in splanchnic microcirculation that may predispose to increased filtration of fluid.

Several lines of evidence indicate that portal hypertension is a major factor in the pathogenesis of ascites. First, cirrhotic patients without portal hypertension do not develop ascites or edema. Although a threshold of portal pressure required for the development of ascites has not been defined precisely, ascites rarely develops in patients who have portal pressure below 12mmHg. Moreover, patients with ascites have significantly higher portal pressure than patients who do not have ascites, and portal pressure correlates inversely with urinary sodium excretion. Secondly, cirrhotic patients treated with surgical portosystemic shunts for the management of bleeding gastroesophageal varices have a remarkably lower long-term probability of developing ascites than do patients treated with procedures that obliterate gastroesophageal varices but do not affect portal pressure (i.e. variceal ablation using banding techniques or sclerotherapy, esophageal transection). Finally, a reduction in portal pressure with side-to-side or end-to-side portocaval anastomosis is very effective in the management of refractory ascites in cirrhosis, although it is associated with high morbidity and mortality.

Recent studies also showed an improvement in renal functional abnormalities together with reduction or elimination of ascites in patients who have cirrhosis treated with a transjugular intrahepatic portosystemic shunt (TIPSS). The mechanism(s) by which portal hypertension contributes to renal functional abnormalities, ascites, and edema formation is not completely understood, but several options have been proposed including:
- alterations in the splanchnic and systemic circulation which would result in activation of vasoconstrictor and antinatriuretic systems and subsequent renal sodium and water retention;
- hepatorenal reflex due to increased hepatic pressure which would directly cause sodium and water retention; and
- substances escaping from the splanchnic area through portosystemic shunts that would have a sodium-retaining effect in the kidney.

Circulatory abnormalities
In human cirrhosis there is a characteristic disturbance in the systemic circulation, which consists of reductions in systemic vascular resistance and arterial pressure and a marked increase in cardiac index. This hyperdynamic circulation is also observed in experimental models of cirrhosis and occurs long before the formation of ascites; it becomes more marked as the disease progresses. The primary site responsible for the reduced vascular resistance in cirrhosis is the splanchnic circulation. As previously discussed, a marked splanchnic arterial vasodilatation occurs in cirrhotic patients and animals with portal hypertension. Whether arterial vasodilatation also occurs in other vascular territories in cirrhosis is still controversial.

Despite extensive investigation, the mechanism(s) of this hyperdynamic circulation in cirrhosis remains unknown. Several explanations have been proposed, including opening of arteriovenous fistulas, reduced sensitivity to vasoconstrictors, and increased circulating levels of vasodilator factors. This latter mechanism has been the most extensively studied. Increased plasma levels of glucagon, vasoactive intestinal peptide, prostaglandins (PGs), substance P, calcitonin-gene-related peptide, or platelet-activating factor have been reported either in cirrhotic patients or in experimental cirrhotic animals, but their role in the pathogenesis of vasodilatation is still unclear.

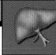

A number of studies have recently focused attention on nitric oxide (NO) as a possible mediator of arterial vasodilatation in cirrhosis. Nitric oxide is a very potent vasodilator agent produced under normal conditions in the vessels, and is believed to play a major role in the maintenance of an active state of vasodilatation in the arterial circulation. Several studies have been reported that suggest an increased synthesis of NO in animals with experimental cirrhosis and ascites. The activity of NO synthase in arterial tissue is increased in rats with cirrhosis and ascites. Consistent with these findings of increased NO production is the observation that the acute administration of an inhibitor of NO synthesis causes a greater increase in arterial pressure in cirrhotic rats with ascites than in normal rats. Furthermore, the chronic administration of orally active NO synthesis inhibitors to cirrhotic rats with ascites is associated with normalization of hemodynamic abnormalities and a marked increase in diuresis and natriuresis, suggesting a role for NO in the pathogenesis of ascites in cirrhosis. Several lines of evidence suggest that NO synthesis is also increased in human cirrhosis. The concentration of NO in serum samples obtained from a peripheral vein is increased in patients with ascites compared with healthy subjects. Nitric oxide production is particularly increased within the splanchnic circulation. Serum nitrite and nitrate, metabolites of NO, and the concentration of NO in exhaled air are also increased in patients who have cirrhosis and ascites. Moreover, the infusion of an inhibitor of NO synthesis into a peripheral artery of cirrhotic patients who have ascites restores the impaired vascular reactivity to vasoconstrictors. Taken together, all these findings in human and experimental cirrhosis suggest that NO synthesis is increased in cirrhosis and plays an important role in the pathogenesis of arterial vasodilatation and ascites.

Pathophysiology of ascites as proposed by the arterial vasodilatation theory

The most widely accepted theory to explain ascites and edema formation in cirrhosis is the arterial vasodilation theory, which considers that sodium and water retention in cirrhosis are secondary events related to a reduction in effective arterial blood volume (EABV) (Fig. 7.1).

As opposed to the classic underfilling theory, the arterial vascular underfilling would not be the result of a reduction in plasma volume, which is in fact increased, but rather the result of a disproportionate enlargement of the arterial tree secondary to arterial vasodilatation. According to the arterial vasodilatation theory, portal hypertension is the initial event with resultant splanchnic arteriolar vasodilation causing underfilling of the arterial circulation. The arterial receptors then sense the arterial underfilling and stimulate the sympathetic nervous system and the renin–angiotensin–aldosterone system, and cause nonosmotic antidiuretic hormone hypersecretion. Renal sodium and water retention are the final consequence of this response to a reduction in EABV. In the early stages of cirrhosis, when splanchnic arteriolar vasodilatation is moderate and the lymphatic system is able to return the increased lymph production to the systemic circulation, the arterial circulation is maintained by transient periods of sodium and water retention. The fluid and sodium retained by the kidneys increase the plasma volume, which helps maintain the EABV within normal limits. The increased plasma volume suppresses the signals that stimulate

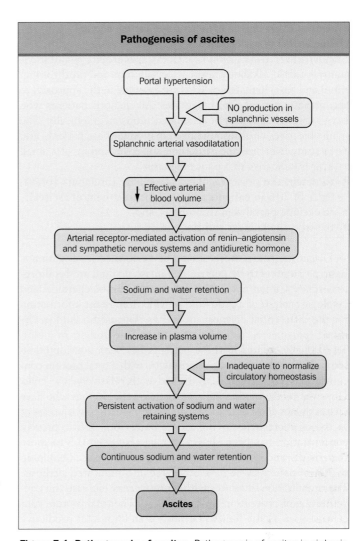

Figure 7.1 Pathogenesis of ascites. Pathogenesis of ascites in cirrhosis as proposed by the 'arterial vasodilatation theory'.

the antinatriuretic systems and sodium retention terminates. Therefore, no ascites or edema are formed at this stage and the relationship between EABV and extracellular volume is still maintained. As liver disease progresses, however, splanchnic arteriolar vasodilatation increases, thus resulting in a more intense arterial underfilling and more marked sodium and water retention. At this time the EABV can no longer be maintained by the increased plasma volume, probably because the retained fluid leaks from the splanchnic circulation to the peritoneal cavity as ascites and/or from the systemic circulation to the interstitial tissue as edema. A persistent stimulation of vasoconstrictor systems occurs in an attempt to maintain EABV. The activation of these systems perpetuates renal sodium and water retention, which accumulates as ascites.

Clinical diagnosis and evaluation

The clinical evaluation of cirrhotic patients who have ascites should be performed after 3–4 days on a low-sodium diet (40–60mmol/day) and without diuretic treatment. The two main objectives are to establish the most appropriate treatment of the ascitic-edematous syndrome and to evaluate the prognosis of the patient and the possible indication for liver transplantation.

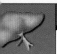

Evaluation of the degree of hepatic dysfunction and the characteristics of ascitic fluid

Standard liver tests (aminotransferases, bilirubin, γ-glutamyl-transpeptidase, alkaline phosphatase, albumin, and prothrombin time) and basic hematology tests are essential in the approach to the cirrhotic patient who has ascites. All cirrhotic patients who have ascites should also be examined ultrasonographically. The main objectives of ultrasound examination in these patients are:

- to study liver size and structure, since the finding of a small liver is indicative of a poor prognosis;
- to detect the presence of hepatocellular carcinoma (prevalence of 20% in patients admitted for treatment of ascites);
- to exclude portal vein thrombosis; and
- to assess the kidneys and the urinary tract.

Diagnostic paracentesis should be performed in all patients. Basic parameters to be determined in ascitic fluid are total protein concentration and white cell count. The biochemical and cytologic analysis of ascitic fluid provides important information for the differential diagnosis of ascites. The ascitic fluid in cirrhotic persons is transparent and yellow/amber in color. Traditionally, ascites in these patients has been considered to show the characteristics of a transudate, with a total protein concentration of less than 2.5g/dL and with relatively few cells. However, recent studies indicate that cirrhotic persons who have ascites do not constitute a homogeneous population with respect to the characteristics of the ascitic fluid. Total ascitic protein concentration has been shown to range between 0.5 to more than 6g/dL, and is greater than 3g/dL ('exudative ascites') in up to 30% of patients who have otherwise uncomplicated cirrhosis. The mobilization of ascites with diuretics may increase the concentration of proteins in the ascitic fluid. The total protein concentration in ascitic fluid in cirrhosis is an important predictive factor of SBP. The ascitic fluid possesses opsonic and bactericidal activity that seems to be mediated by complement and fibronectin. The presence of a neutrophil count greater than 250/mm^3 in ascitic fluid is diagnostic of SBP. It has to be noted that ascitic fluid culture is positive in only 50–80% of patients who have SBP. A total protein concentration greater than 1–1.5g/dL indicates a relatively high concentration of antimicrobial factors (i.e. complement, fibronectin) and a low probability to develop SBP. However, many cirrhotic patients have a total protein concentration lower than 1.5g/dL. In these patients, as discussed later, prophylaxis for SBP should be considered.

The volume of ascitic fluid accumulated may be estimated semiquantitatively for clinical purposes in different grades: mild or grade 1, moderate or grade 2, and severe or grade 3 ascites. The degree of tension of ascites does not only depend on ascitic fluid volume but also on the muscular resistance of the abdominal wall.

Evaluation of the circulatory dysfunction

Mean arterial pressure (diastolic arterial pressure plus one third of the difference between systolic and diastolic pressure) and the measurement of plasma renin activity (PRA) and plasma concentration of norepinephrine are of value in the assessment of circulatory dysfunction in cirrhotic patients who have ascites. These estimate the degree of activation of the renin–angiotensin and sympathetic nervous systems, respectively. The presence of a mean arterial pressure lower than 80mmHg and/or increased plasma renin activity or plasma norepinephrine concentration

indicate a marked circulatory dysfunction, and are associated with a short survival.

Evaluation of renal function and prognosis

Renal function should be evaluated by measuring serum sodium concentration, serum creatinine and blood urea nitrogen (BUN), 24-hour urine volume and sodium excretion, and examining a fresh urine sediment. Serum creatinine is highly specific in the detection of low GFR, but its sensitivity is poor in cirrhotic patients because some patients who have a marked reduction in GFR may have normal or only slightly increased serum creatinine levels. These low creatinine levels relative to GFR have been attributed to the low endogenous production of creatinine, resulting from the poor nutritional status and decreased muscle mass frequently present in these patients. Blood urea nitrogen levels are also not very accurate in the assessment of GFR as they may be lower than expected due to reduced hepatic synthesis of urea or low dietary protein intake. On the other hand, BUN may increase for reasons other than reduced GFR, such as gastrointestinal bleeding. Finally, creatinine clearance may overestimate GFR and is dependent on a very accurate 24-hour urine collection. Hyponatremia is commonly defined as a reduction in serum sodium below 130mmol/L (130mEq/L). The diagnosis of HRS, as discussed later, is based on clinical and laboratory data, but a serum creatinine of more than 200μmol/L (1.5mg/dL) in cirrhotic patients who have ascites indicates an important impairment in renal function.

The appearance of ascites in patients who have cirrhosis carries a poor prognosis. The probabilities of survival 1 and 5 years after the first episode of ascites have been estimated at 50 and 20%, respectively (Fig. 7.2). Among cirrhotic patients who have ascites, those with functional renal failure have the shortest survival time. These patients usually die within weeks or months of the onset of renal failure independent of the degree of hepatic insufficiency as assessed by other parameters (Fig. 7.3). Several studies in nonazotemic cirrhotic patients who have ascites have evaluated the prognostic value of numerous variables based on history, physical examination, hepatic biochemical tests, renal function tests, systemic and splanchnic hemodynamics, and endogenous vasoactive systems (Fig. 7.4). These studies indicate that parameters that estimate systemic and portal hemodynamics and renal function are

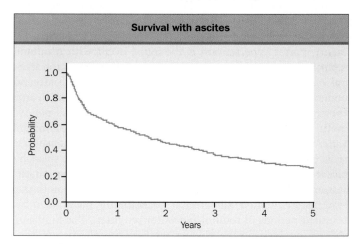

Figure 7.2 Survival with ascites. Probability of survival in a large series of cirrhotic patients who have ascites.

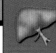

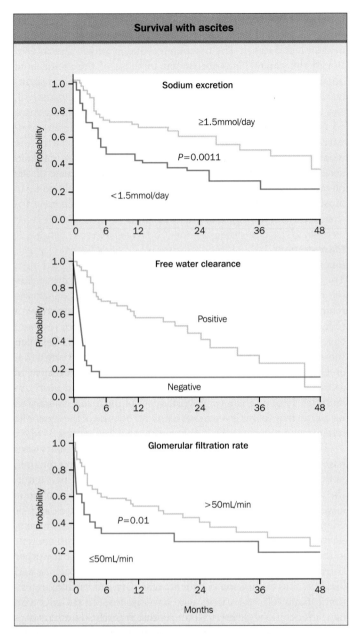

Figure 7.3 Survival with ascites. Probability of survival in cirrhotic patients who have ascites according to renal function.

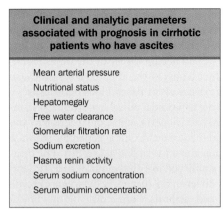

Figure 7.4 Clinical and analytic parameters associated with prognosis in cirrhotic patients who have ascites.

Clinical and analytic parameters associated with prognosis in cirrhotic patients who have ascites

- Mean arterial pressure
- Nutritional status
- Hepatomegaly
- Free water clearance
- Glomerular filtration rate
- Sodium excretion
- Plasma renin activity
- Serum sodium concentration
- Serum albumin concentration

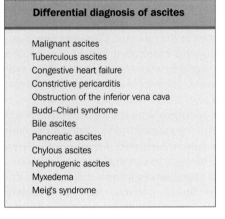

Figure 7.5 Differential diagnosis of ascites.

Differential diagnosis of ascites

- Malignant ascites
- Tuberculous ascites
- Congestive heart failure
- Constrictive pericarditis
- Obstruction of the inferior vena cava
- Budd–Chiari syndrome
- Bile ascites
- Pancreatic ascites
- Chylous ascites
- Nephrogenic ascites
- Myxedema
- Meig's syndrome

better predictors of survival than those used to estimate hepatic function in patients who have cirrhosis and ascites. Serum sodium, serum creatinine and urinary sodium excretion have prognostic value in these patients, as do serum norepinephrine levels and PRA. In particular, the renal capacity to excrete a water load is the most sensitive prognostic factor in cirrhotic patients who have ascites, being better than other parameters of liver disease including the Childs–Pugh score. Median survival time of patients who have normal (>8mL/min), moderately reduced (3–8mL/min), or markedly reduced urine flow after water load (<3mL/min) are 4, 1.5, and 0.5 years, respectively. All these parameters are useful for evaluating cirrhotic patients for liver transplantation.

Differential diagnosis of cirrhotic ascites

Clinical conditions other than cirrhosis are associated with ascites (Fig. 7.5).

The diagnosis of any cause of ascites should be based on clinical, analytic, and exploratory data. Examination of ascitic fluid is an essential tool, but is not always definitive. Malignant ascites is characterized by a total protein concentration of over 30g/L (3.0g/dL) and the presence of neoplastic cells in ascitic fluid. However, when the development of ascites is due to portal hypertension secondary to massive liver metastases with little peritoneal involvement, the total ascitic protein concentration is usually lower than 25g/L (2.5g/dL) and malignant cells are usually absent. The definitive diagnosis should then be achieved by ultrasonography, computed tomography, or laparoscopic examination. Other measurements on ascitic fluid that have proved to be of value in differentiating malignant from cirrhotic ascites include lactic dehydrogenase, total lipids, cholesterol, carcinoembryonic antigen, and fibrin/fibrinogen degradation products.

Chylous ascites is an infrequent feature in patients who have cirrhosis. It has been reported in the postoperative period after splenorenal shunt and after TIPSS occlusion, although in most instances it appears spontaneously. Ascitic fluid is typically turbid and white ('milky' ascites), due to a high concentration of chylomicrons. The diagnosis of chylous ascites is based on ascitic fluid triglyceride concentration, which is usually over 1024mmol/L (110mg/dL) and always higher than the corresponding value in plasma.

The differential diagnosis between cirrhotic ascites and ascites due to tuberculous peritonitis is particularly important since alcoholic cirrhosis may predispose to this condition. Clinically, tuberculous peritonitis is characterized by fever, abdominal pain, anorexia, weight loss, abdominal tenderness, and ascites. The rate of positive cultures of ascitic fluid for *Mycobacterium tuberculosis* varies markedly from 10 to 70%. Among the biochemical parameters, an increased level of lactic dehydrogenase and adenosine deaminase in the peritoneal fluid has been shown to be useful in suggesting this diagnosis. Open peritoneal biopsy during a laparotomy or minilaparotomy, blind needle biopsy of the peritoneum, and laparoscopy with direct biopsy of the affected areas have also been used to confirm the diagnosis of tuberculous peritonitis.

Ascites secondary to postsinusoidal portal hypertension (congestive heart failure, constrictive pericarditis, obstruction of the inferior vena cava, Budd–Chiari syndrome), generally shows a total protein concentration greater than 30g/L (3g/dL). The diagnosis, however, can be established by other clinical, analytic, and exploratory data. The differential diagnosis between chronic Budd–Chiari syndrome and cirrhosis is often difficult on clinical grounds. The ascitic fluid protein concentration may be low in some of these patients as a result of the capillarization of the hepatic sinusoids. On the other hand, these patients may have cutaneous stigmata of chronic liver disease, abnormal liver function tests, splenomegaly and esophageal varices. Computed tomography and ultrasonography may suggest Budd–Chiari syndrome if major hepatic veins are not visualized.

Biliary ascites occurs after biliary tract surgery (mainly cholecystectomy), percutaneous diagnostic procedures (liver biopsy and percutaneous transhepatic cholangiography), and trauma with injury to the gallbladder, common bile duct, hepatic duct or liver. It is often associated with signs and symptoms of peritonitis, including severe epigastric, right upper quadrant or diffuse abdominal pain, rigidity of the abdomen, rebound tenderness, hypotension, tachycardia, oliguria, and marked leukocytosis. Pancreatic ascites occurs in approximately 3% of patients who have chronic pancreatitis as a result of the leakage of pancreatic fluid from a pancreatic duct rupture, or from a pancreatic pseudocyst into the peritoneal cavity. Other less frequent etiologies include acute hemorrhagic pancreatitis and pancreatic cancer. Since most patients who have chronic pancreatitis are alcoholic and may develop massive ascites with little or no abdominal tenderness, the differential diagnosis of pancreatic ascites from cirrhotic ascites may be difficult on clinical grounds. Laboratory analyses are, therefore, essential to establish a correct diagnosis. In virtually all cases, serum and especially ascitic fluid amylase and lipase values are dramatically increased. Other causes of ascites easily differentiated from cirrhotic ascites include nephrogenic ascites, myxedema and Meigs' syndrome, which is due to ovarian carcinoma.

Cirrhotic hydrothorax

Pleural effusions, in the absence of primary pulmonary, pleural or cardiac disease, occur in approximately 5% of patients who have hepatic cirrhosis. Clinical ascites are almost always evident and the pleural effusion is usually right-sided.

Occasionally, however, an effusion develops in the left pleural cavity, on both sides, or in the absence of detectable ascites. The pathogenesis of cirrhotic hydrothorax is, in most cases, the direct passage of ascitic fluid from the abdomen through acquired defects in the diaphragm into the pleural space. The driving force leading to the peritoneal–pleural transfer of fluid is the hydrostatic gradient between the positive intra-abdominal pressure and the negative intrathoracic pressure. In cases of cirrhotic hydrothorax without detectable ascites the transport of fluid into the pleural space probably equals the rate of production of ascites. The presence of direct communications between the peritoneal and pleural cavities can be demonstrated by radioisotopic studies. The

intraperitoneal injection of tracer amounts of [99m]techenetium sulfur colloid is followed by the rapid appearance of the isotope in the pleural cavity. The biochemical and cytologic characteristics of the pleural fluid are similar to those of the ascitic fluid obtained simultaneously. It is not unusual, however, to find slightly higher concentrations of total protein, albumin, cholesterol, and total lipids in pleural fluid than in ascitic fluid, probably related to a higher rate of water reabsorption from the pleural compartment. However, if there are marked differences in the biochemical or cytologic characteristics between the pleural fluid and the ascitic fluid one should search for another cause of the pleural effusion. Although hydrothorax is an incidental finding in most cirrhotic patients, some cases develop massive pleural effusions that lead to respiratory insufficiency.

Management

Bed rest and low-sodium diet

The assumption of an upright posture by patients who have cirrhosis and ascites is associated with a striking activation of the renin–angiotensin–aldosterone and sympathetic nervous systems, a reduction in GFR and sodium excretion, and a decreased response to loop diuretics. Moreover, moderate physical exercise has been shown to impair renal function in cirrhosis with ascites. From a theoretic point of view, bed rest could be useful for the treatment of ascites in cirrhosis, particularly in patients who respond poorly to diuretics. However, this traditional aspect of the management plan for ascites is no longer given much emphasis because of the economic requirement to reduce the duration of hospitalization (Fig. 7.6).

The first step in the management of cirrhotic patients who have ascites is sodium restriction, as the amount of fluid retained in the body depends on the balance between sodium ingested in the diet and sodium excreted in the urine. If sodium excreted is lower than that ingested, patients accumulate ascites and/or edema. Conversely, if sodium excretion is greater than intake, ascites and/or edema decrease. The reduction of sodium content in the diet to 40–60mmol/day (1–1.5g of salt), without any other therapeutic intervention, causes a negative sodium balance and loss of ascites and edema in patients who have mild sodium retention (about 10% of patients who have ascites). In patients who have moderate or severe sodium retention, such sodium restriction is not sufficient by itself to achieve a negative sodium balance, but it may slow the reaccumulation of fluid. These patients would theoretically require a more severe restriction of sodium (less than 20mmol/day). However, such intense sodium restriction is difficult to accomplish and may impair nutritional status.

Diuretic therapy

The pharmacologic treatment of ascites has been based for many years on the administration of diuretics, drugs that increase urinary sodium excretion by reducing the tubular reabsorption of sodium. However, the reintroduction of therapeutic paracentesis has modified markedly the treatment of ascites in cirrhosis. Current indications for use of diuretics in cirrhotic patients include:

- treatment of patients who are not eligible for paracentesis because of low ascites volume;
- prevention of ascites reaccumulation after paracentesis;
- treatment of patients who have edema without ascites; and
- prevention of fluid accumulation in patients who show a positive response to low-sodium diet alone but do not tolerate prolonged sodium restriction.

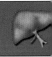

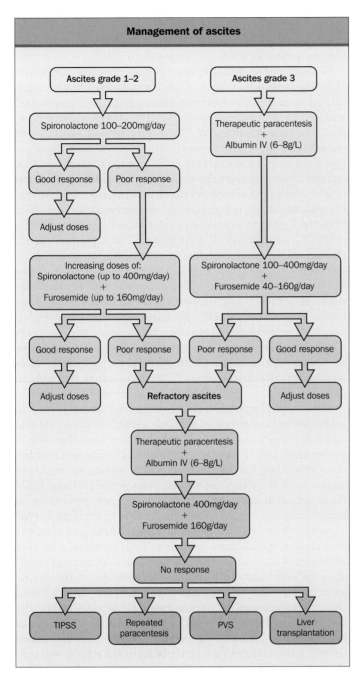

Figure 7.6 Management of ascites. Therapeutic algorithm for the treatment of ascites. PVS, peritoneovenous shunt. (Reproduced with permission of Bataller et al., Drugs. 1997;54:571–80.)

No major advances in the field of diuretic agents have been made in recent years. Diuretic therapy in cirrhosis is based on the administration of spironolactone (50–400mg/day), a drug that competes with aldosterone for the binding to the mineralocorticoid receptor in the collecting tubular epithelial cells, alone or in combination with loop diuretics, especially furosemide (frusemide) (20–160mg/day) or torasemide (10–40mg/day), that act by inhibiting the Na^+–K^+–$2Cl^-$ co-transporter in the loop of Henle. Common complications of diuretic therapy in patients who have cirrhosis include electrolyte disturbances (hyponatremia and hypo-hyperkalemia), hepatic encephalopathy, renal impairment, gynecomastia, and muscle cramps.

Amiloride is used as an alternative to spironolactone when the latter causes painful gynecomastia. The impairment of renal failure during diuretic therapy is due to volume depletion, occurs in patients who have positive response to diuretics, and is usually rapidly reversible after discontinuation of therapy.

Paracentesis

In the past 10 years, therapeutic paracentesis has progressively replaced diuretics as the treatment of choice in the management of large volumes of ascites in patients who have cirrhosis. This change in treatment strategy is based on the results of several randomized studies that compared paracentesis accompanied by plasma volume expansion (either total removal of all ascitic fluid as a single procedure or repeated paracentesis of 4–6L/day) with diuretics in cirrhotic patients who had severe ascites. The results of these studies indicate that paracentesis is more rapid and effective and is associated with a lower number of complications than conventional diuretic therapy. Because paracentesis does not modify the pre-existing renal functional abnormalities of cirrhosis, patients should be given diuretics after paracentesis to avoid reaccumulation of ascites.

The effects of paracentesis on systemic hemodynamics have been delineated in several recent studies. Immediately after paracentesis there are hemodynamic changes that are consistent with an improvement in effective blood volume, with an increase in cardiac output, deactivation of vasoconstrictor and antinatriuretic systems (renin–angiotensin–aldosterone system and sympathetic nervous system), and increase in the plasma concentration of atrial natriuretic peptide. However, this early phase is rapidly followed by reversal of the circulatory changes consistent with a decrease in effective blood volume with reduction in cardiac output, activation of antinatriuretic systems, and reduced plasma atrial natriuretic peptide levels. A recent study has shown that these hemodynamic changes are not reversible and have a negative impact on the evolution of the disease. Patients who develop postparacentesis circulatory dysfunction require higher doses of diuretics to prevent ascites formation, have a greater risk of ascites reaccumulation, and, most importantly, have a shorter survival than patients who do not develop this abnormality. At present, the only effective method to prevent this complication is the administration of plasma expanders. Albumin is more effective than dextran-70 and hemaccel. In patients treated with albumin the risk of postparacentesis circulatory dysfunction is low, and independent of the volume of ascites removed. By contrast, in patients treated with nonalbumin plasma expanders, the risk of postparacentesis circulatory dysfunction is higher than in those treated with albumin, and increases with the volume of ascitic fluid removed. The pathogenesis of postparacentesis circulatory dysfunction is not completely understood, but it is not due to a paracentesis-induced hypovolemia, as plasma volume does not decrease in patients who develope this complication. More likely, this abnormality is due to an arterial vasodilatation that would cause a further impairment in the circulatory function of cirrhotic patients.

Hyponatremia

A low serum sodium concentration in patients who have cirrhosis may reflect extreme water retention or overdiuresis. In either event, the total body sodium is increased and there is almost no role for intravenous sodium supplementation. Hyponatremia in the absence of diuretic therapy is an indicator of a very poor prognosis. The management of ascites in this setting is by paracentesis and diuretics are only introduced if the serum sodium returns to the normal range. The best method to increase the serum sodium is by fluid restriction. A limit of 1.5L fluid intake per day is a standard component of the treatment regimen for ascites, but this may be reduced further to 0.8–1.2L depending on the severity of the hyponatremia (Fig. 7.7). These patients should be assessed for liver transplantation if there are no obvious contraindications to this intervention. However, it is important to bring the serum sodium concentration up to at least 125mmol/L (125mEq/L) immediately before transplantation to reduce the risk of central pontine myelinolysis. This can be achieved with ultrafiltration.

The hyponatremia secondary to diuretic therapy is managed by reducing the dose of diuretics, or stopping all diuretics, depending on the severity (see Fig. 7.7). Hyponatrema is one of the factors that can limit the dose of diuretic long-term and contribute to the diagnosis of intractable ascites. However, diuretic associated hyponatremia may not recur if it developed in association with a reversible deterioration in the clinical status of the patient, for example after a gastrointestinal hemorrhage.

Other therapeutic methods

Peritoneovenous shunting was used frequently in the past in the treatment of ascites in cirrhosis, especially in patients who have refractory ascites. However, its use has declined markedly due to both side effects (shunt occlusion, vena cava thrombosis, peritoneal fibrosis) and introduction of alternative therapies such as paracentesis. It still has a role in patients who are not candidates

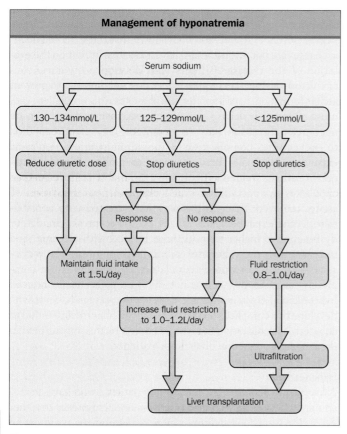

Figure 7.7 Management of hyponatremia. An algorithm for the management of hyponatremia of varying severity.

for transplantation and have a low threshold for encephalopathy or other contraindications to TIPSS. A LeVeen or Denver shunt is most commonly used.

A number of studies have been published recently on the use of TIPSS in patients who have refractory ascites. As with surgical portosystemic shunts, the reduction in portal pressure obtained with TIPSS is associated with favorable effects on renal function. The main advantage of TIPSS over surgical shunts is the reduction of the operative mortality, while the main disadvantage is the frequent obstruction of the prosthesis, which results in increased portal pressure and reaccumulation of ascites. Potential problems of TIPSS are the development of hepatic encephalopathy and impairment in liver function due to the shunting of blood from the liver to the systemic circulation. A recent comparative study in a small series of patients who had refractory ascites showed an increased mortality in patients treated with TIPSS, especially in those patients who had poor liver function, compared with patients treated with paracentesis with albumin infusions. A TIPSS is not recommended in patients who have Childs–Pugh C cirrhosis. The placement of a TIPSS may be followed by the development of cardiac failure, especially in patients who have an underlying cardiomyopathy, for example, alcoholic cirrhosis and iron overload syndromes. Larger controlled studies are required to define whether TIPSS has a role in the management of cirrhotic patients who have refractory ascites (see below).

Liver transplantation has become a standard therapy for patients who have advanced cirrhosis as the 5-year survival rate for adult cirrhotic patients submitted to liver transplantation is greater than 70%. Earlier recommendations suggested that the main indications for liver transplantation in patients who have ascites were refractory ascites, recovery from SBP, and HRS. However, with these guidelines a significant proportion of patients do not reach transplantation because of the short survival expectancy associated with these conditions. A number of factors predictive of survival have been described in patients who have cirrhosis and ascites that may help in the identification of candidates for liver transplantation. The most valuable factors associated with a poor prognosis in these patients are related to abnormalities in renal function and systemic hemodynamics, and include an impaired ability to excrete a water load, dilutional hyponatremia, arterial hypotension, reduced GFR, marked sodium retention, and increased plasma renin activity and norepinephrine concentration. Of interest, in patients who have ascites these parameters are better predictors of prognosis than liver function tests (see Fig. 7.3).

Practical recommendations for the management of ascites

In patients who have mild-to-moderate ascites (grades 1–2), bed rest and sodium restriction (40–60mEq/day) should be indicated initially. In about 20% of cirrhotic patients who have ascites a reduction of sodium intake leads to disappearance of ascites. These patients usually show a relatively high baseline urinary sodium excretion. In nonresponders to sodium restriction, diuretics should be initiated. A useful therapeutic schedule is to start with spironolactone alone (100mg/day). The addition of loop diuretics (i.e. furosemide 40mg/day) may be necessary in some cases to increase the natriuretic effect. If there is no response after 4–5 days, the dosage is increased stepwise up to 400mg/day of spironolactone plus 160mg/day of furosemide (see Fig. 7.6). Cases not responding to this program should be considered as having diuretic-resistant ascites. The best method to assess the effectiveness of diuretic therapy is by monitoring body weight and urine sodium concentration.

The goal of diuretic treatment should be to achieve a weight loss of 300–500g/day in patients who do not have edema and 800–1000g/day in those who have edema. Once ascites has been mobilized, diuretic treatment should be adjusted to maintain the patient free of ascites. A moderate sodium restriction (60–80mmol/day) is advisable to avoid fluid reaccumulation. A frequent cause of failure of diuretic therapy is an inadequate sodium restriction. This should be suspected when body weight and ascites volume do not decrease despite a significant natriuresis. Cirrhotic patients treated with diuretics may develop azotemia due to intravascular volume depletion. A weight loss greater than 500g/day in patients who do not have peripheral edema should be avoided to prevent this complication. Other complications related to diuretic therapy are dilutional hyponatremia, hepatic encephalopathy, gynecomastia, hyperkalemia, and muscle cramps.

Patients who have severe ascites (grade 3) include those who have large volumes of ascites, whether or not the abdomen is tense. The treatment of choice is total paracentesis (total extraction of ascitic fluid in single tap) associated with intravenous infusion of albumin. Paracentesis provides rapid relief of symptoms in these patients. The incidence of hepatic encephalopathy, dilutional hyponatremia, and renal impairment is significantly lower in patients treated with paracentesis than in patients treated with diuretics. However, since paracentesis does not modify the pre-existing renal abnormalities, ascitic fluid reaccumulates after treatment unless patients are treated with diuretics to prevent ascites recurrence. As discussed before, the removal of ascitic fluid has to be associated with the administration of plasma expanders, since large-volume paracentesis without plasma volume expansion constantly induces a reduction in effective intravascular volume, as indicated by marked activation of vasoconstrictor systems, which may result in the development of hyponatremia and/or renal failure in 15–20% of patients. In contrast, paracentesis with intravenous albumin is neither associated with changes in effective intravascular volume nor with alterations in renal function or activity of vasoconstrictor and antinatriuretic systems. Artificial plasma expanders, such as dextran-70 or polygeline, are less effective than albumin in the prevention of postparacentesis circulatory dysfunction, particularly in patients in whom more than 5L of ascitic fluid are removed.

A new definition and diagnostic criteria of 'refractory ascites' have been proposed recently by the International Ascites Club. Refractory ascites is defined as the ascites that cannot be mobilized, or the early recurrence of which (i.e. after therapeutic paracentesis) cannot be satisfactorily prevented by medical therapy. The term 'refractory ascites' includes two different subtypes:
- 'diuretic-resistant ascites' (lack of response to dietary sodium restriction and intensive diuretic treatment); and
- 'diuretic-intractable ascites' (development of diuretic-induced complications that preclude the use of an effective diuretic dosage).

In approximately 10% of patients ascites cannot be controlled despite dietary sodium restriction, bed rest, and maximal diuretic therapy. Most of these patients have severe disturbances of systemic hemodynamics and renal function, as indicated by extremely high levels of renin, norepinephrine, and antidiuretic hormone,

and low renal bloodflow and GFR. These patients can satisfactorily be treated by peritoneovenous shunting and/or paracentesis.

Repeated total paracentesis plus intravenous infusion of albumin is replacing peritoneovenous shunting as the initial treatment of these patients in most centers. Thus, peritoneovenous shunting is only indicated in those few patients who do not accept frequent paracentesis. Although peritoneovenous shunting is more effective than paracentesis for long-term control of ascites, it does not reduce the total duration of hospitalization, does not improve survival, and is associated with an important number of complications, particularly obstruction of the shunt, thrombosis of the superior vena cava, or peritoneal fibrosis. Recently, TIPSS has been proposed as an effective treatment for refractory ascites and is used with increasing frequency as treatment for variceal bleeding in cirrhosis. Its main advantage over the traditional surgical shunts is the decrease in morbidity and mortality that is associated with the procedure. However, TIPSS may also impair hepatic function and induce severe encephalopathy. Moreover, this procedure has the additional problem of a high rate of shunt malfunction due to stenosis of the stent or the hepatic vein segment connecting with the prosthesis. The studies assessing the use of TIPSS in refractory ascites have shown that the insertion of TIPSS is associated with a marked suppression of antinatriuretic systems and an improvement in renal function and in the renal response to diuretics. A significant number of patients remain free of ascites with minimal or no diuretic therapy during follow-up. However, the incidence of hepatic encephalopathy after TIPSS is very high (ranging between 50 and 75%). Moreover, in the only randomized controlled trial so far published, the probability of survival of patients who have refractory ascites treated by TIPSS was significantly shorter than that of patients treated by paracentesis. Multicenter randomized controlled trials in large series of patients are needed to delineate whether TIPSS improves the results obtained with paracentesis or peritoneovenous shunting in terms of quality of life and survival. This technique has also been used for the management of hydrothorax as the dominant manifestation of fluid retention.

At present, no pharmacologic therapy exists for dilutional hyponatremia and the only therapeutic measure that improves or stops the progressive decrease in serum sodium concentration is water restriction. The administration of hypertonic saline solutions is not recommended because it invariably leads to further expansion of extracellular fluid volume and accumulation of ascites and edema. Recently, two types of drug have been developed that selectively increase water excretion: antagonists of the V_2 receptor of antidiuretic hormone and selective κ-opioid agonists. The former group of drugs antagonize selectively the water-retaining effect of antidiuretic hormone in the cortical collecting duct, whereas the latter inhibit antidiuretic hormone release from the neurohypophysis and have also a direct tubular effect. Both groups of drugs induce a dose-dependent increase in urine flow and free water excretion in normal animals as well as in healthy subjects. These renal effects are different from those of classic diuretic agents because the increase in urine volume is associated with only mild or no increase in sodium excretion. Two recent investigations using single doses of nonpeptide V_2 receptor antagonists or the selective κ-opioid agonist niravoline showed that both agents selectively increase water excretion in rats with cirrhosis, ascites, and water retention. Preliminary studies in cirrhotic patients who have ascites have also shown that both drugs increased selective water excretion. Therefore, these compounds offer a novel therapeutic approach for the treatment of water retention and dilutional hyponatremia in cirrhotic patients who have ascites.

SPONTANEOUS BACTERIAL PERITONITIS

Spontaneous bacterial peritonitis is a common and severe complication of cirrhotic patients who have ascites characterized by spontaneous infection of ascitic fluid without an intra-abdominal source of infection. The prevalence of SBP in hospitalized patients with ascites ranges from 10 to 30%. Cirrhotic patients with hydrothorax may also develop a spontaneous infection of pleural fluid.

Pathophysiology

The isolation of aerobic Gram-negative bacteria in the great majority of episodes of SBP suggests that the gastrointestinal tract is the source of bacteria. Although the pathogenesis of SBP is not completely understood, it is generally accepted that it involves three major steps:

- passage of bacteria from the intestinal lumen to the systemic circulation;
- bacteremia secondary to the impairment of the reticuloendothelial system (RES) phagocytic activity; and
- infection of ascites due to defective antimicrobial activity of ascitic fluid.

Studies in experimental animals with cirrhosis suggest that bacterial translocation (i.e. passage of bacteria from the intestinal lumen to mesenteric lymph nodes) is the mechanism by which bacteria from the intestinal lumen reach the systemic circulation. Bacterial translocation may increase under several circumstances, such as hemorrhagic shock. This may explain, at least in part, the high incidence of infections caused by enteric bacteria in cirrhotic patients who have gastrointestinal hemorrhage.

A reduced phagocytic activity of the RES (a system that removes bacteria from the circulation) is another important pathogenic factor in the development of SBP. Cirrhotic patients who have reduced activity of the RES are highly predisposed to develop SBP, whereas this infection is rarely seen in patients who have normal activity of the RES.

Reduced antimicrobial activity of the ascitic fluid also plays a very important role in the development of SBP. Patients who have reduced antimicrobial activity of ascitic fluid have a greater risk of developing ascitic fluid infection than those who have normal antimicrobial activity of the ascitic fluid. As the antimicrobial activity of ascites correlates with total ascitic fluid protein concentration, patients who have low ascites protein content [<10g/L (<1g/dL)] have a greater risk of developing SBP compared with patients who have higher ascites protein concentration.

The most widely accepted theory on the pathogenesis of SBP is shown in Figure 7.8. The initial step involves translocation of bacteria from the gut flora to mesenteric lymph nodes. This translocation would occur either spontaneously or as a consequence of some precipitating events (i.e. gastrointestinal hemorrhage). An increased permeability of the gut is related to histologic changes in the gut mucosa but intestinal bacterial overgrowth may also facilitate bacterial translocation. The bacteria then reach the systemic circulation through the lymphatic system. In cases of SBP not caused by bacteria of enteric origin, the bacteria would reach the systemic circulation from other areas (i.e. respiratory, urinary tracts, or skin). In patients who have normal activity of the RES, bacteria are efficiently removed from the circulation, but persistent bacteremia develops in patients who have impaired activity of the RES. Subsequently, bacteria may reach the ascitic fluid through a hematogenous route. The development of SBP depends on the antimicrobial activity of the ascitic fluid. Infection of ascites does not occur in patients who have good antimicrobial activity of the ascitic fluid. By contrast, patients who have reduced antimicrobial activity of the ascitic fluid develop SBP. Interestingly, a reduced NO production by macrophages present in ascitic fluid has been recently implicated as a mechanism responsible of the reduction in antimicrobial activity of the ascitic fluid in cirrhotic patients who have SBP.

Clinical features and diagnosis

All cirrhotic patients who have ascites should be considered at risk of developing SBP. The prevalence of SBP in unselected cirrhotic patients who have ascites admitted to hospital ranges between 10 and 30%. The clinical spectrum of SBP is very variable. A very high degree of clinical suspicion is required for diagnosis, as only a relatively low percentage of patients show the typical features of an acute peritoneal infection with fever, chills, diffuse abdominal pain, rebound tenderness, and reduced bowel sounds. Fever may be the only clinical sign in a large proportion of patients. In other cases, the infection is manifested by hepatic encephalopathy or septic shock. In 10% of cases SBP may be totally asymptomatic. Renal failure develops in one third of patients who have SBP, it may occur despite the resolution of the infection, and is associated with a poor prognosis. Mechanisms responsible for renal failure during SBP are currently unknown. Patients who survive an episode of SBP are at high risk of developing recurrent episodes of SBP during follow-up. As many as

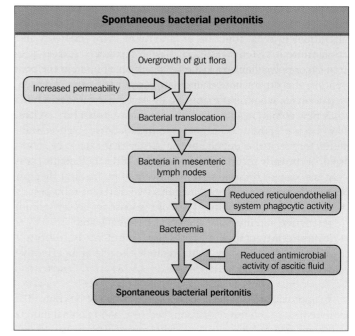

Figure 7.8 Spontaneous bacterial peritonitis. Pathogenesis of spontaneous bacterial peritonitis in cirrhotic patients who have ascites.

70% of patients surviving 1 year after the first episode of SBP will develop a new episode of infection within this period of time. Gram-negative bacteria are the most common isolates in recurrent episodes of SBP regardless of the type of bacteria responsible during the first episode (Fig. 7.9). Factors associated with a greater risk of SBP recurrence are impaired liver function and low protein concentration in ascitic fluid.

The diagnosis of SBP is based upon examination of ascitic fluid. Peritoneal infection is associated with an inflammatory reaction that is responsible for an increased number of polymorphonuclear leukocytes (PMNL) in ascitic fluid. A diagnostic paracentesis should be performed routinely in all patients who have cirrhosis admitted to hospital with ascites and in those hospitalized patients in whom a peritoneal infection is suspected because of fever, abdominal pain, shock, hepatic encephalopathy or renal impairment. It is commonly accepted that the presence of a PMNL count greater than 250/mm^3 in the absence of an intra-abdominal source of infection is indicative of SBP and should prompt the administration of broad-spectrum antibiotics. Some authors use white cell counts of up to twice this level, irrespective of the type of white cell involved. The differential white cell count shows a dominant lymphocytosis in resolving or treated infections. The determination of pH or lactate levels in ascitic fluid are not useful in the diagnosis of SBP. In patients who have bloody ascites the leukocyte count should be evaluated with respect to the total number of red blood cells in ascites and compared with the proportion of leukocytes/red blood cells obtained in the peripheral blood.

The concentration of bacteria in ascitic fluid of patients who have SBP is usually very low (one micro-organism per milliliter or less). This low concentration accounts for the high frequency of culture-negative SBP when using conventional culture methods. It is strongly recommended that culture of ascitic fluid should be performed using blood culture bottles with media for both aerobic and anaerobic bacteria. The minimum amount of ascitic fluid inoculated in each bottle should be 10mL. The rate of identification of the causative bacteria can be increased by performing blood cultures before the administration of antibiotics, and these should be obtained in patients who have increased ascitic fluid PMNL counts before antibiotic therapy is commenced. The most common isolates in ascitic fluid are Gram-negative bacilli from intestinal origin, especially *Escherichia coli*. Pneumococci and other Gram-positive bacteria are less common. Anaerobic and microaerophilic organisms, although very abundant in gut flora, rarely cause SBP. In a significant proportion of patients having SBP, blood cultures are positive. In these cases, as occurs in other infections (i.e. pneumonia or meningitis), bacteria isolated from the peripheral blood are assumed to be bacteria causing SBP. Despite the use of sensitive methods of ascitic fluid culture, between 20 and 40% of episodes of SBP diagnosed by high PMNL count are culture-negative. This condition, known as culture-negative SBP, should be considered as SBP and patients should be managed with antibiotics.

The term bacteriascites refers to the colonization of ascitic fluid by bacteria in the absence of an inflammatory reaction in ascitic fluid. The diagnosis of bacteriascites is currently made when there is positive ascitic fluid culture with a PMNL count <250 cells/mm^3. Patients who have bacterascites represent a heterogeneous population. In some patients this condition represents the colonization of ascites by bacteria that cause a

simultaneous extraperitoneal infection (i.e. bacteriemia, pneumonia, urinary tract infection, or skin infection). These patients usually have signs or symptoms of other sources of infection. In other patients, however, the growth of bacteria from the ascitic fluid may represent a transient and spontaneously reversible colonization of ascites or the first step in the development of SBP. In these latter cases, bacteriascites is usually asymptomatic. As some patients who have bacteriascites may progress to develop SBP, a follow-up paracentesis after 2–4 days or when any clinical change is detected is advisable to rule out persistence or progression of the infection.

The main condition to be considered in the differential diagnosis of SBP is peritonitis secondary to gut perforation or peritoneal abscess, as the latter is also associated with an increased PMNL count in ascitic fluid (Fig. 7.10). Although secondary peritonitis is less common than SBP, the differentiation between the two conditions is very important because surgical treatment is required for secondary peritonitis. The ascitic fluid in cirrhotic patients who have secondary peritonitis is characterized by a markedly high PMNL count, protein levels over 10g/L (1.0g/dL), increased lactate dehydrogenase, and multiple organisms on the Gram stain and/or culture. Nevertheless, the existence of perforation or abscesses causing secondary peritonitis should be confirmed by appropriate methods, such as abdominal radiography, ultrasonography, computed tomography scan, or radioisotope scintigraphy.

Bacteria isolated in 116 cases of spontaneous bacterial peritonitis	
Organism	–
Organisms of enteric origin:	94 (83%)
Escherichia coli	69%
Klebsiella spp.	9
Proteus spp.	4
Enterococcus faecalis	4
Enterobacter serratia	2
Pseudomonas spp.	2
Other	6
Nonenteric organisms	20 (17%)
Gram-positive cocci	17
Other	3

Figure 7.9 Bacteria isolated in 116 cases of spontaneous peritonitis.

Differential diagnosis between spontaneous and secondary bacterial peritonitis		
	Spontaneous	Secondary
PMNL count (cells/mm^3)	250–1200	>1200
pH	>7	<7
Glucose (mg/mL)	>60	<60
LDH (U/mL)	<600	>600
Protein (mg/mL)	<3	>3
Culture	Aerobic (single)	Aerobic/anaerobic (polymicrobial)

Figure 7.10 Differential diagnosis between spontaneous and secondary bacterial peritonitis based on ascitic fluid parameters. LDH, lactate dehydrogenase.

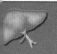
Management

Since SBP is a severe condition that complicates cirrhotic patients who have ascites, empiric antibiotic therapy should be initiated as soon as SBP is diagnosed and before the identification of the causative organisms from culture of the ascitic fluid (Fig. 7.11).

Since Gram-negative aerobic bacteria from the family of Enterobacteriaceae and nonenteroccocal *Streptococcus* spp. are the organisms more frequently causing SBP, the initial empiric antibiotic therapy of SBP should include antibiotic agents capable of covering these organisms. The efficacy and safety of different antimicrobial agents as initial empiric antibiotic therapy in SBP have been extensively investigated in the past decade. The antibiotic treatment should be maintained until the complete disappearance of all signs of infection (fever, abdominal pain, normalization of blood PMNL count) and reduction of PMNL count in ascitic fluid to below 250/mm^3.

The antibiotics of choice as initial empiric treatment for cirrhotic patients who have SBP are third-generation cephalosporins, owing to their broad antibacterial spectrum, high level of efficacy, and limited side effects. Although cefotaxime has been the drug more commonly used, other cephalosporins, such as ceftriaxone, cefonicid, and ceftizoxime, have similar efficacy. In randomized comparative studies, cefotaxime has been shown to be more effective than other types of antibiotics, such as aztreonam or aminoglycosides in combination with ampicillin. Dosage of cefotaxime is 2g given every 6–12 hours. Amoxicillin–clavulanic acid also seems effective, but comparative studies in large series of patients between this antibiotic and third-generation cephalosporins are lacking. Moreover, the possibility of superinfections with the use of amoxicillin–clavulanic acid is not insignificant. In patients who have hypersensitivity to β-lactam antibiotics, the parenteral administration of quinolones, such as ciprofloxacin or ofloxacin, can be recommended. In some instances, patients who have SBP are in a relative good clinical condition and can be treated with oral antibiotics. Recent studies have been carried out using wide-spectrum quinolones, which are almost totally absorbed after oral administration and rapidly diffuse to the ascitic fluid. In a recent randomized controlled trial, oral ofloxacin has been shown to be as effective as intravenous cefotaxime in terms of resolution of infection and survival, and has the additional advantage of oral administration and low cost.

Nevertheless, patients in a severe condition (i.e. septic shock) or who have complications that may impair oral absorption of drugs (gastrointestinal hemorrhage or ileus) should be treated with intravenous antibiotics. Therefore, oral antibiotics, especially ofloxacin, could be given in uncomplicated cases of SBP.

Recent studies have shown that the development of renal failure is the worst prognostic factor for survival and infection resolution in patients who have SBP. In an attempt to avoid this complication, it has been recently reported that volume plasma expansion with albumin administration prevents the impairment of renal function and improves survival in patients who have SBP.

Resolution and prognosis

The resolution of SBP in patients treated with third-generation cephalosporins is obtained in 75–90% of cases. Factors associated with a lack of response to therapy are renal impairment, high blood and ascitic PMNL count, hospital acquired SBP, and high aspartate aminotransferase levels. Despite the high rate of resolution of the infection, the mortality rate of patients who have SBP during hospitalization remains very high at between 20 and 40%. The most important predictor of survival in patients who have SBP is the development of renal impairment during the infection.

Resolution of SBP is achieved in approximately 90% of patients with the initial empiric antibiotic therapy. The resolution of infection is associated with disappearance of all signs of infection, reduction in PMNL count in ascitic fluid to below 250/mm^3, and negative cultures of ascitic fluid. In 10% of patients, clinical and analytic signs of infection do not improve despite the administration of antibiotics. The mortality of these patients is very high. Therefore, monitoring of the evolution of the infection is very important in order to recognize treatment failure early in the course of SBP. A periodic evaluation (i.e. every 48 hours) of ascitic fluid is then highly recommended. Treatment failure is defined when systemic signs of infection have not decreased and/or PMNL count in ascitic fluid is not reduced by at least 25% with respect to pretreatment values after 3 days of therapy. Recognition of treatment failure should prompt the modification of antibiotic therapy. If the causative bacterium has been isolated, the new antibiotic should be given according to the *in vitro* susceptibility. If no causative bacteria have been isolated, imipenem is the recommended empiric antibiotic in these patients.

The long-term prognosis of cirrhotic patients who have recovered from an episode of SBP is poor. The 1-year survival probability is only 40%. Because of this short survival expectation, patients recovering from an episode of SBP should be considered for liver transplantation. The main causes of death in these patients are recurrent episodes of SBP, liver failure, and gastrointestinal hemorrhage.

Prophylaxis

The administration of continuous antibiotic therapy is useful in the prevention of SBP in specific subsets of cirrhotic patients at high risk of developing this complication (Fig. 7.12). Selective intestinal decontamination (with norfloxacin, ciprofloxacin, ofloxacin, or trimethoprim–sulfamethoxazole) is effective in the prevention of the first SBP episode (primary prophylaxis). Cirrhotic patients who have upper gastrointestinal bleeding are at high risk of developing severe bacterial infections, particularly SBP, within the first 5 days after the start of the hemorrhage (20% of patients are already infected at admission and 30–40% develop nosocomial

Antibiotics commonly used for the treatment of spontaneous bacterial peritonitis		
Antibiotic	Administration	Doses
Cefotaxime	Parenteral	2g/8h to 2g/12h
Ceftriaxone	Parenteral	1g/12h
Ceftizaxime	Parenteral	2g/8h
Cefonicid	Parenteral	2g/12h
Aztreonam	Parenteral	1g/8h
Amoxicilin + calvulanic acid	Parenteral/oral?	1g+200mg/6h
Ofloxacin	Oral	400mg/12h

Figure 7.11 Antibiotics commonly used for the treatment of spontaneous bacterial peritonitis.

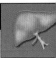

Efficacy of selective intestinal decontamination in patients at high risk of developing spontaneous bacterial peritonitis								
Primary prophylaxis						Secondary prophylaxis		
Patients with low ascitic fluid protein concentration*			Patients with upper gastrointestinal bleeding*			Patients with previous episode of SBP**		
Control patients	Treated patients	Antibiotic used	Control patients	Treated patients	Antibiotic used	Control patients	Treated patients	Antibiotic used
23%	0%	Norfloxacin 400mg/day	17%	3%	Neomycin, colistin and nystatin	68%	20%	Norfloxacin 400mg/day
22%	4%	Ciprofloxacin 750mg/week	21%	9%	Norfloxacin 400mg/day			
8%	0%	Norfloxacin 400mg/day						
27%	3%	Cotrimoxazole 5 x week						

Figure 7.12 Efficacy of selective intestinal decontamination in patients at high risk of developing spontaneous bacterial peritonitis. *Figures represent the percentage of patients developing SBP. **Figures represent the probability of SBP recurrence 1 year after initiation of treatment.

infection during the hospitalization period). Several studies have demonstrated that selective intestinal decontamination with norfloxacin orally or nonselective decontamination with oral, nonabsorbable antibiotics are effective in preventing SBP. Systemic antibiotic therapy has also been used satisfactorily for preventing SBP in these patients. Therefore, prophylactic antibiotics should be given to all noninfected cirrhotic patients who have upper gastrointestinal hemorrhage, regardless of the cause of bleeding. Oral antibiotics are probably more suitable than parenteral because of lower cost. In particular, norfloxacin is recommended during the first 5 days after the onset of hemorrhage.

Hospitalized cirrhotic patients who have low ascitic fluid protein concentration have a high incidence of bacterial infections, especially SBP. It has been demonstrated that cirrhotic patients who have protein concentration in ascitic fluid below 10g/L (1.0g/dL) develop SBP during hospital stay with a significantly higher frequency than those who have a greater protein content. Comparative randomized trials, however, are needed before this can be recommended as an indication for primary prophylaxis. Finally, it has been suggested that long-term primary prophylaxis in cirrhotic patients who have low ascitic fluid protein concentration and/or high serum albumin could be useful for preventing the first episode of SBP. However, further studies should also be performed before this therapy is recommended in clinical practice.

Long-term selective intestinal decontamination, either with norfloxacin, ciprofloxacin, ofloxacin, or trimethoprim–sulfamethoxazole, is also very effective in the prevention of SBP recurrence in cirrhotic patients (secondary prophylaxis). The probability of SBP recurrence at 1 year of follow-up is reduced from 70 to 20% (Fig. 7.13). This reduction is due to a decrease in the probability of developing SBP recurrence caused by Gram-negative bacilli (3% versus 60% at 1 year). The antibiotic prophylaxis does not increase the probability of developing SBP or

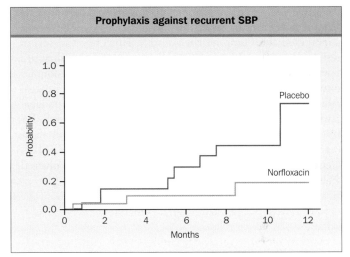

Figure 7.13 Prophylaxis against recurrent spontaneous bacterial peritonitis. Recurrence of spontaneous bacterial peritonitis in cirrhotic patients on long-term secondary prophylaxis with oral norfloxacin compared with placebo. (Reproduced with permission of Ginès et al., Hepatology. 1990;12:716–24 .)

other infections caused by Gram-positive bacteria or Gram-negative resistant organisms. Bacteriologic studies of the fecal flora in patients treated with norfloxacin show a marked reduction or disappearance of Gram-negative bacilli a few days after the initiation of treatment. By contrast, no significant changes in Gram-positive cocci, anaerobic bacteria, and *Candida* spp. occur during treatment. Antibiotic prophylaxis after resolution of SBP should be given to all patients who have SBP, regardless of the type of bacteria responsible for the index episode, because Gram-negative bacteria are the most common isolates in recurrent SBP.

PRACTICE POINT

Illustrative case

A 56-year-old man who had alcoholic cirrhosis presented with abdominal distention. He had been diagnosed 3 years previously and had abstained totally from alcohol since that time. On examination he had moderate ascites and splenomegaly. He was not jaundiced but did have cutaneous stigmata of chronic liver disease. The initial investigations revealed serum sodium 135mmol/L (130mEq/L), serum potassium 4.1mmol/L (4.1mEq/L), serum creatinine 106μmol/L (1.2mg/dL), serum bilirubin 19mmol/L (1.1mg/dL), serum albumin 29g/L, and an international normalized ratio of 1.6. The a-fetoprotein was 11IU/mL. The urinary sodium concentration was 6mmol/L (6mEq/L). The ultrasound examination of the abdomen revealed a small liver, portal vein thrombosis without collateralization, splenomegaly, and moderate ascites.

The patient was put on a 1.5L fluid restriction and was commenced on spironolactone 100mg daily. There was no immediate improvement and the spironolactone dose was increased to 200mg on the 4th day. However, the serum sodium fell to 127mmol/L (127mEq/L) and the diuretics were withdrawn. He then had a 7L paracentesis with albumin supplementation. The following day he had his index variceal bleed and was managed by band ablation of esophageal varices. However, the ascites recurred and on the 11th day after hospitalization he developed encephalopathy. A diagnostic paracentesis was performed and this showed a PMNL count of 560 /mm3 and E. coli was subsequently cultured from the ascites. The protein content of the ascites was 7g/L (0.7g/dL). This was treated with appropriate antibiotics. Over the subsequent 3 weeks he made steady progress and was discharged from hospital on spironolactone 100mg daily and with no clinical evidence of ascites. To prevent further episodes of SBP, he was given norfloxacin (400mg/daily).

Interpretation

This case illustrates the inter-relationship between different complications of cirrhosis. The sudden development of ascites was probably due to the recent thrombosis of the portal vein, which in turn increased the pressure in the esophageal variceal bed. This increased the risk of variceal hemorrhage. The temporal relationship between the paracentesis and the hemorrhage was probably not coincidental and this scenario is frequently seen in clinical practice, even though it has not been definitively described in the literature. The variceal hemorrhage led to worsening of the ascites and increased the risk of SBP. This in turn induced encephalopathy.

The therapeutic options for the ascites were limited in this case. The hyponatremia prevented the aggressive use of diuretics. The fear that paracentesis precipitated the variceal bleed dampened enthusiasm for repeated paracentesis. The portal vein thrombosis precluded the placement of a TIPSS. The satisfactory outcome in this case was fortunate as these patients usually cannot be salvaged by liver transplantation over the time period of the evolution of these complications.

FURTHER READING

Andreu M, Solà R, Sitges-Serra A, et al. Risk factors for spontaneous bacterial peritonitis in cirrhotic patients with ascites. Gastroenterology. 1993;104:1133–8. *Clinical description of risk factors for SBP.*

Arroyo V, Ginès P, Gerbes AL, et al. Definition and diagnostic criteria of refractory ascites and hepatorenal syndrome in cirrhosis. Hepatology. 1996;23:164–76. *International initiative on nomenclature and definitions in ascites.*

Bosch-Marcè M, Jimènez WP, Angeli P, et al. Aquaretic effect of the kappa-opioid agonist RU 51599 in cirrhotic rats with ascites and water retention. Gastroenterology. 1995;109:217–23. *Potential revolutionary advance in the management of water retention.*

Ginès P, Rimola A, Planas R, et al. Norfloxacin prevents spontaneous bacterial peritonitis recurrence in cirrhosis: Results of a double blind, placebo-controlled trial. Hepatology. 1990;12:716–24. *Clinical study establishing role for secondary prophylaxis.*

Ginès P, Arroyo V, Vargas V, et al. Paracentesis with intravenous infusion of albumin as compared with peritoneovenous shunting in cirrhosis with refractory ascites. N Eng J Med. 1991;325:829–35. *Rebirth of paracentesis.*

Ginès A, Fernández-Esparrach G, Monescillo A, et al. Randomized trial comparing albumin, dextran 70, and polygeline in cirrhotic patients who have ascites treated by paracentesis. Gastroenterology. 1996;111:1002–10. *Clinical trial assessing optimal volume expansion regimens in patients with ascites.*

Lebrec D, Giuily N, Hadengue A, et al. Transjugular intrahepatic portosystemic shunts: comparison with paracentesis in patients with cirrhosis and refractory ascites: a randomized trial. J Hepatol. 1996;25:135–44. *Outline of role of TIPS in management of intractable ascites.*

Llach J, Ginès P, Arroyo V, et al. Prognostic value of arterial pressure, endogenous vasoactive systems and renal function in cirrhosis who have ascites. Gastroenterology. 1988;94:482–7. *Clinical correlations with prognosis in patients with ascites.*

Navasa M, Follo A, Llovet JM, et al. Randomized, comparative study of oral ofloxacin versus intravenous cefotaxime in spontaneous bacterial peritonitis. Gastroenterology. 1996;111:1011–7. *Important study in the treatment of spontaneous bacterial peritonitis.*

Schrier RW, Arroyo V, Bernardi M, et al. Peripheral arterial vasodilation hypothesis: a proposal for the initiation of renal sodium and water retention in cirrhosis. Hepatology. 1988;8:1151–7. *An important study of the pathophysiology of ascites.*

Soriano G, Guarner C, Tomás A, et al. Norfloxacin prevents bacterial infection in cirrhotics with gastrointestinal hemorrhage. Gastroenterology. 1992;103:1267–72. *The link between spontaneous bacterial peritonitis and gastrointestinal hemorrhage and its prevention.*

Sort P, Navasa M, Arroyo V, et al. Effect of intravenous albumin on renal impairment and mortality in patients with cirrhosis and spontaneous bacterial peritonitis. N Engl J Med. 1999;341:403–9.

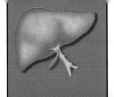

Chapter 8

Hepatorenal Syndrome and Other Renal Diseases

Kevin Moore

INTRODUCTION

The development of renal failure in a patient who has liver disease is not synonymous with hepatorenal syndrome. Renal failure may be due to a variety of causes and these are listed in Figure 8.1. The most common cause in clinical practice is hypovolemia, often due to the use of diuretics.

Hepatorenal syndrome is defined as the development of renal failure in patients who have severe liver disease (acute or chronic) in the absence of any other identifiable cause of renal pathology. It may occur in patients who have cirrhosis and in those with acute liver failure. It is diagnosed after exclusion of other causes of renal failure in patients who have liver disease such as hypovolemia, drug nephrotoxicity, sepsis or glomerulonephritis (Fig. 8.2). For patients developing renal failure in the context of liver disease, the most important question to ask is whether the liver disease is sufficiently severe to cause renal failure, and whether other causes have been excluded.

The prognosis of hepatorenal syndrome is poor with a mortality of 50–95%, depending on the underlying etiology. Survival and recovery of renal function is generally dependent on improvement of liver function due to recovery from the liver insult, effective hepatic regeneration or liver transplantation. Survival is therefore most commonly observed in those who have acute alcoholic hepatitis or acute liver failure, both of which may resolve spontaneously.

PATHOGENESIS

The pathogenesis of hepatorenal syndrome is multifactorial and an outline of the main steps is given in Figure 8.3. The key elements involved in causing renal failure are a reduction of renal blood flow (RBF) (Figs 8.4 & 8.5), and a decrease in the filtration fraction, perhaps as a consequence of mesangial cell contraction (Fig. 8.6). The emphasis of each of the three pathogenic pathways

Causes of liver dysfunction associated with renal abnormalities
Cirrhosis or acute liver failure
Hepatorenal syndrome Hypovolemia Nephrotoxic drugs Nonsteroidal anti-inflammatory drugs (cyclo-oxygenase inhibitors) Sepsis
Cholestatic liver disease
Obstructive jaundice Primary biliary cirrhosis Sclerosing cholangitis
Infectious diseases
Sepsis syndrome Hepatitis B or C virus Malaria Leptospirosis Human immunodeficiency virus Infectious mononucleosis
Toxins
Carbon tetrachloride Other industrial toxins
Systemic diseases
Amyloid Sickle cell disease Connective tissue diseases Hemochromatosis Wilson's disease
Pregnancy
Pregnancy-associated hypertension Acute fatty liver
Polycystic disease

Figure 8.1 Causes of liver dysfunction associated with renal abnormalities.

Criteria for the diagnosis of hepatorenal syndrome
Major criteria
Chronic or acute liver disease with advanced hepatic failure and portal hypertension
Low GFR as indicated by serum creatinine >1.5mg/dL (200μmol/L) or creatinine clearance <40mL/min
Absence of shock, ongoing bacterial infection, and recent treatment with nephrotoxic drugs. Absence of excessive fluid losses (including gastrointestinal bleeding)
No sustained improvement of renal function following expansion with 1.5L of isotonic saline or colloid
Proteinuria <0.5g/day, and no ultrasonagraphic evidence of renal tract disease
Additional criteria
Urine volume <500mL/day Urine sodium <10mmol/L or 10mEq/L Urine osmolality >plasma osmolality Urine RBC <50 per high per field

Figure 8.2 Criteria for the diagnosis of hepatorenal syndrome. The additional criteria relate to factors that are commonly present, but are not required for the diagnosis.

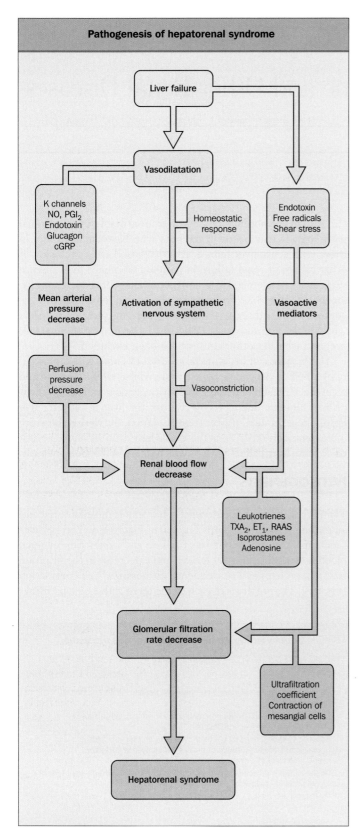

Pathogenesis of hepatorenal syndrome

Liver failure

Vasodilatation

K channels
NO, PGI$_2$
Endotoxin
Glucagon
cGRP

Homeostatic response

Endotoxin
Free radicals
Shear stress

Mean arterial pressure decrease

Activation of sympathetic nervous system

Vasoactive mediators

Perfusion pressure decrease

Vasoconstriction

Renal blood flow decrease

Leukotrienes
TXA$_2$, ET$_1$, RAAS
Isoprostanes
Adenosine

Glomerular filtration rate decrease

Ultrafiltration coefficient
Contraction of mesangial cells

Hepatorenal syndrome

Figure 8.3 Pathogenesis of hepatorenal syndrome. This scheme outlines the major pathophysiologic steps and some of the underlying mechanisms. NO, nitric oxide; PGI$_2$, prostacyclin; cGRP, calcitonin gene-related peptide; TXA$_2$, thromboxane A$_2$; ET-1, endothelin-1; RAAS, renin–angiotensin–aldosterone system.

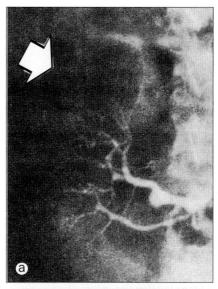

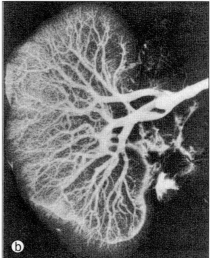

Figure 8.4 Vasoconstriction characteristic of hepatorenal syndrome. Many studies have shown a marked reduction of renal blood flow in patients who have the hepatorenal syndrome. (a) This angiogram shows marked renal vasoconstriction of the lobular, and interarcuate arteries in a patient who has hepatorenal syndrome. Arrow indicates area with no evident arterial flow. (b) A repeat angiogram in the same patient following their death showed relaxation and normal renal vasculature. (From M Epstein et al. Hepatorenal syndrome. 1988;89–118.)

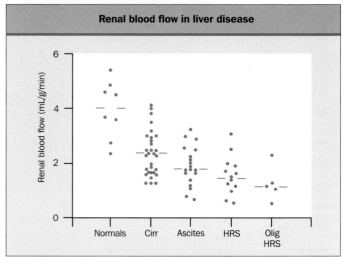

Renal blood flow in liver disease

Figure 8.5 Renal blood flow (RBF) in liver disease. Using Xenon washout studies, Ring-Larsen has shown that there is a progressive reduction of RBF in patients who have decompensated liver disease and hepatorenal syndrome. The most striking aspect of this data, however, is the wide overlap of RBF observed in those who have hepatorenal syndrome (HRS), and those who have ascites, but relatively intact renal function. Cirr., cirrhosis; Olig., oliguric. (Adapted from Ring-Larsen. Gut. 1977;37:635–42.)

Effect of mesangial cell contraction

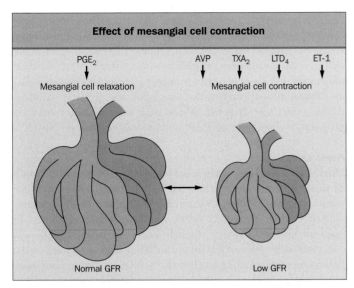

PGE$_2$ → Mesangial cell relaxation

AVP TXA$_2$ LTD$_4$ ET-1 → Mesangial cell contraction

Normal GFR   Low GFR

Figure 8.6 Effect of mesangial cell contraction on the size and surface area of the glomerulus. The glomerulus is a dynamic structure invaginated with mesangial cells, which express actin and can contract in response to agonists such as endothelin-1. This figure shows the effect of mesangial cell contraction on the size and surface area of the glomerulus. Contraction of the mesangial cells decreases the glomerular capillary ultrafiltration coefficient. AVP, arginine vasopressin; ET-1, endothelin-1; LTD$_4$, leukotriene D$_4$; PGE$_2$, prostaglandin E$_2$; TXA$_2$, thromboxane A$_2$.

Factors involved in the pathogenesis of hepatorenal syndrome

Hemodynamic changes causing reduced renal perfusion pressure
Stimulated sympathetic nervous system
Increased synthesis of humoral and renal vasoactive mediators

Figure 8.7 Factors involved in the pathogenesis of hepatorenal syndrome.

Renal autoregulation in hepatorenal syndrome

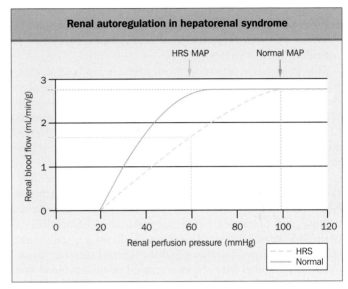

Figure 8.8 Renal autoregulation in hepatorenal syndrome (HRS). Renal autoregulation ensures that there are no major changes in RBF during fluctuations of blood pressure within a reasonably broad physiologic range. However, below about 65mmHg there is a linear fall in RBF with decreasing arterial pressure. In states of sympathetic activation (e.g. HRS) there is a leftward shift in the effector response curve, such that RBF is much more pressure sensitive. Thus, a modest decrease in mean arterial pressure together with an increase in renal sympathetic tone ± renal venous pressure will cause a significant decrease of RBF. MAP, mean arterial pressure.

(Fig. 8.7) probably varies from patient to patient, and between the acute (type 1) and the chronic form (type 2) of hepatorenal syndrome. Each of these pathways are interrelated, and the pathophysiology of this process is complex.

Hemodynamic characteristics

Autoregulation of the renal circulation ensures a stable RBF during changes of renal perfusion pressure (i.e. mean arterial pressure minus renal venous pressure). This normally operates above a mean pressure of 70–75mmHg (Fig. 8.8), and below this level RBF decreases in direct proportion to perfusion pressure. The renal response to decreased blood pressure is, however, altered in severe liver disease in which there is an activated sympathetic system, and increased synthesis of several renal vasoconstrictors. Several animal studies have shown that this causes a rightward shift in the autoregulatory curve, making RBF more pressure-dependent. Thus, as shown in Figure 8.8, even modest decreases in mean arterial pressure may result in a marked fall of RBF. Whether other humoral renal vasoconstrictors that are increased in the hepatorenal syndrome cause a rightward shift in the renal autoregulatory curve is unknown. However, it is likely that any renal vasoconstrictor will make RBF more pressure-dependent. The importance of these comments is clear when it is realized that several studies have consistently shown a progressive decrease in mean arterial pressure with hepatic decompensation, with the lowest values (typically 60–65mmHg) observed in patients who have the hepatorenal syndrome.

The presence of a reduced mean arterial pressure in decompensated patients who have cirrhosis is a risk factor for the development of hepatorenal syndrome. While arterial pressure is decreased there is also an increase in the renal venous pressure. Renal venous pressure (normally less than 5mmHg), may

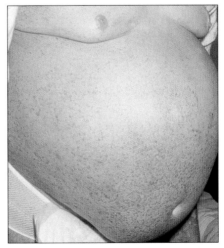

Figure 8.9 Clinical setting for hepatorenal syndrome. The presence of tense ascites in a patient who has cirrhosis can cause a significant increase in renal venous pressure, and intrathoracic pressure. Note this patient also has gynecomastia secondary to the use of spironolactone.

be significantly increased in the presence of tense ascites or as a consequence of cirrhosis itself (Fig. 8.9), and this coupled with a decreased arterial pressure will cause a further decrease of RBF. In normal animals an increase in renal venous pressure causes activation of compensatory pathways. While it is conventional to describe the renal perfusion pressure as being the mean arterial pressure minus the renal venous pressure, there are several vascular beds between the arterial and venous system, such that there is a gradated downward trend in pressure throughout the kidney (Fig. 8.10).

However, it is self-evident that an increase in renal venous pressure must have a negative effect on glomerular plasma flow and hence glomerular filtration rate (GFR). An increase in intra-abdominal pressure has been shown to increase renal production of prostaglandin E_2, which may have an important role in the preservation of renal function, and inhibition of prostaglandin synthesis by cyclo-oxygenase inhibitors causes renal failure in patients who have ascites.

The importance of arterial blood pressure has been demonstrated conclusively in several studies. Infusion of various agonists that increase blood pressure have all been reported to increase urine output, sodium excretion or GFR with variable success. Ornipressin improves renal function acutely, and prolonged administration of ornipressin has a sustained effect in patients developing hepatorenal syndrome (Fig. 8.11).

The presence of modest arterial hypotension raises the question about its cause. It is well established that severe liver disease is characterized by an increase in cardiac output and plasma volume, and decreased peripheral vascular resistance due to peripheral vasodilatation. This is mainly limited to either the splanchnic circulation or that supplying skin and muscular tissue. While some studies have shown increased peripheral blood flow to the limbs, other studies do not support these findings. The primary mechanism is unknown. Splanchnic vasodilatation is partly related to portal hypertension and the opening of portosystemic shunts and minor arteriovenous fistulae, and portovenous shunts within the cirrhotic liver have recently been described. Thus, vasodilatation in cirrhosis is partly related to this shunting of blood from the systemic to the venous circulation. There is general acceptance that vascular reactivity is impaired in cirrhosis since isolated vessels have impaired responsiveness to

vascular agonists. Ultimately several mediators, either singly or in concert, may be responsible for the decreased vascular reactivity, or the opening of these anatomic shunts. Plasma levels of many endogenous vasodilators, as well as vasoconstrictors are elevated in liver failure. In view of the multiple interactions between various vasoactive substances, the search for 'the' primary vasodilator is extremely difficult. More than one mediator may be involved, and several potential mediators have been proposed.

Nitric oxide

Nitric oxide (NO) is synthesized in mammalian cells by a family of three nitric oxide synthases (NOSs). Initially two of these were designated iNOS, or inducible NOS, and cNOS, or constitutive NOS. Inducible NOS was found to be induced in macrophages and vascular smooth muscle cells, and cNOS was constitutively expressed in endothelial and neuronal cells. Following many cloning studies these NOS isoforms have now been redesignated into immunoactivated NOS (iNOS), neuronal NOS (nNOS), and endothelial NOS (eNOS), reflecting their tissue of origin. Neuronal NOS was originally purified in neuronal tissue, but is more widely distributed with an important component in skeletal muscle. Immunoactivated NOS was originally purified from an immunoactivated macrophage cell line, but is present in vascular smooth muscle, and cardiac tissue as well as glial cells. Endothelial NOS was originally described in endothelial cells, but is also present in platelets, cardiac myocytes, hippocampus and elsewhere.

Since NO causes vasorelaxation, it was not long before it was suggested that increased NO synthesis in cirrhosis may account for the vasodilatation of liver disease. Nitric oxide synthesis may be induced by shear stress, or in response to endotoxin-related cytokine expression. The observation that many patients who have decompensated cirrhosis have circulating endotoxemia seemed to provide the missing link. Studies in patients who have decompensated cirrhosis have shown increased plasma nitrite or nitrate indicative of increased NO production. However, it has

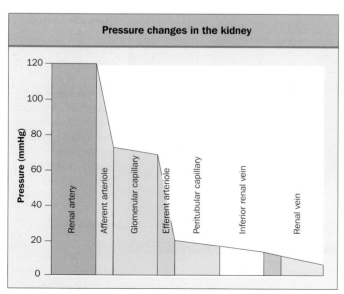

Figure 8.10 Renal pressure gradient. The pressure gradient changes as blood passes from an arterial to a venous circulation.

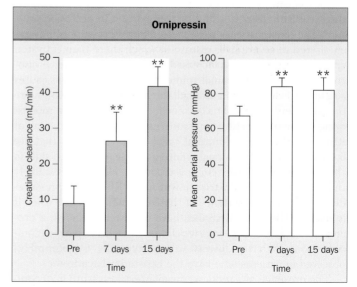

Figure 8.11 Ornipressin. Infusion of ornipressin to patients with the hepatorenal syndrome increases their blood pressure and improves their renal function (GFR) (** signifies $p < 0.05$). (From Guevera et al. Hepatology. 1988;27:35–41.)

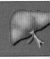

been extremely difficult to demonstrate induction of iNOS in human cells. Cells isolated from the ascitic fluid of patients who have bacterial peritonitis show increased NO synthesis, as do cells isolated from infected urine. Virtually all studies on NOS in liver disease have been carried out in the rat, where the relevance to humans is unclear. In the rat, the studies have yielded a variety of conflicting results in different models. Pharmacologic studies using isolated vascular rings or the mesenteric vasculature have shown decreased vascular reactivity to several agonists, and inhibition of NOS restores or partially restores vascular responsiveness. Likewise studies *in vivo* have shown that inhibition of NO synthesis reverses the systemic and splanchnic circulatory changes in animal models and patients to a greater extent than in controls, suggesting that NO synthesis is increased and contributory. Recent studies in the carbon tetrachloride model of cirrhosis showed increased expression of eNOS in the aorta and mesenteric artery of cirrhotic rats. Administration of L-NG-nitroarginine methylester (L-NAME), an inhibitor of NOS, prevented activation of the neurohumoral systems (vasopressin, renin, and aldosterone system) and normalized sodium excretion. However, studies in the biliary cirrhotic model, which has similar hemodynamic characteristics, do not support the NO hypothesis. Thus, while there still enthusiasm for a primary role of NO in peripheral vasodilatation, there is considerable controversy as to its importance in the hyperdynamic circulation of cirrhosis.

Nitric oxide also circulates or exists in tissues as a vasodilator in other forms such as nitrosothiols, and nitroso–iron complexes. These complexes are formed through undefined mechanisms. While it is known that they may be formed by the reaction of peroxynitrite (itself formed from the reaction of NO with superoxide) with thiol groups on proteins or peptides, it is likely that they are formed through specific pathways. Circulating nitrosothiols may then circulate, functioning as long-acting NO donors.

Glucagon

Plasma glucagon levels are elevated in cirrhosis. Glucagon causes desensitization of the mesenteric circulation to catecholamines and angiotensin II, and causes vasodilatation at pharmacologic doses. Glucagon also elevates intracellular cyclic adenosine monophosphate (cAMP). Recent studies have shown that raised cAMP acts synergistically with endotoxin to induce NOS, and thus NO release by vascular smooth muscle cells. Thus glucagon may enhance NO production in cirrhosis. Whether the therapeutic use of catecholamines to elevate blood pressure, which also elevate cAMP, further enhances NO production when endotoxemia is present is unknown and warrants further study.

Prostacyclin

Prostacyclin is a systemic vasodilatator formed in vascular endothelium. Its secretion might be stimulated by shear stress of the splanchnic arterioles. Urinary excretion of both systemic and renal metabolites of prostacyclin are high in decompensated cirrhosis, and plasma levels (undetectable by available analytic methods), are presumably elevated (Fig. 8.12).

The most convincing evidence to suggest that prostacyclin may be involved in systemic vasodilatation is the observation that administration of indomethacin to cirrhotic patients increases systemic vascular resistance and decreases cardiac output. Likewise, the administration of indomethacin to cirrhotic patients also increases the pressor sensitivity to angiotensin II. Thus,

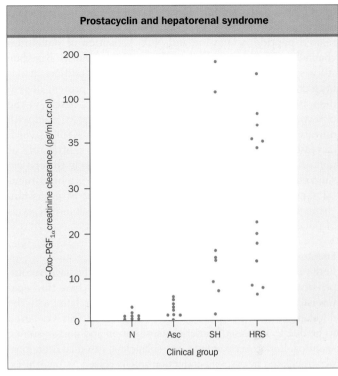

Figure 8.12 Prostacyclin and hepatorenal syndrome. Urinary 6-oxo-$PGF_{1\alpha}$ (a marker of prostacyclin synthesis) is increased in patients who have decompensated liver disease as well as those who have the hepatorenal syndrome. Asc, ascites; SH, severe hepatitis; HRS, hepatorenal syndrome. (From Moore et al. Gastroenterology. 1991;100:1069–77.)

increased endothelial prostacyclin synthesis may be an important pathway causing systemic vasodilatation.

Potassium channels

Small arteries exist in a partially contracted state from which they can constrict further or dilate. Much of this inherent arterial tone is caused by transmural pressure and is termed myogenic tone. The muscle tone in small arteries and arterioles is responsible for peripheral vascular resistance. The membrane potential of arterial smooth muscle cells is regulated by potassium channels. When potassium channels open there is potassium efflux, membrane hyperpolarization, closure of voltage-dependent calcium channels and vasodilatation. Conversely, inhibition of potassium channel opening causes vasoconstriction. There are four distinct types of potassium channel that control the flux of potassium from the intracellular to the extracellular environment. These are designated K_V, K_{Ca}, K_{IR} and K_{ATP}, and represent voltage-dependent, calcium-activated, inward rectifier and adenosine triphosphate (ATP)-sensitive, respectively. Voltage-dependent potassium channels open during membrane depolarization, and are thought to act mainly to limit membrane depolarization. The ATP-sensitive potassium channels are opened during low ATP: adenosine diphosphate (ADP) ratios, or by agonist induced activation of G-protein-dependent pathways. The delayed rectifier channel is opened by membrane depolarization, and the calcium-activated potassium channel is activated by increases in intracellular calcium in a similar manner to that for ATP-dependent potassium channels. Activation of potassium channels can cause vasodilatation due to hyperpolarization of vascular smooth muscle cells. Potentially important activators include tissue hypoxia, prostacyclin, calcitonin gene-related peptide, adenosine and NO. Activation of potassium channels is important in the vasodilatation of cirrhosis. Based on studies with potassium and calcium channel modifiers, it has been proposed that there is an impairment of G-protein-dependent transduction pathways. This hypothesis is based on the observation that hyporeactivity of vessels is not associated with downregulation of receptors, and reactivity to Bay K8644 (which increases intracellular calcium) is normal. The central role of potassium channels in vascular tone makes it likely that potassium channels are important, but whether there is a fundamental abnormality of function of a particular type of potassium channel, or whether function is abnormal due to abnormal levels of potassium channel activators is unresolved.

Endotoxemia and cytokines

Endotoxin levels are usually elevated in patients who have decompensated liver disease and more so in patients who have the hepatorenal syndrome. A higher titer of endotoxin correlated with the development of hepatorenal syndrome (Fig. 8.13). This is believed to be due to increased bacterial translocation and portosystemic shunting. Endotoxemia may cause splanchnic vasodilatation, possibly mediated by cytokine induction and increased NO synthesis. Infusion of lipopolysaccharide into animals causes complement activation, an accumulation of neutrophils in the liver and renal dysfunction. The renal dysfunction that occurs can be blocked by both leukotriene and thromboxane antagonists. These studies, however, used large doses of acute endotoxin, rather than the low-grade endotoxemia observed in hepatorenal syndrome. There are increased circulating levels of several cytokines, including tumor necrosis factor (TNF) and interleukin (IL)-6, particularly in

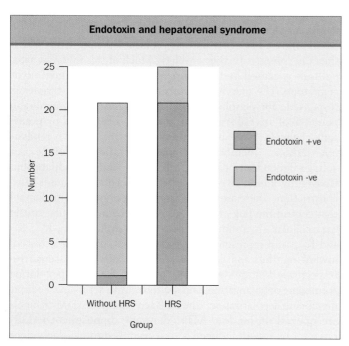

Figure 8.13 Endotoxin and hepatorenal syndrome (HRS). Using the limulus assay, Wilkinson et al. observed that 21 of 25 patients who had HRS were limulus test-positive (i.e. they had detectable endotoxin), whereas 19 of 21 patients who had preserved renal function were normal. (From Wilkinson et al. BMJ. 1976;2:1415–8.)

patients who have alcoholic hepatitis and hepatorenal syndrome, and recent studies in the rat have shown that the systemic vasodilatation observed in the partial portal vein ligated model is blocked by anti-TNF antibodies. The applicability of rat studies, in which iNOS induction by endotoxin and other cytokines is marked, to humans, in which induction of iNOS maybe less marked, is uncertain. In humans it has been very difficult to cause induction of iNOS. Incubation of vessels with endotoxin, TNF-α, or IL-6 are without effect, even when given to isolated blood vessels *in vivo*. However, administration of interferon-α to patients with hepatitis C causes induction of iNOS in circulating monocytes. An alternative pathway that may be involved is the induction of guanosine triphosphate (GTP) cyclohydrolase, which regulates the synthesis of tetrahydrobiopterin, a rate-limiting factor for eNOS. Thus, evidence is now beginning to accumulate that in humans, at least, the upregulation of eNOS may be the main factor responsible for increased generation of NO.

Adenosine

Adenosine is an endogenous nucleoside derived mainly from the intracellular catabolism of ATP. It induces vasodilatation of most vascular beds including the splanchnic circulation. In the kidney, however, it causes renal vasoconstriction, and increases responsiveness to angiotensin II. Administration of dipyridamole, which enhances the action of endogenous adenosine by inhibiting uptake and degradation, to patients who have cirrhosis decreases RBF.

The splanchnic circulation

The changes in the splanchnic circulation in patients who have cirrhosis develop over a considerable period of time, and splenic blood flow increases with the opening up of various portosystemic shunts. Since the systemic vascular resistance (SVR) is derived from the mean arterial pressure divided by cardiac output, then any mechanism that increases cardiac output, with the maintenance of a normal arterial pressure, is bound to decrease SVR. Thus the development of portosystemic collaterals, and secondary increase of arterial blood flow, will clearly lower vascular resistance. While it is tempting to speculate that in cirrhosis a point is reached when compensation cannot be maintained, and thus arterial pressure falls, the argument is less applicable to the decompensation that occurs in acute liver failure or acute alcoholic hepatitis. While one could argue that in cirrhosis the splanchnic vasodilatation develops over a long period of time, the fact that similar changes and renal functional changes occur in acute liver failure or alcoholic hepatitis cannot be ignored. Indeed, portal hypertension can occur acutely, or be exacerbated in such circumstances, but whether this causes the acute development of collaterals sufficient to cause the systemic vasodilatation as observed is unknown.

Implications of vasodilatation

The normal homeostatic response to vasodilatation is the activation of several neurohumoral response mechanisms, primarily aimed at the maintenance of arterial pressure, and should generally be considered beneficial rather than adversarial. These responses may be summarized as:

- activation of the sympathetic nervous system;
- activation of the renin–angiotensin–aldosterone system;
- increased vasopressin release; and
- increased renal production of vasodilatory prostanoids.

Although activations of these neurohumoral mechanisms are essential in maintaining homeostasis, some also induce renal vasoconstriction. This is not surprising since the renal vascular bed normally receives 25% of cardiac output, and is an important regulatory point of blood pressure control. By altering the normal renal autoregulatory response, these mechanisms may contribute to the decreased renal blood flow observed in hepatorenal syndrome.

The renin–angiotensin–aldosterone system (RAAS) is stimulated in 50–80% of patients who have decompensated cirrhosis, and is further elevated in patients who have hepatorenal syndrome. Increased levels of angiotensin II protect renal function by selective vasoconstriction of the efferent glomerular arterioles. Although RBF may fall, GFR is preserved due to an increased filtration fraction. In cirrhosis, inhibition of the RAAS by either saralasin or angiotensin converting enzyme inhibitors (e.g. captopril) causes marked hypotension and decreases GFR, whereas infusion of angiotensin II in cirrhosis has been shown to improve glomerular filtration in some patients, presumably because it may increase arterial pressure, and thus renal perfusion.

Antidiuretic hormone (ADH) or vasopressin levels are elevated due to nonosmolar stimulation, despite the frequent presence of hyponatremia. Vasopressin causes vasoconstriction through V_1-receptors and renal tubular water retention through V_2-receptors in the medullary collecting ducts. This increases volume expansion by water retention, and helps to maintain arterial pressure. Inhibition of V_1-receptors in cirrhotic rats causes profound hypotension. Vasopressin, however, preferentially causes splanchnic rather than renal vasoconstriction. Vasopressin analogs increase blood pressure and presumably systemic vascular resistance, and decrease plasma angiotensin and catecholamine levels. This results in increased urine flow and sodium excretion.

Renal prostaglandins play an important role in the preservation of renal function in all situations with elevated plasma levels of renin, angiotensin, norepinephrine (noradrenaline) or vasopressin, such as dehydration, congestive cardiac failure, shock or decompensated liver disease. In the latter situation urinary excretion of prostaglandin (PG)E_2 and prostacyclin metabolites (6-oxo-$PGF_{1\alpha}$) are increased. The mechanism for increased synthesis of these prostaglandins is unknown, but is likely to be secondary to the increased levels of the vasoconstrictors, many of which have been shown to cause prostaglandin formation *in vitro* or *in vivo*. Administration of cyclo-oxygenase inhibitors (nonsteroidal anti-inflammatory drugs [NSAIDs]) to patients who have ascites frequently cause renal failure, and this usually reverses on cessation of NSAIDs (Fig. 8.14).

Some workers have suggested that hepatorenal syndrome is caused by a deficiency of renal PGE_2 and prostacyclin since urinary excretion of PGE_2 and the prostacyclin metabolite 6-oxo-$PGF_{1\alpha}$ are low in hepatorenal syndrome compared with patients who have ascites but preserved renal function. Other studies, however, have shown that synthesis of prostacyclin is actually increased, but urinary excretion of its metabolite is decreased by the presence of renal failure (Fig. 8.15).

However, the ratio of urinary prostacyclin metabolites to thromboxane A_2 is not correlated with the development of renal failure. Postmortem immunohistochemical studies have shown that prostaglandin endoperoxide synthase is markedly decreased in medullary collecting tubules of patients who have hepatorenal syndrome compared with patients who have liver failure but normal renal function. However, prostacyclin synthase levels

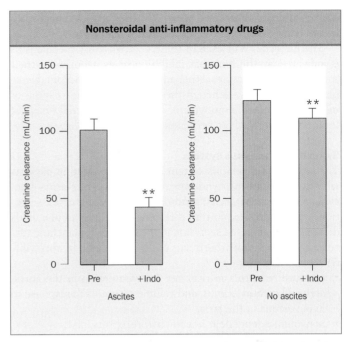

Figure 8.14 Nonsteroidal anti-inflammatory drugs. Administration of nonsteroidal anti-inflammatory drugs such as indomethacin cause a reduction of renal bloodflow and glomerular filtration rate (** signifies $p<0.05$). (Adapted from Boyer et al. Gastroenterology. 1979;77:215–22.)

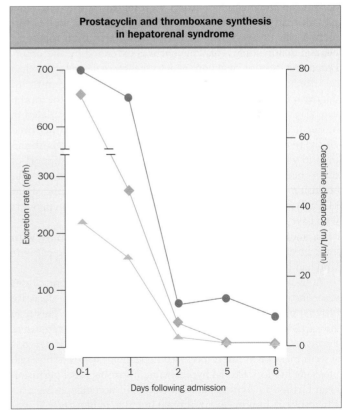

Figure 8.15 Prostacyclin and thromboxane synthesis in hepatorenal syndrome. Urinary excretion of both 6-oxo-$PGF_{1\alpha}$ and TXB_2, markers of prostacyclin and thromboxane synthesis, respectively, decrease in parallel to the fall in creatinine clearance in patients developing the hepatorenal syndrome. Blue circle, creatinine clearance; red diamond, TXB_2; green triangle, 6-oxo-$PGF_{1\alpha}$.

were unaltered. There have been no further histochemical studies to confirm this, and the mechanism is unknown.

The importance of each of these compensatory mechanisms is indicated by the fact that inhibition or antagonism of their actions frequently causes either adverse systemic and/or adverse renal effects. Thus, although they may contribute to some or many of the renal hemodynamic changes, the overall result of their activation tends to be beneficial.

Sympathetic nervous system

The sympathetic nervous system is highly activated in patients who have hepatorenal syndrome. The elevation of plasma catecholamines in hepatorenal syndrome is due to increased secretion, and studies exploiting differences across vascular beds demonstrate increased secretion in the renal and splanchnic vascular beds. The sympathetic axis can be stimulated by three different mechanisms:

- pressure receptors in response to hypotension in the aortic arch and carotid glomus, and volume receptors in response to hypovolemia in the atria;
- nonvolume-dependent hepatic baroreceptors; and
- metabolic changes (c.f secretion in response to hypoglycemia).

All three of these mechanisms might be active in hepatorenal syndrome and with the current available data it is impossible to state which predominates.

The importance of the hepatorenal innervation has been recognized since the 1980s when it was found that increased intrahepatic pressure was associated with increased efferent renal sympathetic nervous system activity. The onset of ascites formation was delayed in dogs with bile duct ligation following hepatic denervation. This concept was extended by the observation that infusion of glutamine into the internal jugular vein had no effect on renal function, whereas it caused a significant decrease of both GFR and RBF when infused into the portal vein (Fig. 8.16). The mechanism is unknown but is postulated to be due to hepatocyte swelling. This effect seemed to be mediated via the renal nervous system since no effect was seen in those animals in which the renal nerves had been severed. In support of this concept in humans, recent studies have shown that acute occlusion of the transjugular intrahepatic portosystemic shunt (TIPSS) is associated with an acute reduction of RBF in patients who have cirrhosis (Fig. 8.17).

In another study, temporary lumbar sympathectomy with local anesthesia increased GFR in five of eight cirrhotic patients who had hepatorenal syndrome.

Activation of the renal sympathetic nervous system causes vasoconstriction of the afferent renal arterioles, with a decrease of renal plasma flow and GFR, and sodium retention. This may also activate renin secretion, resulting in further salt retention. Finally, as discussed above, activation of the sympathetic nervous system makes RBF more pressure-dependent, and α-adrenergic blockade induces arterial hypotension, impairing renal perfusion even further. In contrast, administration of norepinephrine usually results in improvement of renal function in hepatorenal syndrome, probably secondary to improved arterial pressure.

Humoral and renal vasoactive mediators

It is unlikely that the development of hepatorenal syndrome is purely a consequence of renal vasoconstriction. If one examines the relationship between RBF and the presence of hepatorenal

syndrome or hepatic decompensation, there is considerable cross-over in the RBF between these groups. Likewise the presence of an elevated 'resistive index', as determined by duplex Doppler ultrasonagraphy, indicative of renal vasoconstriction was a predictor of the development of hepatorenal syndrome in patients awaiting liver transplantation. While some studies

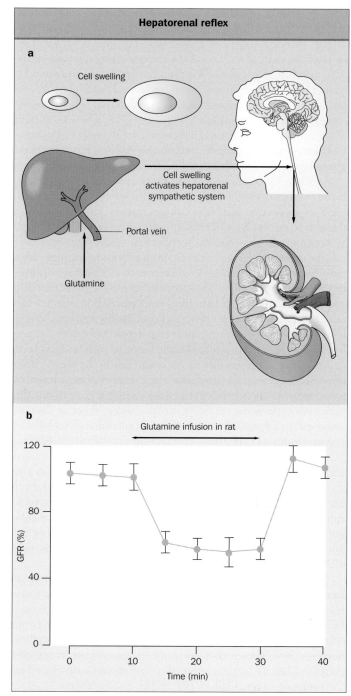

Figure 8.16 Hepatorenal reflex. (a) describes the renal pathway from liver through CNS to kidney. (b) shows the effect of glutamine infusion on glomerular filtration rate (GFR). Infusion of glutamine into the portal vein of a rat causes hepatic cell swelling. This is associated with a sudden reduction of renal blood flow. This response can be prevented by severing the renal sympathetic nerves, which indicates that the sympathetic pathway is involved.

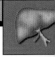

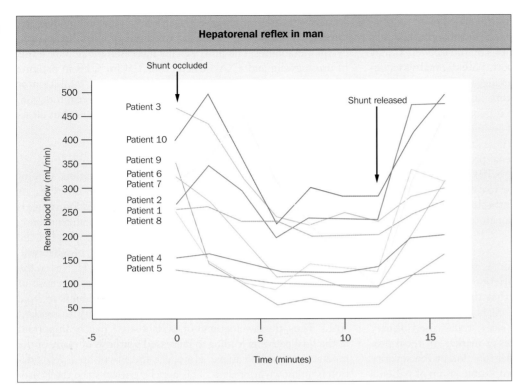
Hepatorenal reflex in man

Figure 8.17 Hepatorenal reflex and glutamine. To confirm the presence of a hepatorenal reflex in humans, Jalan et al. have demonstrated that there is an acute reduction of renal blood flow in cirrhotic patients following the acute inflation of a balloon within a transjugular intrahepatic portosystemic shunt. This causes an acute rise in portal pressure, and a fall in renal blood flow. (With permission from Gut. 1997;40:664–70.)

support the concept of a 'renal blood flow-dependent mechanism', others have noted a marked decrease in RBF in cirrhotic subjects with preserved renal function using intravascular Doppler probes. The observation that two patients may have a comparable decrease of RBF, and yet have either renal failure or 'near-normal renal function' suggests that other factors must be involved that decrease the filtration fraction. The glomeruli within the kidney are dynamic structures, invaginated with mesangial cells that may contract in response to several agonists, and thus reduce the surface area available for glomerular filtration. Many studies have now shown that there is increased synthesis of several vasoactive mediators, which, although renal vasoconstrictors in their own right, also have the important added effect of causing mesangial cell contraction, and therefore lowering the glomerular capillary ultrafiltration coefficient (K_f), and thus the filtration fraction (see Fig. 8.6). Such factors involved may include endothelin, cysteinyl leukotrienes, thromboxane A_2 and F_2-isoprostanes.

Endothelin
This 21 amino acid peptide is a potent vasoconstrictor with preferential renal vasoconstriction, and is a potent agonist of mesangial cell contraction. Endothelin (ET)-1 concentrations are increased in hepatorenal syndrome, and correlate with creatinine clearance in decompensated liver disease (Fig. 8.18). Moreover, the plasma levels observed are comparable with those causing a significant decrease of GFR in normal human volunteers following infusion of ET-1. Immunostaining studies have shown an extensive network of receptors for ET-1 in the kidney, particularly in the medulla. The cause of increased plasma concentrations is unknown. Volume expansion or upright tilt fails to increase plasma ET in patients who have cirrhosis, and there appears to be no correlation with circulating endotoxins. Whether

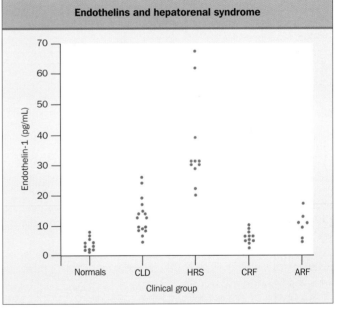
Endothelins and hepatorenal syndrome

Figure 8.18 Endothelins and hepatorenal syndrome. Plasma levels of endothelin-1 are markedly elevated in patients who have hepatorenal syndrome type 1. ARF, acute renal failure; CLD, chronic liver disease; CRF, chronic renal failure; HRS, hepatorenal syndrome. (Adapted from Moore et al. N Engl J Med. 1992;327:1774–9.)

tissue hypoxia or oxidant stress-dependent pathways are important is unknown. Increased lipid peroxidation is known to occur in hepatorenal syndrome, and certain products of lipid peroxidation, namely oxidized low-density lipoprotein (LDL), have been shown to induce ET-1 synthesis *in vitro*, but whether this is significant pathophysiologically is unknown.

Cysteinyl leukotrienes

Leukotrienes (LTs) C_4 and D_4 are produced by inflammatory cells of the myeloid series, and their synthesis by the isolated kidney has been demonstrated. They are both potent renal vasoconstrictors, and cause contraction of mesangial cells *in vitro*. Their synthesis may be stimulated by endotoxemia, activation of complement, or various cytokines. There is good evidence that systemic, and probably renal synthesis of cysteinyl LTs are increased in hepatorenal syndrome. Urinary LTE_4 is markedly elevated, as well as N-acetyl LTE_4 (probably a renal product of LT biosynthesis) in hepatorenal syndrome (Fig. 8.19).

Estimated plasma levels are too low to cause direct effects on the renal circulation, but renal LT synthesis might be an important modulator of renal function in hepatorenal syndrome.

Thromboxane A_2

Thromboxane A_2 (TXA_2) production is stimulated by renal ischemia and causes both vasoconstriction and mesangial cell contraction. It has been suggested that the balance between vasodilatory prostaglandins and TXA_2 might critically favor vasoconstriction. However, many of the early studies used urinary excretion of prostaglandin metabolites as markers of renal production, and failed to control for renal function or the severity of liver disease. When one takes a comparable group of patients who have severe liver disease, but in whom renal failure does not develop, and analyses the urinary excretion of TXA_2 and prostacyclin metabolites, one finds equally increased metabolite levels of prostacyclin and TXA_2, when corrected for GFR in patients who have hepatorenal syndrome. Furthermore, inhibition of TXA_2 synthesis with dazoxiben does not improve renal function. Such studies did not exclude a role for thromboxane, but clearly question its legitimacy as a prime candidate.

F_2-isoprostanes

The F_2-isoprostanes are formed by lipid peroxidation. One of the major F_2-isoprostanes formed *in vivo*, namely 8-iso-$PGF_{2\alpha}$, is a potent renal vasoconstrictor. Synthesis of the F_2-isoprostanes is increased in patients who have type 1 hepatorenal syndrome, which is indicative of increased lipid peroxidation. Whether the F_2-isoprostanes themselves are important mediators of renal vasoconstriction in hepatorenal syndrome is unknown. However, the synthesis of several mediators implicated in the pathogenesis of hepatorenal syndrome are regulated through products of lipid peroxidation or through redox changes secondary to oxidant stress. Thus, the development of oxidant stress may be important as the final pathway leading to increased synthesis of many of the mediators discussed above. However, the site of lipid peroxidation is unknown at present. This may be critical since the F_2-isoprostanes are formed by oxidation of both circulating lipid particles and membrane lipids. In the latter case, their formation as a prostaglandin esterified to a membrane phospholipid causes distortion of the cell membrane (Fig. 8.20), and phospholipases are activated to cleave the offending isoprostane.

CLINICAL FEATURES

There are few clinical features that are specific to hepatorenal syndrome. The characteristic patient will have clinical features of advanced liver disease, with jaundice and ascites being prominent. The renal failure may precipitate or aggravate encephalopathy. Oliguria is a frequent but not a universal finding.

DIAGNOSIS

The diagnosis of hepatorenal syndrome is no longer dependent on the presence of a low urine sodium or high urine:plasma osmolality. The diagnostic criteria currently used are shown in Figure 8.2.

Urinary protein should be less than 500mg/day, which helps to distinguish it from glomerulonephritis, and the urinary sediment is normal or 'near normal'. Urine indices in the early stages typically show a urine sodium below 10mmol/L (10mEq/L), a fractional sodium of <1, a urine:plasma osmolality of >1, and a urine:plasma creatinine ratio of >10. Hepatorenal syndrome is sometimes referred to as functional renal failure, which is indicative of preserved tubular function.

Functional renal failure (as one form of hepatorenal syndrome) may evolve into acute tubular necrosis (ATN), and electron microscopy studies have shown evidence of ATN, even when the urinary indices indicate functional renal failure. In practical terms it is important to distinguish it from the other causes of renal failure such as dehydration, sepsis and the use of nephrotoxic drugs. For those who have viral hepatitis it is important to consider chronic glomerulonephritis, which may complicate both chronic hepatitis B and C virus infection. Rhabdomyolysis can

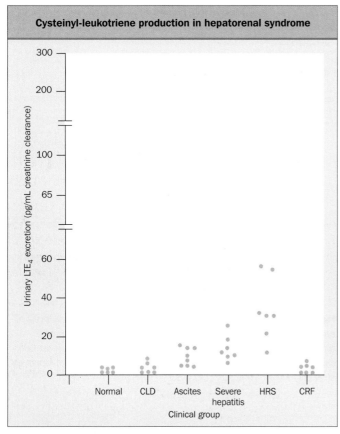

Figure 8.19 Cysteinyl-leukotriene production in hepatorenal syndrome. Urinary LTE_4 excretion is markedly and selectively increased in patients with the hepatorenal syndrome. This indicates that there is increased synthesis of cysteinyl leukotrienes in this condition. LTD_4 is a potent mediator of mesangial cell contraction. CRF, chronic renal failure; CLD, chronic liver disease; HRS, hepatorenal syndrome.

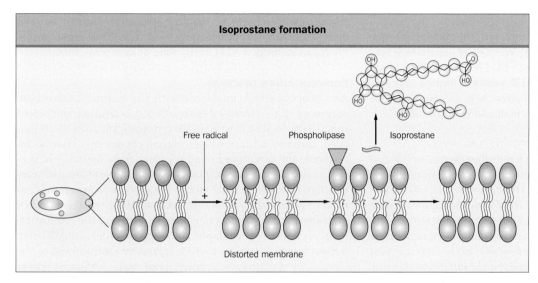

Isoprostane formation

Free radical

Phospholipase

Isoprostane

Distorted membrane

Figure 8.20 Isoprostane formation. When the phospholipid membrane is attacked by a free radical then the arachidonic acid side chain (usually in the sn-2 position) can become oxidized to form an esterified F_2-isoprostane. Molecular modeling studies have shown that when this occurs there is marked distortion of the cell membrane. The isoprostanes are then cleaved by the action of a phospholipase.

cause renal failure and some of its other features can mimic liver disease, for example elevated transaminases and a coagulopathy that is due to due to disseminated intravascular coagulation, rather than to impaired synthesis of coagulation factors.

Two patterns of hepatorenal syndrome are commonly observed in clinical practice. Firstly, there is an acute form, now termed type 1 hepatorenal syndrome, in which renal failure occurs spontaneously, with rapid onset and progressive renal failure. This is defined as a rise in plasma creatinine to >200μmol/L (1.5mg/dL), or a decrease in creatinine clearance to less than 20mL/min. This is most frequently observed in acute liver failure or alcoholic hepatitis, or following acute decompensation on a background of cirrhosis. These patients usually have marked icterus and a significant coagulopathy. There is a more chronic form (now termed type 2 hepatorenal syndrome) in which there is significant renal impairment, and in which renal function staggers towards improvement or deterioration over weeks or months. These patients frequently have refractory ascites, and jaundice may be mild. Patients with chronic liver disease and renal failure are unlikely to have hepatorenal syndrome unless they are severely jaundiced (bilirubin >200μmol/L or 12mg/dL), or have a severe coagulopathy (international normalized ratio [INR] >2.0), or have refractory ascites. The most common cause of apparent hepatorenal syndrome in a patient who has cirrhosis who is not particularly jaundiced is in fact hypovolemia.

MANAGEMENT

Renal function rarely recovers in the absence of hepatic recovery. The key goal in the management of these patients is to exclude reversible or treatable lesions (mainly hypovolemia), and to support the patient until liver recovery (e.g. from alcoholic hepatitis), hepatic regeneration (acute liver disease) or liver transplantation. The summary of patient management is shown in Figure 8.21.

Initial management
In cirrhotic patients, renal insufficiency is frequently secondary to hypovolemia (diuretics or gastrointestinal bleeding), NSAIDs, or sepsis. Precipitating factors should be recognized and treated, and nephrotoxic drugs discontinued.

All patients should be challenged with up to 1.5L of saline or colloid such as human albumin solution to assess the renal response. This should be done with careful monitoring to avoid fluid overload. In practice, fluid overload is not usually a problem, since patients with severe liver disease act as 'fluid sumps' and their vasculature adapts to accommodate the extra fluid by increased venous compliance.

Evidence of sepsis should be sought by blood, ascites, cannulae and urine culture, and non-nephrotoxic broad-spectrum antibiotics commenced.

Optimization of renal hemodynamics
It is important to maximize RBF.

Optimize blood pressure
Mean arterial pressure should be maximized to >75mmHg. Vasopressin, ornipressin (a vasopressin analog), or norepinephrine infusion have all been used with some success. Physiologically, either ornipressin or vasopressin are the most logical first-line therapies.

Paracentesis
Drainage of tense ascites may temporarily improve renal hemodynamics and renal function, by decreasing the renal venous pressure. There may, however. be a modest fall in blood pressure following paracentesis, which may negate any beneficial effects obtained. This can be prevented by careful monitoring of central venous pressures and colloid supplementation.

Management of hepatorenal syndrome

Stop any nephrotoxic drugs including diuretics

Correct any subclinical hypovolemia with 1.5L of saline or colloid, central venous pressure monitoring

Culture blood, urine, sputum, etc. Commence broad-spectrum antibiotics

Optimize blood pressure with colloid, together with glypressin or ornipressin

Consider paracentesis if there is tense ascites

Trial of low-dose dopamine should be considered

Renal support for those who have prospects of liver recovery/liver transplantation

Figure 8.21 Management of the hepatorenal syndrome.

Dopamine

'Low dose' dopamine infusion improves RBF, but in the two small studies in patients who have cirrhosis and hepatorenal syndrome, there was no improvement of GFR, and only one study has shown any improvement of GFR in uncomplicated cirrhosis. Prolonged use may increase catabolism, and if there is no discernible response within 24 hours it should be discontinued.

Renal support

Renal support should only be considered when there is a clear goal of management and potential positive outcome. Thus renal support should only be offered where there is a realistic possibility of hepatic regeneration, hepatic recovery or liver transplantation. Renal support otherwise serves only to protract the terminal illness. Renal support is generally given as continuous hemofiltration when the patients are hemodynamically labile. Intermittent hemodialysis causes marked hemodynamic instability in some patients, but it can be used when the hemodynamic parameters are stable, particularly in the recovery phase of the illness.

Surgical maneuvers and liver transplantation

Transjugular intrahepatic portosystemic shunt has been reported to improve renal function in patients who have refractory ascites after a 4-week interval. Anecdotal reports have also suggested that renal function can improve rapidly in patients who have hepatorenal syndrome. Recent studies have shown that temporary occlusion of the TIPSS by a balloon catheter causes a sudden reduction of RBF consistent with the concept of a hepatorenal reflex arc. There is no role for the LeVeen shunt in hepatorenal syndrome and there has only been one study on lumbar sympathectomy.

The only effective and permanent treatment for hepatorenal syndrome is orthotopic liver transplantation and an early observation in the history of transplantation was the rapid and full recovery of renal function in three patients following liver transplantation. Recovery of renal function was also observed in children with hepatorenal syndrome undergoing liver transplantation. In a recent report comparing survival following liver transplantation in 59 patients who had hepatorenal syndrome and 513 patients who did not have hepatorenal syndrome, only a tendency towards impaired survival was noted with a 1- and 4-year survival of 71 and 60% for hepatorenal syndrome patients, and 83 and 70%, respectively, for patients who did not have hepatorenal syndrome. The same retrospective study also considered the long-term evolution of renal function following liver transplantation on both groups of patients. Both cyclosporine and tacrolimus impair renal function. As a consequence, in 407 non-hepatorenal syndrome patients, GFR decreased from 94.1 to 59.8 mL/min at 1 year following transplantation. In 34 patients who had hepatorenal syndrome, GFR increased from 14.1 to 44mL/min at 1 year following transplantation and GFR remained significantly lower in previous hepatorenal syndrome patients until 4 years following transplantation. Although there was only a tendency towards impaired survival in patients who had hepatorenal syndrome following liver transplantation, the preoperative and postoperative morbidity was much higher. It was also noted that intraoperative hepatic arterial pressure and portal venous resistance was higher in the patients who had hepatorenal syndrome. Dialysis was given to 32% of hepatorenal syndrome patients before liver transplantation, and 10% remained on dialysis following transplantation. Some patients recover renal function within hours of liver transplantation, some take 1–2 days, and a subset recover over weeks. This latter group probably have established ATN at the time of liver transplantation.

Potential future therapies

Any process which interferes with the normal homeostatic responses (i.e. increased sympathetic activation, increased renin–angiotensin-aldosterone system etc.) are unlikely to succeed, and may actually worsen clinical parameters. How do we reconcile the sometimes rapid recovery from hepatorenal syndrome following liver transplantation with some of the pathways that have been described? Firstly, the process of liver transplantation involves the physical severing of the hepatorenal reflex pathways, and in patients in whom activation of the sympathetic nervous system is an important component one would expect a rapid effect. Likewise, there is aggressive management of the circulatory disturbances (namely poor renal perfusion) during liver transplantation, and clinical studies have shown that increasing the renal perfusion improves renal function transiently in hepatorenal syndrome. A well-functioning graft will improve host defense against the multitude of insults that enhance activation of synthesis of many of the circulatory mediators responsible for renal decompensation. Future work must concentrate on those mechanisms that are pathologic, such as increased cytokine production, possibly as a consequence of circulating endotoxins or oxidant stress. Increased plasma concentrations of F_2-isoprostanes have been described and these indicate increased lipid peroxidation, and therefore oxidant stress in patients who have hepatorenal syndrome. Recent publications demonstrating the role of oxidant stress dependent pathways on gene expression of a variety of cytokines suggests that this may be an important pathway in these patients. These mechanisms seem to be primarily deleterious.

OTHER RENAL DISEASES ASSOCIATED WITH LIVER DISEASE

The list of causes of renal failure or renal abnormalities associated with liver disease is shown in Figure 8.1. In some of these disorders, the renal abnormalities may be subtle. For example, aminoaciduria is associated with Wilson's and primary biliary cirrhosis, and may be accompanied by the development of a renal tubular acidosis. Other liver disorders may cause a more insidious renal abnormality such as the development of glomerular lesions causing chronic renal failure. From a clinical point of view those patients who develop renal failure in the absence of severe jaundice usually have either type II hepatorenal syndrome or one of the causes of renal dysfunction outlined below. The exceptions are cholestatic liver disease and leptospirosis. The former is usually diagnosable on imaging and immune studies, and leptospirosis is often characterized by relatively mild enzyme abnormalities and severe jaundice.

Cholestatic liver disease

Renal abnormalities may occur in any form of cholestatic liver disease. These include simple obstructive jaundice due to gallstones or tumor, primary sclerosing cholangitis or primary biliary cirrhosis. A defect in urinary concentrating ability has also been observed in the majority of patients. Decreases in creatinine clearance were observed in 30–70% of patients who had

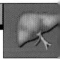

obstructive jaundice of 2–3 weeks duration, although plasma creatinine was within the normal range in all subjects. The average creatinine clearance found in these patients was 60–70mL/minute. The duration of biliary obstruction may influence the severity of renal impairment. In a study of patients who had jaundice of 6 weeks duration due to cholangiocarcinoma, renal impairment was observed in 50%. Renal failure defined as a doubling of serum creatinine occurred in 10% of patients undergoing surgery for obstructive jaundice. The most common cause was postoperative sepsis, and the mortality in the group developing renal failure was 75%. The most important factors in terms of management of such patients is adequate preoperative hydration and prophylaxis against sepsis.

The mechanisms involved are still poorly understood. There is a reduction of RBF. Despite this the response to salt handling may differ between species, with salt retention being rare in patients, but common in the rat. One potential mechanism that has been recently put forward is the idea that oxidative stress may in some way modulate renal function, perhaps as a consequence of bile salt induced injury to mitochondria, with secondary effects on vascular function.

Nonsteroidal anti-inflammatory drugs

Following the discovery of prostaglandins in the late 1960s and early 1970s, it was not long before the role of prostaglandins in the renal abnormalities in cirrhosis were studied. Early investigations of the effect of infused PGA_1, a renal vasodilator, on renal function in three groups of cirrhotic patients subdivided on the basis of the effective renal plasma flow (ERPF) observed that renal function could be correlated with severity of liver disease. PGA_1, increased ERPF, GFR and sodium excretion only in those who have reasonably well-preserved renal function. It was subsequently shown that administration of indomethacin caused a decrease in ERPF and creatinine clearance. Moreover, the decrease in GFR was greatest in those with ascites. Infusion of PGA_1 restored renal function in those given indomethacin, increasing creatinine clearance from 47 to 63mL/min, and ERPF from 355 to 580mL/min. A further observation from these studies was that this was associated with a reduction in the filtration fraction from 14 to 11% (i.e. the amount of glomerular filtration per milliliter of RBF decreased). Filtration fraction depends on efferent arteriolar tone, as well as the glomerular capillary ultrafiltration coefficient (K_f), itself modulated by contraction of mesangial cells.

Indomethacin was also associated with a 60% decrease in plasma renin activity which was restored by infusion of PGA_1. Patients who had cirrhosis with ascites had a 10-fold increase in urinary PGE_2 excretion rate, and in these patients indomethacin caused a decrease in creatinine clearance from 72 to 32mL/min. Renin and aldosterone levels also decreased following indomethacin. However, the impaired pressor response to angiotensin II in patients who had cirrhosis was restored by indomethacin. These two fundamental studies opened the doors to the study of prostaglandins and related compounds in cirrhosis. The most important observation that NSAIDs cause renal impairment in patients who have cirrhosis was of clear practical importance, but moreover indicated that renal prostaglandins are important in the maintenance of renal function in patients who have ascites. Moreover, it was also shown that indomethacin restored sensitivity to angiotensin II. This resulted in a multitude

of studies in which the effect of different prostanoids and other eicosanoids on renal function were studied. The effect of eicosanoids on renal and vascular function are summarized in Figure 8.22.

The use of NSAIDs such as sulindac may possibly be associated with a decreased risk of nephrotoxicity, but the data are not sufficiently robust to support their use with safety in this group of patients. The message from the above studies and those carried out by other groups is that the administration of NSAIDs to patients who have cirrhosis and ascites results in a reduction in free water clearance, a decrease in glomerular filtration rate and an increased risk of gastrointestinal bleeding.

Aminoglycosides

For patients who have pre-existing liver disease, there is increased sensitivity of the kidneys to the nephrotoxic potential of aminoglycosides. Indeed, the presence of liver disease is the most important predictive factor for the development of nephrotoxicity. The mechanism is unknown, but the fact that most patients who have severe liver disease have subclinical renal impairment is likely to be a major factor. The starting dose for gentamicin should never exceed a twice daily regimen of >80mg, and levels should be frequently determined.

Leptospirosis

Leptospirosis represents a spectrum of disease caused by infection with the spirochetes *Leptospira interrogans*. There are different subtypes termed serovars, of which the most well-known is *Leptospira icterohaemorrhagiae*, which causes Weil's disease. High risk groups include workers exposed to contaminated water such as miners, sewer workers, farmers and soldiers. In the Western world, farmers are probably most at risk. Workers who handle animal tissues are also at risk. The reservoir for infection is domestic or wild mammals, especially rodents. In the USA dogs and cattle are important reservoirs. Most spirochetes excreted via the urine do not survive. However, stagnant water and humid but slightly alkaline soil will favor their replication and survival. Organisms enter via abrasions, and the incubation period is around 10 days. There is an early sepsis phase, followed by localization to the liver and kidney. Vasculitic lesions occur widely, and contribute to the development of an erythematous rash and pulmonary hemorrhage. The illness may vary from being asymptomatic to one of severe jaundice, renal failure, and hemorrhage. Anicteric leptospirosis is probably the most common, and often goes undiagnosed. The early phase is characterized by fever, headache, meningism, severe muscular pains, nausea, vomiting,

Ways in which eiconsanoids may affect renal function
Renal vasodilatation
Renal vasoconstriction
Contraction or relaxation of mesangial cells, and modulation of K_f
Altered permeability of collecting ducts to water
Sodium reabsorption in the tubules
Indirectly via systemic effects (e.g. vasodilatation) or via modulation of other mediators
Indirectly by altering gene transcription or enzyme activity

Figure 8.22 Ways in which eicosanoids may affect renal function.

conjunctival suffusion, and prostration. It is often misdiagnosed as aseptic meningitis. Muscle pains are most prominent in the calves. About 70% of these patients have abnormal urinary sediment with proteinuria and hematuria. The second phase follows recovery from the first with the production of antibodies and is referred to as the immune phase.

Severe leptospirosis is characterized by jaundice and renal failure. Severe hyperbilirubinemia (bilirubin >1000μmol/L or >59mg/dL) may occur. However, in contrast the liver enzymes may be normal or only slightly deranged, but increases of aspartate aminotransferase/alanine aminotransferase (AST/ALT) activity by up to 10-fold may occur. Creatine phosphokinase (CPK) is increased in 50% of cases and there is often a mild neutrophilia. It is diagnosed by culture or serology. Treatment should be with a penicillin or doxycycline.

Chronic hepatitis B

It is now well established that chronic hepatitis B virus (HBV) infection can cause glomerulonephritis (Fig. 8.23). Infection with HBV nearly always produces some immune reaction, and circulating immune complexes may be demonstrated in some patients. The predominant renal lesion is membranous glomerulonephritis characterized by basement membrane thickening. Crescentic, mesangioproliferative, membranoproliferative, and focal sclerosing glomerulonephritis have all been described.

Immunostaining reveals the presence of immunoglobulins IgG, IgA, IgM, and C1q and C4 in a coarse granular beaded pattern along the glomerular basement membrane and mesangial areas. Immunofluorescence for antibody to the hepatitis B surface antigen (HBsAg) is positive in the majority with a similar distribution of the immunoglobulins. Thus the primary renal lesions are those of an immune complex-mediated membranous glomerulonephritis. Polyarteritis may also develop in association with chronic HBV infection, and may also lead to renal involvement.

The incidence of renal involvement in HBV infection is unknown. Histologic studies from Poland and elsewhere indicate

a high prevalence of HBsAg in kidney biopsies in patients who have normal liver function, but this is not the experience in the UK. Renal dysfunction may also occur in acute HBV infection, as part of a fulminant presentation or as a modest subclinical decrease in renal function. This may be associated with abnormal urinary sediment. In one study, glomerular abnormalities were noted in 50% of patients who had acute HBV infection with glomerular swelling and focal hypercellularity. Many of the cases are relatively mild, and often do not progress to end-stage renal failure. Whether this reflects an increase in mortality from liver-related problems is not known.

The data on the effects of antiviral therapy on renal disease is limited. Fifteen patients with HBV-related glomerular disease were given interferon-α, and seroconversion occurred in 50%. Of these eight responders, there was a gradual but marked improvement of proteinuria over several years of follow-up. In contrast the seven nonresponders continued to have persistent renal disease. All eight responders had membranous glomerulonephritis, whereas four of the seven nonresponders had membranoproliferative glomerulonephritis.

Chronic hepatitis C

Since the discovery of hepatitis C virus (HCV) in the late 1980s, it has become increasingly apparent that HCV infection gives rise to a variety of autoimmune and immune complex disease processes. These include mixed essential cryoglobulinemia, glomerulonephritis, thyroiditis, antiphospholipid antibodies and porphyria cutanea tarda. Mixed cryoglobulins are immunoglobulins that precipitate reversibly in the cold. The majority are related to connective tissue diseases, lymphoproliferative disease or immunologically mediated glomerular disease. The clinical syndrome of mixed essential cryoglobulinemia is of weakness, arthralgia, and purpura. The renal pattern of injury associated with HCV-related mixed cryoglobulinemia includes typical renal lesions characterized by a particular glomerular monocyte infiltration, a double-contoured appearance of the basement membrane, and the presence of intraluminal hyaline thrombi, due to the deposition of circulating cryoglobulins.

The progression of renal disease is variable with regression of renal symptoms in 35%, but with nephritic or nephrotic episodes in 20%. Uremia occurs in 10% by 10 years after the onset of renal disease, but this figure has to take into account the mortality during this period due to other causes. In a recent study in Saudi Arabia, renal biopsies were carried out in six patients who had HCV-related cirrhosis and proteinuria or elevated serum creatinine. All six patients had some form of glomerulonephritis, with four having membranoproliferative, one focal segmental, and one membranous. In one study, five of eight patients who had membranoproliferative glomerulonephritis associated with HCV had circulating cryoglobulins. Whether treatment of HCV with antiviral therapy has any effect on the prognosis of HCV-related glomerulonephritis is unknown.

While HCV infection can clearly cause glomerular disease, primary renal disease is associated with an increased risk of acquiring hepatitis C. This is most frequently seen in patients undergoing dialysis, who have often had multiple blood transfusions before blood products were screened for HCV. Following the discovery of HCV it became apparent that 10–40% of patients on dialysis had chronic HCV infection. The risk of having HCV is correlated to the number of previous transfusions.

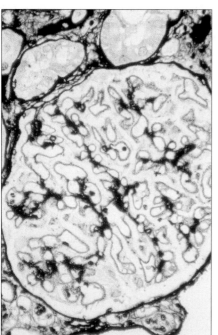

Figure 8.23
Glomerulonephritis.
Hepatitis B typically causes a membranous glomerulonephritis with subepithelial spikes as shown in this figure. This kidney biopsy from a patient with chronic hepatitis B was stained with PAMS (periodic acid–mellanamine silver). (Photograph supplied by Dr M. Jarmulovic, of the Royal Free Hospital, London.)

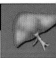

Human immunodeficiency virus

Patients with human immunodeficiency virus (HIV) disease may develop both abnormal liver function tests due to a variety of disorders including tuberculosis and fungal infection. They may also develop an HIV-associated nephropathy characterized by heavy proteinuria, rapidly progressive renal failure, 'collapsing' glomerulopathy and tubulointerstitial abnormalities. Proteinuria is present in 40% of patients with acquired immune deficiency syndrome-related illnesses.

Glomerular abnormalities in cirrhosis

Mild glomerular abnormalities have been noted in many studies in which renal tissue was examined in patients who have cirrhosis. While some of the changes may be etiology-specific (e.g. HBV), it appears that some glomerular lesions simply arise due to the presence of chronic liver disease and are made worse by the presence of portal hypertension. The incidence of renal lesions increases with age and predominates in women. It is associated with increased circulating IgA levels, especially in patients who have alcoholic cirrhosis.

Renal tubular defects in liver disease

Renal tubular acidosis (RTA) comprises a group of clinical syndromes characterized by failure of renal acidification, which is out of proportion to the degree of renal dysfunction. It is associated with chronic liver disease in 25–30% of cases. Distal RTA is subdivided into hypokalemic, normokalemic, and hyperkalemic forms. In the classic hypokalemic form the urine pH is never appropriately low, and acidosis is the result of decreased acid excretion. Distal RTA may be either partial or complete. The partial form is only detectable on formal testing and is present in >30% of patients who have primary biliary cirrhosis (PBC). The complete form which is characterized by hypokalemia, plus or minus a low bicarbonate, and increased serum chloride occurs in approximately 3% of cases of PBC. In proximal tubular RTA, the defect is decreased hydrogen ion secretion in the proximal tubules and is associated with other multiple tubular defects such as Fanconi's syndrome. Renal tubular acidosis has been described in autoimmune hepatitis, PBC, and alcoholic liver disease.

Amyloid

Amyloidosis is a disorder or protein metabolism in which autologous proteins are deposited extracellularly in a characteristic fibrillar form. Amyloid can be focal, localized or systemic in distribution. Amyloid light chain (AL) is associated with lymphoproliferative disease, and amyloid A (AA) is associated with chronic active inflammation. There is also a familial and dialysis-related amyloid. The liver is frequently involved in systemic amyloidosis, occurring in 54% of those who have AL amyloid, 18% of those who have AA amyloid, and hardly if ever in the familial or dialysis-related amyloid syndromes. Early amyloid deposition occurs in the mesangial area and capillary wall of the glomerulus, and around the interstitial fibroblasts and blood vessels. Tubular involvement may also occur. Proteinuria is the commonest renal manifestation and nephrotic syndrome occurs in 65%. Renal involvement is progressive, causing death in the majority of affected patients.

Sickle cell disease

The liver may be involved in sickle cell disease, sometimes with a very marked hyperbilirubinemia and increased transaminases, and occasionally a marked coagulopathy. A variety of functional and structural abnormalities of the kidney have been described. The glomeruli are often enlarged with congested capillary loops that contain sickled red blood cells. These changes are most marked in the juxtamedullary region. The mesangium may also show some degree of hypercellularity, attributed to the accumulation of iron–protein complexes. There is also deposition of immunoglobulins and complement components C1q and C3 along the basement membrane. It appears that the immunoglobulins deposited are directed against renal tubular antigen, and cryoprecipitable complexes of renal tubular antigen–antibody can be detected in the circulation of such patients. Thus, there is good evidence for an immune complex nephritis in sickle cell disease. The net effect of such abnormalities is the development of glomerulosclerosis, interstitial fibrosis, and tubular atrophy. Clinically, approximately 35% have proteinuria, and some develop a nephrotic syndrome. Hematuria is the most common renal abnormality in sickle cell disease and is secondary to congestion of vessels in the pelvic mucosa. Thus sickle cell disease may cause both liver dysfunction and independently cause abnormalities of the kidneys resulting in a variety of disorders ranging from hematuria to glomerulosclerosis, interstitial fibrosis, and nephrotic syndrome.

Connective tissue diseases

Renal lesions are well recognized in the multitude of connective tissue diseases. The liver, however, is rarely significantly involved in connective tissue diseases. Despite the occurrence of antinuclear antibodies in chronic autoimmune hepatitis and systemic lupus erythematosus (SLE), the association of the two conditions is surprisingly rare. The most common abnormality in the liver is steatosis, and hepatomegaly occurs in up to 30% of patients. It may, however, be complicated by a granulomatous hepatitis, nodular regenerative hyperplasia, chronic active hepatitis, and Budd–Chiari syndrome due to the hypercoagulable state that may occur. There has been the occasional report of an association of SLE with PBC and sclerosing cholangitis.

PRACTICE POINT

Illustrative case

A 44-year-old man who had alcoholic cirrhosis was admitted with a history of increasing ascites and oliguria. He had been abstinent from alcohol for 3 years after an initial presentation with acute alcoholic hepatitis. This deterioration occurred after he had taken NSAIDs for gout over a 2-day period. The serum creatinine was 667µmol/L (5.2mg/dL) and the urine output was 350mL over the first 24 hours in hospital. The urinary sodium was 11mmol/L (11mEq/L). He failed to respond to a fluid challenge and a dopamine infusion. He was commenced on hemodialysis and as his liver recovered some of its reserve he remained in renal failure. After being on dialysis for several weeks he was referred for liver transplantation. There was considerable debate as to whether he should have liver transplant alone, or a combined kidney and liver transplant. Renal biopsy was essentially normal, and he eventually received a liver alone after 6 months of hemodialysis. Renal function recovered within hours, and no further dialysis was required.

Interpretation

This is an extreme case which exemplifies the potential for reversal of the hepatorenal syndrome after successful liver transplantation. The lengthy duration of renal failure might suggest morphologic damage to the kidneys, but the normal histology early in the course of the renal failure was an important clue to the potential reversibility. Had the renal failure been due to ATN, return of renal function would have been expected after 6–8 weeks of renal support. Isolated liver transplantation is the preferred operation in these circumstances unless there is convincing evidence of irreversible intrinsic renal pathology. Why the recovery should be so rapid is not clear, but may involve the severing of the hepatorenal neural reflex arc in the course of surgery. Thus, the new liver was unable to maintain an increased sympathetic neural tone to the kidneys.

FURTHER READING

Arroyo V, Gines P, Gerbes AL, et al. Definition and diagnostic criteria of refractory ascites and hepatorenal syndrome in cirrhosis. Hepatology. 1996;23:164–76. *An important paper since it defines the terms, and redefines hepatorenal syndrome.*

Boyer TD, Zia P, Reynolds TB. Effect of indomethacin and prostaglandin A_1 on renal function and plasma renin activity in alcoholic liver disease. Gastroenterology. 1979;77:215–2. *First demonstration that NSAIDs cause renal failure in patients with ascites.*

Cade R, Wagemaker H, Vogel S, et al. Hepatorenal syndrome; studies on the effect of vascular volume and intraperitoneal pressure on renal and hepatic function. Am J Med. 1987;82:427–38. *An interesting study on aspects of paracentesis.*

Dudley F, Kanel G, Wood L, Reynolds T. Hepatorenal syndrome without avid sodium retention. Hepatology. 1986;6:248–51. *The paper that said what we all knew, namely, that urinary sodium is not and should not be a criterion for the diagnosis of the hepatorenal syndrome.*

Epstein M. Hepatorenal syndrome. In: Epstein M, ed. The kidney in liver disease. Baltimore: Williams and Wilkins; 1988:89–118. *An excellent reference source.*

Gonwa TA, Morris CA, Goldstein RM, Husberg BS, Klinthalm GB. Long-term survival and renal function following liver transplantation in patients with and without hepatorenal syndrome-experience in 300 patients. Transplantation. 1991;51:428–30. *Gonwa has the biggest series of patients who have the hepatorenal syndrome, and shows that they do remarkably well after liver transplantation.*

Guevera M, et al. Reversibility of hepatorenal syndrome by prolonged administration of ornipressin and plasma volume expansion. Hepatology. 1988;27:35–41. *This study demonstrates that volume expansion and correction of low blood pressure improve renal function in the hepatorenal syndrome.*

Lang F, Tschernko E, Schulze E, et al. Hepatorenal reflex regulating kidney function. Hepatology. 1991;14:590–4. *A landmark paper that demonstrates the importance of a hepatorenal reflex arc.*

Moore K, Ward P, Taylor G, Williams R. Systemic and renal production of thromboxane A_2 and prostacyclin in decompensated liver disease and hepatorenal syndrome. Gastroenterology. 1991;100:1069–77. *This paper effectively showed the importance of correcting urinary values of prostaglandins for renal function, and generated an entirely new interpretation of studies on renal function and prostaglandin synthesis.*

Navar LG. Renal autoregulation: perspectives from whole kidney and single nephron studies. [Review] Am J Physiol. 1978;234:F357–70. *A nice review of renal autoregulation.*

Ring Larsen H. Renal blood flow in cirrhosis: Relation to systemic and portal hemodynamics and liver function. Scand J Clin Lab Invest. 1977;37:635–42. *The demonstration that there is a wide overlap of values of RBF between those who have hepatic renal syndrome and those who have ascites demonstrates the importance of other factors in its etiology.*

Ring-Larsen H, Palazzo U. Renal failure in fulminant hepatic failure and terminal cirrhosis: a comparison between incidence, types, and prognosis. Gut. 1981;22:585–91. *This paper is one of the few that deal specifically with renal failure in acute liver failure. It also shows the variability of urinary sodium.*

Stein JH. Regulation of the renal circulation. Kidney Int. 1990;38:571–6. *A nice review of the renal circulation.*

Wilkinson SP, Moodie H, Stamatakis JD, Kakkar VV, Williams R. Endotoxemia and renal failure in cirrhosis and obstructive jaundice. BMJ. 1976;2:1415–8. *First demonstration that most patients with HRS had elevated levels of endotoxin.*

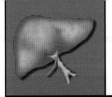

Chapter 9

Hepatic Encephalopathy

Kevin D Mullen

INTRODUCTION

The term hepatic encephalopathy (HE) encompasses a wide spectrum of neuropsychiatric disturbances observed in patients with significant liver dysfunction. The term dysfunction is used rather than disease to include the relatively rare, but well-described group of patients with HE due to portosystemic shunting without intrinsic liver disease. The neuropsychiatric disturbances observed in HE are usually reversible. Three main types of HE are now recognized using a mnemonic system (Fig. 9.1) based on the underlying liver dysfunction. This chapter deals principally with classic type HE occurring in patients with chronic liver disease and/or portosystemic shunts (type C). Encephalopathy in these settings generally falls into a number of discrete clinical patterns (Fig. 9.2). Encephalopathy associated with acute liver failure (type A) is discussed in Chapter 30.

The classification of HE is somewhat confusing in the literature, with some terms used interchangeably by different authors. This reflects the diverse clinical picture and the lack of knowledge as to the precise cause of the neuropsychiatric disturbances. Essentially it is believed that a 'toxin', which is normally metabolized by the liver, reaches the brain and causes the disturbance. Lack of detoxification may be due, in acute liver failure, to virtual absence of liver function, with portal blood flowing through the necrotic liver unaltered. In chronic liver disease structure and function are altered and the development of portosystemic shunting of venous blood allows the liver to be bypassed. This latter mechanism accounts for the rarely encountered encephalopathy in cases with significant portosystemic shunting but without underlying liver disease.

PATHOPHYSIOLOGY

The liver's position in respect of portal venous drainage is perfectly designed for effective detoxification of toxic products of intestinal metabolism and digestion. The high-volume, low-pressure flow through the liver's extensive fenestrated sinusoidal system maximizes contact of portal venous plasma with hepatocytes (Fig. 9.3). This facilitates first pass metabolism of compounds in plasma. Toxic products escaping first pass metabolism or originating in extrasplanchnic sites are also subjected to hepatic clearance via delivery through hepatic arterial bloodflow (second pass hepatic metabolism).

The development of fibrosis and cirrhosis radically alters the detoxification capacity of the liver. Increased resistance to portal venous influx leads to extrahepatic portosystemic venous collateral formation. This alone leads to a reduction in first pass metab-

Classification of HE	
Type	**Definition**
A	**A**cute liver failure associated or 'alfa' HE
B	HE associated with portosystemic **b**ypass and no intrinsic liver disease
C	HE in patients with **c**hronic liver disease/cirrhosis

Figure 9.1 Classification of hepatic encephalopathy (HE). Distinction between acute (type A) and chronic liver disease HE is based on time of 2 months, (i.e. if liver disease present less than 2 months, HE would be classified as type A).

Clinical patterns of HE in chronic liver disease	
Type	**Features**
Subclinical	No easily identifiable clinical features. EEG changes present
Acute*	Discrete episode with full recovery within 4 weeks precipitated or spontaneous
Chronic*	Treatment responsive† Persistent‡ Severe**

Figure 9.2 Clinical patterns of HE in chronic liver disease. *Acute and chronic HE distinguished by length of time mental status changes persist. Greater than 4 weeks: chronic. †A subgroup of patients do very well on treatment, but lapse into HE with cessation of therapy. ‡Persistent neurologic deficits, but patient able to function outside hospital. **Severe, indicates so incapacitated cannot function outside hospital; often fluctuate between moderate (grade I–II) and severe (grade III-IV) with or without identifiable precipitating factor.

olism of 'toxins' in portal venous blood (Fig. 9.4). Compensatory increase in total hepatic bloodflow (mainly mediated by hepatic arterial in-flow) can help maintain hepatic detoxification. Perhaps the most important mechanism leading to a high systemic 'toxin' level and thus HE, is the gradual isolation of hepatocytes from residual portal venous and hepatic arterial perfusion. Hepatocyte isolation results from a number of processes:
- defenestration of hepatic sinusoids;
- subendothelial collagen deposition; and
- intrahepatic portosystemic collateral formation (Fig. 9.4; also, see Fig. 9.3.).

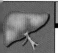

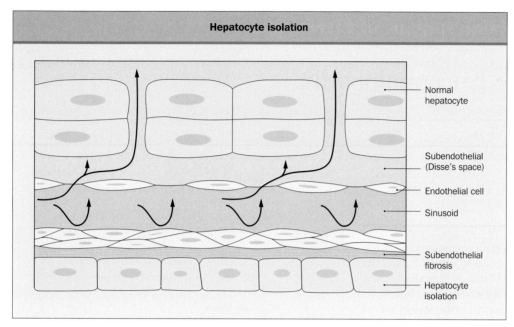

Figure 9.3 The concept of hepatocyte isolation secondary to perisinusoidal fibrosis. In the top half of the figure there is normal diffusion across the endothelial cells into the space of Disse. Due to a free diffusion the products in the sinusoid have direct access to the hepatocyte, and vice-versa. In the lower half of the figure, the result of perisinusoidal fibrosis and vascular distortion results in a poor hepatocyte–sinusoid interaction. This may result in bypass of functioning hepatocytes even in the presence of hepatic bloodflow.

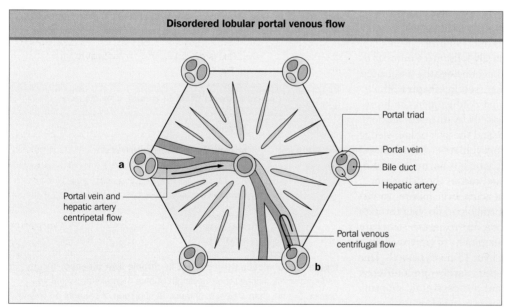

Figure 9.4 Disordered lobular portal venous flow. The normal hepatic lobule with the portal to central flow patterns in the portal vein and hepatic artery shown in (a). In (b), the presence of portal hypertension and a shunted state result in an alteration of the flow dynamics with centrifugal blood flow and disorganized hepatocyte perfusion. This may result in hepatocyte malfunction in both synthetic and detoxifying activities.

Thus, there is both a macroisolation of the hepatocytes by the fibrotic process (see Fig. 9.5), as well as a microisolation due to the hepatocyte sinusoidal barrier caused by the perisinusoidal fibrosis (see Fig. 9.3). This isolation not only reduces hepatic detoxification, but also probably leads to progressive loss of hepatocyte mass and/or function. This may possibly deprive cells of portal venous hepatotropic substances. Ultimately, a point is reached where hepatic detoxification is totally inadequate to prevent accumulation of 'toxins' in the systemic circulation.

Intestinal events play a major role in modulating 'toxin' levels in the systemic circulation of patients with advanced liver disease. Using ammonia as an example of the best known intestinal toxin likely to play a role in HE, a number of points can be made. Although evidence exists that portal hypertension may limit absorption of ammonia from the gut, the reduction in intestinal

motility in portal hypertension enhances ammonia generation and absorption. Large nitrogenous loads from upper gastrointestinal bleeding clearly contribute to intestinal ammonia production/absorption, as may small bowel bacterial overgrowth, constipation, and gastric *Helicobacter pylori* infection. The clinical response of HE to gut cleansing is the strongest evidence available that gut-derived toxins such as ammonia play a major role in HE. Such intestinal events therefore have a significant role in the development of encephalopathy.

Less definite but well accepted is the concept that lean body mass plays a role in the final appearance of clinically evident HE in advanced liver disease. This large mass of metabolically active tissue can provide an alternative site for the handling of intestinal toxins that escape hepatic metabolism. A reduction in lean body mass is frequently observed in the more advanced stages of

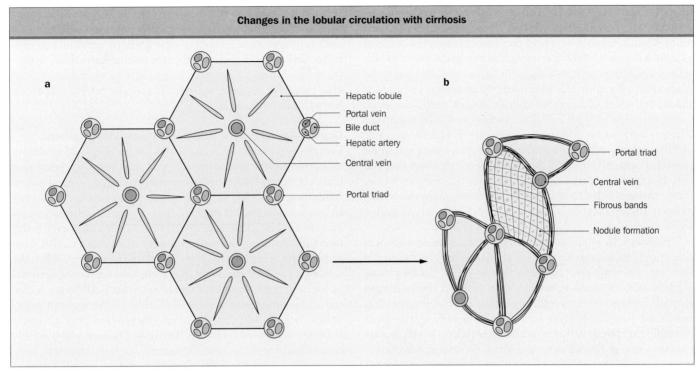

Figure 9.5 Changes in the lobular circulation with the development of cirrhosis. In (a), a normal hepatic lobule with maintained vascular perfusion across the sinusoids in a centripetal direction from the portal triad to the central vein is shown. In (b), loss of lobular architecture, formation of fibrotic bands, and hepatocyte degeneration and regeneration (components of hepatic cirrhosis) result in vascular isolation of hepatocyte clusters. This is macroisolation, in contrast to the microisolation shown in Fig. 9.3.

hepatic decompensation at a time when HE becomes apparent as a major clinical problem.

There was a school of thought which suggested that HE was due to the reduced production of a substance by the diseased liver that 'maintains' brain function. This theory has been largely discounted because of cross circulation studies done in rats many years ago. It is generally accepted that the intestinal toxin hypothesis is correct. The only controversy is whether ammonia alone can explain the whole picture of HE. It is more likely that ammonia in concert with other events or compounds leads to HE.

Finally, the brain itself appears to be sensitized by prolonged exposure to the environment, which leads to HE. The precise molecular mechanism for the 'sensitivity' has not yet been elucidated. Conceivably, it is due to the same toxins that cause alterations in neuronal–astrocyte interactions. Advancement of knowledge would be greatly facilitated by development of an animal model of HE in chronic liver disease more closely reproducing the syndrome as seen in humans.

HYPOTHESES OF PATHOGENESIS

Figure 9.6 lists the various hypotheses proposed over the years to explain the pathogenesis of HE. Rather than discuss these in detail, comments will be made on concepts that have led to treatment possibilities. Figure 9.6 summarizes the various accepted hypotheses and the treatment modalities, both existing and potential. The ammonia hypothesis serves as the paradigm for the various therapeutic possibilities.

Ammonia hypothesis

The primary mechanisms for the role of ammonia in the pathogenesis of encephalopathy are a direct effect on cortical neurons or on postsynaptic inhibitory potentials, and an indirect effect on glutamine/glutamate metabolism with a reduction in excitatory neurotransmitters.

Virtually all effective therapy now available for the treatment of HE can be proposed to mediate its benefit by reduction in blood ammonia levels. Paradoxically, it has been extremely difficult to demonstrate a correlation of the degree of hyperammonemia with the severity of HE. The reasons for this are

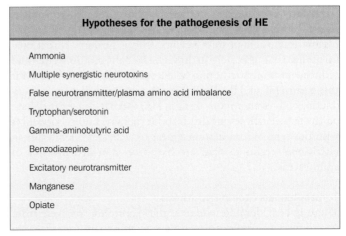

Hypotheses for the pathogenesis of HE

Ammonia

Multiple synergistic neurotoxins

False neurotransmitter/plasma amino acid imbalance

Tryptophan/serotonin

Gamma-aminobutyric acid

Benzodiazepine

Excitatory neurotransmitter

Manganese

Opiate

Figure 9.6 Hypotheses for the pathogenesis of HE.

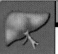
multifactorial. Most studies that attempted to establish a correlation either used venous blood or included patients with multiple simultaneous causes of encephalopathy. Venous blood ammonia levels clearly are inappropriate since they do not reflect brain exposure to this toxin. Many patients with the most severe form of HE have underlying sepsis, circulatory shock, and electrolyte abnormalities, which themselves can cause alteration in brain function. Another potential reason for a lack of correlation of blood ammonia levels and the severity of HE is simply a lack of correlation between blood and brain ammonia concentrations. It should also be emphasized that the only two controlled trials of administration of ammonia to cirrhotic patients failed to induce HE. Moreover, many other gut-derived toxins may be affected by treatments that reduce ammonia generation and absorption from the gut.

The failure to establish correlation between blood ammonia concentrations and the severity of HE may, in fact, be due to the fact that ammonia does not directly cause HE. Studies using modern, more accurate ammonia assays on blood obtained from arterial, arteriovenous, or capillary sites under well-controlled conditions may resolve this issue. In the meantime, the most plausible hypothesis is that ammonia plays a role in HE, but its mechanism may be indirect. Alterations in neuronal–astrocyte interactions or disturbance of other neurotransmitter systems seem the best mechanisms to investigate at present.

Multiple synergistic neurotoxin hypothesis

This hypothesis argues that mercaptans (metabolites or methionine), eight-chain fatty acids (octanoic acid), and possibly phenol accumulate in the systemic circulation in advanced liver disease and synergistically interact with ammonia to cause HE. A considerable component of this hypothesis was questioned when it was determined that the original mercaptan assays used were inaccurate. No specific treatments ever arose from this hypothesis.

False neurotransmitter/plasma amino acid imbalance hypothesis

In this hypothesis, it was originally suggested that amino acid metabolism was disturbed either by colonic bacterial decarboxylation, reduced hepatic deamination, or increased extrahepatic metabolism. These mechanisms resulted in the production of 'false neurotransmitters' and a disturbance in the normal balance of various amino acids.

Essentially there is no evidence supporting the false neurotransmitter part of this hypothesis. Left over from this ingenious hypothesis is a treatment designed to normalize the abnormal plasma amino acid profile seen in cirrhotic persons. Nutritional formulas that are rich in branched-chain amino acids and reduced in aromatic amino acid content were developed for the treatment of HE. Reflecting the major difficulty in conducting clinical treatment trials in HE, there is still great debate on the actual efficacy of this form of therapy. Enteral products with this type of formulation appear to be better tolerated than nutritional regimens that are based on standard profiles of amino acids.

Tryptophan/serotonin hypothesis

There is considerable evidence that serotonin, derived from tryptophan, is produced in excess in presynaptic neurons in HE. Since a whole array of drugs is now available to modulate serotonin actions in the brain at various receptors, we may soon see some definitive work in this field. Interestingly, not only is there some evidence of excessive serotonin neurotransmission in HE, but also there are some hints that a synaptic deficit of serotonin may be present in animal models of HE. However, to date, no specific therapy for HE has arisen from this hypothesis.

Gamma-amino butyric acid/benzodiazepine hypothesis

Gamma-amino butyric acid (GABA) is the principal inhibitory neurotransmitter in the brain. This hypothesis suggested that excess systemic GABA in liver disease produced cerebral neuro-inhibition and the features of encephalopathy. However, although evidence still exists that excessive GABA neurotransmission may be present in HE, there is little evidence for this direct mechanism. The neurotransmitter acts via a GABA–benzodiazepine receptor complex, and rather than just GABA elevations it has been proposed that accumulation of 'endogenous' or 'natural' benzodiazepines would augment GABAergic neurotransmission via the joint receptor. Unlike GABA receptor antagonists, which are highly toxic, benzodiazepine receptor antagonists are well tolerated. The only commercially available benzodiazepine antagonist, flumazenil, has been shown to ameliorate HE in animal models. The efficacy of flumazenil in human HE is somewhat limited. However, unlike just about all other therapy of HE, it has been proven to have greater efficacy than placebo in double-blind randomized controlled trials. Until the source and identity of these endogenous benzodiazepines are clarified, this hypothesis will remain under a question mark and requires further investigation.

Excitatory neurotransmitter hypothesis

In this hypothesis perturbation of the glutamate and aspartate neurotransmitter systems is suggested to play a role in HE. Glutamate is a major excitatory neurotransmitter, and reduced levels or alterations in receptor binding have been described in HE. Alterations in astrocyte interactions may be involved in these changes. The availability of newer drugs to block subtypes of central nervous system glutamate receptors may help to unravel this area. Some effects of ammonia on the brain can be ameliorated by one of these glutamate receptor blockers, mementine. However, no new therapies have yet arisen from this hypothesis.

Manganese neurotoxicity

Recently considerable interest has been generated by the finding of excessive manganese in the brain of patients with HE. This metal appears responsible in a large part for the frequent finding of hyperintensity of the basal ganglia on T1-weighted magnetic resonance images of the brain in cirrhotic patients. The role manganese may play in HE is still uncertain. Potentially chelation therapy could be tested in the near future.

Opiate hypothesis

Opiate accumulation has been proposed to play a role not only in HE, but also in the pruritus of cholestasis. Because of the availability of safe opiate antagonists, it should be feasible to test this hypothesis in humans in the near future. Currently, most supporting information is based on studies in animal models.

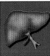

CLINICAL FEATURES

The diagnosis of HE is almost entirely a clinical exercise. As the term implies, a diagnosis of HE requires the recognition of significant liver dysfunction and an alteration in neurologic status. Most of the time, evidence for both is obvious and a key issue is the need to rule out other contributing causes of encephalopathy. Liver dysfunction can be difficult to identify on occasions, particularly in patients with large portosystemic shunts and little or no intrinsic liver disease (so-called type B HE). Mild (subclinical) episodes of HE may be difficult to recognize, especially if the patient has never previously been encountered.

Recognizing significant liver dysfunction

Any change in mental status in a patient with known or suspected significant liver dysfunction is due to HE until proven otherwise. In such a patient a careful search should be made for the factors known to precipitate encephalopathy (Fig. 9.7). It is relatively rare for patients to present with HE in whom clear-cut physical signs or laboratory data do not point to liver dysfunction. However, these rare instances occur often enough in clinical practice to be an important issue. Failure to diagnose HE in these settings may lead to diagnoses as varied as dementia or psychiatric disorders. Treatment for the wrong diagnosis can lead to an aggravation of HE and even to commitment to psychiatric institutions. This was described in the 1950s and still occurs.

Physical findings suggesting chronic liver disease can be missed on cursory examination. The frequency of obesity in the USA makes abdominal examination difficult. Alterations in hepatic size, splenomegaly, and even ascites can be missed. Usually the laboratory evidence of significant liver problems (e.g. reduced albumin, prolonged prothrombin time, elevated bilirubin) counters failure to identify liver disease on examination. However, it is possible to have normal or near normal liver tests and still have HE. The physical findings and other laboratory and radiologic data that may be crucial in the diagnosis of underlying liver dysfunction are listed in Figs 9.8–9.10 (see Chapter 4).

Assessment of neurologic status

There are no truly specific neurologic changes in HE. The clinical picture is complex, and since all parts of the brain may be affected there is marked variability between patients. Essentially, HE consists of varying degrees of change in consciousness and elements of a generalized motor disturbance.

Disturbed consciousness frequently begins with increased sleepiness and reversal of the normal sleep pattern. There is increasing lethargy and lapse into coma that eventually renders the patient unrousable. Accompanying these changes, the patient has a change in personality and intellect. There may be lack of awareness, increased irritability, and short attention span. Inappropriate behavior may occur; writing and speech deteriorates. Progress of deterioration can be assessed by serial use of a

Precipitating factors for hepatic encephalopathy	
Gastrointestinal hemorrhage	Central nervous system active drugs
Hypokalemia	Portosystemic shunt creation (including transjugular intrahepatic portosystemic shunt)
Dehydration	Excessive protein intake
Uremia	Superimposed hepatic injury
Constipation	Noncompliance with therapy
Infection	

Figure 9.7 Precipitating factors for hepatic encephalopathy.

Physical findings in chronic liver disease	
Spider naevi	Splenomegaly
Fetor hepaticus	Ascites
Jaundice	Peripheral edema
Gynecomastia	Dupuytren's contracture
Loss of male hair pattern	Hepatomegaly
Muscle wasting	Parotid enlargement
Caput medusae	Excessive bruising
Palmar erythema	Xanthelasma
Leukonychia	Xanthoma

Figure 9.8 Physical findings in chronic liver disease.

Laboratory findings suggesting underlying liver disease	
Prolonged prothrombin time	Thrombocytopenia
Hypoalbuminemia	Leukopenia
Elevated aminotransferases	Elevated serum globulins
Elevated serum bilirubin	Hyponatremia
Elevated alkaline phosphatase	Hypouricemia
Positive hepatitis serology (especially HCV)	

Figure 9.9 Laboratory findings suggesting underlying liver disease.
HCV, hepatitis C virus.

Radiologic findings suggesting underlying liver disease	
Ascites	Collateral vessels
Irregular liver margins	Splenomegaly
Hyperechoic liver	Dilated bile ducts
Space-occupying lesions	Hepatomegaly
Recanalized umbilical vein	Splanchnic vein and hepatic vein thrombosis

Figure 9.10 Radiologic (CT/ultrasound) findings suggesting underlying liver disease.

number connection test. In such a test, the time taken to join up a series of randomly spaced numbers from 1–25 on a page is measured. This time lengthens or shortens as the patient deteriorates or improves.

Since the clinical course is variable and fluctuates, frequent observations are necessary. A clinical grading system for the stage of encephalopathy has been described and is a useful method for assessing response to treatment (see Fig. 4.14 in Chapter 4).

Evidence of motor disturbances can be helpful in identifying a change in mental status as being due to HE. Several physical signs on neurologic examination can be found (Fig. 9.11). Asterixis is well recognized, but is not specific to HE. However, it is the most characteristic and well-known neurologic abnormality. The 'flapping tremor' ('asterixis') is observed with the patient's arms outstretched, the wrists hyperextended and the fingers separated. There are rapid flexion–extension movements of the hands. Occasionally the arms and head can be involved. The flap is present in stages 1 and 2 of encephalopathy but disappears as coma deepens. As suggested, it is not a specific physical sign and can be present in severe heart, respiratory, or renal failure.

Of the other physical signs, transient asymmetries of findings such as hyper-reflexia and a positive Babinski sign are relatively common. Only when persistently lateralizing do they strongly indicate that other brain disorders may be present. Vivid visual hallucinations, agitated delirium, and sensory disturbances are distinctly uncommon in HE and raise the issue of delirium tremens or some other cause of encephalopathy.

Investigations

Investigations in order to diagnose HE are relatively nonspecific and do not play a major role in the diagnosis of the condition. Sensory evoked potentials are a research tool, and brain scans (CT and MRI) show structural changes related to liver disease rather than changes due to HE.

Electroencephalogram

The electroencephalogram shows some characteristic changes in HE. The normal background waveform is replaced by slower, higher amplititude, and eventually triphasic waves as the condition progresses. These changes begin early, before clinical or biochemical disturbances are present, and may therefore be helpful in diagnosis. The changes are, however, nonspecific and therefore are of low overall sensitivity. Similar changes are found in renal and respiratory failure and hypoglycemia.

MANAGEMENT

It must be emphasized that HE is a manifestation of liver dysfunction and that management should address all aspects of the case. Three areas of management should be considered: the encephalopathy and any precipitating factors; other manifestations of hepatic decompensation; and the underlying liver disease.

Once a diagnosis of HE is considered, supportive measures for a patient in coma are instituted as required (Fig. 9.12). This is followed by gut cleansing, a low protein diet, and lactulose delivered into the gastrointestinal tract. Concurrent precipitating factors for HE (see Fig. 9.7) are sought and specific treatment modalities instituted (Fig. 9.13). Finally, a difficult management issue that arises frequently, especially in severe HE, is whether another cause of encephalopathy or coma is present in the patient (Fig. 9.14). Severe sepsis, accidental or deliberate drug overdose, and intracranial hemorrhage are the most common problems encountered in our hospital. Multiple precipitating factors may occur simultaneously and it is essential to control all of them for clinical response or recovery to occur.

Other treatment options based on the proposed putative toxin hypotheses are shown in Figs 9.15 & 9.16. Of these, reasonably established therapies based on randomized controlled trials include lactitol, acid enemas using either lactulose or acetic acid, rifaximin, vancomycin, metronidazole, sodium benzoate, ornithine L-aspartate, flumazenil, and *Enterococcus faecium* SF 68. Surprisingly, there is little controlled evidence to support the role of lactulose in the therapy of HE, although it is now considered standard therapy and hepatologists, from an empiric point of view, find it effective.

Once effective empiric therapy has been instituted and precipitating factors corrected, one expects most patients to show significant neurologic improvement in 72 hours. Failure to observe this indicates either one or more of the following:

* inadequate empiric therapy;
* failure to identify and correct a precipitating factor;
* another cause of encephalopathy or coma that has been missed; and
* over-aggressive empiric therapy that has caused new problems (e.g. dehydration, electrolyte abnormalities).

General issues that need close attention are gut cleansing and the delivery of lactulose. Failure to obtain free flowing bowel

Physical signs on neurological examination in HE	
Asterixis	Monotonous voice pattern
Hyper-reflexia	Decerebrate posturing
Positive Babinski sign	Decorticate posturing
Saccadic ocular pursuit	Hyperventilation
Parkinsonian features	

Figure 9.11 Physical signs on neurologic examination in HE.

Treatment for encephalopathy	
Treatment aspect	**Measures**
Nutrition and essential elements	Parenteral fluids, amino acids, dextrose
Electrolytes	Potassium, sodium levels
Care of elimination	Bowel, bladder care
Vascular access care	Intravenous cannulas, central lines
Aspiration precautions	Nursing care, physiotherapy
Pressure sore	Prevention, treatment

Figure 9.12 Treatment for encephalopathy. Listed are supportive measures for patients in coma.

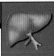

Management of precipiting factors	
Precipitating factor	**Management**
Gastrointestinal bleed	Endoscopic intervention, vasconstrictors (vasopressin, octreotide, somatostatin), prophylaxis for stress ulcers
Sepsis (pneumonia, urinary tract infection, spontaneous bacterial peritonitis)	Antibiotics
Electrolyte abnormalities (hypokalemia, hyponatremia, alkalosis)	Correct abnormality, avoid diuretics, fluid restriction
Exogenous sedatives	Flumazenil, naloxone challenge
Azotemia	Avoid NSAIDs, control sepsis, correct circulating volume abnormalities

Figure 9.13 Management of precipitating factors. NSAID, nonsteroidal anti-inflammatory drugs.

Other causes of encephalopathy or disturbed consciousness in cirrhotic patients	
Respiratory failure	Delirium tremens
Severe sepsis	Wernicke's encephalopathy
Intracranial bleed	Hypoglycemia
Drug overdose	Post ictal
CNS sepsis	Status epilepticus
Severe hyponatremia	Zinc deficiency

Figure 9.14 Other causes of encephalopathy or disturbed consciousness in cirrhotic patients. CNS, central nervous system.

movements delays recovery from HE. Concerns about precipitating variceal bleeding or aspiration by inserting a nasogastric tube and delivering lactulose (30–60mL q2h until bowel movements occur) are unwarranted. However, control of upper gastrointestinal bleeding takes priority over lactulose delivery. The common practice of only using enema treatment in comatose or nearly comatose patients merely prolongs the coma. Getting lactulose into the intestine and right colon is critical to recovery. Only in patients with ileus or bowel obstruction is enema therapy alone warranted. However, in almost all patients an initial enema is effective in beginning colonic cleansing. This is particularly true if firm hard stool is felt on rectal examination and abdominal distension is being noted after multiple doses of lactulose.

Once patients improve, a full diet can be introduced without specific needs for protein restriction unless HE worsens. In patients with clear-cut precipitating factors, it is often feasible to consider stopping lactulose therapy at some point. Correction of precipitating factors alone can correct HE in at least 60% of patients. Nonetheless many physicians continue oral lactulose therapy in the long term after patients have their first bout of overt HE. This is definitely needed in patients who develop HE without a precipitating factor. Compliance with lactulose therapy is poor in many patients because of unpredictable diarrhea (sometimes with incontinence) and a developed aversion to the sweet taste of the syrup. The latter can be overcome by getting patients to add the lactulose to sweetened iced tea, or by substituting lactitol.

Rare cases of intractable HE need additional therapeutic approaches. Oral neomycin in doses of 1–2mg a day may be effective. Higher doses, used in early clinical trials of HE treatment, cause significant toxicity. Short-term oral metronidazole, 250mg three times daily, can be very effective in certain patients but cannot be recommended for long-term treatment. Newer therapies such as rafaximin and sodium benzoate may become routine in the next few years. Oral branched-chain amino acid enriched formulae can be used in patients with

Empiric measures directed towards pulative toxins			
Ammonia			
Substrate reduction	Cathartics, enemas Protein intake reduction/modification		
Decrease ammoniagenesis	Gut bacterial suppression	Antibiotics	
	Non-absorbable disaccharides	Lactulose, lactitol lactose	
	Enteric flora modification	Enterococcus faecium SF 68	
Biochemical neutralization of ammonia	L-glutamic acid Sodium benzoate Ornithine L-aspartate Keto analogs of amino acids Acid enemas		
Endogenous benzodiazepines			
Flumazenil			
? False neurotransmitters			
L-Dopa Bromocriptine Branched-chain amino acids			

Figure 9.15 Empiric measures directed towards pulative toxins.

intolerance to oral protein. Vegetable-based protein diets may also be effective in some cases.

Infrequently, recurrent HE or truly intractable HE is a definite indication for liver transplantation. In patients who are not otherwise candidates for transplantation, attempts at closing or suppressing existing portosystemic shunts may improve HE. Unfortunately, many patients do not have dominant shunts amenable for closure, or closure may precipitate variceal bleeding.

As already stated, other issues that need to be addressed in patients with HE are related to the problems of chronic liver disease (Fig. 9.17). These need to be addressed not only for the continuing care of the patient, but also to prevent further episodes of HE.

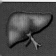
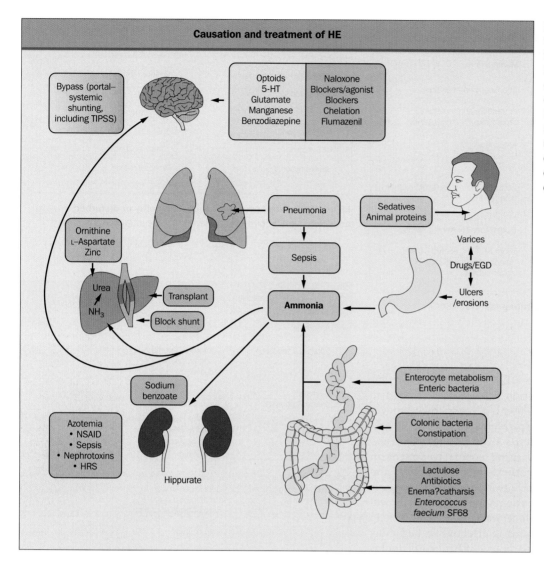

Figure 9.16 Causation and treatment of HE. Pathogenetic factors, clinical events and potential interventions in hepatic encephalopathy. EGD, esophagogastroduodenoscopy; HRS, hepatorenal syndrome; 5HT, 5-hydroxytryptamine; NSAID, nonsteroidal anti-inflammatory drugs. Red boxes signify treatment of HE, whilst blue boxes represent causes of HE.

Management of other manifestations of hepatic decompensation

Control ascites

Avoid hepatorenal syndrome

Manage nutritional deficiencies

Prophylaxis against variceal bleeding

Monitor for hepatoma

Consider transplantation

Figure 9.17 Management of other manifestations of hepatic decompensation (long-term measures).

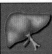

PRACTICE POINT

Illustrative case

A 43-year-old woman was admitted acutely with confusion and disorientation. She was irritable and difficult to manage due to her aggressive behavior. She was known to have drunk an excessive amount of alcohol for 10 years since the death of her husband. There was a history from her neighbor of a recent heavy drinking bout, followed by vomiting. She had been taking large doses of codeine-containing analgesics since she had fractured her ribs in a fall.

On examination there were stigmata of chronic liver disease, with an irregular liver edge on palpation. Her spleen was not palpable, but there was moderate ascites. Rectal examination revealed hard, dark stools.

Investigations showed: hemoglobin 9.5g/dL; white cell count 3.2×10^9/L; platelets 65×10^9/L; mean corpuscular volume 117; sodium 120mmol/L (120mEq/L); potassium 2.5mmol/L (2.5mEq/L); bicarbonate 35mmol/L (35mEq/L); urea 13mmol/L (13mEq/L); creatinine 180μmol/L (2mg/dL); bilirubin 50μmol/L; alanine aminotransferase 45IU/L; alkaline phosphatase 380IU/L; albumin 22g/L and prothrombin time 26s (control 12s).

Initial management was with lactulose, phosphate enemas, chlordiazepoxide, potassium supplements, vitamin K, and a search for infection (chest radiography, blood cultures, ascitic microscopy and culture, and urine microscopy and culture). There was no evidence of infection. Over 2–3 days she became orientated and fully conscious. Two weeks later she was ready for discharge when she was found in the morning to be confused, disorientated and restless. While being assessed, she passed a large melena stool. Central venous access was obtained and emergency endoscopy showed large, esophageal varices with oozing at the cardia and a stomach full of fresh blood. Sclerotherapy was performed and she was monitored closely with appropriate transfusion and fluid replacement. Her condition remained stable. Lactulose via a nasogastric tube was given and after 24–48 hours she was once again fully orientated.

Interpretation

The patient was an alcoholic woman who had evidence of chronic liver disease on examination. She had laboratory evidence of hypersplenism and hepatic decompensation.

The initial assessment suggested symptoms of hepatic encephalopathy and/or alcohol withdrawal. Precipitating factors for HE were constipation (exacerbated by codeine preparations), electrolyte disturbances due to vomiting, and possible hepatorenal syndrome. Sepsis was considered (including spontaneous bacterial peritonitis), as was an intracranial hemorrhage in view of the history of falls. The consensus view was that the majority of her confusion and behavioral disturbance was due to alcohol withdrawal.

The second episode of depressed consciousness was associated with a major variceal hemorrhage, and this precipitated hepatic encephalopathy. Recovery occurred once the bleeding was controlled and the bowel cleared of blood.

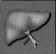

FURTHER READING

Basile AS, Jones EA. Ammonia and GABAergic neurotransmission: inter-related factors in the pathogenesis of hepatic encephalopathy. Hepatology. 1997;25:1303–5. *The authors are well known in the field and have tried to present evidence linking the major hypotheses in the pathogenesis of HE.*

Butterworth RF. The neurobiology of hepatic encephalopathy. Semin Liver Dis. 1996;16:235–44. *One of a series of publications by the author evaluating the evidence for and against various suggested factors in the development of HE. This includes a summary of the data published in this field and is perhaps a must for anyone interested in the evolution of the various theories of the pathogenesis of HE.*

Butterworth RF. Hepatic encephalopathy: disorder of multiple neurotransmitter systems. In: Record C, AL-Mardini H (eds). Advances in hepatic encephalopathy and metabolism in liver disease. Medical Faculty, University of Newcastle upon Tyne; 1997:167–76. *This entire work is the result of a meeting held on HE. In addition to this chapter, each of the chapters in this collection is a state of the art evaluation of the literature in HE.*

Charlton MR. Branched chain revisited. Gastroenterology. 1996;111:252–5. *An interesting commentary on the literature on amino acids in HE, the controversies surrounding this field, and a summary of the conclusions one may draw based on the published data. It is important, because two meta-analyses using the same studies reached different conclusions.*

Cohn R, Castell DO. The effect of acute hyperammonemia on the electroencephalogram. J Lab Clin Med. 1966;68:193–205. *(See Eichler and Bessman below.)*

Conn HO, Leiberthal MM. The syndrome of portal systemic encephalopathy. In: The hepatic coma syndrome and lactulose. Baltimore, MD: Williams & Wilkins; 1978:1–45. *This and the subsequent two books by the senior author (H.O. Conn) are the standard reference texts on hepatic encephalopathy. These books state the past, the present and the expected future in the field of hepatic encephalopathy.*

Eichler M, Bessman SP. A double-blind study of the effects of ammonium infusion on psychological functioning in cirrhotic patients. J Nerv Ment Dis. 1962;134:539–42. *This reference and the work by Cohn and Castell listed above are misquoted often enough in the literature to warrant being quoted separately here. These two studies do not demonstrate the role of ammonia in HE.*

Ferenci P, Herneth A, Steindl P. Newer approaches to therapy of hepatic encephalopathy. Semin Liver Dis. 1996;16:329–38. *A comprehensive review of the literature on the therapeutic options in HE.*

Fessel JM, Conn HO. An analysis of the causes and prevention of hepatic coma. Gastroenterology. 1972;62:191 (abstract). *The abstract quoted perhaps most in HE literature. Brings into prominence the specific role of precipitating factors in the development of HE and hence the importance of controlling these.*

Ito S, Miyaji H, Azuma T, et al. Hyperammonaemia and *Helicobacter pylori.* Lancet. 1995;346:124–5. *H. pylori has intrinsic urease activity that may potentially increase blood ammonia and thus precipitate or contribute to persistence of HE.*

Lockwood AH. Ammonia. In: Lockwood AH (ed.) Hepatic encephalopathy. Boston: Butterworth–Heinemann; 1992:65–72. *A classic book on HE viewed from the perspective of a neurologist. Extensively referenced, critically reviewed literature and illustrated well; a reference book for any worker in this field.*

Mullen KD, Gacad R. Hepatic encephalopathy. Gastroenterologist. 1996;6:188–202. *The key issues of classification and approach to a patient with HE are clarified. The existing confusion and an attempt to clarify many of the issues are briefly reviewed.*

Mullen KD, McCullough AJ. Problems with animal models of chronic liver disease. Suggestions for improvement in standardization. Hepatology. 1989;9:500–503. *A paper suggesting the limitations of available animal models in evaluating HE and the possible strategies to develop models more akin to human HE.*

Norenberg MD. Astrocytic–ammonia interactions in hepatic encephalopathy. Sem Liver Dis. 1996;16:245–53. *A summary of the evidence that astrocyte neuronal interactions influence the development of encephalopathy.*

Pomier-Layrargues G. TIPS and hepatic encephalopathy. Semin Liver Dis. 1996;16:315–20. *An extensive review of the literature with data demonstrating that closure of a portosystemic shunt could potentially reverse encephalopathy.*

Roche-Sicot J, Sicot C, Peignous M, et al. Acute hepatic encephalopathy in the rat: the effect of cross circulation. Clin Sci. 1974;47:609–15. *The classic study showing that the theory that hepatic factors protect the brain against encephalopathy was a myth.*

Rössle M, Piokaschke J. Transjugular intrahepatic portosystemic shunt and hepatic encephalopathy. Digestion. 1996;14:12–19. *The major issues in HE – portal hemodynamics, flow direction and hepatic arterial flow are discussed elegantly. A must for anyone interested in understanding the problems of hepatic hemodynamics and its role in the pathogenesis of HE.*

Seery JP, Taylor-Robinson SD. The application of magnetic resonance spectroscopy to the study of hepatic encephalopathy. J Hepatol. 1996;25:988–98. *A review of the literature on the role of an emerging investigation in HE, magnetic resonance spectroscopy, especially in latent or subclinical encephalopathy.*

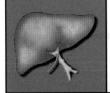

Chapter 10

Associated Systemic Conditions of Liver Disease

Robert S Brown Jr and Steven L Zacks

INTRODUCTION

Patients with liver disease may have a variety of associated extrahepatic conditions. These conditions may not always parallel the course of the liver disease and can be either based on the underlying pathogenesis (e.g. cryoglobulinemia secondary to hepatitis C viremia) or the extent of liver injury (e.g. renovascular changes from cirrhosis). Circulatory and respiratory disorders, in addition to renal diseases (see Chapter 8), are among the most significant. Many of these conditions result from alteration in hepatic bloodflow and portal hypertension that results in changes in hepatic clearance or production of important mediators of the extrahepatic diseases. There are also a number of dermatologic, hematologic, and endocrinologic abnormalities associated with liver disease.

CIRCULATORY AND RESPIRATORY DYSFUNCTION

In liver disease, the major vascular changes occur in the splanchnic and portal circulation, but there are also changes in the systemic circulation. Systemic vascular resistance is decreased and there is a decrease in effective plasma volume. The clinical manifestations of the circulatory derangements are a resting tachycardia, bounding peripheral pulses, low blood pressure, increased cardiac output and index, pronounced cardiac apical impulse, and a midsystolic cardiac murmur at the base of the heart. The decrease in systemic vascular resistance may be from arteriovenous shunting, portosystemic shunting with increased splanchnic flow, and increased levels of circulating vasodilators. Increased levels of nitric oxide as a result of nitric oxide synthase induction in the setting of cirrhosis probably plays a significant role in mediating these changes. Other proposed mediators of the hyperdynamic systemic circulation are bile acids, prostaglandins, glucagon, and bacterial endotoxins. A nonvolume-dependent hepatic baroreceptor may be responsible for the changes in sympathetic tone that contribute to the circulatory changes.

Massive ascites may reduce cardiac output. The amount of ascites may correlate with intra-abdominal and right atrial pressures. Massive ascites results in increased abdominal hydrostatic pressure that pushes on the diaphragm reducing the intrathoracic space and restricts diaphragmatic excursion which, in turn, reduces filling pressure of the heart and increases the right atrial pressure. There is a direct relationship between the amount of ascitic fluid removed during paracentesis and the improvement in cardiac output.

Arterial hypoxemia or abnormal alveolar–arterial oxygen gradients are common in cirrhosis. The prevalence of these abnormalities is as high as 45–56% and an approach to the investigation is outlined in Fig. 10.1. Hypoxemia in liver disease results from a wide range of pulmonary abnormalities including pulmonary vascular dilatation and shunting, pulmonary hypertension, pulmonary vascular leak, pulmonary vasoconstriction, ventilation–perfusion mismatching from hyperdynamic circulation, portal-pulmonary venous communication, pulmonary varices, and adult respiratory distress syndrome (Fig. 10.2). Ascites and pleural effusions can impair diaphragm function, resulting in a restrictive ventilatory defect. Disorders affecting both the liver and lung (e.g. α_1-antitrypsin deficiency) can also contribute to hypoxemia. Clinical manifestations of the pulmonary complications of liver disease are hypoxemia, hyperventilation with a respiratory alkalosis, and clubbing. Spider nevi are frequently associated with the presence of pulmonary vascular abnormalities.

Hepatopulmonary syndrome

Diagnosis of hepatopulmonary syndrome (HPS) requires three components: liver dysfunction, hypoxemia, and intrapulmonary vascular dilatation. The underlying liver dysfunction can range from acute liver failure to cirrhosis. There have also been cases described in patients following liver transplantation with chronic graft rejection. The key link between liver disease and HPS appears to be portal hypertension and it rarely, if ever, occurs in patients without portal hypertension. The etiology of intrapulmonary vascular abnormalities is not completely understood. Nitric oxide may be the most important substance responsible for the vascular dilatation. Angiogenesis factors may also be relevant.

The hypoxemia in HPS is defined as an increased alveolar–arterial gradient [greater than 3kPa (20mmHg)]. It arises from dilatation of the precapillary and capillary beds. Blood in the middle of the dilated beds does not receive oxygen diffusing out of the alveoli. In a phenomenon called orthodeoxia, the hypoxemia is more pronounced when the patient is erect. When a patient with orthodeoxia stands, gravity increases bloodflow through the dilated capillary beds in the lung bases. The hypoxemia can be corrected with oxygen supplementation distinguishing it from other types of pulmonary shunts. The intrapulmonary vascular dilatation of HPS can be documented with contrast-enhanced echocardiography. Microbubbles, induced by contrast, that could not pass through normal capillary beds are able to pass from the right to the left pulmonary circulation. Technetium-labeled, microaggregated albumin, whole body scanning is another noninvasive method of demon-

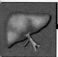

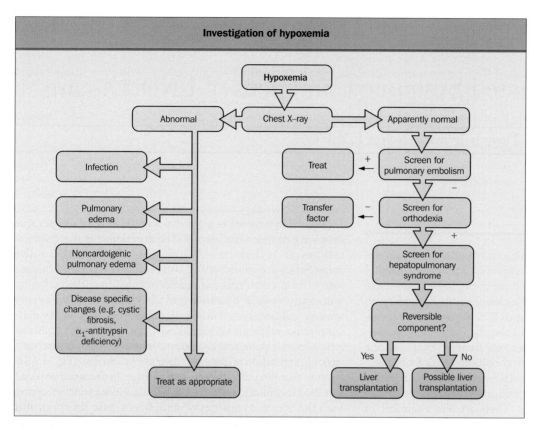

Investigation of hypoxemia

Figure 10.1 Investigation of hypoxemia. A logical approach to the investigation of hypoxemia in patients with chronic liver disease starts with a chest X-ray. The etiology of the hypoxemia is frequently multifactorial in these patients.

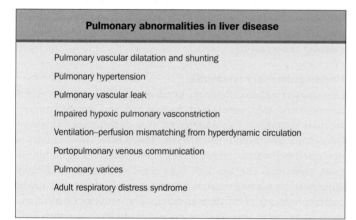

Pulmonary abnormalities in liver disease

Pulmonary vascular dilatation and shunting

Pulmonary hypertension

Pulmonary vascular leak

Impaired hypoxic pulmonary vasoconstriction

Ventilation–perfusion mismatching from hyperdynamic circulation

Portopulmonary venous communication

Pulmonary varices

Adult respiratory distress syndrome

Figure 10.2 Pulmonary abnormalities in liver disease. The main types of pulmonary dysfunction.

strating HPS that works on the same principle as the microbubble study. Detectable radioactivity over vascular beds, such as the kidneys and brain, indicates shunting. Pulmonary angiography is an invasive method of demonstrating the HPS. Angiography demonstrates diffuse and discrete shunt lesions. The presence of HPS is considered an indication for liver transplantation, provided pulmonary hypertension has not developed and adequate oxygenation can be maintained on high flow oxygen in the postoperative period. A reversible element may be demonstrable using prostaglandins or inhaled nitric oxide. Patients with arterial partial oxygen tension (PaO_2) significantly less than 60mmHg on room air or who cannot be maintained above a PaO_2 of 100mmHg on inhaled oxygen are likely to have

adverse outcomes after transplant and may not be a candidate for liver replacement.

Portopulmonary shunts have been described in a small percentage of patients with liver disease. However, these shunts are thought to be too small to produce significant hypoxemia. Furthermore, PO_2 in mesenteric veins is 6.7kPa (50mmHg). Therefore, portopulmonary shunting is not likely to be the major cause of hypoxemia. Pleural vascular anomalies similar to cutaneous spider nevi have been described, but are too small to be a significant cause of hypoxemia.

Pulmonary hypertension

Pulmonary hypertension is characterized by an elevated mean pulmonary arterial pressure and pulmonary vascular resistance with a relatively normal cardiac output. Pulmonary hypertension is considered severe when the mean pulmonary arterial pressure is greater than 6.7kPa (50mmHg). Primary pulmonary hypertension has a prevalence of 0.61–0.73% of patients with cirrhosis. It portends a worse prognosis. The etiology of primary pulmonary hypertension in cirrhosis is not known. A vasoactive substance produced in the gastrointestinal tract that is not cleared because of portosystemic shunting or diminished hepatic function may be responsible. This leads to a plexogenic pulmonary arteriopathy. Recurrent pulmonary emboli are an alternate hypothesis. When considering a patient for liver transplantation, the presence of severe pulmonary hypertension or pulmonary hypertension and limited cardiac reserve is associated with intraoperative right heart failure and early post-transplant death. Post-transplant outcomes are not affected if the mean pulmonary vascular resistance is below 277 dynes/s/cm² or the mean pulmonary arterial pressure is less than 5.9kPa (44mmHg).

Hydrothorax

A right-sided pleural effusion is commonly found in patients with moderate or severe ascites. Occasionally the effusion may develop in patients with no other clinical evidence of fluid retention. Pleural effusions develop from a combination of negative intrapleural pressures drawing ascites up from the peritoneal cavity and increased intraperitoneal pressures pushing ascites up through defects in the diaphragm. Thoracentesis to remove the effusion can improve lung volumes, increase PaO_2, decrease the arterial–alveolar oxygen gradient, and decrease intrapulmonary shunting. However, associated risks include pneumothorax and hemothorax from puncture of thoracic arteries or portosystemic collaterals in the chest wall. Chest tube drainage of a hydrothorax is seldom successful. Fluid will continue to accumulate within the chest cavity and drain via the tube. There is limited experience with pleurodesis to prevent recurrent hydrothoraces. Because the chest cavity continually collects fluid, the parietal and pleural surfaces within the chest cavity may not oppose long enough to allow scarring to develop. A transjugular intrahepatic portosystemic shunt (TIPPS) may be of value in controlling hepatic hydrothorax provided that renal function is adequate [urinary sodium $(U_{Na}) \leq 5mmol/L$, off diuretics]. However, there are limited data on the success of this procedure. Spontaneous bacterial empyema is a recognized complication of hepatic hydrothorax. Organisms leading to the infection are similar to those that cause spontaneous bacterial peritonitis and include *Escherichia coli*, *Clostridium perfringens*, and *Klebsiella pneumoniae*.

Post-transplant right pleural effusions and right lower lobe atelectasis are common and a result of the surgical manipulation of the right upper quadrant. The atelectasis and effusions resolve with time. However, an effusion that does not resolve suggests pulmonary infection or a subdiaphragmatic biloma, abscess, or hematoma. Intraoperative right phrenic nerve injury, which may occur during suprahepatic vena caval clamping, may lead to hemidiaphragm paralysis limiting vital capacity, but not necessarily resulting in prolonged ventilation. Follow-up pulmonary testing suggests that phrenic nerve injury usually resolves in a matter of months.

Other pulmonary manifestations

Encephalopathy associated with a significant decrease in the level of consciousness may lead to aspiration and atelectasis. Intubation and mechanical ventilation can be used to prevent these outcomes. Volume-controlled ventilation is sufficient in the absence of active lung disease as a consequence of the liver disease. Positive end-expiratory pressure should not exceed $8cmH_2O$ because values greater than this may increase intracranial pressure and decrease hepatic bloodflow. Pulmonary infections may be present without infiltrates on radiography due to decreased neutrophil function and resulting decreases in inflammation. Interestingly, as the liver recovers, neutrophil function also recovers, and pulmonary infections may become apparent. The resulting inflammation reduces lung compliance and pressure support ventilation may be required.

Significant liver and pulmonary disease may coexist in diseases such as cystic fibrosis and α_1-antitrypsin deficiency. Granulomatous lung disease may be seen in primary biliary cirrhosis. In Sjogren's syndrome associated with liver disease, pulmonary fibrosis may occur. The fibrosis could be from bronchial gland atrophy from lymphocyte infiltration, causing dryness and the accumulation of inspissated secretions.

Pretransplant assessment

Liver transplantation is the most strenuous of all upper abdominal operations because of operative time and the potential for diaphragmatic injury. Assessment of pulmonary function before liver transplantation detects abnormalities that may result in postoperative complications. Preoperative pulmonary function testing can also detect the presence of pulmonary hypertension and HPS. Most programs require at least an arterial blood gas on room air. Pulse oximetry is rendered inaccurate by hyperbilirubinemia. Measurement of diffusing capacity may be necessary and should be obtained in patients with a history of smoking or an abnormal arterial blood gas. Right heart catheterization may be necessary before liver transplantation to rule out pulmonary hypertension, which can arise from longstanding hypoxemia and be a contraindication to transplantation.

HEMATOLOGIC CHANGES IN LIVER DISEASE

Anemia, neutropenia, and thrombocytopenia are common in advanced liver disease. Approximately 75% of patients with chronic liver disease have anemia. There are many factors that can lead to anemia including the toxic effect of alcohol on the bone marrow, folate deficiency associated with alcoholism, and the anemia of chronic inflammation. Liver disease shortens red blood cell survival, dilutes red blood cells by increasing plasma volume, and impairs the marrow response to the anemia. Red blood cell survival is shortened. Repeated episodes of blood loss (e.g. from variceal bleeding) will lead to a microcytic anemia.

Hemolysis and splenic sequestration also contribute to the anemia. Alloantibodies and alterations in red blood cell metabolism and membranes lead to the hemolysis. There is a reduced capacity for red blood cells to prevent damage from oxidants in the presence of other defects in red blood cells (e.g. glucose-6-dehydrogenase deficiency). Decreased intracellular levels of reduced glutathione and reduced activity of the hexose monophosphate shunt contribute to the inability of red blood cells to tolerate oxidants. Alterations in red blood cell membrane lipid metabolism leads to a spur-cell hemolytic anemia that is seen in approximately 10–15% of patients with liver disease. In advanced liver disease the lipid composition of the red cell is increased by 25–30%, causing the cell to be acanthocytic and macrocytic. Increases in the cholesterol to phospholipid ratio within the red blood cell membrane contribute to the acanthocytosis with decreased membrane flexibility reducing survival. Changes in the surface volume ratio of the red blood cell while in the spleen increases the osmotic fragility. The changes in the lipid composition of the red blood cell are probably induced by changes in plasma lecithin-cholesterol acyltransferase activity or increase in bile acids. When this occurs in the context of alcoholic liver disease it is referred to as Zieve syndrome. Hemolysis is a feature of the acute presentation of Wilson's disease, and there is usually coexisting thrombocytopenia reflecting the underlying cirrhosis and portal hypertension. Autoimmune-mediated hemolytic anemia or thrombocytopenia, or both (Evans' syndrome), may occur in patients with autoimmune chronic hepatitis.

The anemia associated with hypersplenism is typically normocytic or macrocytic with elevations in the reticulocyte count. The hypersplenism associated with portal hypertension may result in sequestration of blood cells leading to neutropenia and thrombocytopenia. About 60% of patients with hypersplenism

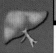
will have a decrease in the white blood cell count. It is important to note that the differential is normal, which can distinguish the leukopenia of hypersplenism from that of other causes. Thrombocytopenia is common in hypersplenism. Hypersplenism rarely requires treatment. However, should pain from massive splenomegaly or cytopenias requiring frequent transfusion develop, TIPSS or surgical shunting may be necessary. Rarely, splenectomy may be required but should be considered high risk.

CUTANEOUS MANIFESTATIONS

Severe pruritus is one of the more common cutaneous manifestations of liver disease. Many substances that are normally secreted in the bile, including those that cause pruritus, are retained in cholestasis. The exact cause of pruritus is not known. Bile acids or a centrally acting opioid agonist have been implicated. Cholestyramine and colestipol, bile sequestering agents, are effective first-line treatments. They may reduce pruritus by sequestering bile salts that would otherwise antagonize opioid receptors. Their activity may involve more than sequestration because they are effective in reducing the pruritus associated with uremia. Ursodeoxycholic acid, a hydrophilic bile acid, is less toxic than natural, hydrophobic bile acids and can also be effective in reducing pruritus. Ursodiol has the other advantage of not further depleting intestinal bile salts that can lead to fat malabsorption. Naloxone and naltrexone, both opioid antagonists, rifampin (rifampicin), ultraviolet light, and ondansetron may be beneficial in some patients.

Chronic liver disease affects the cutaneous vasculature. Spider angiomas are the most common vascular lesions. They frequently occur on the face, upper trunk, and distal upper extremities. A central vessel surrounded by branching, smaller vessels forms the angiomata. Palmar erythema, a reddish pigmentation involving the thenar and hypothenar eminences, is another manifestation of liver disease. Like spider angiomas, palmar erythema may be related to elevated levels of circulating estrogens seen in liver disease. Xanthomas are seen in primary biliary cirrhosis due to hypercholesterolemia. Vitiligo can be seen in a variety of autoimmune diseases, including autoimmune hepatitis and primary biliary cirrhosis.

The nails can be affected in liver disease and may provide some clues into its etiology. Azure lunulae, a bluish discoloration of the white, half-moon, proximal portion of the nail bed, are seen in Wilson's disease. A whitish discoloration of the nail with accentuation of the distal pink portion of the nail plate proximal to the free end of the nail is known as 'Terry's nails' and is seen in cirrhosis, particularly primary biliary cirrhosis. Splinter hemorrhages have been described in hepatitis. Double white transverse lines on the nails, called Muehrcke's lines, are seen in liver failure. Hypertrophic osteoarthropathy, leading to clubbing, can occur in primary biliary cirrhosis.

There are a number of dermatologic diseases seen in association with hepatitis B and C (Figs 10.3 & 10.4, respectively). A necrotizing vasculitis with palpable purpura and petechiae, particularly in the lower extremities, occurs in patients with hepatitis B or C (Fig. 10.5). The course of this skin disease is independent of the hepatitis and is associated with arthralgia, fever, mononeuritis multiplex, and renal disease. Patients with viral hepatitis, particularly hepatitis B, may have twice the risk of developing lichen planus as the general population. Approximately 11.3% of patients with lichen planus have hepati-

tis B. Lichen planus in association with hepatitis C can have a prolonged duration, generalized distribution, and a high incidence of mucosal involvement (Fig. 10.6). It is seen in approximately 5% of patients with hepatitis C. The similarity between the hepatic and dermatologic lymphocytic infiltrate is interesting. However, neither hepatitis virus has been isolated from the skin lesion.

A papular eruption of the trunk and upper extremities has been associated with patients with hepatitis B. Skin biopsy of the eruption shows a perivascular, mononuclear infiltrate. An abnormal cell-mediated host response has been implicated. Papular acrodermatitis is described in children with hepatitis B. It is a papular eruption limited to the face and extremities often associated with inguinal and axillary lymphadenopathy. The eruption may last for 15–30 days and starts to fade as the course of the acute hepatitis peaks. Urticaria and fever has been observed in acute hepatitis B virus infection. Biopsies of the urticarial lesions show deposition of complement, fibrinogen, IgM, and hepatitis B surface antigen. Polyarteritis nodosa has been described in patients with hepatitis B,

---

Dermatologic diseases associated with chronic hepatitis B
Papular eruption of the trunk and upper extremities
Leukocytoclastic vasculitis
Polyarteritis nodosum
Lichen planus
Erythema nodosum
Papular acrodermatitis of childhood
Erythema multiforme
Urticaria
Dermatomyositis-like syndrome
Mixed cryoglobulinemia
Pyoderma gangrenosum

Figure 10.3 Dermatologic diseases associated with chronic hepatitis B. Disorders of the skin seen in association with hepatitis B. (From Parsons ME, Russo GG, Millikan LE. Dermatologic disorders associated with viral hepatitis infections. Int J Dermatol. 1996;35:77–81.)

Dermatologic diseases associated with chronic hepatitis C
Leukocytoclastic vasculitis
Polyarteritis nodosa
Porphyrea cutanea tarda
Lichen planus
Erythema nodosum and panniculitis
Erythema multiforme
Urticaria

Figure 10.4 Dermatologic diseases associated with chronic hepatitis C. Disorders of the skin seen in association with hepatitis C. (From Daoud MS, Gibson LE, Daoud S, El-Azhary RA. Chronic hepatitis C and skin diseases: a review. Mayo Clin Proc. 1995;70:559–64.)

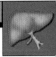
with an estimated prevalence of 0.4%. Angioedema, subcutaneous nodules, urticarial lesions, and ulcerations are seen in polyarteritis nodosa. Leukocytoclastic vasculitis associated with arthralgias and Raynaud's phenomenon have been reported in patients with hepatitis C. Cryoglobulinemia in hepatitis C may present with a number of dermatologic manifestations, including a petechial eruption of the extremities. Purpuric lesions, macules, and papules with ulcerations are described in hepatitis C, while erythema multiforme and erythema nodosum have been temporally associated with hepatitis C virus infection.

Porphyria cutanea tarda, another dermatologic manifestation of hepatitis C, is caused by an enzymatic deficiency in the heme pathway leading to an accumulation of intermediate metabolites, the porphyrins. Specifically, in porphyria cutanea tarda there is a reduction in the hepatic uroporphyrinogen decarboxylase activity, resulting in a reduced conversion of uroporphyrinogen to coproporphyrinogen. The uroporphyrinogen is oxidized to uroporphyrins, which accumulate in the liver and the skin. The porphyrins lead to the biochemical and clinical manifestations of the disease. There is a high prevalence of hepatitis B or C markers in the setting of spontaneous porphyria cutanea tarda (62–76% of patients are hepatitis C-positive). Among the

many manifestations of porphyria cutanea tarda there is hyperfragility of the skin, particularly on the dorsum of the hands; photosensitivity; hyperpigmentation of the face; hypertrichosis; premature aging of the skin; scleroderma-like changes in the thorax, head, and neck; and alopecia (Fig. 10.7). Palmar fibromatosis and ocular photosensitivity are seen in porphyria cutanea tarda. Porphyrins cause the urine to have a reddish fluorescence. Isocoproporphyrin is found in the stool. Treatment of the porphyrias includes phlebotomy and interferon-based treatment for the underlying viral hepatitis.

HORMONAL DERANGEMENTS

In cirrhosis, the reduction of hydrocortisone and glucuronidation of cortisol are impaired. Urinary excretion of corticoids is low. Plasma levels of cortisol are normal or high but lack a circadian rhythm. Production, hepatic clearance, and metabolism of cortisol are impaired. Cortisol is bound to albumin and cortisolbinding globulin, which are both decreased in the setting of cirrhosis. There is debate as to whether the binding activity of cortisol-binding globulin may be increased or decreased. Intrahepatic cholestasis may play a role in the abnormalities of steroid metabolism. Changes in bloodflow to the liver in cirrhosis may play a role in the changes in cortisol metabolism. However, aldosterone metabolism is impaired in part because of changes to hepatic bloodflow in cirrhosis.

There are abnormalities in the circadian rhythm of the anteropituitary, which is responsible for the release of adrenocorticotropic hormone (ACTH), growth hormone (GH), thyroid-stimulating hormone (TSH), follicle-stimulating hormone (FSH), luteinizing hormone (LH), and prolactin. The liver is responsible for the conversion of 85% of thyroxine to triiodothyronine, and circulating levels of the latter are often significantly decreased in patients with cirrhosis. Thyroid antibodies may be found in 15–25% of patients with primary biliary cirrhosis and thyroid dysfunction is the most common extrahepatic manifestation of primary biliary cirrhosis.

The prevalence of impaired glucose metabolism is increased in patients with chronic liver disease, with up to 15% fulfilling criteria for the diagnosis of diabetes mellitus. In most cases this

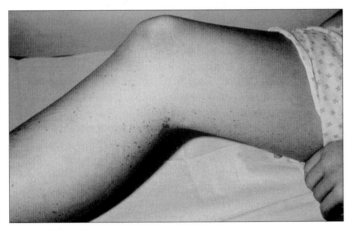

Figure 10.5 Vasculitis. Vasculitic lesions of lower extremities in patient with hepatitis C and cryoglobulinemia. (Courtesy of Eileen Lambroza, MD.)

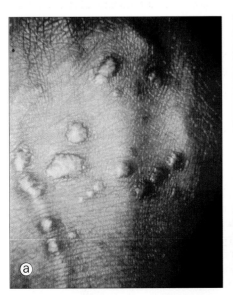

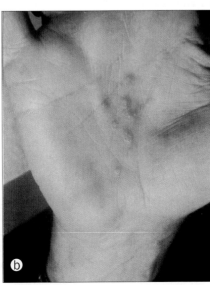

(a)

(b)

Figure 10.6 Lichen planus. This has been reported in association with hepatitis C and primary biliary cirrhosis. (Courtesy of Richard Granstein, MD.)

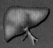
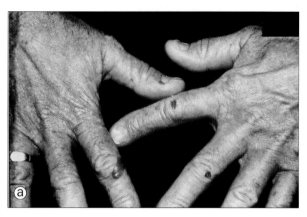
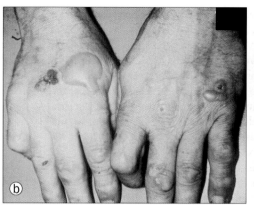
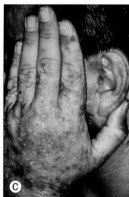

Figures 10.7 Porphyria cutanea tarda. This is the commonest skin condition seen in patients with hepatitis C. (Courtesy of Eileen Lambroza, MD.)

occurs despite increased circulating levels of insulin, which either bypasses the liver through shunts or fails to be extracted by the liver. There is also evidence to suggest that glucose extraction and glycogen synthesis is decreased in muscle. Decreased pancreatic endocrine function may be a feature of alcohol-related chronic pancreatitis or patients with cystic fibrosis who have coexisting liver disease. Hepatitis C virus infection and autoimmune chronic hepatitis appear to be associated with an increased susceptibility to autoimmune diabetes mellitus.

Fertility

Males with liver disease experience feminization and hypogonadism. These changes appear to be independent of the type of liver disease. Some of the changes include loss of body hair, gynecomastia, testicular atrophy, reduced libido, oligospermia, and impotence. The underlying abnormality in the setting of liver disease is in the hypothalamic–pituitary–gonadal hormone axis. At the hypothalamic level, gonadotropic-releasing hormone (GnRH) secretion is impaired. At the pituitary level, there is a decrease in the basal secretion of LH and FSH. At the gonadal level, there is reduced production of sex steroid hormone, 17α-hydroxylase, 3β-hydroxysteroid dehydrogenase, and Δ5,4-isomerase. Changes at the gonadal level and in the production of gonadotropin result in low testosterone levels. At the same time sex hormone binding globulin levels are increased, leading to further reduction in free testosterone levels, the biologically active form of testosterone.

Hyperprolactinemia and hyperestrogenemia that may be seen in males with significant hepatic decompensation further exacerbate feminization. The hyperestrogenemia is due to increased peripheral conversion of androgens to estrogens and decreased hepatic metabolism. In the setting of portal hypertension, adrenal estrogens and androgens in the portal circulation escape hepatic extraction and are aromatized in the peripheral circulation to estrogens. Thus, estrogen levels increase and reduce pituitary LH secretion, leading to a decrease in testosterone levels. The observed sex hormone changes are reversed after liver transplantation.

Unfortunately, there are very few data on hormonal and fertility changes in women with cirrhosis. Despite the proposed explanation for the hormonal changes in males, women experience a masculinization with amenorrhea as a result. Whether this is due to hyperestrogenemia or other factors is unknown.

BONE DISEASE

A decrease in osteoblastic activity and increased osteoclastic activity are seen in cirrhosis of all etiologies. This manifests as osteopenia, which is seen in up to 50% of patients with the cholestatic diseases, primary biliary cirrhosis and primary sclerosing cholangitis, and in 16% of patients with autoimmune chronic hepatitis. Genetic factors and hyperbilirubinemia may be additional factors in the development of the osteopenia. The process primarily affects the hips and vertebrae and atraumatic fractures are common. Calcium supplementation with vitamin D should be used to treat the osteoporosis. Hormone replacement therapy is also beneficial. Ursodeoxycholic acid is not helpful; neither is calcitonin. There are limited but encouraging data on the utility of the bisphosphonates. Osteomalacia caused by vitamin D malabsorption from cholestasis is a rare complication of primary biliary cirrhosis. Osteomalacia is reversible with vitamin D supplementation, but is no longer seen with the availability of liver transplantation. A hypertrophic osteoarthropathy with clubbing is described in patients with liver disease (e.g. primary biliary cirrhosis) (Fig. 10.8).

COAGULOPATHY

Normal coagulation is closely linked to liver function. Most of the coagulation factors, many components of the fibrinolytic system, and some of the important regulatory proteins found in the plasma are made in the liver. The reticuloendothelial system of the liver clears activated clotting factors, activation complexes of both coagulation and fibrinolysis, and the degradation products of fibrinogen and fibrin. Increased levels of these products combined with thrombocytopenia, impaired platelet function, abnormalities in vitamin K-dependent clotting factors, vitamin K deficiency, enhanced fibrinolytic activity, dysfibrinogenemia, and disseminated intravascular coagulopathy (DIC) all contribute to the coagulopathy associated with liver disease (Fig. 10.9). The close link between liver function and coagulation makes the prothrombin time the best indicator of the extent of hepatocellular dysfunction, bleeding risk, and overall prognosis.

There are a number of procoagulants that are affected by liver disease. In biliary cirrhosis and obstructive jaundice there is normal or overproduction of procoagulants. Hepatocellular disease leads to a defect in postribosomal γ-carboxylation, resulting in a decrease in the four vitamin K-dependent procoagulants,

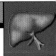

factors II, VII, IX, and X. Hepatocellular damage does not, of itself, lead to vitamin K deficiency. However, malnutrition in association with alcoholic liver disease can lead to vitamin K deficiency. Other causes of vitamin K deficiency include biliary fistula, intrahepatic or extrahepatic cholestasis, cholestyramine use, and fat malabsorption. In fact, the response to administered vitamin K in the setting of liver disease can help distinguish between cholestatic and hepatocellular disease.

In addition to the vitamin K-dependent factors, factor V deficiency is seen in severe liver disease. The degree of deficiency parallels the decrease in levels of albumin. Paradoxically, factor V may be elevated in chronic cholestatic liver disease due to the general increase in protein production that occurs in these diseases. The etiology may be decreased inhibition of factor V by protein C, a vitamin K-dependent protein that is decreased in the presence of cholestasis. Factor VIII is the only factor that is synthesized both within the liver and elsewhere. In the setting of liver disease, factor VIII is increased. It may be that clearance of this factor by the reticuloendothelial system is impaired or that there is increased release by damaged endothelial cells. Thus, factor VIII levels can be difficult to interpret in cirrhosis, and distinguishing DIC and consumption of clotting factors from liver failure and decreased synthesis is difficult. Constituents of the contact activation system (factors XI and XII, prekallikrein, and high-molecular-weight kininogen) may be decreased as part of the general decrease in protein synthesis. Prekallikrein levels can be depressed further because of a low-grade consumptive coagulopathy that can be seen in liver disease in response to transient endotoxemia. Similar to other proteins, factors XI and XII may be increased in cholestatic diseases due to increased protein synthesis. Factor XIII can be decreased in advanced liver disease. However, this factor may also be increased in the setting of cholestatic liver disease. Fibrinogen levels are normal or increased in all forms of liver disease. Dysfibrinogenemia leading to defective polymerization of fibrin is common in liver disease and is detected by an abnormal thrombin time. It is more common in hepatocellular disease than cholestatic disease.

Because plasma inhibitors of coagulation are also synthesized in the liver, levels of these inhibitors may also be abnormal. The liver is the major source of antithrombin III. Levels of antithrombin III may be normal in mild-to-moderate hepatocellular disease. In the setting of cholestasis, levels are normal to increased. In advanced hepatocellular disease and cirrhosis, levels of antithrombin III are decreased. The decreased levels may be a result of consumption due to the low-grade DIC that may accompany advanced liver disease. Alternatively, there may be some transcapillary loss of antithrombin III. However, despite low levels of antithrombin III, thrombosis is rare. The rarity of thrombosis is likely due to many factors including the low levels of procoagulants, the increased fibrinolytic activity associated with liver disease, and possibly normal levels of endothelial-bound antithrombin III, as well as elevations in other antithrombins. Both proteins C and S are synthesized in the liver and are decreased in the setting of advanced liver disease. However, they are not associated with an increased propensity to thrombosis. Although heparin cofactor II, an inhibitor of thrombin, is low in the setting of advanced liver disease, it does not play a role in the abnormalities of hemostasis. Variable levels of α_2-antiplasmin, the primary inhibitor of plasmin, have been found in liver disease. It limits the rate of fibrin degradation by plasmin, thus maintaining the fibrin mesh. A deficiency may contribute to the increased risk of bleeding seen in liver disease. Plasminogen activator inhibitor-1 (PAI-1) is the primary inhibitor of plasminogen activators and limits fibrinolytic activity to the hemostatic plug. Variable levels of PAI-1 have been reported in liver disease; PAI-1 may not increase appropriately and accelerated fibrinolysis may contribute to the bleeding observed. Inhibitors of the contact activation pathway, the plasma protease inhibitors C1-inhibitor, α_1-antitrypsin, and α_2-macroglobulin, are preserved in liver disease.

Plasminogen levels are reduced in liver disease. However, the activity of plasminogen activators is increased. Tissue plasminogen activator (tPA) levels are increased because hepatic clearance is diminished. Bleeding risk is increased further because inhibitors of fibrinolysis (e.g. PAI-1 levels), are decreased. With all the changes in the individual coagulation factors, it is important to recall that all of the individual abnormalities of these factors measured *in vitro* do

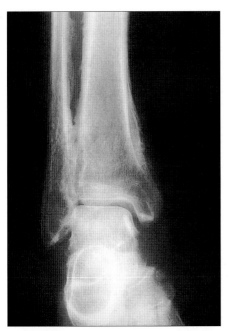

Figure 10.8 Pulmonary osteodystrophy. The periosteal reaction is classical of this condition, which is almost always associated with clubbing.

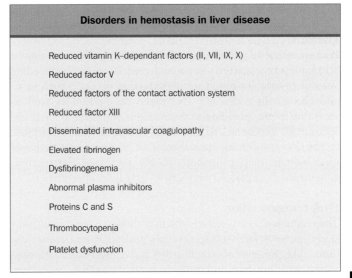

Disorders in hemostasis in liver disease
Reduced vitamin K–dependant factors (II, VII, IX, X)
Reduced factor V
Reduced factors of the contact activation system
Reduced factor XIII
Disseminated intravascular coagulopathy
Elevated fibrinogen
Dysfibrinogenemia
Abnormal plasma inhibitors
Proteins C and S
Thrombocytopenia
Platelet dysfunction

Figure 10.9 Disorders in hemostasis in liver disease. The factors that contribute to the coagulopathy seen with liver disease include coagulation factor synthesis, thrombolysis, and platelet disorders.

not necessarily predispose to clinical risks of bleeding. There is an association between accelerated fibrinolysis and bleeding from mucous membranes and fatal hemorrhage. There is also a relationship between excessive fibrinolysis and fatal gastrointestinal hemorrhage in patients with cirrhosis. Abnormal fibrinolysis is not seen in acute liver disease, with the exception of acute liver failure.

DISSEMINATED INTRAVASCULAR COAGULATION

Disseminated intravascular coagulation is a pathologic coagulative response to an underlying illness in which thrombin is produced and the fibrinolytic system is activated. There is excessive formation of thrombin, which catalyzes the activation and consumption of coagulation factors, fibrinogen, and platelets. Fibrin thrombi form in the microvasculature. The degradation of fibrin and fibrinogen by plasmin produces fibrin degradation products (FDPs). These are cleared by the reticuloendothelial system of the liver. If they are not cleared from the blood, FDPs may circulate and interfere with the cleavage of fibrinogen by thrombin and the polymerization of fibrin monomers. Presentation of DIC ranges from the patient being mildly ill with subclinical laboratory abnormalities, to an acutely ill patient with bleeding and possibly thrombosis. Initiating factors in patients with liver disease may include the release of procoagulants from dying hepatocytes, activation of the intrinsic system by stasis of blood in the expanded portal circulation, and endotoxin from the bowel that is not cleared by the diseased liver. Because the liver has a critical role in maintaining hemostatic balance, the loss of function of the reticuloendothelial system in clearing activated factors and the lack of production of plasma inhibitors could perpetuate or worsen DIC.

Acute DIC is reported to occur in patients with acute fatty liver of pregnancy, acute liver failure, and after the placement of peritoneovenous shunts. Chronic DIC has a pattern of laboratory abnormalities similar to that of chronic liver disease, suggesting that chronic DIC is a manifestation of chronic liver disease or that the two processes are indistinguishable. Patients with chronic liver disease are more susceptible to acute DIC from stresses of surgery, infection, hypotension, and the procoagulant load from the shunting of ascites into the circulation.

Platelets
Both quantitative and qualitative defects in platelets are seen in acute and chronic liver disease and contribute to the bleeding risk due to coagulopathy. Thrombocytopenia occurs in both acute and chronic liver disease. Decreased production as well as increased splenic pooling and destruction contribute to the problem. Drugs, infections, and nutritional deficiencies may contribute to the decreased production. Both DIC and immune-mediated phenomenon may contribute to the increased destruction. Abnormalities in platelet aggregation have been observed.

Liver transplantation
The coagulopathy associated with liver disease is most significant during surgery, liver transplantation, and other invasive procedures. The presence of coagulopathy and hemorrhage were associated with adverse outcomes in patients with liver disease undergoing surgery. The management of the coagulopathy of liver disease is particularly challenging during liver transplantation. During native liver resection bleeding can be significant,

particularly if the patient had previous hepatobiliary surgery. Collateral vessels from portal hypertension contribute to the bleeding. The anhepatic phase of transplantation exacerbates the systemic fibrinolysis and DIC associated with end-stage liver disease. After vascularization of the graft the rate of reversal of the coagulopathy depends on the function of the graft. Hyperfibrinolysis during and shortly after the anhepatic phase has led to the use of antifibrinolytics by some groups. After graft perfusion, particularly if graft function is good, procoagulant factors may return faster than anticoagulants. A hypercoagulable state ensues with a risk of thrombosis. Therefore, some transplant groups contend that inhibitors of thrombin (e.g. antithrombin III) should be used prior to or without the administration of antifibrinolytics after perfusion of the graft. Low-dose heparin and fresh frozen plasma (FFP) are used postoperatively to reduce the risk of thrombosis.

Properly developed guidelines on the management of patients with liver disease and coagulopathy undergoing invasive procedures, such as liver biopsy, placement of central intravenous lines, and paracenteses, do not exist. Patients who require a liver biopsy but have a prothrombin time greater than 3s above control or a platelet count of less than 80,000/mm^3 may face less risk of morbidity and mortality if the biopsy is done via the transjugular route rather than percutaneously. Patients requiring other percutaneous procedures may do well without blood product support if their platelet counts are 100,000/mm^3 or greater and their prothrombin times are not more than 5s above control. Patients who appear to be at risk of bleeding should be given 2–4 units of fresh frozen plasma and platelet transfusions just before commencing the procedure.

Disease-specific associations
A coagulopathy may be seen in patients with hepatocellular carcinoma (HCC), although it is hard to differentiate between the effects of the underlying cirrhosis and the effects of the hepatoma. An abnormal form of prothrombin, des-γ-carboxyprothrombin, is produced in patients with HCC and may contribute to the coagulopathy. Limited data suggest that patients with metastatic disease to the liver have a coagulopathy in the absence of other signs of liver synthetic dysfunction, suggesting that the cause of coagulopathy in malignancy is more than the underlying liver disease. Biliary tract disease results in normal or high levels of coagulation factors, provided that vitamin K levels are normal. Nevertheless, an increased risk of thrombosis is not seen in these patients.

Treatment
Fresh frozen plasma is central to the management of patients with liver disease and coagulopathy, and contains all the procoagulants and anticoagulants found in blood. It can be administered at 12–20mL/kg in attempt to correct the prothrombin time to within 3s of control, although this may not be possible. Vitamin K is only useful in cases of deficiency, particularly in cholestatic liver disease. Intravenous administration is preferable, because intramuscular injection may lead to hematoma and subcutaneous injections may not be reliably absorbed. The historic risk of anaphylaxis is greatly overstated with current vitamin K preparations. Cryoprecipitate, containing factor VIII, von Willebrand factor (vWF), and fibrinogen, and prothrombin complex, containing factors II, VII, IX, and X, are rarely indicated for the management of coagulopathy associated with liver disease. Platelets are of value in the setting of

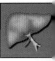

thrombocytopenia, although response to transfusions may be reduced because of splenic sequestration. Heparin and antithrombin III have been used to treat bleeding in patients with liver disease. These agents inhibit thrombin, which decreases procoagulant consumption, leading to normal levels of coagulation factors and normal hemostasis. However, there is no evidence from clinical trials to support their routine use. Desmopressin acetate (DDAVP) can shorten the bleeding time and increase vWF levels, as well as cause transient increases in other factors. However, vWF levels are increased in cirrhosis, so the use of DDAVP is not advocated, except in patients with concomitant renal dysfunction. Antifibrinolytic agents, ε-aminocaproic acid and tranexamic acid, can be used to treat hyperfibrinolysis. However, these agents are contraindicated in patients with DIC because of the risk of thrombosis. Because many patients with advanced liver disease may have an element of DIC and it may be difficult to detect, the use of antifibrinolytics in patients with liver disease is inadvisable.

DRUG METABOLISM

Hepatic clearance of drugs may be influenced by a number of factors (Fig. 10.10). The extent of impairment in drug metabolism in the setting of liver disease is a function of the nature and severity of liver disease. The impairment may be compounded by other factors (e.g. poor nutrition, alcohol or drug use, or the presence of associated drug therapy). Changes in hepatic bloodflow in cirrhosis lead to changes in metabolism of drugs. Liver fibrosis and arteriovenous shunting changes the availability of drugs for hepatic metabolism. The concentration of drugs in the portal and systemic circulation can be altered because of portosystemic shunting. Altered levels of albumin and hepatocyte dysfunction will also alter drug binding in plasma, hepatic uptake, and metabolism. Decreased hepatic enzyme and cofactor levels result from the decrease in hepatic volume, gene expression, and hepatocyte necrosis. The cytochrome P450 system, an important group of enzymes involved in drug metabolism, is impaired in liver disease. The specific isoenzymes known to be impaired are CYP1A2, CYP2A6, CYP2D6, and CYP3A. Uridine diphosphate-glucuronyltransferase, an important enzyme required for the glucuronidation step of biliary excretion, is also impaired in the setting of liver disease. Interleukin-6, which is released in active liver disease, may inhibit cytochrome enzymes. Hepatocyte hypoxia may lead to reduced drug enzyme activity. Cholestasis will impair the elimination of drugs that rely on the enterohepatic circulation for their excretion. In general the net effect of these changes is to reduce drug metabolism and decrease clearance; however, increased clearance of drugs metabolized by the cytochrome P450 system are seen early in alcoholic liver disease due to the induction of these enzymes by ethanol.

IMMUNE MANIFESTATIONS OF LIVER DISEASE

Viral hepatitis has a number of different immune manifestations. Approximately 10–20% of patients with hepatitis C have antinuclear antibodies (ANAs). The antibody titer is low, usually less than 1:100, and has a speckled pattern of immunofluorescence. This is in contrast to type 1 autoimmune hepatitis, in which the ANA titer is greater than 1:100 and homogenous. Anti-smooth muscle antibodies (anti-SMA) in hepatitis have

Factors influencing altered drug metabolism in liver disease
Nutritional deficiency
Shunting, reducing availability for hepatic metabolism
Shunting, changing the volume of distribution
Hypoalbuminemia, reducing drug binding
Reduced levels or function of hepatic enzymes
Altered biliary excretion from cholestasis

Figure 10.10 Factors influencing altered drug metabolism in liver disease. These impact to varying degrees on drug metabolism and care should be taken with all prescribing in patients with chronic liver disease.

low titers, usually less than 1:100, and do not react with actin. The presence of ANAs and anti-SMA antibodies in hepatitis C seems to be clinically unimportant. Anti-liver–kidney-microsomal (Anti-LKM1) antibodies are seen in type 2 autoimmune hepatitis. They may be seen in less than 5% of patients with hepatitis C. In hepatitis C, the titer is usually less than 1:500, in contrast to type 2 autoimmune hepatitis, in which the titer is greater than 1:500. The antigenic sites recognized by the anti-LKM1 antibodies in hepatitis C are different from those of patients with type 2 autoimmune hepatitis, although they are directed against the same isoenzyme of the cytochrome P450 system. The presence of anti-LKM1 antibodies is not associated with severity of liver disease in hepatitis C, although some patients have an increase in their transaminases after starting interferon therapy. Most hepatitis C patients with anti-LKM1 antibodies have anti-GOR antibodies. The presence of anti-GOR antibodies has no pathologic significance, but these antibodies are not present in type 2 autoimmune hepatitis and therefore can be useful diagnostically.

Cryoglobulins are serum proteins that are precipitated below body temperature. There are three types of cryoglobulins, which are determined by the nature of the immunoglobulins that make up the cryoglobulins. Type I is composed of a monoclonal immunoglobulin. Type II consists of a mixture of monoclonal immunoglobulin, usually IgM rheumatoid factor, and polyclonal immunoglobulin. Type III consists of polyclonal immunoglobulin, one of which has rheumatoid factor activity. Complement may be part of type II and III cryoglobulins. Mixed cryoglobulinemia leads to purpura, weakness, Raynaud's syndrome, arthralgias, glomerulonephritis, peripheral neuropathy, sicca syndrome, and vasculitis. The vasculitis arises from the deposition of cryoglobulins in the walls of small vessels.

Many studies report a high prevalence of hepatitis C antibody positivity in the setting of mixed cryoglobulinemia ranging from 30–90%. In fact, some cryoglobulins contain hepatitis C antibodies and RNA. Conversely, 36–54% of patients with hepatitis C have cryoglobulinemia and 70% may have rheumatoid factor. Cryoglobulinemia is not unique to hepatitis C; 15% of patients with hepatitis B and 32% of patients with other liver diseases have been found to have circulating cryoglobulins. In the majority of patients with hepatitis C the concentration of cryoglobulins is low and is type II. Patients may be asymptomatic or have mild symptoms of fatigue and arthralgias. In a small proportion of patients, cryoglobulinemia is associated with vasculitis, arthralgia, skin ulcers, Raynaud's syndrome, purpura, peripheral neuropathy, or glomerulonephritis. The cryoglobulinemia associated with hepatitis C correlates with duration and severity of disease. However, the level of viremia and hepatitis C genotypes do not correlate with the presence of cryoglobulins. Cryoglobulins can be difficult to measure, so careful testing with maintenance of the sample at 37°C is important. Rheumatoid factor, the measurement of which is not temperature-sensitive, can be helpful in suspected cases of cryoglobulinemia when the measured cryoglobulins are negative.

Glomerulonephritis has been associated with hepatitis C and cryoglobulinemia. It is usually the membranoproliferative type. Rarely an endocapillary glomerulonephritis or membranous glomerulonephritis can be seen. The pathogenesis is thought to be the deposition of immune complexes consisting of cryoglobulins and hepatitis C antibodies and RNA in the basement membrane of the glomeruli. Microscopic hematuria and proteinuria, the majority of which is from the immune-mediated renal disease, have been observed in 9 and 27% of patients with hepatitis C, respectively.

Some studies point to an association between hepatitis C and autoimmune thyroiditis. Antihepatitis C antibodies may be seen in 20% of patients with autoimmune thyroiditis. Antihepatitis C antibodies have been found in 7% of patients with antithyroid antibodies without biochemically apparent thyroid disease. Patients with a combination of antihepatitis C and thyroid antibodies have higher levels of anti-GOR antibodies. Antithyroglobulin and antimicrosomal antibodies can be found in 11 and 6%, respectively, of patients with chronic hepatitis C. Other studies suggest the prevalence of either antibody can be as low as 3%. Antithyroid antibodies are more common in hepatitis C than B. However, the connection between hepatitis C and autoimmune thyroiditis is not proven. Thyroid antibody testing is subject to some variability because of the differences in the levels that are considered to be abnormal. In addition, the presence of thyroid antibodies in the general population may be high, with some studies finding a prevalence of up to 30%.

Finally, another possible immune-mediated extrahepatic manifestation of viral hepatitis is sialadenitis. Mild clinical and histologic sialadenitis may be common in hepatitis C patients. The hepatitis C virus may infect the salivary glands directly or cause a lymphocytic sialadenitis. Lichen planus, another immunologically mediated disease, has been associated with a number of different liver diseases, including hepatitis C, autoimmune hepatitis, and primary biliary cirrhosis. Polyarteritis nodosa, pulmonary fibrosis, erythema multiforme, and uveitis have been seen in patients with hepatitis C. However, the presence of these other diseases does not mean they are causally linked to hepatitis C. Rather, because of the increasing prevalence of hepatitis C, these disorders may occur simultaneously.

The autoimmune phenomena are not unique to viral hepatitis. In patients with primary biliary cirrhosis, 25% have a positive rheumatoid factor. Sicca syndrome, with xerostomia and xerophthalmia, can be seen in up to 70% of primary biliary cirrhosis patients. The xerostomia may lead to dysphagia and dental caries. The xerophthalmia can result in corneal ulceration. There are a number of other conditions associated with primary biliary cirrhosis. The 'pack' syndrome is a combination of primary biliary cirrhosis, anticentromere antibody, CREST syndrome, and keratoconjunctivitis sicca.

NEUROLOGIC MANIFESTATIONS OF LIVER DISEASE

Peripheral neuropathy is the most common neurologic manifestation of liver disease. It has been described in up to 45% of patients with cirrhosis, especially when secondary to alcohol. Cholestatic liver diseases (e.g. primary biliary cirrhosis) may lead to vitamin E deficiency and this may manifest as a mixed sensorimotor peripheral neuropathy. A peripheral neuropathy has been described in hepatitis C. Autonomic neuropathy is frequently observed, again more frequently in patients with alcoholic cirrhosis.

Patients with alcoholic cirrhosis may exhibit signs of coexisting Wernicke's encephalopathy or cerebellar disease that are independent of the severity of the liver insult. Similarly, the neurologic manifestations of Wilson's disease vary greatly and do not correlate with the severity of the liver disease.

FURTHER READING

Bach N, Schaffner F, Kapelman B. Sexual behaviour in women with nonalcoholic liver disease. Hepatology. 1989;9:698–703. *An insight into a rarely investigated topic.*

Gordon SC. Extrahepatic manifestations of hepatitis C. Dig Dis. 1996;14:157–68. *A complete review of the extrahepatic diseases associated with hepatitis C.*

Hay JE, Lindor KD, Wiesner RH, Dickson ER, Krom RA, LaRusso NF, et al. The metabolic bone disease of primary sclerosing cholangitis. Hepatology. 1991;14:257–61. *A good study of the issues affecting bone in liver disease.*

Katz SK, Gordon KB, Roenigk HH. The cutaneous manifestations of gastrointestinal disease. Prim Care Clin Office Pract. 1996;23:455–76. *A comprehensive review of the dermatologic manifestations of liver disease.*

Lange PA, Stoller JK. The hepatopulmonary syndrome. Ann Intern Med. 1995;122:521–9. *Good review of topic.*

Marcellin P, Benhamou JP. Autoimmune disorders associated with hepatitis C. Prog Liver Dis. 1995;13:247–67. *A clear, comprehensive review of the autoimmune findings and cryoglobulinemia associated with hepatitis C.*

Paintaud G, Bechtel Y, Brientini MP, Miguet JP, Bechtel PR. Effects of liver diseases on drug metabolism. Therapie. 1996;51:384–9. *A brief review of the subject.*

Parsons ME, Russo GG, Millikan LE. Dermatologic disorders associated with viral hepatitis infections. Int J Dermatol. 1997;36:237–8. *A complete review of the dermatologic diseases associated with hepatitis B and C.*

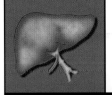
Chapter 11

Viral Hepatitis A and E

John G O'Grady

HEPATITIS A

INTRODUCTION

Hepatitis A is the most common defined cause of viral hepatitis worldwide. In the United States, the number of notified cases annually is around 23,000, but estimates of the real number of cases of clinical disease range up to 75,000 per year. In the 1940s it was called infectious hepatitis (as opposed to serum hepatitis) but was renamed hepatitis A after the causative virus was identified in 1973. A diagnostic test became available in 1975. The hepatitis A virus is a member of the picornavirus family and is an icosahedral particle 28nm in diameter, with a composition of 30% RNA and 70% protein. The hepatitis A virus genome is single stranded, linear, positive sense and contains 7.48kb RNA. The RNA template has one open reading frame (ORF) that produces a polyprotein that is 2227 amino acid residues long and is cleaved to provide the structural and functional proteins of the virus. The hepatitis A virus does not have an envelope but has a capsid comprising 32 subunits, each of which contains four major polypeptides termed VP1–VP4 (Fig. 11.1). Although there is only one serotype of the hepatitis A virus, four genotypes have

been described in human infections with a nucleotide sequence variation ranging from 15 to 25%. However, all the human strains are very closely related antigenically, and infection with one strain confers immunity to the other strains.

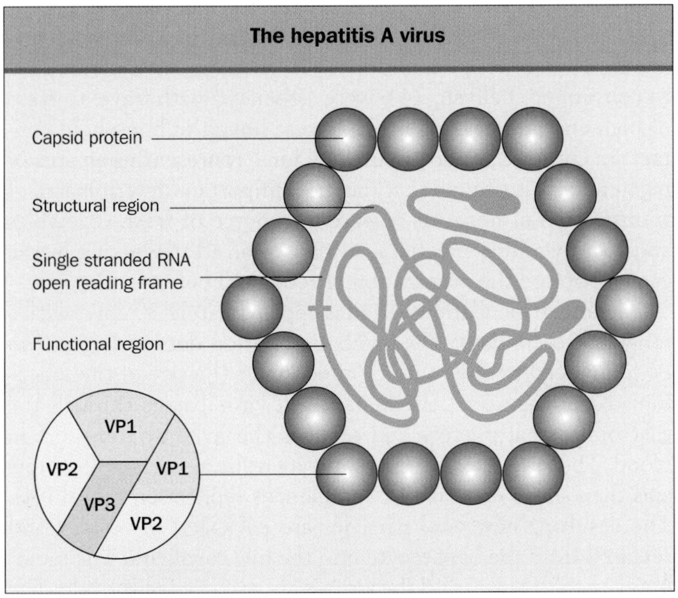

EPIDEMIOLOGY AND PATHOGENESIS

The hepatitis A virus is detectable in blood or feces for 2 weeks before the onset of jaundice and for up to 8 days afterwards. The mode of acquisition is by direct person-to-person contact through the fecal–oral route or by ingestion of contaminated food or water. The secondary strike rate is in the order of 15–20% and person-to-person transmission is most common in situations of prolonged close contact; schools, institutions, and army camps are frequently effected by outbreaks of infection. Contamination of water supplies is still possible in areas that have not developed adequate sewage disposal systems. Infection may result from the consumption of water or ice, as well as uncooked food washed in contaminated water. Uncooked shellfish, including clams, oysters, mussels, and cockles, are a particularly common source of dietary acquisition. A mollusc-related epidemic resulted in over 300,000 infections in Shanghai in 1988.

Some studies suggest that homosexual men are at increased risk of acquiring hepatitis A, especially those practising oral–anal and digital–anal sexual contact. However, sexual transmission through contact with semen or vaginal secretions does not appear to be a significant route of infection. The hepatitis A virus may be detected in blood, and viral transmission has been documented using blood harvested up to 11 days before the onset of symptoms of infection. Hepatitis A transmission has also been documented in hemophiliacs receiving coagulation factors from pooled donors.

Three patterns of endemicity are recognized: low, intermediate, and high (Figs 11.2 & 11.3). In areas classified as high endemicity for hepatitis A, infection is almost universal in early childhood and results in a high level of immunity in the adult population. Epidemiologic studies in North Africa and the Middle East indicate that almost all children have immunity to hepatitis A by the age of 4 years even though most had no clinical infection recognized as hepatitis A. Similar studies in parts of Asia and South America suggest 95–100% immunity before the age of 10 years. The epidemiology of hepatitis A infection is changing in Western countries, with a transition from asymptomatic childhood infections to an increased incidence of symptomatic disease in the 18- to 40-year-old age group. The overall seropositivity rate in the USA is 38% and ranges from 11% in those under the age of 5 years to 74% in those over the age of 50 years. There is also

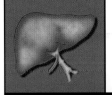

The hepatitis A virus

Capsid protein

Structural region

Single stranded RNA
open reading frame

Functional region

VP1
VP2   VP1
VP3
VP2

Figure 11.1 The hepatitis A virus. Each capsid protein contains four subunits and encloses a single-stranded RNA open reading frame. The virus does not have an envelope.

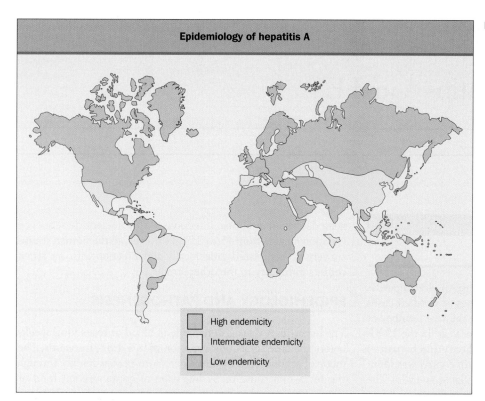

Figure 11.2 Epidemiology of hepatitis A.

Epidemiology of hepatitis A

High endemicity

Intermediate endemicity

Low endemicity

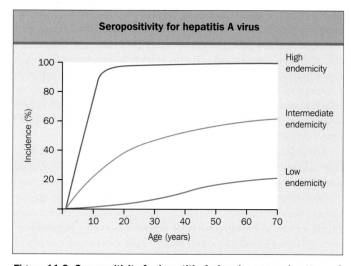

Figure 11.3 Seropositivity for hepatitis A virus by age and pattern of endemicity. High endemicity is associated with acquisition of hepatitis A virus in childhood; infection is delayed and less common in areas of intermediate or low endemicity.

considerable variation based on geography and racial background within the United States. The highest seropositivity rates occur in native Americans, followed by Hispanics, black Americans, white Americans and Asian-Americans.

The improvements in hygiene and sanitation associated with economic growth have reduced the exposure to hepatitis A in early childhood in many parts of the world. In Sweden, the prevalence of seropositivity fell from 69% of subjects born around 1900, to 6% in those born in the 1940s, and just 2% in subjects born after 1950. Non-nationals resident in Sweden had a prevalence of 70–90%, and 42% of all new cases recorded in Sweden were

imported. The incidence of exposure to hepatitis A under the age of 20 years in Hong Kong fell from 29.1% in 1978–1979 to 9.2% in 1987–1989. Groups with a higher risk of acquiring hepatitis A can be identified within countries of low endemicity. These include health care personnel, military and prison populations, and sewage workers. Travellers from low endemicity to higher endemicity areas are at risk of exposure to hepatitis A infection.

The risk factors associated with acquisition of the hepatitis A virus vary in importance in different parts of the world. In the USA, 24% are related to personal contact, 15% to day-care centers, 6% to foreign travel, 5% to an outbreak, and 2% to intravenous drug use. In 40% of cases no risk factor was identified.

A study of acute hepatitis A infection in an area of low endemicity in Europe found that 42% of cases were attributable to consuming shellfish, 24% were associated with travel to areas of high endemicity, and only 1% were linked to household contact. In contrast, a study in urban China, representing an area of high endemicity, found that the most important determinants of transmission of hepatitis A were the source of fresh vegetables and hand-washing practices, in particular after working in the garden, before the preparation of food, and before eating.

The mean incubation period is approximately 30 days, with a range of 15–50 days. The incubation period does not appear to be influenced by the route of infection or the size of the inoculum. After ingestion, the hepatitis A virus passes through the gastrointestinal mucosa and reaches the liver by transport in blood. The virus enters the hepatocyte utilizing surface receptors and then sheds its coat and commences replication (Fig. 11.4). The resulting new viral particles are packaged in vesicles and released from the hepatocyte into the bile canaliculi. The membrane then dissolves and the viruses are excreted in the bile. The hepatitis A virus replicates exclusively in the liver, although the virus has been identified in other sites including lymph nodes, spleen, and kidney.

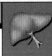

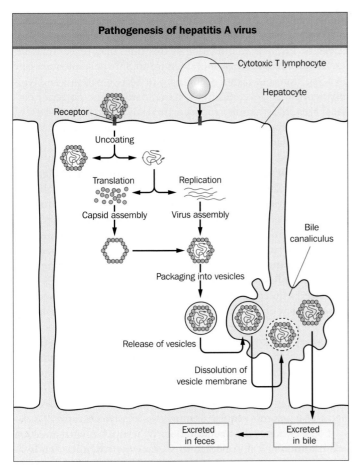

Figure 11.4 Pathogenesis of hepatitis A virus. The cycle of viral replication and shedding of the virus is depicted together with a cytotoxic T lymphocyte, which is the probable mechanism of hepatocyte damage.

The hepatitis A virus was originally assumed to be directly cytopathic, but more recent studies suggest that this may not be the case. The initial phase of viral replication in hepatocytes does not appear to damage the host cells, and an immunologically mediated component to the pathogenesis of hepatocyte necrosis has been suggested. This is thought to involve hepatitis A virus-specific, HLA-restricted cytotoxic T lymphocytes. Clonal analysis of the cellular infiltrates harvested from liver tissue identified antigen-specific CD8+ T lymphocytes. Half of the lymphocytes were hepatitis A virus specific, compared with only 1% of the peripheral lymphocyte clones. There are conflicting studies on the role of natural killer cells in the pathogenesis of hepatitis A.

CLINICAL FEATURES AND DISEASE ASSOCIATIONS

Infection with the hepatitis A virus results in a broad spectrum of sequelae, ranging from subclinical infection, to clinical infections with or without jaundice, to acute liver failure and possible death. The risk of infection with hepatitis A virus being associated with jaundice and clinical disease increases with age (Fig. 11.5). Jaundice is very unusual in children under the age of 4 years. In 4–6 year olds 90% of infections remain anicteric, whereas over the age of 15 years 40–70% of patients infected with hepatitis A virus develop jaundice. Within the anicteric infections, 79% are associated with some symptoms. The incidence of symptomatic

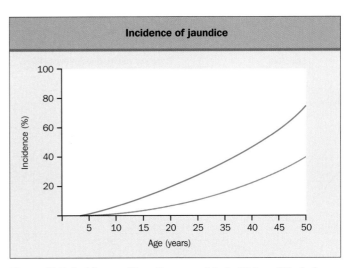

Figure 11.5 Incidence of jaundice associated with hepatitis A virus. The likelihood of developing jaundice after infection with hepatitis A virus increases with age.

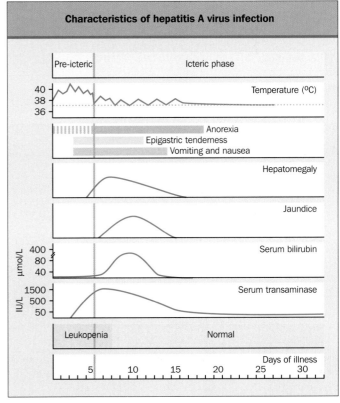

Figure 11.6 Major characteristics of hepatitis A virus infection. The timing of some of the major features is shown in the prodromal and icteric phases of infection with hepatitis A.

disease is 20% higher in males, but there is no evidence to suggest that they are more susceptible to severe hepatitis.

A prodromal syndrome develops in 85% of patients, who ultimately become jaundiced, which can last for up to a week (Fig. 11.6). Typical symptoms include malaise, anorexia, nausea, vomiting, abdominal pain, and fever. Less common prodromal symptoms include myalgia and headaches (see Fig. 11.7). Cigarette smokers tend to lose interest in smoking. The development of dark urine and jaundice marks the beginning of the icteric phase

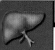

Symptoms of hepatitis A	
Symptom	Range of reported incidences (%)
Jaundice	40–80
Dark urine	68–94
Pale stools	52–58
Malaise	52–94
Anorexia	42–96
Abdominal pain	26–68
Nausea/vomiting	26–87
Fever	18–73
Headache	19–73
Arthralgia	8–40
Myalgia	14–52
Diarrhea	16–25
Respiratory symptoms	20–24
Sore throat	0–20

Figure 11.7 Incidence of the symptoms of hepatitis A.

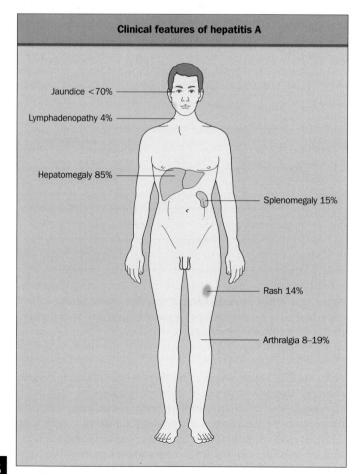

Clinical features of hepatitis A

Jaundice <70%

Lymphadenopathy 4%

Hepatomegaly 85%

Splenomegaly 15%

Rash 14%

Arthralgia 8–19%

Figure 11.8 Clinical features of hepatitis A.

and is typically associated with an improvement in the prodromal symptoms. Jaundice resolves within 2 weeks in 85% of patients. Physical examination at this time may reveal mild-to-moderate tender hepatomegaly in up to 85% and splenomegaly in 15%. Transient rashes occur in up to 14% of patients and lymphadenopathy develops in 4%, particularly in the posterior cervical area. Most studies report arthralgia; it occurs in 8–19% of patients during this phase of the infection but is rarely complicated by an arthropathy (Fig. 11.8).

Prolonged clinical courses have been documented in up to 16% of patients, secondary to either relapsing or cholestatic hepatitis. Relapsing or biphasic hepatitis has been described in 6–10% of patients and occurs at intervals of 4–15 weeks after the original illness. There is no strong correlation between the severity of the initial and the second phase of the illness. However, relapsing hepatitis appears to be associated with a higher incidence of immune-related clinical and laboratory phenomena. A cholestatic phase develops in a proportion of patients and is characterized clinically by deep and protracted jaundice and the development of pale stools and pruritus. Diarrhea and weight loss also develop during the cholestatic phase. Patients with sickle-cell disease appear to be more at risk of developing the cholestatic phase than the general population. Hepatitis A virus infection does not have a chronic phase and does not cause chronic hepatitis. However, it has been suggested that autoimmune chronic hepatitis may be triggered by acute hepatitis A virus infection, and these patients require immunosuppressive therapy.

Some extrahepatic manifestations of hepatitis A virus infection are immunologically mediated. Cutaneous vasculitis tends to involve the buttocks and lower extremities and appears as an erythematous maculopapular or purpuric rash. Immune-complex deposition is demonstrable in skin biopsies, which may also show evidence of vasculitis. Renal dysfunction and failure can occur in acute hepatitis A virus infection that is not complicated by acute liver failure. Most incidents appear to be immune complex-related glomerulonephritis or interstitial nephritis. However, cases of the nephrotic syndrome have also been reported. The risk of renal failure may be higher with cholestatic hepatitis.

Acute pancreatitis is another unusual complication of hepatitis A virus infection that has been described in both adults and children. Cardiac disease is most frequently manifest with bradycardia and associated electrocardiographic changes, including prolongation of the P–R and Q–T intervals, T wave changes, and left axis deviation. Convulsions have been described in a small number of patients, mainly children, in the absence of encephalopathy, fever, or hypoglycemia. Other rare neurologic complications include neuropathies, mononeuritis multiplex, Guillane–Barré syndrome, acute cerebellar ataxia, and transverse myelitis. Aplastic anemia occasionally occurs.

DIAGNOSIS

Laboratory analysis

The serum transaminases alanine aminotransferase (ALT) and aspartate aminotransferase (AST) are the most sensitive markers of hepatocyte necrosis and they increase during the prodromal phase to levels in excess of 500IU/L (see Fig. 11.6). The peak levels may be measured in thousands of units, with ALT levels being higher than AST, but rarely exceeding 5000IU/L. The transaminase levels initially fall quite quickly, at about 10% per

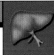

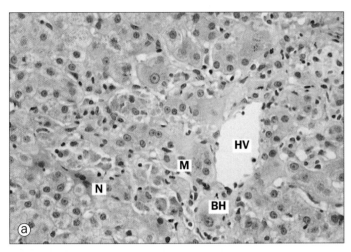

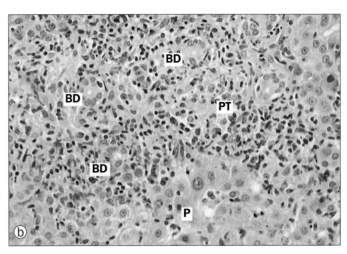

Figure 11.9 Histology of hepatitis A. (a) Lobular cellular infiltration: HV, hepatic venule; BH, ballooned hepatocyte; M, pigment-laden macrophages; N, necrotic hepatocytes. (b) Portal infiltration: BD, bile ducts/ductules; PT, inflamed portal tract; P, lobular parenchyma. (Hematoxylin–eosin.)

day, but may then take many weeks to return to complete normality. The serum transaminases peak before the serum bilirubin does and return to normal in 67% of patients at 2 months, 85% at 3 months, and almost all at 6 months.

A serum bilirubin of around 40μmol/L (2.5mg/dL) is the threshold for differentiating nonicteric from icteric hepatitis. The unconjugated and conjugated fractions of serum bilirubin are both elevated. The serum bilirubin usually peaks at values less than 400μmol/L (25mg/dL) and then falls at a rate of approx-imately 50% per week in uncomplicated infections. Higher serum bilirubin levels are seen in patients with cholestatic hepatitis, coexisting renal failure, sickle cell disease, or glucose 6-phosphate dehydrogenase deficiency. Bilirubin may be detectable in urine before the onset of jaundice. Alkaline phosphatase and γ-glutamyl transferase levels are only modestly elevated unless the disease progresses to either the cholestatic phase or relapsing hepatitis.

Functional or absolute measures of coagulation factors are widely used to screen for the synthetic dysfunction that characterizes severe hepatitis and identifies the cohort at risk of developing acute liver failure. The most common assays used include prothrombin time, prothrombin levels, International Normalized Ratios (INRs) and factor V levels. Serum albumin levels usually remain in the normal range. Mild elevations in both IgG and IgM levels have been reported. Autoantibodies may be transiently positive during acute hepatitis A and persist in the occasional patient who is later diagnosed as having autoimmune chronic hepatitis. Hematologic abnormalities include leukopenia, atypical lymphocytes, and red cell aplasia.

The hepatitis A virus can be detected in stool, serum, and liver by screening for viral antigens or RNA. Viral shedding in the stool usually stops within 30 days of the onset of the infection. The diagnosis of acute hepatitis A is normally confirmed by the detection of the IgM antibody to the hepatitis A virus (IgM anti-HAV) in serum using enzyme-linked immunosorbent assay (ELISA) or radioimmunoassay. The IgM anti-HAV levels reach their peak during the acute and early convalescent phases and become undetectable in 75% of patients 6 months after the onset of the infection. IgM anti-HAV tends to remain detectable throughout the course of relapsing hepatitis. The IgG antibody to the hepatitis A virus (IgG anti-HAV) peaks during the convalescent period and remains detectable for many years.

Histology

Histologic assessment of the liver is rarely undertaken in uncomplicated hepatitis A virus infection. A liver biopsy may be indicated to screen for coexisting liver disease, and some advocate it to assess the degree of hepatocyte necrosis in patients developing acute liver failure. The characteristic histologic features of acute hepatitis A virus infection are random areas of lobular hepatitis with spotty necrosis associated with a mononuclear portal and periportal cell infiltrate (Fig. 11.9). There is a tendency for the lobular changes to be more prominent in the perivenular areas, although a periportal pattern of inflammation and necrosis is often described with hepatitis A virus infection. Confluent necrosis describes larger areas of contiguous necrosis; when this process stretches between acinar structures, usually between a portal tract and a terminal hepatic venule, the term 'bridging necrosis' is applied. More extensive necrosis is described as submassive or massive and these patterns are linked to the clinical syndromes of acute liver failure.

The typical spotty necrosis and associated regeneration give the appearance of hepatocytic plate disarray. The portal tracts are enlarged by the inflammatory infiltrate and associated edema. The cellular infiltrate comprises predominantly lymphocytes and histiocytes but also includes neutrophils and eosinophils. Cholestatic hepatitis is associated with the presence of canalicular bile plugs and possibly a ductular plate transformation.

NATURAL HISTORY AND PROGNOSIS

The age at acquisition of hepatitis A virus infection is a major determinant of the severity of the clinical illness. Acute liver failure is still relatively rare, with fatality rates of 0.14–0.35% for hospitalized patients, which represent only a cohort of the total infected population (Fig. 11.10). Case fatality rates have been calculated at 0.1% under the age of 15 years, 0.4% in 15–39 year olds, and 1.1% in those aged 40 years or greater. The risk of

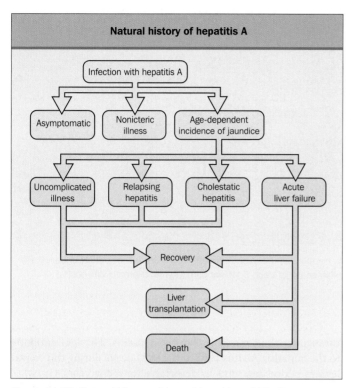

Natural history of hepatitis A

Infection with hepatitis A

Asymptomatic | Nonicteric illness | Age-dependent incidence of jaundice

Uncomplicated illness | Relapsing hepatitis | Cholestatic hepatitis | Acute liver failure

Recovery

Liver transplantation

Death

Figure 11.10 Natural history of hepatitis A. Up to 16% of patients develop relapsing or cholestatic hepatitis. The risk of developing acute liver failure is about 0.35% and this can also occur with relapsing hepatitis.

death from acute hepatitis A in the UK rises in almost a logarithmic fashion after the age of 25 years. Mortality rates in excess of 2% have also been reported in the United States for patients over the age of 40 years.

Amongst those developing acute liver failure, defined by the presence of encephalopathy, the prognosis is also worse with increasing age, and the median age of nonsurvivors in one study was 47 years compared with 33 years for survivors. The King's College Hospital, UK prognostic criteria for acute liver failure identify age greater than 40 years as one of the factors used to select patients for emergency liver transplantation, as well as the presence of jaundice for more than 7 days before the onset of encephalopathy. Older patients with slowly evolving disease have the worst prognosis.

Concomitant infections or disease may lead to an increase in the severity of acute viral hepatitis A. Chronic hepatitis B virus infection has been reported to increase the risk of developing acute liver failure following hepatitis A virus infection. It is not clear whether the degree of liver disease associated with the chronic hepatitis B might be a determinant of outcome. Patients with well-compensated liver disease appear to tolerate hepatitis A virus infections quite well, but those with limited reserve can be expected to be susceptible to more severe disease with hepatitis A. Heavy alcohol consumers, promiscuous homosexual men, and intravenous drug users are more susceptible to severe infections, but this might reflect a higher incidence of chronic liver disease in these populations. Homosexual men are also at risk of multiple viral infections, but there is no evidence that coexisting HIV infection leads to more severe disease.

Pregnancy was associated with more severe disease in the Middle East and India, but not in Western countries. This could be because of unrecognized concomitant infection with hepatitis E virus, which is clearly associated with a poorer prognosis in pregnancy, or malnutrition. Severe exertion and general anesthesia during acute viral hepatitis A have been linked with the development of acute liver failure.

MANAGEMENT

The vast majority of patients who have acute hepatitis A do not require hospitalization. Rest was a traditional feature of the management plan, but although severe exertion has been associated with the development of acute liver failure, there is no evidence to demonstrate that bed rest accelerates the rate of recovery in uncomplicated infections. Patients should be advised to remain ambulant and operate within the confines of their energy levels. Anorexia, nausea, and vomiting may reduce fluid and dietary intake, and a minority of patients may require intravenous fluids if these symptoms are severe. In the majority of patients symptomatic therapy is sufficient. There are no mandatory dietary modifications and the patients should be encouraged to maintain a balanced diet that they consider palatable. The conventional wisdom has also been to prohibit alcohol consumption until the liver function tests return to normal. However, a number of studies have failed to find supporting evidence for this practice, including one that demonstrated that up to 26g alcohol per day was not harmful in patients with acute hepatitis A.

The patients that require hospitalization during the early phase of the infection include those with severe or persistent anorexia or vomiting, those showing any alteration to their mental state, and those exhibiting any deviation of the coagulation factor tests from normal. The latter are at risk of developing acute liver failure and they are best managed in specialist centers with access to liver transplantation. Patients who have cholestatic hepatitis, especially if complicated by ascites, a shrinking liver, or falling albumin levels, should also be hospitalized for assessment. These patients are at risk of subacute liver failure and may also need access to liver transplant services.

There is no specific drug therapy that is useful in patients who have uncomplicated acute hepatitis A virus infection. The hepatitis A virus is resistant to most of the currently available antiviral drugs. Corticosteroids are useful in the management of the cholestatic phase. Prednisolone 40mg/day would be expected to reduce the serum bilirubin by 40% within 4 days and the dose is subsequently tapered over a period of 2–4 weeks depending on the speed of resolution of the cholestasis. Prednisolone 30–40mg/day has also been used in patients who have relapsing hepatitis but with less success and with a longer tapering period of 6–12 weeks. Drug treatment of associated symptoms should be judicious, and sedatives and narcotic drugs should be avoided. Nausea can be treated with metoclopramide, domperidone, or phenothiazines. Acetaminophen (paracetamol) in doses not exceeding 4g/day is the safest analgesic even though it is hepatotoxic in larger amounts. Cholestyramine is the drug of choice for pruritus, as antihistamines are relatively ineffective.

Patients who have severe acute hepatitis are monitored for disturbance of coagulation parameters, which are the best markers of liver failure. A deterioration in these parameters normally precedes the development of encephalopathy, which is the complication that defines the patient as having acute or fulminant liver failure. The coagulation parameters used include prothrombin time, INRs, and factor V levels. Vitamin K is administered intravenously when an abnormal coagulation test is observed to differentiate severe hepatocellular dysfunction from vitamin K deficiency, which may complicate prolonged periods of jaundice. Vitamin K deficiency is especially common during the cholestatic phase of acute hepatitis A virus infection. Serum bilirubin and serum transaminase levels do not discriminate patients who have severe infections from those developing acute liver failure. The blood glucose should be monitored regularly in those who have markedly reduced dietary intake and in any patient who has an altered mental status. Hypoglycemia may precede the development of encephalopathy in patients at risk of acute liver failure, and such patients require intravenous glucose infusions.

PREVENTION

Active and passive immunization are both used for the prevention of hepatitis A virus infection. Passive immunization uses immunoglobulins harvested from patients with natural immunity to hepatitis A. The yield of immunoglobulins from pooled donors has decreased as a result of the lower prevalence of exposure to hepatitis A. An injection of immunoglobulin confers immunity from infection within 3–5 days and this lasts for up to 3 months. Passive immunization remains the intervention of choice for postexposure prophylaxis.

Three approaches to developing a vaccine have been pursued using live-attenuated virus, inactivated vaccines, and recombinant vaccines. The inactivated vaccine is most widely used and is administered in three separate doses at time zero, 1 month, and 6 months. The seroconversion rates are as high as 99% after the second dose, and the third dose results in a marked increase in the circulating amount of antihepatitis A antibody. The third dose lengthens the duration of protection by significantly increasing the antibody titer. The simultaneous administration of active and passive immunization reduces the ultimate antibody level by 50% compared with active immunization alone. The immunity conferred by a full vaccination program would be expected to last between 5 and 10 years. Local irritation at the site of the injection occurs in up to 30% of individuals, and mild fever, headache, and malaise were reported in up to 10%.

In low-endemicity areas, populations to be considered for vaccination include regular travellers from low- to high-endemicity areas, health care and childcare workers, food handlers, military personnel, intravenous drug users, and homosexual men. It has also been suggested that patients who have chronic liver disease and glucose 6-phosphate dehydrogenase deficiency should be vaccinated against hepatitis A.

In intermediate- and high-endemicity areas, more systematic vaccination of young children may become appropriate if it can be justified on cost–benefit analyses. In the United States, the Public Health Service Advisory Committee on Immunization Practices recommended the routine vaccination of young children over the age of 2 years in high-endemicity areas and catch-up vaccination of previously unvaccinated older children. There is also preliminary epidemiologic evidence that vaccination may decrease the magnitude and duration of an outbreak of hepatitis A.

HEPATITIS E

INTRODUCTION

Hepatitis E is an RNA virus measuring 32nm in diameter and classified as belonging to the calicivirus family. The virus is spherical with surface spikes and indentations, and it does not possess an envelope. The genome is single-stranded positive-sense RNA comprising 7.5kb and three ORFs (Fig. 11.11). The largest of the ORFs encodes for nonstructural proteins responsible for viral replication and processing, the second largest for capsid proteins, and the smallest for proteins whose functions are unknown but are recognized as antigenic. A number of different strains of the hepatitis E virus have been identified and the divergence appears to be geographically defined, with clear differences existing between Asian, African, and Mexican strains. However, all the strains share at least one major immune reactive epitope, suggesting that cross-immunity is likely.

Epidemic non-A, non-B hepatitis was described in 1980 and its association with a high mortality rate in pregnant women was observed. Viral particles were isolated from stool in 1983 using immune electron microscopy and the name hepatitis E was given in 1988. The virus was cloned in 1990 and diagnostic tests were developed the following year. Although hepatitis E is very similar to hepatitis A in many respects, it has a different geographic distribution and is associated with a peculiarly high mortality in pregnant women.

EPIDEMIOLOGY AND PATHOGENESIS

Hepatitis E is mainly seen in India, Asia, the Middle East and parts of Latin America, and northeast Africa (see Fig. 11.12). However, endemic areas have been identified in most developing countries where epidemiologic studies have been performed. Hepatitis E

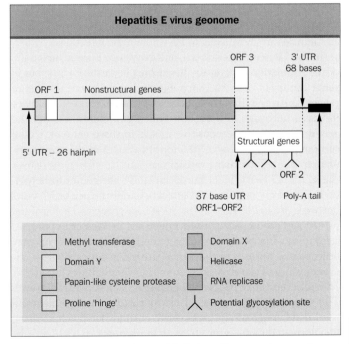

Figure 11.11 Structure of hepatitis E virus. The genomic map of hepatitis E virus is shown with three open reading frames (ORFs).

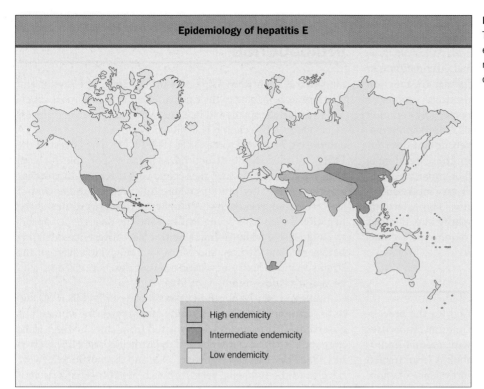

Epidemiology of hepatitis E

High endemicity

Intermediate endemicity

Low endemicity

Figure 11.12 Epidemiology of hepatitis E. The areas of high, intermediate and low endemicity are shown. Intermediate endemicity refers to areas where large epidemics have occurred.

virus has been confirmed as the cause of some huge epidemics of acute viral hepatitis, including ones that involved 29,000 cases in New Delhi in 1955 and over 100,000 cases in Xinjiang in China in 1958. It is estimated that hepatitis E virus causes 90% of all major hepatitis epidemics in India. Major epidemics appear to follow a 10-year cycle, but the basis for this is unclear. Over 90% of cases of epidemic non-A, non-B hepatitis in India have been confirmed as caused by hepatitis E virus infection. Adults account for 75% of clinical cases and tend to be predominantly affected during epidemics. Nevertheless, acute hepatitis E is also a common cause of sporadic infection in children. Children under the age of 15 years and females are most likely to have nonicteric infections.

In the United States, Israel, and Northern Europe, up to 2% of the population have antibodies against hepatitis E virus, but in some European countries such as Spain and Greece this figure ranges up to 6% of the population. In all areas, seropositivity increases with age. In India, less than 5% of children under the age of 10 years are seropositive; this is in sharp contrast to the seropositivity rate of over 90% for hepatitis A in the same population. The seropositivity rate increases to 10–40% in those over the age of 25 years. In an European study, antibodies to hepatitis E virus were not found in subjects under the age of 30 years but were present in 1.4% of the 30–49 age group and 5.7% of the 60–70 age group. Recognized infections in Western countries tend to be associated with travel to endemic areas, but this may reflect a bias towards testing for hepatitis E in patients with a relevant history of travel. A study from the United States found that 38% of seropositive people had no history of international travel. The seropositivity amongst black South Africans was higher in rural dwellers (15.3%), particularly in mud hut dwellers using unchlorinated river water, than urban residents (6.6%).

Studies in the UK and Spain suggest that hepatitis E accounts for a small proportion of cases (up to 6%) of sporadic non-A, non-

B, non-C hepatitis. In China, the equivalent figure was 22%. Higher rates of seropositivity have been identified in some HIV-infected populations and the rates increase further with progression of the disease. Whether this represents a common transmission mechanism or a serologic epiphenomenon is as yet unclear. Higher rates of hepatitis E seropositivity have also been reported in homosexual men (16%) and intravenous drug users (23%) in the United States, but the significance of these findings is again unclear.

The transmission of the hepatitis E virus is through the fecal–oral route. The risk factors for transmission include poor or inadequate hygiene and contaminated water supplies. The incidence of cases of hepatitis E increases during the rainy seasons and in association with flooding. The hepatitis E virus has been identified in rodents and it is possible that rats or mice may play a role in the dissemination of hepatitis E virus infection. Direct contamination does not appear to occur commonly and secondary household strike rates are estimated at 0.7–2.2%. The possibility of maternal–neonatal transfer is disputed, but one study found that six of eight babies of infected mothers were infected with hepatitis E, including one who died from liver failure. In these patients, hepatitis E virus RNA was identified in cord blood using polymerase chain reaction (PCR) techniques. Higher rates of hepatitis E seropositivity have been reported in patients in chronic hemodialysis programs, but properly controlled studies suggest that this observation results from the confounding effects of age and sex. However, the possibility of parenteral transmission cannot be excluded, based on the observed higher seropositivity rates in hepatitis C-positive subjects and in patients developing post-transfusion non-A, non-B hepatitis.

Outbreaks of infection in endemic areas are seen in children and in the 15- to 40-year-old age groups. Some studies have shown a

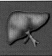

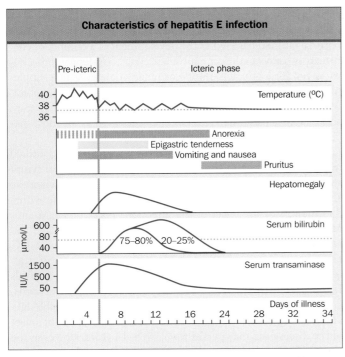

Figure 11.13 Major characteristics of hepatitis E infection. The timing of some of the major features is shown in the prodromal and icteric phases of infection with hepatitis E.

Symptoms of hepatitis E

Symptom	Range of reported incidences (%)
Anorexia	66–100
Malaise	95–100
Nausea/vomiting	29–100
Dark urine	58
Abdominal pain	37–82
Fever	23–97
Diarrhea	Undefined
Arthralgia	Undefined
Pruritus	Common
Urticarial rash	Undefined

Figure 11.14 Incidence of the symptoms of hepatitis E. There are fewer clinical descriptions of confirmed hepatitis E and the incidence of some of the features has not been specified.

male predominance with a typical male:female ratio of 1.0:0.8. However, the greatest impact of hepatitis E is on pregnant females, when it is associated with a high mortality. The overall case fatality at 0.5–4% is higher than that for hepatitis A and increases to 20–25% during the second and third trimesters of pregnancy.

The hepatitis E virus enters the body through the intestine and reaches the liver via the portal vein. The liver appears to be the sole target of infection and once established viral replication occurs, leading to viral shedding in bile. The pathogenesis of hepatitis E may be a combination of direct cytotoxicity and immunologic mechanisms. The cause of the high mortality in pregnant women is poorly understood.

CLINICAL FEATURES AND DISEASE ASSOCIATIONS

Hepatitis E virus is not clinically different from other causes of viral hepatitis (Fig. 11.13). The mean incubation period is 42 days with a range of 15–65 days. Subclinical infection occurs but the extent is unclear because there are limited epidemiologic studies as a result of the lack of widespread serologic testing. Nausea and fever are the usual symptoms during the prodromal phase. The icteric phase commences with the development of dark urine and jaundice. Additional signs and symptoms may include anorexia, abdominal pain, diarrhea, pale stools, arthralgia, pruritus, rash, hepatomegaly, and splenomegaly (Figs 11.14 & 11.15). The symptoms resolve within 6 weeks in most surviving patients. Cholestasis is more common with hepatitis E than with hepatitis A and occurs in 20–25% of infected adults. There is no evidence of chronic infection or related disease in humans.

Acute liver failure characterized by the development of encephalopathy occurs with hepatitis E and the associated clin-

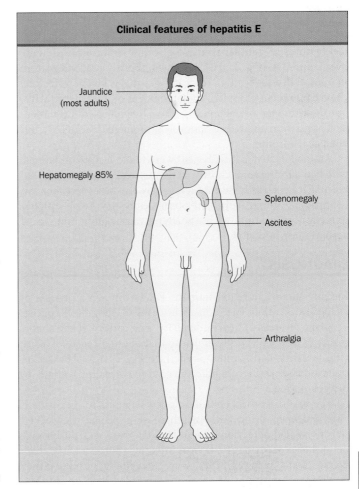

Figure 11.15 Clinical features of hepatitis E.

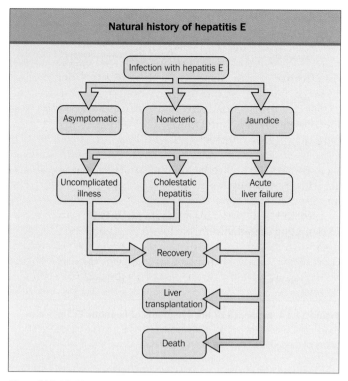

Natural history of hepatitis E

Figure 11.16 Natural history of hepatitis E. Cholestasis occurs in up to 25% of patients. Acute liver failure develops in 1–4% of patients but in up to 25% of women in later pregnancy. Liver transplantation services are not developed in the areas of high endemicity.

ical features are similar to those of other viral causes of acute liver failure (see Fig. 11.16). However, there is a second pattern of clinical disease leading to death and this is characterized by the development of ascites and other signs of liver failure without the presence of encephalopathy. Disseminated intravascular coagulation and sepsis are also prominent features of this clinical syndrome.

Antibodies to hepatitis E virus were found in 13% of patients who had autoimmune chronic hepatitis, again raising the possibility that hepatitis E virus infection may also be a trigger for this condition. Alternatively, this observation may be an epiphenomenon associated with the hypergammaglobulinemia of autoimmune hepatitis.

DIAGNOSIS

Initially the diagnosis of hepatitis E was through a process of exclusion of other viral causes in cases of sporadic hepatitis occurring in areas of high endemicity. The pattern of the abnormality of liver enzymes is similar to that of other causes of acute viral hepatitis and is monophasic (see Fig. 11.13). The serum transaminases and serum bilirubin tend to normalize over a 1- to 6-week period.

The first diagnostic tests developed screened for hepatitis E virus antigen in serum. Although these were specific, they lacked sensitivity, and detection rates of 50–70% were seen during epidemics of acute hepatitis E virus infection. Subsequently, diagnostic tests using ELISA were developed using either recombinant proteins or synthetic peptides representing the immunodominant epitopes of ORFs 2 and 3. Most assays use

domains from at least two geographically defined strains. The ELISA techniques were associated with a relatively high false-positive rate and have led to the development of a number of confirmatory assays to detect neutralizing antibody. One approach is to screen for a broader epitope or range of antigens in a supplementary serologic assay. Another is the use of an immunoblot, while a third approach uses a PCR assessment of reverse transcription in cell culture. This has been proposed as the most specific way of detecting seroneutralizing capability in sera.

Antihepatitis E virus IgM (IgM anti-HEV) has been identified in 95% of patients and as early as 4 days after the onset of symptoms of the infection. IgM anti-HEV titers are highest when the serum transaminases peak, and it is usually undetectable within 4–5 months of the onset of the infection. Therefore, IgM anti-HEV behaves similarly to IgM anti-HAV, and is a reliable and sensitive marker of recent infection. Antihepatitis E virus IgG (IgG anti-HEV) may be less reliable. Although a number of studies found IgG anti-HEV in 90–100% of patients at time intervals ranging from the onset of the infection to 1 year afterwards, another found that 57% of patients did not have detectable IgG anti-HEV. IgG anti-HEV titers peak 30–40 days after the onset of the disease and may persist for up to 8–14 years. However, the titers of IgG anti-HEV tend to be low and their ability to sustain immunity are unproven.

In Indian studies, up to 60% of stool samples contain hepatitis E virus RNA; the yield is highest in samples taken within 7 days of the onset of the disease and transported in liquid nitrogen. Tests have also been developed for the detection of hepatitis E virus RNA in serum and liver using PCR techniques.

Although the liver histology may be indistinguishable from that of hepatitis A virus infection, many patients show a different pattern, especially with prominent cholestasis. One study found that 45% of biopsy specimens showed classic hepatitis, 32% cholestasis, and 17% had bridging collapse. Pseudoglandular acinar transformation, bile ductular proliferation, and cholestasis, particularly in the acinar zone 3, are considered to be typical features of hepatitis E virus infection. The portal and lobular inflammatory cell infiltrate may be less intense than in other types of viral hepatitis and contains a lower proportion of lymphocytes, compensated by an increase in the polymorphonuclear cell component. Focal necrosis, hepatocyte degeneration, and acidophil bodies are all less prominent. Phlebitis involving the central and portal venous radicals may be seen with associated edema.

Liver biopsies in recovered patients show a return to normality.

NATURAL HISTORY AND PROGNOSIS

The outcome of acute hepatitis E virus infection is either death or complete recovery. The predominance of infection in the 10- to 40-year-old age group and relatively low secondary household strike rate are curious features that contrast with the pattern of infection seen with hepatitis A virus. The case fatality rate of 0.5–4.0% is also higher than for hepatitis A and is more in line with the mortality seen with sporadic non-A, non-B, non-C hepatitis in Western countries. Pregnant women are considered to have the highest mortality, especially during the second and third trimesters. The reported mortality rates range from 20 to 25% in India and up to 42% in Ethiopia. No convincing explanation for the pregnancy-related morbidity has been proposed.

Detailed analyses of the early risk factors have not been performed specifically for hepatitis E, as they have for most other etiologies of acute liver failure. However, some indirect data are available from an analysis of prognostic indicators in 423 patients with fulminant hepatitis in India. The etiology of the acute liver failure was not an independent predictor of outcome in this study. Extrapolated data suggest that 38% of this cohort were infected with hepatitis E virus. The strongest early prognostic indicators that were associated with a poor outcome were age of 40 years or older, serum bilirubin greater than 255μmol/L (15mg/dL), and prothrombin time prolonged more than 25 seconds compared with controls. The size of the liver as assessed by clinical examination was a less powerful predictor of outcome. As with many other causes of acute liver failure, the outcome worsened as more complications developed; encephalopathy of greater than grade 2, cerebral edema, and infection were all associated with a higher mortality. This particular study found that pregnant women were more likely to develop acute liver failure, but thereafter the prognosis was similar to that in nonpregnant patients. However, it is not clear whether this observation also applied to the cohort with hepatitis E.

MANAGEMENT

As with hepatitis A, the management is largely supportive. There is no evidence that currently available antiviral agents are effective against hepatitis E. Neither active nor passive immunization is currently available for hepatitis E. Immunogobulin fractions harvested in developed countries lack specific antibodies. Immunoglobulin fractions harvested in countries of high endemicity may contain sufficient antibody, but efficacy has not been established in clinical studies. Monkeys and mice have been successfully vaccinated against hepatitis E, and this has raised hopes that effective vaccines for humans will be developed.

There are no data to indicate that advice on rest and alcohol consumption should differ from that given to patients who have hepatitis A. Good hygiene remains the mainstay of prophylaxis in endemic areas. The hepatitis E virus appears to be inactivated by boiling water but the effect of chlorination is uncertain. Travellers to endemic areas should avoid drinking potentially contaminated water and ice-cooled drinks and eating raw shellfish and uncooked fruit and vegetables.

PRACTICE POINT

Ilustrative case

A 24-year-old male presented to hospital with a 5-week history of jaundice and a 1-day history of confusion. He developed jaundice 3 weeks after returning from a holiday in India and serologic tests carried out by the primary physician showed the presence of IgM anti-HAV. One week prior to admission he developed pruritus and light stools. On examination he was deeply jaundiced, had a palpable spleen and had grade 2 encephalopathy.

The results of preliminary laboratory investigations included serum bilirubin 782μmol/L litre, alanine transferase 154IU/L, alkaline phosphatase 874IU/L, INR 10.1, glucose 3.6mmol/L, serum sodium 131mmol/L, serum potassium 6.8mmol/L, urea 64.2μmol/L, and serum creatinine 754μmol/L. A diagnosis of acute liver failure complicated by renal failure was made and the patient was immediately transferred to a specialist unit.

The initial assessment at the specialist unit supported the diagnosis of acute liver failure but the persistent enlargement of the liver was considered unusual. The patient was established on hemodynamic monitoring and after optimization of intravascular pressures failed to improve renal function he was commenced on hemodialysis. The patient was listed for emergency liver transplantation. He was started on glucose supplementation and antibiotics and given vitamin K parenterally.

The following day the patient's mental state had improved considerably and he was fully alert and orientated. The blood results were serum bilirubin 802μmol/L, alanine transferase 136IU/L, alkaline phosphatase 833IU/L,

INR 1.2, glucose 4.8mmol/L, serum sodium 134mmol/L, serum potassium 4.7mmol/L, urea 32.1μmol/L and serum creatinine 514μmol/L. The patient was removed from the transplant waiting list and after 3 weeks of hemodialysis renal function returned and he was discharged from hospital. The cholestasis resolved over a further 4 week period and the liver function profile returned to normal.

Interpretation

This case illustrates two unusual complications of hepatitis A virus infection – renal failure and cholestasis. These complications independently led to further features, encephalopathy, and coagulopathy. These in combination suggested a diagnosis of acute liver failure. The prothrombin time in this instance was sufficiently deranged to suggest that the patient should be listed for liver transplantation, but more typically a prothrombin time between 50 and 99 seconds (INR 3.5–6.5) combined with a history of jaundice exceeding 7 days before the onset of encephalopathy and a serum bilirubin greater than 300μmol/L would have been the criteria indicating a poor prognosis in a young person with hepatitis A. The coagulopathy in this case was secondary to vitamin K depletion, and all assessments should exclude a vitamin K-responsive element to a coagulopathy. The encephalopathy was secondary to azotemia and this resolved with hemodialysis. The clinical clue that this patient did not have true acute liver failure was the palpable liver, as the liver volume is usually markedly reduced in patients developing encephalopathy after prolonged periods of jaundice.

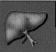
FURTHER READING

Acharya SK, Dasarathy S, Kumer TL, et al. Fulminant hepatitis in a tropical population: clinical course, cause and early predictors of outcome. Hepatology. 1996;23:1448–55. *An analysis of prognostic indicators in acute hepatitis including A and E in India.*

Andre FE, D'Hondt E, Delem A, et al. Clinical assessment of the safety and efficacy of an inactivated hepatitis A vaccine: rationale and summary of findings. Vaccine. 1992;10:S160–8. *The description of the first vaccine against hepatitis A.*

Feinstone SM, Kapikian AZ, Purcell RH. Hepatitis A: detection by immune electron microscopy of a virus like antigen associated with acute illness. Science. 1973;182:1026–8. *The identification of the hepatitis A virus.*

Havens WP Jr. Infectious hepatitis. Medicine. 1948;27:279–326. *An early and detailed account of the clinical features of what later became known as hepatitis A.*

Khuroo MS. Study of an epidemic of non-A, non-B hepatitis: possibility of another human hepatitis virus distinct from post-transfusional non-A, non-B type. Am J Med. 1980;68:818–24. *A detailed clinical and epidemiologic study of an epidemic of hepatitis E.*

Lemon SM. Type A viral hepatitis. New developments in an old disease. N Engl J Med. 1985;313:1059–67. *Overview of the pathogenesis of hepatitis A.*

Mast EE, Krawczynski K. Hepatitis E: an overview. Annu Rev Med. 1996;47:257–66. *This is a succinct review of hepatitis E.*

Mijch AM, Gust ID. Clinical, serologic and epidemiological aspects of hepatitis A virus infection. Semin Liver Dis. 1986;6:42–5. *A good overview of hepatitis A.*

Provost PJ, Ittensohn OL, Villarejos VM, et al. A specific complement-fixation test for human hepatitis A employing CR326 antigen. Proc Soc Exp Biol Med. 1975;148:962–9. *The first diagnostic test for hepatitis A.*

Ramalingaswami V, Purcell RH. Waterborne non-A, non-B hepatitis. Lancet. 1988;i:571–3. *An early account of what later became known as hepatitis E.*

Yarbough PO, Tam AW, Fry KE, et al. Hepatitis E virus: identification of type common epitopes. J Virol. 1991;65:5790–7. *Description of the development of diagnostic tests for hepatitis E.*

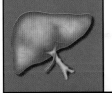

Chapter 12

Viral Hepatitis B and D

Anna Suk Fong Lok and Henry Lik Yuen Chan

HEPATITIS B

INTRODUCTION

Hepatitis B virus (HBV) belongs to the family of hepadnaviruses. The complete virion or Dane particle is 42nm in diameter. It consists of an envelope composed of virus-encoded proteins and host-derived lipid components; and a core particle made up of the nucleocapsid protein, the viral genome, and the polymerase protein. Hepatitis B virus also produces 22nm subviral particles in the form of filaments and spheres that contain only envelope proteins. Such particles do not contain the HBV genome and are noninfectious.

The HBV genome is a circular, partially double-stranded DNA of approximately 3200 base pairs in length (Fig. 12.1). There

are four open reading frames (ORFs) encoding the envelope (pre-S/S), core (precore/core), polymerase, and X proteins. The pre-S/S ORF is divided into pre-S1, pre-S2, and S regions that encode the large (L), middle (M), and small (S) envelope proteins, respectively. The M and S envelope proteins are found in all forms of viral and subviral particles, whereas the L envelope proteins are predominantly found in complete virions. The pre-core/core ORF consists of two regions that encode a precore polypeptide, which is post-translationally modified into a soluble protein, the hepatitis B e antigen (HBeAg) and the core protein (HBcAg). The polymerase protein consists of a protein primer, a spacer, a reverse transcriptase/DNA polymerase, and an RNAase H. The X protein is not required for the replication of the virus. It is a potent transcriptional transactivator of many promotors including HBV and cellular oncogenes. The HBX protein has been implicated in hepatocarcinogenesis.

The replication cycle of HBV begins with attachment of the virion onto the hepatocyte membrane (Fig. 12.2). Inside the hepatocyte nucleus, synthesis of the plus strand HBV DNA is completed and the viral genome is converted into a covalently closed circular DNA (cccDNA). The hepatitis B virus genome replicates by reverse transcription via a RNA intermediate. Transcription of the cccDNA produces a pregenomic RNA that serves both as a template for reverse transcription as well as a messenger RNA for the production of nucleocapsid and polymerase proteins. The pregenomic RNA, and nucleocapsid and polymerase proteins are encapsulated in the virus core particle inside which reverse transcription takes place. A new minus strand HBV DNA is produced followed by the synthesis of a new plus strand HBV DNA. Nucleocapsids with the partially double-stranded HBV DNA can re-enter the hepatocyte nucleus to produce more cccDNA or be secreted as complete virions after coating with envelope proteins.

EPIDEMIOLOGY AND PATHOGENESIS

Epidemiology
Hepatitis B virus infection is a worldwide health problem. It is estimated there are more than 300 million HBV carriers globally, of whom over 250,000 die of HBV-associated liver disease annually.

Prevalence
The prevalence of HBV carriers varies from 0.1–2% in low prevalence areas (USA and Canada, Western Europe, Australia, and New Zealand), to 3–5% in intermediate prevalence areas (Mediterranean countries, Japan, Central Asia, Middle East, and Latin and South America), to 10–20% in high prevalence areas

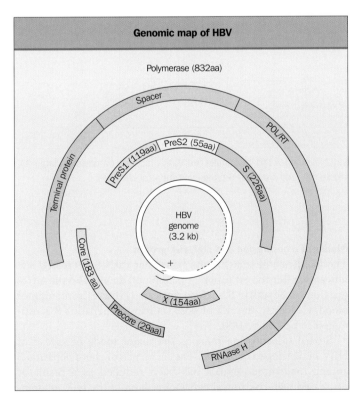

Genomic map of HBV

Polymerase (832aa)
Spacer
PreS1 (119aa)
PreS2 (55aa)
POL/RT
S (226aa)
Terminal protein
HBV genome (3.2 kb)
+
Core (183 aa)
X (154aa)
Precore (29aa)
RNAase H

Figure 12.1 Genomic map of HBV. Map shows the relaxed circular partially double-stranded DNA with four overlapping open reading frames: envelope (preS/S), core (precore/core), polymerase, and X. POL, DNA polymerase; RT, reverse transcriptase; RNAase, ribonuclease.

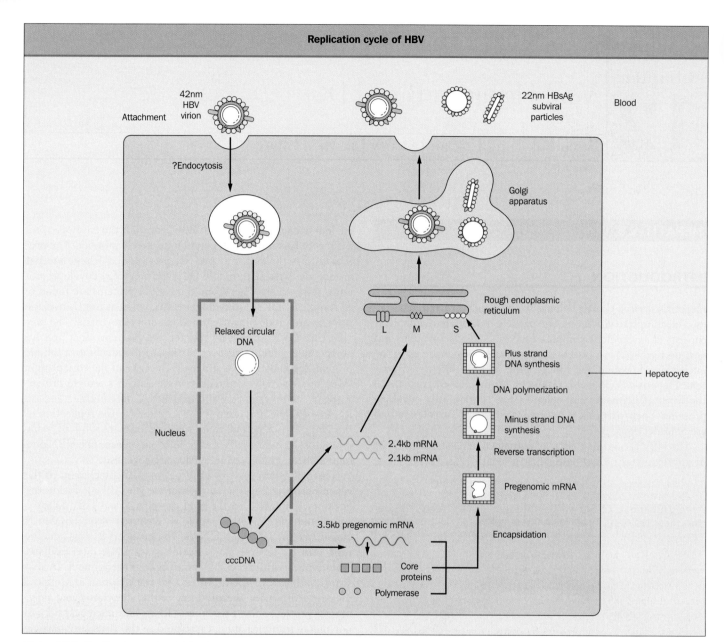

Replication cycle of HBV

Figure 12.2 Replication cycle of HBV. Transcription of cccDNA produces 3.5kb pregenomic RNA which serves as the template for reverse transcription of HBV DNA and translation of core and polymerase proteins; and 2.4kb and 2.1kb messenger (m)RNAs which are translated to large (L), middle (M), and small (S) S proteins of the viral envelope.

(Southeast Asia, China, and sub-Saharan Africa) (Fig. 12.3). The wide range in carrier rate in different parts of the world is largely related to differences in age at infection. The rate of progression from acute to chronic HBV infection is approximately 90% for perinatally acquired infection, 20–50% for infections between the age of 1 and 5 years, and less than 5% for adult acquired infection. Perinatal infection is the predominant mode of transmission in high prevalence areas, probably related to the high prevalence (40–50%) of HBeAg in women of reproductive age. Horizontal transmission, particularly in early childhood, accounts for most cases of chronic HBV infection in intermediate prevalence areas, whereas transmission via unprotected sexual intercourse and intravenous drug use are the major routes of spread in low prevalence areas.

Modes of transmission and high-risk groups

The incidence of transfusion-related hepatitis B decreased significantly after the exclusion of paid blood donors and the introduction of hepatitis B surface antigen (HBsAg) screening of blood. Currently, the risk of post-transfusion hepatitis B is estimated to be 1 in 63,000.

Sexual transmission remains the major mode of spread of HBV in developed countries. The incidence of acute hepatitis B among male homosexuals has been reduced as a result of decreased high-risk sexual behavior related to the HIV epidemic. Heterosexual transmission of HBV infection still occurs. Sexual transmission accounts for approximately 30% of HBV infections in the USA.

Percutaneous inoculation of blood and body fluid, in par-

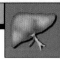

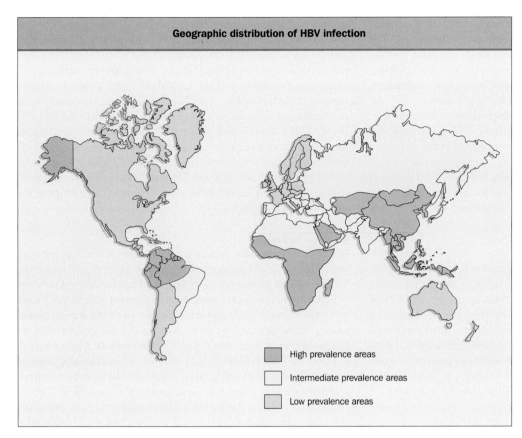

Figure 12.3 Geographic distribution of HBV infection.

ticular needle sharing among intravenous drug users, is an important mode of HBV transmission. Other routes include the reuse of contaminated needles in tattoos, acupuncture, and ear piercing.

Perinatal transmission of HBV occurs in up to 90% of infants born to HBeAg -positive mothers. Transmission takes place at the time of delivery by maternal–fetal transfusion and exposure to maternal blood in the birth canal, as well as postnatally through close mother–baby contact.

Children may acquire HBV infection via minor skin breaks and mucous membranes or close bodily contacts. As HBV can stay outside the human body for a long time, transmission via contaminated household articles such as toothbrushes, razors, and even toys may be possible.

Although HBV DNA has been detected in various bodily secretions of HBV carriers, there is no firm evidence of HBV transmission via body fluids other than by sexual contact.

Health care workers, particularly surgeons, pathologists, and physicians working in hemodialysis and oncology units, have a higher risk of contracting HBV infection via minor skin breaks, cuts, and accidental needle puncture. Patient-to-patient transmission via contaminated instruments and needles may also occur in the health care setting. Institutionalized persons as well as their attendants and family members also have increased risks of HBV infection.

Pathogenesis

The pathogenesis of HBV-related liver disease is largely due to immune-mediated mechanisms. However, in some circumstances HBV can cause direct cytotoxic liver injury.

Immune-mediated liver injury

Liver injury related to HBV is generally thought to be related to cytotoxic T lymphocyte (CTL)-mediated lysis of infected hepatocytes. These cells recognize viral antigens presented in association with class I histocompatibility antigens on the hepatocyte membrane causing apoptosis of the infected hepatocytes. Events that enhance immune clearance as in spontaneous or interferon induced HBeAg seroconversion are often accompanied by exacerbations of liver disease, with flares in serum alanine aminotransferase (ALT) levels and lobular necrosis. Chronic hepatitis B patients who clear HBeAg have been found to have higher levels of interleukin-12, a cytokine that promotes differentiation of Th1 cells and antigen-specific proliferation of CTLs, than those who remain HBeAg-positive. Patients who develop fulminant hepatitis B frequently have no evidence of HBV replication at presentation; some may even be HBsAg-negative. The fulminant course is believed to be due to rapid and aggressive immune clearance. Immune-mediated viral clearance can also occur through noncytolytic pathways via the release of cytokines such as tumor necrosis factor-α and interferon-γ.

Direct cytopathic effects

In general, HBV is not a cytopathic virus. In most patients with chronic hepatitis B, there is no direct correlation between viral load and severity of liver disease. This is particularly true in Asian children and young adults who acquired HBV infection perinatally. These individuals tend to have very high serum HBV DNA levels and abundant intrahepatic virus, but are usually asymptomatic with normal ALT levels and minimal histologic changes. Most patients on hemodialysis also have high serum HBV DNA

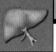

levels but minimal liver disease. Nevertheless, direct cytopathic liver injury can occur when the viral load is very high, as in some patients with recurrent hepatitis B post-liver transplant [orthotopic liver transplantation (OLT)] who develop fibrosing cholestatic hepatitis (FCH). This is characterized by marked cholestasis, minimal necroinflammation, high levels of intrahepatic HBsAg and HBcAg expression, and rapid progression to liver failure. Another form of direct cytopathic liver injury was initially described in transgenic mice that overexpress pre-S antigens, leading to retention of small S proteins, development of ground glass hepatocytes, liver injury, and finally hepatocellular carcinoma (HCC). Similar phenomena have been reported in humans infected with HBV that have mutations in the S gene promoter causing retention of small S protein.

Role of viral mutants

Mutations in all regions of the HBV genome have been found in patients with chronic HBV infection. Some of these mutations, notably the precore stop codon mutation and the T1762/A1764 changes in the core promoter region, have been said to cause more severe liver disease. However, these mutants have also been found in asymptomatic carriers. Thus, these mutations alone are not necessarily pathogenic. However, HBV mutations can potentially modulate the severity of liver disease by altering the level of viral replication or the expression of more immunogenic epitopes.

Hepatocarcinogenesis

Several lines of evidence support an etiologic association between chronic HBV infection and the development of HCC. There is a close correlation between the geographic distribution of HBsAg carriers and the occurrence of HCC. A study of Taiwanese men followed for 9 years found that the relative risk of HCC for HBsAg-positive men was 98. Studies in woodchucks found that chronic infection with hepadnavirus alone is sufficient to cause HCC. Integration of HBV DNA into host chromosomes can be found in the neoplastic liver tissues from most HBsAg-positive patients with HCC. Although HBV is not directly carcinogenic, integration of HBV DNA into the host genome may induce carcinogenesis by activating cellular proto-oncogenes or suppressing growth-regulating genes, or by inducing host chromosomal deletions or translocations. Another mechanism of carcinogenesis may be through chronic liver injury, inflammation, and regeneration.

CLINICAL FEATURES

Infection with HBV has a wide spectrum of manifestations including subclinical hepatitis, anicteric hepatitis, icteric hepatitis, and fulminant hepatitis during the acute phase; and asymptomatic carrier state, chronic hepatitis, cirrhosis, and HCC during the chronic phase.

Acute hepatitis

Approximately 70% of patients with acute HBV infection have subclinical hepatitis or anicteric hepatitis, whereas 30% become icteric. Acute liver failure develops in approximately 0.1–0.5% of patients. The incubation period lasts 1–4 months. A serum sickness-like syndrome may develop during the prodromal period. This is followed by constitutional symptoms such as low-grade fever, malaise, anorexia, nausea and vomiting, and right upper quadrant or midepigastric pain. Jaundice usually appears as the constitutional symptoms begin to subside. Clinical symptoms and jaundice generally disappear after 1–3 months but some patients may have prolonged fatigue, even after normalization of aminotransferase levels. Elevation of ALT and aspartate aminotransferase (AST) levels, up to 1000–2000IU/L, is typically seen during the acute phase, with ALT levels higher than AST levels. Prothrombin time, which reflects hepatic synthetic function, is the best indicator of prognosis. In patients who recover, normalization of aminotransferases usually occurs within 1–4 months, followed by normalization of bilirubin levels. Persistent elevation of ALT levels lasting more than 6 months indicate progression to chronic hepatitis.

Chronic hepatitis

In low or intermediate prevalence areas, only 30–50% of patients with chronic HBV infection have a history of acute hepatitis. The remaining patients in these areas and the majority of patients in high prevalence areas (predominantly perinatal infection) have not experienced acute hepatitis. Many patients are asymptomatic, while others may have nonspecific symptoms such as fatigue and mild right upper quadrant discomfort. Some patients experience exacerbations that may be asymptomatic, mimic acute hepatitis, or manifest as liver failure. Physical examination may be normal or there may be stigmata of chronic liver disease. In patients with cirrhosis, additional findings such as jaundice, splenomegaly, ascites, peripheral edema, and encephalopathy may be present.

Laboratory investigations including liver profile and blood counts may be normal in some patients, but most patients have mild to moderate elevations of AST and ALT levels. During exacerbations, ALT levels may be as high as 50 times the upper limit of normal and α-fetoprotein (AFP) levels of up to 1000IU/L may be seen. Progression to cirrhosis is suspected when there is evidence of hypersplenism (decreased leukocyte and platelet counts) and impaired hepatic function (hypoalbuminemia, prolonged prothrombin time, and hyperbilirubinemia).

Extrahepatic manifestations

Extrahepatic manifestations occur in 10–20% of patients with chronic HBV infection. Mediated by circulating immune complexes, acute hepatitis may be heralded by a serum sickness-like syndrome manifested as fever, skin rashes, arthralgia, and arthritis, which usually subside with the onset of jaundice.

Approximately 10–50% of patients with polyarteritis nodosa are HBsAg-positive. Vasculitis associated with HBV may affect large, medium, and small sized vessels in multiple organs including cardiovascular, gastrointestinal, neurologic, and dermatologic systems. The course is highly variable and the mortality rate is high.

Hepatitis B virus-related glomerulonephritis, most commonly membranous glomerulonephritis, is more often found in children. Approximately 30–60% of children with HBV-related membranous glomerulonephritis undergo spontaneous remission. Remission accompanying HBeAg to anti-HBe seroconversion has also been reported. Interferon has been reported to induce remission in small clinical trials. In adults, the course of HBV-related glomerulonephritis may be progressive and response to interferon is poor.

Other extrahepatic manifestations including essential mixed cryoglobulinemia and aplastic anemia have also been reported.

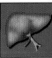

Special patient groups
Pediatric patients
Infants infected perinatally are usually asymptomatic but have a high rate (90%) of progression to chronic infection.

Infection with HBV has been estimated to account for 10–25% of all cases of childhood acute hepatitis. Extrahepatic manifestations including Gianotti's papular acrodermatitis have been reported in 25% of patients. The acute illness is usually mild. Recovery with HBsAg to anti-HBs seroconversion occurs in >80% of children infected after the age of 1 year.

Children with perinatally acquired chronic HBV infection are usually asymptomatic with normal ALT values, despite high serum HBV DNA levels. In contrast, 15–30% of children with childhood acquired chronic HBV infection are symptomatic with elevated ALT levels and chronic hepatitis on liver biopsies. Progression of chronic hepatitis to cirrhosis is rare in children but cases of childhood HCC have been reported.

Immunocompromised patients
Immunocompromised patients may have different clinical manifestations due to increased levels of HBV replication. Abrupt withdrawal of immunosuppressive therapy during cyclic chemotherapy or tapering of steroid treatment may cause a rebound increase in immune clearance and exacerbation of chronic hepatitis B. Although most exacerbations are asymptomatic, fatal hepatic decompensation has been reported. Patients coinfected with human immunodeficiency virus (HIV) and HBV tend to have higher serum HBV DNA levels, lower rate of spontaneous and interferon-induced HBeAg seroconversion, and an increased risk of cirrhosis.

Alcoholics
Alcoholics with HBV infection have been reported to have accelerated liver damage, and an increased risk of progression to cirrhosis and HCC, as well as decreased survival compared with alcoholics who are not HBV-infected.

Coinfection with hepatitis C virus
Acute HBV and hepatitis C virus (HCV) coinfection may delay the onset and shorten the duration of HBs antigenemia as well as lower the peak transaminase levels compared with acute HBV infection alone, suggesting a possible interference of HBV replication by HCV. However, dual infection with HBV and HCV has been reported to be associated with increased risks of acute liver failure.

Most patients who are chronically infected with both HCV and HBV have detectable serum HCV RNA but not HBV DNA, indicating that HBV replication is suppressed by HCV. Nevertheless, liver disease is generally more severe and the risk of developing HCC is higher in patients with dual infections than in those infected with either virus alone.

DIAGNOSIS

The diagnosis of hepatitis B depends on serologic assays for hepatitis B-associated antigens and antibodies (Fig. 12.4). Tests for HBV DNA in serum are used to assess HBV replication. Liver histology is used to determine the severity and stage of liver disease.

Serology assays
Serologic markers of HBV infection are illustrated in Figure 12.5.

Hepatitis B surface antigen and antibody
HBsAg is the hallmark of HBV infection. It is usually detectable 1–10 weeks after an acute exposure to HBV, and approximately 2–6 weeks before the onset of clinical symptoms. Most patients who recover from acute hepatitis B clear HBsAg in 4–6 months. Persistence of HBsAg in serum for more than 6 months implies chronic infection.

Anti-HBs is a neutralizing antibody that confers protective immunity to HBV infection. Recovery from acute hepatitis B is indicated by the disappearance of HBsAg and the development of anti-HBs. However, in some patients there may be a window period lasting several weeks to months when neither HBsAg nor anti-HBs can be detected. Anti-HBs can be detected in individuals who recovered from HBV infection and in those who successfully responded to hepatitis B vaccination.

Hepatitis B virus can be classified into four major subtypes, all of which share a common antigenic determinant 'a'. Antibodies directed against the 'a' determinant confer protection to all HBV subtypes. Coexistence of HBsAg and anti-HBs has been found in some patients. These individuals should be

	HBsAg	HBeAg	Anti-HBc-IgM	Anti-HBc-IgG	Anti-HBs	Anti-HBe	HBV DNA	Interpretation
Serologic markers for HBV infection								
Acute HBV infection	+	+	+		–		+	Early phase
	–		+		–		+/–	Window phase
	–			+	+	+	–	Recovery phase
Chronic HBV infection	+	+		+	–		+	Replicative phase
	+			+	–	+	–	Low (non)replicative phase
	+	+/–	+	+	–		+	Flare-up of chronic HBV infection
	+	–		+	–	+	+	Precore mutants

Figure 12.4 Serologic markers of HBV infection.

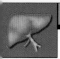

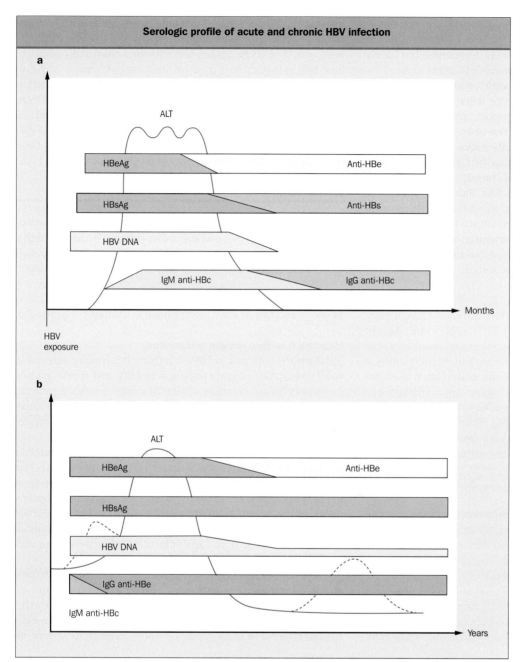

Figure 12.5 Serologic profile of acute and chronic HBV infection. (a) Acute HBV infection and (b) chronic HBV infection.

considered as carriers because the anti-HBs is usually not capable of neutralizing the circulating virus.

Hepatitis B core antigen and antibody

The antigen HBcAg is an intracellular antigen and is not detected in serum. Anti-HBc-IgM is the first antibody to develop during acute HBV infection. It is usually detectable within 1 month after the appearance of HBsAg. It is the only marker of HBV infection detectable during the window period between the disappearance of HBsAg and the detection of anti-HBs. The presence of anti-HBc-IgM usually indicates recent HBV infection. However, the titer of anti-HBc-IgM may increase to detectable levels during exacerbations of chronic hepatitis B, leading to misdiagnosis of acute hepatitis B.

Anti-HBc-IgG is found in association with anti-HBs in indi-

viduals who recover from hepatitis B and with HBsAg in those who have chronic HBV infection. Isolated presence of anti-HBc in the absence of HBsAg and anti-HBs can be detected in approximately 1% of blood donors in low prevalence areas and in up to 20% of blood donors in endemic areas. This situation may occur during the window phase of acute HBV infection, many years after recovery from acute hepatitis B or after many years of chronic HBV infection (Fig. 12.6). Transmission of HBV infection has been reported in blood and organ donors with isolated anti-HBc, but as many as 50% of asymptomatic individuals with isolated anti-HBc may have a false-positive test result.

Hepatitis B e antigen and antibody

The antigen HBeAg is a marker of HBV replication and infectivity. Its presence is usually associated with the detection of

HBV DNA in serum and a high risk of transmission of infection. During acute HBV infection, HBeAg is rapidly cleared, before the disappearance of HBsAg. However, in patients with chronic HBV infection, HBeAg may persist for years to decades. Seroconversion from HBeAg to anti-HBe is usually associated with the disappearance of HBV DNA in serum and remission of liver disease, but a small proportion of anti-HBe-positive patients continue to have active liver disease and detectable HBV DNA in serum. These patients may have residual low levels of wild-type HBV or HBV mutants that prevent the production of HBeAg. The most common mutation is a G–A change at nucleotide 1896, creating a premature stop codon at codon 28 of the precore region (Fig. 12.7). There is a wide variation in the prevalence of the stop codon mutant in different parts of the world with a high prevalence in the Mediterranean basin, an intermediate prevalence in South East Asia and Japan, and a low prevalence in North America and North Europe. The basis for the variable prevalence is related to the fact that the stop codon mutant is restricted to specific HBV genotypes. Other mutations that can decrease HBeAg production include changes in the core promoter region, most commonly A–T and G–A changes at nucleotides 1762 and 1764, respectively, which downregulates transcription of the precore messenger RNA.

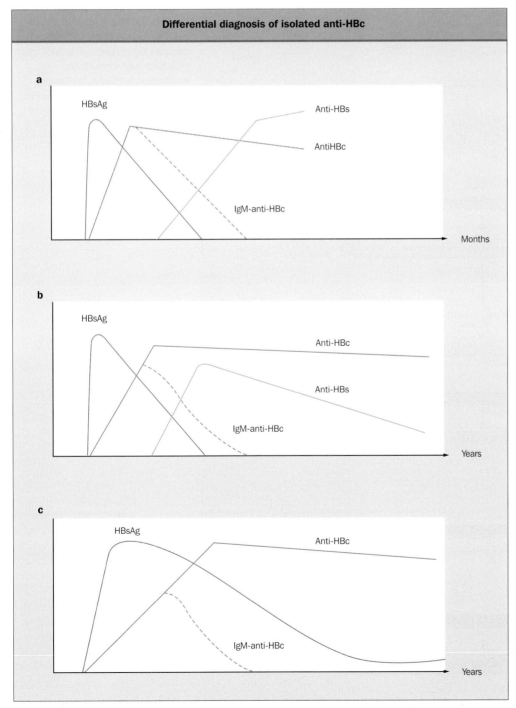

Figure 12.6 Differential diagnosis of isolated anti-HBc. (a) Window period of acute HBV infection, (b) recovered HBV infection, and (c) low level HBV carrier.

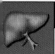

Serum HBV DNA assays

Qualitative and quantitative assays for HBV DNA in serum are used to assess the level of HBV replication. Molecular hybridization assays have a detection limit of 10–50pg/mL or 10^6 viral genome equivalents/mL. The branched DNA (bDNA) assay is more sensitive and can detect HBV DNA levels down to 10^5 genome equivalents/mL. Polymerase chain reaction (PCR) assays are even more sensitive with detection limits of 1–10 genome equivalents/mL. In patients with acute hepatitis B, serum HBV DNA appears early and may precede the detection of HBsAg. In patients with chronic HBV infection, detection of HBV DNA in serum is usually associated with the presence of HBeAg. Seroconversion of HBeAg is in general accompanied by the disappearance of HBV DNA in serum as determined by hybridization or bDNA assays, but HBV DNA frequently remains detectable by PCR assays. The major role of serum HBV DNA assays is to assess candidacy for and response to antiviral therapy in patients with chronic HBV infection. Rarely, tests for HBV DNA in serum may help to identify HBV as the etiology of idiopathic fulminant hepatitis or cryptogenic cirrhosis.

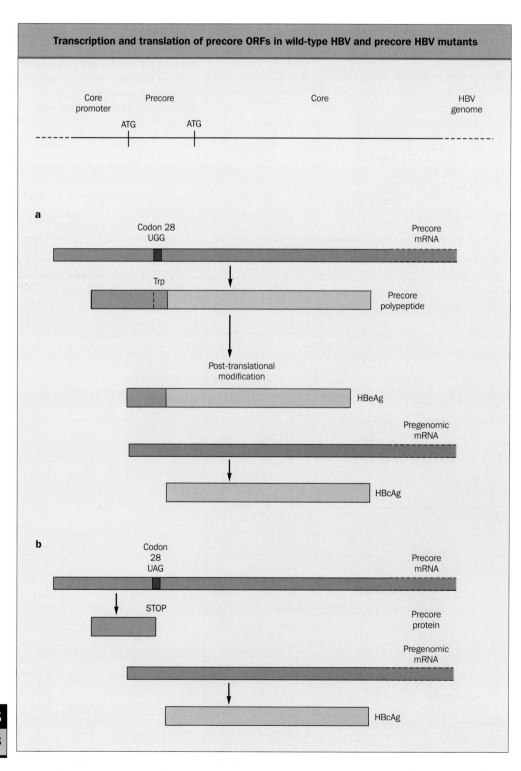

Figure 12.7 Transcription and translation of precore and core ORFs in wild-type HBV and precore HBV mutants. (a) Transcription of precore and core regions of wild-type HBV produces the precore polypeptide which undergoes post-translational modification to HBeAg. (b) Precore mutant with premature stop codon at codon 28 prevents the production of HBeAg, but the translation of pregenomic RNA is not affected.

Liver histology

Liver biopsy is seldom indicated in acute hepatitis B. Histologic changes include lobular disarray, acidophilic degeneration of hepatocytes, focal lobular necrosis, cholestasis, and portal inflammation. Bridging necrosis may be present in patients with severe hepatitis.

Liver biopsy is useful in assessing the severity of liver disease, in predicting prognosis, and in monitoring response to treatment in patients with chronic hepatitis B. The most common features include portal inflammation and periportal necrosis. Periportal necrosis may be severe causing disruption of the limiting plate (piecemeal necrosis or interface hepatitis). As the liver disease progresses, fibrosis, and eventually cirrhosis develops. The histology of chronic hepatitis B is traditionally classified as chronic persistent hepatitis (CPH), chronic active hepatitis (CAH), and cirrhosis. A third form of liver injury, chronic lobular hepatitis (CLH), which is characterized by spotty necrosis and inflammation within the lobules with mild portal inflammation, is seen during exacerbations of chronic hepatitis B. Histologic classification into CPH and CAH was previously used to predict prognosis, but recent studies showed that patients may progress from CPH to CAH and vice versa, suggesting that these two forms of liver injury may be seen during different phases of chronic HBV infection in the same patient.

In recent years, several numeric scoring systems have been developed to provide more objective assessment of liver injury and to permit statistical comparisons of necroinflammation and fibrosis. The best known system, the Knodell Histology Activity Index (HAI), is derived by adding the scores of four components: periportal and bridging necrosis, intralobular degeneration and focal necrosis, portal inflammation, and fibrosis. Recently, an international consensus panel recommended that the reporting of liver histology in patients with chronic hepatitis should include the etiology of chronic hepatitis, the grade of necroinflammatory activity, and the extent of fibrosis.

Immunohistochemical staining reveals the presence of HBsAg. In patients with replicative infection, HBcAg can also be detected.

NATURAL HISTORY AND PROGNOSIS

The natural course of chronic HBV infection is determined by the interplay between virus replication and host's immune response.

Phases of chronic hepatitis B virus infection

In general, chronic HBV infection consists of an earlier replicative phase with active liver disease and a later nonreplicative phase with remission of liver disease (Fig. 12.8). In patients with perinatally acquired infection, there is an additional initial immune tolerance phase when viral replication is not accompanied by active liver disease (Fig. 12.8).

Replicative phase – immune tolerance

Immune tolerance phase is characterized by a high level of HBV replication but inactive liver disease. It usually lasts for 10–30 years. Spontaneous HBeAg clearance rarely occurs during this phase. Tolerance to HBV is believed to be due to transplacental transfer of HBeAg leading to deletion of T cells that can respond to HBeAg/HBcAg (Fig. 12.9).

Replicative phase – immune clearance

Transition from immune tolerance to immune clearance usually occurs between the ages of 15 and 35 years in patients with perinatally acquired HBV infection. During this phase, liver disease is active and spontaneous HBeAg seroconversion occurs at a rate of 10–20% per year. Seroconversion of HBeAg is frequently accompanied by exacerbations of liver disease that are thought to be a result of increased immune-mediated lysis of infected hepatocytes. Most exacerbations are asymptomatic but some are accompanied by symptoms of acute hepatitis, while a small minority progress to liver failure. The transition from replicative to nonreplicative infection may be rapid and smooth or prolonged and fluctuant. Some patients have suboptimal immune response with recurrent exacerbations and intermittent clearance of serum HBV DNA and HBeAg. These patients have a higher risk of developing cirrhosis and HCC due to the repeated episodes of necroinflammation.

In patients with adult acquired chronic HBV infection, the replicative phase is marked by active liver disease. Spontaneous HBeAg seroconversion occurs at a rate of 10–20% per year but exacerbations accompanying HBeAg clearance are less well-described.

Nonreplicative (low-replication) phase

The third phase is generally characterized by the absence of HBeAg and the presence of anti-HBe. In some patients, HBV replication has ceased even though they remain HBsAg-positive. These patients have undetectable serum HBV DNA even by PCR assay. With time, some of them may clear HBsAg. The annual rate of HBsAg clearance in patients with chronic HBV infection is estimated to be 0.5–2%. Most patients, however, remain HBV DNA-positive in serum by PCR assay. These patients usually have inactive liver disease. Reactivation of HBV replication and liver disease may occur when these patients are immunocompromised. A small proportion of patients continue to have moderate levels of HBV replication with detectable serum HBV DNA by hybridization assays and active liver disease. Some of these patients have residual wild-type HBV, especially if they are in the e-window phase between the clearance of HBeAg and appearance of anti-HBe, or have a mutation in the core promotor or precore regions that prevent the production of HBeAg.

Prognosis of chronic hepatitis B virus infection

The sequelae of chronic HBV infection vary from an asymptomatic carrier state to the development of liver cirrhosis, hepatic decompensation, and HCC. The outcome of chronic HBV infection seems to depend on the severity of liver disease at the time HBV replication is arrested.

Long-term follow-up of HBaAg blood donors, most of whom were anti-HBe-positive with normal transaminases, found that they usually remain asymptomatic with minimal risk of developing cirrhosis and HCC. Nevertheless, chronic HBV infection remains an important cause of morbidity and mortality in endemic areas. Progression from chronic hepatitis to cirrhosis, and from compensated cirrhosis to hepatic decompensation and HCC have been estimated to be 12–20%, 20–23%, and 6–15% at 5 years, respectively (Fig. 12.10). Survival after the development of compensated cirrhosis is initially favorable (85% at 5 years) (Fig. 12.11), but decreases dramatically after the onset of decompensation to 55–70% at 1 year and 14–35% at 5 years (Fig. 12.12).

The life-time risk of a liver-related death has been estimated to be 40–50% for men and 15% for women among Chinese patients with chronic HBV infection.

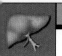

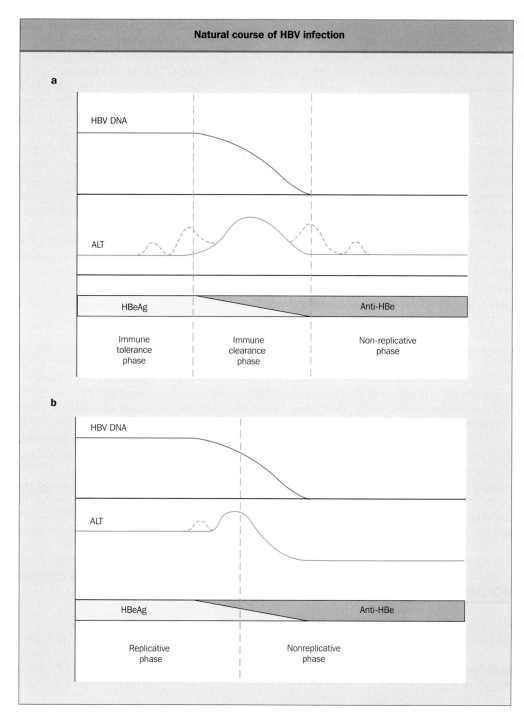

Figure 12.8 Natural course of HBV infection in perinatal infection and adult-acquired infection. (a) Perinatal infection and (b) adult-acquired infection.

Recent studies found that patients with a prolonged replicative phase have impaired survival. This may be related to the increased risks of exacerbations. Recurrent episodes of necroinflammation and regeneration are believed to play a major role in the pathogenesis of liver fibrosis, cirrhosis, and carcinogenesis. In a retrospective study of 366 European patients with HBsAg-positive compensated cirrhosis, the 5-year survival rates of HBeAg-positive and HBeAg-negative patients were 77% and 88%, respectively (P=0.04). Biochemical remission and clearance of HBeAg or serum HBV DNA during follow-up were significantly associated with a higher rate of survival. Even among patients with decompensated cirrhosis, suppression of HBV replication and delayed HBsAg clearance have been shown to result in improved liver function.

MANAGEMENT

The main aim of treatment of chronic HBV infection is to suppress HBV replication before significant irreversible liver damage occurs. The initial goals are to suppress HBV replication (clearance of HBeAg and undetectable serum HBV DNA by hybridization assays) and to induce remission of liver disease (normalization of ALT levels and decreased necroinflammation). The ultimate goals are to eliminate HBV (clearance of HBsAg and undetectable serum HBV DNA by PCR) and to prevent progression to cirrhosis and HCC.

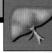

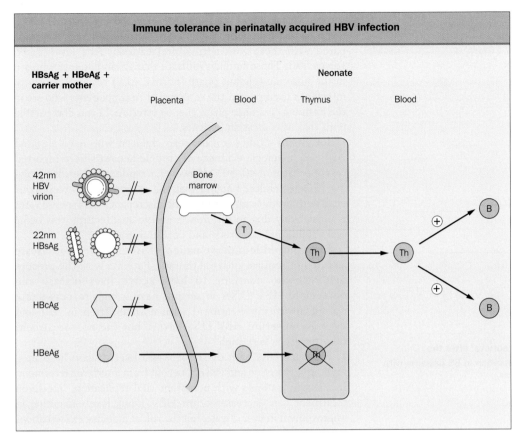

Figure 12.9 Pathogenesis of immune tolerance in perinatally acquired HBV infection. HBV virion particles, 22nm HBsAg subviral particles, and HBcAg are too large to cross the placenta. HBeAg, a small soluble protein, can traverse the placenta resulting in deletion of T cells that can respond to HBeAg. Because HBeAg and HBcAg cross-react at the T cell level, this also results in impaired T cell response to HBcAg. T, progenitor T cells; Th, T helper cells; B, B cells; CTL, cytotoxic T lymphocytes.

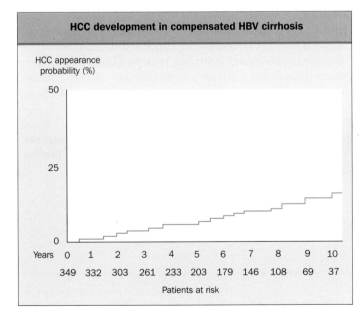

Figure 12.10 Cumulative probability of HCC development in patients with compensated HBV cirrhosis. (Data from Fattovich G, et al., 1995.)

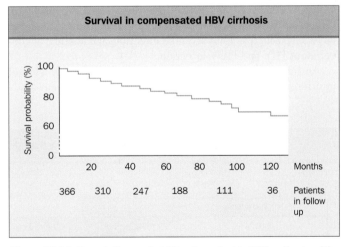

Figure 12.11 Cumulative probability of survival in 366 patients with compensated HBV cirrhosis. (Data from Realdi G, et al., 1994.)

Efficacy

A meta-analysis of randomized controlled trials has confirmed a beneficial effect of interferon-α in patients with chronic hepatitis B (Fig. 12.13). A standard course of interferon treatment involves subcutaneous injections of 5 million units (MU) daily or 10MU three times a week for 16 weeks. Loss of serum viral replication markers (HBeAg and HBV DNA) and HBsAg can be achieved in 30–40% and 5–10% of patients, respectively, within

Interferons

Interferons have antiviral, antiproliferative and immunomodulatory effects. Interferon-α was until recently the only approved treatment for chronic HBV infection in most countries.

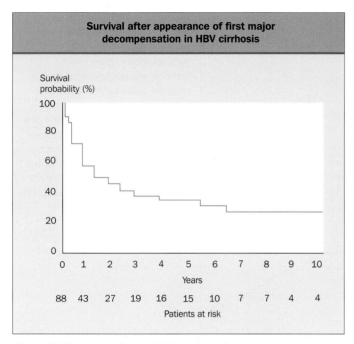

Figure 12.12 Cumulative probability of survival after the appearance of the first major decompensation in 88 patients with HBV cirrhosis. (Data from Fattovich G, 1995.)

12 months of initiation of treatment, compared with 10–15% and 0.5–2%, respectively, in untreated controls. Response is best in patients with low serum HBV DNA levels (pretreatment HBV DNA <200pg/mL) and active liver disease (ALT >100U/L). Other factors associated with a favorable response to interferon include female sex, adult acquired infection, and absence of concomitant HIV and HDV infection.

An initial study in Chinese adults found that only 15% of interferon-treated patients cleared HBeAg. A subsequent study showed that Chinese patients with elevated pretreatment ALT levels had a significantly higher response rate to interferon compared with those with normal pretreatment ALT levels (39% versus 5%). These findings indicate that Asian patients who are in the immune tolerant phase (normal ALT) respond poorly to interferon therapy, but the response of Asian patients who are in the immune clearance phase (i.e. elevated ALT) was comparable with that of Caucasian patients.

Results of studies in European children who have elevated ALT and histologic evidence of chronic hepatitis have reported response rates of 40–50%. However, a randomized study involving Chinese children found that the response rates were poor even with prednisone priming. The discrepancy in response rates is most likely due to differences in age at infection, this being early childhood in Europe and perinatal in Asia.

Most anti-HBe-positive patients have inactive liver disease and do not require antiviral therapy. Patients with the precore mutant, who continue to have active liver disease and detectable HBV DNA in serum, have a high response rate during interferon treatment with normalization in ALT and decrease in serum HBV DNA levels, but the post-treatment relapse rate is very high.

Most patients with decompensated liver disease have non-replicative infection and will not benefit from interferon treatment. In cirrhotic patients with persistent viral replication, interferon treatment can decrease serum HBV DNA levels resulting in improvement in liver disease, but the risk of inducing exacerbations leading to hepatic failure and serious infections is significant, even with low-dose interferon therapy (3MU thrice weekly).

Prednisone priming
Pilot studies suggested that abrupt withdrawal of prednisone may induce a rebound in immune clearance and increase the rate of response to subsequent interferon therapy. However, conflicting results were obtained in large-scale randomized controlled studies. In a meta-analysis of seven studies, the rates of HBsAg, HBeAg and

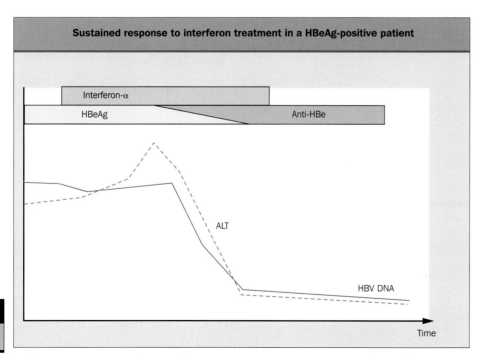

Figure 12.13 Profile of sustained response to interferon treatment in a HBeAg-positive patient.

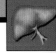

serum HBV DNA clearance were respectively, 6% versus 7%, 41% versus 35%, and 38% versus 36%, in patients who received interferon-α with and without prednisone priming. Based on current data, prednisone priming adds little additional benefit to interferon treatment alone and should not be used as primary therapy.

Long-term outcome

Most responders have a sustained response. Approximately 10–20% of patients who clear HBeAg after interferon treatment experience reactivation of HBV replication, usually within the first year after completing therapy. However, eradication of HBV replication as determined by disappearance of serum HBV DNA by PCR assay seldom occurs in patients who cleared HBeAg only. HBsAg clearance occurs at highly variable rates ranging from 65% in one US study, to 19–24% in European studies, to 9% in a study from Hong Kong. A sustained antiviral response in patients who cleared both HBeAg and HBsAg is invariably followed by a normalization of ALT levels and a decrease in histologic necroinflammation. A recent long-term study found that patients with sustained suppression of HBV replication after interferon treatment have improved overall survival and a reduced likelihood of developing hepatic decompensation and HCC.

Adverse reactions

Interferon therapy is associated with a wide spectrum of side effects. The commonest is flu-like symptoms (fever, headache, malaise, myalgia) during the first 1–2 weeks of treatment. Other adverse effects include fatigue, anorexia, weight loss, and mild alopecia. Mild myelosuppression is common but significant neutropenia ($<1000/mm^3$) or thrombocytopenia ($<60,000/mm^3$) requiring dose reduction or premature termination of treatment is uncommon. Psychiatric problems including anxiety, irritability, depression, and suicidal tendency may occur even in patients without previous emotional problems. Interferon may also induce the development of autoantibodies, but it seldom leads to overt autoimmune disease except for hyper- and hypothyroidism.

Antiviral drugs

Several antiviral drugs have shown early promising results in clinical trials.

Lamivudine

Lamivudine is the (–) enantiomer of 2'3'dideoxy-3'thiacytidine (3TC). It competes with dCTP for incorporation into growing viral DNA chains, thus inhibiting both reverse transcriptase and DNA polymerase activities.

Clinical trials showed that short (4–24 weeks) courses of oral lamivudine at 100mg daily are well-tolerated and effective in decreasing serum HBV DNA to undetectable levels in most patients with chronic hepatitis B (Fig. 12.14). However, serum HBV DNA reappears in the majority of patients after discontinuation of treatment. Very few (0–12%) patients clear HBeAg. Preliminary results of ongoing studies suggest that higher sustained response rates can be achieved with longer duration (1 year) of treatment, but the long-term benefits of lamivudine monotherapy remain to be determined.

Lamivudine resistant mutants have been reported in patients who have been on long-term treatment. The incidence of drug-resistant mutants in patients with chronic hepatitis B is approximately 10–15% after one year of treatment, but appears higher in patients treated for recurrent hepatitis B after OLT. Two major mutations have been described. One involves the substitution of methionine to valine or isoleucine in the highly conserved YMDD motif of domain C. The other involves substitution of leucine to methionine in domain B of the HBV polymerase gene (Fig. 12.15). These mutations lead to breakthrough infection but serum HBV DNA and serum ALT levels usually remain lower than the pretreatment values, suggesting that lamivudine may continue to exert a suppressive effect on the wild-type virus. Nevertheless, flares in liver disease leading to liver failure have also been reported in association with the emergence of the mutants.

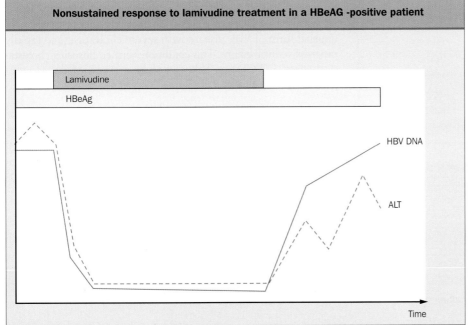

Figure 12.14 Profile of nonsustained response to lamivudine treatment in a HBeAg-positive patient.

Famciclovir

Famciclovir is the oral prodrug of penciclovir. It competes with dGTP for incorporation into the growing HBV DNA chain. In addition to causing chain termination, it also inhibits the priming of reverse transcription.

Preliminary studies have shown that famciclovir in doses of 500mg three times a day is well tolerated and effective in inhibiting HBV replication in patients with chronic hepatitis B, decompensated HBV-related cirrhosis, and recurrent hepatitis B after OLT. However, the effect is not sustained. The efficacy of long-term treatment remains to be established.

Drug-resistant mutants have also been reported with famciclovir treatment. The precise locations of the mutations and their clinical significance are not well defined. The YMDD motif appears to be spared, but the leucine to methionine substitution in domain B of the polymerase gene has been reported, suggesting the potential for cross-resistance with lamivudine (see Fig. 12.15).

Immunomodulatory treatment

Thymic derived peptides (thymosin) stimulate T-cell function. Pilot studies reported promising results. However, a beneficial effect was not confirmed in large randomized clinical trials. The role of thymosin, singly or in combination with interferon, in the treatment of chronic hepatitis B remains to be proved.

T-cell vaccines comprised of peptides that correspond to CTL epitopes of hepatitis B antigens have been shown to induce CTL response and reduce viral antigen production in transgenic mice. Preliminary results of a phase II trial showed that CTL response can be stimulated in patients with chronic HBV infection by inoculation of a vaccine containing an HLA-restricted HBcAg CTL epitope, but the antiviral effect was weak.

Vaccination with plasmid DNA containing HBV S gene has been shown to decrease production of HBsAg and induce an anti-HBs response in transgenic mice that express HBV surface gene, but it remains to be determined whether DNA vaccination can induce anti-HBs response and viral clearance in patients with chronic HBV infection.

Adoptive immunity transfer from bone marrow donors who were anti-HBs-positive has been reported to induce clearance of HBV in recipients with chronic HBV infection. The practical value of bone marrow transplantation as a treatment of chronic hepatitis B is limited due to the high morbidity and mortality.

Future treatment strategy

Based on current experience, monotherapy with interferon or an antiviral drug is unlikely to achieve complete eradication of HBV in most patients with chronic hepatitis B. Combination therapy as in the case of treatment of HIV infection is the logical next step. However, which agents to combine is unclear. Ideally, the two agents should have synergistic, long-lasting effects on HBV clearance; no added toxicity and potential to decrease resistance. Finally, different therapies may have to be designed for different patient populations.

LIVER TRANSPLANTATION

The early results with OLT for chronic hepatitis B were disappointing, with more than 80% of patients experiencing HBV reinfection. Most importantly, in many patients, reinfection was associated with severe and rapidly progressive liver disease.

Factors associated with hepatitis B virus reinfection

The high rate of HBV reinfection after OLT is due to a number of factors including enhanced virus replication resulting from immunosuppression, a direct stimulatory effect of steroid therapy on the glucocorticoid-responsive enhancer region of the HBV genome, and the presence of extrahepatic reservoirs of HBV. Several factors have been associated with a lower rate of reinfection – absence of HBeAg and HBV DNA in the serum before OLT, acute hepatitis B, and coexistent HDV infection.

Diagnosis and clinical course of recurrent hepatitis B

Reinfection with HBV is diagnosed by the reappearance of HBsAg in the serum. Reinfection is almost always accompanied by recurrent liver disease, which can be severe leading to cirrhosis within 1–2 years of reinfection. Some patients develop an unusual form of liver disease with severe cholestasis and rapidly progressive liver failure. This condition, termed fibrosing cholestatic hepatitis (FCH), is believed to be a result of direct cytopathic effects of HBV.

Prevention of recurrent hepatitis B after orthotopic liver transplantation

Various strategies have been evaluated to prevent recurrent hepatitis after OLT. Currently, the most promising prophylactic therapies are long-term high dose hepatitis B immune globulin (HBIG) with or without new antiviral agents such as lamivudine.

Interferon-α

Interferon-α may suppress HBV replication in patients with decompensated cirrhosis, but there is a high risk of serious infections and exacerbation of liver failure. Interferon administered to patients awaiting OLT has been shown to be ineffective in reducing the rate of HBV reinfection after OLT.

Amino acid substitutions in lamivudine- and famciclovir-resistant HBV mutants

	Domain B	Domain C
	528	552
	L	YMDD
Lamivudine-resistant mutants	1 ——— M—	——— V ———
	2 ——— M—	——— I
Famciclovir-resistant mutants	M / — V	

Figure 12.15 Amino acid substitutions in lamivudine- and famciclovir-resistant HBV mutants.

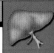

Hepatitis B immune globulin

Initial studies using short-term (i.e. <6 months) HBIG reduced the rate of early reinfection, but many patients became reinfected after cessation of therapy. A retrospective analysis of 372 European patients found a beneficial effect of long-term (i.e. >6 months) HBIG prophylaxis on HBV reinfection and patient survival rates (Figs 12.16a & 12.17a). Multivariate analysis revealed three independent predictors of a lower risk of reinfection: long-term administration of HBIG, HDV superinfection, and acute hepatitis B (Figs 12.16b & 12.17b). Among patients transplanted for HBV-related cirrhosis, the independent predictors of a

lower risk of reinfection were: long-term administration of HBIG, serum HBV DNA, and/or HBeAg-negative before OLT. Although these data support the use of long-term HBIG, HBIG is very expensive and the supply inconsistent. More importantly, significant reduction in the rate of reinfection was only seen in patients who had nonreplicative infection before OLT. In addition, S gene escape mutants have been detected in some reinfected patients. Recent studies suggest that the reinfection rate can be further reduced by maintaining higher anti-HBs titers. While these data are encouraging, the costs would, of course, increase.

Antiviral therapy

Antiviral agents initiated before OLT may prevent graft reinfection by decreasing pre-OLT viral load. Lamivudine and famciclovir have been shown to be well-tolerated in patients with decompensated cirrhosis. Preliminary data suggest that lamivudine alone administered before OLT and continuing after OLT (in the absence of HBIG) can decrease the rate of recurrent hepatitis B. Unfortunately, drug resistant mutants leading to breakthrough infection may occur both before and after OLT. Thus, the

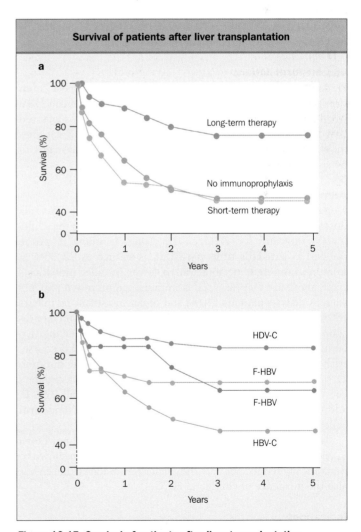

Figure 12.16 Risk of recurrence of HBV infection after liver transplantation. (a) According to duration of HBIG prophylaxis and (b) according to the initial liver disease and pretransplantation viral-replication status. C, cirrhosis; F, fulminant. (Data from Samuel D, et al., 1993.)

Figure 12.17 Survival of patients after liver transplantation. (a) According to duration of HBIG prophylaxis and (b) according to initial liver disease. C, cirrhosis; F, fulminant. (Data from Samuel D, et al., 1993.)

long-term efficacy of antiviral monotherapy in the prevention of recurrent hepatitis B remains to be determined.

Treatment of recurrent hepatitis B

There is currently no established treatment for recurrent hepatitis B after OLT. Interferon therapy is largely ineffective and may be associated with significant side effects such as neutropenia and increased risk of rejection.

Antiviral therapy

Preliminary data indicate that lamivudine and famciclovir are effective in decreasing serum HBV DNA levels and severity of liver disease in patients with recurrent hepatitis B after OLT. Treatment is in general well tolerated. However, these agents have to be administered indefinitely for sustained benefit. Breakthrough infection due to drug-resistant mutants has been reported in 20–25% of patients who have received treatment for one year or more. Thus, the long-term efficacy of antiviral therapy in the treatment of recurrent hepatitis B after OLT remains to be determined.

VACCINATION

Safe and effective hepatitis B vaccines have been available for the prevention of HBV infection in the past 15 years.

Vaccine formulations

Hepatitis B vaccines that are currently available in most countries are genetically engineered and consist of recombinant HBV small S protein (HBsAg) only. Although it has been suggested that incorporation of pre-S antigens into hepatitis B vaccines may increase the immunogenicity, this hypothesis remains to be confirmed.

Administration and efficacy

Hepatitis B vaccine is given intramuscularly, usually in three doses at 0, 1, and 6 months. The dose recommended for adults is 10–20μg and for children 2.5–10μg. Immune response defined as anti-HBs titers >10IU/L is as high as 90–95% in immunocompetent persons, but is lower in older individuals (60% above age 60 years) and in immunocompromised patients such as dialysis patients (40%) and organ transplant recipients (80%). An additional 1–3 doses are recommended for nonresponders. Individuals who fail to respond after receiving two complete courses are unlikely to benefit from a third course. Although the anti-HBs titer decreases with time, the duration of protection is probably life-long, because most responders can mount an amnestic anti-HBs response on rechallenge. In addition, clinical infection is rarely observed during long-term follow-up of responders.

The implementation of universal vaccination of all newborns in endemic areas such as Taiwan and Senegal has been shown to dramatically reduce not only the carrier rate among children but also the incidence of childhood HCC.

Indications

Vaccination is most important for infants, particularly newborns of HBsAg carrier mothers, because of the high risk of progression to chronic infection after perinatal infection. Universal vaccination of all newborns with incorporation of hepatitis B vaccines into the Expanded Program for Immunization in Children is now recommended in most countries. In infants born to carrier mothers, an additional dose of HBIG is administered at birth to provide immediate protection. Catch-up vaccination is also recommended for all children and adolescents who are not previously immunized.

Adults at increased risks of HBV infection such as health care workers, spouses of hepatitis B carriers, patients with chronic liver disease, dialysis patients, male homosexuals, and intravenous drug abusers should also be vaccinated.

Postexposure prophylaxis should consist of the administration of a single dose of HBIG and the simultaneous initiation of a course of vaccination.

Adverse reactions

Adverse reactions are uncommon. Approximately 20% of vaccinees may experience mild reactions at the injection site and a minority may have transient flu-like symptoms.

Vaccine-escape mutant

Mutations in the HBV S gene have been described in infants born to carrier mothers despite adequate anti-HBs response after vaccination. The commonest mutation is a glycine to arginine substitution at codon 145 (G145R) in the 'a' determinant of HBsAg. This mutation has been shown to decrease the binding of HBsAg to anti-HBs, accounting for the breakthrough infection. The exact incidence of this mutant among vaccinees is not clear but is likely to be <5%. There is no evidence to suggest that the efficacy of current vaccines is diminishing. In addition, there is no evidence to suggest that these mutants are transmitted to other family members or the community.

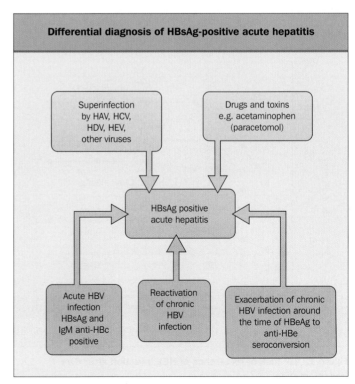

Figure 12.18 Differential diagnosis of HBsAg-positive acute hepatitis. (See Practice Point).

PRACTICE POINT

The diagnosis of acute hepatitis B is based on the detection of HBsAg and anti-HBc-IgM. The differential diagnosis of acute hepatitis in an individual who tests positive for HBsAg should include acute hepatitis B, exacerbations of chronic hepatitis B, and superinfection with other hepatitis viruses such as HCV and HDV (Fig. 12.18). The differentiation of acute hepatitis B from exacerbations of chronic hepatitis B can be difficult because the latter patients may have increased titers of anti-HBc-IgM.

Past HBV infection is diagnosed by the presence of anti-HBs and anti-HBc-IgG. Immunity to HBV infection after vaccination is indicated by the presence of anti-HBs only.

Chronic HBV infection is denoted by the presence of HBsAg for more than 6 months. The evaluation of patients with chronic HBV infection should include tests for virus replication: HBeAg and serum HBV DNA by hybridization assays, and assessment of liver damage by biochemical tests and liver histology. Although PCR assays are more sensitive, the pathogenic significance of minute amounts of HBV DNA that can only be detected by PCR assays is uncertain.

Patients with chronic HBV infection who are positive for HBeAg and serum HBV DNA with elevated ALT levels and chronic hepatitis on biopsy should be considered for antiviral therapy (Fig. 12.19). Response should be monitored by repeat tests for ALT, serum HBV DNA and HBeAg/anti-HBe. Patients who are HBeAg and serum HBV DNA-positive, but have normal ALT levels are unlikely to respond to interferon therapy. The role of new antiviral agents in these patients remains to be determined. Most anti-HBe-positive patients do not require antiviral therapy. Anti-HBe-positive patients who have elevated ALT levels should be tested for serum HBV DNA by hybridization assays to determine if they have active virus replication. In addition, tests for anti-HCV and anti-HDV should be performed to rule out superimposed hepatitis. Anti-HBe-positive patients who remain viremic with active liver disease can be considered for interferon therapy but the rate of sustained response is low. The role of new antiviral agents in these patients is being evaluated.

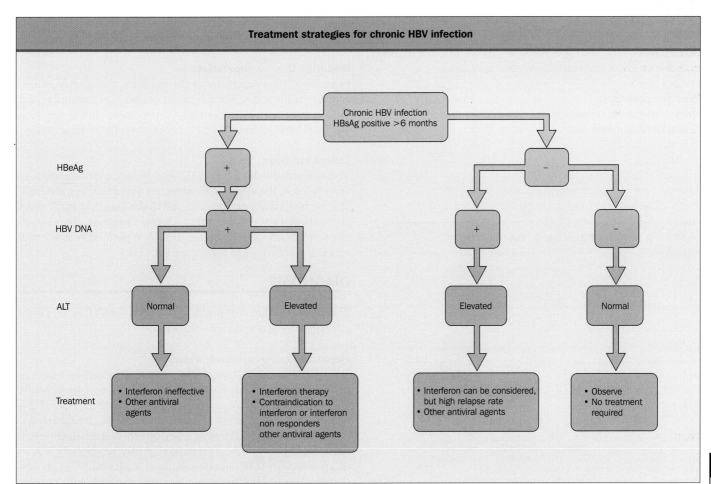

Figure 12.19 Treatment strategy of chronic HBV infection. (See Practice Point.)

HEPATITIS D

INTRODUCTION

Hepatitis D is caused by a defective virus: the hepatitis D virus (HDV). Infection with HDV is closely associated with HBV infection. Although HDV can replicate autonomously, the simultaneous presence of HBV is required for complete virion assembly and secretion. As a result, individuals with hepatitis D are always dually infected with HDV and HBV.

The hepatitis D virion or delta agent comprises a single stranded RNA genome, the hepatitis D antigen (HDAg), and an envelope consisting of HBV envelope proteins (Fig. 12.20).

Hepatitis D virus replicates via its complementary or antigenomic RNA.

EPIDEMIOLOGY

It is estimated that approximately 5% of the HBV carriers worldwide may be infected with HBV. However, the geographic distribution of HDV infection does not parallel that of HBV.

The Mediterranean Basin

Infection with HDV is endemic in these countries. Infection tends to occur early, affecting mainly children and young adults. The main route of transmission is inapparent permucosal or percutaneous spread. Intrafamilial transmission has also been reported.

The Far East

Despite the high prevalence of HBV infection, the prevalence of HDV infection in these countries is, in general, low. Transmission occurs sexually or amongst intravenous drug users.

Western countries

Infection with HDV is uncommon and predominantly confined to intravenous drug users.

Hepatitis D virus virion

HDV RNA → HBsAg

HDAg

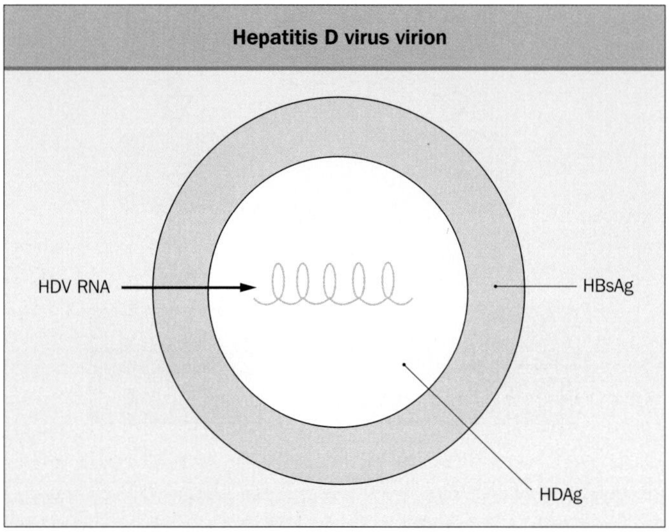

Figure 12.20 Hepatitis D vrus virion. HDAg, hepatitis D antigen.

Outbreaks

Outbreaks of acute hepatitis D with a high incidence of liver failure have been reported among the Yucpa Indians of Venezuela, the Sierra Nevada de Santa Marta in Colombia, some remote areas of the Amazon basin, the Kashmir region, and the Central African Republic.

The incidence of HDV infection has declined in the past 10 years. These changes are most noticable in Italy and are believed to be due to improved socioeconomic conditions, a decrease in high-risk sexual behavior, and vaccination programs against HBV infection.

CLINICAL FEATURES

Due to its dependence on HBV, HDV infection always occurs in association with HBV infection. The clinical manifestations of HDV infection vary from benign acute hepatitis to fulminant hepatitis, and from an asymptomatic carrier state to rapidly progressive chronic liver disease. In most cases of chronic HDV infection, HBV replication is suppressed to very low levels by HDV. Liver damage in these patients is essentially due to HDV only.

Coinfection

Coinfection of HBV and HDV in an individual susceptible to HBV infection results in an acute hepatitis. The clinical picture is indistinguishable from that of classic acute hepatitis B and is usually transient and self-limited. However, a high incidence of acute liver failure has been reported among drug addicts. The rate of progression to chronic HDV infection is not different from that observed after classic acute hepatitis B because persistence of HDV infection is dependent on persistence of HBV infection.

Hepatitis D virus superinfection

Hepatitis D virus superinfection of an HBsAg carrier may present as an unusually severe acute hepatitis in a previously unrecognized HBV carrier or an exacerbation of pre-existing chronic hepatitis B. Progression to chronic HDV infection is almost invariable.

Latent infection

This was initially described in the liver transplantation setting. In this situation, the allograft is reinfected with HDV but not HBV. The antigen HDAg can be detected in the liver, but HDV RNA cannot be detected in the serum. During this phase, there is usually no evidence of liver disease. Infection with HDV is abortive unless the graft is later reinfected with HBV.

DIAGNOSIS

The serum biochemical profiles associated with HDV and HBV infections are given in Figure 12.21.

Hepatitis D virus antibody assays

Total (IgM and IgG) anti-HDV can be detected by enzyme-linked or radioimmune assays. These are the only commercially available tests for HDV infection in many countries. Anti-HDV-IgG appears late in acute hepatitis D. Thus, its clinical value is limited unless repeated testing is performed. Nonetheless, a well-documented anti-HDV seroconversion may be the only way to diagnose acute HDV infection. High-titer anti-HDV-IgG is present in chronic HDV infection. It correlates well with ongoing HDV replication.

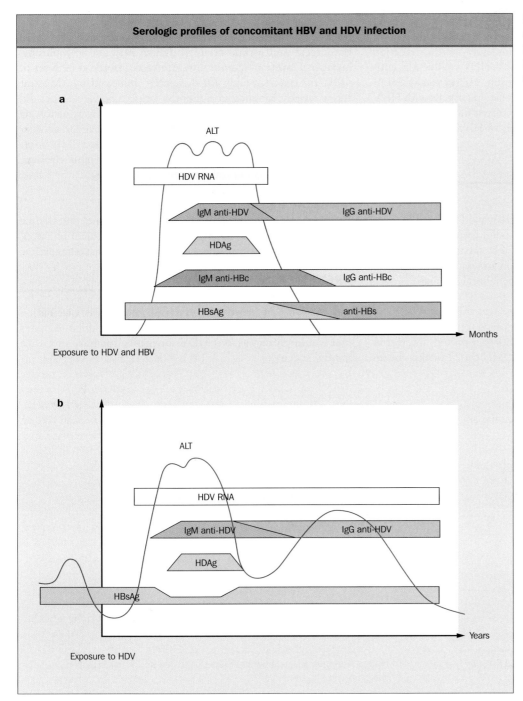

Figure 12.21 Serologic profile of (a) acute HBV and HDV coinfection, and (b) HDV superinfection on chronic HBV infection. HDAg, hepatitis D antigen.

Anti-HDV-IgM is transient and delayed if the course of acute hepatitis D is self-limited. In patients who progress to chronic HDV infection, anti-HDV-IgM is long-lasting and present in high titer. The anti-HDV IgM titer tends to correlate with the level of HDV replication and severity of liver disease.

Detection of serum hepatitis D antigen
In acute HDV infection, serum hepatitis D antigen appears early but is very short-lived and may escape detection if repeated testing is not performed. In chronic HDV infection, hepatitis D antigen may be difficult to detect because of the formation of immune complexes with anti-HDV.

Detection of serum hepatitis D virus RNA
Serum HDV RNA is an early and sensitive marker of HDV infection in acute hepatitis D. In chronic HDV infection, only 70–80% of patients have detectable serum HDV RNA when tested by hybridization assays but most are positive by PCR assays.

Tissue markers of HDV infection
The antigen HDAg can be detected by immunohistochemical staining of liver tissues. The detection of intrahepatic HDAg has been proposed to be the 'gold' standard for the diagnosis of ongoing HDV infection. Hepatic HDV RNA can be detected by *in situ* hybridization.

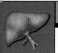

Due to the dependence of HDV on HBV, presence of HBsAg is necessary for the diagnosis of HDV infection. Documentation of the presence of HDV infection relies largely on the detection of anti-HDV. In patients with acute HBV/HDV coinfection, anti-HBc IgM is also present. Tests for serum HDAg and/or HDV RNA should also be performed if available. In patients with HDV superinfection, anti-HDV is usually present in high titers along with serum HDV RNA, while markers of HBV replication may be suppressed.

TREATMENT

Aims
The main goals are to eradicate both HBV and HDV and to ameliorate liver disease. The primary end point is sustained suppression of HDV replication as documented by the undetectability of HDV RNA in serum using hybridization assays and of hepatitis D antigen in the liver using immunohistochemical staining.

Interferon
Interferon-α is at present the only approved treatment of chronic hepatitis D. Based on the limited data reported, interferon needs to be used in high doses up to 9MU thrice weekly for up to one year for optimal results. The overall efficacy is uncertain because of conflicting data from two large controlled studies. In the largest multicenter trial, 61 Italian patients with chronic hepatitis D were randomized to receive interferon-α in doses of $5MU/m^2$ thrice weekly for 4 months, followed by $3MU/m^2$ thrice weekly for another 8 months, or placebo. Treatment did not increase the rate of sustained virus clearance or histologic improvement. More favorable response was achieved in another Italian study in which 50% of patients who received 9MU doses of interferon-α for 48 weeks had biochemical and virologic response as well as improvement in liver histology.

Alternative treatment
Several drugs including ribavirin, suramin, foscarnet and thymic hormones have been evaluated as alternative treatment of chronic hepatitis D. However, the overall results are discouraging.

PREVENTION

The mainstay of prevention of HDV infection is vaccination against its helper virus, HBV. Attempts to produce vaccines that would protect against HDV superinfection have met with limited success.

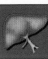

FURTHER READING

Carman WF, Hadziyannis S, McGarvey MJ, et al. Mutation preventing formation of hepatitis B e antigen in patients with chronic hepatitis B infection. Lancet. 1989;ii:588–90. *The first study that reported the detection of premature stop codon in the precore region in patients with HBeAg-negative chronic hepatitis.*

Dienstag JL, Perrillo RP, Schiff ER, et al. A preliminary trial of lamivudine for chronic hepatitis B infection. N Engl J Med. 1995;333:1657–61. *The first report of a randomized double-blind prospective trial demonstrating the efficacy of lamivudine in the treatment of chronic HBV infection.*

Fattovich G, Giustina G, Schalm SE et al. Occurrence of hepatocellular carcinoma and decompensation in western European patients with cirrhosis type B. Hepatology. 1995;21:77–82. *This article reports on the morbidity of 349 European patients with type B cirrhosis.*

Fontana RJ, Lok ASF. Combination therapy for chronic hepatitis B. Hepatology. 1997;26:234–7. *An editorial discussing the new antiviral therapies for chronic HBV infection with particular focus on nucleoside analogs lamivudine and famciclovir and the potential roles and problems of combination therapy.*

Lemon SM, Thomas DL. Vaccines to prevent viral hepatitis. N Engl J Med. 1997;336:196–204. *A comprehensive review of vaccines to viral hepatitis with particular emphasis on HBV and HAV vaccines.*

Lok ASF. Antiviral therapy of the Asian patient with chronic hepatitis B. Semin Liver Dis. 1993;13:360–66. *This review article discusses the mechanisms of immune tolerance in perinatally acquired HBV infection and the role and efficacy of interferon therapy in Asian patients with chronic HBV infection.*

Lok ASF. Natural history and control of perinatally acquired hepatitis B virus infection. Dig Dis. 1992;10:46–52. *This review article compares and contrasts the natural history of perinatally acquired versus adult acquired HBV infection.*

Margolis HS, Alter, MJ, Hadler SC. Hepatitis B: evolving epidemiology and implications for control. Semin Liver Dis. 1991;11:84–92. *A detailed description of worldwide epidemiology and risk factors of HBV infection.*

Perrillo RP, Schiff ER, Davis GL, et al. A randomized, controlled trial of interferon alfa-2b alone and after prednisone withdrawal for the treatment of chronic hepatitis B. N Engl J Med. 1990;323:295–301. *A prospective randomized study comparing the efficacy of interferon plus prednisone withdrawal, interferon alone, and placebo in the treatment of HBeAg-positive chronic HBV infection in the US population.*

Realdi G, Fattovich G, Hadziyannis S, et al. Survival and prognostic factors in 366 patients with compensated cirrhosis type B: a multicenter study. J Hepatol. 1994;21:656–66. *A retrospective study on the database of European Concerted Action on Viral Hepatitis (EUROHEP) project to assess the survival of compensated HBV cirrhosis, primarily in relation to HBV replication and HDV infection, as well as to analyze the prognostic factors for survival.*

Samuel D, Muller R, Alexander G, et al. Liver transplantation in European patients with the hepatitis B surface antigen. N Engl J Med. 1993;329:1842–7. *A retrospective study in 17 European transplant centers to assess the factors associated with HBV recurrence and survival after transplantation. The results showed that long-term HBIG prophylaxis resulted in a significant decrease in rate of recurrent HBV infection.*

Scalioni PP, Melegari M, Wands JR. Recent advances in the molecular biology of hepatitis B virus. Bailliere's Clin Gastroenterol. 1996;10:207–25. *A review of the replication cycle of HBV infection and mechanisms that regulate HBV replication.*

Smedile A, Rizzetto M, Gerin JL. Advances in hepatitis D virus biology and disease. Prog Liver Dis. 1994;12:157–75. *Comprehensive review of the biology of HDV and epidemiology, clinical manifestations and treatment of hepatitis D.*

Thomas HC, Carman WF. Envelope and precore/core variants of hepatitis B virus. Gastroenterol Clin North Am. 1994;23:499–513. *A review article discussing the common genomic variants/mutants of HBV and their implications in clinical practice.*

Wong DKH, Cheung AM, O'Rourke K, et al. Effect of alpha-interferon treatment in patients with hepatitis B e antigen-positive chronic hepatitis B. A meta-analysis. Ann Intern Med. 1993;119:312–23. *A meta-analysis of 15 randomized controlled studies of interferon-α therapy in the treatment of HBeAg-positive chronic hepatitis B.*

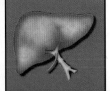

Section 3 Specific Diseases of the Liver

Chapter 13 Hepatitis C and G

George Webster, Simon Whalley, Eleanor Barnes and Geoffrey Dusheiko

HEPATITIS C

INTRODUCTION

Hepatitis C is now recognized as a major public health problem worldwide. The current prevalence is a result of several factors, including the previous inability to diagnose non-A, non-B hepatitis, environmental factors such as lifestyle, in particular injecting drug use, or the use of unsterilized equipment in developing countries, and the high rate of chronic infection that ensues after initial infection. An estimated 150 million people are affected worldwide, with a disease spectrum ranging from mild to severe chronic hepatitis, cirrhosis, and hepatocellular carcinoma. The disease is complex and predictions about long-term prognosis for individual patients remain difficult. There is promise that a proportion of patients who have a sustained response to antiviral therapy with inhibition of viral replication will not develop progressive liver disease. The indications for treatment are currently not exact because the disease appears to progress at variable rates.

The development of specific serologic tests for the diagnosis of hepatitis C, and the considerable research progress that has been made in the past decade, have rapidly enhanced our understanding of this disease and led to improved treatment and prevention.

PATHOGENESIS

The hepatitis C virus
Viral structure
Hepatitis C virus (HCV) is a member of the Flaviviridae family. This family comprises three genera: Flaviviruses, Pestiviruses, and the Hepaciviruses. The latter genus includes a heterogeneous group of RNA viruses known collectively as HCV. Hepatitis C virus is an enveloped virus, and is approximately 50nm in size. The viral genomic RNA is a 9379 nucleotide single-stranded plus sense RNA with a single long open reading frame (Fig. 13.1). The gene product is a viral polyprotein precursor of 3010–3030 amino acids, which undergoes proteolytic post-translational cleavage. The structural proteins are derived from the 5′ end of the genome and the nonstructural proteins from the 3′ end.

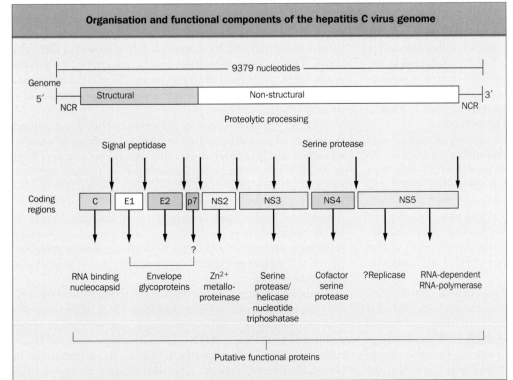

Figure 13.1 Organization and functional components of the hepatitis C virus genome. NCR, noncoding region.

Hepatitis C virus contains several structural proteins, including a basic RNA binding capsid protein, which is membrane-associated but also has a nuclear localized form. E1 and E2 (gp35 and gp70) are putative virion glycoproteins, which may be targets for neutralizing antibodies. These proteins contain hypervariable regions.

Several nonstructural proteins have been identified, which may be important for viral replication. They include a putative NS3 serine protease, RNA helicase, and a NS5a RNA-dependent RNA polymerase. The NS4A polypeptide may function as a cofactor for NS3-mediated cleavage at the 4B/5A site in this reaction.

There are noncoded regions at both the 5′ and 3′ ends of the genome. The 5′ noncoding region of HCV comprises multiple short open reading frames. Experimental evidence indicates the presence of an internal ribosomal entry site within the 5′ noncoding region. Conserved helical structures may also be critical motifs.

Viral heterogeneity, genotypes, and nomenclature

Sequence differences of up to 32% have been found between complete genetic sequences of the most divergent variants of HCV. Sequence variability is found distributed throughout all genes encoded by the genome. The nucleotide and amino acid sequence of the nucleocapsid protein is highly conserved, but there is greater than expected variability of certain regions of the envelope genes. Within the 5′ end there is an untranslated region of at least 341 base pairs that is highly conserved among the isolates sequenced to date. The 3′ end is also highly conserved. The conserved RNA elements favor the possibility that translation control is located in this region.

Provisional classifications of HCV have depended on nucleotide comparisons of complete genomes or subgenomic fragments between variants found in different individuals. The variability of HCV has suggested a two layered classification. This nomenclature, using 'genotypes' that correspond to the major branches of a phylogenetic tree of sequences of genomic or subgenomic regions, and 'subtypes' that correspond to the more closely related sequences within some of the major groups has been widely adopted. The known genotypes have been designated by Arabic numerals from type 1 and the subtypes by letters a, b and c in order of discovery. The current system of nomenclature includes six major genotypes and more than 80 different subtypes. The provisionally named genotypes 7, 8 and 9 are likely to be divergent subtypes of genotype 6.

There may be differences in disease severity associated with different genotypes, but this has been difficult to prove. An inherently greater pathogenicity of type 1 HCV has been implied in patients with cirrhosis, but these data have to be viewed against a background of predominant type 1 infection in older patients in several countries. It is important to point out that severe and progressive liver disease has been found in association with each of the well-characterized genotypes, so that there is little evidence that any variants of HCV are completely nonpathogenic.

Within an individual patient HCV may exist as quasispecies. Clones derived from single patients can show a high degree of sequence heterogeneity when multiple genomes are cloned from the same patient. Sequence changes tend to cluster in the hypervariable regions, but high rates of sequence change have been observed in several parts of the genome as well as the envelope glycoproteins. The mechanisms operating to drive these changes and their clinical or immunologic significance are not well understood.

Pathogenetic mechanisms

Hepatitis C virus is thought to be a noncytopathic virus and liver damage is probably immune mediated. It is not clear why some patients develop mild and stable liver disease while others develop a severe and progressive disease leading to cirrhosis and liver failure. The vast majority of infected individuals develop persistent infection, suggesting that the immune system, while causing liver damage, is unable to mediate viral clearance. The mechanisms of viral persistence and disease pathogenesis are poorly understood but appear to be the result of a complex interaction between the host immune system and the virus.

The ability of HCV to evade the immune response of an infected individual, using the strategy of genetic variation, may be an important mechanism of viral persistence. The viral polymerase has the propensity to introduce random mutations at each replicative cycle, generating continuous variants. The selective force of the humoral and cellular immune response may allow for the emergence of variants that are poorly recognized by the host immune system. It has been suggested that continuous genetic changes in the hypervariable regions of the envelope glycoproteins, which lie on the outside of the virus, may mediate immune escape. This theory does not explain why the immune system appears unable to recognize those areas that are more conserved.

One of the most effective clearance mechanisms against viral infections is the generation of neutralizing antibodies. Evidence that neutralizing antibodies may develop in chronic HCV infection was obtained using the chimpanzee as an experimental model, in which antibodies against both structural and nonstructural HCV proteins can be demonstrated. However, the effectiveness of these antibodies appears to be strain (quasispecies) limited – both chimpanzees and humans may be reinfected several times with different HCV strains and develop a hepatitis each time. Moreover the risk of developing chronic disease is not reduced by a previous infection with a different strain. The presence of multiple quasispecies in HCV infection is a possible mechanism of viral evasion of neutralizing antibodies and presents a critical obstacle to the development of a broadly reactive vaccine.

T-helper (CD4) lymphocyte responses to both structural and nonstructural proteins can often be detected in chronically infected individuals. It has been shown that patients who recover from acute HCV infection develop a more vigorous T-helper response to HCV antigens than those patients who develop chronic disease. It has also been suggested that a stronger T-helper response is associated with a more benign course of infection. Finally, T-helper responsiveness has been associated with viral clearance resulting from interferon therapy. Collectively these studies suggest that T-helper responses are important in HCV clearance and pathogenesis.

Cytotoxic T lymphocytes (CTLs) are thought to be particularly important in viral pathogenesis (Fig. 13.2). They recognize viral antigens on cell surfaces in conjunction with major histocompatibility complex (MHC) class I and lyse infected target cells. Hepatitis C virus-specific CTLs can be demonstrated in chronically infected patients, after stimulation with virus-derived

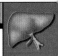
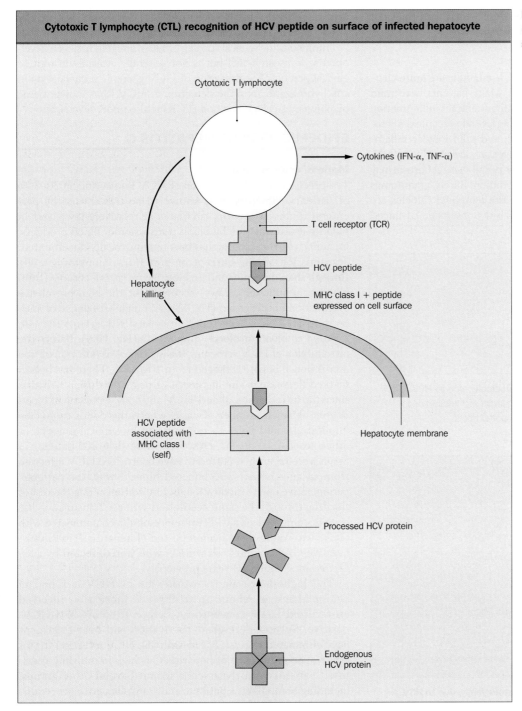

Cytotoxic T lymphocyte (CTL) recognition of HCV peptide on surface of infected hepatocyte

Cytotoxic T lymphocyte

Cytokines (IFN-α, TNF-α)

T cell receptor (TCR)

HCV peptide

MHC class I + peptide expressed on cell surface

Hepatocyte killing

HCV peptide associated with MHC class I (self)

Hepatocyte membrane

Processed HCV protein

Endogenous HCV protein

Figure 13.2 Cytotoxic T-lymphocyte (CTL) recognition of HCV peptide on surface of infected hepatocyte.

peptides, suggesting that, although present, the CTL response cannot clear the virus. It is possible, again, that HCV escapes CTL detection by mutation. However, the HCV CTL response is multispecific (i.e. there is more than one target for the CTL) so that the loss of a single epitope would not provide a method of escape unless that epitope was also immunodominant. To date, no specific HCV peptide has been shown to be dominant for CTL responses.

The CTLs have also been shown to suppress viral replication of certain viruses (e.g. hepatitis B virus) by a noncytolytic pathway through the production of antiviral cytokines such as interferon-γ and tumor necrosis factor-α. Direct analysis of the

susceptibility of HCV to these cytokines must await the development of *in vitro* models of replication.

Most of the studies on HCV infection and cellular immunity have been performed on peripheral blood lymphocytes. In HCV infection cellular immune responses may be compartmentalized to the liver. Intrahepatic HCV-specific CTLs and T helper cells have been reported in increased frequency, when compared with lymphocytes from peripheral blood, and further study of intrahepatic T cells is required.

Other persistent viruses have been shown to evade immune detection by direct interference with antiviral immune responses (e.g. downregulation of MHC or costimulatory molecules) or

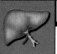

by infection of immune-privileged sites. Thus far, HCV has not been shown to adopt any of these strategies.

Liver pathology

The pathologic features of chronic HCV infection are quite characteristic, albeit not pathognomonic. Many patients have mild hepatitis histologically (Fig. 13.3), with portal tract inflammation with lymphoid aggregates, and mild periportal piecemeal necrosis. Parenchymal steatosis, apoptosis, and mild lobular inflammation may be present. In later stages of disease (Fig. 13.4), portal fibrosis, portal-portal fibrosis, or portal-central fibrosis may be present. Bridging necrosis is not common. Rarely, granulomas can be observed. Although many of the lymphoid follicles are associated with bile ducts, ductopenia is not observed. Advanced

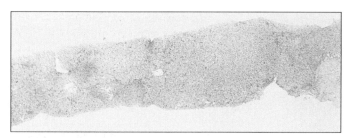

Figure 13.3 Mild chronic hepatitis histologically, due to HCV. A low power view of a core of liver tissue, showing intact architecture and minimal chronic inflammation discernible in portal tracts.

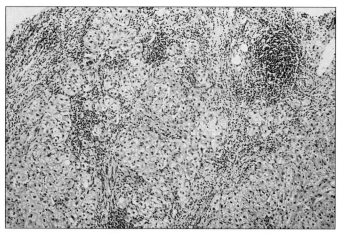

Figure 13.4 Severe chronic hepatitis histologically, due to HCV. A medium-power view showing advanced stage hepatitis, with marked fibrosis and a nodule centrally. Numerous portoseptal lymphoid aggregates are evident, and there is widespread interface and parenchymal inflammation.

disease, with cirrhosis or hepatocellular carcinoma, is generally not associated with features specific to HCV.

Immunohistochemical staining of HCV antigens has been developed as a research tool but is not generally available in routine clinical practice. Identification of HCV genomic sequences by *in situ* hybridization and the detection of HCV RNA in liver tissue by polymerase chain reaction (PCR) is also under investigation.

EPIDEMIOLOGY OF HEPATITIS C

Mode of transmission

The precise mode of acquisition of HCV is uncertain in 20–30% of patients. However, it is known to be transmitted by parenteral routes. The virus circulates at relatively low titers in blood but transmission by blood transfusion or blood products, including clotting factors, has been unequivocally documented. Transmission among current or past intravenous drug users through shared needles and possibly via intranasal cocaine (from blood contaminated straws) accounts for the high prevalence of infection in this group (Fig. 13.5). A high prevalence of antibody to HCV has been found in several risk groups that are exposed to blood or blood components (Fig. 13.6). Before the introduction of HCV screening the incidence of post transfusion non-A non-B hepatitis ranged from 1 to 19%. There has been a marked decrease in the incidence of post-transfusion hepatitis since the introduction of anti-HCV antibody screening of blood donors. A small number of cases where the donor cannot be implicated could point to transmission by surgical practice or other nosocomial means. However, more than 200 patients in Spain were recently reported to have contracted HCV infection from an anesthetist, who injected himself with the patients' perioperative opiate medication, before administering the rest of the drug through the same needle and syringe. Transmission has been documented via anti-D immunoglobulin contaminated with HCV. Two studies have been reported of hepatitis C in Rhesus-negative German and Irish women who were infected by anti-D immunoglobulin 20 years previously.

The highest prevalence worldwide of HCV is found in hemophiliacs, in whom up to 90% of those who received unsterilized factor-concentrates before 1985 are anti-HCV-positive. Solvent detergent inactivation and heat treatment have eliminated the risk of transmitting HCV infection to this group. The prevalence of hepatitis C is high in multiply transfused patients with thalassemia major. Several other groups, including hemodialysis patients and transplant patients requiring frequent blood transfusions, have a higher prevalence of anti-HCV antibody. Health care workers appear to be at relatively low risk.

Means of transmission of HCV.
Transfusion of blood or blood products
Intravenous drug use
Organ transplantation from infected donor
Intranasal cocaine use
Tattooing
Use of unsterilized equipment
Sexual contact
Mother to fetus/infant

Figure 13.5 Means of transmission of HCV.

High-risk groups for HCV infection
Hemophiliac patients
Thalassemia patients
Hemodialysis patients
Transplant recipients
Alcoholics
History of major surgery and transfusion
Intravenous drug users
Persons with multiple sexual partners

Figure 13.6 High-risk groups for HCV infection.

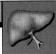

The disease is prevalent in many parts of the world where transmission is probably not caused by blood transfusion or intravenous drug use. Transmission by tattooing, or surgical and medical procedures involving skin-piercing procedures has been reported.

Sexual transmission has been described, but is a relatively inefficient and infrequent route of infection. In the absence of barrier contraception, only 5–10% of regular sexual partners of infected patients are found to be infected. Hepatitis C virus appears much less transmissible sexually than either HIV or hepatitis B virus. However, the overall HCV infection rate is higher in sexually promiscuous groups. Transmission by saliva or saliva containing blood and by a human bite has been reported. Intrafamilial transmission is infrequent. Mother-to-infant transmission has been documented, but occurs in less than 6% of cases. Differences in the rate of maternal infant transmission in different countries remain unexplained. Mother-to-infant transmission rates are higher in patients with higher levels of viremia (greater than 10^7 particles/mL) and in those with HIV infection (up to 36% of cases). The risk of transmission to infants appears virtually zero if the mother is HCV RNA-negative by PCR. It is not clear how important this route is in perpetuating the reservoir of human infection. Although HCV RNA has been found in breast milk, infection of infants by breast-feeding has not been reported.

In several countries a higher prevalence of anti-HCV has been found in patients with alcohol-related liver disease. The prevalence of HCV antibodies correlates with the severity of liver injury and is higher in alcoholic patients with cirrhosis than in those with only fatty change. Human immunodeficiency virus may coexist with HCV, particularly in at-risk groups, such as hemophiliacs and intravenous drug users. The combination may cause aggravated liver disease.

Geographic distribution

The global prevalence of chronic HCV infection is estimated to be 3%, with 4 million HCV carriers in USA, and 5 million in Western Europe. The prevalence of HCV in blood donors has been ascertained in many countries (Fig. 13.7). In the USA 0.5% of blood donors are anti-HCV-positive, but 1.8% of the population are positive on random testing. A higher prevalence has been found in Africa; treatment of schistosomiasis, using unsterilized needles, is considered to be a likely factor in the high prevalence of the disease in Egypt, where up to 15% of the population are anti-HCV-positive.

The geographic distribution of hepatitis C genotypes has been mapped (Fig. 13.8). Blood donors and patients with chronic HCV infection from countries in Western Europe and the USA show frequent infection with genotypes 1a, 1b, 2a, 2b, and 3a, but the frequency of each may vary. There is a trend towards more frequent infection with type 1b in Southern and Eastern Europe. Types 1a and 3a are more common in intravenous drug users in Europe. In the Middle East and parts of north and central Africa, genotype 4a is highly prevalent. Approximately 50% of anti-HCV-positive blood donors in South Africa are infected with type 5a. Type 6a was originally found in Hong Kong.

CLINICAL FEATURES AND NATURAL HISTORY

Acute hepatitis C

Fewer than 15% of patients appear to have an acute icteric hepatitis after infection, although HCV is said to account for about 20% of cases of acute hepatitis in developed countries. The mean incubation period of HCV is 6–12 weeks, but this may be reduced after infection by a large inoculum. The acute course is

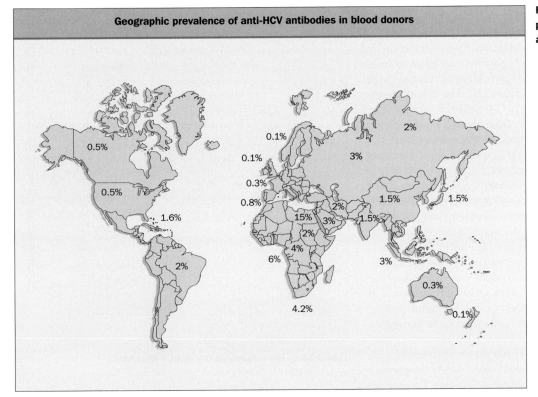

Geographic prevalence of anti-HCV antibodies in blood donors

Figure 13.7 Geographic prevalence of anti-HCV antibodies in blood donors.

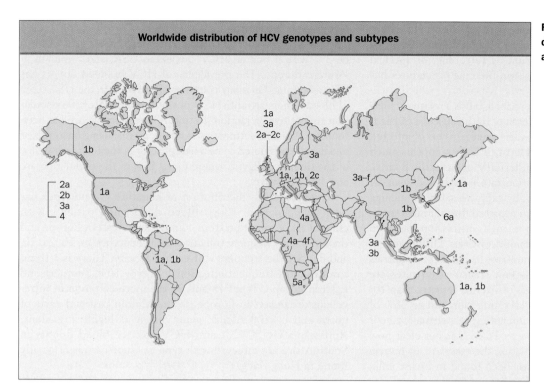

Figure 13.8 Worldwide distribution of HCV genotypes and subtypes.

generally mild and the peak serum alanine aminotransferase (ALT) is less than that typically encountered in type A or B acute hepatitis. Subclinical disease is common and many patients may first present decades later with sequelae of HCV infection such as cirrhosis, without recalling an episode of acute icteric hepatitis. Fulminant hepatitis is a very rare outcome of HCV infection but has been reported in patients when withdrawn from immunosuppression, and in patients superinfected with hepatitis A virus.

Chronic hepatitis C

Both transfusion associated and sporadic hepatitis C have a propensity to progress to chronic infection. Approximately 85% of patients with post-transfusion hepatitis C continue to have abnormal serum aminotransferase levels after 12 months, with chronic hepatitis on liver biopsy (Fig. 13.9). The risk of chronic infection after sporadic hepatitis C is probably similar. The spectrum of clinical disease varies considerably. Most patients with chronic hepatitis C are only mildly symptomatic until the advanced stages of the disease. Fatigue is the most common complaint, but several other relatively nonspecific and minor complaints such as arthralgia are reported. In the early stages of the disease there may be no abnormal physical signs. With the development of cirrhosis, progressive problems may develop, such as weakness, wasting, edema, ascites, and variceal bleeding. Older patients may present for the first time with complications of cirrhosis or hepatocellular carcinoma (HCC). Serum aminotransferases decline from the peak values encountered in the acute phase of the disease, but characteristically remain 2–8 times normal. In patients with chronic viremia the serum aminotransferases may fluctuate over time and may even be normal for prolonged periods.

Progression of disease in individuals may be extremely variable. Many patients have an indolent, only slowly progressive course with little increase in mortality over 20 years. The disease

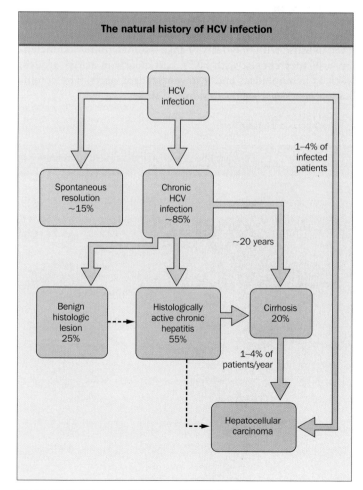

Figure 13.9 The natural history of HCV infection.

is not necessarily benign, however, and rapidly progressive cirrhosis can occur. Up to 30% may develop cirrhosis within 20–30 years. Viral and host factors may be associated with more severe histologic disease (Fig. 13.10). Despite the indolent and slowly progressive nature of the disease, it is apparent from serologic testing for anti-HCV that hepatitis C is a leading cause of morbidity from liver disease in the Western world.

There is a high prevalence of anti-HCV antibodies in patients with HCC. Several controlled studies in Europe have suggested that up to 70% of male patients with HCC are anti-HCV antibody-positive. Unlike hepatitis B, HCC in hepatitis C is extremely unusual in the absence of cirrhosis. However, once cirrhosis is established HCC develops in 1–4% of patients per year.

Extrahepatic disease associations of hepatitis C
A range of extrahepatic conditions have been associated with chronic hepatitis C, but a causative role for some of these conditions is stronger than for others (Fig. 13.11). Of patients with chronic hepatitis C, 36–45% have cryoglobulins in the serum, but less than 10% of these develop the vasculitic syndrome of essen-tial mixed cryoglobulinemia, including a purpuric rash (Fig. 13.12), weakness, arthralgia, and neuropathy. Porphyria cutanea tarda is characterized by the appearance of skin fragility and vesicular rash in sun exposed areas, especially over the back of the hands (Fig. 13.13). Studies have shown marked variations (8–91%) in the frequency of anti-HCV antibodies in this condition. Other associated skin conditions include lichen planus (Figs 13.14 & 13.15). The frequency of HCV in patients with membranoproliferative glomerulonephritis appears high, especially in those with associated cryoglobulinemia.

DIAGNOSIS OF HCV

Hepatitis C virus antibodies
The first diagnostic tests for hepatitis C infection were based on detection of antibodies to expressed proteins of HCV. Most of the initial seroepidemiologic and diagnostic studies of HCV were based on the prevalence of antibodies to c100-3. Current enzyme-linked immunosorbent assays (ELISAs) for antibody to hepatitis C are based on detection of antibody to additional translation products of HCV genes (Fig. 13.16). More recently other antigens have been expressed in yeast or *Escherichia coli*, including the 22kDA core protein of HCV and a second series of nonstructural antigens including c33 and c200 from the NS3, NS4, and NS5a regions. These antigens are included in second- and third-generation solid phase

---

Figure 13.10 Factors associated with increased severity of chronic HCV infection.

Factors associated with increased severity of chronic HCV infection
Host factors
Older patient at time of infection
Long duration of infection
Male sex
Alcohol excess
High liver iron content
Viral factors
High viral load
Quasispecies diversity
Hepatitis B virus/HIV coinfection
? Genotype 1

Figure 13.11 Extrahepatic conditions associated with chronic HCV infection. *Good evidence for causative link with HCV.

Extrahepatic conditions associated with chronic HCV infection
Essential mixed cryoglobulinaemia*
Porphyrea cutanea tarda*
Membranoproliferative glomerulonephritis*
Autoimmune thyroiditis
Sicca syndrome
Idiopathic pulmonary fibrosis
Lichen planus
Focal lymphocytic sialadenitis
B cell lymphoma

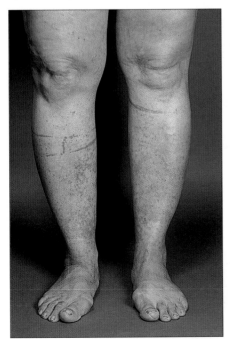

Figure 13.12 Purpuric rash on lower limbs of a patient with essential mixed cryoglobulinemia associated with chronic HCV.

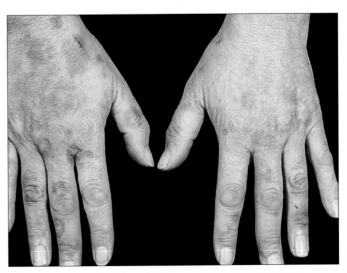

Figure 13.13 Rash of porphyrea cutanea tarda in patient with chronic HCV.

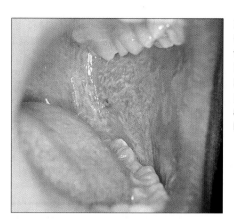

Figure 13.14 Characteristic lacy-white appearance of lichen planus in the buccal cavity (Wickham's striae) in a patient with hepatitis C virus.

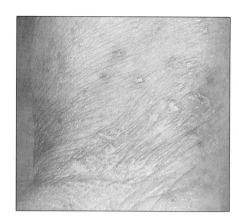

Figure 13.15 Flat-topped, violaceous lesions of lichen planus, in the classic site on the front of the wrist.

ELISAs for antibodies to HCV, which considerably improve the sensitivity of diagnosis. The majority of patients with chronic hepatitis C are anti-c22-positive, indicating a strong anticapsid response.

More recent assays indicate that anti-E2 antibodies are present in the majority of viremic carriers. It is likely that antibodies to the envelope glycoproteins are neutralizing. Immunoglobulin M antibody tests have been developed, but there are no antibody patterns that differentiate persistent viremia from an episode of resolved viremia. The presence of HCV RNA in the absence of anti-HCV antibodies may reflect the lack of immune activity, particularly in immunosuppressed and hemodialyzed patients. A test for HCV core antigen has been developed but the assay remains a research tool. Hepatitis C virus circulates in unconcentrated serum at a concentration that is below the level of detection of antigen by standard immunoassays.

False-positive anti-HCV antibodies have been observed in patients with autoimmune chronic hepatitis. A proportion of patients with chronic hepatitis C have circulating autoantibodies, or have chronic disease with autoimmune features that, of note, can be exacerbated by interferon-α treatment. Up to 50% of patients with type 2 autoimmune hepatitis (anti-LKM1 antibody-positive individuals) are anti-HCV antibody-positive.

Supplemental antibody tests
Early surveys of antibody to HCV in blood donors indicated a high rate of false-positive ELISA assays. This necessitated the development of supplemental assays to confirm a positive test. The most widely used assays are recombinant immunoblot assays (RIBAs), in which four HCV antigens are fixed to a nitrocellulose filter, or a matrix assay, in which HCV antigens are fixed in a matrix pattern along with control proteins. There is a good correlation between RIBA or matrix positive samples and viremia, which can facilitate discrimination between infective and noninfective donors. Although important for confirming the speci-

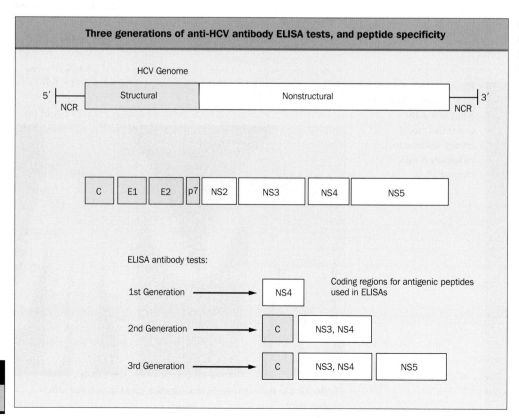

Figure 13.16 Three generations of anti-HCV antibody ELISA tests, and peptide specificity. NCR, noncoding region.

ficity of an anti-HCV test in blood donors, confirmatory tests are almost universally positive in anti-HCV-positive patients with chronic hepatitis and liver disease.

Hepatitis C virus RNA testing

Antibody tests for HCV may confirm exposure to the virus, but cannot distinguish resolved from ongoing infection. Commercial tests are now available that allow the detection of virus in the serum, using qualitative methods, and quantitation of viral concentration. Antigens of HCV are present in very low titers and therefore direct tests for viremia in HCV rely on detection of HCV RNA in serum. Detection of RNA necessitates an amplification of the circulating RNA. Sensitive quantitative assays have been developed based on the PCR. Polymerase chain reaction primers for the 5′-noncoding region are superior to those from NS3 and core, because of the relative conservation of this region.

Improved methods of quantitating HCV RNA are now available, including limiting dilution assays and competitive PCR. One commercially available method uses oligonucleotide probes that are complementary to the 5′-untranslated region and core region to capture HCV RNA, and then branched oligonucleotides subsequently to amplify the signal. The detection limit of this assay is 200,000 copies per milliliter. Recent versions of the branched DNA (bDNA) assay measure genotypes 1–6 with equal efficiency. Other quantitative methods have been utilized and may quantitate HCV to levels of 100 copies per milliliter.

Serologic diagnosis of hepatitis C virus infection

Although approximately one third of seroconversions take place in the acute phase of the disease, sometimes as early as 2 weeks after exposure to HCV, seroconversion can be delayed. The average time from transfusion to seroconversion is of the order of 7–8 weeks with second- and third-generation tests. In some cases with acute self-limiting infection seroconversion may not occur, or antibody titers may wane to undetectable levels. During the early phase of primary HCV infection serum HCV RNA is the only diagnostic marker of infection and RNA testing therefore remains the only means of diagnosis. Serum HCV RNA has been detected within 1–3 weeks of transfusion in patients with hepatitis C.

Hepatitis C virus RNA is usually detectable in patients with abnormal serum aminotransferases and positive anti-HCV antibodies. However HCV RNA can also be found in patients with normal serum aminotransferases. The presence of HCV RNA should be confirmed by PCR in all patients before commencement of antiviral therapy.

Genotyping

Knowledge of HCV genotype is not required for diagnosis, but it is now a useful parameter in the assessment of patients before consideration of treatment. Recent data from trials of combination therapy have shown that different treatment regimens are appropriate for patients with genotype 1 and non-genotype 1 HCV infections.

Several methods of genotyping have been utilized to group isolates of HCV. The most widely used methods are based on restriction fragment length polymorphism, reverse hybridization, type specific PCR, hybridization to type specific oligonucleotides, specific probes, or sequencing. Antibody typing assays have also been used, employing peptides derived from the NS4 region.

Liver biopsy

There is a poor correlation between the extent of histologic disease and either serum ALT or viral load, in patients with chronic hepatitis C virus. Liver biopsy therefore remains a central investigation in the assessment of patients who are being considered for antiviral therapy. It allows the degree of inflammation (grade), and amount of fibrosis (stage) to be determined, and the presence or absence of cirrhosis to be established. Liver biopsy may not be mandatory for patients with persistently normal serum ALT, although 20% of these may have demonstrable histologic disease.

MANAGEMENT

Screening for hepatitis C

The European Association for the Study of the Liver (EASL) International Consensus Conference on Hepatitis C in 1999, concluded that general population screening was not indicated, but should be limited to the following groups:

- persons who may have received blood products prior to 1991;
- hemophiliacs;
- hemodialysis patients;
- children of mothers who have hepatitis C;
- patients with a history of intravenous drug use; and
- organ or tissue donors.

Acute hepatitis C

The serum aminotransferases should be measured periodically in patients with acute hepatitis C together with HCV RNA. At this stage, the determination of true convalescence can be difficult, as some patients may develop normal serum aminotransferases but remain HCV RNA-positive, or may have intermittent viremia. Therapeutic trials of interferon-α for acute hepatitis C have suggested that treatment of the acute disease might lessen the risk of ensuing chronic hepatitis. Thus, if a diagnosis can be made and the patient does not appear to be convalescing 2–4 months after the onset of the infection, interferon-α can be considered at a dose of 3–6 million units three times weekly for at least 6 months. Trials of combination antiviral therapy have not been performed, but if treatment for acute hepatitis C is considered, extrapolation of the impaired response rates for combination therapy in chronic disease to the acute disease favour the use of a combination regimen.

Chronic hepatitis C

Asymptomatic patients identified through blood screening will require a supplemental test to verify that they are anti-HCV antibody-positive, but this is rarely required in a patient with a raised ALT and risk factors for infection. Qualitative PCR for HCV RNA should be performed in all patients, as it may guide further management (Fig. 13.17). If negative, the test may need to be repeated to exclude intermittent viremia at a low level of viral replication. Serum aminotransferases, bilirubin, alkaline phosphatase, albumin, full blood count, and prothrombin time should be measured. Autoantibodies (antinuclear, anti-smooth muscle, anti-LKM1, antimitochondrial, and anti-thyroid antibodies) and thyroid function tests should be performed. Also, in patients whose lifestyle or geographic origin suggest that they are at risk of other forms of viral hepatitis, hepatitis B virus and HIV infection need to be considered.

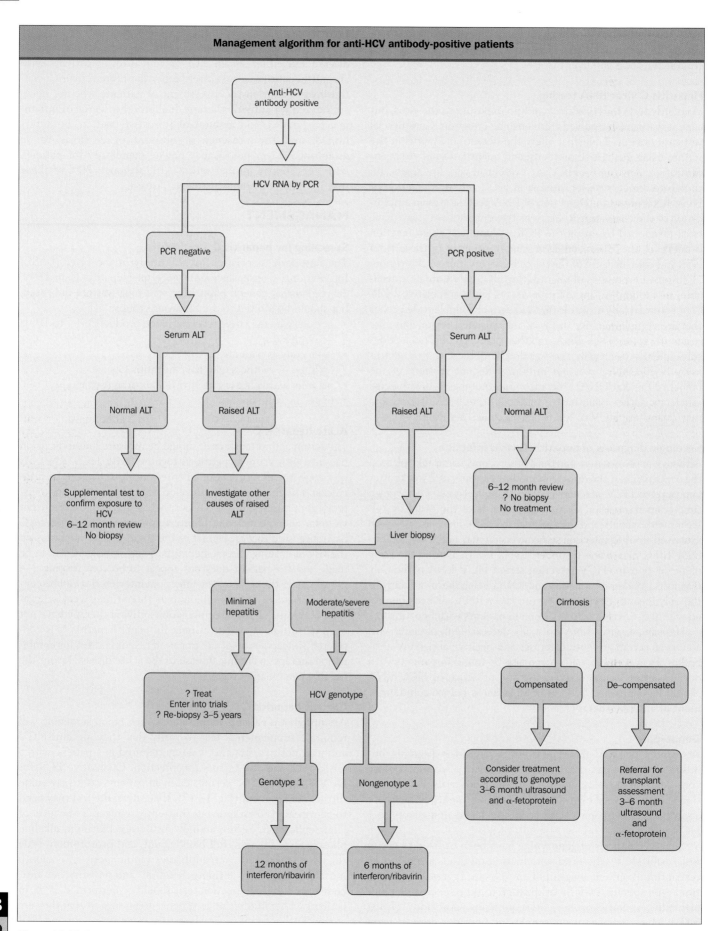

Figure 13.17 Management algorithm for anti-HCV antibody-positive patients.

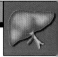
Other causes of chronic hepatitis or diseases of the biliary tract need to be excluded. It is particularly advisable to exclude autoimmune hepatitis as this disease is treated differently. The patient's HCV genotype should be determined, as this determines the appropriate treatment regimen, and allows the patient to be given information regarding likely response to therapy.

A liver biopsy to ascertain the grade and stage of disease should be considered in all patients with established viremia and raised aminotransferases. Individuals with HCV who have elevated ALT and chronic hepatitis histologically should be considered for antiviral therapy. Irrespective of treatment, patients with biopsy-proven cirrhosis should ideally have 3–6 monthly liver ultrasound and α-fetoprotein measurements, in view of the risk of HCC.

ANTIVIRAL TREATMENT

The patient groups appropriate for treatment, and the optimal treatment regimens, are still being established. The US National Institutes of Health consensus document on hepatitis C management concluded that 'treatment is recommended for the group of patients with chronic hepatitis C who are at the greatest risk for progression to cirrhosis'. These patients are characterized by 'persistently elevated ALT, positive HCV RNA, and a liver biopsy with either portal or bridging fibrosis and at least moderate degrees of inflammation and necrosis'. Indications for therapy are less obvious in other groups of patients, including those with less severe histologic changes, (e.g. no fibrosis and minimal necroinflammatory changes). In these patients, progression to cirrhosis is likely to be slow and observation and serial measurements of serum aminotransferases 6 monthly, and liver biopsy every 3–5 years may be an acceptable alternative, unless we learn that responsiveness becomes progressively reduced by delaying treatment. Treatment trials of patients with mild hepatitis due to HCV are underway. The recent EASL International Consensus Conference on Hepatitis C concluded that patients with normal ALT, even if HCV RNA-positive, generally have mild disease, and so should not be routinely treated. In some cases, treatment of patients with persistently normal ALT can be associated with serum ALT abnormalities after treatment.

Definition and time-points of treatment response
It has become conventional to define response to treatment as normalization of ALT (biochemical response) or the development of negative HCV RNA by PCR (virologic response). Virologic response is the best correlate of cleared infection in response to treatment. Although the response during treatment may be categorized ('no response', 'partial response', 'breakthrough', 'complete response'), it is most useful to characterize the long-term response as end of treatment response (ETR), sustained response (SR), or relapse. Sustained response is usually defined as both a biochemical and virologic response 6 months after stopping therapy. Early clearance of virus predicts sustained response, particularly to interferon-α monotherapy. Therefore, patients who do not show a biochemical and virologic response after 3 months of monotherapy should have the course of treatment discontinued. Interestingly, this may not apply to those receiving interferon-α/ribavirin combination treatment, in whom up to 30% of patients who are HCV RNA-positive at 3 months of treatment have been shown to become RNA-negative on continued treatment. However, this may reflect the increasing sensitivity of HCV RNA detection.

Patients who respond usually exhibit histologic improvement. The reduction in histology activity index score in responders is greater than in nonresponders, although histologic improvement has been observed in biochemical nonresponders. The histologic improvement observed in patients who have a decline in, or disappearance of, HCV RNA encourages the concept that viral clearance or at least cessation of active virus replication is advantageous, and may prevent progression to hepatic fibrosis or cirrhosis.

Interferon-α
Interferon-α was the first licensed therapy for chronic hepatitis C, either as monotherapy or in combination with other drugs. The drug is usually given by subcutaneous self-administered injection, and careful history taking and clinical assessment are essential before its use, because of a range of contraindications (Fig. 13.18). Some side effects are experienced by 85% of patients, but therapy only needs to be discontinued in 2–10% of cases. Some, but not all, adverse effects are dose-related, and serious adverse events may occur (Fig. 13.19). Many patients develop flu-like symptoms; some develop severe psychologic side effects, and patients are at risk of developing significant thrombocytopenia and leucopenia. Thyroid abnormalities occur in approximately 3% of treated patients, are much more common in those with anti-thyroid antibodies prior to treatment, and may not normalize after cessation of therapy. A proportion of patients with chronic hepatitis C have chronic disease with features of autoimmune hepatitis that may be provoked by interferon-α treatment.

Response to therapy may depend on a number of factors (Fig. 13.20). Patients with homogenous circulating quasispecies are more likely to respond to treatment. Although this has been incompletely studied, in some cases this mirrors a shorter duration of infection. Recent molecular evidence indicates that an interferon-sensitive determining region (ISDR) may be defined by the NS5a region, where mutations render HCV more sensitive to interferon.

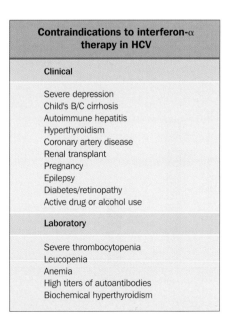

Contraindications to interferon-α therapy in HCV
Clinical
Severe depression
Child's B/C cirrhosis
Autoimmune hepatitis
Hyperthyroidism
Coronary artery disease
Renal transplant
Pregnancy
Epilepsy
Diabetes/retinopathy
Active drug or alcohol use
Laboratory
Severe thrombocytopenia
Leucopenia
Anemia
High titers of autoantibodies
Biochemical hyperthyroidism

Figure 13.18 Contraindications to interferon-α therapy in HCV.

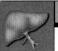

The efficacy of interferon-α therapies has been considered for different patient groups, including:
- 'naive' or untreated patients;
- patients who have shown a biochemical and virologic ETR but have relapsed once treatment has stopped ('relapsers'); and
- patients who have not responded to previous interferon treatment ('nonresponders').

In addition, the efficacy of interferon-α has been assessed in smaller special groups such as children, HIV and HCV coinfected patients with or without reduced CD4$^+$ cell counts, immunosuppressed patients, patients with autoimmune features, and those with extrahepatic manifestations. Transplant recipients, and patients with normal serum aminotransferases are also being studied.

Treatment of interferon-naive patients
Interferon-α monotherapy
Large controlled trials have been performed to evaluate the efficacy of four forms of interferon-α in patients not previously treated with interferon. These are α-2b, α-2a, α-n1, and consensus interferon. The overall experience suggests an equivalent efficacy and safety profile for all forms of interferon-α. It has been suggested that initial response rates vary between interferons, but these differences are generally marginal. In patients who receive a 12-month course of interferon-α monotherapy 3 million units three times per week, up to 50% will have a biochemical ETR, but only 15–25% will have an SR. Meta-analysis has shown that virologic SR is lower than biochemical SR (Fig. 13.21). Higher dose regimens produce more side effects, with minimal improvement in response, except possibly for those infected with HCV genotype 1.

In patients who respond, serum HCV RNA usually becomes undetectable by PCR (<100 copies/mL) in patients after 4–8 weeks of interferon-α treatment. An undetectable HCV RNA at the end of treatment is a prerequisite for sustained response, but does not

Serious adverse reactions to interferon
Clinical
Hepatic decompensation
Neuropsychiatric (depression, psychosis, suicidal ideation)
Bleeding
Cardiac arrythmias
Dilated cardiomyopathy
Hypotension
Acute renal failure
Retinopathy
Hearing loss
Pulmonary interstitial fibrosis
Laboratory
Neutropenia
Thrombocytopenia
Anemia
Hyperthyroidism
Hypothyroidism

Figure 13.19 Serious adverse reactions to interferon.

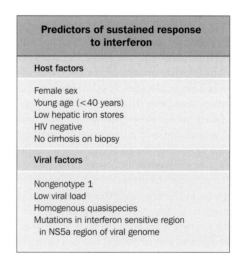

Predictors of sustained response to interferon
Host factors
Female sex
Young age (<40 years)
Low hepatic iron stores
HIV negative
No cirrhosis on biopsy
Viral factors
Nongenotype 1
Low viral load
Homogenous quasispecies
Mutations in interferon sensitive region in NS5a region of viral genome

Figure 13.20 Predictors of sustained response to interferon.

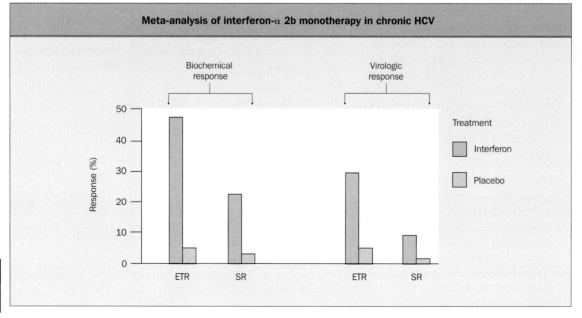

Figure 13.21 Meta-analysis of interferon-α-2b monotherapy in chronic hepatitis C virus. 20 trials; total 552 patients; minimum 24 weeks of treatment. ETR, end of treatment response; SR, sustained response. (Data from Carithers and Emerson, 1997.)

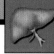

preclude relapse in patients. It is possible that some patients who relapse while on treatment do so because of the development of neutralizing interferon antibodies, or interferon resistance.

Combination therapy

Ribavirin is a guanosine nucleoside analogue that is administered orally. Three randomized, placebo-controlled studies have shown that ribavirin alone results in significant reduction in serum ALT concentrations but does not lead to sustained biochemical and virologic response rates. However, the addition of ribavirin to interferon-α regimens improves treatment responses in chronic hepatitis C. This combination of drugs is now licensed therapy for HCV. The publication in 1998 of several large trials of interferon-α/ribavirin combination therapy as first-line therapy in chronic HCV confirmed significantly better response rates than have been seen with interferon monotherapy. McHutchinson et al. (1998) randomized 912 patients to 6 or 12 months of combination therapy (interferon-α 3 million units three times per week, and ribavirin 1–1.2g/day) or monotherapy (interferon-α 3 million units three times per week). The virologic SR for combination therapy was significantly better than the monotherapy group (Fig. 13.22). Histologic improvement was more common in the combination therapy groups. In a similar study of 832 European patients with chronic HCV, Poynard et al. (1998) showed a virologic SR in 43% of patients receiving combination therapy, compared with 19% receiving interferon-α and placebo. Response rates were worse for those with HCV genotype 1, in whom 12 months combination therapy was clearly shown to have benefit over 6 months. No sig-

nificant differences in SR were seen between 6 and 12 months of treatment in those with nongenotype 1 infection, suggesting that 6 months treatment with combination is as advantageous as 12 months treatment for this group. Recent analysis of patients treated with INF-a/ribavirin has shown that <3% of those who are HCV RNA positive at 6 months will achieve SR after 12 months of therapy. This justifies checking HCV RNA at 6 months in those with genotype 1, and not continuing to 12 months if positive.

Contraindications to ribavirin include end-stage renal failure, anemia, severe heart disease, pregnancy, and inadequate contraception. The major side effect of ribavirin is hemolytic anemia, which can be severe. Cardiovascular disease should be carefully excluded in patients considered for combination therapy, as anemia may lead to angina or heart failure in these patients. Patients require at least monthly monitoring on treatment.

Treatment of relapsers

Different forms of interferon, and combination therapy, have been used in patients who have relapsed following a course of interferon-α monotherapy. Consensus interferon is a synthetic recombinant interferon derived from commonly observed amino acids to provide a consensus sequence. In a multicenter trial, 15μg of consensus interferon given three times a week for 48 weeks, was used to retreat patients who had either relapsed or had not responded to prior α-2b or 9μg of consensus interferon therapy. A total of 58% of patients had sustained virologic response rates.

Hepatitis C virus genotyping was not a component of previous large trials of interferon-α. However, in the recent trial of

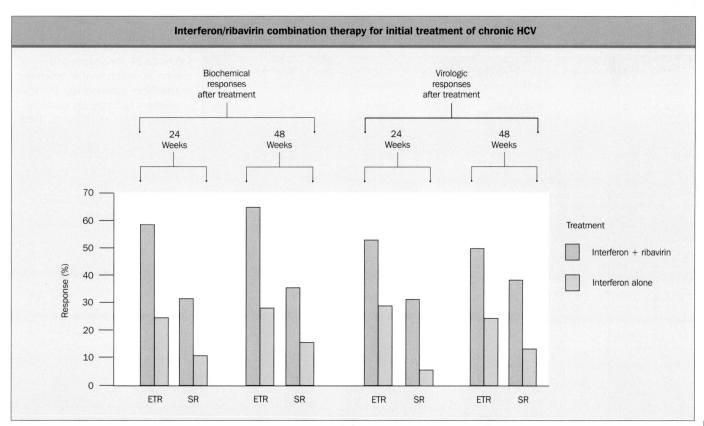

Figure 13.22 Interferon/ribavirin combination therapy for initial treatment of chronic HCV . Results of the biochemical and virologic response to 24 or 48 weeks of either combination or monotherapy. ETR: end-of-treatment response; SR: sustained response. (From McHutchinson JG, Gordon SC, Schiff ER, et al. N Engl J Med. 1998;339:1485–92.)

relapsers to interferon by Davis et al. (1998), none of the 70 patients with genotype 1 and a virus load greater than 2 million copies/mL, who received a further course of interferon monotherapy, demonstrated a virologic SR after 6 months of treatment (Fig. 13.23). Combination therapy has proved promising in patients who have relapsed after monotherapy. In the study by Davies et al., 345 patients who had previously relapsed on interferon were randomized to 6 months' treatment with interferon-α-2b and ribavirin or interferon-α-2b and placebo. Combination therapy produced significantly improved biochemical and virologic SR, and histologic findings, compared with retreatment with interferon-α alone (Fig. 13.24). The EASL International Consensus Conference on Hepatitis C determined that patients who have previously relapsed after interferon monotherapy should be considered for 12 months of combination therapy, or possibly high dose monotherapy for 12 months.

Nonresponders to interferon

Those patients who have shown no response to a previous course of interferon are very unlikely to achieve an SR with a further course, even using combination treatment. The development of new therapies offers the best promise for this patient group. The use of 'suppressive' treatment with interferon-α to reduce histologic progression in nonresponders remains controversial.

Interferon therapy in special groups
Cirrhosis

Antiviral therapy should be targeted to patients before cirrhosis has developed, as patients are at risk of developing sequelae once cirrhosis has developed. Furthermore, interferon therapy may trigger hepatic decompensation in patients with established cirrhosis. However, several small trials have recently suggested that interferon therapy improves liver function and reduces the incidence of HCC in patients with cirrhosis due to hepatitis B or C. There are reservations about the conclusions drawn from this limited experience. There is little information regarding potentially injurious exacerbations of hepatitis C (or hepatitis B) after transient suppression in those given therapy, and information regarding toxicity of interferon and dose response in this group of patients is not fully established. Nonetheless, interferon could be a potentially important treatment, if its antiproliferative, antifibrogenic, and immunomodulatory properties can be proven to play a role in preventing malignant transformation and/or progression of cirrhosis. Treatment of well-compensated cirrhosis appears justified, but the patient should be informed of the poorer predicted response rates, and risk of hepatic decompensation.

Virological SRs after 6 months of retreatment of 'relapsers' to interferon monotherapy		
Treatment for 6 months	Genotype 1 >2×10⁶ copies/ml	Non-genotype 1 <2×10⁶ copies/ml
Interferon + ribavirin	25%	100%
Interferon + placebo	0%	18%

Figure 13.23 Virologic SRs following 6 months of retreatment of 'relapsers' to interferon monotherapy. Stratified according to genotype and viral load. (From Davis GL, et al., 1998.)

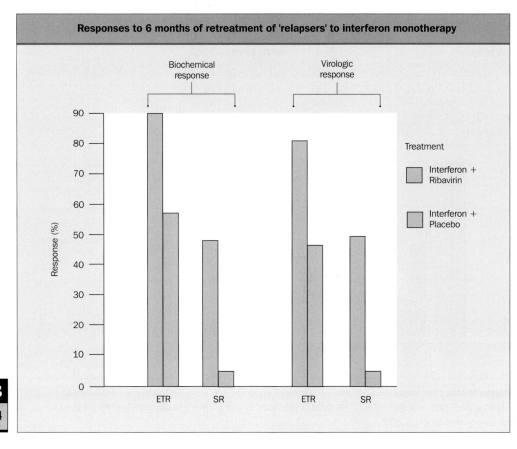

Figure 13.24 Responses to 6 months of retreatment of 'relapsers' to interferon monotherapy. ETR, end-of-treatment response; SR, sustained response. (From Davis GL, et al., 1998.)

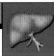

Extrahepatic manifestations

Patients with hepatitis C have been treated with interferon-α in order to alleviate extrahepatic manifestations, including vasculitis, glomerulonephritis, and cryoglobulinemia. Despite beneficial responses during treatment, relapse is very common after cessation, and maintenance therapy may be the way forward in the future.

Children

Few studies of treatment of children with hepatitis C have been performed, and none, to date, of combination therapy. The difficult balance needs to be weighed between the knowledge that histologic disease may progress, with milder disease of shorter duration responding better to treatment, and the fact that serious complications of HCV take 20 years to develop, during which time better therapies may be reasonably predicted to have been developed.

Human immunodeficiency virus-positive patients

Chronic hepatitis C is often found in patients with HIV, and with improved HIV antiviral therapy, HCV threatens to have an increasing impact on morbidity and mortality in this group. There is no consensus regarding the place of treatment in this group. Treatment may be indicated for patients with CD4$^+$ counts >200, but added care is needed in view of potential drug interactions in patients whose HIV has been stabilized by antiretroviral combination therapy.

Liver transplantation

Cirrhosis due to hepatitis C has become one of the most important indications for liver transplantation in most countries, and the number of patients being transplanted for this indication continues to increase. Five and 10-year survivals of 70% and 60% in Europe are similar to those for patients transplanted for other nonmalignant conditions. However, it has become apparent that recurrence of hepatitis C virus in the transplanted liver is almost universal. Although recurrence is usually associated with relatively mild disease, cirrhosis has been reported in about 10% of cases at 5 years, and long-term follow up is not yet available. There is no consensus as to the optimal treatment of HCV in transplant recipients. Combination interferon/ribavirin therapy has often been used in centers where antiviral therapy has been given, but randomized trials are awaited to clarify when antiviral therapy should be commenced, and the importance of concomitant antirejection therapy on HCV progression and response to treatment post-transplant.

Vaccine development

The development of vaccines to prevent hepatitis B virus infection is having a significant effect on the impact of this disease worldwide. The production of a widely available, effective vaccine for HCV is an important, but currently elusive objective. Development is hampered by the inability to culture the virus *in vitro*. The heterogeneity of envelope glycoproteins found with different isolates indicates the existence of a large pool of antigenic variants. The major antigenic differences, particularly in the envelope region, will be an important confounding factor in the development of vaccines for HCV. A polyvalent vaccine will be required. Core-E1-E2 and NS2 genes have been expressed in a recombinant vaccinia vector to infect HeLa cells, and the extracted glycosylated E1 and E2 proteins have been used to vaccinate seven chimpanzees. Recombinant protein was shown to induce neutralizing antibodies. However, despite these encouraging initial results, more cross-challenge and isolate-specific experiments will be required. Interestingly, this measure may also induce resolution of acute infection. Vaccine therapy trials are in progress. Injection of naked DNA to trigger immune response generates antigen for presentation by MHC, and a CD8$^+$ T-cell response. This approach has been explored in several different models. In initial transfection experiments, genomic regions encoding E2 glycoprotein and C protein have been injected into HeLa cells, and injected intramuscularly in mice. A measurable antibody response developed.

Future developments in the treatment of hepatitis C virus infection

The number of patients undergoing antiviral treatment for chronic hepatitis C virus, and the number requiring liver transplantation for hepatitis C cirrhosis is projected to increase over the next 15–20 years, with significant implications on health care provision. Despite the identification of factors that are associated with disease progression, our understanding of the pathogenetic mechanisms that underlie the liver injury in HCV remain incomplete. More research regarding the effect of interferon-α on HCV quasispecies, and of the importance of the putative interferon sensitivity-determining regions within the genome is required. Specific host immune mechanisms may also prove to be an important determinant of response to therapy.

Interferon-α remains inadequately effective therapy for many patients with chronic hepatitis C, but significant improvements for its use in combination with ribavirin have been demonstrated. Improved hepatic histology has been observed in patients with sustained virologic response, which provides a rationale for antiviral treatment in this disease. A possible role of interferon in reducing the risk of HCC in patients with cirrhosis remains intriguing, and potentially important. Treatment regimens may be tailored to the likelihood of response, but this must be more precisely defined. Preliminary data suggest that it could become possible to select patients for therapy based on the major independent factors that influence response to interferon-α therapy.

Despite improvements in therapy, treatment fails to achieve a sustained virologic response in 60% of cases. New antiviral therapies are being developed. Alternative interferons are under evaluation, including pegylated interferon, 'natural' interferon, and interferon-β. The second generation of pegylated (PEG) interferons appear to be more effective interferons, and can be administered once weekly. The advantages of combination therapy have been well demonstrated in the treatment of HIV, and the promising recent results with interferon and ribavirin suggest that this is also the way forward in HCV infection. The use of new combination therapies, including the use of amantadine, nonsteroidal anti-inflammatory agents, or thymosin, in two or three drug regimens, is undergoing evaluation. Drugs to inhibit enzymes of HCV replication (serine protease, helicase or polymerase inhibitors), or HCV translation, are under development. The future development of a vaccine for HCV might be an important advance in limiting further spread of the disease. Improved methods to control HCV in the donor graft would be an important advance in the management of the increasing number of patients who will require liver transplantation for chronic hepatitis C virus in the next 20 years.

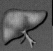
PRACTICE POINT

A 46-year-old businessman is referred to the outpatient clinic by his general practitioner. He has a 3-year history of fatigue and general malaise. His primary care physician found no abnormalities on examination, but routine blood tests revealed mildly elevated serum ALT. On the basis of this an anti-HCV antibody test was performed, and found to be positive. The patient was extremely anxious at this finding. He has been under pressure at work, and described a poor sleep pattern. He recently remarried, and has two teenage children from his first marriage living at home. Further inquiry revealed a brief period of intravenous drug abuse while a university student. He came with a list of questions:

'Am I going to die?'

As in this patient, chronic hepatitis C is often virtually clinically silent, and the diagnosis may therefore come as a huge shock. Many people erroneously believe that progression to end-stage liver disease is inevitable. It is crucial that the patient is informed that this is an important diagnosis, but that disease progression is usually slow, and treatments are improving. An attempt should be made to ascertain the duration of infection, and the natural history of the disease should be outlined (see Fig. 13.9). It is important to explain the factors associated with disease progression (see Fig. 13.10), so that specific behaviors, such as alcohol excess, may be modified.

'How can I pass it on?'

Information about the virus, and its transmissibility should be provided. The patient should be advised not to donate blood. Patients can be advised that the parenteral route is the most important route of transmission and that the virus is not easily transmitted except by this route. Specifically, this man should be fully informed that the risks of sexual transmission to his wife are low, but not zero. It is generally advised that patients with chronic hepatitis C who are in long-term monogamous relationships should not suddenly commence barrier contraception, but that the use of condoms in those having casual sex should be stressed. Patients, preferably with their partners, should be allowed to make their own decisions about testing after being informed of the facts. Considering his teenage children, advice should be given about avoiding virus transmission (e.g. through the sharing of toothbrushes). There is probably no clear indication for them to be tested unless their mother had chronic hepatitis C.

'How bad is my hepatitis C?'

A supplemental antibody test (e.g. RIBA) is not necessary, in view of the presence of raised ALT, and risk factors for HCV infection. HCV RNA detection by PCR should be performed, to confirm ongoing infection, and plan further management (see Fig. 13.17). The patient should be advised of the need for a liver biopsy to grade and stage the extent of histologic

disease, as this information may allow some predictions about prognosis and the need for treatment to be made. Testing for HCV genotype is required, as this may determine the treatment regimen required.

The need for other blood tests to exclude other causes of liver disease (e.g. hepatitis B virus serology), or to identify potential problems with interferon therapy (e.g. thyroid autoantibodies), should be discussed, as outlined above.

'Am I OK to have interferon?'

Contraindications to interferon therapy need to be carefully excluded (see Fig. 13.18). It would be crucial to exclude a depressive illness in this man, who reports a poor sleep pattern and pressures at work. He is recently married, and it is vital that he is informed that his wife should not become pregnant during, or within 6 months of completing a course of interferon therapy (or ribavirin).
Side effects of treatment should be discussed before starting treatment (see Fig. 13.19). It should be explained that most side effects are dose-dependent and resolve after cessation of interferon, but that some effects (e.g. thyroid dysfunction) may persist. This patient is under pressure at work, and he should be aware that interferon therapy commonly causes flu-like symptoms, particularly in the initial few weeks, and that this may affect his performance. The need to attend the clinic for regular follow-up needs to be explained, and a letter from the clinic to the patient's employer, with the patient's consent, may enable further problems to be overcome.
The technique of self-administration of subcutaneous interferon, and its safe storage, should be carefully explained, and initial therapy supervised.

'What treatment regimen will you give me?'

Patients with chronic hepatitis C are often well informed, aided, in part, by the enormous amount of information available on the Internet. A discussion of recent trial results may be required, and the factors that influence response to treatment should be outlined (see Fig. 13.20). The influence of genotype on treatment regimens should be explained. The optimal treatment regimen available at present is interferon-α 3 million units three times per week, and ribavirin 1–1.2g per day. A treatment course of 12 months should be given to patients with genotype 1, but 6 months is sufficient in those infected with genotypes 2 and 3. The definition of response should be clarified, and it should be explained that a sustained virologic response rate in more than 40% of patients treated with combination therapy can be broadly predicted.

'How am I followed up on treatment?'

If combination therapy has been commenced, patients should be seen weekly for the first 4 weeks, to exclude marked falls in hemoglobin, due to hemolysis. Monthly assessment is essential during the rest of treatment, to exclude the development

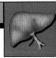

of laboratory (e.g. neutropenia) or clinical (e.g. depression) complications of treatment. In patients receiving combination therapy, treatment should probably be stopped if HCV RNA is still positive at 6 months. Three to six monthly follow-ups after completion of treatment will allow the long-term response to treatment to be defined.

GB VIRUS-C AND HEPATITIS G

INTRODUCTION

GB virus (GBV)-C and hepatitis G virus (HGV) are newly discovered members of the Flaviviridae family. Two isolates of the same virus were discovered in the same year by separate research groups, and given the somewhat cumbersome nomenclature of GBV-C and HGV, respectively. The identification of this virus originated when serum obtained from a surgeon with acute hepatitis (who had the initials GB) induced experimental hepatitis in tamarins. After almost two decades, a molecular search for the GB agent led to the discovery of two flaviviruses by cloning from experimentally infected tamarins. These two agents were given the nomenclature GBV-A and GBV-B, and are now known to be primate viruses. The two clones isolated from tamarins provided the sequence for the construction of degenerate primers to allow the search for a similar agent in human samples. A West African sample proved positive for a similar RNA virus, which was in turn given the nomenclature GBV-C. Independent research by another group also led to the isolation of a similar novel virus designated HGV, which was identified from the plasma of a patient with chronic hepatitis. It is now recognized that GBV-C and HGV are two different isolates of the same virus.

Virology

The genome of GBV-C/HGV is a single-strand RNA with a positive strand polarity and approximately 9392 nucleotides in length (Fig. 13.25). The virus comprises a single large open reading frame that encodes potential polyprotein precursors of 2972 and 2864 amino acids, respectively. The genome of this agent is organized much like those of other pestiviruses and flaviviruses, with genes predicted to encode structural and nonstructural proteins located at the 5′ and 3′ ends, respectively. The nucleotide sequence has 25% identity with hepatitis C virus. Sequences from the 5′-UTR suggest three genotypes correlating with type 1 (West Africa), type 2 (USA), and type 3 (Far East). The degree of sequence difference between these isolates or genotypes is relatively constrained. The E2 region does not contain a hypervariable region. The tissue tropism and sites of replication of GBV-C/HGV remain unclear. It has been difficult to detect GBV-C/HGV minus strand RNA in liver with certainty.

Transmission and epidemiology

GB virus-C virus/HGV has a global distribution and is present in up to 3% of the volunteer blood donor population in Western countries. The prevalence in blood donors is 1–2% in the USA, and GBV-C/HGV is present in approximately 20% of patients receiving chronic hemodialysis. About 14–18% of hemophiliacs who have been treated with untreated factors VIII and IX concentrates are GBV-C/HGV-positive. Inactivation treatments appear to be effective against GBV-C/HGV. A high proportion of hemophiliacs (up to 60%) are anti-E2-positive, indicating recovery from GBV-C/HGV infection. The preoperative prevalence of GBV-C/HGV infection in recipients transplanted for cryptogenic cirrhosis is 26%.

Persistent viremia has been detected for up to 9 years in patients with or, more generally, without hepatitis. Despite the extremely high level of HGV contamination of nonvirus-inactivated blood products, their use has not been associated with

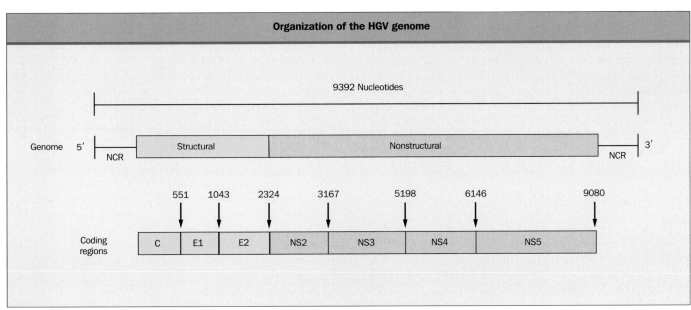

Figure 13.25 Organization of the hepatitis G virus genome. NCR, noncoding region.

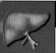

very high rates of persistent infection in recipients. The mean age of patients with persistent infection or coinfection of HCV and GBV-C/HGV has been found to be lower than that of patients with HCV alone, suggesting that clearance of GBV-C/HGV occurs more commonly than HCV.

CLINICAL SIGNIFICANCE

There is currently no clear relationship between GBV-C/HGV infection and progressive liver disease. No definite causal relationship between GBV-C/HGV and chronic hepatitis has been established, and although this human virus may be responsible for some cases of non-A–E hepatitis, surveillance studies in the USA do not implicate GBV-C/HGV as a major etiologic agent of non-A–E hepatitis. Persistent infection with HGV is quite common, but infection does not appear to lead to chronic hepatic disease and does not affect the clinical course in patients with hepatitis A, B, or C virus infection. Most post-transfusion HGV infections have not apparently been associated with classic hepatitis. Most patients with persistent infection have normal serum aminotransferases. Generally most authors have not found significant differences in the degree of fibrosis, presence of portal lymphoid aggregates, steatosis, and hemosiderosis between patients with persistent HCV alone or HCV and GBV-C/HGV coinfection, although we have observed a greater degree of portal inflammation. Infection with GBV-C/HGV does not appear to lead to cirrhosis. It has, however, been difficult to find cases where GBV-C/HGV is the sole infection, but these individuals do not generally have liver disease.

Nonspecific inflammatory bile duct lesions and raised serum alkaline phosphatase and γ-glutamyl transferase levels have been found, but the significance of this lesion has not been validated. GBV-C/HGV does not appear to alter the course of HCV infection of HCV-positive transplant patients. GBV-C/HGV is found infrequently in patients with type 1 autoimmune hepatitis. Overall, the high prevalence in the asymptomatic blood donor population suggests quite frequent, perhaps benign, infection of unknown pathogenic significance.

Higher CD4$^+$ counts have been found in HIV GBV-C viremic persons with better cumulative survival, but again this finding will need validation. Although up to 26% of patients with aplastic anemia are GBV-C/HGV-positive, in most cases this reflects prior multiple transfusions.

Fulminant hepatitis

There are reports of GBV-C/HGV RNA in serum, detected by seminested PCR using primers derived from the NS3/helicase region, of patients with fulminant hepatitis of unknown etiology. It has been suggested that a specific strain of GBV-C may occur in serum of German patients with fulminant hepatic failure. A sequence-motif containing six nucleotide mutations in the NS3 region has been detected in patients with fulminant hepatic failure but is only rarely present in control, nonfulminant infections. The interpretation of these findings requires proof that the virus is not simply a secondary infection as a result of the blood or plasma transfusions received by patients with fulminant hepatitis due to other causes.

DIAGNOSIS

Reverse transcriptase PCR assays for detection of viral RNA have been developed, using primers from the NS3 helicase and 5′ untranslated region; the 5′ untranslated region is highly conserved. Enzyme-linked immunoabsorbent assays have been developed for detection of antibodies to viral envelope proteins (anti-E2). The presence of anti-E2 and HGV RNA are usually mutually exclusive, and development of anti-E2 may be a marker of recovery from GBV-C/HGV.

TREATMENT AND PREVENTION

GBV-C/HGV shares with HCV a susceptibility to interferon-α and HGV RNA concentrations may decline during treatment. However, in view of the lack of data confirming the pathogenicity of this virus antiviral therapy is not advised. GBV-C/HGV coinfection does not affect the responsiveness to interferon-α treatment of patients with chronic HCV infection. Blood products are not now being screened for GBV-C/HGV until further proof of the pathogenicity of this agent has been obtained. Further studies in organ recipients are required.

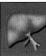
FURTHER READING

Hepatitis C

Alter MJ. Epidemiology of hepatitis C. Hepatology. 1997;26(3):62S–65S. *Review of epidemiology and transmission, as part of NIH Consensus Development Conference.*

Altman JD, Moss P, Goulder P, et al. Phenotypic analysis of antigen-specific T lymphocytes. Science. 1996;274:94–6. *The seminal paper on the development of tetramer technology for defining CTLs.*

Carithers RJ, Emerson SS. Therapy of hepatitis C: meta-analysis of interferon alfa-2b trials. Hepatology. 1997;26:83S–88S. *Paper collating data on monotherapy in chronic HCV.*

Chisari FV. Cytotoxic T cells and viral hepatitis. J Clin Invest. 1997;99:1472–7. *Excellent review of the cellular immune response to HCV.*

Colombo M, Fasani P, Romeo R. Hepatitis C virus and hepatocellular carcinoma. Res Virol. 1997;148:127–34. *A review of the relationship between HCV and HCC.*

Davis GL, Esteban-Mur R, Rustgi V, et al. Interferon alfa-2b alone or in combination with ribavirin for the treatment of relapse of chronic hepatitis C. N Engl J Med. 1998;339:1493–9. *Large multicenter trial showing benefit of combination therapy after relapse on monotherapy.*

Dhillon AP, Dusheiko GM. Pathology of hepatitis C virus infection. Histopathology. 1995;26:297–309. *Review of the liver pathology in HCV.*

Di Bisceglie AM. Hepatitis C. Lancet. 1998; 351:351–5. *Concise, readable overview.*

Dienstag JL. The natural history of chronic hepatitis C and what we should do about it. Gastroenterology. 1997;112:651–5. *A good review of the natural history of HCV and a plea for better treatment in the future.*

Dusheiko G, Simmonds P. Sequence variability of hepatitis C virus and its clinical relevance. J Viral Hepatit. 1994;1:3–15. *A review of the HCV genotypes and how these facilitate our understanding of the disease worldwide.*

Dusheiko G. Side effects of alpha interferon in chronic hepatitis C. Hepatology. 1997;26:112S–21S. *Review of side effects due to range of interferons, as part of NIH Consensus Development Conference.*

EASL International Consensus Conference on Hepatitis C. Consensus Statement. J Hepatol. 1999;Suppl 1:3–8. *Up-to-date consensus statement on management of HCV, at beginning of excellent supplement reviewing all aspects of HCV infection.*

Gane EJ, Lo SK, Riordan SM, et al. A randomized study comparing ribavirin and interferon alfa monotherapy for hepatitis C recurrence after liver transplantation. Hepatology. 1998;27:1403–1407. *A randomized trial of monotherapy regimens post-transplantation.*

Hoofnagle JH. Hepatitis C: The clinical spectrum of disease. Hepatology. 1997;26:15S–20S. *Excellent review of the natural history of HCV as part of NIH Consensus Development Conference.*

McHutchinson JG, Gordon SC, Schiff ER, et al. Interferon alfa-2b alone or in combination with ribavirin as initial treatment for chronic hepatitis C. N Eng J Med. 1998;339:1485–92. *Important, large multicenter trial showing benefit of combination therapy as initial therapy.*

NIH Consensus Development Conference Panel Statement: Management of Hepatitis C. Hepatology. 1997;26:2S–10S. *Recommendations on treatment indications, although treatment regimens require updating following recent trial data.*

Platz KP, Mueller AR, Berg T, et al. Searching for the optimal management of hepatitis C patients after liver transplantation. Transpl Int. 1998;11(Suppl 1):S209–211. *Study of the optimal immunosuppressive regime in HCV transplant recipients.*

Poynard T, Marcellin P, Lee S, et al. Randomised trial of interferon-2b plus ribavirin for 48 weeks or for 24 weeks, versus interferon-2b plus placebo for 48 weeks for treatment of chronic infection with hepatitis C virus. Lancet. 1998;352:1426–32. *Important, large multicenter trial showing benefit of combination therapy as initial therapy.*

Simmonds P, Holmes EC, Cha T-A, et al. Classification of hepatitis C virus into six major genotypes and a series of subtypes by phylogenetic analysis of the NS-5 region. J Gen Virol. 1993;74:2391–9. *Description of the accepted classification of HCV genotypes.*

Springer Seminars in Immunopathology. Immunopathology of hepatitis C infection. 1997;19(1). *Detailed reviews of immune mechanisms involved in viral control or persistence, and mechanism of disease manifestations.*

Zanetti AR, Tanzi E, Paccagnini S, et al. Lombardy Study Group on Vertical HCV Transmission. Mother-to-infant transmission of hepatitis C virus. Lancet. 1995;345:289–91. *Paper demonstrating the marked effect of HIV positivity on maternal transmission of HCV.*

Hepatitis G

Alter MJ, Gallagher M, Morris TT, et al. Acute non-A–E hepatitis in the United States and the role of hepatitis G virus infection. N Engl J Med. 1997;336:741–6. *Study demonstrating minimal role of HGV in post-transfusion hepatitis.*

Berg T, Dirla U, Naumann U, et al. Responsiveness to interferon alpha treatment in patients with chronic hepatitis C coinfected with hepatitis G virus. J Hepatol. 1996;25:763–8. *Study reporting lack of influence of HGV on response of HCV to interferon.*

Bukh J, Kim JP, Govindarajan S, Apgar CL, et al. Experimental infection of chimpanzees with hepatitis G virus and genetic analysis of the virus. J Infect Dis. 1998;177:855–862. *Paper defining organization of HGV genome.*

Charlton MR, Brandhagen D, Wiesner RH, et al. Hepatitis G virus infection in patients transplanted for cryptogenic cirrhosis – red flag or red herring? Transplantation. 1998;65:73–6. *Demonstration of high prevalence of HGV in cryptogenic cirrhosis, and of hepatitis in graft.*

Enomoto M, Nishiguchi S, Fukuda K, et al. Characteristics of patients with hepatitis C virus with and without GB virus C/hepatitis G virus co-infection and efficacy of interferon alfa. Hepatology. 1998;27:1388–93. *Study reports high frequency of previous exposure to HGV in HCV-infected patients, and the effect of interferon.*

Linnen J, Wages J, Jr, Zhang-Keck ZY, et al. Molecular cloning and disease association of hepatitis G virus: A transfusion-transmissible agent. Science. 1996;271:505–508. *Description of HGV genome and virus transmissibility.*

Miyakawa Y, Mayumii M. Hepatitis G virus – a true hepatitis virus or an accidental tourist? N Engl J Med. 1997;336:795–6. *Early editorial debating pathogenicity of HGV.*

Schlauder GG, Pilot-Matias TJ, Gabriel GS, et al. Origin of GB-hepatitis viruses. Lancet. 1995;346:447–8. *A letter describing the then recent description of GBV-A, -B and -C viruses.*

Simons JN, Leary TP, Dawson GJ, et al. Isolation of novel virus-like sequences associated with human hepatitis. Nature Med. 1995;1:564–9. *One of the initial descriptions of HGV.*

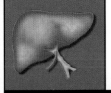

Section 3 Specific Diseases of the Liver

Chapter 14

HIV and the Liver

Johannes Koch and Lawrence S Kim

INTRODUCTION

Human immunodeficiency virus (HIV) has emerged as a major public health problem throughout the world. While initially discovered in Western populations, it has rapidly become one of the most common causes of premature death in many Third World countries, particularly in Africa and more recently Southeast Asia. In the Third World, it has had dramatic micro-economic effects that will likely impact the countries for generations to come.

In the West the news is much better, in that highly effective therapy is now available against HIV. Therapy, however, is limited by the development of acquired drug resistance and by the toxicities of the various therapies, some of which are hepatic.

The liver is a common site of disease among patients infected with HIV. Abnormal liver function tests or clinical features such as hepatomegaly are seen in most patients at some point during the course of their infection. Viral hepatitis [both caused by hepatitis C virus (HCV) and hepatitis B virus (HBV)] was and still is a common comorbidity, so much so that in the early days of the epidemic it was considered to be important for the pathogenesis of disease. We now know that this simply reflects similar routes of acquisition of the viral infections. It does appear that the natural history of hepatitis B and C is more aggressive in the HIV population, although not dramatically so. Once primary biliary processes have been excluded, however, the evaluation and management of these patients is problematic. Most conditions resulting in clinical liver disease represent systemic opportunistic infections or neoplasms; however, the hepatic involvement itself is rarely the cause of death. Instead, the clinical and histologic expression of most diseases of the liver are attenuated because of the impaired immune response. In addition, most liver disorders diagnosed in patients infected with HIV occur late in the natural history of this disease, when immunosuppression is advanced and little can be done to improve the overall outcome.

However, with improvements in HIV treatment, patients who previously died of AIDS before the liver disease advanced to the point of end-stage disease are now finding themselves having their HIV disease controlled through the use of highly active anti-retroviral therapy (HAART), but with the burden of end-stage liver disease. Several liver transplant programs are willing to consider such patients as reasonable candidates for transplantation. This presents several unique problem areas discussed below, where the various drugs used to treat HIV are considered.

EPIDEMIOLOGY

Abnormal liver function tests are nearly universal among patients with HIV at some point during the course of their infection. Abnormal liver tests are found in over 80% of patients with clinical AIDS. Biochemical abnormalities are divided equally between elevations of transaminases and abnormal values of serum alkaline phosphatase activity and/or serum bilirubin levels. However, the pattern of biochemical abnormalities does not reliably predict the etiology of liver disease. Clinical features of liver disease are also prevalent, with hepatomegaly found in up to 75% of patients on physical examination or in autopsy series. Systemic symptoms such as fatigue, anorexia, fever, and weight loss are also very common, especially in patients with clinical AIDS; however, such symptoms may or may not be directly attributable to liver disease. Overt jaundice is relatively uncommon, reported in only 10% of patients at the time of autopsy or liver biopsy.

The presentation of liver disease also varies with respect to geography. This reflects the relative lack of antiviral treatment in the Third World and also epidemiology. For example HBV infection is very common in sub-Sahara Africa and Southeast Asia, while HCV and biliary tract disease appear to be more common in the Western world.

In the West, among patients infected with HIV and abnormal liver function tests, histologic abnormalities are found in over 90% on liver biopsy or autopsy. The most common finding is nonspecific steatosis, followed by portal inflammation, congestion, hepatic granulomas, focal necrosis, and fibrosis or steatosis. A specific etiologic diagnosis may be made in approximately 50% of patients, most commonly mycobacterial infection in the presence of granulomas. A list of the most common pathogens found on liver biopsy is presented in Fig. 14.1.

Results of liver biopsy in patients with AIDS	
Diagnosis	**Prevalence (%)**
No pathogens	50
Mycobacteria	20–40
Cytomegalovirus	10
Kaposi's sarcoma	10
Lymphoma	5–10
Fungal infections	<5
Other	<5

Figure 14.1 Results of liver biopsy in patients with AIDS.

SPECIFIC DISEASE ASSOCIATIONS

Hepatic involvement by HIV

Human immunodeficiency virus can involve the liver directly. The HIV-p24 antigen and HIV messenger RNA have been demonstrated within hepatocytes and Kupffer cells using immunohistochemical staining and *in situ* hybridization techniques. In addition, the presence of viral RNA within whole liver samples has been confirmed using quantitative polymerase chain reaction (PCR). Hepatic macrophages and endothelial cells express the CD4 surface molecule, which serves as the receptor for the HIV gp120 glycoprotein and permits viral infection. It has been shown that human hepatic endothelial cells can indeed be infected with HIV-1 *in vitro*, and that these cells support viral replication. However, it remains as yet unclear whether HIV itself directly damages the liver. No characteristic biochemical or pathologic abnormalities have been found accompanying the presence of HIV within hepatocytes, and normal histology has occasionally been reported. Furthermore, the quantity of stainable HIV antigens in immunohistochemical studies does not correlate with the degree of histologic abnormalities seen.

Mycobacterial infections

Mycobacterium avium-intracellulare (MAI) is the most common opportunistic pathogen found on liver biopsy among patients with AIDS. Infection with MAI occurs late in the natural history of AIDS, with CD4 counts generally less than 50×10^6 cells/mL. The prognosis is correspondingly poor, with median survival 3–5 months from the time of diagnosis. Hepatic involvement occurs in the setting of disseminated disease. The clinical presentation is generally dominated by systemic symptoms, although jaundice can occasionally occur from extrahepatic obstruction secondary to lymphadenopathy. The most prominent biochemical abnormality is a marked elevation of the serum alkaline phosphatase, caused by obstruction of small biliary ductules by granulomas. *Mycobacterium avium-inracellulare* related granulomas are found in 76% of involved histologic specimens. These granulomas are usually poorly formed, probably due to suppressed T-cell activity, and contain numerous acid-fast organisms. However, because histology is not specific, consideration should be given to culturing all liver biopsy specimens to confirm infection with MAI, as opposed to other acid-fast organisms. Treatment with multidrug antibiotic regimens generally produces an initial response; however, because of the advanced nature of immunosuppression in these patients, the long-term outcome remains poor.

Hepatic involvement with MAI must be distinguished from infection with *Mycobacterium tuberculosis*. Patients with acquired immune deficiency syndrome (AIDS) are at increased risk for tuberculosis, with the highest prevalence among patients from low socioeconomic strata and intravenous drug users. Tuberculosis is a particularly important problem in the Third World. Tuberculosis often takes an aggressive course in patients with AIDS, with extrapulmonary involvement in over one-half of cases. In contrast to MAI, histologic specimens in patients infected with *M. tuberculosis* show well-formed granulomas with central caseation, reflecting the fact that infection occurs at less advanced stages of immunocompromise than does MAI. However, because tuberculosis cannot be distinguished from MAI by clinical features or histopathology alone, culture is

required for positive diagnosis. In addition, determination of antimicrobial sensitivities is necessary to guide appropriate therapy. Unless a multidrug-resistant strain is present, response to treatment is good, with a median survival of 16 months.

Rare cases of hepatic involvement with other mycobacterial species, including *M. kansasii*, *M. xenopi*, and *M. genavense*, have been reported. These present with a similar clinical picture of constitutional symptoms, hepatomegaly, and elevated serum alkaline phosphatase. The diagnosis is made by culture of blood or liver biopsy specimens, and response to treatment is variable.

Peliosis hepatis

Early in the AIDS epidemic, a syndrome consisting of dilated, blood-filled hepatic sinusoids and elevated liver function tests was recognized. Histologically, peliosis hepatis consists of numerous blood-filled cystic spaces within the hepatic parenchyma without an endothelial lining. Serum transaminase levels are modestly elevated, with more prominent elevations of serum alkaline phosphatase. This syndrome occurs most commonly in patients with clinical AIDS, in conjunction with cutaneous bacillary angiomatosis. In addition to cutaneous lesions, patients can experience fevers, sweats, rigors, right upper quadrant pain, or pain from bony lytic lesions. Peliosis hepatis has been recognized as a bacterial syndrome following the discovery of its causative agent, *Bartonella hensalae*. Histopathologic studies revealed clumpy granular, purple material within both hepatic and cutaneous lesions, which proved to be bacteria on electron microscopy. Further investigations employing PCR identified the organism as a Gram-negative bacillus closely related to *Rochalimaea quintana*, the causative agent of trench fever. Successful treatment regimens have included erythromycin, doxycycline, ciprofloxacin, and antituberculous regimens, although prolonged therapy for several months may be required.

Fungal infections

Liver involvement with fungal infections occurs in the setting of disseminated disease. A nonspecific clinical presentation is typical, including unexplained fever and/or hepatomegaly. Discrete fungal abscesses are occasionally seen on radiographic imaging studies. Histologically, a nonspecific attenuated granulomatous reaction is characteristic, and special stains and fungal cultures of blood and biopsy tissue are generally required for specific diagnosis.

Liver involvement occurs in up to 20% of patients with cryptococcal meningitis, and reflects disseminated disease. The clinical features are secondary to neurologic and systemic infection. Although serum alkaline phosphatase levels are typically elevated, the hepatic infection itself rarely causes symptoms. The diagnosis of cryptococcal disease is most commonly made by latex agglutination of the capsular polysaccharide antigen in serum or cerebrospinal fluid (CSF). The diagnosis can also be made on tissue using India ink, mucicarmine, or silver stains to detect organisms. The diagnostic yield from liver biopsy material is lower than other sites, including blood, bone marrow, and CSF. In one study, no cases of disseminated cryptococcosis were diagnosed by liver biopsy in cases where diagnostic findings were not present at other sites as well. Treatment with amphotericin or fluconazole may be effective; however, the prognosis was determined mainly by the severity of the neurologic disease. The recent release of a number of liposomal amphotericin products has decreased the toxicity of the drug, particularly in patients on long-term therapy

Hepatic candidiasis is less common among patient with AIDS compared with other conditions where immunosuppression occurs such as intensive cancer chemotherapy or transplantation. This may be due to the relative preservation of neutrophil function among patients infected with HIV. Computed tomography or ultrasound studies typically demonstrate multiple radiolucent microabcesses in the liver and spleen with a characteristic 'bullseye' pattern of central density with surrounding attenuation. Diagnosis is made by histologic demonstration of budding yeast or pseudohyphae within abscesses, surrounded by a neutrophilic infiltrate.

Histoplasma capsulatum is endemic to river valleys in the midwestern USA and may involve the liver in the setting of disseminated infection. Chronic systemic symptoms consist of fever, weight loss, malaise, and bone marrow suppression; however, an acute presentation with shock, multiorgan failure, and disseminated intravascular coagulation has been reported. Biochemical abnormalities consist of moderate elevations of transaminases. On histologic examination of liver biopsy specimens, round-oval yeast with occasional budding can be seen with silver stains. Diagnostic yields are higher from bone marrow than from liver specimens. Treatment of the acute disease is either with amphotericin or itraconazole. In general, long-term treatment is necessary and best accomplished with itraconazole.

A similar nonspecific presentation is seen in infection with *Coccidioides imitis*, which is endemic to the Southwestern USA. In immunocompetent patients, infection produces a mild respiratory illness; however, in the setting of AIDS, disseminated infection with systemic symptoms and liver involvement can occur. Although granulomas may be present in liver biopsy specimens, bronchoscopy has a higher diagnostic yield. As with disseminated histoplasmosis and candidiasis, prolonged treatment with amphotericin is the mainstay of therapy. Hepatic involvement with *Sporothrix* spp. has also been reported in association with fever and weight loss. Other potential manifestations include erythematous, ulcerating cutaneous nodules along peripheral lymphatic drainage routes, chronic erosive arthritis, and osteomyelitis.

Protozoal infections

Pneumocystis carinii is the most common protozoal opportunistic infection among patients with HIV. Although pneumonia is the most common presentation of pneumocystis infection, extrapulmonary involvement may also occur, especially in patients with advanced AIDS. The liver is one of the most common extrapulmonary sites of involvement, occurring in 38% of patients. Pulmonary symptoms dominate the clinical presentation, although isolated cases of primary hepatic involvement with pneumocystis have been reported manifested by constitutional symptoms and abnormal liver function tests. Histologic examination reveals characteristic nodules with a foamy eosinophilic exudate, often in conjunction with necrosis or hemorrhage, as well as peripheral calcification. Cyst forms of the pneumocystis organism can be demonstrated within the exudate by Gomori's methenamine silver stain. Response to treatment with parenteral pentamidine or trimethoprim–sulfamethoxazole is often satisfactory. Moreover, the use of prophylaxis has markedly decreased the rate of death in the West from this infection. The widespread use of aerosolized pentamidine isethionate for prophylaxis against pneumocystis pneumonia may also theoretically increase the incidence of extrapulmonary involvement; since this drug is not absorbed systemically, it may suppress pulmonary disease while permitting the emergence of latent infections at other sites. Currently, trimethoprim–sulfamethoxazole is used most commonly for pneumocystis prophylaxis and this may be more effective against the extrapulmonary sites.

Hepatitis B

The high rate of HBV coinfection seen in patients infected with HIV likely reflects prior lifestyle practices that predispose to both infections. Markers of previous HBV infection, including core antigen (HBcAg) and antibodies to surface antigen (anti-HBsAg), are seen in 90% of patients infected with HIV. The highest coinfection rates are seen among homosexual males and intravenous drug users and in parts of the world where hepatitis B is endemic (i.e. Southeast Asia and sub-Sahara Africa); while other groups such as transfusion recipients and health care workers have a relatively low frequency of coinfection.

Since hepatic injury is mediated by the immune response to HBV, it is not surprising that the natural history of this disease is significantly altered in the presence of HIV coinfection. Following acute HBV infection, the virus is cleared in 95% of immunocompetent patients. In contrast, 50% of HIV-coinfected patients develop chronic infection. However, whether immunosuppression increases the severity of chronic hepatitis remains controversial. Immunosuppressed patients more frequently have markers of HBV replication in serum, including hepatitis B e-antigen (HBeAg) and HBV-DNA. Increased immunohistochemical staining for HBcAg and HBsAg in liver biopsy specimens has also been reported. Despite this, several case controlled series have suggested that HIV-coinfected patients may actually have milder disease, with less pronounced biochemical abnormalities and less inflammation, hepatocellular necrosis, and fibrosis on histologic examination. With regard to mortality from chronic liver disease, Scharschmidt et al. found no difference in survival up to 48 months between 35 patients with HIV–HBV coinfection and 70 patients infected with HIV alone, regardless of whether an AIDS defining condition was present. However similar studies by other authors have yielded contradictory results, with significantly decreased survival among HIV–HBV coinfected patients than among those infected with HIV alone.

Although vaccination against HBV has been recommended for all patients infected with HIV, the response to HBV vaccine appears to be suboptimal in these patients. In normal individuals, protective immunity develops in over 90% following HBV vaccination; however, two-thirds of HIV-infected patients have an absent, delayed, or inadequate immune response. The protection afforded by vaccination is also suboptimal among these patients, with a higher rate of loss of protective antibody to HBsAg over time compared with immunocompetent patients.

Historically, HIV rather than HBV infection was the major determinant of life expectancy for most patient, resulting in little enthusiasm or rationale for treatment of HBV in HIV-coinfected individuals. As the prognosis of patients infected with HIV improves due to rapid advances in antiretroviral therapy and disease management, the impetus to treat HBV infection in coinfected patients will increase. Unfortunately, treatment options remain limited. Interferon-α was until recently the only drug currently approved for treatment of chronic HBV. Human immunodeficiency virus-coinfected patients, however, have been identified in a meta-analysis as a subgroup with poor response to interferon. This finding was confirmed in a small controlled trial, in which an 8% response was seen in HIV-positive subjects, compared with 39% in controls.

The good news is that several antiviral drugs of the nucleoside analog class, such as lamivudine, also directly inhibit HBV replication. Thus, one can 'kill two birds with one stone' with these drugs. Moreover, in contrast to interferons, lamivudine is extremely well tolerated, with few side effects. Modulating the immune response in an immunosuppressed patient never held much promise. However, exactly how effective the antiviral drugs will be over the long term remains to be determined. The major limitation to their long-term use in HIV patients with hepatitis B is similar to the problem with their use in treating HIV: the development of viral mutations that encode for resistance to the antiviral. In the case of lamivudine, this occurs in the YMDD motif of the polymerase molecule, with an incidence of as high as 30% per year. While the mutant virus is relatively replication deficient, it remains unclear as to whether this translates into less severe clinical disease. Like the treatment of HIV, the use of multidrug combinations, using drugs with either different mechanisms of action or sites for the development of resistance, hold more promise for effective treatment of these patients in the future.

Hepatitis C

Hepatitis C virus coinfection is seen more commonly among intravenous drug users than in other risk groups for HIV, probably secondary to a shared parenteral mode of transmission. In immunocompetent patients, HCV follows a relatively indolent course, with progression to liver failure in a minority of patients over a time span that is measured in decades. However, an acceleration of this natural history is seen among patients coinfected with HIV. Similar to HBV, viral load, as measured by HCV-RNA levels, is greater among patients with HIV coinfection, and a higher risk of developing liver failure has been reported for coinfected hemophiliacs. Whether these patients are at increased risk for the development of hepatocellular carcinoma is unclear.

The risk of developing clinical liver disease increases with progression of the HIV infection as measured by p24 antigenemia and decreasing CD4 counts. However, in a cross-sectional study of 512 HIV-infected patients, Wright et al. found no difference in mortality among those with and without HCV, suggesting that, as with HBV, it is the still HIV infection rather than HCV that ultimately determines outcome in these patients. It also is important to point out that this study was performed in patients before the development of HAART. It is likely that the efficacy of HAART will increase the number of HCV-positive patients who develop clinically apparent liver disease, by decreasing the risk of death from HIV.

Another potential problem in patients with HIV–HCV coinfection is interaction with new antiretroviral therapies. Several cases of acute hepatic decompensation occurring in patients with underlying viral hepatitis have been reported in association with protease inhibitor therapy. Although it remains unclear whether hepatic decompensation was due to exacerbation of viral hepatitis itself or *de novo* hepatotoxicity (see below), such reports have led to recommendations by some authorities to avoid certain protease inhibitors in patients with HCV coinfection pending the results of more definitive studies.

As with HBV, treatment of HCV in HIV-coinfected patients remains problematic. Short-term response to interferon treatment in HIV-coinfected patients has been addressed by two small uncontrolled studies that suggested a reduction in levels of HCV-RNA and improved histology. However, the rate of sustained virologic responses is very low. Whether the combination if interferon and ribavirin will be more efficacious remains to be determined. Since many of these patients suffer from anemia, ribavirin will likely be difficult to give in full dose, given that its major side effect is hemolysis. With the absence of any clearly effective regimens and the questionable impact of HCV infection on the overall prognosis of patients with HIV, aggressive treatment cannot be recommended at the present time outside clinical research trials.

Neoplasms

Kaposi's sarcoma

The description in 1981, of cutaneous Kaposi's sarcoma among young, gay men was among the first clues leading to the recognition of the epidemic soon to be known as AIDS. It was later discovered that Kaposi's sarcoma was not merely a cutaneous process among patients with AIDS, but could disseminate in up to one-half of patients. The liver proved to be a common site of involvement, with hepatic nodules found in approximately one-third of patients on autopsy, generally in the setting of widespread visceral disease.

Kaposi's sarcoma appears to occur almost exclusively in homosexual men with AIDS, as opposed to other risk groups. Visceral disease occurs in the presence of cutaneous lesions and is often asymptomatic, although elevations of alkaline phosphatase may be seen when there is extensive involvement. Therefore, the diagnosis of hepatic Kaposi's sarcoma is most often made at the time of autopsy. Visceral involvement is associated with a poor prognosis, with less than 20% of patients surviving at 2 years. The presence of systemic symptoms is a particularly ominous prognostic factor. Histologically, the lesions are easily identified as solid dark red to purple nodules, filled with densely packed spindle-shaped endothelial cells that form slit-like vascular channels. Nodules are generally multifocal, occurring most commonly in the portal regions. Although lesions may respond to radio- or chemotherapy, hepatic disease is usually not treated unless symptomatic, since the nodules in themselves rarely are a direct cause of death or severe morbidity.

Non-Hodgkin's lymphoma

Reports of unusual cases of undifferentiated non-Hodgkin's lymphoma (NHL) occurring in homosexual men were another early manifestation of the AIDS epidemic. These neoplasms are primarily of B-cell origin. High-grade morphologic variants predominate, including large cell lymphoma, Burkitt's, and immunoblastic subtypes. Evidence implicating prior infection with Epstein–Barr virus (EBV) in the pathogenesis of NHL in patients with AIDS includes the documentation of EBV genomic fragments within tumor cells by DNA hybridization, as well as the universal presence of anti-EBV antibodies in patients with NHL.

Acquired immune deficiency virus-associated NHL is characterized by aggressive clinical behavior. Extranodal presentation is the norm, with the gastrointestinal tract following the bone marrow as the most common site of involvement. Although rare cases of primary hepatic lymphoma have been reported, liver involvement typically occurs in the setting of multiorgan disease. Three-quarters of patients with NHL in the setting of HIV infection experience systemic symptoms; however, the hepatic lesions themselves are generally asymptomatic. Dull right upper quadrant pain or jaundice can occasionally be seen with bulky tumors. Serum alkaline phosphatase elevations are most sensitive for hepatic involvement, with elevated transaminases and bilirubin in advanced disease. Prognosis is poor with a median survival of 5–6 months. Although approximately 50% of patients have been reported to respond to various chemotherapeutic regimens, disease-free intervals have been short and recurrence rates high. Overall survival, however, is no worse than that in AIDS patients without lymphoma, most likely because NHL usually accompanies advanced immunocompromise.

Drug-induced hepatotoxicity

Hepatotoxicity secondary to medications is a particularly important cause of abnormal liver function tests and clinical liver disease among patients infected with HIV. Risk factors for drug-induced hepatotoxicity include polypharmacy, as well as the poor nutritional status that often accompanies advanced disease. Fig. 14.2 lists common medications used in the treatment of patients infected with HIV that have been associated with hepatotoxicity. Trimethoprim–sulfamethoxazole is commonly used for treatment or prophylaxis of pneumocystis pneumonia. Elevations of liver enzymes are common with this drug, occurring in up to 50% of patients. A hepatitis-like pattern of transaminase elevation occurs most commonly; however, a cholestatic pattern may also be seen, especially in the setting of coexisting hepatic involvement with infection or neoplasm. Although discontinuation is rarely necessary, granulomatous hepatitis can occur. Antituberculous drugs including isoniazid and rifampin (rifampicin) are another common source of hepatotoxicity. Pentamidine also has been associated with elevated transaminases in approximately 15% of patients. Among antifungal agents, ketoconazole has traditionally been described as a common cause of hepatotoxicity; however, fluconazole is currently more widely prescribed. This agent has been associated with abnormal liver function tests in 16% of treated patients, but most patients can be retreated without recurrence.

Finally, antiretroviral agents, including protease inhibitors, have been associated with reports of severe acute hepatotoxicity and occasional acute liver failure. In terms of the nucleoside analogs, D4T may cause elevated liver tests. In terms of the protease inhibitors, hepatoxicity is a major complication. Indinavir, amprevavir, ritonavir, and saquinavir can all produce abnormal liver tests. In particular, indinavir commonly causes jaundice. All three of the non-nucleoside reverse transcriptase inhibitors delaviridine, efavirenz, and nevirapine may cause elevated liver tests. It is important to point out that in most cases the abnormalities are of little consequence. However, in the setting of pre-existing liver disease they can cause confusion. When feasible, a trial of medication withdrawal may uncover potential drug-induced hepatotoxicity in patients with abnormal liver enzymes. If liver biopsy is performed, the presence of eosinophilic granulomas without organisms also suggests a drug-induced etiology.

Liver transplantation

Human immunodeficiency virus is an important topic in liver transplantation for two reasons. First, before adequate screening of blood and organ donors, HIV acquisition was not uncommon before and during the transplant procedure. However, at present, this is of historic interest, as this is now an extremely rare occurrence. Second, while HIV infection has been regarded as an absolute contraindication to liver transplantation, the success of HAART has lead some programs to reconsider this position.

The rationale for offering liver transplantation to HIV-positive patients is as follows. Most programs believe that if a patient has less than 50% chance of surviving 5 years after orthotopic liver transplantation (OLT), OLT is contraindicated. If you accept this, and that the expected survival rate for even the very best candidates is 75% at 5 years, any comorbid condition that carries an independent mortality of greater than 30% within 5 years represents a contraindication to OLT. Human immunodeficiency virus treatment experts have stated that HIV-positive patients with no diagnosis of AIDS, who are HIV RNA-negative on antiviral therapy and who have a CD4 count greater than 300/mL likely meet these criteria.

However, others have questioned the wisdom of transplanting such patients for the following reasons. First, HAART utilizes drugs with a high potential for drug interactions with immunosuppressive medications or hepatotoxicity. Second, an adequate CD4 count does not preclude deletions of specific T-cell populations (e.g. against CMV), that may predispose these patients to certain opportunistic infections after liver transplantation. Finally, post-transplant T-cell activation could lead to enhanced HIV replication, which may increase the chance of developing drug resistance or developing AIDS.

The metabolism of the drugs used to treat HIV infection is complex and varies by the class of drug. Nucleoside analogs are most commonly renally excreted. Zidovudine (azidothymidine) undergoes glucuronidation. Several of these drugs interact with medications commonly used prophylactically against common post-transplant infections, including trimethoprim–sulfamethoxazole, dapsone, and gancyclovir.

Both of the calcineurin inhibitors cyclosporine and tacrolimus, which generally represent the cornerstone of most immunosuppressive regimens, undergo hepatic metabolism by the cytochrome P450 protein CYP 3A4. Drugs that either induce or inhibit P450 activity may effect the metabolism of these medications, which may impact the patient's level of immunosuppression. Most of the protease inhibitors used against HIV, including amprenavir, indinavir, nelfinavir, and ritonavir, are CYP 3A4 metabolized. Similarly

Common hepatotoxic drugs in AIDS
Trimethoprim–sulfamethoxazole
Isoniazid
Pentamidine
Rifampin (rifampicin)
Fluconazole/ketoconozole
Zidovudine (azidothymidine)
Didanosine

Figure 14.2 Common hepatotoxic drugs in AIDS.

most of the non-nucleoside reverse transcriptase inhibitors, including delaviridine, efavirenz, and nevirapine, are CYP 3A4 metabolized. Thus, one will need to closely monitor cyclosporine and tacrolimus blood levels when administering these in the presence of the HAART medications. This issue of drug interactions occurring as a result of changing P450 activity applies not only to immunosuppressive medications, but also to other P450 metabolized drugs that are dose-critical , such as coumadin (warfarin).

Not only are there interactions with the calcineurin inhibitors, one also needs to be of aware of interactions with other immunosuppressive agents (i.e. mycophenolate mofetil and azathioprine), most notably in terms of synergistic bone marrow depression.

There have been several reports of HIV patients who have undergone liver transplantation. One such report is of 26 men with hemophilia underwent OLT between 1982 and 1996; 23% were HIV-positive. In terms of the liver disease these patients suffered from, 69% had hepatitis C alone, 12% hepatocellular carcinoma, and 15% HBV. In this group, liver transplantation was very effective for hemophilia as the median time to normal factor VIII activity was 24 hours. While the survival rates in the in the HIV-negative subset was 90 and 83% at 1 and 3 years respectively, the 1- and 3-year survival rates in the HIV-positive subset were only 67 and 23%. In the patients with hepatitis C, the disease reportedly recurred in only six of 20.

A second report detailed the course of 88 HIV transplant recipients, 22 were HIV-positive before transplantation, while the rest acquired HIV as a result of the transplant procedure. A total of 28% developed AIDS after transplantation; 80% of those died of AIDS-associated complications after a mean of 37 months. The mean time to AIDS in patients with pretransplantation HIV infection was 17 months. It is important to emphasize that these patients were untreated.

The number of HIV–HCV coinfected patients referred for OLT will only increase. Whether HIV infection, in the absence of a diagnosis of AIDS, should be an absolute contraindication for OLT, remains to be determined. If liver transplantation is judged appropriate for HIV-positive patients, drug interactions and the potential for hepatotoxicity will be real problems and will require careful monitoring of drug levels.

DIAGNOSIS AND MANAGEMENT

Several tenets should guide the evaluation of patients infected with HIV who present with abnormal liver function tests and/or clinical manifestations of liver disease. First, although hepatic abnormalities are nearly ubiquitous among these patients, they rarely cause significant morbidity in and of themselves, and are virtually never directly responsible for death. Second, hepatic involvement by opportunistic infections or neoplasms generally occurs in the setting of disseminated, multiorgan disease. In the majority of cases, such processes can more readily be diagnosed from extrahepatic sites as opposed to by liver biopsy. Finally, many of these disseminated processes are poorly amenable to treatment. In contrast, primary biliary processes in patients infected with HIV are frequently symptomatic, may be fatal, and often are amenable to curative or palliative intervention. As such, they require an aggressive diagnostic and therapeutic approach.

An algorithm for the clinical evaluation of liver function test abnormalities in patients infected with HIV is presented in

Fig. 14.3. A cholestatic pattern should prompt evaluation of the patency of the biliary tree. In most situations, this will be accomplished most expeditiously and cost-effectively by transabdominal ultrasound. Patients with dilated bile ducts should be evaluated with cholangiography, and if a focal cause of obstruction is found endoscopic or surgical intervention is indicated (Fig. 14.4).

In the presence of a normal biliary tree, or if a hepatocellular pattern of biochemical abnormalities is present, a diligent search for reversible etiologies of liver disease should be performed. This includes a review of all medications for potential hepatotoxins, as well as careful history and physical examination to search for manifestations of opportunistic infection or neoplasm in other organ systems. The role of liver biopsy in these patients remains controversial. Histologic abnormalities are found in almost all patients who undergo biopsy; however, the majority of these are nonspecific and do not lead to significant changes in management or prognosis. Schneiderman et al. reported abnormal histologic findings in 89% of 103 patients undergoing biopsy or autopsy at San Francisco General Hospital. The prevalence of such abnormalities led to initial enthusiasm regarding liver biopsy; however, subsequent series have shown that the yield of specific *treatable* diagnoses is low. Furthermore, many of the diagnoses that are made from liver biopsy could be made by less invasive means, such as blood cultures and aspirates of bone marrow or lymph nodes. In the San Francisco General Hospital study, only 8% of liver biopsies resulted in a new diagnosis. Because liver biopsy rarely provides unique information to influence management or improve survival, it is not recommended for routine

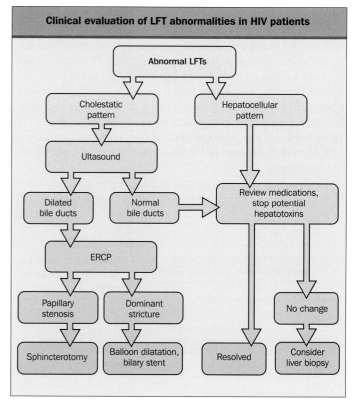

Figure 14.3 Clinical evaluation of liver function test (LFT) abnormalities in HIV patients. ERCP, endoscopic retrograde cholangiopancreatography.

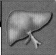

evaluation of abnormal liver function tests among patients infected with HIV. Its use should be restricted to situations where severe symptoms and marked biochemical abnormalities are present and less invasive tests have proved unrevealing.

SUMMARY

Hepatobiliary disease is common in patients with HIV. This often reflects coexistent disease with similar modes of acquisition (e.g. hepatitis B and C). However, the liver disease may also reflect the presence of one the AIDS-defining complications. An emerging problem is drug toxicity, associated the ever growing number of antiretroviral medications, generally used in various combinations. The evaluation of HIV-positive patients with liver test abnormalities should focus on identifying reversible causes of liver and biliary tract disease. Finally, as patients with HIV infection live longer, the treatment of liver diseases such as hepatitis C will take on greater importance. This likely will include liver transplantation for those patients who develop end-stage liver disease.

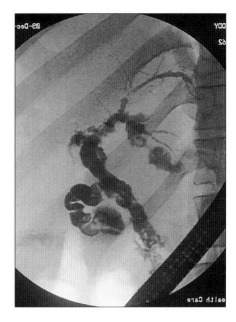

Figure 14.4 Aids cholangiopathy. ERCP demonstrates a diffuse stricturing of the intrahepatic and extrahepatic bile ducts similar to primary sclerosing cholangitis.

FURTHER READING

Bonacini M, Nussbaum J, Ahluwalia C. Gastrointestinal, hepatic, and pancreatic involvement with *Cryptococcus neoformans* in AIDS. J Clin Gastroenterol. 1990;12:295–7. *Small case series of disseminated cryptococcosis.*

Cohen O, Stoeckle M. Extrapulmonary pneumocystis carinii infection in the acquired immune deficiency syndrome. Arch Intern Med. 1991;151:1205–14. *Review of 39 reported cases of extrapulmonary pneumocystis infection in patients with AIDS.*

Goldin R, Fish D, Hay A. Histological and immunohistochemical study of hepatitis B virus in human immunodeficiency virus. J Clin Pathol. 1990;43:203–5. *Compared markers of replication and histologic findings in 20 patients infected with HIV, and 30 controls.*

Knowles D, Chamulak G, Subar M. Lymphoid neoplasia associated with the acquired immune deficiency syndrome. Ann Intern Med. 1988;108:744–53. *Large case series of 105 patients with HIV-associated lymphoma.*

Krogsgaard K, Lindhardt B, Nielson J. The influence of HTLV-III infection on the natural history of hepatitis B virus infection in male homosexual HbsAg carriers. Hepatology. 1987;7:37–41. *Longitudinal study of markers of HBV replication in homosexual men.*

Lebovics E, Thung S, Schaffner F, Radensky P. The liver in the acquired immune deficiency syndrome: a clinical and histologic study. Hepatology. 1985;5:293. *Case series of liver biopsy results in patients with AIDS.*

Perkocha L, Geaghan S, Yen T. Clinical and pathological features of bacillary peliosis hepatitis in association with human immunodeficiency virus infection. N Engl J Med. 1990;232:1581–6. *Early study linking the causative agent of HIV-associated peliosis hepatitis to that of cutaneous bacillary angiomatosis.*

Scharschmidt B, Held M, Hollander H. Hepatitis B in patients with HIV infection: relationship to AIDS and patient survival. Ann Intern Med. 1992;117:837. *Compared survival among patients with chronic HBV infection, with and without HIV coinfection.*

Schneiderman D, Arensen D, Cello J. Hepatic disease in patients with the acquired immune deficiency syndrome (AIDS). Hepatology. 1987;7:925. *Large series of liver biopsy and autopsy results from patients with AIDS at San Francisco General Hospital.*

Wong D, Colina Y, Naylor C. Interfon alpha treatment of chronic hepatitis B: randomized trial in a predominantly homosexual male population. Gastroenterology. 1996;108:165–71. *Randomized trial of interferon therapy in patients with HBV and HIV coinfection.*

Wright T, Hollander H, Pu X. Hepatitis C in HIV-infected patients with and without AIDS: prevalence and relationship to patient survival. Hepatology. 1994;20:1152–5. *Cross-sectional study of mortality patients infected with HIV, with and without HCV coinfection.*

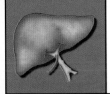

INTRODUCTION

Infectious agents frequently involve the liver, either as the primary target organ or as part of multiorgan infection. The portal venous circulation and the biliary tract provide convenient routes of invasion for pathogens emanating from the gastrointestinal tract. Furthermore, the rich vascular supply to the liver renders it susceptible to secondary infection as a consequence of severe systemic infections. Parasitic infections of the liver were once relatively uncommon in Western countries, but with the increasing number of immigrants from developing nations, the frequency of these infections appears to be on the rise. This chapter reviews the important nonviral hepatobiliary infections, with an emphasis on clinical diagnosis and management.

PYOGENIC LIVER ABSCESS

Historic background

The first case of pyogenic liver abscess was described in 1846 and was secondary to appendicitis. In the preantibiotic era, pyogenic liver abscess typically occurred in young individuals with appendicitis and associated pylephlebitis. In recent years, most cases of pyogenic liver abscess have been attributed to biliary tract disease or a cryptogenic etiology. The first successful use of an antibiotic, sulfanilamide, in conjunction with surgical drainage for multiple hepatic abscesses was in 1938. In 1953 successful treatment of pyogenic abscess by percutaneous drainage was reported. The mortality from pyogenic liver abscess has decreased from almost 100% in preantibiotic era to 10–25% in recent reports.

Epidemiology

Pyogenic liver abscess is responsible for approximately 8–15 per 100,000 hospital admissions. Worldwide, amebic liver abscesses are more common, whereas in Western countries pyogenic abscesses are more frequently seen. Pyogenic abscesses most often occur in patients over 40 years of age, with a peak incidence in the sixth decade. This is in contrast to early reports in which a majority of cases occurred in young adults. This change in presentation appears to be a direct result of the changing etiology, with biliary tract disease accounting for many more cases in recent years than acute appendicitis. Liver abscess occurs slightly more often in males, but all races appear equally affected.

Etiology and pathogenesis

In the preantibiotic era, pyogenic liver abscess typically occurred in the setting of severe appendicitis with associated pylephlebitis. Bacterial pathogens can enter the liver via both the hepatic arterial or portal venous circulation. Hepatic arterial dissemination results from a systemic bacteremia, whereas portal venous spread more often complicates intra-abdominal infections, such as diverticulitis, peritonitis, or postoperative infections.

Recent studies implicate the biliary tract as the most common source of pyogenic liver abscess. Cholangitis, occurring as a result of either benign or malignant biliary obstruction or as a consequence of endoscopic, radiologic or operative intervention, as well as gallstone disease, are frequent predisposing factors. In these cases multiple abscesses are typically present. Penetrating wounds may lead to solitary, or less commonly multiple liver abscesses. Included within this category would be iatrogenic causes, such as liver biopsy and surgical procedures. Cases of pyogenic abscess without an apparent cause, cryptogenic abscess, seem to be more frequent now than in the past.

Parasitic invasion of the biliary tree by roundworms or flukes may be associated with biliary infection and pyogenic abscess. Likewise, secondary infection of an amebic abscess, hydatid cyst, hematoma, biloma, or liver metastasis can also occur. Liver abscess after embolization of hepatic tumors has also been described.

Microbiology

Escherichia coli is the most frequently isolated organism in cases of pyogenic liver abscess. Other Gram-negative bacilli, including species of *Klebsiella*, *Proteus*, and *Pseudomonas*, and Gram-positive enteric organisms such as *Enterococcus faecalis* and *Enterococcus faecium* are also frequently isolated. *Staphylococcus aureus* and *Streptococcus pyogenes* are uncommon isolates, except in patients with penetrating trauma. *Yersinia* spp. have been reported in patients with hemochromatosis. Recurrent pyogenic cholangitis due to *Salmonella typhi* is an infrequent cause. Infections with anaerobic organisms are increasingly recognized as a cause of pyogenic abscess. The most commonly isolated anaerobic organisms include the following: *Bacteroides* spp., *Fusobacterium* spp., *Actinomyces* spp., and rarely *Clostridia* spp. Some authors consider the microaerophilic streptococci to be among the most important causes of liver abscess. Polymicrobial infections are often present (Fig. 15.1).

Pathology

The liver may contain one or more abscesses. Multiple abscesses are typically seen in blood-borne infections and in infections occurring as a result of cholangitis. Liver abscesses are more commonly seen in the right lobe of the liver. When there is an associated pylephlebitis, the portal vein and its branches may contain pus and blood clots. The abscess typically is composed of necrotic

Microbiology of pyogenic liver abscess

Gram-negative organisms: *E. coli*, *Klebsiella* spp., *Proteus* spp., *Pseudomonas* spp.

Gram-positive organisms: *Enterococcus* spp., *Staphylococcus* spp., *Streptococcus* spp.

Anaerobic organisms: *Bacteroides* spp., *Fusobacterium* spp., anaerobic streptococci (*Peptostreptococcus* and *Peptococcus* spp.), and rarely *Clostridium* spp.

Micro-aerophilic organisms: *Streptococcus milleri*

Miscellaneous: *Haemophilus* spp., *Yersinia* spp., and *Actinomycosis* spp.

Figure 15.1 Microbiology of pyogenic liver abscess. The main causative organisms fall into five main categories and culture techniques should reflect the diversity of potential causes.

liver tissue with a marked polymorphonuclear cell infiltrate surrounded by a fibrous capsule.

Clinical features

The clinical history may reveal previous biliary tract disease, abdominal pathology, or a history of surgery or instrumentation. Abdominal pain and fever are the two most common symptoms. The onset may be acute, but more commonly is subacute with malaise, anorexia, nausea, vomiting, and weight loss. Individuals harboring multiple abscesses may present with more severe symptoms. The pain is usually localized to the right upper quadrant, but diffuse abdominal pain is also common. Large abscesses and those involving the dome of the liver result in subdiaphragmatic irritation; these patients often present with right shoulder pain and coughing. Elderly or immunosuppressed patients may present with a paucity of symptoms. Fever with right upper quadrant tenderness or a tender right upper quadrant mass may be present on physical examination, but their absence does not exclude the diagnosis. Jaundice is generally a late finding, unless the abscess

Signs and symptoms of pyogenic liver abscess

Symptoms and signs	No. (%) of patients (total number = 89)
Abdominal pain	74 (89)
Fever 38°C	56 (67)
Chills	40 (48)
Anorexia	22 (27)
Malaise	14 (17)
Weight loss	11 (13)
Mental confusion	6 (7)
RUQ tenderness	58 (70)
Jaundice	20 (24)
Hepatomegaly	6 (7)

Figure 15.2 Signs and symptoms of pyogenic liver abscess. The frequency of the main signs and symptoms are shown. RUQ, right upper quadrant.

occurs as a result of biliary obstruction. The relative frequency of signs and symptoms in patients presenting with pyogenic abscess are listed in Fig. 15.2.

Diagnosis

Routine blood tests are often abnormal, but the abnormalities are nonspecific. Almost half the patients have hemoglobin below 12g/dL. Leukocytosis with left shift and elevated sedimentation rates are seen in more then 75% of patients. Nonspecific liver enzyme abnormalities are common and include hyperbilirubinemia, as well as mild elevations of alkaline phosphatase and aminotransferases. A poor outcome has been associated with patients presenting with an elevated prothrombin time and a serum albumin <2g/dL (20g/L).

Diagnostic imaging plays a key role in establishing the diagnosis, although distinguishing amebic abscess from a pyogenic abscess may not be possible (Figs 15.3 & 15.4). Computed tomography scanning has a sensitivity of 95–100% for detecting liver abscess. A pyogenic abscess typically appears as a hypodense lesion with smooth margins on CT imaging. Ultrasonography is slightly less sensitive but appears to have a higher specificity.

Blood cultures may be positive in 50–90% of cases depending on culture techniques and specimen handling. Diagnostic aspiration of the abscess cavity is recommended when blood cultures are negative and in the absence of an adequate response to empiric antibiotic therapy. The aspirated material should be cultured for aerobic, anaerobic, and microaerophilic organisms.

Prognosis

The mortality without treatment approaches 100%. The combination of needle aspiration and antibiotic therapy has reduced the overall mortality to between 10 and 25%. The survival for patients with a solitary pyogenic abscess is better (90%) than for patients with multiple abscesses (40%). Poor prognostic signs include the following: delayed diagnosis, old age, hyperbilirubenemia, coexisting medical conditions, multiple abscesses, pleural effusion, and hypoalbuminemia. Cryptogenic abscesses appear to have a better prognosis and lower mortality rate (5%).

Treatment

Antibiotics are the mainstay of therapy for pyogenic liver abscess and should be started as soon as the diagnosis is suspected. Combination antibiotic therapy consisting of ampicillin, aminoglycoside, and metronidazole is the most frequently employed regimen. In many centers, however, the prevalence of resistant strains of Enterobacteriaceae has resulted in the use of either a third- or fourth-generation cephalosporin, a fluoroquinolone, or at β-lactam/β-lactamase inhibitor antibiotic combination (i.e. ampicillin/sulbactam, ticarcillin/clavulinic acid, piperacillin/tazobactam) in place of ampicillin and an aminoglycoside for initial empiric therapy. Subsequent antibiotic therapy should be adjusted according to the results of bacterial culture and sensitivity reports. In most situations, patients require a prolonged course of antibiotics, consisting of an initial 2–3 week course of intravenous antibiotics, followed by 2–6 additional weeks of a suitable oral antibiotic.

While many patients respond to treatment with antibiotics alone, patients with large or complex abscess cavities often fail to respond to antibiotics. Thus, antibiotic therapy should be combined with a drainage procedure in most cases. Before the

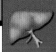

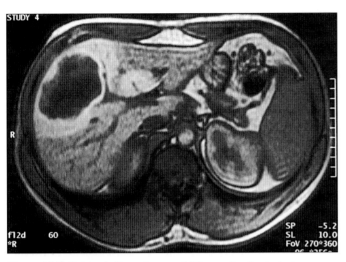

Figure 15.3 Pyogenic liver abscess. MRI scan showing typical appearances of solitary pyogenic liver abscess.

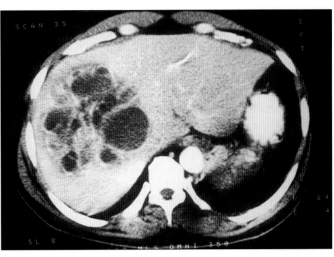

Figure 15.4 Pyogenic liver abscess. CT scan of a *Klebsiella* liver abscess with the complex matrix and internal septation typical of this organism.

widespread availability of CT and ultrasound imaging, surgical drainage was considered the treatment of choice. Ultrasound- or CT-guided percutaneous abscess drainage has largely supplanted surgical drainage in recent years. The success rate of percutaneous drainage combined with antibiotic therapy is now greater than 90%. Ultrasound- and CT-guided drainage work best in patients with a solitary abscess. Radiologic drainage procedures can be used successfully in patients with multiple abscesses cavities and in those with cavities containing necrotic material. In cases where percutaneous drainage fails to drain the abscess cavity adequately, surgical drainage may be necessary.

A combined approach utilizing antibiotics and percutaneous drainage appears to be the most effective treatment for patients with pyogenic liver abscess. Antibiotic therapy alone is best suited for patients with multiple small abscesses that are not amenable to percutaneous drainage. Surgical therapy should be reserved for selected cases where percutaneous drainage is unsuccessful, when there is coexisting intra-abdominal disease requiring surgery, and is situations where abscesses are complicated by rupture or extension into adjacent structures.

HEPATIC AMEBIASIS

The first case of amebic liver abscess was described in 1890. In 1912, emetine was introduced as the first drug active against amebiasis. The major breakthrough in the treatment of amebiasis came in 1966 with the introduction of metronidazole therapy.

Lifecycle
The amebic lifecycle is simple and consists of two stages: the cyst and trophozoite stages. Amebic disease is generally acquired by ingesting food or water contaminated with feces containing the cyst (Fig. 15.5). In the small intestine the cyst wall undergoes digestion allowing the amebae to develop into invasive trophozoites. The trophozoites travel to the proximal colon where they take up residence, dependent on the presence of bacteria for survival. Under the influence of triggering mechanisms that are as yet unknown, the trophozoites become large and invade the mucosa causing invasive colonic disease (i.e. amebic dysentery). In some cases the invasive

trophozoites are carried via the portal circulation to the liver, resulting in the formation of an abscess. Humans are the only known host for *Entamoeba histolytica*. As trophozoites are not always invasive, the mere presence of trophozoites or cysts in stool does not confirm the diagnosis of amebic liver abscess.

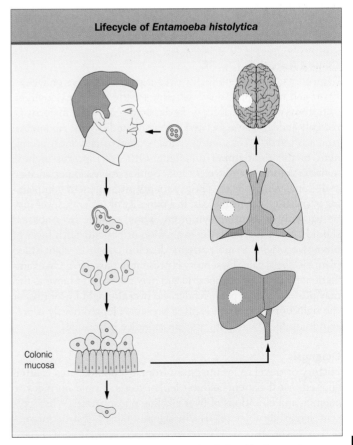

Figure 15.5 Life cycle of *Entamoeba histolytica*. The ingested organism proliferates in the colon (dysentery) and leads to systemic invasion (abscess formation) and/or fecal shedding.

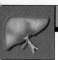

Epidemiology

It has been estimated that *E. histolytica* is responsible for about 40,000 deaths worldwide annually. The disease is very common in developing tropical and subtropical countries, mainly due to poor sanitary and hygienic conditions. High rates of amebic infection have been reported from India, sub-Saharan regions of Africa, and within areas of South and Central America. Amebiasis occurs with equal frequency in men and women; however, amebic abscesses and extraintestinal disease occurs 3–10 times more often in men. Infections occurring in developed countries are usually confined to certain high-risk groups, including travelers, immigrants, prisoners, and homosexual males. Even though the intestinal occurrence of *E. histolytica* is much higher in homosexuals, the incidence of amebic dysentery or liver abscess is not increased in patients with acquired immune deficiency syndrome. This may be due to the fact that majority of homosexuals are infected with nonpathogenic strain of amebae.

Pathology

The right lobe of the liver is more often involved than the left. Most often the abscesses are found under the dome of the diaphragm. There may be one or more abscess cavities present. The abscess typically has a necrotic center containing material resulting from the lysis of liver cells, red blood cells, and connective tissue. This gives the abscess fluid its typical 'anchovy paste' appearance. Leukocytes are usually absent, which is in contrast to pyogenic abscess in which leukocytes are found in large numbers. Amebae are typically absent from the abscess fluid, but can be found adjacent to the fibrinous wall of the abscess invading normal liver tissue. Secondary bacterial infections occur in 20% of cases, resulting in the presence of green or yellow pus.

Clinical features

Symptoms develop gradually, over a period of days or weeks. Fever and right upper quadrant pain are the two most common symptoms of amebic abscess. Fever is present in the majority of patients and is often associated with chills and sweats. Abdominal pain is often dull, constant in character, and usually most prominent in the right upper quadrant. Other symptoms include malaise, vomiting, and weight loss. Some patients experience no abdominal pain or fever. These patients often present complaining of malaise and weight loss. In a minority of patients, fever may be the only presenting symptom. Thus, amebic liver abscess should be considered in the evaluation of patients with fever of unknown origin. Some patients develop cough or right-sided pleuritic chest pain. Dysentery is present in only 10%. On examination, patients often appear ill and may not want to move as this may provoke severe pain. Tenderness over the right lower ribs, or the right upper quadrant is often present. Hepatomegaly is present in up to 50% of patients, but jaundice is unusual.

Diagnosis

History of travel to, or migration from an endemic area is often elicited. Most patients exhibit leukocytosis, a mild normocytic anemia, and elevations of liver alkaline phosphatase. When present, hyperbilirubinemia usually signifies biliary obstruction secondary to the abscess or bacterial superinfection. Abnormal chest radiographs are common and may mimic a right lower lobe pneumonia. Technetium 99m sulfur colloid scans and gallium scan lack specificity. Ultrasound and CT scans are useful in localizing the abscess as well as following the response to treatment, but distinction from pyogenic abscess may be difficult. Aspiration of the abscess is now rarely necessary for establishing the diagnosis due to the high sensitivity of serologic tests. Both, the indirect hemagglutination test and enzyme-linked immunosorbent assay (ELISA) are sensitive and positive in over 90% of cases. An amebic abscess is unlikely if these tests are negative, except early in the course of infection. These antibodies may persist for years following an acute infection, and a positive test should be correlated with the clinical and radiologic findings in patients from endemic areas. Newer tests employing recombinant antigens, detection of IgM antibodies, and DNA probes may offer improved sensitivity for the diagnosis of acute infections.

Treatment

Metronidazole, 750mg three times a day for 5–10 days is curative in over 90% of cases. Clinical improvement is usually seen within 3–5 days, although the abscess cavity may take weeks or even months to disappear. A single dose of tinidazole is effective but this drug is not currently available in the USA. Alternative agents include dehydroemetine and chloroquine phosphate. Unlike pyogenic abscesses, needle aspiration or abscess drainage offers no additional therapeutic benefit. Aspiration may be indicated for very large abscesses, for abscesses involving the left lobe, where rupture is believed to be imminent, and in those patients with persistent symptoms after 5 days of metronidazole treatment in whom bacterial superinfection must be excluded. Surgical drainage is indicated when percutaneous drainage fails or cannot be effectively performed. A luminal amebicide, paramomycin or iodoquinol, is often used to eradicate intestinal carriage of the organism. Metronidazole alone may eradicate luminal amebae when used for 10 days or more.

Complications

Rupture is the most common complication and can occur into the pericardial, peritoneal, and pleural cavities, as well as into other intra-abdominal organs. Patients may present with symptoms of pericardial effusion or pericarditis. Rupture into the chest often occurs on the right side and can result in an hepatobronchial fistula or amebic empyema. However, sterile sympathetic effusions are far more common than the effusion secondary to rupture, however. The formation of an hepatobronchial fistula may present as hemoptysis. Rupture into the peritoneal cavity often results as peritonitis. Other complications are rare and include hemobilia and reversible portal hypertension.

Prognosis

With early diagnosis and management, the mortality in uncomplicated cases is less then 1% with an overall mortality of 2–18%. Predictors of poor prognosis include: hyperbilirubinemia, encephalopathy, hypoalbuminemia [serum albumin level less then 2.0g/dL (20g/L)], and multiple abscesses.

Prevention

Contaminated food or water is the most common source of infection. Travelers to endemic areas should follow general guidelines for avoiding enteric infections. The efforts to develop a vaccine against *E. histolytica* appear promising, with recombinant versions of three amebic antigens having shown protective efficacy in animal models.

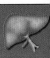

ECHINOCOCCOSIS (HYDATID DISEASE)

Epidemiology

Four species are recognized within the genus *Echinococcus*. The most clinically relevant form is cystic echinococcosis (hydatid disease) caused by *Echinococcus granulosus*. This species is endemic to many parts of the world including sheep-raising areas of South and Central America, Mediterranean countries, the Middle east, Central Asia, and Northern China, as well as certain areas of New Zealand, Australia, and Canada. The incidence varies according to geographic region and ranges from as low as 13/100,000 in Greece to as high as 220/100,000 in the Turkana district of Kenya. The parasite has been eradicated from Iceland. Infection in the USA is most often imported from endemic areas. Echinococcosis involves patients of all ages but peak incidence is seen in young adults between the ages 20 and 40 years.

Lifecycle

The adult tapeworm, which measures about 3–4mm in length, inhabits the small intestine of dogs, the definitive host (Fig. 15.6). The adult worm produces eggs that are released to the environment. Sheep, cattle, and men are intermediate hosts. Infection of the intermediate host, including humans, occurs through eating food contaminated with dog feces containing the infectious eggs. After ingestion of eggs, the oncospheres hatch in the stomach or small intestine, become activated, penetrate the epithelial layer, and migrate via blood and lymphatic vessels to the visceral organs, primarily the liver, where they develop to another larval stage, the metacestode. The definitive host acquires the infection by eating

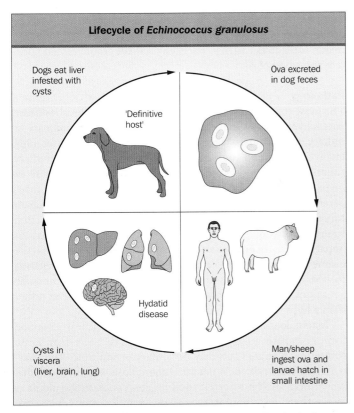

Lifecycle of *Echinococcus granulosus*

Dogs eat liver infested with cysts

Ova excreted in dog feces

'Definitive host'

Cysts in viscera (liver, brain, lung)

Hydatid disease

Man/sheep ingest ova and larvae hatch in small intestine

Figure 15.6 Lifecycle of *Echinococcus granulosus*. The dog is the definitive, but not exclusive, host and the liver lung and brain are the main target organs affected by abscesses.

organs from the intermediate host containing the metacestode, completing the lifecycle. *Echinococcus* spp. require two mammalian hosts for completion of the lifecycle and direct transmission from human to human does not occur.

Pathology

Cyst size usually ranges between 1 and 15cm, although larger cysts have been reported. Each cyst has an outer membrane known as an endocyst. The endocyst consists of an outer layer and an inner germinal layer. The germinal layer gives rise to protoscolices. The cysts containing protoscolices are known as fertile, while the cysts without protoscolices are sterile. Rupture or accidental opening of fertile cysts can cause dissemination of echinococcosis. Within large cysts, smaller daughter cysts of various sizes may be formed. The thin layer of host tissue surrounding the hepatic cysts is the pericyst.

Clinical features

Echinococcus granulosus commonly involves the liver, but other organs, including the lungs, kidneys, spleen, bone, and brain, may also be involved. Most patients have single organ involvement and harbor a solitary cyst. The simultaneous involvement of two organs is seen less often. The right lobe of the liver is affected more often then the left lobe.

Small *E. granulosus* cysts (<5cm) are almost always asymptomatic. As the cysts grow, they may cause pressure-related symptoms. Patients usually present with a low-grade fever and vague abdominal pain. The diagnosis is often delayed due to subtle symptoms. An enlarged, tender liver may be found on examination. Acute immunologic reactions, such as asthma or anaphylactic shock, may be the first, often life-threatening clinical manifestation of hydatid disease. Rupture of a cyst into the biliary tree may mimic biliary colic, or present with symptoms of cholangitis, biliary obstruction, or acute pancreatitis. If the cyst becomes infected, the presenting features are identical to those seen with a pyogenic liver abscess. Membranous glomerulonephritis is an uncommon complication of hydatid disease.

Diagnosis

In cystic echinococcosis (CE) routine tests are often nonspecific. Liver chemistries may be normal or suggestive of cholestasis. Hypergammaglobulinemia is observed in approximately 30% of cases and eosinophilia in less then 15%. Ultrasonography may show solitary or multiple round or spheric cystic lesions (Fig. 15.7). Typically the cysts appears anechoic with well-defined margins. This may be difficult to distinguish from benign serous cysts. Some cysts may exhibit echodense areas within the cyst and be difficult to differentiate from an abscess or neoplasm. In most cases, CT scanning allows for better definition of the location, size, and morphology of the cysts than does ultrasonography. In one study, CT alone allowed for a correct diagnosis in 61% of 120 patients with CE involving the liver, lung, kidneys, and spleen. When combined with serologic testing, CT scanning will establish the correct diagnosis in more than 90% of cases. Magnetic resonance imaging appears to offer no major advantage over CT in the diagnosis of hydatid cyst.

Immunodiagnostic tests are available to detect specific serum antibodies or antigens. The indirect hemagglutination test (IHAT) and the ELISA are the most widely used methods for the detection of echinococcal antibodies. Approximately 10% of patients

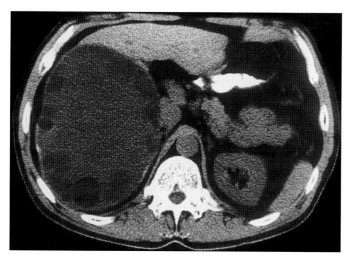

Figure 15.7 Hydatid cyst. Typical CT appearances of hydatid cyst with characteristic 'daughter cysts'.

with hepatic hydatid cyst and up to 40% of patients with extra-hepatic disease may fail to produce detectable serum antibodies, resulting in a false-negative IHAT test. Enzyme-linked immunosorbent assay appears to offer similar sensitivity to that of IHAT. False-positive results may be seen due to cross-reactivity with noncestode parasites. The arc-5 test for the detection of cestode-specific antibodies can be used to exclude cross-reactions caused by noncestode parasites.

Diagnostic puncture of the cyst is not recommended and carries the risk of anaphylactic reactions or dissemination. Ultrasound- or CT-guided needle aspiration may be performed for diagnosis if the serologic studies are negative for echinococcosis and the radiologic studies are inconclusive.

Treatment

Surgery remains the treatment of choice in CE. The perioperative instillation of protoscolicidal agents (ethanol, hypertonic saline) to prevent recurrence is controversial and carries the risk of inducing sclerosing cholangitis as a late complication in patients harboring a communication between the cysts and the biliary tree. Favorable results have been reported with the preoperative administration of albendazole. In recent years there have been reports of laparoscopic treatment of hydatid cyst with mixed results. The benefits of this approach over conventional surgery have yet to be determined.

The PAIR method (Puncture of cyst percutaneously, Aspiration of fluid, Introduction of protoscolicidal agent, and Re-aspiration) has been described recently as an alternative to surgery. Albendazole is used before and after the aspiration. Studies have shown results comparable to those of cystectomy with shorter hospital stays and reduced costs in patients undergoing PAIR therapy. The incidence of anaphylaxis in patients undergoing aspiration was negligible in the recent studies. Currently the World Health Organization (WHO) recommends this technique for patients who are not candidates for surgery or who refuse surgery. Even though this technique needs further evaluation, it appears to be a promising alternative to surgery.

Chemotherapy with benzimidazoles (mebendazole or albendazole) is clinically effective in about 30% of cases. The WHO recommends that chemotherapy should be reserved for patients with inoperable disease or after incomplete surgery. It is also indicated for prevention of secondary echinococcosis after spontaneous or traumatic rupture of cyst.

HEPATIC TUBERCULOSIS

Tuberculosis was almost eradicated from the USA following World War II. However, in the 1970s and 1980s mass migration from countries where tuberculosis is endemic, together with the emergence of a new and uniquely susceptible group of immuno-compromised individuals due to human immunodeficiency virus (HIV) infection, has radically changed the picture.

Epidemiology

The true incidence of hepatic tuberculosis is unknown, but in a study of patients with pulmonary tuberculosis, 75% were found to have histologic abnormalities on liver biopsies, including granuloma formation in 25%. In another series, hepatic involvement was found in up to 80% of patients dying from pulmonary tuberculosis. The impact of the HIV epidemic on the overall incidence of hepatic tuberculosis is unclear, but extrapulmonary disease is much more common in HIV-positive patients and a number of recent case reports suggest it may be significant.

Pathogenesis

Hepatic involvement most likely occurs as a consequence of hematogenous spread from the primary source, in most cases the lungs. Pulmonary involvement can be demonstrated in up to 90% of patients presenting with hepatic tuberculosis. *Mycobacterium bovis* infection of the liver is rare, even in developing countries where pasteurization is not routinely performed. Involvement of the liver in tuberculosis has been reported to occur in several forms that can be broadly classified into two major categories: diffuse parenchymal tuberculosis and focal hepatic tuberculosis

Pathology

The most common presentation of hepatic tuberculosis is diffuse parenchymal involvement, as seen in patients with pulmonary or miliary tuberculosis. Less commonly, the liver is the only involved organ and the condition is known as primary miliary tuberculosis of the liver. The later is thought to be due to hematogenous spread of tuberculosis to the liver from an inapparent extrahepatic source. Diffuse hepatic tuberculosis (miliary tuberculosis) is characterized by granulomas of less then 1mm found throughout the hepatic parenchyma. Granulomatous hepatitis has been reported after vaccination with bacille Calmette–Guerin (BCG) and also after BCG bladder instillation for the treatment of bladder cancer. This is now thought to be a result of mycobacteremia and BCG infection of the liver rather than a hypersensitivity reaction.

Tuberculous liver abscess, or tuberculoma, is the least common form of hepatic tuberculosis. The lesions are larger than 2mm (often much larger) and may be solitary or multiple. The characteristic lesion of focal hepatic tuberculosis is a tuberculoma, which may also be referred to as an abscess. A tuberculoma is larger than the granulomas seen in granulomatous hepatitis. Histologically, tuberculomas consist of granulomas that enlarge and develop a fibrous capsule. Caseous material with abundant bacilli is found within the tuberculoma. The biliary tract may be

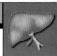

involved and biliary tract involvement in the absence of liver involvement has also been reported. Tuberculous involvement of other organs is often present.

Clinical features
Many cases of diffuse hepatic involvement are asymptomatic and are often diagnosed on liver biopsy performed for the evaluation of abnormal liver chemistries. Chronic low-grade fever and hepatomegaly are common and hepatic tuberculosis should be included in the differential diagnosis of fever of unknown origin. Other symptoms are nonspecific and may include malaise and weight loss. Symptoms due to extrahepatic disease may also be present. Jaundice is uncommon.

Focal hepatic tuberculosis presents in two distinct clinical forms (Fig. 15.8). Patients with the most common form present with hepatomegaly, fever, and weight loss in the absence of jaundice. These patients may have a hard, nodular liver on examination resembling patients with cirrhosis or hepatic neoplasm. They may also have one or more large caseating granulomas throughout the liver and lympadenopathy. Less frequently, patients present with chronic or relapsing jaundice, resembling the clinical illness seen in patients with common bile duct stones, strictures, or malignancy. Fever, abdominal pain, and weight loss may also occur. These individuals have direct biliary tract involvement with granulomas and strictures, or develop jaundice as a consequence of biliary obstruction secondary to enlarged, extrinsic lymph nodes.

Diagnosis
Nonspecific abnormalities of liver chemistries are common with diffuse disease, but normal liver tests do not exclude the diagnosis. Plain abdominal films may show hepatic calcifications. Chest radiographic abnormalities consistent with pulmonary tuberculosis are present in the majority of patients. Liver biopsy is usually diagnostic. Culture of liver obtained from biopsy is recommended, although cultures for *M. tuberculosis* are often negative.

The diagnosis of focal disease may be difficult as the presentation mimics that of other conditions, particularly liver abscess and neoplasm. The diagnosis should be considered in patients with HIV infection, history of intravenous drug abuse, and in patients from endemic areas of the world. The majority of patients with focal hepatic tuberculosis have normal liver function. The most consistent abnormality in these patients is an elevation in alkaline phosphatase. Patients with biliary tract involvement often present with elevated aminotransferases, bilirubin, and alkaline phosphatase. Tuberculin skin tests are positive in a majority of patients. Abnormal chest radiographs are common and pulmonary tuberculosis is seen in approximately 80% of cases. Plain abdominal radiographs may demonstrate calcifications. Ultrasound and CT findings are usually nonspecific.

Peritoneoscopy combined with liver biopsy is accurate in making the diagnosis in almost 100% of cases with focal disease. The liver lesions appear as cheesy white, irregular nodules of varying sizes on the liver surface. The yield of acid-fast material from biopsy specimen on staining is variable and reported to be between 9 and 59%. In patients with jaundice and signs of extrahepatic obstruction, endoscopic retrograde cholangiopancreatography (ERCP) or percutaneous cholangiogram may show extrinsic compression or biliary strictures with or without bile duct dilatation. Larger abscesses may mimic pyogenic abscess on imaging studies. Needle aspiration of these lesions is often negative for acid-fast bacilli. Occasionally, cultures are positive for other organisms, leading to the mistaken diagnosis of pyogenic abscess.

Treatment
Treatment of hepatic tuberculosis employs a combination of antituberculous drugs, usually isoniazid, rifampin (rifampicin), and pyrazinamide. In areas of isoniazid resistance, ethambutol or streptomycin may be used. The response to treatment is generally excellent with almost no long-term sequelae. The duration of treatment is not well-established but generally 12 months of treatment is adequate.

The treatment of focal hepatic tuberculosis in the absence of jaundice or other signs of extrahepatic biliary obstruction is similar to that of diffuse parenchymal tuberculosis. In patients with biliary involvement the response rate after 3 months of therapy with triple antituberculous drugs is only 25%, as compared with 75% in nonjaundiced patients. Surgical or endoscopic drainage of the biliary system, along with antituberculous therapy, is the mainstay of treatment in the group with extrahepatic biliary obstruction. There are no established guidelines for the duration of treatment and relapse, even after a year without symptoms, has been reported. Some authors recommend life-long treatment with suppressive antituberculous drugs.

LEPTOSPIROSIS

Leptospirosis is a zoonosis that is endemic in the tropics and infects a variety of wild and domestic animals. Human infection, often an acute febrile illness, has been described under many different names including swineherd's disease, mud fever, Fort Bragg fever, 7-day fever, and autumn fever. Weil's disease is the name given to icteric leptospirosis, which accounts for about 10% of cases of leptospirosis, and is the focus of this section.

Historic background
The first description of the disease came in 1883 when it was associated with work in sewers. In 1886 Weil differentiated the severe icteric form of this disease from other icteric illness. He described four cases, each having a febrile illness with neurologic

Hepatobiliary tuberculosis		
Type	With jaundice	Without jaundice
Abdominal pain	Common	Common
Fever	87%	54%
Hepatomegaly	100%	94%
Tranaminase elevation	90%	5%
Alkaline phosphatase	Almost 100%	50–60%
Splenomegaly	40%	18%
Ascites	16%	6%

Figure 15.8 Hepatobiliary tuberculosis. The signs and symptoms of the two presentations differ in frequency.

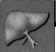

symptoms, jaundice, hepatomegaly, and renal involvement. In 1914, spirochetes were seen in the liver of a guinea pig that had been inoculated with blood from a patient with Weil's disease. In retrospect, it was learned that the organism had been identified in 1905 in sections of kidney taken from a patient in New Orleans who was believed to have died of yellow fever. This was the first case on record of leptospirosis in the USA. In 1917, a new genus was created for the organism named *Leptospira*.

Microbiology

Leptospires are coiled, motile spirochetes with bent ends often resembling question marks. Each organism is about 0.1μm wide and 6–20μm long. There is only one species, *L. interrogans*, in the genus *Leptospira*. There are many antigenic variations and 240 serotypes have been identified. These serotypes are arranged under 23 serogroups. At least 27 serotypes of leptospira occur naturally in the USA. The three clinically most important serogroups are *L. icterohaemorrhagiae*, *L. canicola*, and *L. pomona*. The serogroup *L. icterohaemorrhagiae*, initially found in rats but later found in dogs, cattle, and swine, is responsible for about 50% of the cases of Weil's disease. The other two serogroups that are also found in dogs, cattle, and swine usually cause nonicteric illness.

Epidemiology

Leptospirosis occurs throughout the world. The disease is endemic in tropical regions where up to 30% of the population is seropositive for leptospirosis. In the USA the disease has been reported from all regions. The disease occurs in a wide range of domestic and wild animals. Rats are the most common host for *L. icterohaemorrhagiae*. The serotype *L. canicola* is principally found in dogs, whereas *L. pomona* is found in livestock. Interspecies spread of specific serotypes among animal hosts is frequent. Asymptomatic host animals carry high numbers of leptospires in their kidneys. The organism is shed in the urine of these animals.

Human infection can occur either by direct contact with urine, contaminated water, or soil. The organisms enter the human body through abraded or cut skin. Contact with mucous membranes and swallowing infected water can also result in human infection. The disease involves both sexes and individuals of all ages but is more common in young males. The male to female ratio is 4:1. The disease is more common during the summer.

Clinical features

The incubation period usually varies between 7 and 14 days, with a mean of 10 days. Typically, leptospirosis is a biphasic illness and can be divided into septicemic and immune phase. During the first or septicemic phase, which lasts 4–7 days, leptospires are present in blood and cerebrospinal fluid (CSF). This phase is characterized by an acute onset of influenza-like illness. The symptoms include fever, chills, myalgia, headache, and nausea. The headache is often frontal and less commonly temporal or diffuse. Severe muscle pain typically involving the thighs and lower back is common and muscle tenderness is often significant. Cutaneous hyperesthesia may also be present. One characteristic symptom is severe leg pain on walking. Cough with chest pain and dyspnea due to pulmonary involvement may also be seen. Pulmonary hemorrhage is common in certain countries such as Korea. Patients often appear toxic with high spiking fevers. Conjuctival suffusion

is very common. Disturbances of sensorium are seen in some patients. Weil's disease has similar clinical features during the first stage, although jaundice is common by the end of first stage. The first phase ends with clinical improvement and disappearance of leptospires from the circulation.

The second or immune phase starts after an asymptomatic period of 1–3 days. Circulating antibodies appear in the circulation and most of the symptoms are due to immune-mediated injury. The fever recurs and is more pronounced in Weil's disease. Signs of meningeal irritation are common. Eye involvement is manifested by iritis or iridocyclitis. Less common symptoms include transient ischemic attacks, encephalitis, and neuropathy. Weil's disease is often associated with hemorrhages and renal involvement. Patients are often deeply jaundiced. Right upper quadrant tenderness and hepatomegaly are common. Splenomegaly was described in all four patients in Weil's initial description, but later studies found it to be uncommon. The hyperbilirubinemia is often marked with only minimal elevation of transaminases. Renal manifestations of Weil's disease may vary from mild proteinuria to acute tubular necrosis and renal failure. Vasculitis manifested by hemorrhages at multiple sites including subarachnoid hemorrhage has been reported in severe cases of Weil's disease. Death commonly occurs due to renal, pulmonary or cardiac complications, but death due to liver failure is extremely unusual.

Pathogenesis and pathology

The disease appears to be the result of both the direct damage caused by leptospires, as well as damage secondary to immune response. The primary lesion is a cell membrane defect of small blood vessel endothelium that leads to hemorrhage, ischemia, and secondary degenerative changes in organs. Grossly, the liver may be slightly enlarged. Hemorrhages involving multiple organs including kidneys, adrenals, liver, muscle, and lungs are frequently seen on autopsy of patients who died from Weil's disease.

Hepatocellular necrosis is mild, which correlates with minimal elevation of transaminases. Biliary stasis is the most prominent feature, and probably results from excessive hemolysis and inability of hepatocytes to excrete bilirubin. Intra- and extrahepatic bile ducts appear normal. Proliferation of hepatocytes is commonly seen with mitotic figures. Kupffer cells appear swollen and contains leptospiral debris. Characteristic histologic changes are seen in kidneys, skeletal muscles, and lungs on autopsy.

Diagnosis

Even though the clinical diagnosis of leptospirosis is almost always a challenge, the laboratory diagnosis is usually simple (Fig. 15.9). During the initial phase of the disease, leptospires can be easily cultured from the blood or CSF. The culture may take as long as 30 days to show any growth, and therefore prolonged incubation is essential. A positive culture is diagnostic. During the second phase the organism can be seen in the urine, by dark field microscopy, which may remain positive for months. Serologic diagnosis is more commonly employed. The microagglutination test (MAT) is the generally recognized basis for serodiagnosis. This test is available only from the US Centers for Disease Control and Prevention. The MAT can recognize specific serovars. The macroagglutination test or slide test is the most commonly used screening test for leptospirosis. A case is presumed if the slide test is positive after onset of symptoms, but confirmatory tests are often needed due to low

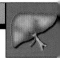

Leptospirosis		
Laboratory test	**Nonicteric leptospirosis**	**Weil's disease**
Complete blood count	Leukopenia or leukocytosis, often mild Anemia is uncommon Thrombocytopenia may be seen	Severe leukocytosis Anemia common Thrombocytopenia common
Chemistry	Renal functions are usually normal Phosphokinase elevated 4–5 times in 50%	Azotemia is common Phosphokinase levels similarly raised
Liver chemistry	Transaminases normal or mildly elevated Bilirubin less than 3mg/100ml Mild hypoalbuminemia may be seen Alkaline phosphatase is normal	Transaminases elevated Severe hyperbilirubinemia Albumin slightly decreased Alkaline phosphatase is often normal Coagulopathy seen in severe disease
Urinalysis	Proteinuria common but mild Casts and blood may be present	The abnormalities are more prominent and often last much longer depending on the degree of renal involvement
Chest radiography	Abnormal in up to 70% – patchy lesions, focal consolidation, pleural effusion and cardiomegaly	Similar to patients with anicteric disease
Cerebrospinal fluid	Proteins very high between 100–200mg/dL Lymphocyte predominance Normal glucose	Same

Figure 15.9 Leptospirosis. The pattern of laboratory abnormalities differs between nonicteric leptospirosis and Weil's disease.

specificity of this test. Dark field examination lacks sensitivity and specificity, and therefore should not be used if other methods are available. Dot-ELISA has been shown to be similar to MAT in terms of sensitivity and specificity, and is much easier to perform. The IgM titers rise early in the disease and can be readily identified by ELISA. The ELISA is now commercially available. Leptospiral RNA can be detected by polymerase chain reaction (PCR), which is highly sensitive and specific, but is not available commercially.

Treatment

Oral doxycycline given in the first 3 days of illness decreases severity and duration of symptoms, and may prevent complications and mortality. In severe cases penicillin G is effective even when treatment is delayed. Doxycycline, 200mg orally once a week, is highly effective prophylaxis. Empiric therapy with doxycycline or penicillin G is appropriate if the diagnosis of leptospirosis is considered clinically and epidemiologically. Other antibiotics that are effective against leptospires are streptomycin, erythromycin, and other tetracyclines. The choice of antibiotic is not as important as the fact that patients with severe disease need optimum supportive treatment. This is especially true for patients with hepatic or pulmonary involvement and patients with hemorrhage and renal disease. The response to antibiotics is generally good in the presence of good supportive care. Early bed rest may minimize subsequent morbidity. Azotemia and jaundice require meticulous attention to fluid and electrolyte therapy. Dialysis should be considered in patients with azotemia.

HEPATOBILIARY ASCARIASIS

Ascariasis is caused by the nematode *Ascaris lumbricoides*; the earliest recorded human helminth. The disease commonly presents with intestinal or pulmonary symptoms, but a significant proportion of patients may present with hepatobiliary involvement. The infection is acquired by the ingestion of eggs.

Lifecycle

The fertilized eggs are passed in the feces. The eggs require moist soil to survive and embryonate. Children are often infected while playing on infected soil. Geophagia is another common mode of acquisition among children, as is ingestion of food and water contaminated by eggs. In dry, windy weather, ascaris eggs can become airborne and can be ingested. After swallowing, the eggs hatch in the proximal small intestine. The larvae, each about 200–300μm in length, migrate to cecum and penetrate into the mucosa, and are transported by the portal venous system to the liver. In the liver the larvae can be seen in the sinusoids. In heavy infections, passage of larvae through the liver may cause an acute illness. This illness is characterized by right-sided abdominal pain, hepatomegaly, and generalized toxicity. From liver the larvae migrate via hepatic veins into the heart and thence into the lungs. The larvae eventually enter the alveolar space. From there they gradually move into the tracheobronchial tree and eventually ascend to the hypopharynx where they are swallowed. On reaching the small intestine the larvae attain sexual maturity in about 3–4 months and begin producing fertilized eggs.

Epidemiology

Ascariasis is endemic in China, South East Asia, Latin America and some European countries, with prevalence as high as 90%. In the USA, ascariasis is the third most common helminth infection. It has been estimated that about 4 million people are infected in the USA. People of all ages are infected but the highest prevalence is seen among children between ages 2 and 14 years. The prevalence of ascariasis is high in crowded, rural areas with poor sanitary conditions. The parts of the world where human feces are still utilized for cultivation of vegetables have high rates of infectivity. The hepatobiliary ascariasis is three times more common in females than in males, and pregnant females are highly susceptible to migration of worms to the gallbladder.

Clinical features

Hepatobiliary ascariasis has been recognized as an important clinical entity during the past two decades, mostly because of better imaging modalities and overall awareness of the disease. It is caused by entry of ascarides into the biliary tree through the ampullary orifice. In addition to blocking the common bile duct, the worm can enter and block the cystic and pancreatic ducts as well, resulting in a variety of clinical conditions. Normally the ascarides live in jejunum, but high parasite load may result in migration into the duodenum and subsequently into the biliary tree. Even though ascariasis commonly affects children, hepatobiliary disease is uncommon in children probably due to small size of ampullary orifice. In one study of 109 patients from India with pancreatobiliary disease, ascariasis was the cause in 36.7% of cases and was as common as gallstones as the cause of the biliary disease.

In its mildest form, the disease presents with biliary colic characterized by right upper quadrant pain associated with nausea and vomiting, lasting from hours to days. The pain may be recurrent in nature. This condition results from the invasion of ampullary orifice by the ascarides. The worm often moves in and out of the orifice, causing intermittent symptoms. The condition may be distinguished from cholangitis by the absence of fever, jaundice, and leukocytosis. Obstruction of cystic duct by adult worm can result in acalculous cholecystitis, characterized by right upper quadrant pain that radiates to the back and shoulder, low-grade fever, and a palpable gallbladder in right hypochondrium. On ultrasound, the gallbladder is often distended with thickened walls. Sometimes, the worms can be seen in the gallbladder.

The blockage of distal common bile duct by an adult worm can result in acute cholangitis or pancreatitis, similar to common bile duct obstruction by gallstones. Patients with acute cholangitis present with right upper quadrant pain, high fever, jaundice and leukocytosis, and often appear toxic. In the absence of appropriate antibiotics and drainage of biliary tree the patients often proceed to shock and even death in severe cases.

Diagnosis

In endemic areas, the presence of ova of *A. lumbricoides* in the stool is not diagnostic of hepatobiliary ascariasis. Ultrasonography and ERCP are two modalities commonly used to confirm the diagnosis (Fig. 15.10). Ultrasonography is quick, easy to perform, noninvasive, and has high sensitivity and specificity for detection of worms within the gallbladder and bile ducts. The worms usually appear as hyperechoic, linear structures. Often movement of the worm can be detected on ultrasonography. As worms actively move in and out of the bile ducts the ultrasound may not be positive in some cases. Ultrasound can show hepatic abscesses as well as changes in the pancreas in patients with acute pancreatitis. An additional advantage of ERCP is that it can identify the worms in the duodenum, and movement in and out of ampullary orifice can often be seen. In addition, ERCP can be used to remove the worms from the bile duct.

Treatment

Mebendazole, a benzimidazole, is the most commonly used drug. It inhibits the formation of the worm's microtubules and blocks the uptake of glucose by the parasite. The dose is 100mg of mebendazole twice a day for 3 days. Albendazole, a newer benzimidazole,

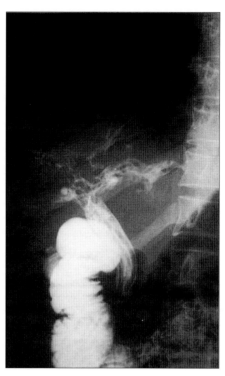

Figure 15.10 Ascaris. ERCP appearances of ascarides within the biliary tract.

is highly effective and can be taken as a single 400mg dose. Imidazoles are teratogenic and should not be used during pregnancy. Pyrantel pamoate, a neuromuscular blocking agent, is effective as a single dose of 10mL/kg. Gastrointestinal side effects are common with this drug. Piperazine, although no longer used in the USA due to occasional neurotoxic reactions, is highly effective and very cheap. This drug is widely used in developing countries. The worms often respond to the medical therapy and leave the bile ducts within days. In patients with cholangitis, early drainage should be achieved by placement of a nasobiliary catheter to prevent sepsis and shock. Endoscopic removal of worms from the bile ducts is recommended in patients who do not respond to conservative management or in those who continue to have worms in the bile ducts 2–3 weeks after treatment. Pancreatitis should be managed conservatively. Consideration should be given to ERCP in patients with pancreatitis in whom there is a high likelihood of common bile duct obstruction.

HEPATOSPLENIC SCHISTOSOMIASIS

Hepatosplenic schistosomiasis is a disease caused by certain species of the genus *Schistosoma*. The three species associated with liver disease are *S. mansoni*, *S. japonicum*, and *S. mekongi*. *Schistosoma haematobium* causes urinary schistosomiasis, but does not affect the liver. The disease, in its chronic form, is characterized by hepatosplenomegaly and other signs of portal hypertension.

Epidemiology

It has been estimated that over 200 million people worldwide harbor schistosomal infection. *Schistosoma mansoni* is endemic in Africa, South America, and Caribbean; *S. japonicum* in Far East, and *S. mekongi* in southeast Asia. Of those infected, a small proportion develops serious chronic disease. Hepatosplenic schistosomiasis affects both sexes and all age groups, including children.

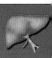

Lifecycle

The ova are excreted in the feces of infected individuals. The ova hatch immediately in water, liberating free-swimming miracidia. The miracidia penetrate a specific snail host and become cercariae within 4–6 weeks. The cercariae pass into water and remain infective for 2–3 days. Humans are infected by contact with fresh water containing cercariae. The cercariae penetrate the unbroken skin, sometimes causing intense itching (swimmer's itch), and within 24–48 hours migrate to the lungs via peripheral veins and lymphatics. Two to three weeks later they migrate to intrahepatic portal veins where they remain until they mature. It is during this initial migration that the syndrome of acute schistosomiasis (Katayama fever) usually begins. After 6–12 weeks, the adult worms migrate to their final habitat. At this stage each worm measures about 10–20mm in length. *Schistosoma mansoni* and *S. japonicum* inhabit tributaries of inferior and superior mesenteric veins, respectively, producing symptoms of intestinal schistosomiasis. Each female worm lays 300–3000 eggs daily. The eggs are laid in the terminal venules draining into the superior and inferior mesenteric veins. From there the eggs either re-enter the liver via portal vein or enter the lumen of the intestine and are passed in the feces.

Pathology

The pathology seen in schistosomiasis mainly results from the inflammatory changes, and subsequent fibrosis induced by the passage of eggs through the walls of the vessels and organs. Initially the migrating eggs cause severe a necrotizing and inflammatory reaction leading to granuloma formation in the involved tissue, the liver, intestine or urinary bladder, depending on the species. These granulomas are rich in eosinophils but lymphocytes, macrophages, and plasma cells are abundant as well. In the liver, ova are seen in the portal and periportal regions, surrounded by granulomata. This is followed by fibrosis in chronic cases. Grossly the liver is enlarged but may be normal or even small in the later stages. The surface is often irregular and left lobe may be disproportionately enlarged. The characteristic lesion of chronic hepatosplenic schistosomiasis is 'clay pipestem' lesion (Fig. 15.11). This is described as wide bands of fibrosis around portal veins. On cut surface, this lesion appears as a cross-section

through the stem of a clay pipe. The parenchyma between the areas of fibrosis is usually well preserved. This is reflected by normal liver function in most patients with hepatosplenic schistosomiasis. Schistosomiasis does not cause cirrhosis.

Pathogenesis

Genetic factors may play a role in the development of hepatosplenic schistosomiasis. Another, probably more important factor in the development of hepatosplenic schistosomiasis is the intensity of infection, with patients with high worm loads being more prone to develop hepatosplenic disease. The pathogenesis of portal hypertension is not well understood. There is sufficient evidence that the obstruction to portal bloodflow occurs at the level of smaller portal tracts at presinusoidal level. What induces the fibrosis is controversial. Some researchers believe that granulomatous reaction to eggs initiate the fibrosis. Those who do not agree claim that the fibrosis is often seen far from granulomas, and in chimpanzees the fibrosis preceded the egg deposition in the portal tract. Furthermore the excess collagen may be deposited independent of any granuloma in the space of Disse, producing fibrosis at the level of the sinusoids.

Clinical features

There are three main clinical presentations of schistosomiasis: acute dermatitis, acute schistosomiasis, and chronic schistosomiasis.

Acute dermatitis is also known as swimmer's itch and may develop within minutes of coming in contact with water infected with cercariae. It presents with severe itch with erythema followed by a papular rash. The rash and symptoms may last for a few days. Acute dermatitis is seen almost exclusively in travelers who have never previously been exposed to the parasite.

Acute schistosomiasisis is also known as Katayama fever and is also almost exclusively seen in patients exposed to the schistosome for the first time. The symptoms starts 3–6 weeks after the larval invasion and coincides with early egg-laying. The clinical manifestations may vary considerably from general malaise to a very severe illness. The intestinal symptoms are more common during the acute stage and include abdominal pain and diarrhea. The diarrhea may be accompanied by blood and mucus, and later develops into frank dysentery. Other symptoms include myalgia, hepatomegaly, splenomegaly, and eosinophilia. The fever lasts many weeks and may be difficult to distinguish from fever caused by typhoid, malaria, or acute fascioliasis. The history of exposure to water may not always available. The eggs are often absent from the stool in the acute stages and diagnosis is often made by serologic tests.

Chronic schistosomiasis results from untreated acute disease. The symptoms in this stage of schistosomiasis are secondary to an inflammatory response of the body to the eggs and subsequent fibrosis. Patients usually complain of dysentery, although this feature may be absent. Pseudopolyps may develop in the colon of the affected individuals and protein-losing enteropathy with subsequent anasarca has been seen. Most of the patients with chronic schistosomiasis may remain asymptomatic for years. The severe periportal fibrosis leads to portal hypertension and subsequent development of splenomegaly, esophageal varices, and ascites. The splenomegaly in this stage results from portal hypertension, while in acute disease the splenomegaly is due to reticuloendothelial hyperplasia. Liver failure is rare and stigmata of chronic liver dysfunction such as gynecomastia, spider

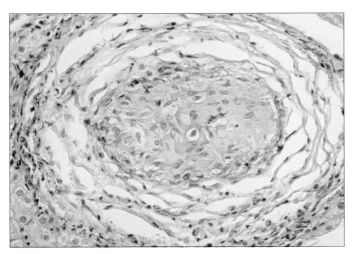

Figure 15.11 Schistosomiasis. The characteristic pattern of portal fibrosis described as 'pipestem'.

angiomas, and palmer erythema, are usually absent. Similarly, jaundice and encephalopathy is not seen except in terminal cases. The anemia is unusual and if present is due to slow gastrointestinal blood loss secondary to portal hypertensive gastropathy. Variceal bleeding is often well-tolerated in schistosomiasis due to the absence of liver failure.

Diagnosis

The acute disease (Katayama fever) should be suspected in any individual with a history of possible exposure to infected water who presents with fever, dysentery, and peripheral eosinophilia. The chronic disease is more difficult to diagnose. The patients usually present with tender hepatomegaly or splenomegaly. Other symptoms of acute disease are often absent. The differential diagnosis should include other causes of hepatosplenomegaly. In early phase the stools may be negative for ova. A high IgM titer is diagnostic of acute schistosomal infection. Eosinophilia is almost always seen and may be a useful clue to the correct diagnosis. Multiple stool specimens should be obtained in patients suspected of having acute or chronic schistosomiasis. Sigmoidoscopy with biopsy of rectal valve may show ova in patients with negative stool studies and improves the yield. Multiple biopsies should be obtained and the specimen should be compressed between two glass slides and examined under direct microscopy. Liver biopsy is often nondiagnostic due to the small size of tissue obtained, although it may be helpful in excluding other causes of liver disease. The presence of schistosome eggs in the biopsy specimen is no more revealing than positive findings on stool examination or rectal biopsy. There is a high incidence of hepatitis B in patients with schistosomiasis, and therefore the liver biopsy should be interpreted carefully.

Treatment

Chronic active hepatosplenic schistosomiasis should be treated with antischistosomal therapy. This will prevent progression of the disease, but will not reverse the Symmer's fibrosis or portal hypertension. Praziquantel and oxamniquine are two oral drugs that are very effective against *S. mansoni*. Praziquantel is used as a single dose of 30mg/kg. In heavy infections, 60mg/kg divided in three doses and administered over 1 day is indicated. Oxamniquine is also given orally in a dose of 20–30mg/kg for 3 days. Cure rates of up to 90% have been reported with these drugs. In *S. japonicum* and *S. mekongi*, praziquantel is the drug of choice. The drug is given at a dose of 20mg/kg three times a day for 3 days, although the dose described above for heavy *S. mansoni* infection may be equally effective. Appropriate treatment should be provided for any complications of hepatosplenic schistosomiasis, although these complications are uncommon since the introduction of praziquantel.

The acute schistosomal disease should be treated symptomatically. Steroids (prednisone 0.5mg/kg three times a day) should be used for 2–3 days to control the acute phase before administering the more specific therapy. Praziquantel is effective against all three species. The dose is same as for chronic hepatosplenic schistosomiasis (60mg/kg in three divided doses given over 1 day). The treatment of acute disease will not alter the course of acute illness but it will prevent the development of chronic hepatosplenic schistosomiasis and its complications.

LIVER FLUKES

There are many different flukes that infect the hepatobiliary system in human beings. The best known is sheep liver fluke or *Fasciola hepatica*. *Clonorchis sinensis* and *Opisthorchis viverrini* are common in Asia and commonly known as oriental fluke. *Opisthorchis felineus* and *Dicrocoelium dendriticum* are common in Russia and certain parts of Africa.

Fasciola hepatica

The common sheep fluke is common in certain parts of Europe including England. The snail *Lymnaea trunculata* is the intermediate host. The metacercaria from these snails survive on the vegetation and human infection occurs as a result of eating contaminated watercress. The metacercaria excyst in the small intestine and the flukes penetrate through the wall of the intestine into the peritoneal cavity. They penetrate through the liver capsule into the hepatic parenchyma and eventually enter the biliary tree. The mature worms produce eggs in the bile duct that enters the small intestine with bile and excreted in stool.

Mild infections are usually asymptomatic. Heavy infections usually present with an acute illness that closely mimics acute cholangitis. The eggs released by adult flukes in the bile ducts cause severe inflammatory reaction followed by fibrosis. The patients usually present with right upper quadrant pain, fever, and eosinophilia. Jaundice is present in patients with bile duct obstruction. Physical examination usually reveals enlarged tender liver. Secondary bacterial infections may develop and these patients often have high spiking fever and leukocytosis. Elevation of alkaline phosphatase is commonly seen.

The acute disease closely resembles Katayama fever and other acute febrile illnesses. Eosinophilia is a consistent finding. The diagnosis is usually confirmed by documenting the ova in the stool. However, these may no be detected until 12 weeks after the infection. Immunodiagnosis with counter immune electrophoresis (CIEP) and ELISA is both sensitive and specific. Computed tomography scan may show peripheral filling defects in the liver due to the migrating fluke. Multiple linear filling defects or stricture are shown by ERCP, and bile aspirate often yields flukes (Fig. 15.12). Liver biopsy is often unnecessary to make the diagnosis.

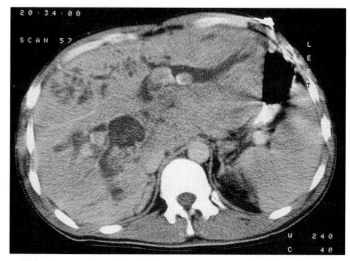

Figure 15.12 Fluke. MRI showing segmental intrahepatic duct dilatation and calculi after liver fluke infestation, so-called 'oriental cholangitis'.

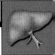

Praziquantel, a very effective antihelminthic, is not effective against *Fasciola hepatica*. The drug of choice is bithionol in a dose of 50mg/kg per day for 10 doses. Parentral, 1mg/kg per day for 14 doses is an alternative. Bacterial cholangitis should be treated aggressively with intravenous antibiotics, as the mortality is high. Complications like biliary stricture and obstruction should be managed accordingly.

Clonorchis sinensis

Commonly known as Chinese liver fluke, *Clonorchis sinensis* is common in China, Japan, and other parts of Asia. This fluke is very similar to *Opisthorchis viverrini*, a common fluke in Thailand. Both C. *sinensis* and O. *viverrini* infection occurs by eating raw, contaminated fish. The adult flukes live in the bile ducts of the host and release eggs that cause severe inflammation and fibrosis. Heavily infested individuals may have as many as 20,000 flukes. The clinical features are similar to those of fascioliasis and diagnosis is often made by documenting the ova in the stool. The intrahepatic stones are seen in chronic infections. Many reports have shown a higher incidence of cholangiocarcinoma. The drug of choice is praziquantel, but the response is suboptimal and relapses are common.

PRACTICE POINT

Illustrative case

A 56-year-old man presented with right upper quadrant pain, fever, and diarrhea of 10 days' duration. There was a history of altered bowel habit for 6 months before the development of these symptoms. He worked as a sheep farmer in the Welsh mountains and there was no history of travel beyond his normal environment. Physical examination revealed a fever of 38°C and mildly tender hepatomegaly. An ultrasound of the abdomen confirmed the presence of a mass in the right lobe of the liver that was consistent with a liver abscess. Serologic testing for *Echinococcus* spp. was submitted, but there was a 2-week interval before the result was reported as negative. Colonoscopic examination was limited by the presence of severe diverticular disease in the sigmoid colon. A barium enema was performed and identified a constricting carcinoma in the ascending colon. The tumor was removed surgically and a drain was inserted into the abscess cavity. He was treated with intravenous antibiotics for 6 weeks and made an uneventful recovery.

Interpretation

Although this man had a classic background for hydatid disease, this ultimately proved to be a 'red herring'. The delay in obtaining the result of serologic tests for *Echinococcus* spp. can be problematic, and in this case other features of the clinical picture precipitated the appropriate investigations and treatment. The liver lesion was a pyogenic liver abscess consequent to the carcinoma of the bowel. Cursory examination of the bowel might have concluded that the diverticular disease was the cause of the liver abscess. A comprehensive screen should be performed for all potential causes, especially in older patients and where the primary site of infection is equivocal. The prolonged course of antibiotics is typical of these patients.

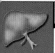
FURTHER READING

Alvarez SZ, Carpio R. Hepatobiliary tuberculosis. Dig Dis Sci. 1983;28:193–200. *A good review of this condition.*

Bissada AA, Bateman J. Pyogenic liver abscess: a 7 years experience in a large community hospital. Hepatogastroenterology. 1991;138:317–20. *Extensive clinical experience.*

Centers for Disease Control and Prevention. Outbreak of leptospirosis among white water rafters, Costa Rica. JAMA. 1997;278:808–9. *CDC report on interesting outbreak affecting 36% of party of white-water rafters.*

Chu KM, Fan ST, Lai EC, Lo CM, Wong J. Pyogenic liver abscess: an audit of experience over the past decade. Arch Surg. 1996;131:148–52. *Study of 83 cases.*

Gosh KL, Pathmanathan R, Chang KW, Wong NW: Tuberculous liver abscess. J Trop Med. 1987;90:255–7. *Good clinical description.*

Greenstein AJ, Sachar DB. Pyogenic and amebic abscesses of the liver. Semin Liver Dis. 1988;150:120–7. *Detailed clinical review.*

Khuroo MS, Wani NA, Javid G, et al. Percutaneous drainage compared with surgery for hepatic hydatid cysts. N Engl J Med. 1997;337:881. *Randomized trial of 50 patients demonstrating efficacy of nonsurgical treatment.*

Leebeek FWG, Ouwendijh RJTh, Kolk AHJ, et al. Granulomatous hepatitis caused by Bacillus Calmette–Guerin (BCG) infection after BCG bladder instillation. Gut. 1995;38:616–18. *Novel case report.*

Lightowlers MW, Gottstein B. Echinococcosis/hydatidosis: Antigens, immunological and molecular diagnosis. In: Thompson RCA, Lymbery AJ, eds. Echinococcus and hydatid disease. Wallingford: CAB International; 1995:9335. *Authoritative review.*

Ochsner A, De Bakey, Murray S. Pyogenic abscess of the liver. An analysis of forty-seven cases with review of the literature. Am J Surg. 1938;40:292–319. *Historic interest.*

Ribeiro MA, Souza CC, Almeida SHP. Dot-ELISA for human leptospirosis employing immunodominant antigen. J Trop Med Hyg. 1995;98:452–6. *Description of development of diagnostic test.*

Schwartz DA. Cholangiocarcinoma associated with liver fluke infection: A preventable source of morbidity in Asian immigrants. Am J Gastroenterol. 1986;81:76–9. *Describes linkage of fluke infestation and cholangiocarcinoma.*

Soong CG, Kain KC, Abd-Alla KA, et al. A recombinant-cysteine rich section of the *Entamoeba histolytica* galactose-inhibitable lectin is efficacious as a subunit vaccine the gerbil model of amebic liver abscess. J Infect Dis. 1995;171:645–51. *Basis for potential development of vaccine.*

Stimson AM. Note on organism found in yellow-fever tissue. Public Health Rep. 1907;22:541–5. A description of the First case of heptospirosis in the USA.

Symmers W St. C. Note on a new form of liver cirrhosis due to the presence of ova of *Bilharzia haematobium*. J Pathol Bact. 1903;9:237–9. *Historic interest.*

Tazawa J, Sakai Y, Maekawa S, et al. Solitary and multiple pyogenic liver abscesses: Characteristics of the patients and efficacy of percutaneous drainage. Am J Gastrol. 1997;92:271. *Extensive clinical study.*

Turkcapar AG, et al. Surgical treatment of hydatidosis combined with perioperative treatment with albendazole. Eur J Surg. 1997;163:923–8. *Clinical description of role of albendazole.*

WHO Informal Working Group on Echinococcosis. Guidelines for treatment of cystic and alveolar echinococcosis in humans. Bull World Health Organ. 1996;74:231–42. *Authoritative policy document.*

Zhang Y, Li E, Jackson TFHG, et al. Use of a recombinant 170-kilodalton surface antigen of *Entamoeba histolytica* for serodiagnosis of amebiasis and identification of immunodominant domains of the native molecule. J Clin Microbiol. 1992;30:2788–92. *Diagnostic test.*

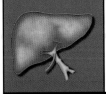

Section 3 Specific Diseases of the Liver

Chapter 16

Autoimmune Hepatitis

Michael P Manns and Christian P Strassburg

INTRODUCTION

Autoimmune diseases of the liver potentially affect two epithelial target tissues, hepatocytes and biliary cells or cholangiocytes, and lead to three principle disease entities. Primary biliary cirrhosis (PBC) and primary sclerosing cholangitis (PSC) target the proximal and distal biliary tree. Autoimmune hepatitis (AIH) targets the hepatocyte and results in a chronic inflammatory disease, predominantly affecting the periportal hepatocellular compartment of the liver. Despite the fact that the autoimmune reaction of all three disease entities leads to the destruction of different defined microanatomic structures, these autoimmune diseases all share some clinical and laboratory characteristics. All three diseases are chronic inflammatory conditions and AIH and PBC predominantly affect the female sex. They are characterized by circulating serum autoantibodies, although the specifics of this association are less clear for PSC. The frequently found criterion of a favorable response to immunosuppressive therapy to establish a diagnosis of autoimmune hepatitis, however, only convincingly applies to AIH. The classic forms of the disease are readily identifiable, but in the early stages of disease misdiagnosis is common. Histologic features suggestive of autoimmune hepatitis are frequently seen in early PBC, and patients who have PSC are not infrequently treated as autoimmune hepatitis if cholestasis is not a prominent feature and cholangiography has not been performed. To complicate matters further, overlap syndromes have been described.

Historically, AIH was first described in 1950 when a form of chronic hepatitis was recognized in young women featuring jaundice, elevated gammaglobulins and amenorrhea, and this eventually progressed to cirrhosis. This form of chronic hepatitis was later noted in combination with other extrahepatic autoimmune syndromes. Due to the striking similarities to the clinical picture of systemic lupus erythematosus (SLE) and the presence of antinuclear antibodies (ANAs), it was initially termed lupoid hepatitis. However, liver involvement is not a prominent feature of SLE, and subsequent systematic evaluation of the cellular and molecular immunopathology, the clinical symptoms, and the laboratory features established autoimmune hepatitis as a separate clinical entity distinguishable from other forms of chronic hepatitis. It has been subclassified on the basis of the pattern of autoantibodies present and it is treated by a specific therapeutic strategy that involve immunosuppression with corticosteroids and other drugs. A recently established scoring system allows for a reproducible and standardized approach to diagnosing and consequently treating AIH. The use and interpretation of seroimmunologic and molecular biologic tests permits a precise discrimination of autoimmune hepatitis from other etiologies of chronic hepatitis, in particular from chronic viral infection, which is the most common cause of chronic hepatitis worldwide.

DEFINITIONS

Autoimmune hepatitis is a chronic inflammatory disease of the liver that has usually been present for more than 6 months at the time of diagnosis. It is defined as a chronic, mainly periportal hepatitis, is associated with hypergammaglobulinemia and serum autoantibodies, and responds to immunosuppressive treatment in most cases. There is a significant predisposition of the female sex and a significant association with the presence of HLA DR3 and DR4 alleles among affected patients. Autoimmune hepatitis is associated with numerous extrahepatic autoimmune syndromes such as autoimmune thyroiditis, vitiligo, nail dystrophy, ulcerative colitis, alopecia, and rheumatoid arthritis, but also glomerulonephritis and diabetes mellitus. The diagnosis of classic AIH depends on the absence of evidence of chronic viral hepatitis, and other causes of chronic liver disease such as metabolic disorders (especially Wilson's disease), and genetic and toxic causes must be excluded (Fig. 16.1).

The outlined global definition of AIH shows that the diagnosis of AIH cannot be reached through the determination of a single parameter or the presence of an individual symptom. On the contrary, AIH is diagnosed as the result of precise and methodic exclusion of other diseases. This process is greatly facilitated by a recently established scoring system, which incorporates characteristic features of AIH and contradictory features into the calculation of a probability score (Fig. 16.2).

Apart from its use as a precise diagnostic tool, this provisional scoring system also provides a basis for the scientific evaluation and comparison of patient groups from different centers as well as from different parts of the world.

The single most significant finding in AIH is the presence of circulating autoantibodies. The discovery of autoantibodies directed against different cellular targets, including endoplasmic reticulum membrane proteins, nuclear antigens, and cytosolic antigens, has led to a suggested subclassification of AIH based upon the presence of three specific autoantibody profiles (Fig. 16.3).

According to this approach, AIH type 1 is characterized by the presence of antinuclear antibodies and/or anti-smooth muscle antibodies (SMAs); AIH type 2 is characterized by anti-liver–kidney microsomal autoantibodies (LKM-1) directed against cytochrome P450 2D6; and AIH type 3 is characterized by autoantibodies against soluble liver antigens (SLA) which are

Differential diagnosis of autoimmune hepatitis and diagnostic tests	
Disease	**Exclusion by**
Hepatitis C virus (HCV) infection	Anti-HCV, HCV RNA
Hepatitis B and D virus (HBV, HDV) infection	HBsAg, anti-HBc, HBV DNA Anti-HDV antibody, HDV RNA
Hepatitis A virus (HAV) Hepatitis E virus (HEV) Ebstein–Barr virus (EBV) Herpes simplex virus (HSV) Cytomegalovirus (CMV) Varicella-zoster virus (VZV)	Antibodies, serology: immunologulins G and M
Drug-induced hepatitis	History, withdrawal of drug LKM-2, LM autoantibody
Primary biliary cirrhosis (PBC)	Antimitochondrial antibodies (anti PDH-E2, BCKD-E2) Liver histology: copper deposition Unresponsive to steroids
Primary sclerosing cholangitis (PSC)	Cholangiography
Wilson's disease	Ceruloplasmin, urine copper, eye examination, copper in liver
Hemochromatosis	Serum ferritin, serum iron, transferrin, liver histology: iron staining
α_1-antitrypsin deficiency	Serum α_1-antitrypsin (if abnormal isoelectric focusing for PiZZ/PiSS/PiMZ/PiSZ genotype)

Figure 16.1 Differential diagnosis of autoimmune hepatitis and diagnostic tests.

Scoring system for diagnosis of autoimmune hepatitis: minimum required parameters		
	Parameter	**Score**
Gender	Female	+2
	Male	0
Serum biochemistry	Ratio of elevation of serum alkaline phosphatase versus aminotransferase	
	>3.0	–2
	<3.0	+2
Total serum globulin, γ-globulin or IgG	Times upper normal limit	
	>2.0	+3
	1.5–2.0	+2
	1.0–1.5	+1
	<1.0	0
Autoantibodies (titers by immunofluorescence on rodent issues)	Adults ANA, SMA or LKM-1	
	>1:80	+3
	1:80	+2
	1:40	+1
	<1:40	0
	Children ANA or LKM-1	
	>1:20	+3
	1:20	+2
	<1:20	0
	or SMA	
	>1:20	+3
	1:20	+2
	<1:20	0
	Antimitochondrial antibody	
	Positive	–2
	Negative	0
Viral markers	IgM anti-HAV, HBsAg orIgM anti-HBc positive	–3
	Anti-HCV positive by ELISA and/or RIBA	–2
	HCV positive by PCR for HCV RNA	–3
	Positive test indicating active infection with any other virus	–3
	Seronegative for all of the above	+3
Other etiological factors	History of recent hepatotoxic drug usage or parenteral exposure to blood products	
	Yes	–2
	No	+1
	Alcohol (average consumption)	
	Male <35 gm/day; female <25 gm/day	+2
	Male 35-50 gm/day; female 25-40 gm/day	0
	Male 50-80 gm/day; female 40-60 gm/day	–1
	Male >80 gm/day; female >60 gm/day	–2
	Genetic factors: HLA DR3 or DR4	
	Other autoimmune diseases in patient or first degree relatives	+1

Figure 16.2 Scoring system for diagnosis of autoimmune hepatitis: minimum required parameters. Interpretation of aggregate scores: definite AIH, greater than 15 before treatment and greater than 17 after treatment; probable AIH, 10 to 15 before treatment and 12 to 17 after treatment. (From Johnson and McFarlane, 1993.)

directed against cytokeratin 8 and/or 18 and other cytosolic hepatocellular proteins. In AIH type 3, antibodies against liver–pancreas antigen (LP) are also found. In addition, many cases of AIH display autoantibodies that show reactivity towards the asialoglycoprotein receptor (ASGPR) and some reactivity with the liver cytosolic antigen 1 (LC-1).

Among the aforementioned subclasses, AIH type 1 represents the most common form of AIH, whereas AIH types 2 and 3 are rare entities. Type 2 displays a regionally very divergent prevalence, with a very low occurrence in the USA, but accounting for up to 20% of AIH cases in Western Europe. Whether AIH type 3 is a separate subentity is a matter of debate. However, the recognition of SLA and LP autoantibodies as markers of AIH in cases of ANA and LKM negativity justifies recognition of this subset of patients and increases the accuracy of diagnosing all cases of AIH, irrespective of clinical presentation. Although the subclassification into these three groups is a matter of ongoing discussion and refinement, it does appear to reflect a true clinical and prognostic difference that is relevant to the course of the disease in individual patients. Type 2 patients are younger and more frequently display an acute onset of hepatitis with a severe clinical course and more rapid disease progression than patients who have AIH type 1.

EPIDEMIOLOGY AND PATHOGENESIS

Epidemiology of autoimmune hepatitis

Autoimmune hepatitis is a rare disorder. Based on limited epidemiologic data, the prevalence is estimated to range between 50 and 200 cases per 1 million in Western Europe and North America among the Caucasian population. The prevalence of

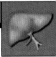

Classification of chronic hepatitis					
Hepatitis type	HBsAg	HBV DNA	anti-HDV (HDV RNA)	anti-HCV (HCV RNA)	Autoantibody
HBV	+	±	–	–	–
HDV	+	–	+	–	~10% anti-LKM-3
HCV	–	–	–	+	~2% anti-LKM-1
Autoimmune hepatitis type 1	–	–	–	–	ANA
type 2	–	–	–	–	LKM-1
type 3	–	–	–	–	SLA/LP
Drug-induced	–	–	–	–	some ANA, LKM, LM
Cryptogenic	–	–	–	–	–

Figure 16.3 Classification of chronic hepatitis. (Adapted from Desmet et al., 1994.)

AIH is similar to that of SLE, PBC, and myasthenia gravis, all of which share an autoimmune pathogenesis. Among the North American and Western European Caucasian populations, AIH accounts for up to 20% of patients who have chronic hepatitis. However, chronic viral hepatitis remains the major cause of chronic hepatitis in most Western societies. In countries in which viral hepatitis B and C are endemic, such as in Asia and Africa, the incidence of AIH appears to be significantly lower. Meaningful epidemiologic data from these countries are unfortunately not yet available. Interestingly, AIH in Japan is associated with the HLA DR4 allele, which is in contrast to findings in Europe and the USA where an association with HLA DR3 has been conclusively demonstrated. The relative incidence of AIH among patients with chronic hepatitis is also lower and is estimated to be around 5%. Additional epidemiologic analyses are required to comprehensively elucidate the prevalence and geographic distribution of AIH.

Immunopathogenesis of autoimmune hepatitis

There is no doubt that a loss of self-tolerance is the pathophysiologic process driving AIH, and this leads to the observed sequelae. However, the precise cause of this disease remains elusive and a number of concepts have been pursued to elucidate the causative agents or mechanisms leading to AIH. On the one hand, the prominent feature of serum autoantibodies has lead to the determination, characterization, and evaluation of humoral autoimmunity in AIH. On the other hand, evidence has pointed to a viral etiology of AIH, potentially resulting in either a virus-triggered, sustained autoaggressive immunologic reaction, or an autoimmune reaction directly induced by hepatotropic viruses. Other investigations point to a dysregulation of cellular immunity, in particular those studies using animal models such as the experimental autoimmune hepatitis (EAH) model in mice. Genetic factors appear to represent a mandatory component of the pathogenesis of AIH, as has been demonstrated through the prevalence of selected HLA alleles in patients suffering from AIH.

Autoantibodies in autoimmune hepatitis

Circulating autoantibodies are the hallmark of AIH. Autoantibodies are the single most important finding determining diagnosis, treatment and discrimination of autoimmune disease from chronic viral infections. The identification, molecular cloning and recombinant expression of hepatocellular autoantigens has enabled the implementation of precise testing systems and the scientific evaluation of humoral autoimmunity associated with AIH. Autoantibodies of significance for AIH are: ANAs, SMA, LKM, SLA, LC-1, LP, and ASGPRs.

Antinuclear antibodies

Antinuclear antibodies are directed against functional and structural components of both the membrane, structural and genomic components of the cell nucleus. The target antigens are a heterogeneous and incompletely defined group of cellular proteins. Antinuclear antibodies are also detected in PBC, and investigations have been aimed at identifying target antigens that are specific for AIH. Antinuclear antibodies are determined by indirect immunofluorescence on cryostat sections of rat liver and on Hep-2 cell slides. Most commonly, a homogeneous or speckled immunofluorescence pattern is encountered. Antinuclear antibodies have been found to be reactive with centromere, ribonucleoproteins, and cyclin A. They represent the most common autoantibody in AIH and occur in high titers usually exceeding 1:160 (Fig. 16.4).

Antismooth muscle antibodies

Anti-SMA are directed against components of the cytoskeleton such as actin, troponin, and tropomyosin. They frequently occur in high titers and are usually associated with coexisting ANAs. However, SMA autoantibodies also occur in advanced diseases of the liver of other etiologies, in infectious diseases, and in rheumatic disorders. In these cases titers are often lower than 1:80. Antismooth muscle autoantibodies are determined by indirect immunofluorescence on cryostat sections of rat stomach (Fig. 16.5).

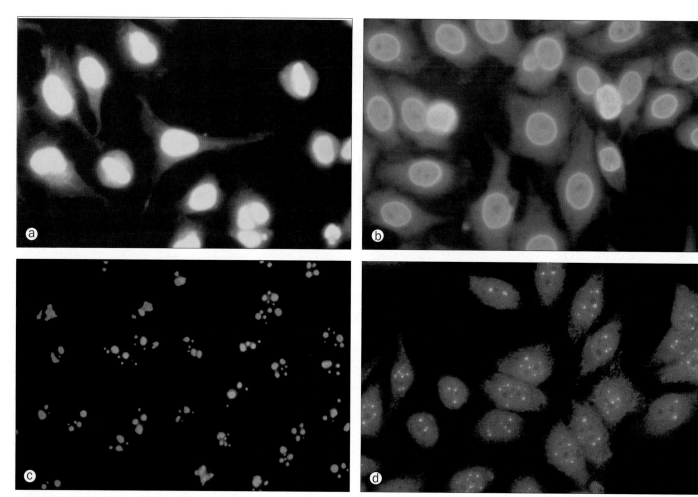

Figure 16.4 Antinuclear antibodies. Indirect immunofluorescence micrographs of ANAs found in autoimmune hepatitis and other autoimmune diseases, and detected on immobilized Hep-2 cells. (a) Typical aspect of homogeneous nuclear staining found in a patient who has autoimmune hepatitis type 1 with titers exceeding 1:160. These autoantibodies are frequently directed against double stranded DNA and histones and are a typical finding in type 1 autoimmune hepatitis. (b) Aspect of the nuclear membranous (rim) immunofluorescence pattern found in a patient who has autoimmune hepatitis type 1 at titers exceeding 1:160. In this pattern autoantibodies are directed against lamins (lamin B, but also lamin A and C). Membranous immunofluorescence is not a frequent finding and can indicate the existence of mixed immune syndromes including vasculitis and other features of SLE. (c) Indirect immunofluorescence study showing a nucleolar ANA fluorescence pattern. This pattern is rarely seen in autoimmune hepatitis, but is common in rheumatologic diseases such as scleroderma and polymyositis. If present in autoimmune hepatitis type 1, it can be indicative of overlap syndromes with rheumatologic disorders. (d) Indirect immunofluorescence study showing multiple nuclear dots. This pattern is not typical for autoimmune hepatitis and is mainly found in about 20% of patients who have PBC. Usually AMA are present at the same time but can also be missing in cases of ANA-positive, AMA-negative PBC. These autoantibodies are directed against the sp100 nuclear antigen (100kDa).

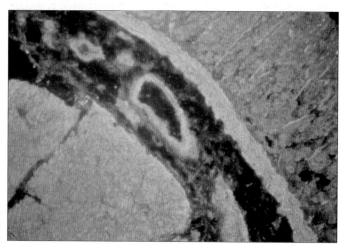

Figure 16.5 Anti-smooth muscle antibodies. Typical immunofluorescence pattern of SMA autoantibodies detected on rat stomach cryostat sections. This serum shows immunoreactivity with the muscularis mucosae and muscularis propria layers of rat stomach. Note that the mucosa is excluded from reactivity. This autoantibody is often detected in conjunction with ANA in autoimmune hepatitis type 1.

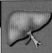

Liver–kidney microsomal antibodies

First described in 1973, LKM are directed against proteins of the endoplasmic reticulum (microsomal protein). Detection is by indirect immunofluorescence and the autoantibodies are reactive with the proximal renal tubules and the hepatocellular cytoplasm (Fig. 16.6).

These autoantibodies termed LKM-1 were associated with a second form of ANA-negative AIH. Between 1988 and 1991 the 50kDa antigen of LKM-1 autoantibodies was identified as cytochrome P450 2D6 (CYP 2D6). These autoantibodies recognize a major linear epitope between amino acids 263 and 270 of the CYP 2D6 protein. These autoantibodies inhibit CYP 2D6 activity *in vitro* and are capable of activating liver infiltrating T-lymphocytes. This indicates a combined humoral and cellular immune mechanism leading to the development of LKM autoantibodies. In addition to linear epitopes, LKM-1 autoantibodies have also been shown to recognize conformation dependent epitopes. However, the recognition of epitopes located between amino acids 257 and 269 appears to be a specific autoimmune reaction of autoimmune hepatitis and is discriminatory against LKM-1 autoantibodies associated with chronic hepatitis C virus infection. The cytochrome CYP 2D6 has been found to be expressed on the hepatocellular surface and its expression appears to be regulated by cytokines.

Antibodies against microsomal proteins form a heterogeneous group spanning several immune-mediated diseases including AIH, drug-induced hepatitis, autoimmune polyendocrine syndrome type 1 (APS-1), and chronic hepatitis C virus (HCV) and hepatitis D virus (HDV) infections (Fig. 16.7).

Liver–kidney microsomal autoantibodies against CYP 2A6 are found in patients who have APS-1 with hepatic involvement. Anti-CYP 2A6 autoantibodies also occur in HCV infection. Liver–kidney microsomal autoantibodies, which are characterized by an immunofluorescence pattern that selectively stains the hepatocellular cytoplasm but not kidney, have been found to be directed against CYP 1A2. These autoantibodies are also found in APS-1 with hepatic involvement and occur in dihydralazine-induced hepatitis. A second type of LKM autoantibodies, LKM-2, are directed against CYP 2C9 and are induced in ticrynafen-associated hepatitis. A third group of LKM autoantibodies, LKM-3, as identified in 6–10% of patients who had chronic hepatitis D virus infection (HDV). These autoantibodies are directed against family 1 UDP-glucuronosyltransferases (UGT1A), which are also a superfamily of drug metabolizing proteins located in the endoplasmic reticulum. Autoantibodies of the LKM-3 group have been identified in HDV infection, but also in AIH type 2 patients. They can also occur in LKM-1-negative and ANA-negative AIH.

In addition, LKM-positive sera display reactivity with a number of as yet undefined antigens with molecular weights of 35kDa, 57kDa, 59kDa, and 70kDa. These autoantibodies are predominantly found in AIH, HCV infection, and halothane hepatitis. Liver–kidney microsomal autoantibodies are visualized by indirect immunofluorescence on rodent cryostat sections. Subclassification is achieved by enzyme-linked immunosorbent assay (ELISA) and Western blot, preferably using recombinant antigens.

Antibodies against soluble liver antigens

Soluble liver antigens were detected in a patient who had ANA-negative AIH and have been reported to be directed against cytokeratins 8 and 18 and other autoantigens of the cytoplasm. They are highly specific for AIH. In about 75% of cases they occur simultaneously with other autoantibodies such as SMAs and antimitochondrial antibodies. Those patients who are ANA-positive additionally have SLA autoantibodies in 11% of cases. Soluble liver antigen autoantibodies are detected by ELISA. Recently, reactivity of SLA autoantibodies with glutathionesulfotransferases (GSTs) as the cytosolic target antigen, and a novel 50kDa protein from activated lymphocytes, has been reported.

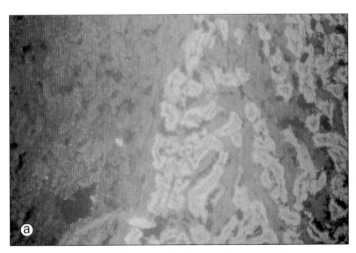

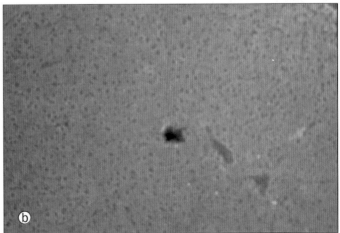

Figure 16.6 Anti-liver–kidney antibodies. Indirect immunofluorescence showing LKM-1 autoantibodies on rat kidney and liver cryostat sections. Serum of a patient who has autoimmune hepatitis type 2. (a) Typical indirect immunofluorescence pattern of LKM-1 autoantibodies detecting the proximal (cortical) renal tubules (left of micrograph) but excluding the distal tubules (right of micrograph), located in the renal medulla, which corresponds to the tissue expression pattern of the autoantigen CYP 2D6. (b) Using rat hepatic cryostat sections a homogeneous cellular immunofluorescence staining is visualized excluding the hepatocellular nuclei (LKM-1).

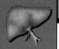

Heterogeneity of antibodies directed against endoplasmic reticulum antigens (microsomal antigens) in liver diseases			
Antibody	kDa	Target antigen	Disease
LKM-1	50	Cytochrome P450 2D6	Autoimmune hepatitis type 2, hepatitis C
LKM-2	50	Cytochrome P450 2C9	Ticrynafen-induced hepatitis
LKM-3	55	UGT1A	Hepatitis D-associated autoimmunity Autoimmune hepatitis type 2
LKM	50	Cytochrome P450 2A6	Autoimmune polyendocrine syndrome type 1 (APS-1) Hepatitis C
LM	52	Cytochrome P450 1A2	Hydralazine-induced hepatitis Hepatitis with autoimmune polyendocrine syndrome type 1 (APS-1)
	57	Disulfidisomerase	Halothane hepatitis
	59	Carboxylesterase	Halothane hepatitis
	35	?	Autoimmune hepatitis
	59	?	Chronic hepatitis C
	64	?	Autoimmune hepatitis
	70	?	Chronic hepatitis C

Figure 16.7 Heterogeneity of antibodies directed against endoplasmic reticulum antigens (microsomal antigens) in liver diseases. LKM, liver–kidney microsomal autoantibodies; kDa, molecular weight in kilodaltons; UGT1A, family 1 uridine diphosphate-5'-glucuronosyltransferases.

Other autoantibodies

Other antibodies have been described in AIH. The ASGPR is a liver-specific glycoprotein located in the cell membrane. Autoimmunity targeting this antigen is observed in 88% of all patients who have AIH. However, anti-ASGPR antibodies are also found in chronic HBV and HCV infections, alcoholic liver disease, and PBC. The levels of anti-ASGPR antibodies fluctuate according to inflammatory activity of the disease and can be viewed as an additional marker to monitor therapeutic efficacy. Anti-ASGPR antibodies appear to be a general marker of liver autoimmunity.

Antibodies against a cytosolic protein showing immunofluorescence with liver and pancreas have been identified and termed anti-LP antibodies. The antigen of these autoantibodies is not cytokeratin. Liver–pancreas antibodies are present in about 33% of patients who have AIH and their significance is presumably similar to that of SLA autoantibodies, allowing a differentiation of ANA-negative AIH. Anti-cytosol antibodies type 1, anti-LC-1 antibodies, often occur in conjunction with ANA and SMA autoantibodies in AIH type 1, but are also detectable in chronic HCV infection. The clinical significance is not yet completely defined.

Predisposing and triggering mechanisms

Conclusive evidence for a single unifying pathogenetic mechanism of AIH has not yet been presented. Many observations point towards a viral etiology and this has been investigated in numerous studies. However, the concept that viral infection is the etiology of AIH remains a matter of controversy. In anecdotal reports, hepatitis A virus, HBV, Epstein–Barr virus, and herpes simplex virus (HSV) have all been implicated in triggering autoimmune hepatitis. As a potential underlying mechanism, molecular mimicry between viral and body proteins has been suggested. In this respect, it was shown that the B-cell epitope of CYP 2D6, which is targeted by LKM-1 autoantibodies, displays homology with the immediate early antigen IE175 of HSV. A case has been reported in which the only difference in HLA identical twins with discordant manifestation of AIH was HSV exposure.

Hepatitis C virus infection is associated with a broad array of serologic markers of autoimmunity and immune-mediated syndromes. Liver–kidney microsomal autoantibodies are present in 3–5% of cases. However, this serologic autoimmunity differs with respect to recognition of antigen targets (CYP 2D6 and CYP 2A6), recognition of epitopes (AIH mainly 257–269, HCV more diverse, and also more conformation-dependent epitopes), and the clinical presentation. These considerations suggest that it is unlikely that HCV is etiologically responsible for AIH.

Apart from viral agents, a genetic predisposition must be regarded as a mandatory prerequisite of AIH. Certain HLA haplotypes have been identified to confer a high risk for the development of AIH. Caucasian subjects characteristically display the HLA A1, B8, DR3 phenotype, which has also been found to be associated with a number of other autoimmune diseases including diabetes mellitus. In contrast, Japanese patients display a predominance of the HLA DR4 haplotype. The impact of genetic traits become evident when the natural history of the disease is analyzed. Patients who have the DR3 allele have an earlier onset of AIH, a more severe course, are less

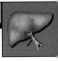

likely to attain remission, and have a higher rate of relapse. All of these characteristics lead to a greater need for liver transplantation. Carriers of the DR4 allele in contrast have a more benign course of AIH (Fig. 16.8). These findings provide evidence for a genetic component in the etiology of AIH.

In LKM-1-positive patients an association with the null allele of complement factor C4A has been found (C4AQ0). Complement factor C4A has been proposed to exert a role in virus neutralization that may contribute to the development of immune-mediated diseases. The molecular analysis of HLA antigens has demonstrated that HLA DR3 and DR4 have a common amino acid sequence between positions 67 and 72 of the DRb protein, which is present in 94% of patients who have AIH. The DRb molecule has an important impact on peptide antigen binding by the HLA class 2 molecule and can therefore exert an influence on the immune-mediated attack on the hepatocyte.

The presence of autoantibodies, the association of specific HLA alleles with AIH, and the observation of a lymphocytic infiltrate in the liver in AIH led to the establishment of an immunopathogenetic model for AIH. However, the significance of T-cell immunity has now been recognized as paramount for the development and maintenance of chronic AIH. In the model of experimental autoimmune hepatitis (EAH) in mice, transplantation of T cells can initiate AIH-like disease in naive animals.

Although the potential role of T-cell and B-cell mechanisms in autoimmune hepatitis has been outlined, the exact mechanism of hepatocellular toxicity remains undefined (Figure 16.9).

Autoantigen peptides and aberrantly expressed antigens such as ASGPR, CYP 2D6, and UGTs can be presented together with HLA class 2 antigens to a CD4$^+$ T$_H$0 cell. This activated cell can differentiate to a T$_H$1 cell under the influence of interleukin (IL)-12 and elaborate interferon (IFN)-γ and IL-2. Interferon-γ leads to an increase of hepatocellular HLA class 1 expression and to an activation of cytotoxic T lymphocytes, which increases the risk of class 1 restricted hepatocellular cytotoxicity. Interferon-γ also induces hepatocellular HLA class 2 expression. Under the influence of IL-4, the T$_H$0 cell can also differentiate in the direction of a T$_H$2 cell and begin to elaborate IL-10, IL-4, and IL-5. This can lead to B-lymphocyte activation and potentially to autoantibody production. In principle, hepatocellular toxicity can therefore be achieved through cytotoxic T cells, direct cytokine mediated cytolysis or by autoantibody and complement-mediated killer cell activity, or a combination of these factors. Studies have shown CD4$^+$ lymphocytes in the area of piecemeal necrosis, or interface hepatitis as it is now called. In addition, T lymphocytes from AIH patients are capable of stimulating autoantibody production of B cells, and liver infiltrating T cells can be stimulated by treatment with known autoantigens.

A possible connection to viral infections may be the ability of viruses to perform cytokine mimicry. It has been shown that Epstein–Barr virus is capable of elaborating a viral IL-10, which is 70% homologous with human IL-10. This may enact B-cell stimulation without prior cascade activation.

CLINICAL FEATURES

Autoimmune hepatitis is part of the syndrome of chronic hepatitis, which is characterized by sustained hepatocellular inflammation of at least 6 months duration and elevation of the transaminases alanine aminotransferase (ALT) or asparate aminotransferase (AST) to at least 1.5 times the upper limit of normal. About 49% of patients who have AIH have an acute clinical presentation with an hepatic illness and jaundice, and occasional cases of acute liver failure have been reported. In most cases, however, the clinical presentation is not spectacular and is characterized by fatigue, right upper quadrant pain, and jaundice. Palmar erythema and spider nevi may be present. In the later stages, the consequences of portal hypertension dominate, with ascites, bleeding esophageal varices and encephalopathy. A specific feature of AIH is the association of extrahepatic immune-mediated syndromes including autoimmune thyroiditis, vitiligo, alopecia, nail dystrophy, ulcerative colitis, rheumatoid arthritis, diabetes mellitus, and glomerulonephritis (Fig. 16.10).

Immunoserologic parameters assume a central role in the subclassification of AIH (Fig. 16.11) and allow the discrimination of clinically different groups of patients.

Autoimmune hepatitis type 1 is characterized by seropositivity for ANA and in most cases SMA autoantibodies. In 97% of patients hypergammaglobulinemia with elevated immunoglobulin G is present. Representing 80% of the cases of AIH, this form is the most prevalent subclass and was historically first described as lupoid, classic, or idiopathic AIH. About 70% of patients are female with a peak incidence between ages 16 and 30 years, but 50% of patients are older than 30 years. An association with other immune syndromes is observed in 48%, with autoimmune thyroid disease, synovitis, and ulcerative colitis being the commonest manifestations. The clinical course is often unspectacular and a presentation with acute liver failure is rare. About 25% have cirrhosis at the time of diagnosis.

Autoimmune hepatitis type 2 is characterized by the presence of LKM-1 autoantibodies against CYP 2D6. In 10% of cases LKM-3 autoantibodies against UDP-glucuronosyltransferases are also present. In contrast to AIH type 1, additional organ-specific autoantibodies are present such as antithyroid, antiparietal cell, and anti-Langerhans cell autoantibodies. Extrahepatic immune syndromes such as diabetes, vitiligo, and autoimmune thyroid disease are also more prevalent. Serum immunoglobulin levels are moderately elevated, but there is

Classification of autoimmune hepatitis based on genetic markers		
HLA	DR3	DR4
Genotype	DR B1*0301	DR B1*0401 (DR B1*0405 in Japanese)
Age at onset	<30 years	>40 years
Disease activity	+++	+
Treatment response	++	++++
Relapse after treatment	+++	+
Liver transplantation	+++	+
DRb chain amino acid as risk factor	Lysine at AA71	?

Figure 16.8 Classification of autoimmune hepatitis based on genetic markers.

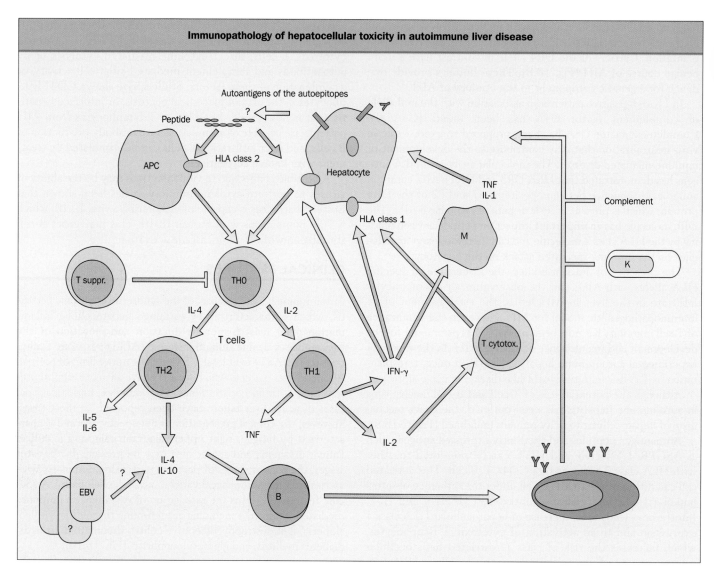

Immunopathology of hepatocellular toxicity in autoimmune liver disease

Figure 16.9 Immunopathology of hepatocellular toxicity in autoimmune liver disease. Diagram explained in text. (Adapted from Mieli-Vergani and Mieli-Vergani, 1996.)

often a reduction in IgA levels. AIH type 2 is a rare disorder that affects 20% of AIH patients in Europe, but only 4% in the USA. There is a female predominance. The peak age is around 10 years, but AIH type 2 is also observed in adults, especially in Europe. Autoimmune hepatitis type 2 carries a higher risk of progression to cirrhosis and is much more likely to present with the clinical features of acute liver failure.

Autoimmune hepatitis type 3 is characterized by SLA (and LP) autoantibodies, but 74% also have other serologic markers of autoimmunity, including SMA and AMA. Autoimmune hepatitis type 3 has a lower prevalence than AIH type 2, affects female patients in 90%, and has a peak age between 20 and 40 years at presentation. The validity of this subclass of AIH is a matter of debate and further evaluations will have to determine whether it represents an entity in itself or is a variation of AIH type 1.

DIAGNOSIS

The profile of liver function tests does not discriminate AIH from other liver disorders. The acute presentation with jaundice is asso-

ciated with high transaminases, but in a pattern similar to that of acute viral hepatitis. Occasionally these patients have an associated autoimmune hemolytic anemia that can lead to serum bilirubin levels in excess of 800μmol/L (47mg/dL). The more indolent presentations show varying degrees of elevation of the transaminases, but any impairment of synthetic function should point to the possibility that cirrhosis has already become established. The role of autoantibodies and immunoglobulin levels in the diagnosis has already been described. Ultimately, the diagnosis of AIH is part of the differential diagnosis of chronic hepatitis and is reached through the exclusion of other causes of hepatitis (see Fig. 16.1).

The diagnosis can also be reached with the aid of a scoring system devised by the International Autoimmune Hepatitis Group and the International Association for the Study of the Liver (IASL), which describes the probability of AIH. The validity of this model has been confirmed in clinical evaluations. As has been elaborated in the previous sections of this chapter, the positive criteria for AIH include sex, inflammatory activity, autoantibodies, HLA type, histology, the absence of viral infection and ethanol abuse, and a response to corticosteroid treatment. The

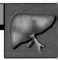

Autoimmune hepatitis: associated extrahepatic syndromes

Autoimmune thyroid disease	Diabetes mellitus
Ulcerative colitis	Autoimmune thrombocytopenic purpura
Synovitis	Vitiligo
Rheumatoid arthritis	Nail dystrophy
Lichen planus	Alopecia
CREST syndrome	

Figure 16.10 Autoimmune hepatitis: associated extrahepatic syndromes.

Comparison between genuine and virus-induced autoimmunity

	Autoimmune hepatitis	Viral hepatitis
Autoantibody titer	↑ ↑ ↑	↑
Linear autoepitopes	+ + +	+
Conformational epitopes	+	+ + + +
Inhibitory antibodies	+ +	+ +
Autoimmune response	Homogenous	Heterogeneous
Treatment	Immunosuppression	(Antiviral)

Figure 16.11 Comparison between genuine and virus-induced autoimmunity.

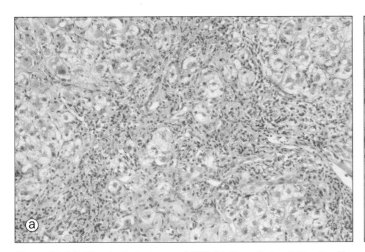
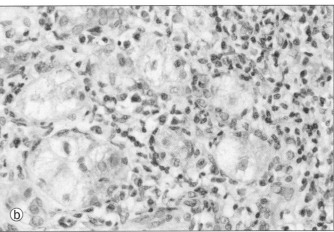

Figure 16.12 Histologic features of AIH. (a) Expanded portal tracts with chronic inflammatory cell infiltration that largely invades the parenchymal limiting plate. Note the isolated and pale staining hepatocytes deeply enmeshed within the new portal boundaries. (b) Higher magnification of the interface showing single or rosette-forming hepatocytes surrounded by lymphocytes and plasma cells. (Courtesy of Professor B Portmann.)

determination of autoantibodies using state of the art techniques including indirect immunofluorescence, ELISA, and recombinant antigen Western blot is paramount for a precise definition of AIH. The probability of AIH decreases whenever signs of bile duct involvement are present, such as elevation of alkaline phosphatase, histologic signs of cholangiopathy and detection of AMA. If one or more components of the scoring system are not evaluated, only a score pointing to a probable diagnosis can be compiled. Significantly, this approach also permits the rational characterization of patients who have unclear or overlap syndromes and facilitates a scientific comparison of patient populations worldwide.

Histology

Although AIH is not characterized by a disease-specific histologic feature, percutaneous liver biopsy should be performed when coagulation studies allow this to be performed with safety. Usually, the histology in the untreated patient shows a portal and periportal hepatitis with lymphocytic and plasma cell infiltrates (Fig. 16.12).

When the inflammation erodes the parenchymal limiting plate, interface hepatitis is said to be present. This descriptive term has replaced piecemeal necrosis, and the more general descriptions of chronic active hepatitis and chronic persistent hepatitis, which were previously based on the presence or absence of piecemeal necrosis, have also been abandoned. Liver morphology is now described by a score for both the degree of inflammatory activity and of fibrosis, so that the morphology in this situation may be described as autoimmune chronic hepatitis, stage 3, grade 11 (equivalent to extensive fibrosis with marked necroinflammatory activity). Cirrhosis may be present at the time of the first clinical presentation. A lobular hepatitis may also be present, but is only indicative of AIH in the absence of copper deposits or biliary inflammation. In addition, the presence of granulomas or iron deposits argues against the diagnosis of AIH. The response to treatment should be assessed histologically as continued necroinflammatory activity may not be reflected in abnormal liver function tests.

Differentiation of cryptogenic hepatitis and overlap syndromes

Cryptogenic hepatitis is an etiologically undefined chronic hepatitis. It is unclear how many of these patients in fact suffer from AIH without the presence of serum autoantibodies detectable with the available state of the art techniques. In about 13% of these patients, who had initially been tested by indirect immunofluorescence for ANA, SMA and LKM, it was possible to detect SLA autoantibodies and thereby contribute to diagnostic clarity by assigning them to the autoimmune category of hepatitis. Clinically this group of cryptogenic hepatitis resembles AIH type 1 with respect to age and sex distribution, HLA antigen types, inflammatory activity, and response to therapy.

Overlap syndromes are conditions in which the features are very suggestive of AIH, but additional markers or symptoms point to other diseases within the differential diagnosis of AIH. Among these are PBC in 8% with serum AMA and histologic signs of cholangitis, PSC in 6% with typical changes on cholangiography, and autoimmune cholangitis in 10% with ANA, SMA, and histologic inflammation of the biliary system. Hepatitis has also been described in 10–15% of patients who have APS-1. This syndrome is characterized by a triad of mucocutaneous candidiasis, hypothyroidism, and Addison's disease. In these patients autoantibodies to CYP 1A2 and CYP 2A6 have been detected as serologic markers of autoimmunity.

A clinically significant association is virus-associated autoimmunity, which describes the coexistence of autoantibodies and virus infection. The most important associations are HCV infection and HDV infection in which LKM autoantibodies can be detected in 2–5% and 6–12%, respectively. Autoimmune hepatitis type 2 and HCV infection with LKM autoantibodies are clinically distinct entities (see Fig. 16.11). Liver–kidney microsomal autoantibodies in virus infection are present at lower titers and recognize more conformational and diverse epitopes than in genuine AIH. This discrimination is relevant since it forms the basis for mutually exclusive therapeutic strategies: immunosuppression in AIH and interferon in chronic viral hepatitis.

NATURAL HISTORY AND PROGNOSIS

The natural history and prognosis of AIH are largely defined by the inflammatory activity present at presentation and by the presence or development of cirrhosis. With a 5- to 10-fold elevation of AST and two-fold gammaglobulin elevation, mortality without treatment is 90% in 10 years. Approximately 17% of patients who have periportal hepatitis develop cirrhosis in 5 years, but this figure increases to 82% when bridging necrosis or necrosis of multiple lobules is present. The presence of cirrhosis indicates a mortality of 58% in 5 years. The course of AIH is also strongly influenced by the HLA antigen profile of the affected individual. The presence of HLA B8 is associated with severe inflammation at presentation and a higher likelihood of relapse after treatment. Individuals who are DR3 have a lower probability of reaching remission, have more frequent relapses, and require transplantation more often. The HLA DR4 positive subgroup is characterized by a higher age of onset and a more benign outcome.

MANAGEMENT

The indication for treatment of AIH is based on the inflammatory activity and to a lesser extent on the presence of fibrosis or cirrhosis. In the absence of inflammatory activity immunosuppressive treatment has only limited effects.

Independent of the clinically or immunoserologically defined type of AIH, treatment is implemented with predniso(lo)ne alone or in combination with azathioprine. The therapeutic benefit of corticosteroids was established in the 1970s in controlled trials and azathioprine was mainly used as a 'steroid-sparing' drug. The use of prednisone or its metabolite prednisolone is equally effective as chronic liver disease does not seem to have an effect on the synthesis of prednisolone from prednisone. It is important to accurately differentiate viral infection from autoimmune hepatitis. Treatment of replicative viral hepatitis with corticosteroids must be prevented, as must the administration of interferon in AIH as this can lead to a dramatic exacerbation of the disease.

An indication for treatment is present when aminotransferases are elevated 1.5-fold, gammaglobulin levels are elevated two-fold, and histology shows moderate-to-severe periportal hepatitis. Symptoms of severe fatigue are also an indication for treatment. An absolute indication exists in cases with a 10-fold or higher elevation of aminotransferase levels, histologic signs of severe inflammation and necrosis, and those who have evidence of disease progression.

The treatment regimen and suggested follow-up examinations are summarized in Fig. 16.13.

Therapy is usually administered over the course of 1–2 years. The decision between monotherapy and combination therapy is guided by a number of principles. Long-term steroid therapy leads to cushingoid side effects and it has been shown that cosmetic side effects decrease patient compliance considerably (Fig. 16.14).

Serious complications such as steroid-induced diabetes, osteopenia, avascular necrosis of bone, psychiatric symptoms, hypertension, and cataract formation also have to be anticipated in long-term treatment. Side effects are present in 44% of patients after 12 months and in 80% of patients after 24 months of treatment. However, predniso(lo)ne monotherapy is possible in pregnant patients. Azathioprine, on the other hand, leads to a decreased dose of prednisone. It bears a theoretic risk of teratogenicity. In addition, abdominal discomfort, nausea, cholestatic hepatitis, rashes, and leukopenia can be encountered. These side effects are seen in 10% of patients receiving a dose of 50mg per day. From a general point of view, a postmenopausal woman with osteoporosis, hypertension and elevated blood glucose would be a candidate for combination therapy. In young women, pregnant women or patients who have hematologic abnormalities, prednisone monotherapy may be the treatment of choice.

Treatment is initiated according to the regimen in Fig. 16.13. Continuous treatment is essential since most cases of relapse are the result of erratic changes of medication and/or dose. Dose reduction is aimed at finding the lowest possible maintenance dose. Since histology lags 3–6 months behind the normalization of serum parameters, therapy has to be continued beyond the normalization of aminotransferase levels. Usually, maintenance doses of prednisone range between 2.5 and 10mg daily. After 12–24 months of therapy predniso(lo)ne may tapered and withdrawn over the course of 4–6 weeks.

The outcome can be classified into four categories: remission, relapse, treatment failure, and stabilization. Remission is a complete normalization of all inflammatory parameters, including histology. This is achieved in 65% of patients after 24 months of treatment. Remission can be sustained with azathioprine monotherapy of 2mg/kg body weight. This prevents cushingoid side effects. However, side effects such as arthralgia (53%), myalgia (14%), lymphopenia (57%), and myelosuppression (6%) have been observed. Relapse is characterized by a three-fold increase

Chapter 16

Autoimmune Hepatitis
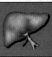

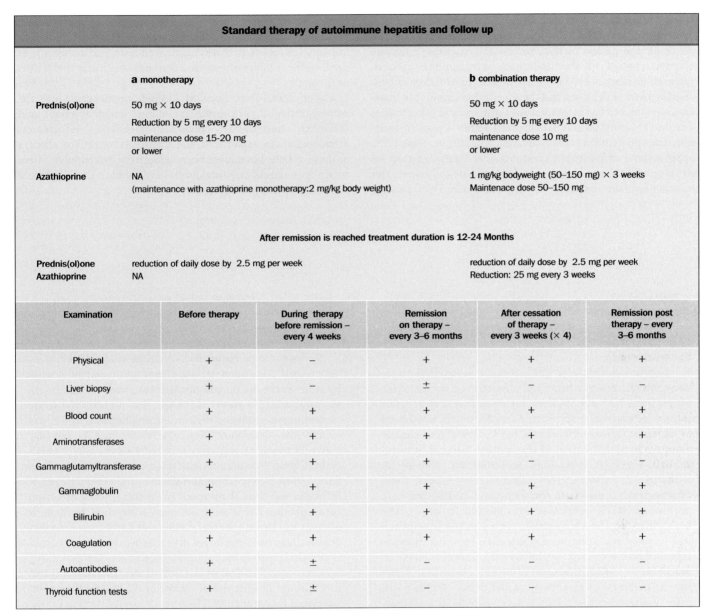

Standard therapy of autoimmune hepatitis and follow up					

a monotherapy

Prednis(ol)one — 50 mg × 10 days
Reduction by 5 mg every 10 days
maintenance dose 15-20 mg
or lower

Azathioprine — NA
(maintenance with azathioprine monotherapy:2 mg/kg body weight)

b combination therapy

50 mg × 10 days
Reduction by 5 mg every 10 days
maintenance dose 10 mg
or lower

1 mg/kg bodyweight (50–150 mg) × 3 weeks
Maintenace dose 50–150 mg

After remission is reached treatment duration is 12-24 Months

Prednis(ol)one — reduction of daily dose by 2.5 mg per week
Azathioprine — NA

reduction of daily dose by 2.5 mg per week
Reduction: 25 mg every 3 weeks

Examination	Before therapy	During therapy before remission – every 4 weeks	Remission on therapy – every 3–6 months	After cessation of therapy – every 3 weeks (× 4)	Remission post therapy – every 3–6 months
Physical	+	–	+	+	+
Liver biopsy	+	–	±	–	–
Blood count	+	+	+	+	+
Aminotransferases	+	+	+	+	+
Gammaglutamyltransferase	+	+	+	–	–
Gammaglobulin	+	+	+	+	+
Bilirubin	+	+	+	+	+
Coagulation	+	+	+	+	+
Autoantibodies	+	±	–	–	–
Thyroid function tests	+	±	–	–	–

Figure 16.13 Standard therapy of autoimmune hepatitis and follow-up. All drug doses are daily doses.

of aminotransferase levels and the reoccurrence of clinical symptoms. Relapse is present in 50% of patients within 6 months of treatment withdrawal and in 80% after 3 years. Relapse is associated with progression to cirrhosis in 38% and liver failure in 14%. The occurrence of a relapse calls for reinitiation of standard therapy and perhaps a long-term maintenance dose with predniso(lo)ne or azathioprine monotherapy. Treatment failure characterizes a progression of clinical, serologic, and histologic parameters during standard therapy. This is seen in about 10% of patients. In these cases the diagnosis of AIH has to be carefully reconsidered to exclude other etiologies of chronic hepatitis. In these patients experimental regimens can be administered or ultimately liver transplantation becomes necessary. Stabilization is the achievement of a partial remission. Since 90% of patients reach remission within 3 years, the benefit of standard therapy has to be re-evaluated in this subgroup of patients. Ultimately, liver transplantation provides a definitive treatment option.

Side effects of predniso(lo)ne and azathioprine	
Predniso(lo)ne	**Azathioprine**
Acne	Nausea
Moon-shaped face	Vomiting
Striae	Abdominal discomfort
Dorsal hump	Hepatotoxicity
Obesity	Rash
Weight gain	Arthralgia
Osteoporosis	Myalgia
Avascular necrosis of bone	Leukocytopenia
Psychiatric symptoms	Teratogenicity?
(euphoria, psychosis, depression)	Oncogenicity?
Diabetes mellitus	
Cataract	
Hypertension	

Figure 16.14 Side effects of predniso(lo)ne and azathioprine.

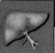

Liver transplantation is the definitive treatment option for unresponsive disease, including the presentation as acute liver failure, or clinical disease as the consequence of cirrhosis despite effective control of the underlying autoimmune process. However, no marker for the reliable prediction of failure of conservative treatment exists, and the specific indications for transplantation tend to be the general ones that apply to other causes of cirrhosis. If remission is not achieved within 4 years of treatment, the option of liver transplantation is usually necessary. The 5-year survival of patients undergoing liver transplantation for AIH is up to 92%, and as such there is no difference between this and other favorable indications for transplantation. These patients carry a higher risk of developing rejection after transplantation. Recurrence of AIH in the transplanted liver has been reported, but this appears to be easily controlled with corticosteroids as used for the primary disease and does not frequently lead to loss of the graft.

Experimental strategies with limited experience include the administration of cyclosporin, tacrolimus, ursodeoxycholic acid (UDCA), budenoside, phosphatidylcholine, intravenous immunoglobulin, rapamycin, and thymus extracts. The efficacy of these options has not yet been definitively determined. These treatments should only be administered within the context of controlled and approved studies.

PRACTICE POINT

Illustrative case

An 11-year-old Caucasian girl is brought to medical attention with an apparent history of elevated transaminase levels between 100 and 300IU/L for more than 2 years. The history indicated the administration of a blood transfusion as an infant. Immunoglobulin A and G levels were slightly elevated; immunoglobulin M was normal. Clinical, serologic, and histologic evaluations indicated the absence of hepatitis A virus, HBV, Epstein–Barr virus, and cytomegalovirus infection. Anti-hepatitis C antibodies were positive but HVC-RNA was not detected in serum. The biopsy showed chronic hepatitis with a mixed plasma cell and lymphocytic infiltrate and interface hepatitis. Routine autoantibody screening by immunofluorescence failed to detect ANA, AMA, SMA, or LKM autoantibodies. There was no evidence of α_1-antitrypsin deficiency, Wilson's disease, of any other metabolic, genetic or toxic liver disease. Interferon treatment was commenced in a dose of 3 million units thrice weekly.

After 4 weeks a picture resembling acute hepatitis emerged with a 20-fold increase in serum ALT levels. Interferon treatment was immediately discontinued. A re-analysis of the autoantibodies demonstrated the presence of LKM immunofluorescence on cryostat sections, LKM-1 reactivity upon ELISA analysis, and the presence of a 50kDa band using Western blot assays. Therapy with 40mg of prednisolone daily was initiated and ALT levels fell to normal levels for the first time.

Interpretation

The discrimination of chronic viral hepatitis and autoimmune hepatitis is possible using refined seroimmunologic and molecular biological methods such as indirect immunofluorescence, ELISA, Western blot, and RT-PCR. While it appears unlikely that virus infections cause AIH, the overlap of chronic virus infection and latent AIH can be a diagnostic problem.

Markers of viral hepatitis A–E can be readily and reliably determined. Also the determination of serum autoantibodies by state of the art techniques will accurately detect serum autoantibodies. In cases where low titer autoantibodies are present in patients who have chronic viral hepatitis, these may indicate the coexistence of genuine but latent AIH, but may also reflect virus-associated or induced serologic autoimmunity. Interferon is contraindicated in genuine AIH. Here, interferon will have to be administered with cautious monitoring of serologic and clinical parameters. In the absence of serum autoantibodies latent AIH, although a very rare problem, is difficult to diagnose. In the presence of LKM autoantibodies before treatment, one could differentiate the recognition of CYP 2D6 epitopes. Recognition of the major epitope located between amino acids 257 and 269 of the CYP 2D6 protein may indicate a higher risk of coexisting AIH rather than virus-associated autoimmunity. However, a carefully administered and closely monitored therapeutic trial following adequate diagnostic measures can be a more rational diagnostic tool.

The decision is between immunosuppression, standard therapy of AIH, and IFN-α, standard therapy of chronic viral hepatitis but contraindicated in genuine autoimmune hepatitis. Virus-associated autoimmunity in chronic viral hepatitis has to be differentiated from coexisting chronic viral hepatitis and AIH to prevent interferon-related exacerbation of AIH. If this is not possible by seroimmunologic or molecular biological methods, a cautiously administered therapeutic trial with interferon can be the only option.

In the above mentioned scenario, normalization of ALT levels is achieved with prednisolone administration. In cases with replicative HCV infection and coexisting AIH this decision is more difficult and will have to be based on the clinical response and the course of the disease. Fortunately, genuine AIH in chronic viral hepatitis is a very rare condition. The treatment of patients with chronic HCV infection which display low titer virus-associated autoantibodies is possible in many cases without severe disease exacerbation.

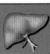

FURTHER READING

Beaune PH, Dansette PM, Mansuy D, et al. Human antiendoplasmatic reticulum autoantibodies appearing in a drug induced hepatitis directed against a human liver cytochrome P450 that hydroxilates the drug. Proc Natl Acad Sci USA. 1987;84:551–5. *The first cytochrome P450 enzyme identified as autoantigen.*

Czaja AJ, Carpenter HA. Validation of a scoring system for the diagnosis of autoimmune hepatitis. Dig Dis Sci. 1996;4:305–14. *Application of a scoring system to the diagnosis of autoimmune chronic hepatitis.*

Desmet VJ, Gerber M, Hoofnagle JH, et al. Classification of chronic hepatitis: diagnosis grading and staging. Hepatology. 1994;19:1513–20. *New and current histologic classification of chronic hepatitis.*

Homberg JC, Abuaf N, Bernard O, et al. Chronic active hepatitis associated with anti-liver/kidney microsome antibody type 1: a second type of 'autoimmune' hepatitis. Hepatology. 1987;7:1333–9. *Description of a second variant of anti-liver–kidney microsomal antibodies associated with autoimmune chronic hepatitis.*

Johnson PJ, MacFarlane IG, Alvarez F, et al. Meeting report: International Autoimmune Hepatitis Group. Hepatology. 1993;18:998–1005. *Considerations on definitions and nomenclature in autoimmune chronic hepatitis.*

Johnson PJ, McFarlane IG, Williams R. Azathioprine for long-term maintenance of remission in autoimmune hepatitis. N Engl J Med. 1995;333:958–63. *Demonstration of the role of monotherapy with azathioprine in maintaining remission.*

Mackay IR, Taft LI, Cowling DC. Lupoid hepatitis. Lancet. 1956;2:1323–6. *Further description of distinct form of hepatitis termed 'lupoid' although the distinction from lupus was clearly made.*

Manns MP, Krüger M. Immunogenetics of chronic liver disease. Gastroenterology. 1994;106:1676–97. *Overview of the immunogenetics of autoimmune chronic hepatitis.*

Manns MP, Gerken G, Kyriatsoulis A, et al. Characterization of a new subgroup of autoimmune chronic active hepatitis by autoantibodies against soluble liver antigen. Lancet. 1987;1:292–4. *Another link to AIH not identified by classic autoantibodies.*

Manns MP, Griffin KJ, Sullivan KJ, et al. LKM-1 autoantibodies recognize a shot linear sequence in P4502D6, a cytochrome P450 monooxygenase. J Clin Invest. 1991;88:1370–78. *Further progress to understanding the molecular basis of autoimmune hepatitis.*

Mieli-Vergani G, Mieli-Vergani D. Autoimmune hepatitis. Arch Dis Childhood. 1996;74:2–5. *Important description of the spectrum of disease in the pediatric population.*

Philipp T, Durazzo M, Straub P, et al. Recognition of uridine diphosphate glucuronosyltransferase by LKM-3 autoantibodies in chronic hepatitis D. Lancet. 1994;344:576–81. *Another clue to the molecular basis of the pathogenesis of the disease.*

Rizzetto M, Swana G, Doniach D. Microsomal antibodies in active chronic hepatitis and other disorders. Clin Exp Immunol. 1973;14:331–4. *Original description of autoimmune chronic hepatitis with anti-liver–kidney microsomal antibodies.*

Strassburg CP, Obermayer-Straub P, Alex B, et al. Autoantibodies against glucuronosyltransferases differ between viral hepatitis and autoimmune hepatitis. Gastroenterology. 1996;111:1576–86. *Experimental evidence helping to understand differences between pure autoimmune disease and viral-related autoantibodies.*

Strassburg CP, Obermayer-Straub P, Manns MP. Autoimmunity in hepatitis C and D virus infection. J Viral Hepatitis. 1996;3:49–59. *An overview of viral-related autoimmunity.*

Tan EM. Antinuclear antibodies. Diagnostic markers for autoimmune diseases and probes for cell biology. Adv Immunol. 1991;44:93–151. *Excellent overview of ANAS.*

Waldenström J. Leber, Blutproteine und Nahrunseiweiss. Deutsche Z f Verd u. Stoffwechselkr. 1950;15:113–21. *First clinical description of autoimmune chronic hepatitis.*

Zanger UM, Hauri HP, Loeper J, et al. Antibodies against human cytochrome P450 dbl in autoimmune hepatitis type 2. Proc Natl Acad Sci USA. 1988;27:8256–60. *Link between anti-liver–kidney microsomal antibodies and cytochrome P450.*

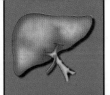

Chapter 17   Primary Biliary Cirrhosis

James Neuberger

INTRODUCTION

Primary biliary cirrhosis (PBC) is a chronic, progressive cholestatic disorder, principally affecting middle-aged women and reported most frequently in Europe and North America. At the end-stage of the disease, patients can be treated satisfactorily by hepatic transplantation.

EPIDEMIOLOGY AND PATHOGENESIS

Epidemiology
It has been difficult to achieve an accurate assessment of the prevalence and incidence of PBC. The published studies have shown marked variation, which, in part, is due to differences in methodology, as indicated below.

Case definition
During the past decade, it has been realized that the spectrum of disease is far greater than previously appreciated. As a consequence, the definition of PBC has changed so that part of the variation in the reported disease incidence and prevalence may reflect changes in recognition of the syndrome.

Case finding
Depending on the methods used to identify cases of PBC, different conclusions may be drawn. For example, those tertiary referral units reporting on their own experience will deduce lower rates than those based on screening a defined population. The recognition that antimitochondrial antibodies (AMAs) are associated with PBC allows screening of large numbers of blood samples such as those from blood donors and may give a far higher incidence of PBC.

Incidence studies
These are difficult to interpret in diseases such as PBC in which the onset of the disease is insidious and the date of onset cannot readily be defined.

These caveats should be remembered when the findings of different studies are considered (Fig. 17.1).

From the published studies, several conclusions can be drawn:
- Although PBC is described throughout the World, the disease is more common in Northern Europe and in North America than in Africa, the Indian subcontinent and South America.
- The distribution of patients is patchy and there is no consensus regarding whether PBC is more common in urban or rural environments.
- The reported prevalence and incidence of PBC appears to be increasing.

Unlike other autoimmune diseases, there is no close association between the disease and any human leukocyte antigen (HLA) genotype. Although there is an association with HLA B8, this is weak in patients from Europe and North America, but stronger in Japanese patients, in whom this allele is more prevalent. In European and North American patients there is a weak association with DRB1*0801; in Japanese patients, a weak association has been reported both for DPB1*0803 and the linked allele DPB1*0501. There is increasing evidence of a family predisposition for the disease: the prevalence of disease amongst first degree relatives is markedly increased compared with that of the general population, possibly up to 500-fold. Affected family members are often siblings rather than different generations. Where different generations are affected, the second generation usually presents earlier and tends to have a more rapid progression.

Reported incidence and prevalence of PBC in different countries where centers have published on more than one occasion		
Location	Incidence/10^6	Prevalence/10^6
Sheffield (UK)	38	54
Dundee (UK)	10.6	40
Newcastle upon Tyne (UK)	41	392
Malmo (Sweden)	24	92
Glasgow (UK)	15	93
Ontario (Canada)	3	22
Victoria (Australia)	–	19
Estonia (Russia)	2	27
Quebec (Canada)	3.9	25
Spain	7.5	46
Denmark	1	–
Germany	–	0.7
Portugal	–	74

Figure 17.1 Reported incidence and prevalence of primary biliary cirrhosis (PBC) in different countries where centers have published on more than one occasion.

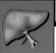
Pathogenesis

The pathogenesis of PBC remains controversial. Different etiologies have been suggested.

Autoimmune disease

There are many features which suggest that PBC may be an autoimmune disease. Histologic findings (see below) indicate involvement of the immune system. Lymphocytes infiltrating the biliary epithelial cells are predominantly CD4⁺, although occasional CD8⁺ lymphocytes and B cells are seen. There is an increase in γ-δ cells within the portal tract. Analysis of T-lymphocyte clones derived from livers of patients with PBC shows a slight preponderance of Th-1 cells. There is considerable heterogeneity of T-cell receptor V-β usage. The damaged bile duct cells show overexpression of a variety of immune molecules (Fig. 17.2) including adhesion molecules, major histocompatibility complex (MHC) class II antigens, mitochondrial autoantigens and interleukin-2 receptors. These biliary epithelial cells also express tumor necrosis factor and γ-interferon. However, it is difficult to distinguish those factors which arise as a consequence of cholestasis from those which are central to the pathogenesis of disease. For example, increased expression of class II MHC antigens is common in obstructive cholestasis and it is probable that both class II expression and expression of the co-stimulatory ligands B7-1 and 2 occur late in the disease. However, there are other features which suggest that PBC has an immune pathogenesis. As shown in Fig. 17.3, there is widespread disturbance of both the cellular and humoral immune system. The association of PBC with other autoimmune diseases again is consistent with an autoimmune pathology.

Infection

A variety of infectious agents have been suggested to trigger PBC. These include bacterial infections with *Escherichia coli* and with mycobacteria, especially *Mycobacterium gordonae*. Patients with PBC have a greater incidence of recurrent bacteriuria, and those with *E. coli* urinary tract infection have detectable but low titers of AMAs. Others have shown that the feces of patients with PBC may contain a greater number of rough forms of *E. coli*; however, both observations have been disputed. While some have reported the presence of mycobacterial nucleic acid in the livers of patients with PBC, others have been unable to confirm their findings. Convincing evidence of a pathogenic role for any of these infectious agents is still lacking. There is a possibility that molecular mimicry may account for the development of PBC.

Viral-like particles have been found in the biliary epithelial cells of patients with PBC, but again their relevance to pathogenesis remains uncertain and these particles have not yet been defined.

Drugs

Drugs including chlorpromazine have been implicated in the cause of PBC, but it remains to be seen whether the drug causes it, triggers it or merely unmasks it.

Genetic factors

The family and HLA associations are reported above. Recent studies have shown that patients with PBC have reduced levels of the anion transporter AE2, both in lymphocytes and bile duct cells. This transporter is implicated in the chloride bicarbonate

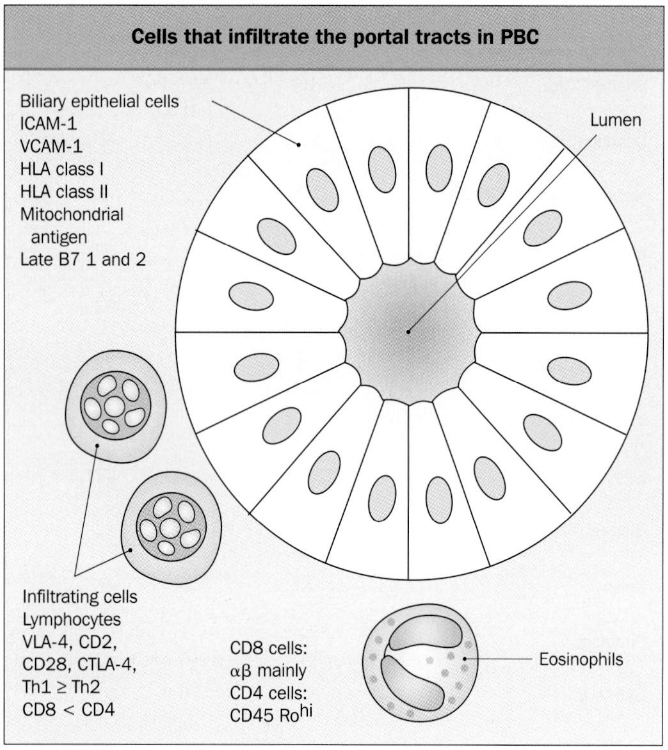

Cells that infiltrate the portal tracts in PBC

Biliary epithelial cells
ICAM-1
VCAM-1
HLA class I
HLA class II
Mitochondrial antigen
Late B7 1 and 2

Lumen

Infiltrating cells
Lymphocytes
VLA-4, CD2,
CD28, CTLA-4,
Th1 ≥ Th2
CD8 < CD4

CD8 cells:
αβ mainly
CD4 cells:
CD45 Ro^hi

Eosinophils

Figure 17.2 Cells that infiltrate the portal tracts in PBC with the commonly expressed receptors and ligands. HLA, human leukocyte antigen; ICAM, intercellular adhesion molecule; VCAM, vascular cell adhesion molecule; VLA, very late antigen.

Immune abnormalities in patients with PBC	
Clinical	Association with autoimmune diseases
Serologic	Raised immunoglobulins (especially IgM and IgG) Autoantibodies: PBC specific (AMAs and some ANAs) PBC nonspecific Increased circulating immune complexes Adhesion molecules (e.g. ICAM-1, VCAM-1 and E-selectin) Peripheral esinophilia Increased complement metabolism
Cellular	Impaired T-cell responses to exogenous antigen Impaired T-cell secretion of cytokines Impaired suppressor T-cell function Reduced NK activity Reduced switching from IgM to IgG production Altered Th1/Th2 balance
Histologic	Granulomas Infiltration with esinophils and CD4⁺ cells and plasma cells infiltrating the portal tracts Increased expression of HLA class I and II Increased biliary expression of HLA class II, adhesion molecules, co-stimulatory molecules

Figure 17.3 Immune abnormalities in patients with PBC. AMA, antimitochondrial antibodies; ANA, antinuclear antibodies; HLA, human leukocyte antigen; ICAM-1, intercellular adhesion molecule 1; Ig, immunoglobulin; NK, natural killer cell; VCAM-1, vascular cell adhesion molecule 1.

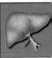

anion exchanger: it has been suggested that reduced activity of AE2 could contribute to the pathogenesis of disease.

Animal models

There have been a few animal models of PBC reported, although none has yet been convincingly shown to resemble PBC. Graft versus host disease (GvHD), both in humans after bone marrow transplantation and in animal models, shows some features of nonsuppurative destructive cholangitis, and rarely AMAs may be present. However, the natural history of the two conditions is quite different and the histologic features of GvHD show less cellular infiltration. One study has shown that inoculation of severe combined immunodeficiency (SCID) mice with lymphocytes from patients with PBC is associated with a greater degree of bile duct damage and infiltration than when mice are injected with peripheral blood lymphocytes from normal individuals.

In Faenze, a region of Italy, wild rabbits are reported to show hepatic histologic features resembling PBC, although these naturally occurring animals have not been fully studied.

While immunization of laboratory animals with the pyruvate dehydrogenase complex (the main target recognized by AMAs) results in the appearance of AMAs, there are no features suggestive of PBC on histology.

In conclusion, the pathogenesis of PBC remains uncertain, and without a clear etiology it is difficult to develop a logical strategy for therapy. None of the postulated hypotheses readily explains many of the clinical features of the syndrome, including the association with other autoimmune diseases, the close correlation with AMA, the female preponderance, the very slow progression, the lack of a similar syndrome in children, the recurrence after transplantation, the fact that only middle-sized bile ducts are the major targets of damage and the family association. Many in the field consider that there is a trigger which, in susceptible individuals, leads to progressive damage, but the nature of the trigger and the factors determining susceptibility are not defined.

CLINICAL FEATURES AND DISEASE ASSOCIATIONS

The symptoms of patients with PBC vary from no symptoms at all to end-stage liver disease. Although 90% of patients are female, the rate of progression is similar in men and women. Unlike most other autoimmune diseases, PBC has not been described in children. The characteristic features associated with PBC include lethargy and itching, although patients may present in many ways.

Presymptomatic disease

A recent study from the University of Newcastle (UK) examined the liver histology of people found to have AMAs, but normal liver function tests. Of 29 patients, the liver histology was normal in only two, the remainder showing histologic features compatible with or diagnostic of PBC. Over the period of follow-up, of a median of 18 years, five died, but none from liver disease. The median period from detection of AMAs to the first abnormality of liver tests was 6 years. Three-quarters developed symptoms of PBC and over 80% developed abnormal liver tests. At present, relatively few patients are detected in this stage.

Asymptomatic disease

About 15% patients with PBC present during the asymptomatic stage. Patients with asymptomatic disease present with symptoms unrelated to PBC (such as arthritis, sicca syndrome or with abnormal liver tests found during a routine medical examination). Such patients have the clinical, serologic and histologic features of PBC. It used to be believed that asymptomatic patients had a better prognosis, but this is largely an artifact associated with lead-time bias and selection bias. Studies suggest that patients with asymptomatic PBC develop symptoms about 5 years after diagnosis. The median time from diagnosis to liver failure is 10–15 years.

Symptomatic disease

Patients present with the characteristic symptoms of PBC – lethargy and pruritus. The median time to liver failure, before the use of ursodeoxycholic acid (UDCA), was 5–10 years, but may now be greater.

Decompensated primary biliary cirrhosis

Patients present with symptoms of decompensated liver disease such as bleeding esophageal varices or ascites. The median time to liver failure is 2–5 years.

Symptoms

The main symptoms of PBC are pruritus and lethargy.

Pruritus

It used to be considered that pruritus was due to retention of bile acids associated with cholestasis. However, recent work has discounted this theory and has concentrated on the importance of naturally occurring opioid agonists. There is an increased opioid tone characterized by an increase in the concentration of endogenous opioid receptors together with upregulation of the receptors. The itching in PBC, therefore, has been considered analogous to the itching in those patients addicted to opioids. This has led to an increase in understanding of possible mechanisms of pruritus and introduction of new therapies.

Lethargy

Lethargy associated with PBC varies considerably between patients, but in some cases it may be so debilitating that transplantation is the only effective therapy. The lethargy of PBC must be differentiated from other causes of tiredness that may present in any patient. These include:
- depression;
- unrecognized thyroid disease or adrenal disease;
- side effects of medication, in particular, drugs such as antihistamines given in an attempt to control itching.

Lethargy affects to up to 85% of patients and is the worst symptom in nearly half.

The cause of lethargy is unknown, but some recent work has indicated the possibility of altered neurotransmission. Studies in animals with bile duct ligation has suggested that cholestasis is associated with reduced concentration of the hypothalamic corticotropin-releasing hormone, leading to decreased levels of physical activity. Therapeutic studies of buspirone, a serotonin 1 α-receptor agonist that increases corticotropin-releasing hormone, results in stimulating serotonin release and may improve symptoms.

Other clinical features of the disease

Bone disease

Osteomalacia occurs rarely and responds to vitamin D replacement. Risk factors for osteomalacia include:

- malabsorption;
- intrinsic bowel disease (such as celiac disease);
- sequestration of vitamin D by concomitant drugs such as cholestyramine.

Osteopenia, in contrast, is a greater problem. The female sex, age, poor nutritional intake and malabsorption all contribute to osteopenia. Furthermore, bilirubin itself directly affects osteoblastic activity. There is controversy as to whether the osteopenia of PBC arises primarily from a high turnover state with increased free absorption of bone, or a low turnover state. In PBC the osteopenia affects primarily axial rather than peripheral bones and therefore is best assessed in the vertebral bodies.

Periostitis

Periostitis is seen in association with finger and toe clubbing and rarely gives rise to severe pain in the wrists and ankles. Some develop hypertrophic pulmonary osteoarthropathy.

Endocrine associations

As shown in Fig. 17.4, there is a strong association of PBC with other autoimmune diseases. Thyroid dysfunction is one of the most common with up to one-quarter of patients with PBC having thyroid antibodies. Biochemical and clinical hypothyroidism is less common, but it is important to screen patients for thyroid dysfunction. Hyperthyroidism is unusual.

Abdominal pain

Right upper quadrant pain is a significant feature in up to 20% of patients with PBC. The cause is unknown and does not relate to the severity of disease. There is an increased association of gallstones in patients with PBC, although these are generally asymptomatic. Occasionally right upper quadrant pain is associated with cholangitis or rarely hepatocellular carcinoma.

Rheumatologic associations

Rheumatoid factor

Rheumatoid factor occurs in up to one-quarter of patients with PBC, and this may be associated with features of rheumatoid arthritis.

Sicca syndrome

Sicca syndrome is characterized by a dry mouth, dry eyes and often with a dry vagina. It may be found in up to 100% of cases, but most series report an incidence of around 70%.

Raynaud's phenomenon

Raynaud's phenomenon occurs in a smaller proportion of patients. Rarely there is the full blown CREST syndrome (calcinosis, Raynaud's disease, esophageal dysmotility, sclerodactyly and telangiectasia) and occasionally scleroderma is present.

Pulmonary disorders

Patients with PBC, as with other chronic liver conditions, may develop primary hepatopulmonary syndrome. There is an overlap with sarcoid disease; however, granulomatous lung involvement may be seen in PBC. Pulmonary fibrosis may also occur.

Renal abnormalities

Many patients with PBC have renal tubular acidosis. The cause of this is not clear, but may be related to chronic copper retention.

Urinary tract infection

Urinary tract infections (UTIs) are found in patients with PBC. There is controversy as to whether UTIs are more common in women with PBC compared with women with other causes of liver disease. Glomerulonephritis rarely occurs and is associated with circulating immune complexes.

Skin disorders

Xanthoma and xanthelasma may occur. Vitiligo is rarely seen.

Other features of PBC are those associated with chronic cholestasis of any cause. The development of jaundice and skin pigmentation, symptoms of portal hypertension such as ascites and fluid retention are not specific to the disease and are discussed in greater detail elsewhere (see Chapters 4–10).

Cancer

There does appear to be an increased association of patients with PBC with cancer, notably cancer of the breast. Furthermore, patients with PBC are at increased risk of developing primary liver cell cancer [hepatocellular carcinoma (HCC)]; risk factors include duration of cirrhosis and male sex. It seems appropriate, therefore, to screen all cirrhotic patients with PBC with serum α-fetoprotein estimations every 6 months and to carry out an annual ultrasound examination.

Examination

On examination, the patient may look very healthy and there may be no abnormal physical signs. However, many patients have skin pigmentation; this is often most prominent on the face around the temporal areas. It used to be thought that the pigmentation was a consequence of excoriation, but this does not appear to be the case. Jaundice is a late feature. The classical cutaneous stigmata of chronic liver disease (such as spider nevi) are often absent. On the face, xanthomata may be seen around

Diseases associated with PBC	
Common (up to 80%)	Sicca syndrome
Frequent (about 20%)	Thyroid disease Arthralgia Raynaud's syndrome Sclerodactyly Fibrosing alveolitis
Rare (less than 5%)	Addison's disease Glomerulonephritis Renal tubular acidosis Myasthenia gravis Vitiligo Thrombocytopenic purpura Systemic lupus erythematosus Hypertrophic pulmonary osteoarthropathy

Figure 17.4 Diseases associated with PBC.

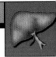

the eyes. Scratch marks may be present on the arms or the thorax. Clubbing of the fingers may be present. Most patients (up to 75%) will have hepatomegaly at diagnosis, and up to 50% will have splenomegaly. Ascites is seen late (Fig. 17.5).

DIAGNOSIS

Laboratory tests

The liver function tests may be normal in those with presymptomatic disease. However, characteristically liver function tests show a cholestatic pattern with elevation of serum alkaline phosphatase, 5′ nucleotidase and γ-glutamyl transpeptidase. Serum aminotransferases are usually raised only moderately and rarely exceed five times normal. As the disease progresses, liver function tests become more deranged and serum bilirubin starts to rise. The standard liver function tests are not specific for PBC (Fig. 17.6).

The red cells are usually normal, although hypersplenism may be present; a macrocytosis, possibly a consequence of liver disease, should lead to further investigations including measurement of folate and vitamin B_{12} and thyroid function.

Hypercholesterolemia

Hypercholesterolemia, often associated with elevation of lipoprotein X, is common. However, lipoprotein concentrations are low, and high-density lipoprotein cholesterol concentrations are usually increased in the early stages but tend to fall with disease progression.

Hepatic synthetic function

Hepatic synthetic function is usually well-preserved until the late stages, so serum albumin and prothrombin time are usually normal. An elevated prothrombin time may indicate malabsorption of vitamin K.

Immune abnormalities

There are many disturbances of the immune system of which hyper-γ globulinemia and autoantibodies are the best described. Serum immunoglobulins (Igs) are usually increased, particularly serum IgM and to a lesser extent IgG. Serum IgA levels are usually normal. Although levels of complement are within the normal range, there is evidence of increased complement activation as suggested by a raised C3d level. Circulating immune complexes are present in the blood and levels correlate with the presence of arthralgia. There may be a circulating esinophilia. Lymphocyte counts are usually normal although there is functional disturbance with a failure of B lymphocytes to switch from IgM to IgG synthesis.

Autoantibodies

A variety of autoantibodies are found in patients with PBC (Fig. 17.7). Those characteristic of PBC are components of the nuclear pore complex antibodies and AMAs.

Antibodies to nuclear pore proteins are found in about 25% of patients with PBC. These antibodies are directed against a 210kDa transmembrane protein (Gp210) and are specific to patients with PBC. In those who have histologic features of PBC but are negative for the AMAs, these antinuclear antibodies are present in nearly half. The major epitope is a short 15-amino-acid stretch in the cytoplasmic C-terminal domain of the transmembrane protein.

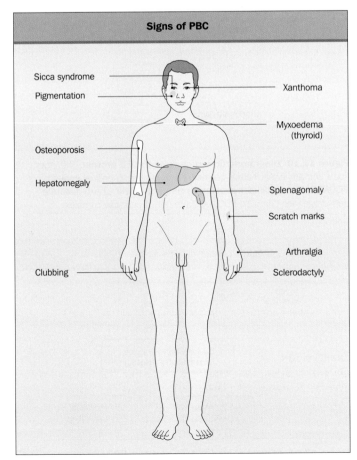

Figure 17.5 Signs of primary biliary cirrhosis PBC. (Note that signs of decompensated liver disease, such as ascites, are not shown.)

Liver function tests in PBC		
	Early	Late
Albumin	N	↓
Bilirubin	N	↑↑↑
Alkaline phosphate	↑↑↑	↑↑↑
AST/ALT	N or ↑	N or ↑
Prothrombin time	N	↑

Figure 17.6 Liver function tests in PBC. AST/ALT, aspartate aminotransferase/alanine aminotransferase.

Autoantibodies in PBC
*Antimitochondrial
*Antinuclear pore gp120
Thyroglobulin
Acetylcholine receptor
α-Enolase
Ro-La
Centromere
Antinuclear
Antiplatelet

Figure 17.7 Autoantibodies in PBC. *Specific to PBC.

Another PBC-specific nuclear pore complex antibody that is present in approximately 1% of patients with PBC reacts with an inner nuclear membrane protein. The significance of these nuclear pore complex antibodies is uncertain. These antibodies are seen more commonly in patients with autoimmune cholangitis.

Anticentromere antibodies are usually seen in association with sclerodactyly.

Antimitochondrial antibodies

Antimitochondrial antibodies are found in approximately 95% of patients with PBC. There are various subtypes of AMA, some of which are found in other conditions such as drug-induced diseases, cardiomyopathy, systemic lupus erythematosus and some infections including tuberculosis, hepatitis C viral infection and syphilis.

The AMAs specific to PBC react with components of the 2-oxo-acid dehyrogenase complex, which comprises three main enzyme complexes: pyruvate dehydrogenase complex (PDC), 2-oxo-glutarate dehydrogenase complex (OGDC) and the branch-chain 2-oxo-acid dehydrogenase complex (BCOADC) (Fig. 17.8).

The enzymes are composed of multiple copies of subunits. The E2 subtype of PDC is most closely associated with PBC. These enzymes are involved in intermediary metabolism (Fig. 17.9).

These antigens of the inner mitochondrial multienzyme complex, although located in the mitochondria, are encoded in the nucleus and assembled in the cytoplasm. The major B-cell autoreactivity is with the noncatalytic portion, in a lipoyl domain of the E2 component (dihydrolipoamide acetyl transferase of pyruvate dehydrogenase). In contrast, a T-cell epitope includes the whole E2 protein (Fig. 17.10).

Antibodies to components of 2-oxo-acid dehydrogenase complex

Component of 2-oxo-acid dehydrogenase	Antigenic domain	Prevalence in PBC (%)
Pyruvate dehydrogenase complex (PDC)	E2	95
	X	95
	E1α	40
	E1β	5
2-oxo-glutarate dehydrogenase complex (OGDC)	E3	75
2-oxo-acid dehydrogenase complex (BCOADC)	E2	60

Figure 17.8 Antibodies to components of 2-oxo-acid dehydrogenase complex.

Biochemical function of the 2-oxo-acid dehydrogenax complex

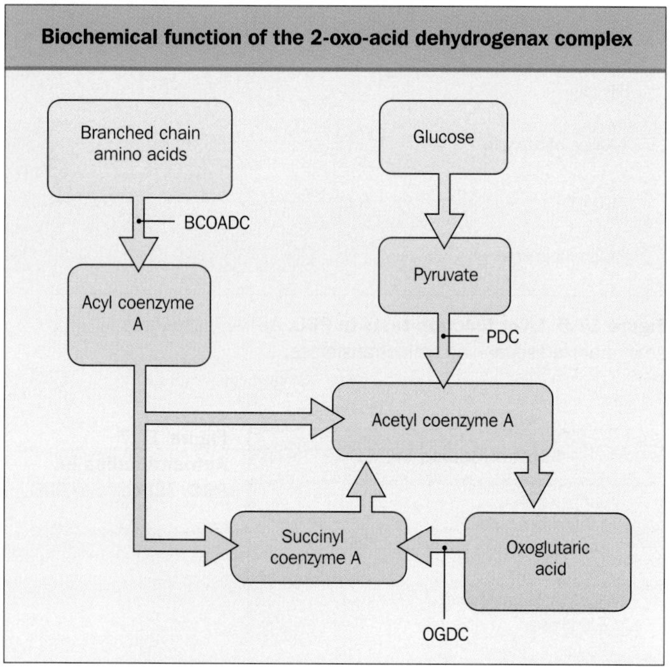

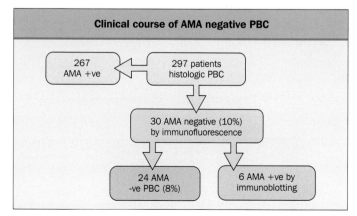

Figure 17.9 Biochemical function of the 2-oxo-acid dehydrogenase complex (BCOADC). OGDC, 2-oxo-glutarate complex; PDC, pyruvate dehydrogenase complex.

Diagramatic structure of E2 protein

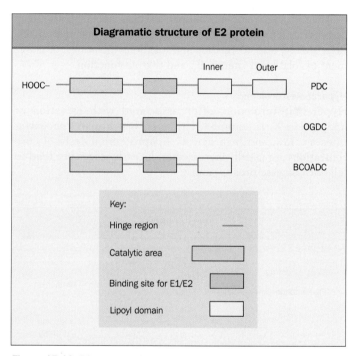

Figure 17.10 Diagrammatic structure of the E2 protein. The inner lipoyl domain is the main B-cell epitope of antimitochondrial antibody. BCOADC, 2-oxo-acid dehydrogenase complex; OGDC, 2-oxo-glutarate dehydrogenase complex; PDC, pyruvate dehydrogenase complex.

Clinical course of AMA negative PBC

297 patients histologic PBC → 267 AMA +ve

30 AMA negative (10%) by immunofluorescence

24 AMA -ve PBC (8%)   6 AMA +ve by immunoblotting

Figure 17.11 Clinical course of AMA-negative PBC. There was no difference in clinical outcome between AMA-positive and AMA-negative patients. (Adapted from Invernizzi *et al.*, Hepatology 1997;25:1090–5.)

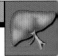

Nuclear-type sequence analysis of human monoclonal and recombinant antibodies suggests that these antibodies are derived from clonal selection of a restricted set of somatically mutated immunoglobulin germ lines. The role of these antibodies in the pathogenesis remains unclear. However, it has been shown that the antigen is present on the surface of biliary epithelial cells and so may play a role in the genesis of disease.

A small proportion of patients with PBC histologically have no AMAs detectable by standard immunofluorescent techniques. In about 10%, AMAs are detectable by immunoblotting and in about 5% AMAs become detectable as the disease progresses. Others remain consistently negative. These patients with 'autoimmune cholangitis' tend to have a higher level of antinuclear antibodies (especially antibodies to gp210) and serum IgG. There is

often an initial biochemical response to corticosteroids, but the disease pattern resembles that of PBC; most believe that autoimmune cholangitis is a variant of PBC (Fig. 17.11).

There is a very close association between the presence of PBC and E2-specific AMAs. Indeed AMAs may be detectable in the serum of patients even at a time when liver tests and liver histology is normal.

Radiology

Radiology has little part to play in the diagnosis of PBC. The liver is usually enlarged. Ultrasound and computed tomography (CT) scanning may show the presence of large lymph nodes in the porta hepatis. The significance of these enlarged nodes is uncertain.

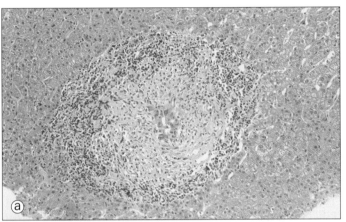

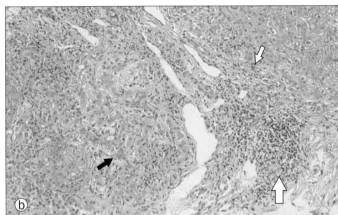

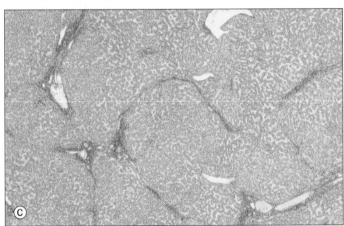

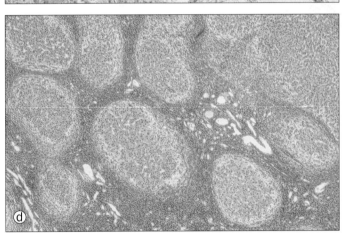

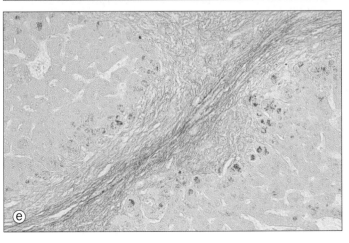

Figure 17.12 Histologic features of PBC. (a) Stage 1: needle biopsy showing granulomatous cholangitis; there is bile duct damage, but no fibrosis or ductular proliferation is seen. (Hematoxylin and eosin). (b) Stage 2: needle biopsy showing lymphoid aggregates (large white arrow), an expanded portal tract with marginal ductular proliferation (small black arrow), and interface hepatitis (small white arrow); there is no appropriately sized bile duct in the portal tract. (Hematoxylin and eosin). (c) Stage 3: hepatectomy specimen showing periportal fibrosis with portal–portal linkage; normal vascular relationships are maintained and nodules are not yet present. (Hematoxylin and van Gieson). (d) Stage 4: hepatectomy specimen showing an established micronodular cirrhosis. (Hematoxylin and van Gieson). (e) Stage 4: cirrhotic PBC liver-copper-associated protein typical of the chronic cholestasis of PBC is stained positive by orcein in the periseptal hepatocytes. (All courtesy of Dr SG Hubscher, University of Birmingham, UK.)

Histology

The characteristic histologic feature of PBC is the granulomatous cholangitis or nonsuppurative destructive cholangitis.

Histologically, PBC is divided into four stages (Figs 17.12 & 17.13):

- Stage 1 is characterized by a florid bile duct lesion and necrotic bile ducts with shrunken and vacuolated bile ducts surrounded by granulomatous lesions. These granulomas consist of lymphocytes, plasma cells, eosinophils and giant cells. Biliary epithelial cells are often shrunken. Lymphoid aggregates may be present.
- Stage 2 is where inflammation spreads out from beyond the portal tract. There is so-called biliary piecemeal necrosis characterized by periportal vacuolated hepatocytes, often surrounded by foamy macrophages. Bile ducts become more damaged and there is an increase in the number of portal tracts devoid of bile ducts.
- Stage 3 shows the fibrosis has progressed, resulting in scarring with adjacent portal tracts being linked by fibrous septa. Cholestasis is becoming increasingly evident and deposition of

copper-associated protein starts.
- Stage 4 is characterized by an established cirrhosis.

The histologic staging of PBC is of limited use: portal hypertension may develop before the onset of cirrhosis; the different features may be distributed patchily so that sampling errors may give misleading information as to progression; and the histologic features of early PBC may be seen in those with an established cirrhosis.

NATURAL HISTORY AND PROGNOSIS

As can be deduced from the patterns of presentation, symptoms on presentation vary greatly; the increasing use of automated laboratory investigations and wider screening for autoantibodies means that more cases are being diagnosed at the asymptomatic or presymptomatic stages. Of those who present with symptomatic disease, about half will present with pruritus. There is often a considerable delay between the onset of pruritus and the diagnosis of PBC. One-quarter will present with hepatic symptoms such as jaundice, gastrointestinal bleeding or ascites and one-quarter will present with nonspecific features such as fatigue (up to 20%), abdominal pain, weight loss, gastrointestinal disturbance or with one of the collagen diseases, such as arthralgia, scleroderma, sicca syndrome or osteopenia.

The natural history of PBC is well-characterized from a number of studies (Fig. 17.14).

Prognostic models

The increasing use of liver transplantation for the management of PBC, has highlighted the need for accurate assessment of prognosis. Several prognostic models have been developed. These in general have been derived from Cox regression analysis on follow-up of patients usually carried out in tertiary centers. In these models, those variables which have, on multivariate analysis, an independent statistically significant association with survival are weighted and the factors applied in a score; from this score the median survival probability or the probability of surviving a given length of time can be calculated.

All models have shown that the serum bilirubin is the most important prognostic factor (Fig. 17.15).

Histologic stages of PBC	
Stage	**Characteristics**
1	Portal hepatitis Bile duct damage Granulomas Florid duct lesion
2	Periportal fibrosis ± periportal hepatitis Prominent enlargement of portal tracts Intact newly formed limiting plates Ductular proliferation
3	Septal fibrosis Scarring Bridging necrosis
4	Cirrhosis

Figure 17.13 Histologic stages of PBC.

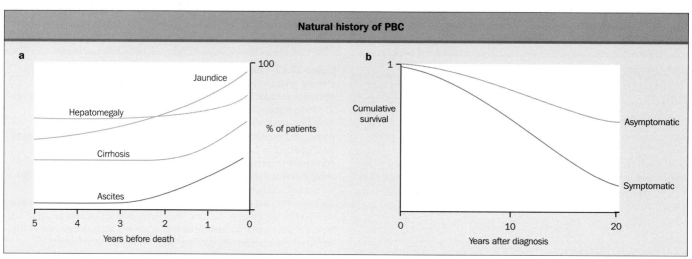

Figure 17.14 Natural history of PBC. (a) Progression of jaundice, hepatomegaly, cirrhosis and ascites prior to death, and (b) survival after diagnosis of PBC to death/transplantation.

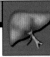

Clinical variables in different prognostic models				
European	Yale	Mayo	Glasgow	Oslo
Age	Age	Age	Age	Variceal bleeding
Bilirubin	Bilirubin	Bilirubin	Bilirubin	Bilirubin
Albumin	Hepatomegaly	Albumin	Variceal bleeding	
Cirrhosis	Fibrosis	Prothrombin	Fibrosis	
Cholestasis		Edema	Cholestasis	
			Mallory's bodies	

Figure 17.15 Clinical variables in different prognostic models.

Mayo Clinic model for prognosis in PBC

R = 0.987 log$_e$ (serum bilirubin mg/dL)
  −2.53 log$_e$ (albumin g/dL)
  +2.38 log$_e$ (prothrombin time, seconds)
  +0.059 (if edema present)

Figure 17.16 Mayo Clinic Model for prognosis in PBC.

Different prognostic models have evolved with different variables. The most widely used are the Mayo Clinic models (Fig. 17.16).

These models are very useful for assessing the prognosis of populations of patients, but are less valuable when applied to the individual since confidence limits are so large. The most widely used and most simple to use model is that of the serum bilirubin. Once bilirubin approaches 170µmol/L (10mg/dL) prognosis is usually limited to 18 months or less.

MANAGEMENT

Making the diagnosis

In many cases of PBC the symptoms are vague and nonspecific. Presence of abnormal cholestatic liver function tests and a normal liver on ultrasound will raise the possibility of liver disease. The demonstration of AMAs and elevation of serum immunoglobulins will often lead to the diagnosis.

Whether a liver biopsy is necessary to confirm the diagnosis is a matter of debate. The close association between PBC and the presence of AMAs suggests that liver biopsy is not always necessary. The presence of cirrhosis on liver histology and of other histologic features (such as central cholestasis) carry relatively little prognostic weight. However, where there is doubt as to the diagnosis, all other complicating diseases need to be excluded, and liver biopsy is indicated. An algorithm for the diagnosis is shown in Fig. 17.17.

The diagnosis of PBC is usually easy. However, the differential diagnosis may pose some problems: there is an overlap with autoimmune hepatitis in those who are AMA negative; and sarcoidosis may affect the liver and may coexist with PBC. Sarcoidosis usually affects the lungs and is AMA negative; the granulomas are usually distributed in sarcoid throughout the liver parenchyma, whereas in PBC they are usually centered around the portal tracts. Other causes of granulomatous hepatitis include drugs and infections (bacterial, mycobacterial, viral and protozoal).

Treatment of symptoms

Many of the symptoms relating to portal hypertension and liver disease are not unique to PBC, and therefore their treat-

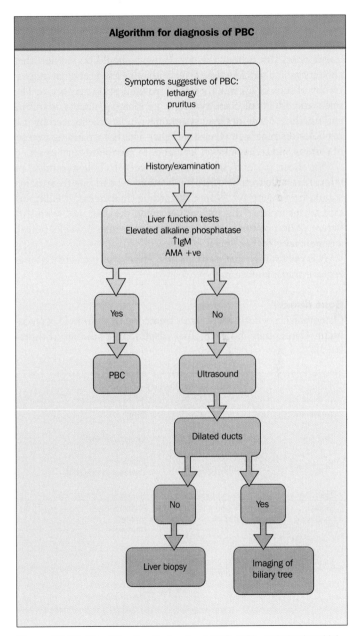

Figure 17.17 Algorithm for diagnosis of PBC. AMA, antimitochondrial antibody; IgM, immunoglobulin M.

ment will not be discussed here. Because there is a strong element of pre-sinusoidal portal hypertension, signs and symptoms of portal hypertension often develop before the onset of a true cirrhosis.

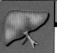
Lethargy

The lethargy associated with PBC may be disabling. As indicated above, it is important to exclude other treatable causes of lethargy. Otherwise, the patient should be given symptomatic advice.

Pruritus

The mainstay of treatment of pruritus is cholestyramine (Fig. 17.18).

Most patients will respond to cholestyramine provided they can tolerate enough. It may take several weeks before the treatment is effective. A dose of 4g four times a day should be started. Once the pruritus is under control the dose should be gradually reduced. It is most effective when taken before and after breakfast with subsequent doses throughout the day. Patients should be warned that cholestyramine should not be taken with other medication as sequestration of such drugs and, therefore, malabsorption may occur. The main side effects of cholestyramine are bloating, nausea, vomiting and diarrhea. Many of these symptoms can be ameliorated by use of cholestyramine light (Questran light). This has aspartame instead of sorbital and so has a lower incidence of gastrointestinal upset.

For those patients who are intolerant of cholestyramine or who are unable to take other medication, second line treatments should be considered. Before discarding treatments, it is important to ensure that the patient has taken the drug and for a sufficient period of time; cholestyramine may take 3 weeks before a beneficial effect is noted.

It is only rarely that patients are refractory to treatment and require transplantation.

Bone disease

Osteomalacia occurs rarely and is treated with vitamin D replacement. Osteopenia, however, may respond to a number of thera-

pies. Calcium supplements should be given and calcium is best absorbed when taken last thing at night. In pre- and postmenopausal women, hormone replacement therapy is effective and is not associated with increased cholestasis. Other treatments that are effective include biphosphonates, such as cyclical etidronate, with calcium supplements. Calcitonin, ursodeoxycholic acid (UDCA) and sodium fluoride are of limited benefit.

DRUG THERAPY

In the absence of a defined etiology, it is difficult to develop a logical strategy for treatment. Furthermore, a number of features of the disease make clinical therapeutic studies difficult to undertake.

Natural history

The natural history of disease is prolonged and, therefore, to demonstrate any significant effect on survival, a large number of patients needs to be studied for a long period of time.

Choice of end points

Most of the earlier studies used death as the end point of therapeutic studies; this is clearly clinically relevant and objective! However, this is now much less of a relevant end point since most patients with end-stage disease will be considered for liver replacement.

Lack of surrogate end points

Although, as indicated above, serum bilirubin remains an excellent prognostic marker, it does not necessarily follow that alteration of prognostic markers implies alteration in prognosis. The advent of liver transplantation for patients with end-stage disease has made survival to death an inappropriate end point. Survival to death or transplantation is limited as the indications for transplantation may vary considerably between patients.

Specific drugs

A variety of medical approaches to treatment have been assessed (Fig. 17.19).

These include immunosuppressive and antifibrotic drugs. The number of drugs tried in the treatment of PBC is ample testimony to the overall lack of effect. It may be that the natural history of progression of disease means that different treatments are required at different stages.

Of the drugs studied, only ursodeoxycholic acid (UDCA) is currently indicated for treatment of PBC.

Ursodeoxycholic acid

Ursodeoxycholic acid is an endogenous tertiary bile acid found in small amounts in humans. It is synthesized in the liver from 7-ketolithocholic acid, a product of bacterial oxidation of chenodeoxycholic acid. In the normal situation UDCA comprises less than 5% of the bile acid pool.

Several randomized prospective double-blind studies have shown that UDCA is associated with improved liver function tests and retards progression of the consequences of portal hypertension such as the development of esophageal varices.

The effect on survival, however, is less clear-cut, although some studies have suggested there may be a delay in the requirement for transplantation. Interestingly, use of UDCA is associated with improvement in not only biochemical abnormalities, but

Treatment for pruritus of PBC		
Treatment type		Drug
First line	Standard therapy	Cholestyramine
Second line	Often effective	Rifampicin Ursodeoxycholic acid
Third line	Some benefit shown in early studies	Naloxone Nalmefene Propofol Naltrexone
Fourth line	May be effective in a few patients, but some side effects	Stanozolol Antihistamines Corticosteroids Phenobarbitone
Fifth line	Effective, but invasive with adverse effects	Plasmaphoresis External biliary diversion Transplantation
Little or no effect		Ondansetron S-adenosyl methionine Oil of evening primrose Sunlight and ultraviolet light

Figure 17.18 Treatment for pruritus of PBC.

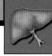

Figure 17.19 Drugs used in the treatment of PBC. It is recognized that the classification is somewhat arbitrary as some drugs have multiple effects, (e.g. antifibrotic and immunosuppression).

Drugs used in the treatment of PBC			
	Drug	**Type**	**Benefit**
Drugs with some documented benefit	Bile acids	Ursodeoxycholic acid	Improves symptoms and biochemistry, probably improves survival
	Immunosuppressive	Corticosteroids	Some biochemical improvement, but osteoporosis may occur
		Cyclosporin	May improve symptoms and survival, but toxic (especially renal)
		Azathioprine	May improve survival
		Tacrolimus	May improve survival, toxic (especially renal)
		Methotrexate	Improves biochemistry and histology; pulmonary toxicity
	Antifibrotic	Colchicine	May improve biochemistry, histology, and survival
Drugs shown to have little or no effect		d-penicillamine Rifampin (rifampicin) Thalidomide Malotilate Chorambucil (toxic)	

also in immune abnormalities (Fig. 17.20).

Furthermore, AMAs may no longer become detectable in this serum. There is no clear-cut demonstrable effect on either the symptoms of PBC or the liver histology.

Ursodeoxycholic acid should be given at a dose of 10–15mg/kg. It is effective when given as a single daily dose. A reduction in serum alkaline phosphatase within 6 months of therapy is a good predictor of response to therapy.

There is little doubt that UDCA is safe. The major side effects are diarrhea and bloating.

The mode of action of UDCA in PBC is not clear. A number of mechanisms have been postulated. These include:
- A cytoprotective effect whereby the normal toxicity of endogenous retained bile acids to hepatocytes and biliary epithelial cells *in vitro* is mitigated by the introduction of UDCA.
- Immunomodulatory effects (see Fig. 17.20).
- Suppression of bile acid-induced cytotoxicity.

Glucocorticoids
Glucocorticoids have usually been avoided in patients with PBC because of fears of exacerbating osteoporosis. However, in combination with therapy such as biphosphonates, this may be less of a problem than previously feared. There are few long-term prospective, double-blind, placebo-controlled studies in PBC; at a dose of prednisolone of 30mg/day, some symptomatic improvement was noted with a small improvement in liver tests; there was no change noted in survival or liver histology.

Azathioprine
In one multicenter, prospective study, azathioprine at a dose of 1–2mg/kg/day was found to be associated with an improvement in survival (60% reduction in mortality at 5 years), after adjust-

ments were made for the difference in severity of disease in the two groups of patients.

Drug toxicity was not a problem. Interpretation of the findings was made more difficult by the high drop-out rate.

d-Penicillamine
Although an initial study suggested a possible therapeutic benefit, several larger studies have failed to document any benefit; d-penicillamine has the distinction of being the only drug that has been convincingly shown to have no therapeutic benefit in PBC.

Cyclosporine and tacrolimus
These drugs, which both act by inhibiting interleukin-2 production, have been tried and shown to have some effect on improving liver tests and reducing mortality. However, they are not widely used because of long-term nephrotoxicity.

Immunomodulatory effects of ursodeoxycholic acid noted in patients with PBC	
Serologic	Fall in IgM Reduction/abolition of AMAs Normalization of eosinophilia Reduction in serum soluble ICAM-I
Histologic	Reduction in HLA class I and II overexpression by hepatocytes Reduction in class II expression by biliary epithelial cells

Figure 17.20 Immunomodulatory effects of ursodeoxycholic acid noted in patients with PBC. AMA, antimitochondrial antibody; HLA, human leukocyte antigen; ICAM-1, intercellular adhesion molecule.

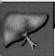

Colchicine

Several short-term studies have suggested that colchicine (1.2mg/day in two divided doses) may improve liver function tests and may reduce mortality. Some patients have less inflammation on liver histology but long-term studies in a larger number of patients are required to show any convincing effect.

Methotrexate

Methotrexate historically has been avoided in patients with liver disease because of fears of hepatic toxicity (fibrosis and liver cell damage). In open-label studies, methotrexate (15mg/week in three divided doses) was shown in a small number of patients to improve liver function tests and liver histology greatly. Double-blind studies have been reported with variable results; few cases of hepatic toxicity have been reported, although some studies have shown that pulmonary damage may be a significant side effect. Lower doses are ineffective.

Other drugs

Thalidomide, S-adenosyl methionine and malotilate have not been shown to be effective. Chlorambucil use has been abandoned as it was considered too toxic.

Combination therapy

The success of UDCA has led researchers to evaluate the combination of UDCA with other drugs such as methotrexate or corticosteroids. At present, there are no convincing data that combination therapy offers any additional advantage.

LIVER TRANSPLANTATION

Liver transplantation remains the only effective therapy for patients with end-stage disease. Indications for transplantation include either symptomatic disease that is making the patient's life intolerable (such indications include intractable pruritus or lethargy) or signs and symptoms of end-stage disease (Fig. 17.21).

In general patients should be considered for liver transplantation when the life expectancy in the absence of transplantation is 1 year or less. However, it must be remembered that those factors that predict survival prior to transplantation differ from those that predict survival after transplantation.

Results following transplantation are good. Most centers

Indications for liver transplantation in patients with PBC
Estimated survival < 1 year
Increasing jaundice, with serum bilirubin >170µmol/L (>10mg/dL)
Intractable ascites
Encephalopathy
Falling serum albumin <3g/dL (<30g/L)
Progressive muscle loss
Recurrent, spontaneus bacterial peritonitis
Increasing osteoporosis
Hepatopulmonary syndrome
Early, incidental hepatocellular carcinoma
Unacceptable quality of life (as intractable pruritis or extreme lethargy)

Figure 17.21 Indications for liver transplantation in patients with PBC.

report survival rates in excess of 80% at 5 years. There is rapid resolution of pruritus and lethargy and bone loss slows substantially. The quality of life, while never being totally normal, is usually excellent.

Recurrence of disease

For many years, whether PBC recurred in the allograft remained controversial. There was general agreement that serum IgM became elevated and that AMAs persisted. These features do not, however, prove recurrence and the diagnosis has to be made on histologic criteria. Several centers have now reported histologic features of PBC in the allograft. Furthermore, the aberrant distribution of E2 seen in the native PBC liver is also found in the allograft whether or not there are histologic features of recurrent PBC. It is not known what factors are associated with disease recurrence, but immunosuppression appears to play a significant role.

The proportion of patients with histologic features of recurrence varies, but up to 20% of patients will have histologic evidence of recurrent disease at 5 years. Whether this adversely affects survival remains to be established.

GENERAL MANAGEMENT

It is important to remember that patients with PBC may well develop malignancy both within the liver and extrahepatically. Thus, all patients with cirrhosis, particularly men, should be screened with regular ultrasound measurements every year and measurement of α-fetoprotein every 6 months. Thyroid function tests should be done annually and the presence of elevated thyroid-stimulating hormone should lead to the consideration of the introduction of thyroxine.

Diet

The patient should be encouraged to take a normal diet; fat should only be reduced if it is associated with bloating or diarrhea.

Drug therapy

Since hepatocellular function is usually well-preserved, patients can tolerate most medications safely. Even hormone replacement therapy is rarely associated with exacerbating liver dysfunction. As with patients with other types of liver disease, nonsteroidal anti-inflammatory drugs should be used with caution.

People with PBC should not be made into patients, and unnecessary medication should be avoided. However, especially in middle-aged women, consideration should be given to prevention of osteoporosis. Fat soluble vitamins (A, D, E and K) should be given to those who are jaundiced.

Monitoring

Patients who are not jaundiced and whose symptoms are well-controlled require infrequent monitoring, perhaps every 6 months. In the presence of cirrhosis, consideration should be given to the use of β-blocker therapy to reduce the risk of variceal bleeding; male patients should also be monitored for the development of hepatocellular carcinoma since early detection should lead to consideration of liver transplantation. As the jaundice progresses, patients should be seen more frequently with a view to consideration of the timing of liver transplantation, early recognition and treatment of complications.

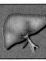

Illustrative case

A typical patient is a middle-aged woman who presents with lethargy, itching and has abnormal liver function tests. The diagnosis is usually readily confirmed by documenting cholestatic liver function tests, raised immunoglobulins and circulating AMA. In such a situation liver biopsy is rarely necessary. The patient should be counseled as to the nature of the disease and warned that it is likely to be progressive. Most patients respond well to the introduction of UDCA, and this should be maintained in the long term.

Asymptomatic patient with positive antimitochondrial antibody

In these cases the optimal management is uncertain. In the view of the author, these patients should be followed up on an annual basis in order to detect early symptoms and institute therapy. There is little benefit from liver biopsy in these patients. There has been no evidence that UDCA therapy is of any clinical benefit.

Antimitochondrial antibody-negative primary biliary cirrhosis

Many of these patients have autoimmune features such as raised transaminases, elevated immunoglobulin and high titer autoantibody. If the liver biopsy shows classical features of PBC, there is uncertainty regarding whether corticosteroids are of benefit. The author's practice, in the presence of elevated titers of antinuclear factor antibody and immunoglobulin and the presence of piecemeal necrosis on liver biopsy, is to offer such patients corticosteroids. Patients should be treated as for autoimmune hepatitis, but the effect of steroids on bones should be ameliorated by the use of cyclical etidronate and calcium supplements. In general, however, most of these patients develop classical PBC.

FURTHER READING

Addison T, Gull W. On a certain affection of the skin. Guy's Hosp Rep. 1851;7:265. *An early description of PBC.*

Ben Ari Z, Dhillon AP, Sherlock S. Autoimmune cholangiopathy: part of the spectrum of autoimmune chronic active hepatitis. Hepatology. 1993;18(1):10–15. *Good description of antimitochondrial negative PBC or autoimmune hepatitis.*

Berg PA, Doniach D, Roitt IM. Mitochondrial antibodies in primary biliary cirrhosis. I. Localization of the antigen to mitochondrial membranes. J Exp Med. 1967;126:277–90. *Historic description of antimitochondrial antibody in PBC.*

Burroughs AK, Butler P, Sternberg MJE, Baum H. Molecular mimicry in liver disease (letter). Nature. 1992;358:377–8. *Discussion of molecular mimicry in PBC.*

Christensen E, Neuberger J, Crowe J, et al. Beneficial effect of azathioprine and prediction of prognosis in primary biliary cirrhosis. Final results of an international trial. Gastroenterology. 1985;89:1084–91. *Multicentre clinical trial of azathioprine in PBC: earliest study to use Cox regression analysis to develop a prognostic model.*

Coppel RL, McNeilage LJ, Surh CD, et al. Primary structure of the human M2 mitochondrial autoantigen of primary biliary cirrhosis: dihydrolipoamide acetyltransferase. Proc Natl Acad Sci USA. 1988;85:7317–21. *Description of auto antibodies in patient with chronic liver disorder.*

Dickson ER, Grambsch P, Fleming TR. Prognosis in primary biliary cirrhosis: model for decision making. Hepatology. 1989;10:1–7. *A discussion about the use and abuse of prognostic model.*

Doniach D, Roitt JM, Walker JG, Sherlock S. Tissue antibodies in primary biliary cirrhosis, active chronic (lupoid) hepatitis, cryptogenic cirrhosis and other liver diseases and their clinical implications. Clin Exp Immunol. 1966;1:237–62. *One of the initial descriptions of antibodies in clinical practice.*

Fussey SP, Ali ST, Guest JR, et al. Reactivity of primary biliary cirrhosis sera with Escherichia coli dihydrolipoamide acetyltransferase (E2p): characterization of the main immunogenic region. Proc Natl Acad Sci USA. 1990;87:3987–91. *Characterization of AMAs: First identification of E2 as the major autoantigen in PBC.*

Gershwin ME, McKay IR. Primary biliary cirrhosis: paradigm or paradox for autoimmunity? Gastroenterology. 1991;100:822–4. *An excellent discussion about the role of autoimmunity in PBC.*

Gershwin ME, MacKay IR, Sturgess A, Coppel RL. Identification and specificity of a cDNA encoding the 70kd mitochondrial antigen recognized in primary biliary cirrhosis. J Immunol. 1987;138:3525–31. *Important immunological study.*

Heathcote EJ. Autoimmune cholangitis. Gut. 1997;30:440–2. *A review of autoimmune cholangitis.*

Jones EA, Bergasa N. Why do cholestatic patients itch? Gut.1996;38:644–5. *A review of the possible mechanisms of pruritus in patients with PBC.*

Joplin R, Lindsay JG, Johnson GD, Strain A, Neuberger J. Membrane dihydrolipoamide acetyltransferase (E2) on human biliary epithelial cells in primary biliary cirrhosis. Lancet. 1992;339:93–4. *First demonstration that E2 is present on the plasma membrane of human biliary epithelial cells in PBC.*

Kaplan M. Primary biliary cirrhosis. N Engl J Med. 1996;335:1570–80. *A personal review of PBC.*

Manns M, Kruger M. Immunogenetics of chronic liver diseases. Gastroenterology. 1994; 106:1676–9. *An excellent review of the immunogenetics of PBC (and other liver diseases).*

Metcalf JV, Mitchison H, Palmer J, Bassendine M, James OF. Natural history of early primary biliary cirrhosis. Lancet. 1996;348:1399–402. *An excellent account of early PBC and its natural history.*

Mysor M, James OFW. The epidemiology of primary biliary cirrhosis in north east England: an increasingly common disease? Q J Med. 1990;75: 877–85. *A useful review of the epidemiology of PBC.*

Neuberger J. Primary biliary cirrhosis. Lancet. 1997;350:876–9. *A recent review of PBC.*

Poupon RE, Lindor K, Cauch-Dudeck K, et al. Combined analysis of randomised, controlled trials of ursodeoxycholic acid in primary biliary cirrhosis. Gastroenterology. 1997;113:884–90. *Analysis of three placebo-controlled trials showing a therapeutic benefit of UDLA in PBC.*

Swain M, Maric M. Defective corticotrophin-releasing hormone mediated neuroendocrine and behavioural responses in cholestatic rats: implications for cholestatic disease-related sickness behaviour. Hepatology. 1995;22:1560–64. *One of the first papers to look at the mechanisms of lethargy in patients with PBC.*

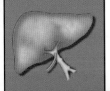

Section 3 Specific Diseases of the Liver

Chapter 18 Primary Sclerosing Cholangitis

Russell H Wiesner

INTRODUCTION

Primary sclerosing cholangitis (PSC) is a chronic cholestatic syndrome of unknown etiology that is characterized by chronic cholestasis and diffuse inflammation and fibrosis that involve the entire biliary tree. The pathologic process obliterates intrahepatic and extrahepatic bile ducts, which ultimately leads to biliary cirrhosis, portal hypertension, and hepatic failure.

The syndrome PSC was first described by Delbet in 1924, and as of 1980 only 100 cases were documented in the English language/literature. It was therefore considered a rare disease before the widespread application of endoscopic retrograde and percutaneous transhepatic cholangiography in the late 1970s, which allowed the diagnosis of PSC to be made without surgery (Fig. 18.1). The recognition of the association between PSC and inflammatory bowel disease coupled with the use of routine screening with biochemical liver tests as part of the routine general examination has further increased the frequency with which PSC is diagnosed. Today, the identification of abnormal liver function tests in patients with inflammatory bowel disease leads to an earlier diagnosis of PSC, frequently when the patient has minimal or no symptoms related to liver disease. These advances

in the diagnosis of PSC have led to a better understanding of the hitherto seldom diagnosed syndrome; particularly, its diagnostic features and natural history.

Despite these advances, the etiology remains unknown and no curative therapy has been identified. Immunopathogenic mechanisms seem likely to play a major etiologic role based on strong associations of PSC with human leukocyte antigens (HLA haplotypes), presence of autoantibodies, a close relationship with other autoimmune diseases, and the presence of multiple immunologic abnormalities. However, to date, target antigens have not been identified and, surprisingly, immunosuppressive therapy has had minimal impact on disease progression.

EPIDEMIOLOGY

Although the prevalence of PSC in the USA is unknown, it can be estimated because of its frequent association with chronic ulcerative colitis (CUC). Studies have shown a 2.4–7.5% prevalence of PSC in patients with CUC. Because the incidence of CUC ranges from 40 to 225 cases per 100,000 population, the incidence of PSC in the USA is estimated to be between two and seven cases per 100,000 population. This estimate was recently supported by the results of epidemiologic studies from Sweden and Norway in which the incidence of CUC and PSC was noted to be 171 and 6.3 cases per 100,000 population, respectively. These results, however, probably underestimate the actual incidence of PSC because the disease can occur in patients with normal serum levels of alkaline phosphatase, and 20–30% of patients with PSC did not have associated inflammatory bowel disease. Therefore, PSC seems to be more common than previously suspected, and may have a frequency similar to that reported for primary biliary cirrhosis (PBC).

PATHOPHYSIOLOGY

The cause of PSC remains unknown despite extensive investigation into various mechanisms related to bacteria, toxins, viral infections, genetic predisposition, and immunologic mechanisms, all of which have been postulated to contribute to the pathogenesis and progression of this syndrome (Fig. 18.2).

Bacteria toxin theory

The close association of inflammatory bowel diseases, especially CUC, with PSC has been intriguing and led several investigators to postulate that portal bacteremia or absorption of toxins or toxic bile acids from the inflamed colon may play a major role in the pathogenesis of PSC. It was postulated that the primary

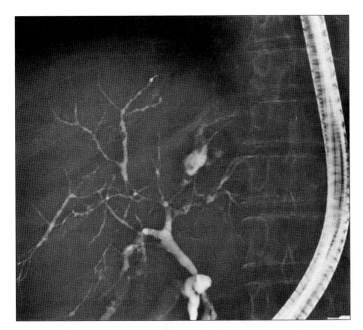

Figure 18.1 Cholangiogram. Classic cholangiographic findings in the setting of PSC are noted including strictures, beading, and irregularities of the intrahepatic and extrahepatic biliary system.

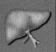

Pathophysiology of PSC		
Causal factor	Supportive features	Contradicting aspects
Colonic bacteria or toxins	Association with UC Bacterial peptides induce changes seen in PSC	Portal bacteremia not a feature of severe PSC Clinical association with quiescent PSC
Viral	Some viruses (e.g. CMV) can cause duct damage	No direct link between any virus and PSC has been established
Genetic	Strong HLA associations reported	Associations are not totally consistent
Immunologic	Hypergammaglobulinemia Autoantibodies Circulating immune complexes Complement activation Abnormal cell mediated immunity	No clinical response to immunosuppressive therapy

Figure 18.2 Pathophysiology of primary sclerosing cholangitis (PSC). The pathophysiology is probably multifactorial involving some or all of these proposed causative factors. UC, ulcerative colitis; CMV, cytomegalovirus; HLA, human leukocyte antigen.

event in PSC was a chronic, low-grade portal vein bacteremia that caused chronic biliary tract inflammation and fibrosis. Other investigators were unable to demonstrate a significant incidence of portal vein bacteremia in patients undergoing surgery for severe, uncontrolled CUC. Furthermore, detailed hepatic histologic analysis revealed that portal phlebitis, the hallmark of portal vein bacteremia, was mild or absent in most patients with PSC. Thus, little evidence supports the hypothesis that portal bacteremia has a major pathogenic role in this syndrome.

It has been postulated that PSC is caused by a reaction to toxic bile acids, such as lithocholic acid, arising from the bacterial action in the diseased colon that allows absorption of the toxin directly into the portal blood. This hypothesis has also been refuted because multiple studies have been unable to demonstrate major abnormalities in bile acid metabolism in patients with PSC or CUC.

Proinflammatory bacterial peptides synthesized by colonic bacteria in a rat model caused portal inflammation and neutrophilic cholangitis similar to the histopathologic lesion seen in early PSC. Animals that had experimentally induced colitis experienced an eight-fold increase in biliary excretion of these proinflammatory bacterial peptides. In another study, investigators demonstrated that intestinal bacterial overgrowth in rats is associated with hepatic inflammation similar to that seen in PSC. Thus, further investigation into the potential role that proinflammatory bacterial peptides may play in the pathophysiology of PSC seems warranted.

On the other hand, evidence suggests that an increased absorption of toxins by way of an inflamed colon does not play a major part in the pathophysiology of PSC. This possibility is supported by the observation that the severity of CUC does not appear to be related to the risk of PSC developing, since most patients with PSC have mild or quiescent inflammatory bowel disease. Furthermore, PSC has been known to develop years before the onset of CUC and may develop years after proctocolectomy for CUC. In addition, PSC is diagnosed in a substantial number of patients who have no past or present clinical or histologic evidence of CUC. These findings suggest that colonic disease associated with increased absorption of bacterial products or toxins is not a major factor in the pathogenesis of this syndrome.

The remaining toxin worthy of notation in relation to the pathophysiology of PSC is copper. It has been shown that PSC leads to an excess accumulation of hepatic copper. This probably represents an epiphenomenon that is related to cholestasis since it has now been well demonstrated that increased hepatic copper levels are found in all patients with chronic cholestasis regardless of the cause. Furthermore, D-penicillamine therapy, which is known to be associated with a reduction in hepatic copper levels, was not shown to have a beneficial effect in PSC in a controlled clinical trial. Therefore, there is little evidence to support hepatic copper toxicity as a major factor in the pathophysiology or disease progression of PSC.

Viral infection

Infection of biliary epithelial cells by viral agents has been postulated by some to be involved in the pathogenesis of PSC. The results of several studies have essentially excluded hepatitis A, B, and C viruses as causative factors in PSC. Cytomegalovirus infections have also been implicated in the pathophysiology of PSC. It can cause intralobular bile duct destruction and has been implicated in causing a decrease of intralobular bile ducts. Fibrosis and destruction of large ducts, however, have never been associated with cytomegalovirus infection. More importantly, inclusion bodies, typical of cytomegalovirus infection, have never been demonstrated histologically in bile duct epithelial cells or in hepatocytes from patients with PSC.

Other reports suggesting that reovirus type 3 can induce cholangitis and biliary atresia in weanling mice and primates raises the possibility that this virus may also be a causative factor in PSC. More recent data have shown that neither the prevalence nor the titers of antibodies to reovirus type 3 differ between normal adult control patients and patients with PSC. Thus, there is no evidence to support the hypothesis that the pathophysiology of PSC is related to a viral infection.

Familial and genetic predisposition

Familial and genetic factors have been proposed to contribute to the pathogenesis of PSC. Familial occurrence of PSC has been reported. Multiple studies have shown a strong association between PSC and HLA haplotypes suggesting genetic susceptibility. Initially, the associations of PSC with the HLA haplotypes B8, DR3, DR2, and A1, B8, DR3 were noted. In 1990 an investigation reported a 100% association of PSC with the HLA-DRw52a (or DRB3*0101). Subsequent studies did not confirm this observation but demonstrated that only 52–55% of PSC patients were positive for the HLA-DRw52a haplotype. Later, HLA haplotypes DR3 and DR6 were also found to be highly associated with PSC. In addition, the strong association of PSC with the DRB1*1301, DQA1*1301, and DQB1*0603 alleles were demonstrated. Meanwhile, investigators began to examine the correlation between patients' HLA antigens and PSC prognosis. One study revealed those HLA-DRw52a-positive PSC patients had a significantly diminished estimated median survival compared with the HLA-DRw52a-negative group. Recently, two studies have reported that PSC patients with HLA-DR4 haplotype demonstrated an aggressive disease progression. In contrast, another report concluded that HLA-DR and HLA-DQ haplotypes do not represent a hall-

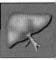

mark for a more rapid PSC deterioration. Analysis of the characteristics of each population included in those studies and further investigations are needed to clarify this issue.

Immunologic cause

To date, the most attractive hypothesis for the pathogenesis of PSC postulates immune-mediated damage of bile ducts. Genetic information as well as abnormal humoral and cellular immune profiles that have been described in PSC patients, although inconclusive, support the evidence. For example, the HLA haplotypes related to PSC (i.e. HLA-B8, HLA-DR3) are also associated with known autoimmune disorders.

The immunohumoral abnormalities reported in PSC patients include:

- hypergammaglobulinemia, often with a disproportionate rise in serum IgM levels;
- increased titers of antismooth muscle, antinuclear, anticolonic, antiportal tract, perinuclear antineutrophil cytoplasmic (pANCA), and antiendothelial cell antibodies;
- increased levels of circulating serum and bile immune complexes; and
- activation of the complement system and abnormal clearance of immune complexes from the circulation.

In an interesting study, a shared and specific epitope was detected on human colon and biliary epithelium. Moreover, circulating autoantibodies against this specific epitope were detected in the serum of two-thirds of PSC patients. Recent interest has focused on the high prevalence of pANCA in PSC patients with or without CUC. Currently, pANCA is considered a marker of PSC despite the variation in its specificity and sensitivity reported in studies due to methodologic differences. Nevertheless, pANCA is not suggested for screening of PSC since it is not pathognomonic and its titer widely fluctuates during the course of the disease. The pattern of pANCA staining in PSC has been characterized as atypical perinuclear and is distinct from the one seen in Wegener's granulomatosis, possibly reflecting the difference in the target antigen. The antigen(s) that react with pANCA in PSC remain unknown. Proposed antigens include cathepsin G, a chymotrypsin-like protease, and the bactericidal/permeability increasing protein, an endotoxin-binding protein of polymorphonuclear granulocytes. To investigate the prognostic significance of pANCA in PSC, a number of studies have been conducted. These reports revealed that the titer of pANCA in PSC patients does not correlate with liver histology, clinical activity, and biochemical profiles. Of interest, the pANCA titer can persist after liver transplantation and proctocolectomy. The presence of pANCA in PSC patients has been associated with more extensive biliary disease. Further studies are needed to identify the antigenic determinants of pANCA in PSC in order to understand the role of these antibodies in PSC.

In an early study, the inhibition of leukocyte migration by biliary antigens in PSC suggested the presence of a cellular-mediated immune mechanism in its pathogenesis. The cellular-mediated immune abnormalities described in PSC patients are the following:

- significant decline in the total number of circulated T cells due to a disproportionate decrease in CD8 (suppressor/cytotoxic) cells leading to an increase in the ratio of $CD4^+$ to $CD8^+$ cells;
- significantly increased ratio of $CD4^+$ to $CD8^+$ T cells in the blood of cirrhotics compared with noncirrhotics;
- elevation in the absolute number and percentage of peripheral B cells;
- increase in the absolute number and percent of $\gamma\delta$-T cells in the peripheral blood and portal areas; and
- dominant usage of the $V\beta3$ gene segment of the T-cell receptor only in the T lymphocytes infiltrating the liver.

These findings suggest altered immunoregulation in PSC. Further studies on the characterization and activation of T lymphocytes infiltrating the liver are necessary to elucidate their role in the pathogenesis of PSC.

The enhanced expression of HLA class II antigens on the biliary epithelial cells of patients during the early stages of PSC and after extrahepatic biliary obstruction has been reported. Although this finding may suggest an autoimmune activation of host lymphocytes by the bile duct epithelia that became capable of presenting self or foreign antigens, it most likely reflects an epiphenomenon of the disease since it is not distinct for PSC.

Adhesion molecules such as the intercellular adhesion molecule (ICAM)-1, a ligand for the leukocyte adhesion receptor lymphocyte function-associated antigen (LFA)-1, is involved in the communication between T lymphocytes and antigen-presenting cells (APCs). Intercellular adhesion molecule -1 has been detected on bile duct epithelia in cirrhotic-stage PSC; increased serum levels of circulating ICAM-1 have also been found in PSC. The fact that the expression of HLA-DR predates the expression of ICAM-1 in bile ducts of PSC patients suggests minimal participation of the latter in the initiation of PSC. Nevertheless, LFA-1 is overexpressed in intrahepatic lymphocytes, implying that additional unidentified adhesion molecules may exist in the bile ducts of patients with PSC. Proinflammatory cytokines induce the expression of ICAM-1, and HLA class I and II molecules on human bile duct epithelia. However, the importance of cytokines in the pathogenesis of PSC remains unclear and further studies are needed.

It has been proposed that PSC is the consequence of an environmental insult that leads to the autoimmune destruction of biliary epithelia in a genetically inclined individual. Understanding the molecular basis of the genetic and autoimmune milieu involved in PSC is a prerequisite to clarifying the pathogenesis of PSC and devising rational and effective medical therapies.

CLINICAL FEATURES

The syndrome PSC can effect any age group and any race, but it appears to occur predominantly in young Caucasian males. In the Mayo Clinic series of 174 adult PSC patients, two-thirds were male and the mean age at the time of diagnosis was 39 years. The syndrome can occur in infancy and childhood. The clinical presentation of PSC can range from the finding of an increased serum alkaline phosphatase level in an asymptomatic patient undergoing a general examination to a complication of portal hypertension, such as the onset of ascites, variceal bleeding, or portosystemic encephalopathy. With increasing frequency, PSC is being diagnosed in patients with established inflammatory bowel disease who have abnormal biochemical liver function tests. However, patients with advanced-stage PSC can have normal liver tests.

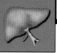

Symptoms and signs

Many patients are asymptomatic at the time of presentation and diagnosis; however, most of these have a cholestatic biochemical profile that is characterized by an increased serum alkaline phosphatase level. Seventy-five per cent of patients who are symptomatic will present with a variety of symptoms including progressive fatigue, pruritus, or jaundice. Ascending cholangitis secondary to bacterial infection of the biliary tree, characterized by pain, fever, and jaundice, is an unusual feature unless the biliary tree has a stricture or has been previously surgically manipulated. Other symptoms are similar to those that occur in patients with other chronic liver diseases such as weight loss, ascites, variceal bleeding from an esophageal or stomal source, and hepatic encephalopathy (Fig. 18.3). On physical examination, nearly one-half of PSC patients will have hepatomegaly or jaundice at the time of diagnosis. Other common signs include splenomegaly, hyperpigmentation, and xanthomas (see Fig. 18.3).

Frequency of symptoms and signs of PSC	
Symptom/sign	Frequency (%)
Fatigue	66
Puritis	59
Jaundice	59
Hepatomegaly	48
Weight loss	34
Splenomegaly	34
Cholangitis	28
Hyperpigmentation	14
Ascites	7
Variceal bleed	6
Xanthoma	4
Hepatic encephalopathy	2

Figure 18.3 Frequency of symptoms and signs of PSC. Profile of the signs and symptoms present at the time of diagnosis.

Complications associated with chronic cholestasis and PSC
Complications associated with chronic cholestasis
Fatigue Pruritis Steatorrhea Fat malabsorption Fat-soluble vitamin deficiency
Complications characteristic of PSC
Bacterial cholangitis Gallbladder and biliary stenosis Dominant bile duct strictures Cholangiocarcinoma Hepatocellular cancer

Figure 18.4 Complications associated with chronic cholestasis and PSC. These are a combination of the complications common to all causes of chronic cholestasis and those characteristic of PSC.

Complications of chronic cholestatic liver disease

These include fatigue, pruritus, steatorrhea, and fat-soluble vitamin deficiencies and associated consequences (Fig. 18.4). Fatigue, although a nonspecific symptom, is a frequent complaint of PSC patients. Fatigue of notable severity can manifest early during the course of PSC and generally parallels progression of the liver disease. While little is known about the specific cause of fatigue, a recent study has suggested that fatigue associated with cholestasis may be attributable to altered serotoninergic neurotransmission in the brain. However, at this time, no specific therapy is available for this symptom.

Pruritus, another common symptom of PSC, can be debilitating and can lead to severe excoriations and diminished quality of life. Although the pathogenesis of pruritus remains unknown, several hypotheses have been suggested, the most recent of which implies that pruritus may be related to increased availability of endogenous opiate ligands at the central opiate receptors. The theory that endogenous opiates are involved in the pathogenesis of pruritus associated with cholestasis is supported by the fact that exogenous opiates induce pruritus, cholestasis is associated with increased opiate neurotransmission, and pruritus, in the setting of cholestasis, can be ameliorated by using opiate antagonists.

In general, the severity of pruritus tends not to parallel disease progression in PSC; in fact, during the end stages of PSC, pruritus tends to diminish. Various therapies have been used to treat pruritus (Fig. 18.5). In most patients, pruritus can be readily controlled; however, in a small number of patients, pruritus is associated with a marked diminished quality of life and, in rare cases, can be an indication for liver transplantation.

Steatorrhea associated with fat-soluble vitamin deficiency has also been described in patients with PSC. Fat malabsorption in PSC, like that seen in PBC, is most often related to diminished intestinal concentration of bile acids. In PSC, however, steatorrhea also can be caused by chronic pancreatitis, bacterial overgrowth, or celiac disease, all of which can be associated with PSC. These causes of steatorrhea should be considered in the differential diagnosis if steatorrhea occurs in a PSC patient who is not jaundiced and does not have cirrhotic-stage disease on liver biopsy. Patients who have cirrhosis, jaundice, or both should be

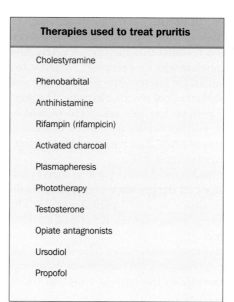

Therapies used to treat pruritis
Cholestyramine
Phenobarbital
Anthihistamine
Rifampin (rifampicin)
Activated charcoal
Plasmapheresis
Phototherapy
Testosterone
Opiate antagonists
Ursodiol
Propofol

Figure 18.5 Therapies used to treat pruritus. Treatment options for pruritus, including nonpharmacologic approaches.

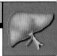

Treatment of osteopenia associated with PSC
Avoid alchohol
Avoid smoking
Increase ambulation
Vitamin D (maintain serum hydroxyvitamin D levels)
Calcium
Estrogen
Calcitonin
Fluoride
Bisphosphonates
Liver transplantation

Figure 18.6 Treatment of osteopenia associated with PSC. Factors that may improve bone density in patients with PSC.

Bone mineral densities of the lumbar spine in general do not correlate with serum levels of bilirubin, 25-hydroxyvitamin D levels, fecal fat excretion, or the presence or absence of inflammatory bowel disease. Histomorphometric examination of bone from several PSC patients has shown increased bone reabsorption, reduced bone formation, and moderate-to-severe osteopenia with little or no evidence of osteomalacia.

The pathophysiology of osteopenia remains unknown and currently no effective therapy has been found to prevent or manage osteopenia associated with chronic cholestatic liver disease. One hypothesis suggests that there is suppression of osteoblast function by a substance retained in cholestatic plasma, such as serum bilirubin. In a recent *in vitro* study, serum bilirubin was shown to inhibit the activity in human osteoblast-like cells, suggesting a possible pathogenic role of hyperbilirubinemia as the cause of osteoporosis in PSC patients. Further studies will be needed to confirm these findings.

Treatment for bone disease associated with PSC often includes supplemental vitamin D and calcium, along with adequate exercise and avoidance of excessive alcohol and tobacco consumption (Fig. 18.6). Overall, this approach does not appear to be of major benefit to patients with cholestatic-induced osteoporosis. Other treatments such as the use of calcitonin, which inhibits bone reabsorption, and the use of sodium fluoride, which can enhance spine density and increase bone formation, have been shown to be of limited benefit in a small number of PSC patients.

The use of estrogen therapy, which has been shown to be of benefit in the treatment of postmenopausal osteoporosis, has also been shown to be of benefit in patients with osteoporosis associated with cholestasis. Furthermore, bisphosphonate compounds have been shown to be of value in the treatment of

screened for fat-soluble vitamin deficiency by determining levels of vitamin A, D, and E, as well as a prothrombin time on a 6-monthly basis. Patients who have fat-soluble vitamin deficiency should receive adequate supplemental therapy.

Metabolic bone disease, particularly osteoporosis, has recently been shown to be a frequent complication in patients with advanced PSC who are undergoing assessment for liver transplantation. Indeed, bone mineral density levels are often severely decreased in this group of patients. Despite the fact that two-thirds of patients with PSC are of male gender, 50% have bone mineral density levels that are below the fracture threshold.

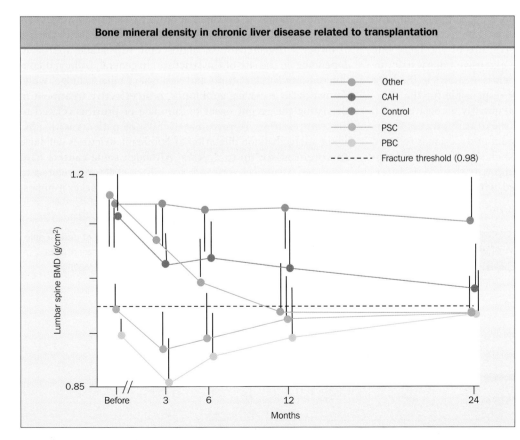

Figure 18.7 Bone mineral density in chronic liver disease related to transplantation. Measurements (mean ± SD) of the lumbar spine using dual photon absorptiometry pretransplantation, at 3 months, 6 months, 12 months, and 24 months after liver transplantation in patients with chronic liver disease and in an age- and sex-matched control population. CAH, chronic active hepatitis. (Reproduced with permission from Porayko MK, et al. Bone disease in liver transplant recipients: incidence, timing, and risk factors. Transplantation Proceedings. Elsevier Science, 1991;23:1462–5.)

osteopenia associated with both chronic cholestatic liver disease and post-transplant bone disease. However, caution should be exercised with the use of oral bisphosphates in patients with portal hypertension because of the potential for esophageal ulceration.

Following liver transplantation for PSC, the rate of bone loss is accelerated in the PSC patient. This is probably due to a combination of factors, including immobilization and the use of high doses of corticosteroids. Recent studies from the Mayo Clinic have shown that bone mineral density of the lumbar spine decreases for the first 3–6 months post-transplant, during which time there is an increase in pathologic fractures (Fig. 18.7). One year post-transplantation, however, bone mineral density seems to increase; generally by 2 years post-transplantation density has been shown to rise above pretransplantation levels.

The use of antireabsorptive drugs, such as calcitonin and bisphosphonates, have been shown to be effective not only in preventing corticosteroid-induced osteoporosis, but also in preventing bone loss after liver transplantation. Further studies are obviously needed to determine the true efficacy of these agents in preventing post-transplant bone loss.

A high incidence of avascular necrosis in PSC patients post-transplant, which frequently requires joint replacement, has also been reported. Avascular necrosis is most likely related to the use of high-dose corticosteroids, but the advent of new and more powerful immunosuppressive agents and the trend toward early steroid withdrawal should reduce the incidence of both pathologic fractures and avascular necrosis in the early post-transplant period.

Complications characteristic of primary sclerosing cholangitis

These are included in Fig. 18.4. Bacterial cholangitis is an unusual presenting symptom of PSC, but frequently appears in patients who have had previous biliary surgical treatment or in whom intervention with radiologic dilatation has been carried out for an obstructing dominant stricture of the large bile ducts. Back pressure resulting from extensive biliary stricturing and the presence of concurrent debris or stones in the large bile ducts is believed to be partially responsible for the deterioration in liver function and is frequently associated with bacterial cholangitis. Progression of the disease process to cirrhosis and liver failure may be delayed if obstruction is relieved during the early stages. In treating such situations, endoscopic decompression is an attractive, temporary therapeutic alternative because it can be performed with relative ease, can

facilitate dilatation of multiple strictures at the same time the procedure is performed, and eliminates surgical therapy that might prevent future complications related to liver transplantation. The results of trials suggest that balloon dilatation and stenting can alter the usually protracted course of PSC and may delay the timing of, or even the necessity for liver transplantation (Fig. 18.8). Patients undergoing endoscopic decompression, or who have severe intrahepatic disease associated with bacterial cholangitis, should receive prophylactic broad-spectrum antibiotic therapy to prevent recurrent bouts of bacterial cholangitis. Preference is for quinolone antibiotics because of their high biliary concentration and broad-spectrum action against both Gram-positive and Gram-negative bacteria. In addition, one study has suggested that the combination of ciprofloxacin and ursodeoxycholic acid may be beneficial in preventing sludge formation in those patients undergoing biliary dilatation with stent placement.

Cholelithiasis and choledocholithiasis occur in up to 30% of patients with PSC. Chronic cholestasis predisposes to the formation of cholesterol gallstones and bacterial cholangitis causing bile stasis, which predisposes to the formation of pigment stones. Indeed, diagnosing choledocholithiasis can be extremely difficult in patients with PSC. Therefore, a cholangiogram is essential for eliciting the cause of new onset jaundice or bacterial cholangitis. If choledocholithiasis is documented, stone extraction or surgical intervention is indicated.

Approximately 20% of patients with PSC develop an obstructing dominant stricture of the biliary tree. Frequently, the site of the stricture is in the biliary hilum, but strictures can also occur in the common bile duct and the common hepatic duct. This complication is often associated with the acute onset of jaundice, pruritus, and/or fever related to bacterial cholangitis. If a dominant stricture is found on cholangiography, cytologic specimens should be obtained in order to exclude bile duct carcinoma, and balloon dilatation should be performed with the use of either a transhepatic or endoscopic retrograde approach, depending on the site of the stricture. In general, balloon dilatation of dominant strictures and removal of biliary sludge, while the patient is receiving antibiotics, is an effective treatment in alleviating the recent onset of jaundice or pruritus related to this complication. Approximately 50% of patients with PSC who undergo balloon dilatation of dominant strictures will have improvement for up to 2 years. Although some centers have advocated a surgical approach for biliary strictures related to PSC, the absence of prospective controlled data makes it impos-

Summary of endoscopic therapy for PSC				
Year	n	Procedure	Follow up (months)	Result
1997	23	Balloon dilation and ursodiol	45	Improved survival
1996	25	Dilation and stenting	29	Improved symptoms 57%
1995	53	Dilation and stenting	31	Improved symptoms 77%
1993	42	Dilation and stenting	52	Improved symptoms 70%
1991	35	Dilation and stenting	35	Improved symptoms 85%

Figure 18.8 Summary of endoscopic therapy in PSC. Summary of the outcome of five studies reported between 1991–97.

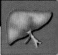

sible to assess the affect of biliary surgical treatment on the natural history of PSC. Because PSC is generally a progressive disease, biliary surgical intervention should be considered only as a palliative measure aimed at relieving symptoms and excluding a concomitant diagnosis of cholangiocarcinoma. Biliary surgical treatment has little or no value for patients with PSC who have cirrhosis or for those who have severe intrahepatic bile duct disease on cholangiogram. Biliary operations also seem to increase the difficulty and risk of liver transplantation and should be avoided if possible.

A number of recent long-term studies are now revealing that cholangiocarcinoma may develop in 6–30% of patients with PSC if they are followed over a period of 10–30 years (Fig. 18.9). The syndrome PSC should therefore be considered a premalignant condition of the biliary tree just as CUC is considered a premalignant condition of the colon. Bile duct carcinoma in the setting of PSC has been difficult to diagnose because of the lack of serologic markers and the fact that biliary cytologic and histologic studies for the most part have been insensitive in diagnosing early cholangiocarcinoma. A chronic increase in the serum bilirubin level in PSC patients may be an indication of the development of cholangiocarcinoma.

At least 10% of patients with PSC undergoing liver transplantation were found to have an unsuspected cholangiocarcinoma. Patients with concurrent PSC and cholangiocarcinoma that was diagnosed before transplantation have an overall poor prognosis with less than 10% surviving for more than 2 years after liver transplantation. Even patients in whom an incidental cholangiocarcinoma is found at the time of transplantation have a 2-year survival rate of approximately 40%, which is far below that of PSC patients who do not have a concurrent cholangiocarcinoma (Fig. 18.10). Thus, most liver transplant centers consider a diagnosis of cholangiocarcinoma a relative

or even an absolute contraindication to proceeding with liver transplantation. However, a number of centers are employing multimodal adjuvant therapeutic protocols (i.e. radiation and chemotherapy) to try to improve the results of liver transplantation and preliminary results have been encouraging. Operative management (hepatic resection), chemotherapy, and radiotherapy have been shown not to be useful in the treatment of bile duct cancer.

Because of the serious implications of a concomitant cholangiocarcinoma in the PSC patient, it has been important to try to identify which patients are at a high risk for developing this complication. There are conflicting data on the correlation between the duration of CUC or cirrhotic-stage PSC and the risk of developing cholangiocarcinoma. The use of tumor markers, such as CA 19-9, and cytologic techniques are helpful in diagnosing an existing cholangiocarcinoma, but have not been shown to date to be helpful in the early diagnosis or in screening for cholangiocarcinoma in PSC patients. Clearly, further studies will be needed to better identify those PSC patients at high risk for developing cholangiocarcinoma.

Hepatocellular cancer can also develop during the course of PSC. The patients at risk appear to be those who have advanced-stage PSC with extensive fibrosis, cirrhosis, and diffuse nodular regeneration of the liver. The question of screening PSC patients for hepatocellular cancer has arisen; however, in the absence of well-established advanced cirrhosis, screening for hepatocellular cancer in PSC patients cannot be recommended at this time.

Complications of portal hypertension

The end stages of PSC are often associated with complications of portal hypertension. One special complication is the development and bleeding from peristomal varices in patients who have

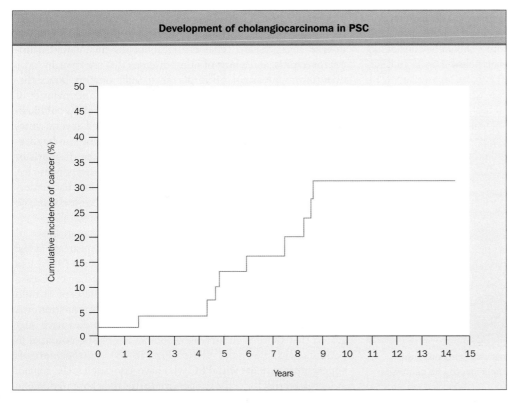

Figure 18.9 Development of cholangiocarcinoma in PSC. Cumulative actuarial incidence of cholangiocarcinoma from the time of onset of PSC. (Reproduced with permission from Farges O, et al. Primary sclerosing cholangitis, liver transplantation, or biliary surgery. Surgery. Mosby-Year Book, 1995;22:451–7.)

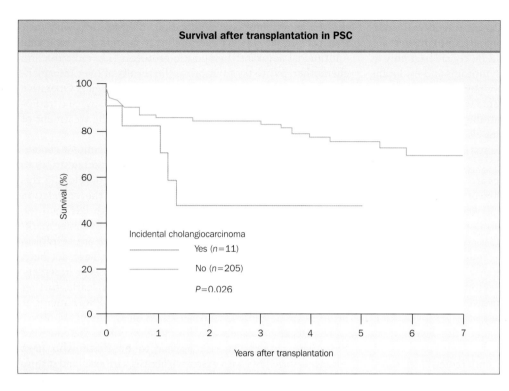

Figure 18.10 Survival after transplantation in PSC. Kaplan–Meier survival plot after transplantation in patients with PSC with and without detection of an incidental cholangiocarcinoma in the excised liver. The difference was statistically significant. Five-year survival rates 0.47 ± 0.17 and 0.75 ± 0.04, respectively. (Reproduced with permission from Abu-Elmagd KM, et al. Surgery, Gynaecology, and Obstetrics. American College of Surgeons, 1993;177:335–44.)

undergone proctocolectomy with the creation of an ileostomy (Fig. 18.11). Treatment for bleeding peristomal varices has been the creation of a transjugular intrahepatic portosystemic shunt, which has usually been quite successful in decreasing the number and severity of bleeding episodes. As in other forms of chronic liver disease, esophageal variceal bleeding is best managed by variceal band ligation or sclerotherapy. Another option is the use of a transjugular intrahepatic portosystemic shunt. If possible, surgical shunting procedures should not be performed to avoid the risks associated with a subsequent liver transplant if indicated.

Ascites is best treated with large-volume paracentesis and diuretic therapy. Administration of albumin should be considered in patients who have serum albumin levels below 2.6g/L. In PSC,

spontaneous bacterial peritonitis is a complication often related to biliary sepsis and cholangitis. In this situation, the use of oral selective bowel decontamination solution or chronic antibiotic therapy should be especially appropriate to prevent recurrence of this severe life-threatening complication. Hepatic encephalopathy is managed with the use of lactulose and dietary protein restriction only if absolutely necessary.

Associated diseases

The syndrome PSC is associated with a variety of autoimmune-type diseases (Fig. 18.12). These include inflammatory bowel disease, celiac disease, retroperitoneal fibrosis, rheumatoid arthritis, thyroiditis, and a host of other diseases that are thought to be of autoimmune origin. Of importance, inflammatory bowel disease occurs in up to 80% of patients with PSC. The majority of these patients have CUC and a minority have Crohn's colitis. In general, inflammatory bowel disease is diagnosed several years before PSC. However, inflammatory bowel disease can be diagnosed simultaneously with PSC or years after the diagnosis of PSC is made. In fact, the onset of inflammatory bowel disease has been demonstrated up to 6 years after a PSC patient had undergone liver transplantation, and PSC has been diagnosed for the first time many years after a proctocolectomy for CUC.

In patients with PSC and CUC, the mean age at onset of inflammatory bowel disease was 25 years and the mean age at the time of diagnosis of PSC was 39 years. Most patients (94%) had experienced symptoms related to inflammatory bowel disease at the time the diagnosis of PSC was made. Quiescent or mild disease based on symptoms and colonoscopic examination was found in 80% of patients with PSC. Recent studies have suggested that there is an increased colonic neoplastic potential in patients with PSC and CUC (Fig. 18.13). Furthermore, it appears that patients with PSC who have associated CUC remain at increased risk for colon cancer even after they have undergone

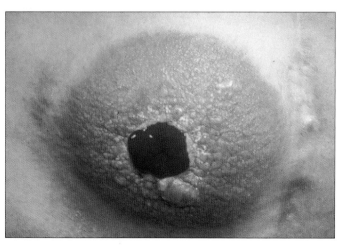

Figure 18.11 Peristomal varix. A peristomal varix surrounding the abdominal ileostoma in a patient with PSC. (Reproduced with permission from Mayo Clinic Proceedings,)

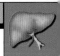

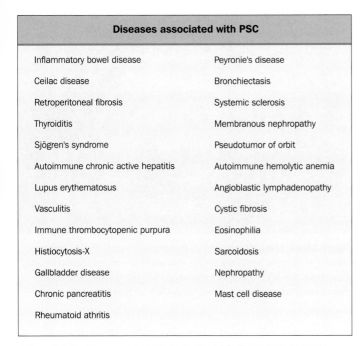

Diseases associated with PSC	
Inflammatory bowel disease	Peyronie's disease
Ceilac disease	Bronchiectasis
Retroperitoneal fibrosis	Systemic sclerosis
Thyroiditis	Membranous nephropathy
Sjögren's syndrome	Pseudotumor of orbit
Autoimmune chronic active hepatitis	Autoimmune hemolytic anemia
Lupus erythematosus	Angioblastic lymphadenopathy
Vasculitis	Cystic fibrosis
Immune thrombocytopenic purpura	Eosinophilia
Histiocytosis-X	Sarcoidosis
Gallbladder disease	Nephropathy
Chronic pancreatitis	Mast cell disease
Rheumatoid athritis	

Figure 18.12 Diseases associated with PSC. These include many autoimmune diseases, diseases linked to biliary disease, and miscellaneous associations.

liver transplantation. A recent study suggests that immunosuppressive therapy in patients suffering from PSC and CUC does not alter the course of colon disease. These patients remain at increased risk for developing colon cancer and should undergo yearly colonoscopic surveillance and screening because CUC is frequently quiescent, particularly in patients receiving immunosuppression, and because CUC can develop for the first time following liver transplantation. If moderate or severe dysplasia is found after transplantation, a total proctocolectomy has been recommended as a prophylactic measure.

In addition to inflammatory bowel disease, as listed above, PSC can be associated with a number of other diseases, most of which are thought to be autoimmune diseases and are related to abnormalities in immune regulation.

DIAGNOSIS

Criteria used to diagnose PSC have evolved with time. Originally, the diagnosis of PSC was established only with laparotomy, palpation of a fibrotic common bile duct, and a biopsy of the common bile duct performed to exclude bile duct cancer. Later, operative cholangiography revealed beading and irregularity of the extrahepatic and intrahepatic bile ducts, which today are the characteristic radiologic findings and are diagnostic of PSC in the appropriate clinical setting. The development of endoscopic retrograde cholangiopancreatography (ERCP) and transhepatic cholangiography (THC), both of which became technically feasible in the late 1970s, have had the greatest impact in diagnosing PSC. With ERCP, the spectrum of PSC rapidly expanded to patients with isolated intrahepatic disease alone, and the number of cases of PSC diagnosed per year increased 2–3-fold at most centers. In addition, the important relationship between PSC and the development of cholangiocarcinoma was confirmed using serial cholangiograms in patients with PSC. Therefore, cholangiocarcinoma, once considered an exclusionary criterion for the diagnosis of PSC, was shown to be within the spectrum of complications that developed during the course of PSC.

Currently, the diagnostic criteria for PSC are centered on characteristic cholangiographic findings, which are by no means entirely specific for PSC; however, in the appropriate clinical setting are useful in establishing the diagnosis of PSC. Cholangiographic changes similar to those found in PSC can be seen in other conditions and can cause difficulty in making the correct diagnosis. In general, these conditions also can be readily diagnosed by obtaining a detailed history and by carefully

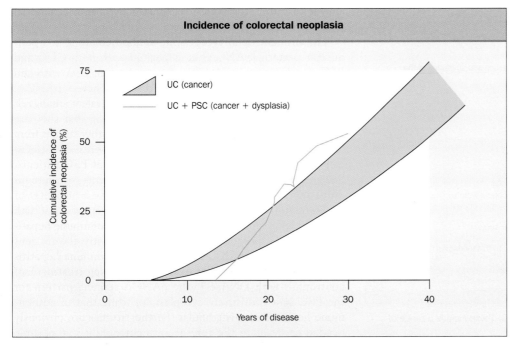

Figure 18.13 Incidence of colorectal neoplasia. Cumulative incidence of colorectal neoplasia (carcinoma and dysplasia) over time in ulcerative colitis (UC) patients with PSC compared with the range of cumulative incidence of cancer over time in UC patients alone. (Reproduced with permission from Devrroede G. Colorectal Cancer. In: Winawer S, et al (eds). Prevention, epidemiology, screening. Raven Press;1980.)

evaluating the cholangiographic and histologic findings, which are frequently helpful in excluding causes of secondary sclerosing cholangitis.

The diagnostic inclusion and exclusion criteria for PSC are outlined in Fig. 18.14.

These include:

- a cholestatic biochemical profile (alkaline phosphatase level of more than 1.5 times the upper limits of normal for 6 months or more);
- a cholangiogram showing strictures in the intrahepatic, or extrahepatic biliary tree, or both (Fig. 18.1);
- a liver biopsy specimen that reveals inflammatory fibrosis of interlobular and septal bile ducts, as well as early evidence of obliteration (Fig. 18.15) in the absence of evidence of other causes of chronic liver disease; and
- exclusion of causes of secondary sclerosing cholangitis (see Fig. 18.14).

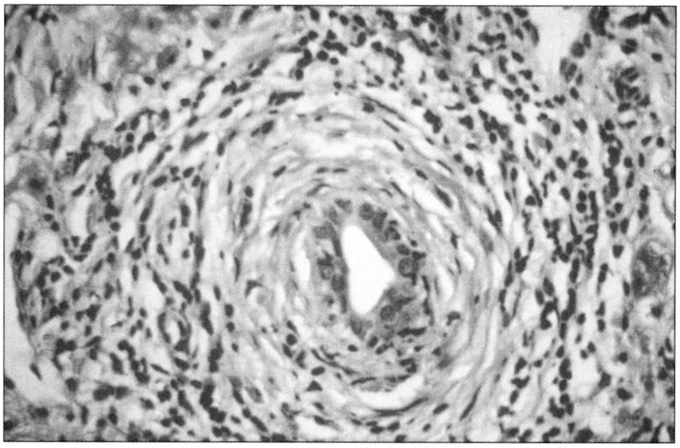

Biochemical and immunologic testing

Biochemical abnormalities are in no way specific for the diagnosis of PSC. However, a cholestatic profile of 6 or more months' duration is the hallmark of PSC, and most patients have at least a two-fold increase in serum levels of alkaline phosphatase activity. Nevertheless, patients with cholangiographically documented PSC in whom alkaline phosphatase levels were normal have been described. A number of these patients had advanced histologic-stage disease on liver histology.

Serum levels of aminotransferase are similarly increased in 92% of patients, but are usually less than five times the upper limits of normal, except in children, and the mean increase is about three times the upper limits of normal. In patients with the highest aminotransferase levels, histologic features of auto–immune chronic active hepatitis have been noted, and an

Figure 18.15 Liver biopsy. Photomicrograph of a liver biopsy specimen showing concentric peribiliary fibrosis that leads to early obliteration of the intralobular bile duct during late stages of PSC. Hematoxylin and eosin. (Reproduced with permission from Mayo Clinic Proceedings.)

overlap between the histologic features of PSC and chronic active hepatitis has been reported by a number of investigators.

While serum bilirubin levels are typically elevated in patients with advanced PSC, they tend to fluctuate widely during the course of the disease. At the time of diagnosis, serum albumin levels were decreased and prothrombin times were increased in 17 and 16% of patients, respectively. Hypergammaglobulinemia occurred in approximately 30% of patients, and IgM levels were increased in 45% of patients. Antinuclear antibodies and anti-smooth muscle antibodies were found to occur in 55 and 35% of adult patients, respectively, in a single study. Other studies have found a much lower prevalence of these antibodies, and the titers are often lower than those observed in patients with typical autoimmune chronic active hepatitis type I. Antimitochondrial antibodies in low titer occurred in less than 5% of patients, but the antigenic epitopes specifically recognized by antimitochondrial antibodies in patients with PSC appear to differ from those recognized by antimitochondrial antibodies in patients with PBC.

The antineutrophil cytoplasmic antibody binding in a perinuclear pattern (pANCA) is associated with both CUC and PSC. Approximately 65–85% of patients with PSC with and without inflammatory bowel disease have pANCA. Furthermore, pANCA was also found to be prevalent among relatives (25%) of patients with PSC, indicating that they are linked to familial immunogenetics. However, other studies from the UK have been unable to confirm the presence of antineutrophilic cytoplasmic antibodies in relatives of PSC patients. Recently, a study has revealed that 92% of patients with autoimmune hepatitis type I were also found to have a high titer of pANCA. However, the pANCA in PSC were composed of both IgG_1 and IgG_3 subclasses while those with autoimmune hepatitis had an IgG_1 predominance. More importantly, the antigens recognized by the pANCA in PSC and autoimmune hepatitis appear to be different. For example, following treatment of neutrophils with DNAse-1, the pANCA staining pattern for the PSC sera is diffusely cytoplasmic, while that of autoimmune hepatitis sera is granular. Further studies are obviously needed to evaluate the role of antineutrophilic cytoplasmic

Diagnostic criteria for PSC
Inclusion criteria
Chronic cholestatic biochemical profile (serum alkaline phosphatase level >2 times upper limits of normal for >6 months)
History of inflammatory bowel disease
Typical cholangiographic abnormalities; beading and stricturing of the extrahepatic bile ducts, or both
Liver histology compatible with PSC:
Fibro-obliterative duct lesion
Periductal fibrosis
Ductopenia
Biliary cirrhosis
Presence of pANCA (nonspecific)
Exclusion criteria
Biliary calculi (unless secondary to bile stasis)
History of biliary tract surgery other than cholecystectomy
Congenital abnormality of the biliary tree (Caroli's disease)
Cholangiopathy associated with acquired immune deficiency
Ischemic stricturing secondary to trauma or surgery
Bile duct neoplasm
Exposure to biliary toxin (floxuridine, formalin, thiabendazole)
Evidence of concurrent liver disease
(PBC, autoimmune chronic active hepatitis,
drug-induced cholestatic hepatitis)

Figure 18.14 Diagnostic criteria for PSC. These include a range of inclusion and exclusion criteria.

antibodies, but to date they appear to be nonspecific as a diagnostic marker for PSC and there is little evidence that they play a major etiologic role.

Radiology

Visualization of the biliary tract is essential to confirm the diagnosis of PSC. The method of choice is ERCP, but adequate cholangiographic studies can be obtained using the percutaneous transhepatic approach in those patients in whom ERCP is unsuccessful.

The typical cholangiographic findings in PSC reveal multifocal stricturing and beading involving both the intrahepatic and extrahepatic biliary tree (see Fig. 18.1). Involvement may be of the intrahepatic bile ducts alone, extrahepatic bile ducts alone, or both. These strictures typically are short and annular with interbeading segments of normal or slightly dilated bile ducts and are diffusely distributed, which produces the classic beaded appearance. Pathologically, this corresponds to the intrahepatic cholangiectasis and bile duct obliteration typically seen in PSC.

The gallbladder and cystic duct can be involved in up to 15% of cases. In a large series of patients with PSC, 81% had involvement of both the intrahepatic and extrahepatic bile ducts, 11% had involvement of the intrahepatic bile ducts alone, and 8% had involvement of only the extrahepatic bile ducts without involvement of the intrahepatic bile ducts. A variation of PSC termed 'small duct PSC' affects bile ducts that are too small to be seen on cholangiography; thus, cholangiograms are normal and the diagnosis is made on the basis of liver histology.

Cholangiographic findings have also been noted to be of prognostic importance in PSC. Patients having high-grade and diffuse stricturing of the intrahepatic bile ducts were found to have an overall poor prognosis (Fig. 18.16). Therefore, therapeutic intervention aimed at relieving extrahepatic bile duct obstruction with balloon dilatation or surgical choledochojejunostomy may not have a significant impact on survival if the patient has severe intrahepatic disease. Such procedures probably should be avoided in such patients.

Markedly dilated bile duct segments, a polypoid mass within the bile duct, or progressive stricture formation on serial cholangiograms were features highly suggestive of the development of a concurrent bile duct carcinoma. In such cases, multiple biopsy specimens and brushings from the bile duct should be obtained at the time the cholangiogram is performed in an attempt to make the diagnosis of cholangiocarcinoma. However, such techniques are usually diagnostically insensitive and positive in only up to 40–60% of cases in which bile duct cancer is present. A recent report suggested that severe cholangiocarcinoma in PSC patients may be detected using positron emission tomography.

Histology

The advent of liver transplantation has allowed the morphologic findings of both the extrahepatic and intrahepatic bile duct pathology to be more thoroughly studied. Gross biopsy specimens of PSC from the extrahepatic bile ducts show a thickened fibrous wall, often with mixed inflammatory infiltrates, which tend to cluster around biliary glands. These changes are nonspecific and do not allow the pathologist to distinguish between a benign localized postoperative biliary stricture and a stricture that is associated with PSC. The changes in the cholangiographically demonstrable large intrahepatic bile ducts resemble the findings in the extrahepatic bile ducts in PSC. Fibrosed bile duct segments may alternate with areas of cholangiectasis to produce the beaded appearance seen on cholangiograms.

In the early stages of PSC, histologic changes typically consist of bile duct proliferation, edema in some portal tracts, and ductopenia in others, often associated with fibrous cholangitis (pericholangitis). Therefore, if a liver biopsy specimen displays histologic features of extrahepatic biliary obstruction in some portal tracts and periductal fibrosis in others, the diagnosis of PSC should be entertained when other clinical features are present. Although helpful in establishing the diagnosis of PSC, these histologic findings are in themselves not diagnostic of PSC. A clinical correlation is essential in establishing the diagnosis of PSC. Fibrous obliterative cholangitis is occasionally present in histologic

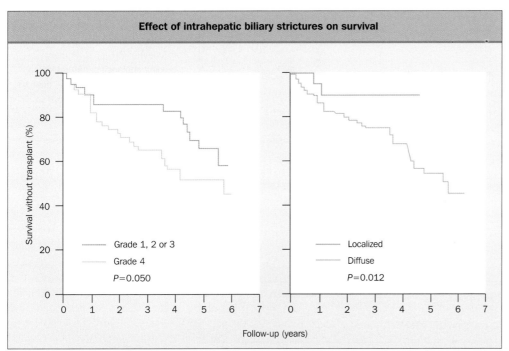

Figure 18.16 Effect of intrahepatic biliary strictures on survival. Effects of (a) intrahepatic stricture grade, and (b) extent of intrahepatic strictures on survival curves for patients with PSC. End point was either death or liver transplantation. (Reproduced with permission from Craig DA, et al. Primary sclerosing cholangitis: value of cholangiography in determining the prognosis. Am J Roentgenology. 1991;157:959–64.)

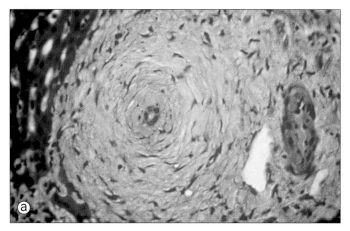

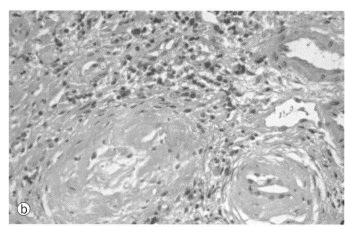

Figure 18.17 Liver biopsy. (a) Periductal fibrosis and early obliteration typically seen in patients with PSC and (b) complete bile duct obliteration.

(Reproduced with permission from Wiesner RH, et al. Current Concepts in Primary Sclerosing Cholangitis. Mayo Clinic Proceedings. 1994;69:969–82.)

specimens. It represents transformation of bile ducts to a solid fibrous cord and is nearly diagnostic of PSC (Fig. 18.17). This histologic finding is present in fewer than 7% of percutaneous liver biopsies obtained from PSC patients.

Although hepatic parenchymal manifestations of PSC are often not diagnostic, we have found them important for staging the disease and in determining the prognosis. Similar to the histologic staging established for PBC, four histologic stages have been defined for PSC (Fig. 18.18). Survival based on histologic stage is shown in Fig. 18.19. Patients with cirrhotic-stage disease clearly have a diminished survival as compared with patients with noncirrhotic-stage disease.

Differential diagnosis

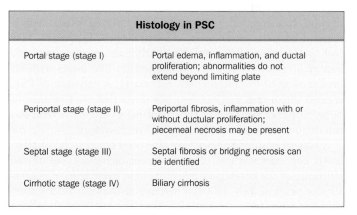

Histology in PSC	
Portal stage (stage I)	Portal edema, inflammation, and ductal proliferation; abnormalities do not extend beyond limiting plate
Periportal stage (stage II)	Periportal fibrosis, inflammation with or without ductular proliferation; piecemeal necrosis may be present
Septal stage (stage III)	Septal fibrosis or bridging necrosis can be identified
Cirrhotic stage (stage IV)	Biliary cirrhosis

Figure 18.18 Histology in PSC. The histologic staging of PSC.

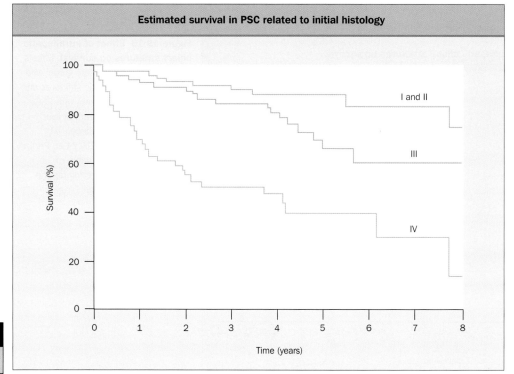

Figure 18.19 Estimated survival in PSC related to initial histology. Kaplan–Meier estimated survival by histologic stage on liver biopsy at study entry. (Reproduced with permission from Wiesner RH, et al. Primary sclerosing cholangitis: natural history, prognostic factors and survival analysis. Hepatology. 1989;10:430–6.)

The differential diagnosis of liver disorders that can present with cholestasis and the presence of ductopenia on liver histology includes PBC, sarcoidosis, chronic graft-versus-host disease, idiopathic adulthood ductopenia, drug-induced ductopenia, and liver allograft rejection. In addition, other disorders that can present with cholestasis alone include alcoholic hepatitis, drug-induced hepatitis, viral hepatitis, and autoimmune chronic active hepatitis. The latter disorders generally can be differentiated on the basis of clinical history, liver biochemistry, viral serology, histology, and cholangiography.

The most useful test in distinguishing PBC from PSC is a cholangiogram. The extrahepatic bile ducts are not involved in PBC and radiographic abnormalities present in the intrahepatic ducts in patients with cirrhotic PBC are usually distinguishable from those seen in classic PSC. Other causes of chronic cholestasis include hepatic involvement with histiocytosis and drug-induced ductopenia associated with drugs such as phenothiazine. Ductopenia in adults is labeled as idiopathic when serum studies are negative for antimitochondrial antibody, a cholangiogram is normal, inflammatory bowel disease is absent, and viral injury can be excluded.

Investigation of HIV-infected patients has led to the recognition of a condition termed 'AIDS-related sclerosing cholangitis'. Typically, these patients have right upper quadrant pain and a cholestatic biochemical profile. An ultrasound examination may show thickened bile ducts and less often bile duct stricturing and/or dilatation. Features on cholangiography are essentially indistinguishable from those of PSC. In a study examining the natural history of AIDS-related sclerosing cholangitis, the median CD4+ lymphocyte count was low in all patients. Cryptosporidiosis with or without cytomegalovirus infection has been identified as a potential infective cause of 'AIDS-related sclerosing cholangitis' in 75% of cases.

Other diseases that can mimic PSC include histiocytosis-X, cystic fibrosis, amyloidosis, and sarcoidosis. All these entities can present with intrahepatic bile duct stricturing, typical of that seen in PSC.

NATURAL HISTORY AND PROGNOSIS

The majority of PSC patients who are asymptomatic at the time of diagnosis develop symptoms of fatigue and pruritus within a number of years. Several recent studies show that PSC is usually a progressive disease. The largest of these studies comes from the Mayo Clinic in which 174 PSC patients were followed for 6 years. Median survival from the time of diagnosis of PSC was 11.9 years, and both symptomatic and asymptomatic patients at the time of diagnosis had a decreased survival as compared with a US population matched for age, sex, and race (Fig. 18.20). These findings have been confirmed by several other centers, which have reported the median survival from the time of diagnosis of PSC to be between 9 and 17 years.

A subgroup of 45 PSC patients who were asymptomatic at the time of diagnosis warrants special mention. These patients were prospectively followed for a mean of 6.25 years. During this period of time, 76% experienced progression of liver disease based on clinical and/or pathologic findings (Fig. 18.21). Furthermore, 31% developed liver failure resulting in either death or the need for a life-saving liver transplant.

In contrast, some studies found PSC to be a more benign disease. Studies from Norway estimated the mean survival of patients with PSC to be 17 years after the initial diagnosis was made. Reasons for these differences have recently been put into perspective. First, PSC progresses silently for several years and can be detected only by prospective follow-up with serial liver function tests and hepatic histologic examinations, which were not performed in all studies. Secondly, early detection of PSC

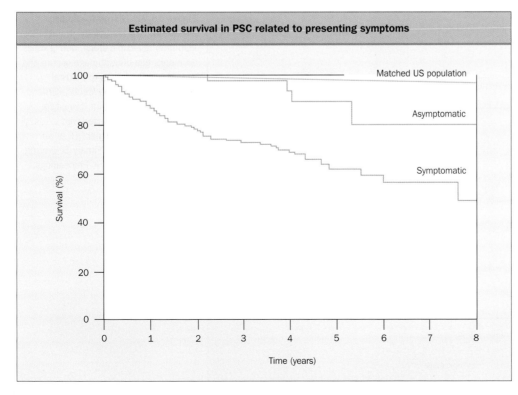

Estimated survival in PSC related to presenting symptoms

Survival (%) vs Time (years)

Figure 18.20 Estimated survival in PSC related to presenting systems. Kaplan–Meier estimated survival curves for asymptomatic and symptomatic patients with PSC. For comparison, survival curves in US population matched for age, sex, and race to asymptomatic patients are also shown. Difference in survival: asymptomatic versus control subjects, $P<0.001$; symptomatic versus asymptomatic patients, $P<0.003$. (Reproduced with permission from Wiesner RH, et al. Primary sclerosing cholangitis: natural history, prognostic factors and survival analysis. Hepatology. 1989;10:430–6.)

would appear to influence favorably the mean survival estimates, such as in the Norwegian studies in which patients with inflammatory bowel disease who had minimal abnormalities in liver function tests were aggressively assessed with cholangiography and diagnosed early in the course of their disease. Thirdly, the starting point for survival analysis is important for determining the overall survival time. The comparison of one group of patients in whom follow up began at the time of cholangiographic diagnosis of PSC and a second group of patients in whom the diagnosis of PSC was back-dated to the time of the first onset of symptoms or biochemical abnormalities will provide different survival times. Therefore, when these differences in study design are taken into account, the weight of evidence indicates that PSC in most patients is a progressive disease.

Histopathologically, PSC evolves into a ductopenic syndrome in which there is progressive stricturing of both large and small bile ducts. The overall result is that the interlobular and septal bile ducts become obliterated and functionally lost. In the histopatho-

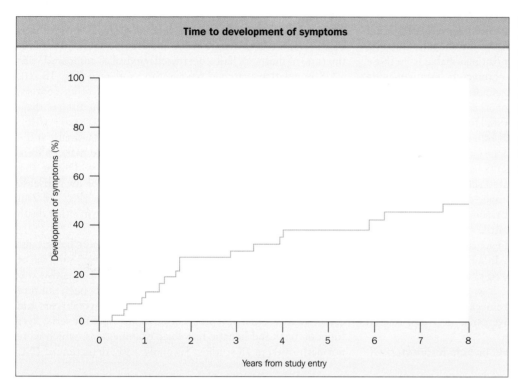

Figure 18.21 Time to development of symptoms. The estimated time to development of symptoms using the Kaplan–Meier method with Mayo Clinic diagnosis of PSC as the starting point. (Reproduced with permission from Porakyo et al. Patients with asymptomatic primary sclerosing cholangitis frequently have proferrive disease. Gastroenterology. 1990;98:1594–602.)

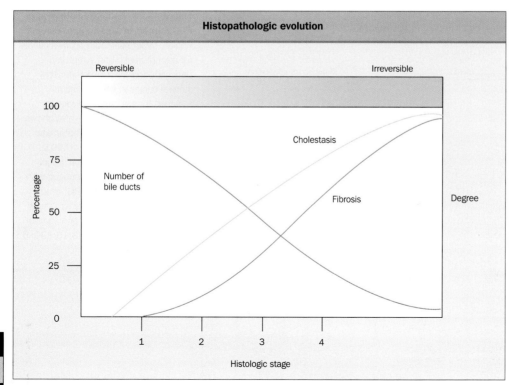

Figure 18.22 Histopathologic evolution. Histopathologic evolution of PSC from reversible stage, during which time early bile duct damage occurs and which should respond to medical therapy, to irreversible fibrotic–cirrhotic stage, which is resistant to medical intervention. (Reproduced with permission from Wiesner RH, et al. Current Concepts in Primary Sclerosing Cholangitis. Mayo Clinic Proceedings. 1994;69:969–82.)

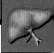

logic evolution of PSC (Fig. 18.22), when a critical number of interlobular bile ducts are lost, ongoing cholestasis occurs and leads to portal fibrosis and eventually irreversible biliary cirrhosis. Thus, it seems logical that therapeutic intervention would be most successful when it is instituted early in the course of the disease before severe ductopenia and irreversible damage to the liver occurs. Unfortunately, at this time there is no medical, radiologic, or surgical therapy of proven efficacy.

Prognostic survival models

A better understanding of the history of PSC is important in determining the rate of disease progression and the estimated survival for an individual patient at any specific time during the course of PSC. Predicting survival on the basis of clinical, bio-

chemical, and histologic features is important for monitoring therapeutic intervention and as an aid for the timing of liver transplantation in PSC patients. The use of sophisticated statistical approaches, most notably Cox multivariate regression analysis, has facilitated the development of a prognostic model based on independent clinical variables in which a survival risk score can be calculated and translated into a survival function for estimating survival for an individual PSC patient (Fig. 18.23). Several models have been developed based on long-term follow-up of a large number of PSC patients in whom important clinical predictors of prognosis have been determined (Fig. 18.24). In the Mayo model, patient age, serum bilirubin level, hemoglobin concentration, hepatic histologic stage, and presence or absence of inflammatory bowel disease was identified as independent prognostic vari-

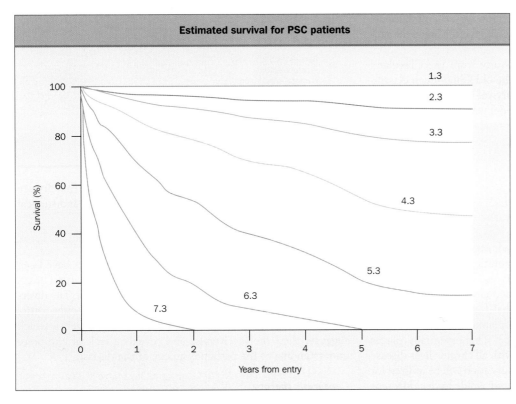

Figure 18.23 Estimated survival for PSC patients. Estimated survival for PSC patients by translating Mayo PSC risk score into a survival function. Increasing risk score leads to decreased survival. (Reproduced with permission from Wiesner RH, et al. Liver transplantation for primary sclerosing cholangitis: impact of risk factors on outcome. Liver Transplantation and Surgery. 1996;2:99–108.)

Prognosis of PSC					
Mayo clinic	Multicenter	New Mayo	Kings College	Norway	Sweden
Bilirubin	Bilirubin	Age	Heptomegaly	Age	Age
Age	Histologic stage	Bilirubin	Splenomegaly	Bilirubin	Bilirubin
Histologic stage	Age	Albumin	Alkaline phosphatase		Histologic stage
Hemoglobin	Splenomegaly	Variceal bleed	Histologic stage		
Inflammatory bowel disease		Aspartate amniotransferase			

Figure 18.24 Prognosis of PSC. The prognostic models have identified a range of variables, but histologic criteria were not used in all models.

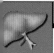

ables. In the King's College model, the presence of hepatomegaly, splenomegaly, degree of elevation of alkaline phosphatase, and histologic stage were found to be independent predictors. In Norway, investigators using multivariate analysis have found that patient age and serum bilirubin levels were independent risk factors for survival. In a fourth model, based on the data from five major liver transplant centers throughout the world (Mayo Clinic in Rochester, MN; Oxford, UK; King's College, UK; Tufts University, Boston, MA; and Thomas Jefferson University, Philadelphia, PA), 426 PSC patients with a mean follow-up of 3 years were studied. In this study, serum bilirubin level, histologic stage, patient age, and splenomegaly were identified as independent prognostic variables. With these variables, a severity risk score can be determined and translated into a survival function so that survival of any PSC patient at any point in the disease process can be estimated. Subgroup analysis from these various liver transplant centers indicates that this model is generalizable to a wide spectrum of patients who have PSC. However, the new model also requires the need for a liver biopsy, which often limits the utility of the model as a clinical tool.

This deficit was addressed in a study from the Cleveland Clinic where the authors evaluated the old Child–Pugh classification as a prognostic indicator for survival in PSC. The authors further compared the Child–Pugh model with the Mayo disease-specific PSC model. The Child–Pugh model utilizes the following clinical factors:

- serum bilirubin level;
- serum albumin level;
- prothrombin time;
- presence or absence of ascites; and
- grade of portosystemic encephalopathy.

The study demonstrated that the age-adjusted Child–Pugh model predicted survival before liver transplantation with accuracy similar to that of the Mayo PSC model. It also had the advantage of not requiring a liver biopsy and avoided complex mathematical computations. Furthermore, it is ideal for use in formulating minimal listing criteria for liver transplantation for the United Network for Organ Sharing (UNOS). This essentially places PSC patients on a level playing field with all chronic liver disease patients in whom the Child–Pugh classification will be utilized for liver transplantation listing purposes and avoids having different criteria for each disease.

However, there are obvious shortcomings with regard to all of these models in that none of them have been prospectively evaluated, they all use historic data, and they do not take into account certain risk factors that are important in determining the timing for liver transplantation in the PSC patient, such as variceal bleeding, quality of life, and the possibility of developing a hepatobiliary malignancy. Nevertheless, these models have been useful in counseling patients and have been important in advising the appropriate timing for liver transplantation for patients with this disease. Additional ongoing studies will be needed to assess prospectively the models and their applications toward further optimizing the timing of liver transplantation, particularly with waiting times for liver transplantation now approaching 2 years at many centers. In addition, the challenge remains to refine further these models so that they might be applied to monitoring the effect of experimental therapy on disease progression.

Figure 18.25 Treatment of PSC. The traetments include drugs, radiologic, and surgical approaches. All are aimed at retarding disease progression.

Treatment of PSC
Medical
Cupruretic: D-penicillamine
Immunosuppressive: Prednisone, Azathioprine, Cyclosporine, Methotrexate, Tacrolimus
Antifibrotic: Colchicine
Choleretic: Ursodeoxycholic acid
Radiological
Cholangioplasty, Biliary infusion therapy
Surgical
Reconstructive surgery, Proctocolectomy, Liver transplantation

MANAGEMENT

Primary therapy for PSC aimed at interrupting the disease process can be subdivided into medical, radiologic, and surgical approaches (Fig. 18.25).

Medical therapy

Over the past 20 years, various medical treatments have been used in PSC patients in the hope of improving the natural history of the hepatobiliary disease and improving survival. The diversity of medical therapies includes the use of cupruretic, immunosuppressive, antifibrogenic, and choleretic agents, which suggests their ineffectiveness and reveals a lack of complete understanding of the pathophysiology of the disease.

Cupruretic therapy

The evidence of increased hepatic copper in PSC provided the main rationale for evaluating D-penicillamine as a therapeutic agent for PSC. In a prospective randomized, double-blind, placebo-controlled trial, D-penicillamine had no favorable effect on PSC progression and patient survival. This was determined after 36 months of follow-up based on careful analysis of clinical and biochemical profiles, radiologic findings, liver histology, and survival data between the two groups of PSC patients. Furthermore, major adverse effects of D-penicillamine including proteinuria and thrombocytopenia, led to the discontinuation of the drug in 20% of treated patients.

Immunosuppressive therapy

The use of immunosuppressive agents in the therapy of PSC was based on the concept that PSC is an autoimmune disease. In uncontrolled observations, oral corticosteroids have been shown to improve the biochemical profile in PSC patients; however, long-term or controlled studies of corticosteroids are lacking. In a small, controlled study in PSC patients, topical corticosteroid application in the biliary tree via nasobiliary lavage provided no advantage over placebo. Other immunosuppressive agents that have been employed in the treatment of PSC include:

- azathioprine – the experience has been mostly anecdotal;
- cyclosporine – the results were negative;
- methotrexate – a randomized, double-blind, placebo-controlled trial showed no benefit in the treatment group; and
- tacrolimus – a small open-label study showed only improvement in liver enzymes.

These attempts at immunosuppressive therapy lead to the conclusion that further studies are needed to define the immunosuppressive effects in PSC patients. In addition, an open trial of prednisone and colchicine in PSC patients demonstrated no benefit on progression of hepatic histology and liver biochemical tests over a 2-year period. A pilot study combining ursodeoxycholic acid and methotrexate for the treatment of PSC was associated with toxicity, without improvement in liver function tests compared with ursodeoxycholic acid therapy alone.

Antifibrotic therapy

Due to the fact that PSC leads to liver cirrhosis, antifibrotic agents, such as colchicine, were suggested as a therapeutic option for PSC. Recently, in a prospective, double-blind study, 84 PSC patients were randomized to received 1mg of colchicine versus placebo daily for a period of 3 years. The results of this multicenter study revealed that colchicine had no beneficial effect on patient symptoms, liver biochemistry, hepatic histology, or survival.

Choleretic therapy

The enthusiasm for the use of ursodeoxycholic acid, a hydrophilic bile acid, in the treatment of PSC emerged from favorable data on its use for PBC and from promising clinical

and biochemical improvement reported in PSC patients receiving ursodeoxycholic acid in small uncontrolled studies. Subsequently, a prospective, randomized, double-blind, placebo-controlled trial involving 14 PSC patients was performed to examine further the efficacy of ursodeoxycholic acid. The authors of that study concluded that PSC patients treated with ursodeoxycholic acid at 13–15mg/kg of body weight per day for 1 year demonstrated marked improvement in serum liver tests and histology on liver biopsy. The proposed benefit of orally administered ursodeoxycholic acid in cholestatic patients is thought to be related to:

- its accumulation in the endogenous bile pool which leads to replacement of endogenous potentially toxic bile acids in the cholestatic liver;
- its protective effect at the cellular and subcellular levels of the hepatocyte and cholangiocyte;
- its hypercholeretic activity; and
- its immunomodulatory effect.

However, in the recently published largest randomized, double-blind, placebo-controlled trial of ursodeoxycholic acid treatment for PSC, no clinical benefit was found. The study included 105 patients with well-established PSC given ursodeoxycholic acid 13–15mg/kg of body weight per day compared with placebo. The mean follow-up was 2.2 years. In this study, ursodeoxycholic acid, but not placebo, demonstrated improvement in liver function tests at 1 and 2 years of treatment. Nevertheless, the primary outcome (time to treatment failure), as defined by the authors, and survival were not significantly different in the two groups of PSC patients (Fig. 18.26). In another randomized, controlled study involving 59 PSC patients treated for 2 years with either ursodeoxycholic acid (300mg twice a day) or colchicine (0.6mg twice a day), the outcome was not better than the untreated control group.

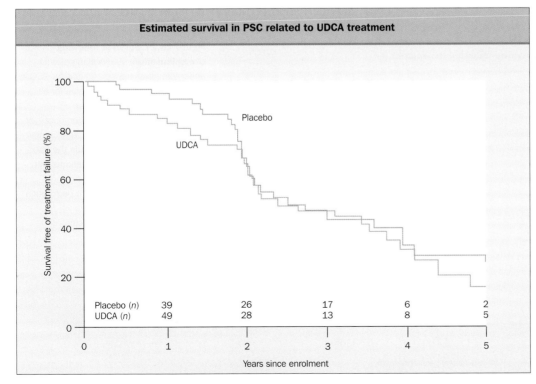

Figure 18.26 Estimated survival in PSC related to UDCA treatment. Kaplan–Meier analysis of survival free of treatment failure among study patients. Treatment failure was defined as one or more of the following: death, liver transplantation, histologic progression by two stages, progression to cirrhosis, development of esophageal varices, development of ascites or encephalopathy, sustained quadrupling of the serum bilirubin concentration, marked worsening of fatigue or pruritus, inability to tolerate the drug, and voluntary withdrawal from the study. UDCA, ursodeoxycholic acid. (Reproduced with permission from Lindor KD, et al. Ursodiol for Primary Sclerosing Cholangitis. N Eng J Med. 1997;336:691–5.)

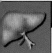

In summary, to date, effective pharmacologic treatment for the underlying hepatobiliary disease in PSC is lacking. The data do not support the use of any mentioned agent except in the context of well-designed experimental studies. Future therapeutic trials for PSC must be centered on the asymptomatic patient because, when ductopenia occurs, the disease appears to be irreversible since bile duct epithelial cells are unable to regenerate.

Surgical therapy
Until the advent of liver transplantation, surgical therapy for PSC was focused on alleviation of pruritus and jaundice, exclusion of cholangiocarcinoma, and the prevention of colonic adenocarcinoma by performing a proctocolectomy in patients with concurrent PSC and CUC.

Biliary surgery
Since PSC is a progressive disease, biliary surgery was introduced primarily to improve symptoms. Biliary enteric anastomoses with biliary stenting and reconstruction of the hepatic duct bifurcation with long-term transhepatic stents have been performed. In two retrospective studies evaluating biliary tract reconstructive surgery, the cirrhotic group of PSC patients showed a significantly higher mortality rate compared to the noncirrhotic group. Thus, it is now widely accepted that biliary surgery should be avoided in PSC patients with cirrhosis or severe, diffuse intrahepatic disease. Instead, these patients should be considered for liver transplantation.

Although biliary reconstruction may benefit noncirrhotic PSC patients with extrahepatic disease, the lack of prospective, controlled data makes it impossible to assess the long-term effects of this procedure on the natural history of PSC and the subsequent risk of developing cholangiocarcinoma. In our view, the value of biliary surgery is limited to selected PSC patients without cirrhosis who are not candidates for liver transplantation when extrahepatic dominant strictures are not amenable to endoscopic or transhepatic dilatation.

Proctocolectomy
In patients with both PSC and CUC, proctocolectomy is frequently performed due to indications relevant to inflammatory bowel disease. The possible effect of proctocolectomy on the natural history of PSC was examined in a retrospective analysis involving 45 patients with coexisting PSC and CUC, of whom almost half had undergone proctocolectomy and the rest had not. This study revealed that the clinical signs, biochemical profile, histologic progression on liver biopsy, and survival were not different in the two groups. Moreover, the fact that PSC can occur years after proctocolectomy argues against any beneficial effect of this procedure on the progression of PSC. Nonetheless, patients with both PSC and CUC remain at high risk for the development of adenocarcinoma of the colon; thus, an annual surveillance colonoscopy is strongly indicated, particularly in patients with PSC who have undergone liver transplantation. Proctocolectomy should be performed for intractable symptoms of inflammatory bowel disease that are not amenable to medical treatment and for colonic dysplasia and malignancy. In patients with PSC and CUC, if proctocolectomy is indicated, an ileal pouch anal anastomosis is the procedure of choice since this procedure prevents the development of peristomal varices. Of note, a complication of the ileal pouch anal anastomosis is pouchitis, a nonspecific inflammation of the ileal reservoir that occurs more frequently in patients with coexisting PSC and CUC than in CUC patients alone. Frequently, treatment with metronidazole or other antibiotics will effectively control this condition.

Orthotopic liver transplantation
Currently, the only suitable life-saving treatment for patients with end-stage PSC is orthotopic liver transplantation. Over the past decade, the outcome of liver transplantation in PSC patients with end-stage disease has improved significantly, and liver transplantation has emerged as the treatment of choice for these patients. Indeed, retrospective analysis of PSC patients using the Mayo PSC natural history model has shown that liver transplantation significantly improves the survival rate at all risk stratifications com-

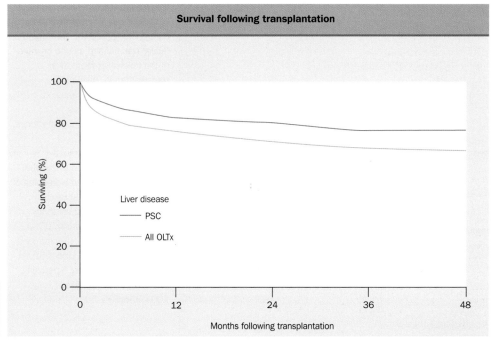

Figure 18.27 Survival following transplantation. Survival in patients undergoing liver transplantation for PSC in comparison with overall survival for all indications for orthotopic liver transplantation. Patients undergoing liver transplantation for PSC had significantly improved survival ($p<0.01$) on the basis of 1992 data from UNOS. Patients with PSC ($n=499$); other indications ($n=4332$). (Reproduced with permission from Agean Communications. Contemporary Internal Medicine. 1994;6:37–46.)

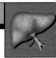

pared with the estimated survival and the absence of liver transplantation. Recently, the 1-year and 5-year patient survivals after liver transplantation for PSC have been reported to be between 90 and 97%, and 85 and 88%, respectively (Fig. 18.27), based on independent studies from three major liver transplant centers. In patients with end-stage PSC, one of the major clinical challenges is selecting the ideal time for liver transplantation. It is known that patients with high Mayo PSC risk scores have an increased risk of death after orthotopic liver transplantation compared with patients with low Mayo risk scores. In addition, risk factors specific to PSC that affect the outcome of liver transplantation have been recognized. Recently, a prognostic model to predict the post-liver transplant morbidity in PSC and PBC has been described. In PSC patients, the guidelines for liver transplantation should include intractability of symptoms, signs, and complications of portal hypertension. However, careful consideration of each patient's needs and quality of life remain important in this disease.

Despite a favorable outcome, liver transplantation for PSC is associated with specific complications. Post liver transplant complications include an increased incidence of acute and chronic rejection frequently leading to graft loss, biliary strictures and leakage, hepatic artery thrombosis, and lymphoproliferative disease. Recurrence of PSC after liver transplantation has been controversial primarily due to the lack of gold standard criteria for the diagnosis of recurrent PSC. When a cohort of patients was evaluated for recurrent disease based on biochemical, cholangiographic, and histologic criteria, 20% were found to have evidence of recurrent disease at a mean of 55 months after liver transplantation. A number of these patients have required retransplantation, and the impact of the recurrence of PSC is yet to be determined.

PRACTICE POINT

Case history

A 37-year-old man presented to the gastrointestinal clinic with a 7-week history of progressive jaundice associated with features suggestive of obstructive jaundice. He developed ulcerative colitis at the age of 25 years and a diagnosis of PSC was made at the age of 31 years. The diagnosis of PSC was made on the basis of changes documented at an ERCP performed because of an alkaline phosphatase that was twice the upper limit of normal. He was treated with ursodeoxycholic acid 750mg/day. He had no previous symptoms related to the PSC and the colitis was quiescent.

The investigations revealed serum bilirubin 276μmol/L (16.2mg/dL), alkaline phosphatase 1093IU/L, serum aspartate aminotransferase 112IU/L, albumin 31g/L (3.1g/dL), and INR 1.3. The CA 19.9 was ten times above the upper limit of normal. The ultrasound showed no evidence of duct dilatation, but the gallbladder was enlarged and contained multiple calculi. At ERCP, a tight dominant stricture was noted at the hilum. This was dilated using a balloon with a moderate degree of success. Brush cytology subsequently revealed dysplastic cells. A subsequent CT scan showed no mass lesion around the hilum. He was listed for transplantation and received a graft 5 months later. The examination of the explanted liver confirmed the diagnosis of cholangiocarcinoma and he died of recurrence of this malignancy 17 months later.

Interpretation

This case illustrates the difficulties inherent in monitoring patients with PSC. The first clinical symptoms can be due to malignant transformation and cholangiocarcinoma is not exclusive to patients with long-standing symptomatic disease. There are no satisfactory methods to screen for malignant change before the potential for cure is lost. In this case, the decision to proceed to transplantation was mainly driven by the detection of dysplastic cells in the absence of proof of the existence of cholangiocarcinoma. The cholangiocarcinoma escaped detection at surgery highlighting the difficulty that may exist in making the diagnosis, even when the index of suspicion is high. The outcome was typical of patients transplanted with cholangiocarcinoma, even when the tumor bulk was low. Malignant transformation changed this man from being a perfect candidate for transplantation to one that was not amenable to any therapy. Patients with PSC should be very carefully monitored and early involvement with a transplant program is prudent.

FURTHER READING

Abu-Elmagd KM, Malinchoc M, Dickson ER, et al. Efficacy of hepatic transplantation in patients with primary sclerosing cholangitis. Surg Gynecol Obstet. 1993;177:335–44. *A large series of patients with PSC demonstrating improved survival with liver transplant as compared with survival as estimated by the Mayo Survival Model.*

Ahrendt SA, Pitt HA, Kalloo AN, et al. Primary sclerosing cholangitis: resect, dilate, or transplant? Ann Surg. 1998;227:412–23. *A retrospective analysis of patients with primary sclerosing cholangitis who underwent endoscopic or radiologic dilatation, surgical resection, or transplantation. The authors concluded that resection is associated with a decrease in long-term occurrence of hepatocellular cancer and, in patients with noncirrhotic disease, a better overall outcome.*

Bansi DS, Fleming KA, Chapman RW. Importance of antineutrophil cytoplasmic antibodies in primary sclerosing cholangitis and ulcerative colitis: prevalence, titer, and IgG subclass. Gut. 1996;38:384–9. *Evaluation of antineutrophil cytoplasmic antibodies in PSC and ulcerative colitis and the potential role they may play in etiopathogenesis.*

Bergquist A, Glauman H, Persson B, et al. Risk factors and clinical presentation of hepatobiliary carcinoma in patients with primary sclerosing cholangitis: a case-control study. Hepatology. 1998;27:311–6. *An assessment of risk factors and clinical presentation of patients with hepatobiliary carcinoma in patients with primary sclerosing cholangitis.*

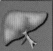
Boberg KM, Fausa O, Haaland T, et al. Features of autoimmune hepatitis in primary sclerosing cholangitis: an evaluation of 114 primary sclerosing cholangitis patients according to a scoring system for the diagnosis of autoimmune hepatitis. Hepatology. 1996;23:1369–76. *A description of patients having components of both autoimmune chronic active hepatitis and PSC; scoring system for the diagnosis of each entity.*

Broome U, Lofberg R, Veress B, Eriksson LS. Primary sclerosing cholangitis and ulcerative colitis: evidence for increased neoplastic potential. Hepatology. 1995;22:1404–8. *An important study showing an increased potential for the development of colorectal dysplasia and cancer.*

Craig DA, MacCarty RL, Wiesner RH, Grambsch PM, LaRusso NF. Primary sclerosing cholangitis: value of cholangiography in determining the prognosis. Am J Roentgenology. 1991;157:959–64. *A study evaluating the impact of a variety of cholangiographic findings on overall prognosis.*

Farges O, Malassagne B, Sebagh M, Bismuth H. Primary sclerosing cholangitis, liver transplantation, or biliary surgery. Surgery. 1995;22:451–7. *A review of a large group of patients who either underwent liver transplantation or biliary surgery. The authors conclude that liver transplantation is the treatment of choice.*

Graziadei IW, Wiesner RH, Batts, et al. Recurrence of primary sclerosing cholangitis following liver transplantation. Hepatology 1999;29:1050–6. *A large group of patients with well-characterized PSC who developed nonanastomic biliary strictures following liver transplantation highly suggestive of recurrence of disease. These findings were not seen in a control group of patients who underwent a Roux-en-Y anastomosis for indications other than PSC.*

Hay JE, Lindor KD, Wiesner RH, Dickson ER, Krom RAF, LaRusso NF. Metabolic bone disease in primary sclerosing cholangitis. Hepatology. 1991;14:257–61. *A study of a large group of patients with PSC indicating that osteoporosis is a common complication.*

Lee YM, Kaplan MM. Primary sclerosing cholangitis. N Engl J Med. 1995;332:924–33. *An excellent overall review of PSC with regard to diagnosis, treatment, epidemiology, and overall outcome.*

Ludwig J, Barham SS, LaRusso NF, Elveback LR, Wiesner RH, McCall JT. Morphologic features of chronic hepatitis associated with primary sclerosing cholangitis and chronic ulcerative colitis. Hepatology. 1981;1:632–40. *A description of the morphologic features of PSC in early- and late-stage disease.*

Ludwig J. Small duct primary sclerosing cholangitis. Semin Liv Dis. 1991;11:1791–6. *A description of small duct PSC involving only the interlobular and septal bile ducts with complete sparing of the large bile ducts.*

Mayo PSC Study Group. Ursodiol for primary sclerosing cholangitis. N Engl J Med. 1997;336:691–5. *A prospective randomized trial evaluating Ursodiol in the treatment of PSC, indicating that Ursodiol is of little benefit in preventing progression of disease.*

Rosen CB, Nagorney DM, Wiesner RH, Coffey RJ Jr, LaRusso NF. Cholangiocarcinoma complicating primary sclerosing cholangitis. Ann Surg. 1991;213:21–5. *A large group of patients with PSC who developed cholangiocarcinoma. The study indicates a poor prognosis with any type of therapeutic intervention.*

Stiehl A, Rudolph G, Sauer P, et al. Efficacy of ursodeoxycholic acid treatment and endoscopic dilation of major duct stenoses in primary sclerosing cholangitis. An 8-year prospective study. J Hepatol. 1997;26:560–6. *An evaluation of ursodeoxycholic acid and endoscopic dilatation of major duct stenoses in patients with PSC. This is an 8-year prospective study, which was uncontrolled, but did suggest there may be a benefit from this dual therapy.*

Wiesner RH, Grambsch PM, Dickson ER, et al. Primary sclerosing cholangitis: natural history, prognostic factors and survival analysis. Hepatology. 1989;10:430–6. *A large group of patients in whom multivariate regression analysis was performed to formulate a model to estimate survival for the individual PSC patient.*

Wiesner RH, Porayko MK, Dickson ER, et al. Selection and timing of liver transplantation in primary biliary cirrhosis and primary sclerosing cholangitis. Hepatology. 1992;16:1290–9. *A review assessing the PBC and PSC survival model and its potential use in the selection and timing of liver transplantation for optimal outcome.*

Wiesner RH, Porayko MK, Hay JE, et al. Liver transplantation for primary sclerosing cholangitis: impact of risk factors on outcome. Liver Transpl Surg. 1996;2:99–108. *An assessment of clinical risk factors that may have a major effect on outcome of patients transplanted for PSC.*

Wilschanski M, Chait P, Wade JA, et al. Primary sclerosing cholangitis in 32 children: clinical, laboratory, and radiographic features with survival analysis. Hepatology. 1995;22:1415–20. *A large study of children with PSC describing their clinical, laboratory, radiographic features, and the impact of the disease on long-term survival.*

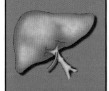

Section 3 Specific Diseases of the Liver

Chapter 19 Alcoholic Liver Disease

Nick Sheron

INTRODUCTION

Social indulgence in alcohol, whether in the form of a fine Bordeaux, or New Zealand Sauvignon Blanc, a pint of English beer or a bottle of Swedish vodka, is a fundamental and important part of Western European culture. Moderate indulgence in alcohol also brings health benefits in the form of a 50% reduction in ischemic heart disease compared with teetotallers. However, alcohol taken irresponsibly is a major cause of physical and mental ill health. In high doses over prolonged periods alcohol is toxic to the brain, vasculature, heart, and above all the liver. The link between alcohol intake and liver disease was known to both the Ancient Greeks and the Ayervedic physicians of India. It was, however, lost to Western medicine until relatively late in this century, with the prevailing view for much of this time that liver damage was a result of dietary deficiency – despite the development of significant liver injury in many affluent and clearly well-nourished individuals over the years.

Alcohol remains the single most significant cause of liver disease throughout the Western world, responsible for between 40 and 80% of cases of cirrhosis in different countries. Many of the factors underlying the development of alcoholic liver injury remain unknown, and significant questions remain about the value of even very basic therapeutic strategies. Alcohol-induced liver disease forms a spectrum: at one end lies the relatively benign lesion of fatty liver, and even very heavy drinkers will in the majority of cases not progress from this to the more severe forms of liver injury. At the other end of the spectrum, a proportion of heavy drinkers will develop alcoholic hepatitis, a disease that may begin acutely with no preceding clinical features. This has an immediate mortality of 30–60%. Around 20% of heavy drinkers develop progressive liver fibrosis, culminating finally in alcoholic cirrhosis, after perhaps 10–20 years of heavy indulgence.

EPIDEMIOLOGY AND PATHOGENESIS

The average annual *per capita* consumption of alcohol in Europe varies from approximately 4L in Norway to 13L in France, and it is 7L in the USA. Average alcohol consumptions are more usually reported as the number of units per week (1 unit = one glass of wine, half a pint or 270 mL of 3.5–4.0% beer, or a small measure of spirits containing 37–40% alcohol) or as the number of grams per day. A unit of alcohol approximately equates to 7g of alcohol. The relationship between alcohol intake and the development of alcoholic cirrhosis is not a simple dose-related toxicity. There is a clear relationship between the overall intake of alcohol and death rates from cirrhosis, as illustrated by the marked rise in cirrhosis-related mortality following the repeal of wine rationing in France following the Second World War (Fig. 19.1) and the gradual increase in cirrhosis as alcohol consumption has increased in most of the developed world since the 1950s. There appears to be a threshold for the development of alcoholic cirrhosis at around 40 units/week. The most recent estimates of the relative risk of developing cirrhosis suggest that with alcohol intakes of 28–41 units/week, 3% of men and 4% of women will develop clinically evident cirrhosis over 12 years. These figures rise to around 6–8% with intakes over 42 units/week. Similar studies in the past have found marked increases in the development of cirrhosis with alcohol intakes exceeding 40 units/week. Once within this window of toxicity, the rate of development of cirrhosis is around 2% per year up to a ceiling of 20–30%, irrespective of the level or previous duration of alcohol consumption (Fig. 19.2). This finding that a maximum of 20–30% of lifelong alcoholics will develop significant liver disease has been confirmed by many biopsy and autopsy cross-sectional studies.

Liver cirrhosis was the ninth leading cause of death in the USA in the late 1980s, and the sixth leading cause of death in the age group 45–64 years. Determining exact death rates as a result of alcohol intake is difficult, because of the marked under-reporting of alcohol as a cause of death. Combining data from longitudinal studies (Fig. 19.3) does, however, provide information

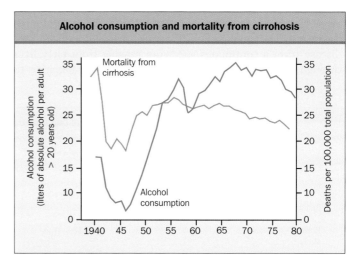

Figure 19.1 Alcohol consumption (adults) and mortality from cirrhosis in France: 1939–1980. (Data from Lelbach WK. Epidemiology of alcoholic liver disease. In: Hall P, ed. Alcoholic liver disease. New York: Wiley and Sons; 1985:130–66.)

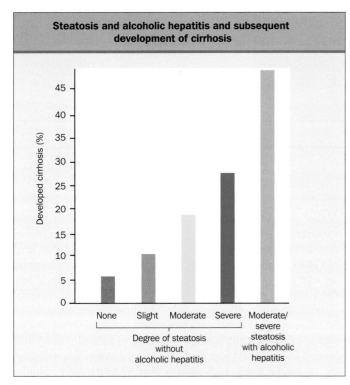

Figure 19.2 Steatosis and alcoholic hepatitis and subsequent development of cirrhosis. Taken over a mean 12 year period.

established cirrhosis. More than 80% of heavy drinkers (>40 units/week) will develop alcohol-induced fatty liver. Of these, a proportion (10–35%) will develop acute alcoholic hepatitis and 20–30% will eventually develop cirrhosis.

Genetic susceptibility to alcohol-induced liver injury

A number of twin studies have examined the potential link between alcohol and liver damage (Fig. 19.5). The interpretation of these studies has been hampered by the fact that alcoholism itself clearly has a genetic component, and thus very large twin studies are needed to differentiate this component from a susceptibility to liver disease within populations of alcoholics. The biochemical determinants of alcoholism are as yet unknown, but their existence raises important ethical considerations about the nature of addiction as a disease as opposed to an open choice of lifestyle. A seminal study of nearly 13,000 twin pairs found a clear genetic trait in the development of liver injury, in addition to that determining alcohol consumption.

This genetic trait is clearly multifactorial, and a number of studies have aimed to identify candidate genes. Most investigators have concentrated on the enzymes of the metabolic pathway, many of which are polymorphic. A mutation in the enzyme acetaldehyde dehydrogenase is very common in Oriental populations. This leads to low enzyme activity and a classic flushing reaction following alcohol ingestion, due to an inability to metabolize acetaldehyde, one of the major toxic metabolites of ethanol. Individuals who have this mutation tend not to drink to excess, but interestingly there is some evidence to suggest that they have a higher incidence of alcoholic cirrhosis if they do. Associations between polymorphisms in the genes coding for acetaldehyde dehydrogenase, alcohol dehydrogenase, and cytochrome P4502E1, and the development of alcohol-induced cirrhosis have all been sought, but so far no consistent associations have been demonstrated. More recently polymorphisms in genes of the pro- and anti-inflammatory cytokine cascades have been associated with the development of inflammatory disease, and preliminary evidence suggests that polymorphic tumor necrosis factor (TNF) loci may be associated with the development of alcoholic hepatitis. Although these results have not yet been conclusively confirmed, they suggest an avenue for future studies.

It is likely that some of the newer techniques in the analysis of multifactorial genetic traits will provide a series of candidate genes for the development of alcoholic liver injury over the next few years, and interesting insights may develop from the increasing use

about associations between levels of alcohol intake and death rates from all causes, showing a J-shaped curve due to the protective effect of moderate drinking against heart disease. These studies give a calculated annual excess death rate due to alcohol consumption for the UK of up to 28,000, or approximately 46/100,000 population. In comparison, estimated death rates from reported cases of alcohol-induced cirrhosis are currently between 5 and 10/100,000 population in Western Europe and the USA (Fig. 19.4).

The epidemiologic data show that alcohol is one of several permissive factors for the eventual development of cirrhosis; the other factors are unknown but may be both genetic and environmental. The three pathologic forms of alcohol-induced liver disease form a continuous spectrum ranging from fatty liver through various degrees of fibrosis and alcoholic hepatitis to

Deaths due to alcohol consumption				
	Duration of follow-up (years)	Sample size	Estimate of excess deaths	95% Confidence interval
Honolulu heart study	8	8006	4462	3807–5463
Civil servant study	10	1422	6645	6019–6875
Kaiser–Permanente study	10	6336	13909	12,863–15,341
Chicago Western Electric study	17	1832	14117	13,164–14,729
Framingham study	22	2106	3806	3640–3934

Figure 19.3 Deaths due to alcohol consumption among men aged 35–64 in England and Wales. (Anderson P, Br Med J. 1988;297:825.)

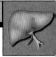

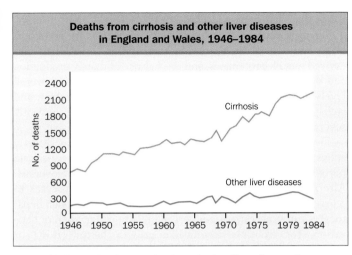

Figure 19.4 Deaths from cirrhosis and other liver disease in England and Wales, 1946–1984. Source: OPCS Mortality Statistics. HMSO: London; 1986

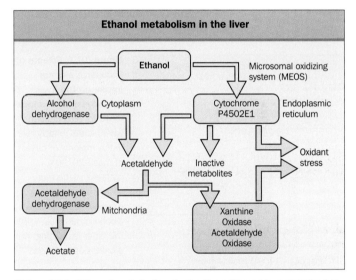

Twin pairs (n)	Monozygotic (%)	Dizygotic (%)	Ratio
12,898	–	–	1.5–2.1
174	71	32	2.2
15,924	26	13	2
86 (men)	59	36	1.6

Summary of twin studies on alcohol-drinking behaviour and alcoholism

Figure 19.5 Summary of twin studies on alcohol-drinking behavior and alcoholism. There is a clear excess in monozygotic twins, suggesting a genetic trait.

Figure 19.6 Ethanol metabolism in the liver. Ethanol is metabolized in the liver via two pathways, alcohol dehydrogenase and cytochrome P4502E1 leading to the production of acetaldehyde, and a number of other metabolites including free radicals leading to oxidative stress.

of transplantation in alcoholic liver disease. Patients transplanted for alcoholic liver disease who continue to drink may prove to be unwitting subjects in an as yet unstructured experiment, which in time will provide valuable data as to whether the risk of redevelopment of alcoholic liver disease is modulated by host or donor genes. It is entirely possible that the donor organ may display a different susceptibility to alcohol toxicity, although the testing of this hypothesis would not be something that one would necessarily wish to encourage.

Alcohol-induced fatty liver
The causation of alcohol-induced fatty change is relatively well-understood. Alcohol is metabolized via two major enzyme pathways (Fig. 19.6), resulting acutely in increases in ratios of hepatic reduced and unreduced nicotinamide adenine dinucleotide (NADH and NAD, respectively), with resulting decreased fatty acid oxidation and increased triglyceride synthesis. In addition acetaldehyde, a potentially toxic metabolite, is generated and this may affect microtubular function. These combined effects are sufficient to explain the dose-related acute development of swollen hepatocytes containing excessive fat, protein, and water following heavy alcohol intake over a period of weeks or months. Fatty liver is seen in both humans and animals fed relatively high levels of alcohol for periods of weeks to months, and resolves completely when alcohol intake ceases.

Animal models of alcoholic liver injury
The interpretation of many of the animal studies of alcohol-induced liver disease are fraught with difficulty. Most animals, with the curious exception of baboons, have a natural aversion to alcohol. In order to give alcohol to rats, for example, it must be administered either as a component of a liquid diet or given as a direct intragastric infusion via a stainless steel cannula, an experimental model with significant ethical considerations. When these rats are fed both alcohol and a high fat diet for several weeks they develop macrovesicular fatty change, focal necrosis and inflammation, and ultimately fibrosis. They do not develop disease with a pathologic resemblance to human alcoholic hepatitis. Manipulation of the balance of saturated fats in

the diet of these animals is reflected in changes in levels of fat, focal inflammation, and necrosis. The focal necrosis seen in these animals is similar to the injury induced by experimental administration of endotoxin, and may in part be endotoxin-related. Antibiotic treatment has been shown to ameliorate the level of liver injury in these fat- and alcohol-loaded animals. This effect is hypothesized to reflect changing intestinal flora, and thus the quantity or quality of bacterial endotoxin loading on the liver reticuloendothelial system. It is generally accepted that the fat/alcohol model induces oxidant stress and lipid peroxidation within the liver, and that this, combined with possible effects of endotoxin, may in turn then result in the liver pathology seen in these animals.

A series of experiments has been performed using a colony of alcohol-drinking baboons; over 5 years, 13 of 63 animals developed fibrosis. The typical clinical and histopathologic lesion of alcoholic hepatitis was seen, suggesting that alcohol-induced fatty liver may progress directly to fibrosis and subsequently cirrhosis. The theory that fat infiltration of the liver may lead directly to fibrosis in a proportion of individuals is supported by data from humans who have nonalcoholic fatty liver and steatohepatitis, in whom approximately 10% may ultimately develop cirrhosis. Very occasionally these individuals may develop the classic picture of alcoholic hepatitis, with ballooned hepatocytes, Mallory's hyaline, and florid parenchymal neutrophil infiltration. In humans the picture of alcohol-induced fibrosis is complicated by the development of alcoholic hepatitis, which, while perhaps not always necessary for the development of fibrotic liver injury, is clearly critical in enhancing the process in the majority of human clinical cases (Fig. 19.7).

Alcohol-induced fibrosis

Probably the key event in the development of hepatic fibrosis is the transformation of vitamin A-containing hepatic stellate cells, to a myofibroblastic phenotype in which they secrete matrix proteins into the space of Disse, producing pericellular fibrosis. This process, coupled with hepatocyte cell death and the collapse of liver cell plates, gives rise eventually to the micronodular fibrotic

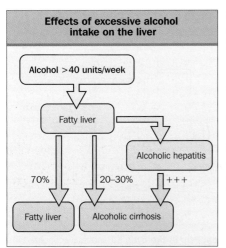

Figure 19.7 Effects of excessive alcohol intake on the liver. Excessive alcohol intake (>40 to 70 units per week) leads to fatty liver in the majority of cases; of these 20–30% will progress to the more severe lesions of alcoholic cirrhosis and alcoholic hepatitis, with the latter facilitating progression to fibrotic injury.

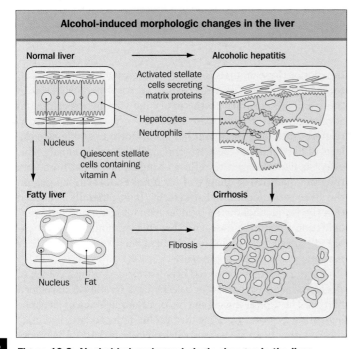

Figure 19.8 Alcohol-induced morphologic changes in the liver. Morphologic changes are associated with the progression of normal liver to fatty liver, alcoholic hepatitis and subsequently alcoholic cirrhosis.

bands that characterize alcoholic cirrhosis (Fig. 19.8).

There is a balance between matrix production by myofibroblasts and matrix degradation by macrophage and stellate cell-derived metalloproteinases, and this balance of matrix production and degradation may also be important in determining overall levels of fibrosis. The link between excess alcohol intake and stellate cell activation remains unclear, and there are currently several hypotheses, none of which are mutually exclusive.

First, it has been suggested alcohol metabolism may directly activate stellate cells via acetaldehyde or oxidative stress/lipid peroxidation, although the concept remains controversial. Alternatively, alcohol metabolism may cause hepatocytes to release factors that activate stellate cells directly. Although hepatocytes can synthesize mediators of stellate cell growth or activation, for example insulin-like growth factor (IGF) or transforming growth factor (TGF)-α, there is so far relatively little evidence to support this hypothesis. A third hypothesis suggests that alcohol metabolism causes stellate cell activation via other cells, for example macrophages, neutrophils or lymphocytes. Inflammatory cells can activate stellate cells directly through cytokine release and perhaps indirectly via matrix degradation, and it is highly likely that interactions between stellate cells, resident macrophages, and inflammatory cells may result in stellate cell activation.

The mechanisms of stellate cell activation are currently the focus of intensive basic research in hepatology, and it is highly likely that these mechanisms will be detailed over the next few years, raising the exciting prospect of new therapies aimed directly at reducing matrix production or inducing matrix degradation. A number of pharmaceutical companies currently have biologically active compounds that look very promising in experimental models.

Alcoholic hepatitis

Epidemiologic data suggest that alcohol is only one of several permissive factors for the development of alcoholic cirrhosis, and twin studies would support the hypothesis that some of these factors are genetic. There is as yet, however, no explanation for the development of acute alcoholic hepatitis; in order to be at risk of developing this disease, one must have had a very high alcohol intake for a relatively long period of time. The mean alcohol intake in the largest reported study was approximately 250g/day, with a mean duration of 25 years – in other words, a staggering cumulative alcohol intake of 2.28 metric tons of alcohol or 3800 cases of rum. In some cases these patients may be perfectly well with no signs or symptoms of liver disease, until they suddenly develop jaundice. They then become deeply jaundiced over a period of a few weeks, often with ascites, encephalopathy, and acute portal hypertension. Following admission to hospital, they cease alcohol consumption, but the clinical condition continues to deteriorate over 2 or 3 weeks, and up to half will die during this hospitalization. Following an episode of severe alcoholic hepatitis (in patients without pre-existing cirrhosis), half of the survivors will have established cirrhosis on follow-up biopsy, and a small proportion have evidence of continuing inflammation in the absence of demonstrable alcohol intake.

The key pathologic features of alcoholic hepatitis, are ballooned hepatocytes with or without Mallory's hyaline, neutrophil infiltration, and pericelluar fibrosis. Mallory's hyaline is not specific to alcoholic liver disease and reflects cellular injury. Neutrophils are often clustered around hepatocytes containing Mallory's hyaline; this is termed satellitosis, and this is considered to be a very characteristic feature of alcoholic hepatitis. One explanation for this phenomenon is that Mallory's hyaline may be chemotactic for neutrophils. Another is that the neutrophils may be participating in the process of hepatocellular injury. There is now good evidence that the release of neutrophil chemotactic cytokines by hepatocytes plays a role in mediating the neutrophilic hepatitis. High tissue and circulating levels of the neutrophil chemokine interleukin (IL)-8 correlate with the intensity of parenchymal neutrophil infiltration and with mortality. In addition, infection of hepatocytes by retroviruses expressing murine neutrophil chemokines leads to a neutrophilic hepatitis with liver damage.

There is also good evidence of a general activation in the proinflammatory cascade in alcoholic hepatitis. Circulating levels of proinflammatory cytokines are elevated and correlate with mortality. Levels of the inflammatory marker and mediator of liver regeneration, IL-6, are almost as high as those found in endotoxic shock, suggesting widespread and uncontrolled levels of macrophage activation. There are potential links between alcohol metabolism, oxidant stress, and cytokine induction. The majority of the proinflammatory cytokines and chemokines, including IL-8, are controlled by redox-sensitive nuclear transcription factors. There is as yet no direct evidence that neutrophilic inflammation modulates liver damage in human alcoholic hepatitis. However, data from clinical studies have indicated that neutrophil infiltration was the only marker of corticosteroid responsiveness, and this is of interest as one of the major mechanisms of corticosteroid action is believed to be through suppression of cytokine synthesis. It is possible that the presence of neutrophils and other inflammatory cells may be an epiphenomenon, and the curiously low levels of liver enzymes found in even very severe alcoholic hepatitis suggest either that this is the case or that more complex processes are involved, for example the facilitation of hepatocyte apoptosis by interactions with inflammatory cells.

The critical question as to how these processes are initiated remains unsolved. It has been suggested that alcoholic hepatitis is an autoimmune disease, with the autoantigens being acetaldehyde-modified liver proteins. Acetaldehyde is highly reactive, may induce antigenic modifications in proteins, and circulating antibodies to these modified proteins are found in alcoholic liver disease. The development of an autoimmune process would help to explain many features of the timing of alcoholic hepatitis, and the persistence of liver inflammation in cases where alcohol intake has been assumed to have stopped. Against an autoimmune hypothesis is the fact that the morphology of inflammation in alcoholic hepatitis is very different from the classic portal tract infiltration and interface hepatitis found with classic immune-mediated liver damage in autoimmune chronic active hepatitis and chronic hepatitis B virus infection, or in other drug-mediated liver disease with a presumed autoimmune origin. The need for such prolonged and heavy alcohol intake would also be more in favor of some form of cumulative toxic process than an autoimmune etiology. Another theory results from the previously detailed animal studies. Ethanol may induce increased gut permeability to endotoxin, and it has been hypothesized that endotoxin-induced Kupffer cell activation may then induce widespread inflammation and tissue damage.

The focal necrosis seen in experimental models of fat and alcohol-induced liver injury is highly characteristic of endotoxin-induced liver injury, but these histopathologic features are not generally seen in alcoholic hepatitis.

It seems very likely that very high levels of ethanol intake may prime hepatocytes (and to some extent stellate cells) both for injury, via fat accumulation, oxidant stress, and tubular damage, and for chemokine synthesis through changes in the balance of intracellular transcriptional factors. In this condition, the liver can be likened to a loaded gun in which a further environmental trigger may then be capable of inducing local Kupffer cell activation, with release of the proinflammatory cytokine cascade, and hepatocyte chemokine production. A self-perpetuating cycle of inflammation, tissue damage and fibrosis, may then ensue and in the absence of ethanol this will initially intensify (ethanol generally has a direct suppressive action on cytokine release) before gradually subsiding. It is likely that these environmental triggers may be multifactorial, including infective, toxic, and immune factors in individuals who have different genetic backgrounds.

CLINICAL FEATURES AND DISEASE ASSOCIATIONS

The diagnosis of alcoholic liver disease may be suggested by either the presence of liver disease of uncertain etiology or the consideration of liver injury in acknowledged high alcohol consumers. A patient may present with any of the features of liver disease, in which case alcohol must always be suspected as a possible factor in the etiology. Alternatively the presence of liver disease may be suspected as a result of high alcohol intake. In either case a careful alcohol history is essential. The alcohol history should give a clear picture of the underlying drinking pattern, including the type of alcohol, the amount, where it is consumed, and features of dependence (Fig. 19.9).

The type of alcohol consumed is critically important. A patient regularly drinking two pints of cider, beer, lager or alcopop a day may be consuming anything from 28 to 85 units per week (or up to 85g/day) depending upon the strength of the drink, which may vary from 3 to 9% alcohol by volume. In patients who have drinking patterns predominantly at home, it may be more revealing to ask how many bottles of wine or spirits a patient buys each week, rather than enquire about average daily intakes.

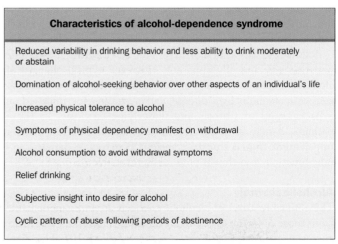

Characteristics of alcohol-dependence syndrome
Reduced variability in drinking behavior and less ability to drink moderately or abstain
Domination of alcohol-seeking behavior over other aspects of an individual's life
Increased physical tolerance to alcohol
Symptoms of physical dependency manifest on withdrawal
Alcohol consumption to avoid withdrawal symptoms
Relief drinking
Subjective insight into desire for alcohol
Cyclic pattern of abuse following periods of abstinence

Figure 19.9 Characteristics of alcohol-dependence syndrome.

The spectrum of alcoholic liver disease includes three separate pathologic diagnoses, fatty liver, alcoholic hepatitis or cirrhosis. These may coexist in any combination. It is also entirely possible for alcoholic cirrhosis to be present in the absence of any abnormal clinical or biochemical features.

Fatty liver

Fatty liver occurs in a majority of heavy drinkers and is usually asymptomatic or associated with very nonspecific features, for example fatigue, nausea or right upper quadrant discomfort. On examination hepatomegaly may be present, and liver enzymes, may be mildly elevated. Fatty liver resolves completely after several weeks of abstinence. However, it is not a completely benign disease, as in the longer term fibrosis and cirrhosis will develop in up to 10% of those continuing to consume alcohol. There is good evidence that the more severe the fatty infiltration, the higher the likelihood of progression to more significant disease (see Fig. 19.2). Very occasionally, heavy binge drinkers may present with liver failure secondary to an acute fatty liver. In this case the clinical picture is identical to that of alcoholic hepatitis except that there is no histologic evidence of hepatitis on biopsy. The degree of hepatomegaly may be massive, and the liver may occupy more than half of the abdominal cavity.

Alcoholic hepatitis

The clinical syndrome of acute alcoholic hepatitis is distinctive, with a mortality rate of up to 60% in severe cases. This very common and potentially reversible disease is often unrecognized. The 'catch all' diagnosis of alcoholic liver disease is unhelpful and misleading, and should serve only as a step towards a comprehensive classification of the underlying liver problem. Clinical alcoholic hepatitis typically occurs in a heavy drinker (40–70 or more units/week) of several years duration. Sometimes the onset of alcoholic hepatitis may be associated with a particularly heavy binge, but often there is no obvious predisposing cause. There is an acute onset of malaise and jaundice, often with nausea, anorexia, vomiting, or diarrhea. There may be florid stigmata of chronic liver disease, with spider nevi and facial telangiectasia, and the presence of ascites and encephalopathy. Disease severity is determined by the combination of the level of jaundice and the degree of coagulopathy. These parameters often deteriorate for 2–3 weeks after admission and cessation of alcohol intake, suggesting the existence of an uncontrolled cascade of inflammation within the liver. Death occurs as a result of liver failure often associated with renal failure or uncontrolled sepsis, or following variceal hemorrhage. Not all episodes of alcoholic hepatitis are clinically apparent. However, typical changes of alcoholic hepatitis are seen in the majority of patients hospitalized with alcoholic liver disease, and are often superimposed on a background of fibrosis and underlying cirrhosis. In these patients, it may be impossible to estimate the degree of liver impairment that is due to transient hepatocyte damage and inflammation, and thus is potentially reversible.

Alcoholic cirrhosis

The clinical features of alcoholic cirrhosis are indistinguishable from those of cirrhosis of other etiologies, and represent a wide spectrum of clinical presentations (see Fig. 19.10). The diagnosis of alcoholic cirrhosis rests upon the characteristic biopsy appearances of micronodular cirrhosis, in the presence of suitable evidence of excess alcohol intake (>40 units/week) over a suitably long period of time (10 or more years), having excluded other causes of chronic liver disease. The clinical features of alcoholic cirrhosis are variable, and may resolve to a surprising degree with prolonged abstinence, even in advanced cases. However, as with other causes of cirrhosis, an irreversible decline in liver function may continue despite the absence of continued alcohol consumption.

Extrahepatic manifestations
Cardiovascular

A number of cross-sectional studies have shown that with a reported average alcohol consumption of 3 or 4 units per day, there are very slight increases in both systolic and diastolic blood pressure, suggesting a dose relationship between mild hypertension and alcohol consumption. The mechanisms are unclear, but are thought to lead to a slight increase in the incidence of cerebrovascular events (strokes) in people who have moderate alcohol intake in the order of 3–6 units per day. In contrast, with the establishment of significant liver injury and cirrhosis a hyperdynamic circulation can develop with relatively low blood pressure, tachycardia, low peripheral resistance, and increased chronic output.

It has been known for some time that chronic excessive alcohol consumption can lead to congestive cardiomyopathy. While initially this was attributed to nutritional deficiencies, the prevailing opinion now is that excessive alcohol intake over a period of many years can lead to the development of an alcoholic cardiomyopathy, with evidence of right and left ventricular failure. The clinical onset is usually insidious and laboratory and electrocardiogram findings are no different to those of the congestive

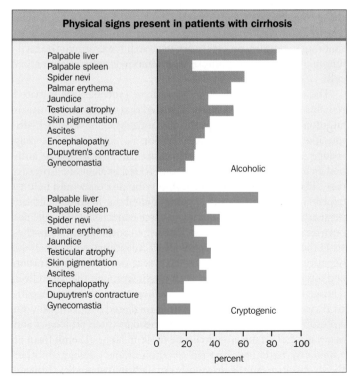

Figure 19.10 Physical signs at presentation in patients with alcoholic and cryptogenic cirrhosis. Adapted from Powell et al. Med Australia. 1971;945.

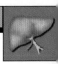

cardiomyopathy of other etiologies. The diagnosis is predominantly that of exclusion. Cardiomyopathy is associated with depressed cardiac output, elevated left and right ventricular filling pressures, and decreased ventricular contractivity. A variety of conduction abnormalities can occur with bundle branch blocks, atrioventricular blocks, and ventricular arrhythmias which can in some cases lead to sudden death.

Skeletal muscle disease

A particularly heavy bout of drinking in association with chronic alcohol intake can lead to acute muscle damage varying from mild transient elevations of muscle enzymes to rhabdomyolysis with myoglobinuria. In the latter case a sudden onset of muscle pain, edema, and weakness associated with elevations of serum creatinine kinase and myoglobinuria may occur, last for several days, and resolve over a period ranging from days or weeks after cessation of alcohol consumption. In addition to an acute alcoholic myopathy, chronic alcohol intake can lead to progressive painless wasting and weakness, particularly of proximal muscle groups in the legs and this is often associated with a coexisting peripheral neuropathy. Histopathology reveals type II muscle fiber atrophy. The etiology of either form of myopathy is currently unknown.

Pulmonary disease

Hypoxia is not unusual in cirrhosis of any etiology and the pathogenesis of this is often unclear. However, in many cases with normal clinical and radiologic examinations, hypoxia is probably related to a ventilatory perfusion mismatch with intrapulmonary arteriovenous shunting. Pulmonary hypertension is a complication in approximately 2% of patients who have severe portal hypertension, and it is an important complication to recognize in the context of liver transplantation.

Nervous system

Both acute and chronic excessive alcohol intake have profound effects on the nervous system. In addition, nutritional deficiencies result in a variety of specific syndromes of liver system damage.

Chronic alcohol abuse is associated with cortical atrophy, usually documented by computed tomography (CT) scan, and the incidence of dementia is higher than in the nonalcoholic population. Wernicke–Korsakoff syndrome caused by thiamine deficiency is characterized by oculomotor disturbance (nystagmus, Gay's palsy or ophthalmoplegia), cerebellar ataxia affecting the trunk and lower extremities, and mental confusion sometimes leading to stupor or coma. This can lead to Korsakoff's psychosis characterized by antegrade and retrograde amnesia. Features of both Wernicke encephalopathy and Korsakoff's psychosis are potentially reversible by treatment with intravenous thiamine, but in the case of Korsakoff's psychosis, the recovery may be incomplete in up to 50% of cases. Chronic alcohol intake can be associated with cerebellar degeneration characterized by gait and truncal ataxia evolving over a period of many years. Central pontine myelinolysis is a rare complication, often related to acute changes in serum sodium concentrations in the context of chronic liver disease. The clinical features include progressive quadriparesis, pseudobulbar palsy, and partial ophthalmoplegia, but frequently the diagnosis is made at autopsy. The Marchiafava–Bignani syndrome occurs almost exclusively in chronic alcoholics and is characterized by demyelination of the corpus callosum, with associated frontal and hemispheric damage.

Peripheral neuropathy associated with malnutrition is seen in the context of chronic excessive alcohol intake. It usually takes the form of a progressive painful distal sensory neuropathy affecting the legs associated with pain, paresthesia, and weakness. Treatment consists of correction of nutritional deficiencies, particularly those of vitamin B complex, and abstinence from alcohol. Recovery occurs over many months, but may be incomplete.

Acute alcohol withdrawal syndrome

The acute alcohol withdrawal syndrome begins with tremor as the most common symptom, and this can occur within a few hours of stopping drinking after a period of prolonged alcohol dependence. Associated symptoms include nausea, sweating, irritability, and alcohol craving 24–48 hours after cessation of alcohol intake. Transient auditory or visional hallucinations may occur in up to 25% of patients and these resolve over 2–3 days. Treatment of the acute alcohol withdrawal syndrome is with benzodiazapines, and the use of chlormethiazole in this syndrome is no longer considered justifiable.

Endocrine abnormalities

Endocrine abnormalities are not uncommon in alcoholic liver disease and occur both as a consequence of excessive and prolonged alcohol ingestion and the development of liver disease. Alcohol may induce gonadal dysfunction with hypoandrogenization, decreased libido, and impotence, possibly as a direct effect on testicular function. Alcoholics may also have low plasma gonadal hormone levels and hyper estrogenization with associated cutaneous vascular changes and gynecomastia. In the latter situation total estradiol concentrations are usually normal. Chronic alcoholics may develop a pseudo-Cushing's syndrome, in which the clinical features are typical of those of Cushing's syndrome with moonface, muscle wasting, abdominal stria, weight gain, fatigue, bruising, and hypertension. The syndrome is indistinguishable from true Cushing's syndrome on biochemical testing. Diagnosis is made on the basis of the reversal of symptoms with abstinence and appears to be due to a direct affect of alcohol stimulating adrenocortocotropic hormone (ACTH) secretion. Hypoglycemia may occur in alcoholics, usually after a period of prolonged fasting in malnourished individuals, and glucose levels should be checked in all patients who have hepatic encephalopathy, stupor, or coma. Alcoholic ketoacidosis may occur as a complication of the acute withdrawal syndrome, and is associated with a moderate metabolic acidosis, and elevated serum ketones and serum lactate levels.

Biochemical complications

Moderate alcohol intake is associated with an increase in serum triglyceride levels, and heavy alcohol abuse may be associated with grossly elevated levels caused by increased concentrations of very-low-density lipoproteins. These changes probably occur as a direct result of alcohol metabolism. Hyperuricemia is common in alcohol abuse, and this is thought to be both a direct result of alcohol metabolism and the indirect effect of lactic acidemia.

Gastrointestinal tract

Acute and chronic alcoholic intake produce both mucosal and motor dysfunction in the gastrointestinal tract. Esophagitis and

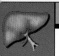
Clinical and biochemical data in asymptomatic alcoholics				
Histologic groups	No. of patients	No. with liver enlargement	No. with one or more biochemical abnormality	No. with no clinical or biochemical changes
Normal liver	38	3	5	30
Alcoholic hepatitis	11	5	6	2
Cirrhosis	9	5	6	2
Chronic hepatitis	12	3	7	5
Fatty liver	50	11	25	21
Hemosiderosis	21	3	2	18
Portal fibrosis	10	1	4	7
Other changes	3	1	3	0
Total	154	32	58	85

Figure 19.11 Clinical and biochemical data in 154 asymptomatic alcoholics admitted to an acute detoxification clinic. Data from Bruguera et al. Arch Pathol Lab Med. 1977;101:647.

gastritis are common features of both acute and chronic excessive alcohol intake, although chronic alcoholics do not have a higher incidence of peptic ulceration. Motor abnormalities include a reduction in lower esophageal sphincter pressure and decreased esophageal peristalsis. These changes may be associated with a peripheral neuropathy in chronic alcoholism. Alterations in small intestinal function also occur with mucosal changes to duodenal and jejunal villi, and these may lead to a mild degree of malabsorption.

Pancreatic disease

Chronic alcohol intake is an important cause of chronic pancreatitis, through mechanisms that are currently unknown. The clinical course may consist of attacks of acute pancreatitis occurring against the background of chronic pancreatitis, and these attacks are often precipitated by acute alcohol abuse. Repeated attacks lead to a chronic calcific pancreatitis associated with chronic abdominal pain and exocrine pancreatic failure.

DIAGNOSIS

Laboratory

Biochemical tests may raise the suspicion of underlying alcoholic liver disease, but it is not possible to grade the severity, or indeed exclude the presence of liver disease biochemically (Fig. 19.11). Levels of aspartate transaminase (AST) may be moderately elevated in all forms of alcoholic liver disease, but are usually only in the range of 2–5 times normal even in severe alcoholic hepatitis (Fig. 19.12).

Alanine transaminase (ALT) levels are usually lower, in contrast to chronic viral or autoimmune hepatitis, and may be normal or 2–3 times elevated in severe alcoholic hepatitis, a surprising finding in view of the degree of neutrophilic inflammation and fibrosis often seen in these cases. The presence of high transaminase levels in alcoholic liver disease should raise the possibility of an alternative diagnosis.

Levels of alkaline phosphatase (ALP) are often normal or minimally elevated in alcoholic fatty liver, and may be moderately elevated (2–4 times normal) in alcoholic hepatitis and decompensated cirrhosis. In contrast, levels of γ-glutamyl transferase (γ-

GT) are commonly elevated in heavy drinkers, irrespective of the presence of liver disease. This enzyme is induced by ethanol, and a number of other drugs including, for example, phenytoin, and levels may return to normal within a few weeks of abstinence. The presence of high levels of γ-GT are not a helpful predictor of the presence of significant liver disease. An elevation in bilirubin in the absence of duct obstruction is suggestive of either alcoholic hepatitis or more advanced liver disease. The combination of a high bilirubin and an increase in prothrombin time is the best marker of disease severity in alcoholic hepatitis and is predictive of mortality. The cumbersome but widely used discriminant function (DF) analysis [4.6 × prolongation in prothrombin time (seconds) + bilirubin (μmol/L)/17], is helpful in assessing the severity of liver disease (severe disease has a DF of 32 or more), but does not differentiate between patients who have reversible (alcoholic hepatitis) and end-stage liver damage. Repeated episodes of alcoholic hepatitis, or encephalopathy or

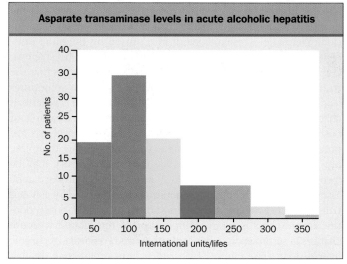

Figure 19.12 Aspartate transaminase levels in 90 patients admitted with acute alcoholic hepatitis. Note the relatively low levels of AST in this disease.

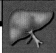

ascites are more suggestive of the latter, but a liver biopsy is required to assess the degree of inflammation and fatty change.

Of the other biochemical tests, a low serum sodium is often suggestive of severe underlying cirrhosis. Patients who have severe alcoholic hepatitis are highly likely to develop the hepatorenal syndrome. In these cases the degree of liver failure may prevent significant increases in urea levels, and serum creatinine estimations should be used routinely to monitor for renal dysfunction. Alcoholic hepatitis is usually associated with an elevated peripheral neutrophil count. An elevated neutrophil count should always provoke a search for sepsis, but even in the presence of very high counts there may be no evidence of bacterial or fungal infection and the neutrophil count remains unaltered by antimicrobial therapy. This reflects the intense neutrophilic hepatitis pathognomonic of this condition. Serum immunoglobulin (Ig)A levels are frequently elevated in patients who have acute alcoholic hepatitis, and the levels do not necessarily fall following withdrawal from alcohol. Ferritin is an acute phase protein and may be markedly elevated in acute alcoholic hepatitis, with levels falling over several months following cessation of alcohol consumption. However, hemochromatosis is not an uncommon disease and all patients who have elevated ferritins should be carefully evaluated with repeat testing, followed by iron studies, genotyping, or liver biopsy where appropriate. Macrocytosis is a feature of heavy alcohol intake, seen in 60–80% of heavy drinkers, irrespective of the degree of underlying liver disease or concomitant vitamin B_{12} or folate deficiency. A number of other biochemical tests have been proposed to detect covert alcohol intake, the most specific of these being carbohydrate deficient transferrin (Fig. 19.13), but none of these tests is a substitute for a careful and detailed alcohol history.

Radiology

Abdominal ultrasound is a helpful first step in the evaluation of patients who have suspected liver disease and is mandatory in the presence of clinical evidence of disease. Ultrasound serves to exclude partially the present of extrahepatic duct obstruction, and is a relatively sensitive (94%) but less specific (84%) guide to the presence of fatty liver. The presence of a small irregular liver on ultrasound is diagnostic of advanced cirrhosis. Similarly, features of portal hypertension, splenomegaly or varices may be

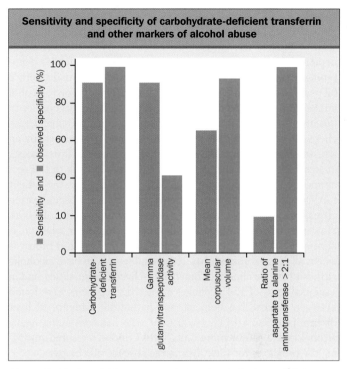

Figure 19.13 Sensitivity and specificity of carbohydrate-deficient transferrin and other markers of alcohol abuse. Data from Bird et al. Br J Addict. 1991;86:697.

evident, but otherwise ultrasound is a very poor guide to the presence of parenchymal disease and fibrosis. Doppler ultrasound may be used to assess the patency of the portal vein. Portal vein occlusion is not uncommon in advanced cirrhosis and may be a cause of explained deterioration in liver function or ascites. Both ultrasound and CT scanning are helpful in the diagnosis of primary hepatocellular carcinoma, which may eventually supervene in 5–15% of patients who have alcoholic cirrhosis. Computed tomography scanning will also confirm the presence of fatty infiltration, but other than for the investigation of focal lesions (Fig. 19.14) it may not have a major role in the diagnosis of alcoholic liver disease. Similarly, magnetic resonance imaging may be helpful in isolated cases.

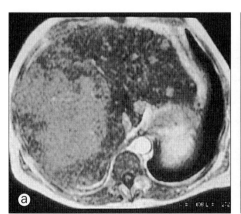
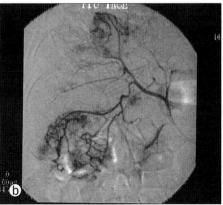
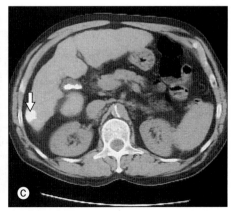

Figure 19.14 Hepatocellular carcinoma superimposed on alcoholic cirrhosis imaged by three different mechanisms. (a) Magnetic resonance image showing the diffuse multifocal hepatocellular carcinoma post-contrast with resovist. (b) Digital subtraction angiography of a multifocal hepatocellular carcinoma. (c) Hepatocellular carcinoma shown on CT scan after angiography, showing lipiodol concentrated in the hepatocellular carcinoma in the left lobe (arrow).

Histology

Older studies found that around 10–20% of liver disease in heavy alcohol abusers was unrelated to alcohol. With the advent of hepatitis C serology, and more recently hemochromatosis genotyping, many of the alternative diagnoses can be made before biopsy. However, in the presence of a history of heavy alcohol intake for a prolonged duration, it is not possible to diagnose or to quantify the degree of alcohol-induced liver injury on clinical, biochemical, or radiologic criteria. This can only be achieved by an assessment of liver histology. In the absence of clinical liver disease, in a patient who is capable of reducing alcohol intake to the recommended levels it may not be necessary to investigate the patient further with a liver biopsy. A liver biopsy requires hospitalization at least as a day-case, and has a mortality of around 1:10,000. However, where continued alcohol intake occurs, or where it is necessary to investigate the etiology of liver disease, liver biopsy is essential. It is estimated that 10% of subjects who have alcoholic cirrhosis have no clinical or biochemical liver abnormalities, and in a seminal study of 154 alcoholics marked discrepancies were found between clinical, biochemical, and pathologic evidence of liver disease (see Fig. 19.11). No patient who has continuing heavy alcohol intake (40 or more units/week) can be reassured regarding the prognosis for their liver in the absence of a biopsy.

Fatty liver occurs within days of alcohol binge and resolves over weeks. The hepatocytes are distended by lipid droplets, usually a single droplet per cell, with little inflammatory infiltrate. The distribution of the fat is predominantly perivenular, extending across the acinus with increasing severity. Occasional lipogranulomata may be seen, and rarely a microvesicular pattern of steatosis is observed.

The cardinal features of alcoholic hepatitis include balloon dilatation, Mallory's bodies, and neutrophil infiltration of the parenchyma. The ballooning degeneration or necrosis is often seen with aggregates of eosinophilic intermediate filament proteins within hepatocytes termed Mallory's hyaline (Fig. 19.15).

The cytoplasm of ballooned hepatocytes often appears wispy and cobweb like (Fig. 19.16). Cells contain excess fluid and protein, probably as a result of disturbed microtubular function. Patchy parenchymal inflammation occurs comprising predominantly neutrophils, with smaller numbers of macrophages and lymphocytes – the typical neutrophilic hepatitis characteristic of alcohol-induced liver inflammation. Neutrophils may be seen to cluster around individual hepatocytes termed 'satellitosis'. Fibrosis with a characteristic pericellular or 'chicken wire' distribution is often present. Within the acinus more pronounced fibrosis may be found in a perivenular distribution, and the presence of this lesion is associated with an increased risk of progression to cirrhosis.

The typical appearances of both fatty liver and of mild alcoholic hepatitis may be seen in the absence of alcohol intake. This is the lesion of steatohepatitis, and may occur in association with poorly controlled diabetes, obesity, rapid weight loss, a drug reaction (e.g. to amiodarone), or as a cryptogenic finding. It is not entirely a benign lesion and around 10% of cases will progress to cirrhosis over 5 years.

Alcoholic cirrhosis is the end of the spectrum of alcoholic liver disease in which bands of fibrosis link central veins, forming spheric micronodules around 2–4mm in diameter. This is called micronodular cirrhosis (Figs 19.17, 19.18 & 19.19). Bands of fibrosis are thought to be a result of both hepatocyte loss and

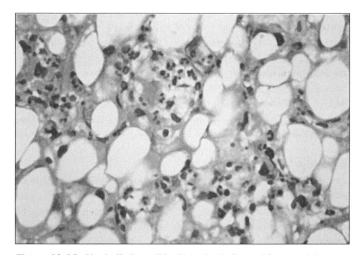

Figure 19.16 Alcoholic hepatitis. Note the ballooned fat-containing hepatocytes with pericellular infiltration by neutrophils.

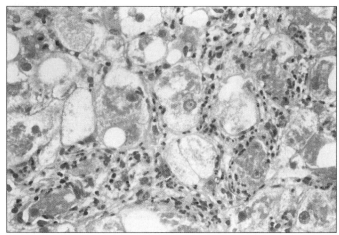

Figure 19.15 Alcoholic hepatitis. Note the swollen hepatocytes containing Mallory's hyaline, and surrounded by an infiltrate of inflammatory cells consisting of macrophages and neutrophils.

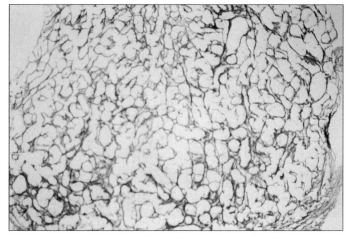

Figure 19.17 Reticulin stain of a micronodule from a patient who has alcoholic micronodular cirrhosis. Note the pericellular fibrosis in the typical chicken wire distribution pattern.

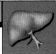

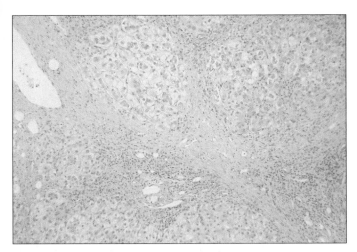

Figure 19.18 Hematoxylin and eosin stain of a liver with micronodular cirrhosis showing broad bands of fibrosis.

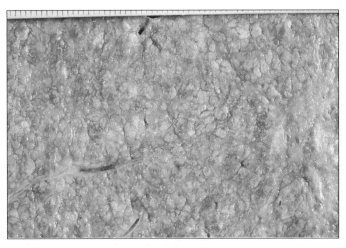

Figure 19.19 Micronodular cirrhosis. Visual appearance of micronodular cirrhosis.

collapse of intervening basement membrane and new collagen synthesis by hepatic stellate cells within the space of Disse. All the features of fatty liver and of alcoholic hepatitis may be superimposed upon a background of cirrhosis, suggesting an 'active cirrhosis' with continued liver damage, and probable continued alcohol intake. Following prolonged abstinence, cirrhosis is likely to be inactive with fibrotic bands containing mature collagen, and a tendency for larger macronodules to form.

NATURAL HISTORY AND PROGNOSIS

Fatty liver will be found in around 80% of heavy drinkers, and will resolve providing alcohol intake is reduced to safe levels. If heavy alcohol intake continues a proportion of subjects will progress to develop alcoholic hepatitis and/or cirrhosis, with some evidence that this may be related to the severity of fatty liver. In the seminal study of 258 alcoholics followed for over 10 years, 11–27% developed cirrhosis depending upon the degree of fatty change (see Figs. 19.2 & 19.20).

The outcome, following an episode of alcoholic hepatitis, is dependent upon the severity of liver injury and subsequent drinking patterns. Overall, approximately 50% of patients will develop cirrhosis over a 10-year period. Of these up to half will have developed cirrhosis within 2–3 years. However, in practice, cirrhosis will already be present in a large proportion of patients presenting with alcoholic hepatitis for the first time. The development of cirrhosis is more likely after severe (70%) compared with mild (30%) alcoholic hepatitis, and with continued heavy drinking as opposed to abstinence. The mortality rate following an episode of acute alcoholic hepatitis is also different in those who continue to consume alcohol as compared with those who moderate (Fig. 19.21), with a 1-year survival in continuing drinkers of around 85% and a 5-year survival of 60%.

Once alcoholic cirrhosis has developed, the overall survival is dependent upon two major factors: the degree of impairment of liver function and continued alcohol intake. Of these the former is the most immediate determinant of survival. In the presence of ascites, the 5-year survival rate for patients who have diagnosed alcoholic cirrhosis varies from 16 to 25%, with an overall 1-year survival rate of 40–80% (Fig. 19.22).

Continued alcohol intake has a major impact on survival with most series agreeing that complete cessation of alcohol intake reduces mortality by around 50% at 5 years, irrespective of the severity of liver damage at the time of presentation (Figs 19.23).

The presence of hepatic encephalopathy is a very poor prognostic sign with a 1-year survival rate of around 20%, and a zero 5-year survival rate in the absence of transplantation (see Fig. 19.22).

The situation regarding prognosis following an episode of variceal hemorrhage is slightly more difficult to predict and 5-year survival rates in the older series varied from 0 to 60%. These data also suggested that cessation of alcohol intake had relatively little impact on these figures, and at least one more recent study supports this view. Survival following variceal hemorrhage is to some extent dependent upon the likelihood of further bleeding, which in turn is dependent upon the size of varices. There is also some evidence that the portal pressure is an independent predictor of survival in alcoholics, with cirrhosis prior to the index variceal hemorrhage. More recent data on 5-year survival following variceal hemorrhage that take into account the impact of sclerotherapy and β blockade therapy suggest a 5-year survival rate of around 40%, but again these figures are completely dependent upon the underlying level of liver dysfunction with 5-year survivals of 52, 32, and 3% in Child's grades A, B, and C, respectively.

MANAGEMENT

Outpatient management of early alcoholic liver disease
These patients comprise two groups, those who have abnormal liver function and a high alcohol intake, and those who have normal liver function despite the high alcohol intake. The management of both groups is essentially identical, with the exception that other causes of liver disease should be considered and excluded in the first group (Fig. 19.24). In each case a very careful history must establish the pattern and the underlying reasons for excessive alcohol intake, with the aim of complete cessation or reduction of alcohol intake to safe levels. In the absence of features of alcohol dependency, counseling may be all that is required. In the presence of alcohol dependency more concentrated support and input may be required, including a psychiatric assessment, or specialist alcohol counselling and referral to specialist support agencies.

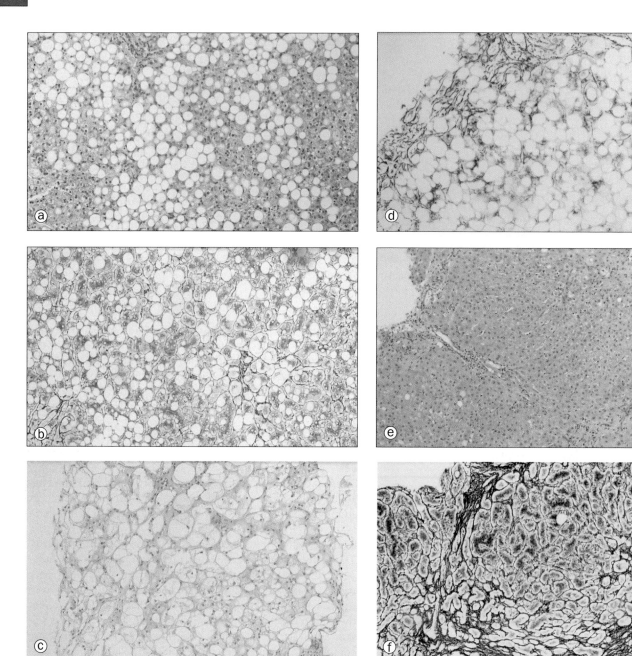

Figure 19.20 Histological liver sections showing the progress of alcoholic liver disease in a single patient over a 14 month period. The patient presented in September 1993 with unexplained jaundice, a liver biopsy revealed grade 4 fatty change and some mild pericellular and perivenular fibrosis (a) H&E section, (b) reticulin stain showing black collagen fibers. After a further biopsy in June 1994 showed the typical features of alcoholic hepatitis, it was finally discovered that the patient was secretly drinking over one bottle of spirits per day. (c) H&E section reveal- ing typical alcoholic hepatitis with fatty and ballooned hepatocytes, with Mallory's hyaline and occasional neutrophils, (d) reticulin staining shows increased fibrosis. The patient was treated with Prednisolone for one month and made a good recovery. A final biopsy was performed during the course of the investigation of a pyrexia of unknown origin (e and f) after the patient had cut their alcohol intake. It shows little fatty change remaining but severe pericellular fibrosis/micronodular cirrhosis (case courtesy of Prof M Arthur).

In the presence of severe physical dependency, admission to hospital for acute detoxification may be required, in which case the symptoms of physical withdrawal should be treated where necessary with a benzodiazepine, for example chlor-diazepoxide 10–30mg q6h, reducing over 3–6 days. Assuming that a liver biopsy is not required to exclude another diagno-sis, the patient should then be reviewed after a period of time, and providing alcohol intake is reduced, no further action is necessary. This represents the majority of cases encountered in a typical liver clinic. Patients continuing to drink high levels of alcohol should undergo liver biopsy to confirm the diagnosis and to stage the degree of alcohol-induced liver damage for prognostic purposes. The experience of a liver biopsy may help the patient to focus on the message that a level of alcohol intake in excess of 50 units/week is associated with a 20% risk of the development of liver cirrhosis over a 10-year period. In patients who continue to drink excessively despite medical advice, the liver biopsy should be repeated at intervals of around 5 years to assess progression of the disease.

Acute alcoholic hepatitis
General issues
Acute alcoholic hepatitis is a devastating disease with a hospital mortality of up to 50% in severe cases. In relatively young patients, it will occur as the first presentation of alcoholic liver disease. The apparent level of complacency and ignorance about

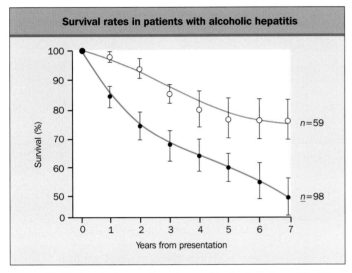

Figure 19.21 Survival rates in patients with alcoholic hepatitis. The figure shows the survival of two groups of patients: those who significantly reduced their alcohol intake (white circle), and those who continued to drink (black circle). Data from Alexander, Am J Gastroenterol. 1971;56:515.

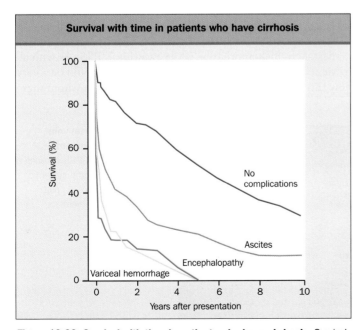

Figure 19.22 Survival with time in patients who have cirrhosis. Survival is related to clinical status at presentation as modified by subsequent alcohol consumption. Data from Saunders JB et al. Br Med J. 1981;282:265.

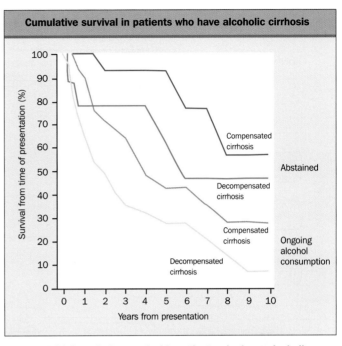

Figure 19.23 Cumulative survival in patients who have alcoholic cirrhosis according to clinical features at presentation and ongoing alcohol consumption. Data from Saunders JB et al. Br Med J. 1981;282:265.

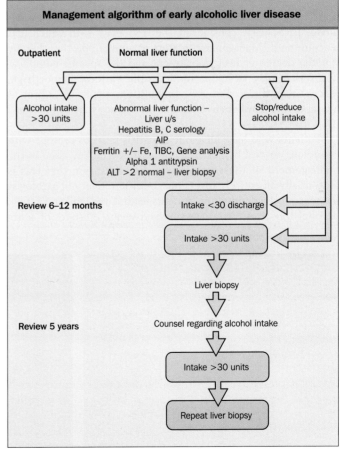

Figure 19.24 Management algorithm of early alcoholic liver disease. U/S, ultrasound; AIP, autoimmune profile; ALT, alanine transaminase; TIBC, total iron binding capacity (transferrin saturation).

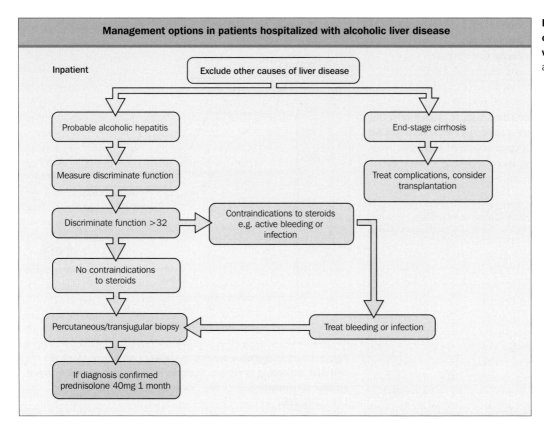

Management options in patients hospitalized with alcoholic liver disease

Inpatient

Exclude other causes of liver disease

Probable alcoholic hepatitis

End-stage cirrhosis

Measure discriminate function

Treat complications, consider transplantation

Discriminate function >32

Contraindications to steroids e.g. active bleeding or infection

No contraindications to steroids

Percutaneous/transjugular biopsy

Treat bleeding or infection

If diagnosis confirmed prednisolone 40mg 1 month

Figure 19.25 Management options in patients hospitalized with alcoholic liver disease. AH, alcoholic hepatitis.

the management of this disease is therefore difficult to comprehend, particularly considering the frequency with which it is encountered. Management centers around supportive therapy for the degree of liver impairment and the specific complications that may develop, for example variceal hemorrhage, encephalopathy, and ascites. In addition, a specific subset of patients who may benefit from specific therapy may be identified (Fig. 19.25).

Patients who have alcoholic hepatitis tend to present with jaundice, variceal hemorrhage, or ascites. The key issue in the management of these patients is the realization that this is potentially an entirely reversible condition. Every hepatologist has encountered numerous patients leading very full and active, alcohol-free lives, who have survived severe episodes of acute

alcoholic hepatitis, as well as the occasional nihilism of some nonspecialist physicians. Aspects of the general management which require particular attention in alcoholic hepatitis are given below.

Variceal hemorrhage should be treated acutely with endoscopic banding or sclerotherapy depending upon prevailing expertise, once the patient is hemodynamically stable. Increasingly, patients rebleeding following one session of endoscopic therapy are shunted, via a percutaneous transhepatic portal systemic shunt (TIPSS) (Fig. 19.26). It may be necessary to stabilize the patient using a 4-lumen Sengstaken–Blakemore tube while awaiting TIPSS. As with all patients who have variceal hemorrhage, there should be a very low threshold for electively ventilating patients in whom there

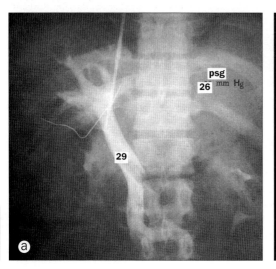
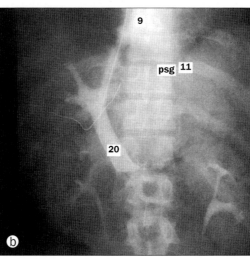

Figure 19.26 Portal vein pressure measurements. (a) Pre- and (b) post-TIPSS showing a reduction in the portal systemic gradient from 26 to 11. psg, portal systemic gradient.

is any worry about protecting the airway during endoscopy or Sengstaken–Blakemore tube insertion. Once hemorrhage has been controlled, more specific therapy may be considered.

Jaundice is the cardinal feature of acute alcoholic hepatitis, and the level of bilirubin combined with, to a lesser extent, the degree of coagulopathy forms the basis of the DF analysis, which is predictive of mortality (see Page 19.8). Patients who have a DF <32 will generally survive. However, it should be remembered that patients usually deteriorate for up to a further 2–3 weeks following cessation of alcohol intake and thus the DF will often rise following admission. The key management issues during this time are the general support of the patient, with prompt recognition and treatment of infective and metabolic problems.

In common with patients suffering from acute liver failure, patients who have acute alcoholic hepatitis are effectively highly immunocompromised, with a very high rate of clinically significant bacterial and fungal infections. The presence of fever, elevated white cell count, or other clinical or microbiologic evidence of infection should be an indication for prompt broad-spectrum antibiotic cover. There is currently no evidence to support the use of antibacterial prophylaxis, in either alcoholic or acute liver failure. In the event that fever or white count elevation persists despite antibiotic treatment, systemic antifungal treatment with either fluconazole or amphotericin should be considered. Although infection is a very frequent and often fatal complication of alcoholic hepatitis, the disease process itself often mimics infection, with occasionally extremely high circulating neutrophil counts. These can only be safely ascribed to the disease process once infection has been comprehensively excluded.

Patients who have acute alcoholic hepatitis have a very high incidence of renal problems, including the hepatorenal syndrome. Urine output and serum creatinine levels must be monitored carefully and aggressive colloid and fluid replacement under the cover of a central line should be used. It is particularly important to avoid over-diuresis in a vain attempt to reduce ascites during the acute period. Hepatorenal syndrome is diagnosed when patients develop low urine output and rising creatinine in the presence of adequate central volumes. Urinary sodium and urea concentration may mimic those found in dehydration, although a normal or high urinary sodium does not preclude the diagnosis. Prompt recognition and treatment of impending renal failure will very often reverse the process. However, when fully established hepatorenal syndrome carries a very poor prognosis, which is entirely dependent upon that of the underlying liver disease. It should therefore be recognized that in many cases, acute alcoholic hepatitis is a reversible disease and renal support should be actively considered in those cases where a reversible lesion is suspected. Hyponatremia is also extremely common in acute alcoholic hepatitis, although the clinical suspicion is that these patients are more likely to have coexisting end-stage liver disease. On the whole, hyponatremia reflects the level of underlying liver impairment and aggressive fluid restriction is often complicated by the development of renal impairment. Hyponatremia is rarely a fatal complication of alcoholic hepatitis, but renal failure very often is and consequently the balance of clinical decisions should favor preservation of renal function rather than correction of serum sodium levels.

The development of ascites is often a feature of acute alcoholic hepatitis, and aggressive diuresis should not be attempted for the reasons outlined above. Moderate levels of ascites are best left untreated until the underlying disease process improves. If necessary severe ascites is best treated by paracentesis with colloid replacement.

Levels of encephalopathy reflect the underlying degree of liver dysfunction and may also be a useful clinical sign of an acute deterioration, for example as a result of unrecognized infection. Mild levels of encephalopathy will often respond to lactulose, but protein intake should never be restricted as patients who have acute alcoholic hepatitis are invariably catabolic, and protein restriction may paradoxically aggravate the encephalopathy. Patients who have alcoholic liver disease are very often nutritionally depleted, including vitamin, antioxidant, trace element, protein, and calorie deficiencies. Levels of malnutrition have been identified as a prognostic factor in alcoholic hepatitis, and there are theoretic reasons and experimental evidence suggesting that antioxidant deficiencies in particular may exacerbate the disease process. Patients should undergo a formal nutritional assessment and adequate nutrition is a key element of therapy. In the event that adequate intake cannot be ensured using a normal diet together with nutritional supplements, nasogastric (NG) tubes should be inserted to facilitate nutrition at an early stage. It is very rarely necessary to use parenteral access in these patients, and fine-bore NG tubes have been shown to be safe despite the occurrence of recent variceal hemorrhage.

Specific drug therapy

Prednisolone therapy for alcoholic hepatitis has been the subject of a number of randomized clinical trials since 1971 (Fig. 19.27), and these trials have in turn been subjected to five separate meta-analyses. The majority of the clinical trials have found no overall benefit from corticosteroid treatment, whereas the majority of the meta-analyses have found a slight benefit of corticosteroid therapy. The major problem with the meta-analyses has been the lumping together of heterogenous trial protocols. This includes the most recent and currently widely quoted meta-analysis, which found no benefit for corticosteroids. In that meta-analysis, the second highest statistical weight was accorded to a trial of 3 days of corticosteroid therapy, whereas the majority of protocols used at least 1 month of therapy, and this supports the maxim regarding 'lies, damned lies, and meta-analyses'. There are however three well-performed and conflicting clinical trials that enable one to construct a rational basis for therapy in this condition. The largest trial published to date compared placebo ($n=88$), oxandrolone ($n=85$), and prednisolone ($n=90$), and the mortality in each of these groups was identical at all time points. The exact entry criteria for this trial were not clearly defined, and relied on the clinical diagnosis of alcoholic hepatitis. The trial would thus have included a proportion of patients who had irreversible end-stage alcoholic liver disease as opposed to alcoholic hepatitis. The clear message from this large study is that on the basis of a purely clinical diagnosis of possible alcoholic hepatitis, corticosteroid therapy cannot be justified.

There has been only one randomized clinical trial in which all patients had a pathologic diagnosis of alcoholic hepatitis histologically proven in all cases, using transjugular biopsy where necessary, and this has been the subject of two reports. The second included an open-treatment prednisolone group ($n=61$), in addition to the placebo ($n=29$) and randomized prednisolone ($n=32$) groups. The overall survival at 6 months in the two treated groups was 73% and 84%, compared with 41% in the placebo group

Prednisolone therapy compared to placebo therapy							
Prednisolone			Placebo				
Died	Total	%	Died	Total	%	p	
1	20	5.0	6	17	35.3	<0.01	
6	11	54.5	7	9	77.8	ns	
7	20	35.0	9	25	36.0	ns	
6	12	50.0	5	16	31.3	ns	
2	7	28.6	2	7	28.6	<0.01	
6	12	50.0	7	15	46.7	ns	
1	24	4.2	6	31	19.4	ns	
7	15	53.3	7	13	53.8	ns	
17	27	63.0	16	28	57.1	ns	
22	94	23.4	25	93	26.9	ns	
2	35	5.7	11	31	35.5	0.006	
4	32	12.5	16	29	55.2	0.001	
Total 82	309	26.5	117	314	37.3		

Figure 19.27 Cumulative results of 12 clinical trials in which therapy with prednisolone was compared with placebo therapy. ns, not significant.

($p=0.02$). However, by 2 years the mortality in all three groups was identical. Thus, prednisolone was clearly associated with a short-term improvement in mortality in patients who had histologically proven alcoholic hepatitis. In view of the overall lack of effect when all comers are treated, these results also suggest that prednisolone may have increased mortality in patients who had irreversible end-stage liver disease in previous trials. The only feature predictive of a treatment response in this trail was the level of neutrophil infiltration in the biopsy. In conclusion, steroids effectively reduce mortality in the subset of patients who have biopsy-proven alcoholic hepatitis. These patients should be managed in centers where transjugular biopsy and appropriate therapy can be used.

Absolute contraindications to corticosteroid therapy include uncontrolled infection and uncontrolled variceal hemorrhage. Relative contraindications include a subacute course suggestive of end-stage disease, or repeated admissions with alcohol-related problems which would preclude consideration for transplantation in due course.

Many other treatments have undergone controlled trials in alcoholic hepatitis and cirrhosis. These include anabolic steroids, colchicine, propylthiouracil, cyanidanol, silymarin, thioctic acid, polyunsaturated phosphatidyl choline, and malotilate. There is no good evidence that any of these treatments are effective. A number of promising approaches are currently the subject of clinical trials. Pentoxifyllene is a drug that has been used in the past for vascular conditions, and it is a relatively potent inhibitor of proinflammatory cytokine release, in particular TNF release from macrophages. There is good theoretic and experimental evidence to suggest that antagonism of TNF may intervene in the proinflammatory cascade thought to be involved in alcoholic hepatitis, and preliminary studies in the use of pentoxifyllene have been promising. However, larger multicenter studies are needed.

N-acetyl cysteine (NAC) has been shown to be of benefit to survival in acute liver failure, in addition to its specific use in acetaminophen (paracetamol)-induced liver failure. *N*-acetyl cysteine replenishes liver glutathione stores, thus restoring the oxidant balance away from oxidant stress. There is also evidence that NAC may have more direct actions on intracellular signaling. Similarly *S*-adenosylmethionine may modulate oxidant stress. Clinical trials of

both these substances are currently underway in alcoholic hepatitis. Ursodeoxycholic acid is under investigation for the treatment of cholestatic disease, predominantly primary biliary cirrhosis, and again there are some intriguing insights as to how this may have effects at an intracellular level. It is likely that future studies may explore the role of this substance in alcoholic hepatitis. Finally, our knowledge of the cytokine pathways important in the regulation of inflammation and fibrosis is increasing rapidly and it is highly likely that this knowledge will provide targets for specific antagonists. Many pharmaceutical companies are exploring these areas, but very few candidate drugs are currently available for clinical trials.

Alcoholic cirrhosis

Many patients presenting with acute alcoholic hepatitis will already have a degree of cirrhosis on liver biopsy, and the management is essentially very similar. Even in the presence of cirrhosis a substantial degree of improvement in liver function is often seen if the patient is able to cease alcohol intake. In patients who have diuretic-resistant ascites, jaundice, or encephalopathy which persists for at least 6 months into a period of complete abstinence, transplantation should be considered as a therapeutic option.

Transplantation

The issues surrounding the use of liver transplantation in alcoholic liver disease are largely ethical and psychologic. Patients transplanted who have alcoholic liver disease have an equivalent survival to those with other indications; elective transplantation in a good center is associated with a 5-year survival of 80–90%. The problem is that each year there are approximately 26,000 cirrhosis deaths in the USA, and only around 2500 livers available for transplantation. There is thus a perceived reluctance to use liver transplantation for what could be described as a self-induced disease, depending upon one's point of view about the origins of alcoholism. It is vitally important that these issues are debated by society as a whole and not just by the medical profession. In the UK all transplant centers will offer transplantation for alcohol-induced liver disease in patients who have given evidence of a clear commitment to abstinence, and in whom transplantation is clearly necessary. Evidence of the former is generally taken to include at least a 6-month period of abstinence, with no further

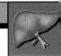

psychologic contraindications. Evidence of the latter is generally similar to the indications for transplantation in other diseases with the very important proviso that even in end-stage cirrhosis considerable clinical improvement can follow abstinence from alcohol intake.

A few centers have transplanted patients who have acute alcoholic hepatitis, often where there has been no warning of impending liver failure. Results of transplantation in this situation have so far been mixed and difficulties in the selection of these patients and the surrounding ethical issues have yet to be resolved. However, in cases where a relatively otherwise fit person, with little prior warning of impending liver failure, has severe liver (and usually renal) failure, it is most definitely worthwhile discussing the case with a transplant unit.

PRACTICE POINT

Illustrative case

A 36-year-old woman was referred to a gastroenterology clinic with abdominal pain, a week long history of jaundice, increasing tiredness, and dark urine. There was no previous history of liver disease and there were no risk factors for viral hepatitis. The stated alcohol consumption was half a bottle of wine per day. She did not smoke and there was no history of exposure to recreational drugs. She had been divorced 6 months previously and was caring for two teenage children. Since her divorce she had given up her employment as a waitress. The only medication was acetaminophen 2–4g daily for headaches. On examination she was mildly jaundiced, had few cutaneous stigmata of chronic liver disease, and had no splenomegaly or ascites.

The results of preliminary laboratory investigations performed that day included: serum bilirubin 6.6mg/dl (112μmol/L), alanine transferase 54IU/L, alkaline phosphatase 164IU/L, γ-glutamyl transferase 334IU/L, international normalized ratio (INR) 1.1, and serum creatinine 1.2mg/dl (102μmol/L). An ultrasound of the liver showed a 'bright' liver consistent with fatty infiltration. She was advised to abstain from alcohol, use nonsteroidal anti-inflammatory drugs rather than acetaminophen, and was given a review appointment in 2 weeks.

She returned on schedule but was now very tired, deeply jaundiced, had ascites, and was passing very little urine. The blood results were serum bilirubin 3.2 mg/dl (544μmol/L), alanine transferase 83IU/L, alkaline phosphatase 224IU/L, INR 1.6, serum sodium 128mmol/L, and serum creatinine 5.7mg/dl (473μmol/L). She was hospitalized and commenced on hemodialysis and prednisolone 40mg daily. Two days later she bled from esophageal varices. After stabilization of her condition she was referred to the liver transplant service. She was not considered suitable for transplantation because of her alcohol history and she died 16 days later.

Interpretation

The clinical diagnosis of alcoholic hepatitis was likely on the basis of the history of alcohol consumption, minimal elevation of the transaminases, elevated γ-glutamyl transferase, and the ultrasonic appearance of the liver. It is valid to suspect the possibility of the development of alcoholic liver disease in any individual who has an intake in excess of 40 units/week, but in this case the true alcohol intake was not admitted initially and there were circumstances in the social history that suggested she might have been drinking more heavily.

Prevention of alcoholic liver disease is practically achievable in many cases by simple intervention and advice at an early stage. This patient did stop drinking after the initial consultation, but typically the liver disease continued to deteriorate. The acetaminophen was misguidedly stopped as it is one of the safest analgesics in patients who have liver disease and the low transaminase level excluded significant hepatotoxicity. Furthermore, the nonsteroidal anti-inflammatory drug may have contributed to a deterioration in renal function.

The clinical course of alcoholic hepatitis was very typical in this patient. The presence of renal failure indicated a poor prognosis, but the decision to hemodialyse was justified on the grounds of age, first presentation, and a possible contribution from the nonsteroidal anti-inflammatory drug to the renal dysfunction. The assessment of the transplant program was typical of current practice, although some centers are considering young patients on their first presentation more favorably. This is in part due to the belief that refractory alcoholism cannot be diagnosed in these patients, and they will not live to receive treatment for their alcohol abuse patterns unless they survive the medical illness.

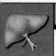

FURTHER READING

Alexander JF, Lischner MW, Galambos JT. Natural history of alcoholic hepatitis 2. The long term prognosis. Am J Gastroenterol. 1971;56:515–25. *Data on the long-term prognosis of acute alcoholic hepatitis.*

Becker U, Deis A, Sorensen TI, et al. Prediction of risk of liver disease by alcohol intake, sex, and age: a prospective population study. Hepatology. 1996;1006;23:1025–9. *Good data on risk of developing cirrhosis as a function of quantity and duration of alcohol consumption.*

Brenner DA, Chojkier M. Acetaldehyde increases collagen gene transcription in cultured human fibroblasts. J Biol Chem. 1987;262:17690–5. *A laboratory model linking alcohol with fibrosis.*

Bruguera M. Comparison of clinical, biochemical and histological findings in 154 individuals chronically abusing alcohol. Arch Pathol Lab Med. 1977;101:644. *Good clinicopathologic study.*

Christensen E, Gluud C. Glucocorticoids are ineffective in alcoholic hepatitis: a meta-analysis adjusting for confounding variables. Gut. 1995;37:113–18. *Influencial meta-analysis.*

Gines A, Escorsell A, Gines P, et al. Incidence, predictive factors, and prognosis of the hepatorenal syndrome in cirrhosis with ascites [see comments]. Gastroenterology. 1993;105:229–36. *Informative study of the hepatorenal syndrome.*

Gressner AM, Lahme B, Brenzel A. Molecular dissection of the mitogenic effect of hepatocytes on cultured hepatic stellate cells. Hepatology. 1995;22:1507–18. *Work implicating activation of stellate cells in liver disease.*

Harrison DJ, Burt AD. Pathology of alcoholic liver disease. Baillieres Clin Gastroenterol. 1993;7:641–62. *Good review of pathologic changes.*

Koskinas J, Kenna JG, Bird GL, Alexander GJ, Williams R. Immunoglobulin A antibody to a 200-kilodalton cytosolic acetaldehyde adduct in alcoholic hepatitis [see comments]. Gastroenterology. 1992;103:1860–67. *Autoimmune component in the pathogenesis of acute alcoholic hepatitis.*

Lieber C S. Aetiology and pathogenesis of alcoholic liver disease. Baillieres Clin Gastroenterol. 1993;7:581–608. *Excellent review.*

McCormick PA, Morgan MY, Phillips A, et al. The effects of alcohol use on rebleeding and mortality in patients with alcoholic cirrhosis following variceal haemorrhage. J Hepatol. 1992;14:99–103. *Recent study failing to find a benefit in survival from abstention from alcohol after variceal bleeding.*

Maher JJ, Scott MK, Saito, JM, Burton MC. Adenovirus mediated expression of cytokine induced neutrophil chemoattractant in rat liver induces a neutrophilic hepatitis. Hepatology. 1997;25:624–31. *Experimental model with interesting observations on function of neutrophils.*

Mathurin P, Duchatelle V, Ramond MJ, et al. Survival and prognostic factors in patients with severe alcoholic hepatitis treated with prednisolone. Gastroenterology. 1996;110:1847–53. *Study of major clinical interest.*

Mendenhall CL, Anderson S, Garcia-Pont P, et al. and Veterans Administration Cooperative Study on Alcoholic Hepatitis. Short-term and long term survival in patients with alcoholic hepatitis treated with oxandrolone and prednisolone. N Engl J Med. 1984;311:1464–9. *Seminal work.*

Pinto HC, Abrantes A, Esteves V, Almeida H, Correia JP. Long-term prognosis of patients with cirrhosis of the liver and upper gastrointestinal bleeding. Am J Gastroenterol. 1989;84:1239–43. *Clear data on the impact of the degree of liver dysfunction on prognosis.*

Powell EE, Cooksley, WG, Hanson R, et al. The natural history of nonalcoholic steatohepatitis: a follow-up study of forty-two patients for up to 21 years. Hepatology. 1990;11:74–80. *An interesting description of an entity that shares some histologic features with alcoholic liver disease.*

Ramond MJ, Poynard T, Rueff B, et al. A randomized trial of prednisolone in patients with severe alcoholic hepatitis. N Engl J Med. 1992;326:507–12. *Best study to date of corticosteroids.*

Sheron N, Bird G, Koskinas J. Circulating and tissue levels of the neutrophil chemotaxin interleukin-8 are elevated in severe acute alcoholic hepatitis, and tissue levels correlate with neutrophil infiltration. Hepatology. 1993;18:41–6. *Study integrating some of the pathogenetic elements of acute alcoholic hepatitis.*

Simpson KJ, Peters TJ. Animal models of alcoholic liver disease. Baillieres Clin Gastroenterol. 1993;7:609–25. *Study of correlation between alcohol consumption and fat infiltration in liver.*

Tsukamoto H, Matsuoka M, French SW. Experimental models of hepatic fibrosis: A review. Semin Liver Dis. 1990;10:56–65. *Illustrates the difficulty in establishing animal models of alcoholic liver disease.*

Vorobioff J, Groszmann RJ, Picabea E, et al. Prognostic value of hepatic venous pressure gradient measurements in alcoholic cirrhosis: a 10-year prospective study. Gastroenterology.1996:111:701–709. *A comprehensive clinical study of the importance of portal pressure.*

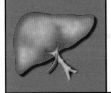

Section 3 Specific Diseases of the Liver

Chapter 20 Hemochromatosis

Martin Lombard

INTRODUCTION

Iron is essential to all biologic systems, being a cofactor of many important enzymes such as ribonucleotide reductase and having the ability to bind reversibly with oxygen as heme. It is thought that iron played an important role in the genesis and evolution of early life forms by forming iron–sulfur proteins and being incorporated into ligands such as porphyrin, which was a prerequisite for photosynthesis. The particular properties that render iron so useful in this context also account for its biologic toxicity. Thus all biologic systems have had to evolve mechanisms first to acquire iron, which is most abundant in an insoluble form, and second to limit its toxicity. The importance of iron to humans is underscored by the enormous health burden posed worldwide by iron deficiency anemia. Iron excess can also cause considerable health problems and its importance in relation to infection and carcinogenesis has also recently received much attention.

In this chapter the problem of iron excess is considered as it presents to the clinician, particularly in hepatology. Although hemochromatosis is the commonest cause of iron overload, many patients are referred with high ferritin levels or iron deposits in the liver who may not be considered to have hemochromatosis and the issues of distinction and investigation are discussed here.

Definition and terminology

Hemochromatosis is a term that denotes iron overload. The term was first used by von Recklinghausen over 100 years ago. Subsequently, 'primary' or idiopathic hemochromatosis has been distinguished from hemochromatosis secondary to other causes and some pathologists have made a distinction between hemochromatosis (a clinical syndrome of iron overload) and hemosiderosis (tissue deposition of iron). Since the 1970s when nonsecondary iron overload was found to be associated with human leukocyte antigen (HLA), the term 'hereditary hemochromatosis' has been coined; this has become 'genetic hemochromatosis' (GH). To avoid confusion, many clinicians now restrict the term hemochromatosis to this entity of GH and other iron overload syndromes are referred to in the context of their underlying disorder. Siderosis is restricted to the observation of iron deposition, usually in the liver, detected by Perl's potassium ferrocyanide stain (giving a Prussian blue reaction) and hyperferritinemia should be the preferred term when ferritin is elevated but a definitive diagnosis of iron overload is uncertain.

Historic perspective

Hemochromatosis was probably first recognized in 1865 and its association with cirrhosis and diabetes was appreciated at an early stage. By the early 20th century, familial cases were described and Sheldon suggested that it may be an inborn error of metabolism that was inherited. Controversy over whether it was in fact inherited or acquired, in particular whether it was due to alcohol, reigned until its association with the HLA complex was described in the mid-1970s, and the putative gene responsible was only recently identified in the mid-1990s.

In parallel with these developments, the pathologic sequelae of iron overload were well-documented in the first half of this century and attention turned to discerning the normal physiology of iron, its absorption, and its regulation in tissue. Treatment for hemochromatosis by venesection was attempted in the 1950s and has been established and accepted since the mid-1960s. Much has still to be learned about iron metabolism and its abnormalities and recent attention has focused on the synergistic pathologic role of iron in a number of diverse conditions such as rheumatoid disease, viral hepatitis, alcoholic liver disease, myocardial disease, cancer and even dementia (Fig. 20.1).

EPIDEMIOLOGY AND PATHOGENESIS

Prevalence and heredity

Genetic hemochromatosis (GH) is inherited in an autosomal recessive pattern. The gene responsible has a prevalence in populations of North-West European descent of approximately 10%. It has been postulated, with some circumstantial evidence, that the original mutation may have been in a Celtic population. The observed prevalence of the clinical entity of hemochromatosis has varied from 0.1 to 0.5%, depending on the criteria used for

Historic milestones in hemochromatosis		
1865	Trousseau	'Bronze diabetes'
1871	Troisier	Pigment cirrhosis
1889	von Recklinghausen	'Haemochromatose'
1927	Sheldon	Hereditary inborn error
1955	Finch and Finch	Familial cases
1957	Brick	Probably first venesection
1969	Bomford and Williams	Phlebotomy series
1975	Simon	HLA association
1985	Niederau	Survival figures
1996	Feder	Cys282Tyr mutation

Recent issues		Iron contribution to other pathology
		  Alcoholic liver disease
		  Porphyria cutanea tarda
		  Viral liver disease
		  Rheumatoid disease
		  Ischemic heart disease
		  Dementia

Figure 20.1 Historic milestones in hemochromatosis.

diagnosis (Fig. 20.2). Thus, hemochromatosis is the most common inherited potentially lethal metabolic defect in these populations. There are other iron overload conditions described in other ethnic populations that are considered later.

The gene has been identified in the past by allelic association with an HLA class I antigen, particularly type A3 (present in 70%) and by linkage disequilibrium with B7 and B14. This association, useful in the past for screening relatives of affected individuals, has recently been superseded by identification of a gene mutation that is present in approximately 90% of all series so far reported. The mutation is a single substitution of tyrosine for cysteine at position 282 of the *HFE* gene (sometimes incorrectly referred to as 'HLA-H') which is 5Mb telomeric to the HLA-A complex on chromosome six and displays some similarities to HLA gene products (Fig. 20.3). The C282Y mutation is easily detected and is now used for family screening. It is presently being assessed for population screening, although it is already clear that not all individuals homozygous for C282Y develop iron overload. A second his63asp mutation in the same gene has been described less commonly and its relevance to the pathogenesis of GH is unclear.

Pathophysiology of hemochromatosis

Iron content in the body and in specific cells is tightly regulated by iron transport and storage proteins working in concert, presumably to prevent toxicity. The average daily intake on a normal diet is 10–20mg, but there are many factors that affect the amount available for absorption (Fig. 20.4a). There is no specific excretory mechanism, although daily losses of 1mg occur through desquamation of skin and gastrointestinal epithelium,

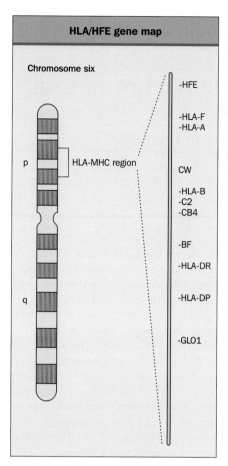

Figure 20.3 Diagram of the HLA/HFE gene map. An expanded area of the short arm of chromosome six is shown, which contains the HLA region and where the search for the GH gene has been concentrated. The HFE gene was discovered to be 5Mb telomeric to HLA-A.

Prevalence studies				
Study	Year	Population (n)	Initial criteria	Prevalence (%)
Finch and Finch. Medicine 34:381–430	1955	Hospital admissions		0.005
Mac Sween and Scott. J Clin Pathol 26:936–42	1973	Post mortem (520)	Liver Bx	0.1
Dadone, et al. Am J Clin Pathol 78:196–207	1982	Pedigree (537)	Model	0.005
Olsson, et al. Acta Med Scand 213:145–50	1983	Employees (623)	Sat >70%	0.5
Borwein, et al. Can Med J131:895–901	1984			0.3
Olsson, et al. Acta Med Scand 215:105–12	1984	Blood donors (1311) Hospital out pt. (4079) Hospital in pt. (5122)	Sat >70%	0.23 0.24 0.07
Tanner, et al. Gut 26: A1139	1985	Blood donors (1600)	Ferritin >N	0.5
Elliot, et al. Aus NZ J Med 16:491–5	1986	WW2 veterans (343)	Sat >55%	1.2
Karlsson, et al. Acta Med Scand 224:299–304	1988	General pop (22070)	Sat >70%	0.05
Edwards, et al. N Engl J Med 318:1355–62	1988	Blood donors (11065)	Sat >55%	0.45
Hallberg, et al. J Intern Med 225:249–55	1989	General pop (23355)	Sat >70%	0.073
Leggett, et al. Br J Haematol 74:525–30	1990	Employees (1968)	Sat >45%	0.36
Jonsson, et al. J Clin Epidemiol 44:1289–97	1991	General pop (2588)	Ferritin >N	0.37
Wiggers, et al. J Intern Med 230:265–70	1991	Blood donors (4302)	Sat >70%	0.37
Balan, et al. Gastorenterology 107:453–9	1994	Hospital patients (12258)	Serum iron > 180µg/dL	0.033
Smith, et al. Hepatology 25:1439–46	1997	Employees (2294)	Sat > 55%	0.25
Bell, et al. J Hepatol 26:272–9	1997	Blood donors (10552)	Ferritin > N	0.34

Figure 20.2 Prevalence studies. This table summarizes published series that attempted to find the 'true' prevalence of hemochromatosis in the population by various means. The prevalence varies with the screening parameters used, the regional location and type of population studied. The 'average' prevalence figure in these studies is 0.33%. This figure gives a prevalence of expression of 3–4 cases per 1000 population and is approximately half of the predicted homozygous frequency for the C282Y mutation in the *HFE* gene. Sat, transferrin saturation; liver Bx, liver biopsy; n, numbers studied.

and in females 30–50mg per month extra is lost by menstruation. Absorption of iron is an active process in the proximal small intestine and this is regulated by a unique negative feedback system operating at this site, resulting in 1–1.5mg per day of iron normally being absorbed (Fig. 20.4b). Absorption is controlled by body iron stores that are believed to convey information, by an as yet unknown mechanism, to intestinal cells in the crypts of Leiberkuhn, thus programming them for absorption. When the cells migrate to functional positions on the villus they take up luminal iron and transfer it according to how they have been programmed. If the body is iron replete, these cells retain iron, rather than transfer it to plasma, and the iron is lost (excreted) when the intestinal cell is shed, and vice versa.

All cells in the body, including intestinal epithelial cells, acquire transferrin-iron from plasma by receptor-mediated endocytosis (Fig. 20.4c). Iron in the cytosol is utilized by enzymes or incorporated into ferritin protein. Transferrin-receptor and ferritin are reciprocally regulated so that excess iron stimulates ferritin synthesis

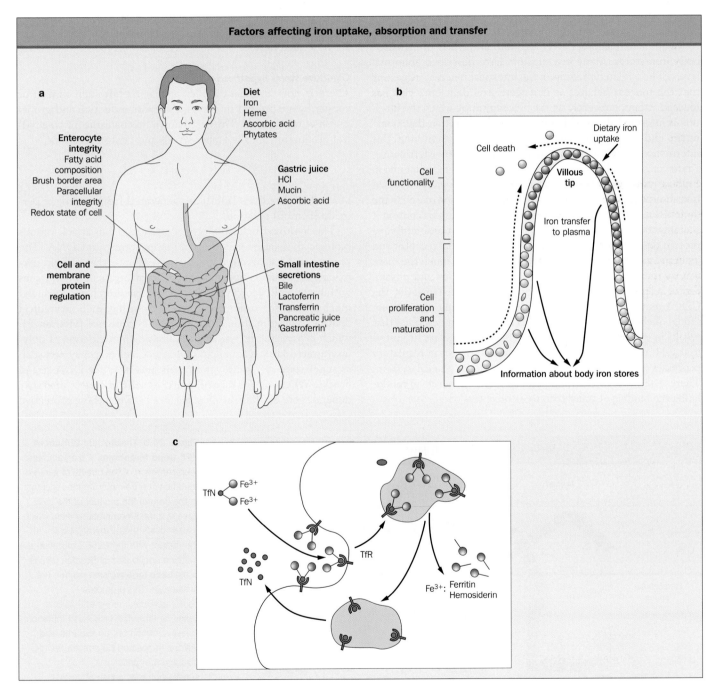

Figure 20.4 Factors affecting iron uptake, absorption and transfer. (a) Factors affecting iron uptake. There are many factors in the diet, gastric and intestinal lumina and epithelial layer that affect uptake. (b) Regulation of iron absorption. The normal life span of enterocytes from crypt to villous tip is 3–5 days. It is thought that cells are 'primed' in the crypts so that they respond to exposure with dietary iron at the villous tip in a way that is appropriate for the prevailing level of body iron. (c) Transfer of iron into a cell. Transferrin is a glycoprotein that binds and transports two ferric iron molecules. The TfR–TfN complex is internalized in an endosome, the iron removed and the apo-TfN returned to the plasma. The HFE protein (see later) may influence this process. TfN, transferrin; TfR, transferrin receptor.

and downregulates transferrin-receptor expression, thus limiting further inflow of iron. If the cell is iron deficient, transferrin-receptor is expressed and ferritin is repressed. Hemosiderin is believed to be a form of degraded ferritin. Serum ferritin level is a good indication of body iron stores.

Although the precise details of the regulatory mechanisms for iron absorption are not yet clear, in normal iron replete individuals iron absorption is limited to a low steady state to maintain an average total body iron content of 3–4g. As described above, if this limit is exceeded iron absorption is reduced; if iron deficiency is present, iron absorption is conversely increased. This regulatory process is abnormal in hemochromatosis so that iron absorption continues at an inappropriately high rate in the face of increased body iron stores. Many investigators have described abnormal levels of iron-related proteins in the intestinal mucosa, suggesting that the mucosa behaves as if it were iron deficient. This has focused attention recently on the mechanism by which the intestine is informed about body iron stores. A suggestion that transferrin and its receptor may be involved in conveying this information has gained some credence because atransferrinemia, a rare congenital disorder in humans, and hypotransferrinemia in a mouse model, are both associated with inappropriately increased iron absorption, which results in pathologic deposition of iron in the same tissue pattern as seen in hemochromatosis. In this context it is of interest to note that the *HFE* gene encodes a transmembrane protein that is known to bind β₂-microglobulin. The receptor and its ligand are internalized in an endocytic cycle in much the same way as transferrin and its receptor, but its function and physiological relevance to iron metabolism is unknown. However, the C282Y mutation prevents binding of β₂-microglobulin and a mouse model of abeta-2-microglobulinemia has also been described that results in iron overload (Fig. 20.5). Other evidence has suggested that GH may be due to a more generalized defect in regulatory processes affecting the liver or the reticuloendothelial system. There is also evidence that the HFE product has a role in modulating the binding of transferrin to its receptor.

Thus, although the precise reasons for iron loading are not yet clear, the recent identification of the *HFE* gene and its product have brought us much closer to understanding this condition. The strongest evidence points to a defective conveyance of information about body iron stores to intestinal cells in order that the regulatory mechanisms controlling iron absorption can be primed.

Mechanisms of iron toxicity

Iron is important in biologic systems because of its oxidation-reduction behavior and its ability to bind oxygen. It is also because of these same biochemical properties that iron is potentially toxic. The principal hypotheses by which iron can cause damage are described here.

Oxidative stress hypothesis

There is now abundant evidence that metals such as iron or copper, when present in excess, can cause induction and propagation of oxyradicals. The best known mechanisms for free radical production are the Haber–Weiss and Fenton reactions:

$$Fe^{++} + H_2O_2 \rightarrow Fe^{+++} + OH^\bullet + OH^-$$

i.e. hydroxyl radicals (OH⁻) are generated from hydrogen peroxide (Fenton) reaction.

The hydroxyl radical is very reactive and can attack various biologic molecules including lipids, proteins, and DNA. The process that has received greatest attention is that of lipid peroxidation, which is postulated to disrupt organelle membranes within the cell. However, all biologic systems have advanced mechanisms for minimizing and preventing such oxyradical damage. These include glutathione; α-tocopherol (vitamin E), which is particularly important in limiting peroxidation of polyunsaturated fatty acid in lipid bilayers; scavenging enzymes, such as superoxide dismutase; and repair processes for DNA strand breaks. Whether free radical injury actually occurs *in vivo* may depend more on the prevailing balance between these protective

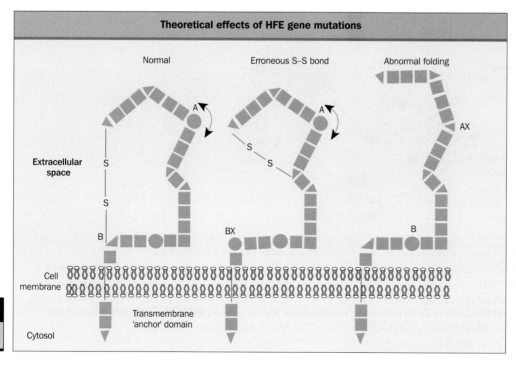

Figure 20.5 Theoretical Effects of HFE Gene Mutations. A diagrammatic representation of the effects of genetic mutations on transmembrane receptors. In the normal the product of the HFE gene is a transmembrane protein which usually binds beta-2 microglobulin. In the patient with the C282Y mutation the cysteine amino acid at position 282 is substituted for a tyrosine residue (i.e. position B). This promotes conformational change and affects ligand binding. The his63-asp mutation is less common but an aspartic acid residue at position 63 substitutes for histidine (i.e. position A). This substitution may cause abnormal folding, but its functional significance is unclear.

Theoretical effects of HFE gene mutations

Normal — Erroneous S–S bond — Abnormal folding

Extracellular space

Cell membrane

Transmembrane 'anchor' domain

Cytosol

Iron toxicity

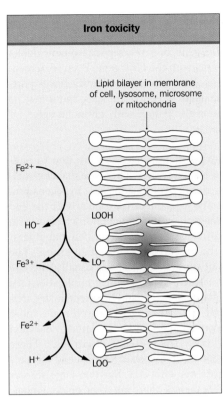

Lipid bilayer in membrane of cell, lysosome, microsome or mitochondria

Fe^{2+}

HO^-

LOOH

Fe^{3+}

LO^-

Fe^{2+}

H^+

LOO^-

Figure 20.6 Iron toxicity. Illustration of how iron plays a role in the production and propagation of free radicals to produce peroxidation in the lipid bilayer. A Fenton type reaction produces hydroxyl radicals (HO^-) which can attack polyunsaturated fatty acid in the lipid bilayer to produce a lipoyl radical, yielding conjugated dienes and lipid peroxyl (LOO^-) radicals. A chain reaction produces further peroxyl and hydroperoxide radicals (LOOH) disrupting the membrane and interfering with trans-membrane protein function.

mechanisms and the peroxidation process. There is evidence in patients with iron overload and GH that vitamins C and E and glutathione stores are depleted or deficient, and that oxyradical products are formed (Fig. 20.6).

Lysosomal fragility hypothesis

Excess accumulation of iron in lysosomes may result in increased fragility, allowing release of hydrolytic enzymes into the cytoplasm in much the same way as occurs in lysosomal storage diseases. This process and the oxyradical lipid peroxidation hypotheses are not mutually exclusive, as there is evidence that lysosomal membrane peroxidation leads to fragility and enzyme leakage. Experimental work has demonstrated that this can be induced by iron excess. It has also been observed that there are increased numbers and larger sized lysosomes in patients with iron overload. Lysosomal enzyme activity is increased in such patients and this has also been shown in at least one study to correlate with fibrosis.

Impairment of cellular function

Various studies have shown that vital enzyme activity is disturbed in the presence of iron overload, although the mechanisms remain unclear. Mitochondrial cytochrome oxidase activity is reduced, leading to impairment of oxidative metabolism and to disturbances in cellular calcium homeostasis.

DNA damage and mutagenesis

The observation that significant numbers of patients with established cirrhosis due to hemochromatosis develop hepatocellular carcinoma has stimulated interest in mechanisms of DNA damage. Several investigators have demonstrated DNA strand breaks in cell and animal models of iron overload induced by oxidative damage.

Fibrogenesis

The development of fibrosis has been regarded as a secondary effect of peroxidation tissue damage. Indeed there is experimental evidence that collagen gene transcription can be increased by artificially driven peroxidation with iron. However, this is not a straightforward process as it is difficult to induce fibrosis in animal models of iron overload, and other factors may be necessary. There is some evidence of a direct fibrogenic effect of iron, by increasing hepatic hydroxyproline content and prolyl hydroxylase activity.

CLINICAL FEATURES AND DISEASE ASSOCIATIONS

The classic presentation of hemochromatosis in a middle-aged man, pigmented with diabetes and hepatomegaly or possible cirrhosis, is now unusual, but still occurs. Occasional patients present

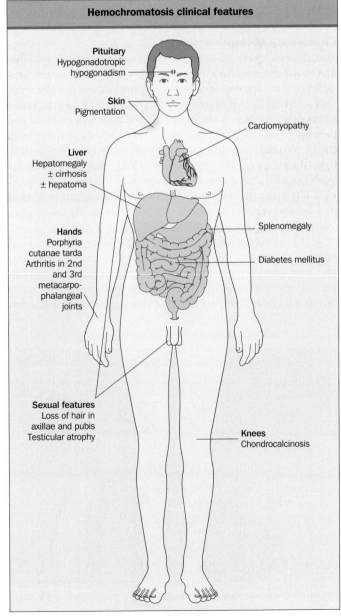

Hemochromatosis clinical features

Pituitary
Hypogonadotropic hypogonadism

Skin
Pigmentation

Cardiomyopathy

Liver
Hepatomegaly
± cirrhosis
± hepatoma

Hands
Porphyria cutanae tarda
Arthritis in 2nd and 3rd metacarpo-phalangeal joints

Splenomegaly

Diabetes mellitus

Sexual features
Loss of hair in axillae and pubis
Testicular atrophy

Knees
Chondrocalcinosis

Figure 20.7 Hemochromatosis clinical features.

with arthritis or sexual dysfunction and the alert clinician follows a line of investigation leading to a diagnosis of hemochromatosis. More frequently, abnormal liver enzymes or serum ferritin are detected on routine automated screening and patients are referred for further investigation in the 'preclinical' phase. This latter mode of presentation often produces difficulty in reaching a definitive diagnosis, as hyperferritinemia is not uncommon in other chronic inflammatory or metabolic conditions.

There are no diagnostic features that can be said to be specific for a diagnosis of hemochromatosis unless they occur in the context of a syndrome such as cirrhosis in association with diabetes mellitus, pigmentation, hypogonadotropic hypogonadism and metacarpo-phalangeal arthritis (Fig 20.7). Various clinical features may be present as outlined. In several large series, up to 50% of males and 25% of females have end-organ damage at the time of presentation.

In established hemochromatosis, pigmentation (Fig. 20.8) and hepatomegaly are common, and the other features are variable. Jaundice is most unusual and the presence of ascites or jaundice is indicative of other disease or complications such as hepatoma or hepatic failure.

Clinical and pathologic correlates

Hepatic iron stores are normally cumulative with time, possibly due to a slight imbalance in favor of absorption over losses. This difference is exaggerated in hemochromatosis, but it is apparent that a threshold level of iron (5mg/g wet weight liver), 10 times greater than normal, is associated with fibrosis and cirrhosis and presumably damage in other organs. This age effect is the basis for the hepatic iron index (μmol/L iron per gram dry weight liver divided by age in years; normal <1.9), which can be useful to distinguish hemochromatosis from other causes of iron overload. Concomitant hepatic injury due to viral hepatitis or alcohol may be exacerbated by higher levels of iron, as discussed elsewhere in this chapter (page 20.7).

It has been generally assumed that the later presentation of female patients is due to a protective effect of menstrual blood loss. However, a small subgroup of patients may present at a much earlier age with reproductive (hypogonadotropic) problems or cardiomyopathy, and this subgroup appears to have an equal sex

incidence and higher levels of iron at presentation. It is not yet clear whether these patients represent a genetic subgroup with a different mutation in the *HFE* gene, or have a separate genetic defect perhaps operating in synergy with the *HFE* gene. Even so, screening studies in healthy populations seem to identify fewer postmenopausal females than males of equivalent ages, and it may be that rates of iron absorption also reduce with advancing age.

Complications

The principle complications of iron overload are due to end-organ damage in the iron-loaded tissues. These are diabetes mellitus (iron overload in pancreas); hypogonadotropic hypogonadism (iron overload in the pituitary); arthritis (particularly of the 2nd and 3rd metacarpo-phalangeal joints); and chondrocalcinosis (in the knees). Cardiomyopathy has also been described, but at least in some cases this may be exacerbated by alcohol excess. The symptoms and severity of these complications usually improve following phlebotomy treatment. The hepatic complications are those of cirrhosis (see Chapters 4–10), and hepatocellular carcinoma (HCC). As with HCC in other liver diseases, males more frequently develop this complication, and it is related to duration and degree of iron overload in the presence of cirrhosis. There have been preliminary reports of increased incidence of colorectal and lung cancer in patients with GH, but two large studies failed to confirm this. Nonetheless, there are some epidemiologic data to suggest that these cancers may be associated with increased exposure to dietary or environmental iron.

Disordered iron metabolism in other conditions
'Non-HLA' iron overload

Genetic (HLA-linked) hemochromatosis appears to be confined to Caucasian ethnic groups. Iron overload of dietary origin has been well-described in black Africans particularly among the Bantu (Bantu siderosis). It has been thought that this is due to increased amounts of bioavailable iron in a traditional beverage fermented in steel drums. However, recent studies have found that even in communities where no such tradition exists, iron overload can occur. In addition, in parts of Asia an iron loading condition causing arthropathy, Kashin–Beck disease, has been recognized for many years and is confined to Asian groups. A small Melanese population with iron overload has also been described. None of these conditions is associated with HLA and the relative contributions of other genetic factors or environmental factors such as hepatitis B and C remain uncertain.

Perinatal hemochromatosis not due to atransferrininemia has also been recognized. This condition is almost invariably fatal and is not known to be HLA-associated. It is unclear whether it represents a more severe dysfunction of the *HFE* gene product or is due to an entirely different genetic defect.

A French group of investigators has recently suggested that a homogenous entity of iron overload with normal transferrin saturation occurs in association with insulin resistance and hyperlipidemia. These associations have been observed frequently as described below, but an explanation remains elusive.

Hyperlipidemia and coronary heart disease

Serum ferritin is increased in many patients with ischemic heart disease. Studies, particularly in Finland, have indicated a strong correlation and it has even been suggested that serum ferritin is a better predictor of coronary artery disease than serum choles-

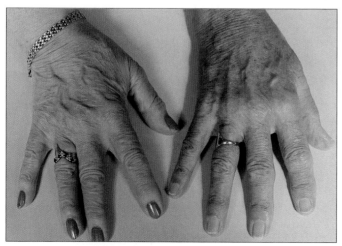

Figure 20.8 Classic hemochromatosis. Brown discoloration of the skin in an elderly male presenting with classic hemochromatosis (diabetes with cirrhosis and pigmentation). His wife's skin is shown for comparison (left).

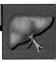

terol. This and other evidence has been used to generate an intriguing hypothesis that iron may play a central role in ischemic heart disease. However, this appears to be no more common in patients with GH or their relatives than other populations, and the hyperferritinemia is likely to reflect metabolic derangement or oxidant stress rather than iron storage level.

For the clinician, the importance of this observation is that it will produce problems in interpreting screening results in a general population.

Steatosis

Many patients referred with hyperferritinemia and mild abnormalities of liver enzymes are found to have fatty liver or steatosis. Both hyperferritinemia and steatosis are common to a number of pathologic entities including diabetes mellitus and alcoholic liver disease. The reason for elevation of serum ferritin in this situation is not clear.

Diabetes

In published large series, up to 60% patients presenting with GH had diabetes mellitus and there is some evidence that its prevalence in also increased in their relatives. There is no evidence that iron accumulates in patients with diabetes mellitus in the absence of GH or other iron-loading predisposition. However, hyperferritinemia at a level up to 50% above normal is common in diabetic patients. There is also evidence that the level of serum ferritin may correlate with hyperglycemia or glycemic control. The mechanisms for this are unclear, but are likely to be related to oxidoreductant changes related to insulin deficiency or resistance in the liver. The phenomenon can produce difficulties of interpretation in situations where diabetes or lipid clinics are included in screening programs.

Alcoholic liver disease

Hepatic siderosis is seen in approximately 20% of patients with alcoholic liver disease and hyperferritinemia is even more frequent. Additionally, in published series of patients with GH, up to 70% drink excessive amounts of alcohol (in some studies more than 50g daily) and a significant proportion have stigmata of alcohol damage on liver biopsy. Small wonder then that for years, until the HLA association was confirmed, there was controversy regarding whether alcohol was the principal cause of hemochromatosis. Even now, this relationship can pose diagnostic problems.

Clinically, liver enzymes are usually normal in hemochromatosis alone, but can also be normal in alcoholic liver disease. Transferrin saturation or ferritin may be raised in alcoholic liver disease, but it is unusual to find both elevated simultaneously and they are not usually commensurately raised as they would be in hemochromatosis. Perl's stain usually demonstrates only grade 1 or 2 siderosis in alcoholic liver disease and rarely grades 3 or 4 as in hemochromatosis. Powell and colleagues have devised the hepatic iron index (μmol iron per gram dry weight liver divided by age in years) to help with this problem. An index greater than 1.9 is considered diagnostic of hemochromatosis. The recently described HFE mutation may help further with this differentiation.

Porto-systemic shunting

Approximately 15% patients with portal hypertension have some evidence of excessive iron deposition, usually in the periportal hepatocytes. Undoubtedly some of this may be related to conditions such as preceding steatosis or alcoholic liver disease. It is not known whether shunting *per se* can result in iron deposition.

Porphyria (see also Chapter 22)

Iron stores are commonly increased in both hereditary and acquired forms of porphyria and there is good evidence both that the iron exacerbates the clinical manifestations of disease and that these can be ameliorated by iron depletion. Iron in the liver induces 5′-aminolaevulinic acid (ALA) synthase and hemoxygenase and inhibits uroporphorynogen decarboxylase. The net effect of these changes is to increase the tissue levels of porphyrins and reduce the feedback inhibitory effect that heme would normally exert on this pathway, thus further increasing tissue levels of porphyrins.

Hepatic siderosis has been observed in liver biopsies of up to 100% of patients with porphyria cutanea tarda (PCT), but additional features on liver biopsy have long suggested that alcohol also plays an important role in this condition. There is recent evidence that the HFE gene C282Y mutation is more common in patients with PCT and that removal of iron can ameliorate the clinical effects of excess porphyrins.

Thalassemias and other anemias

In thalassemia major and other dyserythropoietic anemias (sideroblastic anemia and pyruvate kinase deficiency), excessive iron absorption occurs probably directly or indirectly as a result of relative hypoxia. The iron loading that occurs as a consequence is identical in distribution and effect to that seen in GH, but is exacerbated commonly by the requirement for blood transfusions that lead to parenteral iron overload in addition. Iron loading and damage occur at an earlier age, particularly in thalassemia and warrants aggressive prophylactic use of oral and parenteral iron chelators with close monitoring. Some of these patients succumb to cardiac problems before liver complications become clinically manifest.

Other iron loading anemias include congenital and acquired sideroblastic anemias, congenital dyserythropoietic anemia, refractory hypoplastic anemia, severe hemolytic anemia, and any recurrent anemia that requires repeated blood transfusion. In adult dyserythropoietic anemias, the degree of iron loading is often disproportionately greater than would be expected from the anemia alone. It is not yet known whether heterozygosity of GH may play a role in some of these conditions.

Chronic inflammatory disease

It has long been recognized that normochromic normocytic anemia commonly occurs in anemia of chronic disease, of which perhaps rheumatoid disease is a good paradigm. In this condition, serum iron is low, iron absorption is reduced, marrow iron stores are replete, and serum ferritin is raised. Serum ferritin, often more than twice normal levels, correlates with inflammatory disease activity.

Ferritin is an acute phase protein and its transcription appears to be inducible by proinflammatory cytokines such as interleukin-1β and tumor necrosis factor-α. It has been postulated that these are evolutionary phenomena to protect against toxic effects of iron released when tissue is damaged, or to make that iron less available to infective agents. The importance of this observation to clinicians is to be aware that ferritin in inflammatory conditions is a poor guide to iron storage levels. Distinguishing features between hyperferritinemia in inflammatory disorders and

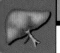
hemochromatosis are that in the former, plasma iron is usually normal or low and the ferritin level is rarely above 700µmol/L. C-reactive protein is usually normal in GH.

Viral hepatitis

An association between excessive iron deposition in the liver and progression of hepatitis B has been recognized for many years. More recently, since the identification of hepatitis C virus (HCV) as the agent responsible for most cases of non-A non-B hepatitis, it has become more evident that iron may play a role in the pathology of virus-mediated liver disease.

To date much of the evidence is circumstantial: hyperferritinemia and hepatic iron deposition are more common in patients with advanced disease; hyperferritinemia correlates with a lower response to interferon treatment, and lowering iron stores can improve the response; iron depletion on its own can normalize plasma liver enzymes in patients with HCV infection. It has also been suggested that differences in iron levels may explain gender differences in HCV infection such as responsiveness to interferon, progression of disease, and development of HCC.

Hyperferritinemia may simply reflect inflammatory activity as seen in other conditions or oxidant stress in the liver. Iron deposits in the liver, perhaps due to hepatic necrosis, are more difficult to explain. Iron absorption in these patients has not been studied but there seems to be no association between presence of the C282Y mutation and progression of HCV.

DIAGNOSIS

'Hemochromatosis' signifies the accumulation of excessive iron stores or the genetic susceptibility to do so. The clinical diagnosis of hemochromatosis rests on confirming iron overload in tissues with or without associated clinical features. At the present time, most authorities would insist on iron overload being present on a liver biopsy (Fig. 20.9). The place of the C282Y mutation in diagnosis has not yet been clearly delineated. For example some persons homozygous for this mutation do not have identi-fiable iron overload, although they must be considered susceptible. Conversely there are subjects with confirmed and sometimes severe iron overload not secondary to an identifiable cause who have only one or even no copies of this mutation.

Investigation

Hemochromatosis should be suspected in anyone with a serum ferritin outside the normal range (males: 300µg/L; females 200µg/L)

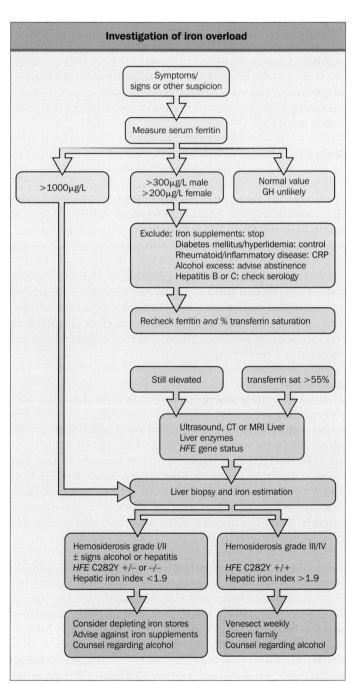

Figure 20.10 Investigation in iron overload. Iron overload can present in many different ways but serum ferritin is a useful starting point for investigation. Any abnormality should be interpreted in the context of conditions known to be associated with hyperferritinemia as described. It is worthwhile rechecking a second time, particularly after a period of abstinence from alcohol. Persisting abnormality can be pursued as shown in the algorithm.

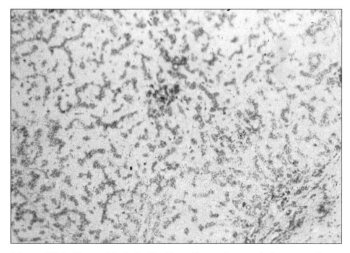

Figure 20.9 Hemosiderin in the liver. Photomicrograph demonstrating hemosiderin in the liver by Perl's potassium ferrocyanide stain (Prussian blue). Note that staining is heaviest in the periportal areas and concentrated in hepatocytes. Biliary epithelium is also iron-loaded. This patient was not cirrhotic.

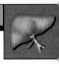

or a transferrin saturation over 55%. These results warrant explanation either by exclusion of associated conditions as discussed above, or by confirmation of iron overload by further investigation (Fig. 20.10). The *HFE* gene test at this stage of investigation will be useful in confirming suspicion that iron overloading is due to GH, but a negative or heterozygous result is not sufficient to exclude a diagnosis of clinically significant iron overload. Computed tomography of the liver with densitometry or MRI scanning can be useful in certain circumstances to decide whether a biopsy is indicated. However, although their specificity is high, the sensitivity of these tests is poor, particularly when steatosis is present in the liver, which commonly occurs if diabetes or excess alcohol consumption are associated. A liver biopsy with Perl's stain and grading of siderosis or chemicophysical estimation of iron concentration are the gold standards of diagnosis (see Fig. 20.9). Where a biopsy is not obtainable or the results are equivocal, a trial of venesection can be very useful and prove diagnostic. A standard unit of blood (450ml) contains approximately 250mg elemental iron. As total body iron is normally 3–4g, patients with hemochromatosis are likely to tolerate consecutive weekly venesection of 25–30 units of blood without becoming anemic. By convention, removal of a 'body's worth' of iron (4g or 16 sequential units) is also regarded as diagnostic. Other investigations may be indicated depending on the patient and his/her symptoms as listed.

Differential diagnosis

Any abnormality of serum ferritin or iron indices warrants explanation, and as discussed in the previous section siderosis on liver biopsy occurs in certain circumstances. The commonest difficulty is differentiating iron overload due to hemochromatosis from that seen in alcoholic liver disease, particularly as many patients with true GH drink excessive alcohol. There is some correlation between the severity and distribution of Perl's hemosiderin stain and diagnosis of hemochromatosis. Grade III or IV siderosis is common in hemochromatosis and much less common in alcoholic liver disease. A hepatic iron index (μmol iron per g dry weight liver tissue divided by age in years) greater than 1.9 has been demonstrated to differentiate reliably between these two conditions in the pre-*HFE* era. Detection of the C282Y mutation of the *HFE* gene should prove useful in such cases and lesser degrees of iron overload should be assessed in the light of the *HFE* gene status and concomitant medical conditions (see Fig. 20.10).

Other investigations
Glucose
Glucose levels should be checked in all patients in view of the frequency of diabetes mellitus.

Liver enzymes
Liver enzymes are usually normal in GH. Elevated aspartate aminotransferase (AST) or alanine aminotransferase (ALT) should alert the clinician to the possibility of associated problems such as alcohol, hepatitis B and C, or fatty liver. Gamma-glutamyltransferase (GGT) is very nonspecific, but also may be a marker of other liver pathology.

Liver function tests
Albumen, prothrombin time, and bilirubin are usually normal, except in end-stage disease. Any abnormality in these results should be investigated.

Gonadotropin profile
Both luteinizing hormone (LH) and follicle-stimulating hormone (FSH) are reduced in patients with symptomatic sexual dysfunction. The response to gonodotropin-releasing hormone is reduced, but in contrast pituitary–adrenal and pituitary–thyroid responsiveness is usually normal.

Alpha-fetoprotein
This is always normal unless hepatoma is present. In cases of established cirrhosis it should be measured frequently.

Imaging
Ultrasound usually demonstrates an echobright liver. If cirrhosis is present, the border and echotexture may be irregular. It is a useful screening test for hepatoma. Computed tomography scan has the advantage of allowing densitometry measurements in comparison to other tissue standards (water, fat). Several studies have reported densitometry measurements of greater than 60 Hounsfield units being relatively specific for iron overload. Unfortunately the presence of steatosis reduces the average densitometry reading and due to the frequency of diabetes and alcohol excess in particular, CT has not been found to be sensitive enough to be useful as a screening tool. Magnetic resonance scanning shows a prolonged relaxation at T2 and has been used as a research tool to differentiate primary and secondary iron overload. Like CT it is relatively specific, but not sensitive enough to be used routinely for screening or diagnosis.

NATURAL HISTORY AND PROGNOSIS

It is essential to consider the prognosis of this condition in the context of the stage of disease at the time of diagnosis.

In genetic iron overload, iron absorption is increased and iron accumulates relentlessly for at least five decades. There is some evidence that accumulation, and perhaps absorption may decline after the sixth decade. As discussed earlier, most patients are now diagnosed in the preclinical stages, having been identified through abnormal automated tests or by family or targeted population screening. For those who are not identified in this way, iron deposition in liver, pancreas, pituitary, heart, and synovium will result respectively in cirrhosis, diabetes mellitus, hyopgonadotropic hypogonadism, cardiac failure or arthritis, usually from the fourth decade onwards. Occasionally iron accumulation has been sufficient to produce these features in younger patients, and sexual dysfunction or cardiomyopathy may present earlier, more frequently and seem equally common in both sexes. Neonatal hemochromatosis is discussed in Chapter 23.

Usually, once any of these end-organ diseases occurs, they are irreversible, although it has been reported that their functional effects can be ameliorated by depleting the excessive iron stores. Otherwise the organ damage tends to follow the same course whatever its cause, that is, cirrhosis continues to pose a risk from portal hypertension. Hepatoma may arise in up to 30% of male patients with GH. There have been occasional reports of reversal of fibrosis following depletion of iron stores.

In the past, most patients died from the complications of end-organ failure. The first major breakthrough in reversing this trend was the introduction of insulin in the 1950s. This improved survival from time of diagnosis at that time from an average of 1 year to 5 years. The main improvement in survival

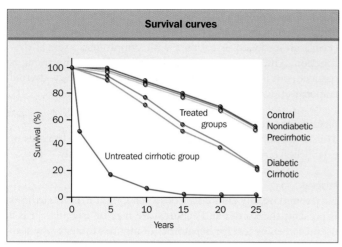

Figure 20.11 Survival curves. Prognosis depends on the degree of iron loading at presentation and the presence or absence of established complications, particularly diabctcs or cirrhosis. There has not been a controlled trial of venesection and the untreated group is historic data. (These survival curves were constructed from cumulative published data in: Williams et al., Quart J Med. 1969;38:1–16; Bomford & Williams, Quart J Med. 1976;180:611–23; Niederau et al., N Engl J Med. 1985;313:1256–62; Adams et al., Gastroenterology. 1991;101:368–72. Figure previously published in 'Pancreatic disease and diabetes mellitus', O'Toole P, Lombard M. In: Pickup J, Williams G, eds. Textbook of diabetes. Oxford: Blackwell Science; 1997.)

in this condition was realized with the introduction of venesection to remove iron stores in the late 1950s and was widely accepted a decade later. Cumulative evidence shows that once iron excess has produced irreversible end-organ damage, the prognosis depends on the organ affected and whether other factors are at play (Fig. 20.11). However many studies have now shown that removal of excess iron improves longevity whether or not end-organ damage is present.

The observation that patients without end-organ damage, for example precirrhotic hemochromatosis, have a normal life expectancy with prevention of complications if iron stores are removed has been confirmed in several studies. Prognosis in these patients is excellent. This has given impetus to the imperative of preclinical diagnosis and screening.

MANAGEMENT

Once a diagnosis has been confirmed, management can be considered under the headings of removal of excess iron, monitoring iron status, amelioration and monitoring of end-organ damage, and screening relatives of the index case.

Treatment
Removal of excess iron
Iron is most easily and conveniently removed by weekly venesection of a standard unit of blood (usually 450ml), each of which contains approximately 250mg iron. In some countries, the national blood transfusion service may agree to use this blood or plasma and may undertake liver phlebotomy. Some patients may not tolerate this frequency and fortnightly or monthly venesection may be better tolerated. However, patients can often have

in excess of 20g of iron and less frequent than weekly venesection will take a considerable amount of time to deplete fully their iron stores.

Very occasionally, elderly patients with angina or heart failure may not tolerate venesection. In these circumstances deferoxamine (desferrioxamine infusion; 2g overnight three times weekly) can be used to increase urinary iron excretion. Oral chelators have not been evaluated in these patients, but the occasional patient may benefit. Ascorbic acid has been used to mobilize iron stores in some patients and enhances excretion of iron by deferoxamine. However, there have been case reports of serious toxicity and cardiac deaths with its use in this context, possibly resulting from a rapid redistribution of iron, and its use cannot be recommended.

Monitoring iron status
During the venesection program, depletion of iron stores is best monitored by measuring serum ferritin and hemoglobin at intervals every 4–6 sessions, and perhaps more frequently when approaching normal levels. Some clinicians have used CT densitometry or MRI to follow progressive depletion of iron stores in the liver. Sequential liver biopsy is unnecessary unless indicated for other reasons.

The aim of treatment is to remove excess iron stores from all tissues. To be certain of this objective many investigators deplete iron stores to a level bordering on deficiency using a target hemoglobin of 11g/dL (female) or 12g/dL (male) or serum ferritin below 50µg/L. Once this level is achieved, much less frequent venesection (3 or 6 monthly) is required to keep iron stores at a low or normal level and the patient should continue to be monitored both for accumulation of iron or complications of end-organ damage. In general serum ferritin declines gradually during venesection, whereas transferrin saturation level can be erratic or not fall precipitously until iron stores are almost depleted. Conversely, transferrin saturation rises earlier and more dramatically with re-accumulation of iron stores and is possibly a better monitoring test in this context (Fig. 20.12).

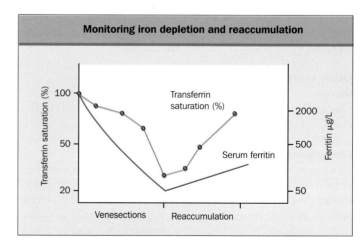

Figure 20.12 Monitoring iron depletion and reaccumulation. Serum ferritin falls gradually during venesection and is a useful guide to predicting duration of venesection. Transferrin saturation increases more rapidly with reaccumulation of iron following cessation of venesection and may be a more useful guide to requirement for further venesection after initial treatment.

Amelioration and monitoring of end-organ damage
Clinically significant end-organ damage should be managed in the usual way. Most patients with established diabetes are insulin dependent and will require close monitoring for complications of diabetes with examination of eyes by fundoscopy, renal function by serum creatinine, and assessment of peripheral neuropathy.

Arthritis is managed by simple analgesia or nonsteroidal anti-inflammatory drugs. These are usually only necessary in the short-term. Arthralgia is often worse during periods of greatest iron flux such as during venesection.

Hypogonadotropic hypogonadism usually warrants hormone replacement therapy. If fertility is an issue, pulse therapy with gonadotropins given subcutaneously either by injection or by pump infusion may be necessary. Where male sexual dysfunction is the clinical issue, testosterone can be given, either by monthly intramuscular depot injection or, more recently, by daily skin patches. There has been a theoretic concern about contribution of testosterone to development of HCC in cirrhotic males, but there is little evidence of this in practice.

The indications for orthotopic liver transplantation are the same as for those in other chronic liver diseases, namely development of hepatic failure or decompensation or the discovery of a small hepatoma during follow-up screening. Studies of patients who have been transplanted for GH have not helped to resolve the question of site of the metabolic defect, perhaps because the latency period to build up iron stores is so long. Because the condition is relatively common, iron loaded livers can be and have been inadvertently grafted into patients requiring transplants for other reasons. The physiologic evidence accumulated in these patients has been confusing. The discovery of the *HFE* gene marker will help to clarify some of the observations in these patients, and of course will ultimately lead to the identification of the tissue specification of the gene product.

SCREENING FOR IRON OVERLOAD
Relatives of the index case
The identification of the C282Y mutation in the *HFE* gene should make screening of family members much more reliable and has superseded the usefulness of HLA typing in this respect. More than 90% of index cases should be homozygous for the C282Y marker. Their siblings have a 50% chance of carrying one mutation allele (i.e. carrier status) and a 25% chance of carrying both (homozygous affected) or neither (homozygous normal). However, several families are known in which the genetics do not 'run true', and it is still essential that indices of iron overload (at least serum ferritin) are also checked.

Up to 25% of individuals thought to be heterozygous for this condition are known to have evidence of excessive iron accumulation, either by elevated serum ferritin or increased siderosis on liver biopsy.

Offspring of affected individuals are obligate carriers (heterozygous for the gene mutation). With a gene frequency of 10% in the general population, there is a 5% chance that offspring will have inherited a second mutation from the other parent. As there is some evidence that hererozygotes can have intermediate levels of excess iron, it is important that iron indices are checked in this group also. Because iron accumulates with age and significant iron overload is uncommon in children, it would seem sensible to recommend measurement of serum ferritin every 5 years from the age of 15 or 20 years to perhaps age 50 years. Usually

thorough counseling of the individual is sufficient to inform them of this requirement.

Parents of affected individuals should also be obligate carriers with an additional 5% risk that they are homozygous for the condition and should be assessed accordingly. Extending family screening beyond this immediate family will yield approximately 10% cases based on experience. This is certainly justifiable on health economic grounds, but often requires a dedicated screening system (Fig. 20.13).

Screening other populations
Various studies have undertaken population screening in different populations. The most extensive of these has been aimed at determining the prevalence of GH in a healthy population and has targeted blood donors or adults employed by corporate institutions. Both approaches have used biochemical indices only for screening (predating identification of the *HFE* mutation) and have demonstrated prevalence rates of 1:200–1:1000 (see Fig. 20.2). The test used at initial screen plays an important role in determining the effectiveness of subsequent detection and avoidance of excessive recall. Transferrin saturation is generally thought to be the more sensitive test but the cut-off value taken to be significant varies between 45 and 70%. Ferritin, when used as the initial screening test, is generally used to recall subjects with

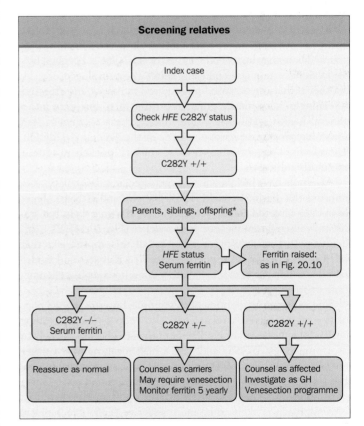

Figure 20.13 Screening relatives. Screening of the relatives of an index case can be extended through the larger kindred. The most important group to screen are siblings as these have the greatest risk of homozygosity for the mutation. If the index case does not have the common *HFE* mutation, biochemical screening of the family should be carried out with appropriate counseling. *When children are very young, the other parent may be tested, if C282Y –/– (90% cases), the children need not be tested until adulthood.

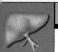

Prevalence of hemochromatosis in specific subpopulations				
Study	Population	*n*	Initial parameter used	% Discovery
Phelps, et al. 1989 Lancet. 2:2133–4	DM	418	Ferritin > normal	0.96
O'Brien, et al. 1990 Diabetes Care. 13:532–3	DM	572	Ferritin > normal	0.5
Singh, et al. 1992 Diabetic Med. 9:730–1	DM	406	Saturation >62%	0.49
George, et al. 1995 Ann Rev Biochem. 32:521–6	DM	1194	Saturation >55%	0.84
Turnbull, et al. 1997 Q J Med. 90:271–5	DM	727	Saturation >55% Ferritin > normal	0.13
Olynyk, et al. 1994 Aust NZ J Med. 24:22–5	Rheum	339	Saturation >55% Ferritin >500 µg/L	1.5

Figure 20.14 Prevalence in specific subpopulations. This table summarizes published series that sought to determine whether the prevalence of hemochromatosis was increased in certain subpopulations because their disease occurred more frequently in association with hemochromatosis. DM, diabetes mellitus; RA, rheumatoid arthritis.

levels outside the normal laboratory reference range (usually 300µg/L male; 200µg/L female), but it is likely to be less sensitive, particularly in younger patients and females, and less specific if used in a general population that includes categories of patients in whom hyperferritinemia can also occur. Some studies have used combination approaches.

It has also been argued that this approach is cost-effective but it has not been incorporated into widespread screening programs. There may be several reasons for this. One is a general lack of awareness amongst clinicians about the prevalence of GH; another is that the organization required to mount any effective screening or surveillance program is difficult to integrate into a general health service provision; finally, there is concern that screening programs provoke anxiety in the general population. The advent of a genetic marker for screening is unlikely to address these difficulties.

Attempts have been made to target specific subpopulations to improve the diagnostic yield. Thus, diabetes and arthritis clinics have been targeted and most studies have shown a slight but statistically insignificant increase in prevalence (Fig. 20.14). One difficulty with the widespread adoption of this approach is that ferritin may be raised in poorly controlled diabetes and is also raised nonspecifically in inflammatory conditions such as rheumatoid arthritis.

The widespread adoption of this approach to the general population, as opposed to a relatively healthy population selected by health (blood donors) or employment (health checks), is likely to prove much less specific and have a high recall rate for further investigation. It is not yet clear what will be the general usefulness and general applicability of using the *HFE* mutation in screening populations other than family pedigrees of affected individuals. This approach is likely to be more sensitive than a biochemical approach, but the specificity for iron overload is not yet certain. Using genetic tests for screening has additional problems of provoking anxiety unnecessarily and perhaps leaving individuals exposed to scrutiny of risk or stigma by insurance companies. At the moment, until these issues are resolved, more widespread population screening for GH is unlikely to be adopted.

Economics of screening

Several investigators have attempted to assess the economic benefits of screening taking into account the costs to a health service of potential complications of undiagnosed hemochromatosis and days of employment lost. There have been two such studies in North America, one in a hospital outpatient setting using serum iron as the preliminary screening parameter and the second using percentage transferrin saturation in males aged 30 years and over undergoing routine health checks. In addition, the economics of screening have been modeled in the hypothetic situations of screening blood donors or restricting screening to males aged 30 years or more.

The conclusions from these types of analysis is that screening is cost-effective, namely, it is less expensive than the potential costs of complications of hemochromatosis developing in those undiagnosed cases. One study suggested that screening would be economic as long as the initial screening test (the most expensive in volume terms) could be kept below US$10.

The problem with these analyses is that they cannot be generalized to screening wider populations and they cannot take into account the fact that some patients do not go on to develop complications, because they present and are subsequently diagnosed and treated or are identified as a result of family screening. Nonetheless, they confirm that failure to diagnose GH can be extremely costly.

PRACTICE POINT

Illustrative case

A 64-year-old man is referred by his doctor for your opinion. His younger brother aged 55 years was found to have hemochromatosis when he presented with hematemesis secondary to cirrhosis and liver cancer. The patient referred to you is extremely anxious. His doctor performed some blood tests which show: Hb10 4g/dL, MCV76fL, serum ferritin <5µg/L, ALT 30IU/L, alkaline phosphatase 120IU/L, γ-glutamyl transferase 34IU/L, AFP 4g/L. In his past history he had a partial gastrectomy at age 20 years for duodenal ulcer disease.

His daughter aged 35 years, on hearing that he was being screened for a genetic disease, had her own doctor run some tests and her ferritin level is 520µg/L. Her only medical history is that she suffers from rheumatoid arthritis and is on methotrexate. She is concerned for her own children and has accompanied her father to your clinic.

Physical examination of the patient reveals a fairly healthy, but thin 64-year-old male. He has no hepatomegaly and no stigmata of liver disease or of hemochromatosis. You arrange investigations which confirm the results of the general practitioner's tests and his liver ultrasound is reported as normal. You also tested his *HFE* gene status which is reported as M/M for the C282Y mutation (i.e. homozygous for hemochromatosis), his daughter's status is later shown to be M/n.

Interpretation

1. Anxiety in families is common when genetic disorders first surface. This is apt to be more so in the context of a dramatic presentation such as hemorrhage and cancer in a relation seen to be in the prime of his or her life. The best way to deal with this anxiety is to give a simple explanation of hereditary principles. The following facts need to be conveyed.

- Hemochromatosis is a recessively inherited condition; it requires two abnormal genes for the condition to become manifest.
- The gene prevalence for hemochromatosis in the general (Caucasian) population is 10%.
- For an affected individual, it can be assumed that both parents had at least one abnormal gene each, and that all of his/her offspring received one of his/her abnormal genes.
- For his/her siblings, there is a 1:4 chance of them having two abnormal genes, a 1:4 chance of them having two normal genes or a 1:2 chance of having one abnormal gene (based on the assumption that the parents were only carriers). There is a 1:100 chance that either parent had two abnormal genes (homozygous); in that case siblings of the index patient have a 1:2 chance of being homozygous, or will definitely be heterozygous.
- There is a 1:10 chance that the affected individual's spouse is a carrier so that his/her offspring have a 1:20 chance of being homozygous and affected (as compared with 1:100 chance for the general unrelated population).

2. The 55-year-old brother presented with hematemesis secondary to cirrhosis and hepatoma. Although presentation with end-stage hemochromatosis is now rare, it would characteristically occur in males in the 5th or 6th decade. Up to 30% males with cirrhosis and hemochromatosis may develop a hepatoma. Hematemesis is an unusual presentation of hemochromatosis.

3. The patient referred to you does not have iron overload. The results of his full blood count and serum ferritin actually show that he is iron deficient. His iron deficiency is due to the fact that he has been achlorhydric for 44 years since his partial gastrectomy. Gastric secretion of hydrochloric acid and ascorbic acid is necessary to make dietary iron bioavailable for absorption. The iron deficiency is likely to be even more pronounced if he had a type of gastrectomy involving bypass of the proximal duodenum where iron absorption takes place. Of course, occult blood loss will need to be excluded. The patient is found to be homozygous for the common mutation in the *HFE* gene, so he has the genetic defect but he has been spared the phenotypic expression of this disease fortuitously by his previous operation!

4. As the patient has 'genetic' hemochromatosis but not 'phenotypic' iron overload, there is no advantage to him in performing a liver biopsy. Now that *HFE* can be used to differentiate hyperferritinemia associated with hemochromatosis from other causes, it could be argued that liver biopsy is a defunct investigation for any patient homozygous for C282Y (in much the same way that M2-specific mitochondrial antibody may obviate the need for liver biopsy to diagnose primary biliary cirrhosis). However, liver biopsy remains the only reliable way of assessing end-organ damage in hemochromatosis and it is this rather than the amount of iron overload that determines prognosis.

5. The daughter's genotype would be predicted to be at least heterozygous once her father's status was known. There was a 1:20 chance that she may have got a second abnormal gene from her mother (who in turn had a 1:10 chance of being a carrier given that the gene frequency in the general population is 10%). She was indeed found to be a heterozygote.

Although early reports (before gene tests) indicated that up to 25% of putative heterozygotes may have some biochemical expression of the condition (raised serum ferritin), in fact this is very unusual in practice and even less so in women. Other causes of hyperferritinemia in the daughter should be considered. These include active inflammation, alcohol excess, prior blood transfusion or prolonged dietary iron supplementation, hyperlipidemia, obesity, or diabetes mellitus. In inflammatory conditions such as the rheumatoid arthritis, which the daughter has, serum ferritin behaves as an acute-phase protein possibly to help limit free radical damage mediated by inflammation. This can also occur with HCV infection. Typically the ferritin reaches a level of 400-600µg/L, as in this case. C-reactive protein is usually also raised and transferrin saturation is normal. These patients commonly have a normocytic normochromic anemia with a Hb of about 8–10g/dL.

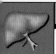
FURTHER READING

Bacon BR, Britton RS. The pathology of hepatic iron overload: a free radical-mediated process? Hepatology. 1990;11:127–37. *Thorough discussion of the mechanisms of iron toxicity in relation to the liver.*

Bonkovsky HL, Banner BF, Rothman AL. Iron and chronic viral hepatitis. Hepatology. 1997;25:759–68. *Reviews the evidence that iron excess can cause synergistic damage in the presence of chronic viral hepatitis.*

Brock JH, Halliday JW, Pippard MJ, Powell LW. Iron metabolism in health and disease. London: Saunders; 1994. *Excellent text book (480 pages in 14 chapters, thousands of references) on all aspects of iron metabolism and disorders.*

Burnt MJ, Halliday JN, Powell LW. Iron and coronary heart disease. Br Med J. 1993;307:575–6. *Commentary on an intriguing proposal that iron excess is a significant contributory factor to ischemic heart disease.*

deSousa M, Brock JH. Iron in immunity, cancer and inflammation. Chichester: John Wiley; 1989. *Wide-ranging discussion of iron in the context of systemic disease.*

Feder JN, Gnirke A, Thomas W, et al. A novel MHC class I-like gene is mutated in patients with hereditary haemochromatosis. Nature Genet. 1996; 13:399–408. *Landmark paper identifying the common genetic mutation near HLA which is thought to result in hemochromatosis.*

Hallbeg L, Asp N. Iron Nutrition in health and disease. London: John Libbey; 1996. *Good overview of nutritional and other aspects of iron metabolism in relation to conditions other than GH.*

Irving MG, Halliday JW, Powell LW. Association between alcoholism and increased hepatic iron stores. Clin Exp Res. 1988;12:7–13. *Experimental attempts to explore and explain the observed relationship between alcoholic excess and iron accumulation.*

Koeppen AH. The history of iron in the brain. J Neurol Sci. 1995;134:Suppl. 1–9. *Discussion of the role which iron has in brain chemistry and how it may be involved in brain development, Parkinson's disease and Alzheimers disease.*

Milder MS, Cook JD, Stray S, Finch CA. Idiopathic hemochromatosis: an interim report. Medicine. 1980;59:34–49. *Excellent review of the clinical features and characterization of hemochromatosis in 1980 – most of the information still pertains 20 years later.*

Niederau C, Fisher R, Sonnenberg A, Stremmel W, Tampish HJ, Strohmeyer G. Survival and causes of death in cirrhotic and non-cirrhotic patients with primary hemochromatosis. N Engl J Med. 1985;31:1256–62. *Landmark paper describing the survival patterns of subjects with hemochromatosis.*

Niederau C, Fisher R, Sonnenberg A, Stremmel W, Tampish HJ, Strohmeyer G. Long term survival in patients with hereditary hemochromatosis. Gastroenterology. 1996;110:1107–1019. *An update of the 1985 report.*

Rothschild MA, Berk PD, Tavill AS, Bacon BR. Metals and Free-radical induced liver injury. Semin Liver Dis. 1996;16(no.1). *An excellent update on the scientific background of hepatotoxicity of iron and other metals is included.*

Simon M, Bourel M, Genetet B, Fauchet R. Idiopathic hemochromatosis. Demonstration of recessive transmission and early detection by family HLA typing. N Engl J Med. 1977;297:1017–21. *Landmark paper identifying for the first time a confirmed association between hemochromatosis and HLA and setting the scene for a genetic expedition to find the gene almost 20 years later.*

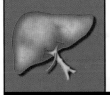
Chapter 21 Wilson's Disease

M Stuart Tanner

INTRODUCTION

Wilson's disease is an autosomal disorder of copper metabolism. The gene, *ATP7B*, encodes a copper carrier that both exports copper from hepatocyte to bile and enables ceruloplasmin synthesis. Wilson's disease may present with almost any variety of liver disease in the age range of 3–12 years or with psychiatric and/or neurologic disease in adolescence. Young adults present with combined hepatic and neurologic problems, or less commonly with hemolysis or arthritis. Asymptomatic disease is frequently diagnosed after presentation of an index case within a family. Low plasma ceruloplasmin, a positive penicillamine challenge test, and raised hepatic copper concentration suggest the diagnosis. However, there are numerous diagnostic pitfalls. Molecular methods are now being used to aid diagnosis, but this approach poses new management dilemmas. If diagnosed early, it is readily treatable with zinc or chelators, and has a good long-term prognosis. Fulminant hepatic disease has a poor outcome without transplantation.

In 1902 and 1903 Kayser and Fleischer independently described a pigmented corneal ring in a patient with multiple sclerosis and in two other neurologic patients, respectively. Wilson described four patients in 1911 with dysarthria, tremor, and progressive movement disorder who at autopsy had cavitation of the lenticular nucleus and cirrhosis. The term hepatolenticular degeneration was first used in 1921 and the autosomal recessive inheritance pattern was recognized at that time. The association with low plasma levels of the blue protein ceruloplasmin followed in 1952, but attempts to treat the disease with plasma proved fruitless. Attempts at chelation therapy started in the 1950s and penicillamine became the treatment of choice from 1956. Treatment with zinc sulfate started in 1961 but was slow to achieve therapeutic respectability, until in 1979 resolution of Kayser–Fleischer (KF) rings was demonstrated with zinc. Triethylenetetramine hydrochloride was also introduced in the late 1960s when it was used for patients intolerant of penicillamine.

The molecular biology of Wilson's disease began to be elucidated in 1985 when the Wilson's disease gene locus was shown to be linked to esterase D on chromosome 13 following a study of three Middle East kindreds. This demonstrated that it was distinct from the loci for ceruloplasmin on chromosome 3 and the metallothionein cluster on chromosome 16. In 1993 the identity of the Menkes' disease gene (*ATP7A*) was published. In a rare female patient with this X-linked condition, characterization of the chromosomal break point and analysis of the coding region revealed a putative transmembrane protein resembling the bacterial cationic transport ATPases. Ten months later three groups reported an homologous gene for Wilson's disease (*ATP7B*).

EPIDEMIOLOGY

Wilson's disease occurs worldwide and has been identified in almost every race. The prevalence of the disease is approximately 1:30,000 births with reported incidences ranging from 5 to 30 per million population. The gene carrier rate is 0.3–0.7%. The highest incidences are seen in areas characterized by high levels of inbreeding (e.g. Sardinia and isolated Japanese islands). Phenotypic variability and molecular epidemiology are considered later.

PATHOPHYSIOLOGY

Copper metabolism

Copper is essential to life. Copper-containing enzymes are fundamental to cellular respiration (cytochrome c oxidase), free radical defence (superoxide dismutase), neurotransmitter function (dopamine β-monooxygenase), connective tissue synthesis (lysyl oxidase), melanin synthesis (tyrosinase), and iron metabolism (ceruloplasmin). Copper's unique electron structure allows these cuproenzymes to catalyze redox reactions, but causes ionic copper to be very toxic, readily participating in reactions that promote the synthesis of damaging reactive oxygen species.

Dietary copper intake is approximately 1–2mg/day. Quoted copper contents of foods are unreliable. While some foods, such as organ meats and shellfish, have consistently high concentrations, others such as dairy produce are consistently low in copper. However, the copper content of cereals and fruits varies greatly with soil copper content and the method of food preparation. Estimates of copper intake should include water copper content, and the permitted upper copper concentration for drinking water is 2mg/L. The recommended intake in the first 6 months of life is 80μg/kg per day. Clinical effects from dietary deficiency in infancy comprise anemia, neutropenia, and bone changes and are reported in infants suffering from malnutrition and chronic diarrhea. Acute ingestion of copper salts either accidentally (e.g. chemistry set poisoning) or with suicidal intent causes gastrointestinal fluid loss and ulceration, shock, and intravascular hemolysis. Chronic copper dietary excess is associated with Indian childhood cirrhosis.

Approximately 10% of dietary copper is absorbed. This fraction varies with the nature of the diet, being for example higher in breast-fed infants than in formula-fed or weaned infants. It is influenced by other dietary constituents such as zinc, which reduces absorption by inducing enterocyte metallothionein. Percentage absorption is higher from a low than a high copper diet. The unabsorbed remainder remains bound to metallothionein in the enterocyte and is lost as villous cells are desquamated into the gut lumen – a so-called 'mucosal block' to absorption.

Absorbed dietary copper travels to the liver in portal blood complexed to albumin, histidine, and possibly a high molecular weight protein transcuprein (Fig. 21.1). Hepatic copper uptake is avid. Copper is reduced to Cu^+ and transported across the plasma membrane by Ctr1. Within the hepatocyte it is chaperoned to its site of action by a series of carrier proteins. These include the chaperone protein Hah1, which carries copper to the Wilson's disease protein (WDP) situated in the trans-Golgi. Copper is transferred from Hah1 to the copper-binding sections of WDP by a carefully orchestrated sequence of shifting sulfydryl bonds, so ensuring that at no stage is ionic copper free to cause damage. Other chaperones carry copper to the mitochondrion (Cox17) and to superoxide dismutase (lys7). Any copper within the cytoplasm is bound to glutathione and then metallothionein, and thence taken up by lysosomes where it exists as an insoluble copper- and sulfur-rich polymer that is excreted into bile canaliculi. Copper bound to WDP is transported across the trans-Golgi membrane and is inserted into apoceruloplasmin. Copper leaves the hepatocyte either by being secreted into plasma tightly embraced within ceruloplasmin or carried to the bile canalicular membrane by WDP and excreted into bile. Biliary copper is nonreabsorbable.

Whereas iron status is controlled by regulating its absorption, copper status is controlled by regulating its biliary excretion. Iron overload is caused by defects in control of absorption, which may be genetic (hemochromatosis) or acquired (hemosiderosis). Copper overload is caused by defects in biliary excretion, which may also be genetic (Wilson's disease) or acquired (cholestatic states).

Wilson's disease protein

Wilson's disease protein (WDP) (Fig. 21.2) is a transmembrane protein, situated in the trans-Golgi membrane, which binds and transports copper. It belongs to a class of cation transporters known as P-type ATPases because, during the transport cycle, there is reversible protein phosphorylation by ATP at an invariant aspartate residue, forming a covalent phosphoprotein intermediate. Wilson's disease protein contains the following functional domains: eight transmembrane sequences (1–8), in one of which (region 6) is the cys-pro-cys sequence found in all P-type ATPases and thought to form an ion channel; six copper binding regions [Cu] containing cys-X-X-cys motifs at the amino terminal end; and ATP binding, aspartyl kinase and phosphorylation domains. Alternatively spliced forms of WDP lacking transmembrane sequences 3 and 4 (exon 8) are expressed in brain.

ATP7B is 57% homologous with the ATP7A, with higher homology in functional regions. Both may be regarded as cellular copper pumps, differing principally in their tissue distribution. Boys with Menkes' syndrome cannot pump copper out of the enterocyte into portal blood; they therefore cannot absorb copper and have a systemic copper deficiency. Because the same defect is present in all tissues except liver, Menkes' syndrome is not corrected by systemic copper administration.

Much of the information about the intracellular location and function of WDP comes from studies of animal and tissue culture models and by extrapolation from knowledge about the

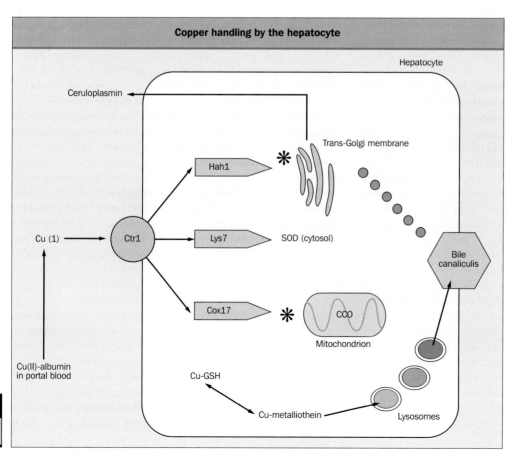

Copper handling by the hepatocyte

Figure 21.1 **Copper handling by the hepatocyte.** Copper is a highly reactive ion, necessary for synthesis of cytochrome c oxidase (CCO), superoxide dismutase (SOD), lysyl oxidase, and ceruloplasmin. It is capable of catalysing oxygen free radical mediated damage if not bound to specific proteins. It is internalized (Ctr1), chaperoned to its site of activity (e.g. by Hah1 to WDP), linked to apoceruloplasmin by WDP, and then either secreted into plasma tightly embraced within ceruloplasmin or carried to the bile canalicular membrane by WDP and excreted into bile. Glutathione and metallothionein bind copper in the cytosol, before it is internalized into lysosomes. GSH, reduced glutathione.

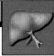

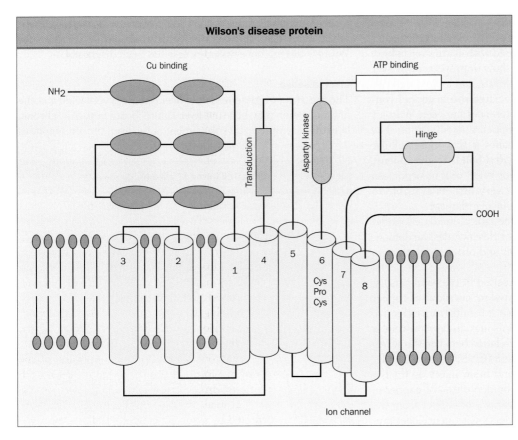

Figure 21.2 The Wilson's disease protein. The WD gene, *ATP7B* at 13q14.3, is 7.5kb in length. It encodes a copper transporting ATPase, the WDP. 21 exons encode six copper binding regions (Cu1–Cu6); transmembrane regions; an energy transduction region; an aspartyl kinase region containing an invariant aspartate residue that is reversibly phosphorylated during the transport cycle; and large ATP-binding and hinge loop at the carboxy terminal end. The gene and its product bear close resemblance to the Menkes' disease gene and product, and differ in tissue location – WDP is found only in liver, brain, and kidney. WDP resides in the membrane of the trans-Golgi apparatus and is bifunctional. It passes copper to ceruloplasmin, and it is carried in secretory vesicles to the bile canalicular membrane for copper export.

Menkes' protein, so must be interpreted cautiously. Present data indicate the following:

- WDP is principally located in the trans-Golgi membrane. There its function is to pass copper into cisternae of the Golgi where it joins apoceruloplasmin to form holoceruloplasmin.
- In situations of high intracellular copper WDP may traffic to vesicles adjacent to the canalicular membrane and be involved in copper excretion.
- A shortened 140kDa WDP probably lacking one or two copper binding sites resides in the mitochondrial membrane where it presumably passes copper into the mitochondrion to be incorporated into cytochrome oxidase.
- Little is known about WDP in the brain.
- Studies of Wilson cDNA in fibroblasts deficient in the Menkes

copper transporter show that expression of wild-type Wilson gene caused WDP to be synthesized, to localize to the trans-Golgi, and to traffic to the plasma membrane while cDNA carrying the most common Wilson' disease mutation, H1069Q, caused synthesis of a WDP, which did not localize to the trans-Golgi, had a short half-life, and was not functional.

Mechanisms of cell injury

The lack of the WDP copper exporter in the liver cell explains the principal biochemical features of Wilson's disease (Fig. 21.3). Copper is cytotoxic to isolated hepatocytes as it is to bacteria, fungi, and algae. Nevertheless the relationship between copper storage and tissue damage is not straightforward. There is, for example, no clear relationship between liver copper concentra-

Biochemical features of Wilson's disease	
Biochemical abnormality	**Explanation**
Low serum ceruloplasmin	Failure to incorporate copper into ceruloplasmin Apoceruloplasmin has a very short half-life
Low serum copper (but note that in particular clinical circumstances serum copper can be normal or high, see below)	A consequence of low ceruloplasmin because most copper in the serum is ceruloplasmin-bound 'free' (i.e. non-ceroplasmin copper is raised, particularly in liver failure, see below)
Raised hepatic copper	Failure of biliary secretion
Disturbed liver function tests	A consequence of hepatic copper storage (but note that other factors must contribute, see below)
Raised urine copper	Increased clearance of serum 'free' copper
Renal Fanconi syndrome	Renal tubular copper deposition

Figure 21.3 Biochemical features of Wilson's disease. The main biochemical changes seen in Wilson's disease and the underlying mechanism.

tion and liver damage: the presymptomatic toddler with Wilson's disease but minimal histologic abnormality may have a higher liver copper concentration than the child with acute liver failure. Some penicillamine-treated patients show improvement of liver function without falling liver copper levels, and a rapid deterioration on its cessation without an associated rise in copper concentration. There are phenotypic differences between Wilson's disease patients with similar liver copper concentrations. The probable explanation of these anomalies is that most cellular copper is either safely bound by sulfydryl bonds to glutathione, metallothionein, copper-chaperones, or WDP, or is incorporated into cuproenzymes. This means that very little is available to cause free radical-mediated macromolecular damage.

In vitro, copper is able to cause free radical-mediated oxidative DNA damage. *In vivo*, evidence for this includes the demonstration of bulky nuclear DNA lesions and of large deletions in mitochondrial DNA.

In the brain, copper is mainly deposited in the basal ganglia. While this has previously been attributed to 'overflow' of copper from liver to brain, it is more likely that it results from defective action of the WDP in neurones. Wilson's disease protein is expressed in the brain. There is no correlation between the severity of hepatic and central nervous system (CNS) damage. Similar questions exist about brain copper and brain injury as for the liver. Kayser–Fleischer rings, caused by deposition of copper in the iris, probable represent simple overflow of copper from the liver. They are usually present in patients with neurologic presentation, but not in younger children with hepatic presentation. They do not cause visual impairment. There is no correlation between the presence or absence of KF rings and the degree of abnormality of urine copper or serum ceruloplasmin.

Animal models

The Long Evans rat with a cinnamon coat (LEC rat) develops hepatitis and cirrhosis with high liver copper concentrations. There is a partial deletion at the 3′ end of the Wilson's disease gene. While resembling human Wilson's disease biochemically, it differs from humans in:

- having excess iron storage in the liver – this may be a separately inherited trait;
- also developing hepatocellular carcinoma; and
- not showing neurologic features.

The toxic milk mouse was discovered because pups suckled on affected dams die from copper deficiency. This is due to reduced copper in the milk. The human equivalent of this scenario has not been reported. The recessively inherited copper toxicosis of the Bedlington terrier is not a model of Wilson's disease, but demonstrates that other genetic mechanisms may lead to a copper-related cirrhosis.

CLINICAL FEATURES AND DISEASE ASSOCIATIONS

Wilson's disease has protean clinical presentations (Figs 21.4 & 21.5). Approximately 40% present with liver disease usually between the ages of 3 and 12 years. Approximately 50% have a psychiatric or neurologic presentation, usually in adolescence or early adult life, and about half of this group will have clinically detectable liver disease. The remainder present with skeletal,

renal or hemolytic disease, and these features may also be present in the other clinical categories. Siblings should be screened for Wilson's disease once an index case has been diagnosed.

Liver disease

The spectrum of presentation of liver disease is very wide and the first indication may be acute liver failure, acute hepatitis, chronic hepatitis, asymptomatic enlargement of the liver, the serendipitous

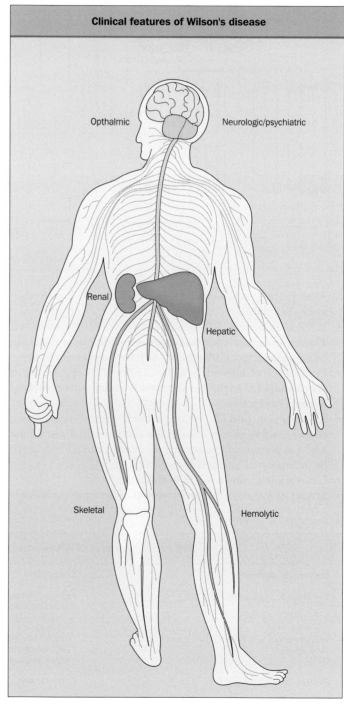

Figure 21.4 Clinical features of Wilson's disease. Wilson's disease affects liver, brain, kidney, hemopoietic system, eye, and bone. Wilson's is a multisystem disease, but the majority of patients present either with liver disease in childhood, psychiatric or neurologic abnormalities in adolescence or adult life, or a combination of these.

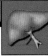

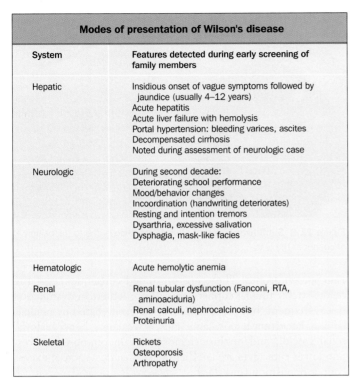

Figure 21.5 Presentation of Wilson's disease. Wilson's disease usually presents with hepatic or neurologic conditions, but some present in other ways. RTA, renal tubular acidosis.

Modes of presentation of Wilson's disease	
System	Features detected during early screening of family members
Hepatic	Insidious onset of vague symptoms followed by jaundice (usually 4–12 years)
	Acute hepatitis
	Acute liver failure with hemolysis
	Portal hypertension: bleeding varices, ascites
	Decompensated cirrhosis
	Noted during assessment of neurologic case
Neurologic	During second decade:
	Deteriorating school performance
	Mood/behavior changes
	Incoordination (handwriting deteriorates)
	Resting and intention tremors
	Dysarthria, excessive salivation
	Dysphagia, mask-like facies
Hematologic	Acute hemolytic anemia
Renal	Renal tubular dysfunction (Fanconi, RTA, aminoaciduria)
	Renal calculi, nephrocalcinosis
	Proteinuria
Skeletal	Rickets
	Osteoporosis
	Arthropathy

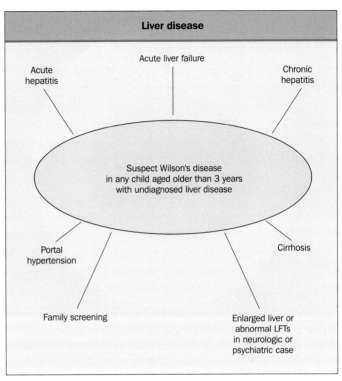

Figure 21.6 Liver disease. Suspect Wilson's disease in any child aged older than 3 years with undiagnosed liver disease. LFT, liver function tests.

finding of abnormal liver function tests, variceal hemorrhage from unsuspected portal hypertension, or signs of decompensated chronic liver failure (Fig. 21.6). Since Wilson's disease may present with almost any clinical variety of hepatic abnormality, it is vitally important that it should be suspected in any child or young adult with undiagnosed liver disease. Other patients are discovered to have silent liver disease after they have presented with the neurologic, ophthalmic, hemolytic, skeletal or, rarely, renal manifestations. Clinical awareness of Wilson's disease is therefore important and must be multidisciplinary.

Acute liver failure, characterized by the development of encephalopathy, usually occurs without antecedent illness but occasionally seems to be precipitated by another illness such as hepatitis A or E, chicken pox or measles. Previous episodes of hemolysis or hepatitis may have occurred. In a child with acute liver failure, Wilson's disease must always be considered, and is a likely diagnosis if hepatitis A IgM is negative, there is no history of ingestion of paracetamol, amanita or other relevant xenobiotic, and autoantibodies are negative. The presence of an associated Coomb's negative hemolytic anemia is a very strong pointer to the diagnosis of Wilson's disease. The hemolysis contributes a large amount of unconjugated bilirubin to the total serum bilirubin and these patients are disproportionately jaundiced, often having serum bilirubin levels in excess of 800μmol/L (47mg/dL) (Fig. 21.7).

Older children and adults usually have cirrhosis at the time of presentation with the clinical picture of acute liver failure. This may be manifest by a liver that is reduced in size, splenomegaly and ascites, or dependent edema earlier in the course of the illness than might be expected for other causes of acute liver failure. A very similar presentation may be seen in patients diagnosed with Wilson's disease who abandoned penicillamine therapy 6–18

months previously. It has been suggested, but not universally confirmed, that the alkaline phosphatase is unusually low in acute liver failure due to Wilson's disease.

An acute hepatic illness, which may resolve and be attributed to non-A–E viral hepatitis, may be the first presentation. In developed countries, an acute hepatitis for which a viral etiology cannot be determined in the age group at risk is sufficiently uncommon to suggest that the ceruloplasmin should always be measured in such cases. Once again, associated hemolysis is highly suggestive of Wilson's disease. Chronic hepatitis in Wilson's disease may be impossible to distinguish on clinical grounds from autoimmune hepatitis. The histologic appearances in these cases may also show features commonly seen in autoimmune chronic hepatitis, including interface hepatitis. The presence of steatosis, in particular, should trigger the search for Wilson's disease in

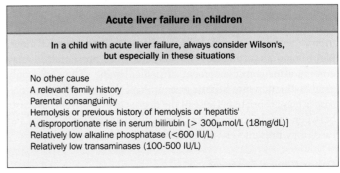

Acute liver failure in children
In a child with acute liver failure, always consider Wilson's, but especially in these situations
No other cause
A relevant family history
Parental consanguinity
Hemolysis or previous history of hemolysis or 'hepatitis'
A disproportionate rise in serum bilirubin [> 300μmol/L (18mg/dL)]
Relatively low alkaline phosphatase (<600 IU/L)
Relatively low transaminases (100-500 IU/L)

Figure 21.7 Acute liver failure in children. The diagnosis of Wilson's disease should always be sought in a child with acute liver failure, but especially in these situations.

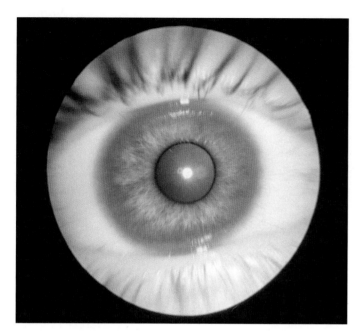

Figure 21.8 Kayser–Fleischer rings. The brown-green discoloration around the periphery of the cornea is best seen when looking at the eye from the side. Slit-lamp examination is recommended if it is apparent in any patient suspected of having Wilson's disease.

such cases. The issue is easily resolved if KF rings (Fig. 21.8) are present, but in their absence the diagnosis or exclusion of Wilson's disease will rest upon laboratory tests.

Among neuropsychiatric patients with Wilson's disease, the reported prevalence of hepatic abnormalities varies widely, probably because of observer variation.

Neurologic disease

It is important to have a high index of suspicion for Wilson's disease in teenagers and young adults presenting with deteriorating school performance, psychiatric abnormalities, or neurologic features. Copper deposition is predominantly in the lenticular nuclei, cerebellum and substantia nigra, and the most common neurologic manifestations are dystonia and parkinsonism. Cognitive ability initially remains intact. The neurologic manifestations are easily misdiagnosed and deteriorating performance at school, worsening handwriting, and behavioral problems are often misguidedly attributed to adolescence. Among children with a neurologic presentation, it is common to detect asymptomatic hepatosplenomegaly, and/or abnormal liver function tests, and histologic abnormalities on liver biopsy. While KF rings may not be detectable in patients with hepatic presentations, it is very unusual for patients with motor symptoms due to Wilson's disease not to have KF rings. Neurologic abnormalities not detectable at presentation may emerge after commencement of penicillamine. The commonly used distinction into hepatic or neurological cases of Wilson's disease is inappropriate because of the degree of cross-over that exists between the clinical features. This is also true within families and cases may present very differently within the same sibship.

Other Clinical Features

Renal tubular abnormalities are frequently found in Wilson's disease and these include glycosuria, aminoaciduria, renal tubular acidosis, impaired phosphate reabsorption, or a full blown renal

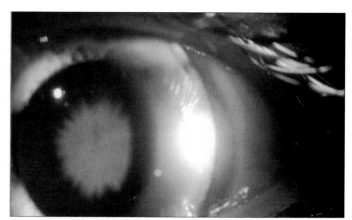

Figure 21.9 Sunflower cataract. This appearance is due to deposition of copper in the lens.

Fanconi syndrome. These are presumed consequence of the demonstrable tubular copper deposition. Glomerular dysfunction is less frequent, but proteinuria may be exacerbated by penicillamine. Recurrent hypokalemic muscle weakness, hyperoxaluria, renal calculi, and nephrocalcinosis are uncommon features. Sunflower catarracts are another ocular manifestation of excess copper deposition (Fig. 21.9).

Skeletal manifestations include copper-mediated oxidative damage to collagen and this probably underlies the arthritis that occurs in a small number of patients with Wilson's disease. The secondary effects of renal tubular phosphate leak and hepatic osteodystrophy are likely to be the cause of the radiologic abnormalities such as rickets or osteoporosis that occur in a larger percentage. Pigmentation of the skin, particularly on the shins, and blue discoloration of the bases of the fingernails are other features occasionally seen.

DIAGNOSIS

Biochemistry

The first essential in making the diagnosis of Wilson's disease is to consider it in the first place. A biochemical diagnosis is made by finding two of the following three abnormalities (Fig. 21.10):
- low plasma ceruloplasmin, below 200mg/L (20mg/dL);
- raised urinary copper, greater than 25μmol (155μg)/24 hours following penicillamine administration; and
- hepatic copper greater than 250μg/g dry weight.

Alternatively, the diagnosis may be made on one of the following molecular bases:
- haplotypic identity with a biochemically proven sibling; and
- Wilson's disease mutations.

These approaches are useful in clarifying the diagnosis in difficult patients.

The penicillamine challenge is one of the most useful tests in the diagnosis of Wilson's disease. Basal urine copper is an unreliable parameter, showing both poor sensitivity and poor specificity, although values greater than 5μmol/24h (320μg/24h) are highly suggestive. A penicillamine challenge test gives greater discrimination. Following penicillamine 0.5g 12-hourly × 2, urine copper exceeds 25μmol/24h (1600μg/24h) in 88% patients with Wilson's disease and 2% of those with other liver disorders.

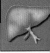

Isotopic copper incorporation studies may be helpful. Following an oral dose of labeled copper, two peaks in plasma activity are seen. The first, peaking at around 4 hours, represents newly absorbed copper that is associated with albumin. The second, a slower rise, represents copper incorporation into ceruloplasmin. Failure of this secondary rise suggests Wilson's disease.

The difficulty with this investigation is the short half-life and limited availability of the radioactive isotopes ^{64}Cu and ^{67}Cu, and the difficulty of assay of the stable isotope ^{65}Cu. In confusing cases this test may be discriminatory. A 24:4 hour activity ratio >1 demonstrates normal ceruloplasmin synthesis and makes Wilson's disease unlikely.

Diagnosis of Wilson's disease		
Parameter	**Normal**	**Wilson's disease**
First line tests		
Plasma ceruloplasmin	>200mg/L (>20mg/dL)	<200mg/L in 85–90% cases
Penicillamine challenge:		
Urine copper pre-penicillamine	>1.25μmol (>80μg)/24h	>3μmol (>192μg)/24 h in 65% cases
Urine copper after penicillamine	<25μmol (<1600μg)/24h	<25μmol/24 h in 90% cases
Hepatic copper	<50μg/g dry weight	>250μg/g dry weight
Contributory tests		
Kayser–Fleischer rings	Absent	Present in neurologic cases
Serum copper	11–24μmol/L	Low, normal, or high (see text)
Serum free copper	<1.6μmol/L (<100μg/L)	>7μmol/L suggests WD
Haplotypes and mutations		See text
Isotopic copper studies		See text
Liver histology		See text

Figure 21.10 Diagnosis of Wilson's disease. Diagnostic parameters for Wilson's disease.

Diagnostic pitfalls in Wilson's disease	
Parameter	**Difficulties in interpretation**
General	Failing to consider the diagnosis
KF rings	Usually absent in children with hepatic presentation At an early stage only detected by slit-lamp examination Difficult to see in brown or green eyes Not pathognomonic – can occur in chronic cholestasis

Serum copper	May be low, normal or high:
	  Low because serum caeruloplasmin is low
	  High if free copper released from necrotic liver

Ceruloplasmin	May be >200mg/L (>20mg/dL) in10% cases, particularly in
	  chronic hepatic inflammation
	May be <200mg/L in 5–10% heterozygotes
	May be <200mg/L in acute liver failure or decompensated
	  cirrhosis from other causes
	Aceruloplasminemia, a cause of dementia in middle
	  adult life

Urine copper	Baseline urine copper values poorly discriminatory
Penicillamine challenge 500mg 12 hourly x 2	Urine copper >25μmol/24 hours gives diagnostic sensitivity and specificity around 90%
Liver histology	Hematoxylin and eosin appearances are suggestive but not diagnostic Copper stains characteristically negative despite high copper
Haplotype analysis	No diagnostic haplotype in UK population Haplotype useful for family screening, but not for primary diagnosis
Mutations	3 commonest mutations only account for 30% alleles
Isotopic copper studies	Radioactive isotopes ^{64}Cu and ^{67}Cu half-life too short for diagnostic use Stable isotope ^{65}Cu difficult to assay

Figure 21.11 Diagnostic pitfalls in Wilson's disease. There are numerous possible pitfalls in the interpretation of tests and the diagnosis of Wilson's disease.

There are numerous pitfalls in the diagnosis of Wilson's disease (Fig. 21.11). The biochemical parameters are robust in the presymptomatic patient and in most neurologic patients, but in those presenting with liver disease there are a number of weaknesses and different clinical scenarios pose different diagnostic traps. Plasma ceruloplasmin is low in the neonatal period, rising to adult levels by 3–6 months of age. Neonatal hepatic copper is raised to values of the order of 400μg/g dry weight (normal <50), falling to adult values by 6 months. The newborn may be described as having temporary functional Wilson's disease. Therefore, in the newborn sibling of a proband Wilson's disease cannot be diagnosed or excluded on biochemical grounds until 6 months of age.

In acute liver failure due to Wilson's disease, rapid diagnosis is essential because of the need to list urgently for transplantation. However, each of the biochemical parameters may be misleading. Hypoceruloplasminemia may be obscured by plasma administration or partially 'corrected' because ceruloplasmin is an acute phase reactant and is temporarily raised. On the other hand a low ceruloplasmin may be found in other causes of acute liver failure because of impaired protein synthesis. Serum copper, low in the Wilson's disease patient before hepatic necrosis, may be elevated, because free (nonceruloplasmin) copper may leak from the necrotic liver. Coagulopathy precludes liver copper estimation. The most valuable measurement is the urine copper concentration, often greatly raised because serum free copper is high. In the patient with acute liver failure suspected to be due to Wilson's disease, a 24h urine collection should be started immediately, proceeding to a postpenicillamine collection in the second 24h.

In Wilson's disease presenting as a chronic hepatitis, the principal difficulty is that chronic inflammation may raise plasma ceruloplasmin to near-normal levels. Histologic appearances in liver may mimic autoimmune hepatitis, while histochemical stains for copper or copper-associated protein may be negative despite high liver copper concentrations. The two most valuable biochemical measurements in this group of patients are the penicillamine challenge and the liver biopsy copper estimation. Liver copper, normally below 50μg/g dry weight, will be elevated in autoimmune hepatitis, but values rarely exceed 250μg/g dry weight, whereas in Wilson's disease it is rare to find values below

250μg/g dry weight. When a liver biopsy is performed in a patient in whom Wilson's disease is a possibility, it is essential that a piece of the biopsy is saved in a sterile dry plastic copper-free container and frozen for subsequent analysis.

Liver histology

The earliest abnormalities in presymptomatic cases comprise ultrastructural changes to the mitochondria, which are pleomorphic, show increased matrix density, separation of the normally apposed inner and outer membranes, and widening of intercristal spaces. The earliest histologic changes comprise microvesicular and macrovesicular fatty deposition, and glycogen-containing vacuoles in the nuclei of periportal hepatocytes; peroxisomes are dense and enlarged. As the disease progresses, portal fibrosis and inflammation develop.

Cases presenting with clinical liver disease may show a histologic picture indistinguishable from chronic aggressive hepatitis with interportal fibrous bridging or frank cirrhosis (Figs 21.12 & 21.13).

Features suggestive of Wilson's disease are:
- fatty change;
- Mallory hyaline;
- glycogen-containing vacuoles in the nuclei;
- lipofuscin;
- copper staining; and
- iron deposition in Kupffer cells in patients who have had hemolysis.

In well-established liver disease, copper may be demonstrable by rhodanine or rubeanic staining (Fig. 21.14). The elastin stains orcein and aldol fuchsin will then usually show granular staining thought to represent lysosomal copper–protein polymer. It cannot be emphasized too strongly that these methods are negative in early cases, presumably because at that stage the copper is cytosolic and in low molecular weight complexes.

Liver copper is elevated to greater than 250μg/g dry weight. In presymptomatic children values may be higher than in older symptomatic cases, which contradicts the common view that in Wilson's disease copper builds up in the liver to a level that causes damage. Rather, it suggests that some other factor initiates damage in the copper-laden liver.

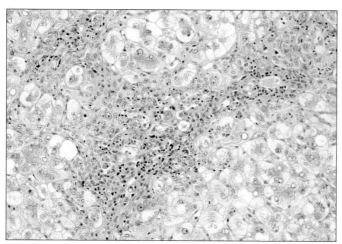

Figure 21.12 Histology of Wilson's disease. The portal tract is inflamed and expanded with some interface hepatitis. The hepatocytes are large, pale staining, and have clear cytoplasm. The nuclei show vacuolation.

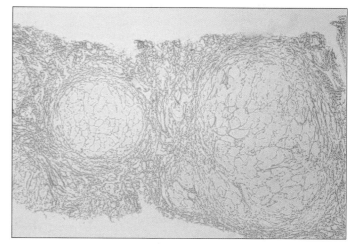

Figure 21.13 Histology of Wilson's disease. The presence of cirrhosis is confirmed using the reticulin stain.

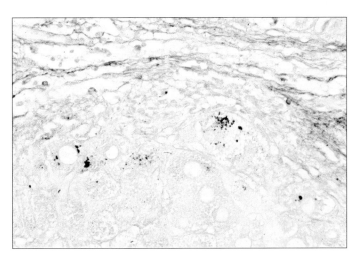

Figure 21.14 Histology of Wilson's disease. The dark granules are copper deposits. Note that the copper staining greatly underestimates the excess of copper in the liver, which should be assessed by weight per gram of dry tissue.

Molecular diagnosis

Haplotype analysis

Through the identification of polymorphic microsatellite markers near to the Wilson's gene, a haplotype may be constructed. Haplotype analysis is only of value in primary diagnosis in those inbred communities among which Wilson's disease is caused by a single mutation or small number of mutations. For example, the eight Wilson's disease patients in three families identified in Iceland (population 265,000) share a common ancestry, a single mutation (2010del7), and the haplotype 11-5-7 or 11-5-4. In the heterogeneous population of north Europe, a large number of haplotypes are found in association with Wilson's disease. The real value of haplotype analysis in the UK is in family studies (see Fig. 21.15). In an informative family, it is possible to determine with certainty whether the siblings of a case are presymptomatically affected, heterozygote carriers, or unaffected, so enabling treatment of cases to commence before damage occurs and avoiding unnecessary treatment of siblings.

Mutation analysis

The Wilson's disease gene has been identified (Fig. 21.16). More than 100 mutations are now recognized, scattered throughout the gene. There is considerable ethnic variability and particular mutations predominate in particular populations. Examples include the 2010del7 Icelandic mutation; two mutations at the same site in exon 8 in Taiwanese families; Arg778Leu and Arg778Gln; and Asn1270Ser in Costa Rica and Sicily. The commonest mutation worldwide is His1069Gln in exon 14, which disrupts the ATP-binding site. At least 40 mutations have been identified in the UK. The three commonest UK mutations, His1069Gln, Gly1266Arg, and Met769Val, only account for 32% of chromosomes.

Most Caucasian patients are compound heterozygotes, while immigrant patients from ethnic minorities where consanguinity is common are frequently homozygous. Mutations vary between ethnic groups; for example, the common mutation His1069Gln is absent in Asian patients. His1069Gln is only found in 12% UK patients compared with 38% in North American, Russian, and Swedish patients.

There is some evidence of a genotype/phenotype relationship. Patients with the 2010del7 Icelandic mutation are quite

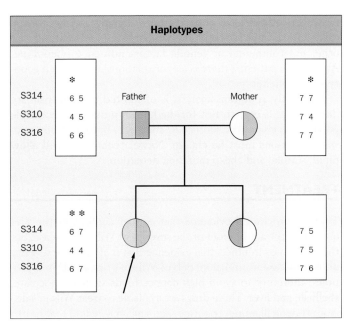

Figure 21.15 Haplotypes. Haplotype analysis in a family with Wilson's disease. The affected child has Wilson's disease genes on chromosomes bearing the markers 6-4-6 and 7-4-7, and has inherited one each of these from each parent. Her sister has inherited neither affected chromosome.

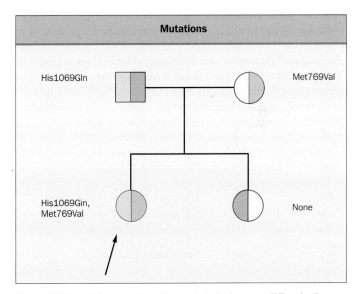

Figure 21.16 Mutations. Mutation analysis in the same Wilson's disease family as shown in Fig. 21.15. The affected child has two Wilson's disease mutations, His1069Gln and Met769Val. She, like most UK Caucasian patients, is a compound heterozygote, whereas many Wilson's disease patients from inbred communities are true homozygotes. She has inherited one mutation from each parent. Her sister has inherited neither mutation.

clinically homogeneous, having a neurologic onset at age 14–25 years. In 10 Dutch patients homozygous for the His1069Gln neurologic presentation occurred at 20.3 years (SD 6.1 years), while six compound heterozygotes with His1069Gln and another mutation presented at 17.8 years (SD 5.8 years) with neurologic or hepatic disease. Costa Rican patients (Asn1270Ser) have a high incidence of acute liver failure.

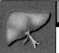

However, others have observed both hepatic and neurologic cases among their His1069Gln homozygotes, and contend that other environmental or genetic factors influence phenotype. Among UK patients, there is a poor relationship between genotype and phenotype.

Currently, mutation analysis is of limited value in primary diagnosis. It is easy to test for the known mutations by simple polymerase chain reaction (PCR) methods, but ethnically relevant mutations must be chosen. Newer technology will allow rapid, simple, and cheap mutation detection.

TREATMENT

There is no clinical evidence that copper content of the diet influences the age of onset or the severity of Wilson's disease, but there is some circumstantial evidence that it affects the severity of liver disease in animal models of Wilson's disease. It is appropriate therefore to avoid high copper foods such as chocolate, shellfish, and liver. Three drugs are available to treat Wilson's disease: D-penicillamine, trientine, and zinc (Fig. 21.17). A fourth agent, ammonium tetrathiomolybdate, remains experimental.

Penicillamine
Although the initial rationale for using penicillamine was to achieve 'decoppering', it is clear that it does not act in this way. Treatment does not cause liver copper levels to fall to normal and cessation of treatment may be associated with clinical relapse with rise in liver copper. Penicillamine 'detoxifies' the copper possibly by inducing metallothionein as a consequence of augmenting the bile pool or by a direct anti-inflammatory action. The dose should be titrated to achieve a significant capriuresis but to avoid toxicity. The toxic effects include:
- skin rash, usually urticarial occurring soon after commencing treatment, and responding to cessation of treatment;
- proteinuria, in most cases mild and not requiring cessation of treatment, but in a small number of patients proceeding to immune complex nephrotic syndrome; and
- bone marrow depression.

Pyridoxine deficiency is a theoretic risk in childhood. A more serious and fortunately rare side effect is systemic lupus erythematosus (SLE).

Trientine
Trientine was initially introduced as a second-line drug for patients intolerant of D-penicillamine. The majority of the side effects associated with penicillamine do not recur when trientine is used, with the exception of SLE. The most commonly reported side effect is sideroblastic anemia. Colitis resolving on cessation of trientine has also reported. Both penicillamine and trientine may cause initial deterioration of neurologic function on commencement of treatment.

Zinc
Zinc, by inducing metallothionein in intestinal cells, reduces absorption and, by inducing metallothionein in hepatocytes, binds copper. It is of low toxicity and cheap, but its principal disadvantage is palatability.

Treatment strategies and outcomes
The initial management of Wilson's disease must be tailored to the clinical presentation (Fig. 21.18). Patients with acute liver failure have a poor prognosis, and must be transferred to a center where they can be listed for liver transplantation. A prognostic score has been found to be helpful in deciding upon the need for transplantation (Fig. 21.19). Serial evaluation distinguishes those patients who are developing irreversible failure and should be listed for transplantation from those in whom medical treatment should be continued. The initial management, and while awaiting a donor organ, includes standard care of the child with liver failure. Acetylcysteine has therapeutic logic since maintenance of glutathione must be important in binding released copper. Chelation with penicillamine and zinc is usually insufficient to rescue the patient with acute liver failure due to Wilson' disease. Attempted physical removal of copper by peritoneal dialysis, exchange transfusion, and hemodialysis have all been tried without great success. Ultrafiltration is probably the most effective technique.

For other presentations of liver disease, there is controversy regarding the optimal treatment. Penicillamine is tried and tested and remains the first-line therapy, a change being made to trientine if side effects occur. Increasingly, however, the

Management of Wilson's disease	
Clinical category	**Management**
Acute liver failure	Transfer to liver transplant center Management of liver failure (chapter *) Acetyl cysteine Hemofiltration Use clinical score to decide about transplant (see Fig. 21.19)

Chronic hepatitis
Acute hepatitis not proceeding
  to liver failure
Hemolysis
	Penicillamine with pyridoxine
	  or trientine
	When liver function improves, zinc

Neurologic presentation	Ammonium tetrathiomolybdate for 8 weeks then penicillamine or zinc
Presymptomatic	Zinc

Figure 21.18 Management of Wilson's disease. This must be tailored to the clinical presentation.

Drugs used in the treatment of Wilson's disease	
Drug	**Dose**
D-penicillamine	20mg/kg per day with pyridoxine 25mg/day
Triethylene tetramine dihydrochloride (trientine)	300mg three times a day
Zinc sulfate or acetate	150–300mg three times a day
Ammonium tetrathiomolybdate	30mg twice a day

Figure 21.17 Treatment of Wilson's disease. Drugs used in the treatment of Wilson's disease.

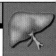

Prognostic index in acute liver failure in Wilson's disease					
Score in points	0	1	2	3	4
Serum bilirubin μmol/L (mg/dL)	<100 (<6)	100–150 (6–9)	150–200 (9–12)	200–300 (12–18)	>300 (>18)
Serum AST IU/L	<100	100–150	150–200	200–300	>300
Prothrombin time: seconds prolonged	<4	4–8	8–12	12–20	>20

Figure 21.19 Prognostic index in acute liver failure in Wilson's disease. A serum bilirubin of 170μmol/L (10mg/dL), an asparate aminotransferase (AST) of 220IU/L, and a prothrombin time 21 seconds prolonged would score 2+3+4=9. A score >7 is an indication to consider transplantation while commencing therapy. Deterioration of serial estimates of the score confirms the need for transplantation.

availability, competitive pricing, and freedom from side effects is being seen as a justification to consider trientine as an appropriate first-choice therapy. Monitoring the effectiveness of, and compliance with chelation therapy is more difficult. Urine copper levels will rise to high values in the first 3 months. With continued treatment the levels decline after 1 year, even though liver copper remains high. After this time, urine copper should be measured 6 monthly. A falling value suggests that the patient may have discontinued the drug, while an unexpectedly very high value may suggest that the patient has restarted it recently in anticipation of the clinic visit. Effectiveness of therapy is monitored by biochemical liver function tests, which should improve steadily over the first months of treatment, and by serial liver biopsy. It is difficult to interpret liver copper levels in follow-up biopsies, since two effects are operative: penicillamine removes that fraction of liver copper which is mobilizable, thus reducing liver copper but both penicillamine and zinc induce metallothionein, which binds copper and may therefore cause liver copper concentration to rise. For this reason, changes in hepatic inflammation are of more significance than changes in liver copper concentration. Likewise, the histologic appearances may deteriorate rapidly despite no significant change in hepatic copper concentration in the patient who discontinues treatment.

With therapy, the prognosis for Wilsonian chronic hepatitis is good; even those with cirrhosis usually remain well and achieve normal liver function tests within 1 year. In contrast to the iron storage disease hemochromatosis, Wilson's disease is rarely associated with hepatoma. Patients with neurologic presentation often deteriorate on commencement of penicillamine. Acute generalized dystonia and akinetic rigid syndrome following penicillamine may be associated with MRI lesions of the thalamus and brainstem that resolve on cessation. In this group, ammonium tetrathiomolybdate has been recommended for 8 weeks followed by penicillamine or zinc. This regimen has not been generally adopted, and is limited by the availability of a ammonium tetrathiomolybdate. Other groups report resolution of this neurologic exacerbation with zinc.

Neurologic abnormalities stabilize and continue to improve with prolonged treatment.

Liver transplantation

Liver transplantation is indicated for patients with acute liver failure and an adverse prognostic score, and for those patients who do not respond to therapy, or who have advanced liver failure and/or intractable portal hypertension. Severe neurologic disease in the absence of liver failure is a controversial indication. While there are reports of significant neurologic improvement after transplantation, in other cases psychiatric changes have worsened.

The results of liver transplantation in Wilson's disease are good. In a series of 39 patients transplanted between 1981 and 1991, survival was 79.4%, although the outcome in those with acute liver failure was less good (73% survival) than those with chronic disease (100%). In another series of patients with acute liver failure, those with Wilson's disease had better results than the group as a whole. Successful live-related donation from the mother is reported. A successful liver transplant restores biochemical indices of Wilson's disease phenotype to normal. There are varied reports of improvement or lack of improvement in neurologic disease after liver transplantation

Pregnancy

Treatment must be continued throughout pregnancy, because of the risk of acute liver failure if it is stopped. The danger of discontinuing treatment during pregnancy has been amply demonstrated. There are numerous reports of successful pregnancy in women treated with penicillamine and trientene. Theoretic considerations suggest that zinc may be a safer option during pregnancy because of possible effects upon collagen synthesis in the fetus. Infants of Wilson's disease mothers present no particular problems. Assuming that there is no parental consanguinity, the risk that the baby had Wilson's disease is approximately 1:300, although all will of course be obligate heterozygotes. In the mouse model of Wilson's disease, pups suckling upon a Wilson's disease mother develop copper deficiency, but this has not been observed in humans.

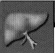

PRACTICE POINT

Clinical case

A 13-year-old male was admitted as an emergency with a 2-week history of jaundice and abdominal distension. He was mildly confused. He had no previous illnesses, but an 11-year-old brother was been seen by a behavioral psychiatrist. The investigations were as follows: serum bilirubin 896μmol/L (53mg/dL) [unconjugated fraction 433μmol/L (25mg/dL)]; aspartate aminotransferase 112IU/L; alkaline phosphatase 110IU/L; albumin 26g/L; international normalized ratio (INR) 2.9; serum creatinine 210μmol/L; and serum sodium 122mmol/L (122mEq/L). Kayser–Fleischer rings were detected on slit lamp examination. The ultrasound examination revealed a small nodular liver, splenomegaly, and ascites.

He was treated with vitamin K, but there was no improvement in the INR. Therefore, he was transferred to a transplant center and was successfully transplanted 2 days later. Four years later he is well and the KF rings have disappeared.

Interpretation

The diagnosis of acute liver failure due to Wilson's disease was apparent from the coexisting anemia and the evidence of hemolysis. Kayser–Fleischer rings were sought on slit lamp examination as they are frequently missed on clinical examination. The radiologic investigations suggested the presence of cirrhosis and portal hypertension, which are usually present with this clinical presentation. Once encephalopathy develops, even in its mildest form, it is an indication for emergency transplantation as medical therapy is ineffective. The excellent outcome is typical of the results of liver transplantation for Wilson's disease. The younger brother was confirmed as suffering from Wilson's disease and his behavioral problems resolved in first 12 months of therapy with penicillamine.

FURTHER READING

Bellary S, Hassanein T, Van Thiel DH. Liver transplantation for Wilson's disease. J Hepatol. 1995;23,373–81. *Results of liver transplantation in a sizeable cohort.*

Berghella V, Steele D, Spector T, Cambi F, Johnson A. Successful pregnancy in a neurologically impaired woman with Wilson's disease. Am J Obstet Gynecol. 1997;176:712–4. *Describes an approach to the management of pregnancy.*

Brewer GJ, Johnson V, Dick RD, et al. Treatment of Wilson disease with ammonium tetrathiomolybdate: II. Initial therapy in 33 neurologically affected patients and follow-up with zinc therapy. Arch Neurol. 1996;53:1017–25. *Authoritative paper on the use of ammonium tetrathiomolybdate in Wilson's disease.*

Bull PC, Thomas GR, Rommens JM, Forbes JR, Cox DW. The Wilson disease gene is a putative copper transporting P-type ATPase similar to the Menkes gene. Nature. Genet. 1993;5:327–37. *Landmark study in the hunt for the gene linked to Wilson's disease.*

Da Costa CM, Baldwin D, Portmann B, et al. Value of urinary copper excretion after penicillamine challenge in the diagnosis of Wilson's disease. Hepatology. 1992;15:609–15. *The penicillamine challenge in the diagnosis of Wilson's disease.*

Dening TR, Berrios GE. Wilson's disease: clinical groups in 400 cases. Acta Neurol Scand. 1989;80:527–34. *Large and valuable clinical study.*

Faa G, Nurchi V, Demelia L, et al. Uneven hepatic copper distribution in Wilson's disease. J Hepatol. 1995;22:303–3. *A reminder that liver copper may vary between biopsies taken from different lobes of the liver.*

Hoogenraad TU. The history of Wilson's disease. In: Warlow CP, van Gijn J, eds. Wilson's disease, major problems in neurology, 30. London: Saunders, 1996:1–13. *Good review of early history, and of population studies.*

Hoogenraad TU, Howen RHJ. Prevalence and genetics. In: Warlow CP, van Gijn J, eds. Wilson's disease, major problems in neurology, 30. London: Saunders; 1996:14–24. *Another good review of epidemiology and genetics.*

Lyon TDB, Fell GS, Gaffney D, et al. Use of a stable copper isotope (^{65}Cu) in the differential diagnosis of Wilson's disease. Clin Sci. 1995;88:727–32. *Description of radioisotope techniques in the diagnosis of Wilson's disease.*

Maier-Dobersberger T, Mannhalter C, et al. Diagnosis of Wilson's disease in an asymptomatic sibling by DNA linkage analysis. Gastroenterology. 1995;109:2015–18. *Use of haplotype analysis for diagnosis in siblings.*

Nagano K, Nakamura K, Urakami KI, et al. Intracellular distribution of the Wilson's disease gene product (ATPase7B) after *in vitro* and *in vivo* exogenous expression in hepatocytes from the LEC rat, an animal model of Wilson's disease. Hepatology. 1998;27:799–807. *Interesting animal model for Wilson's disease.*

Sallie R, Chiyende J, Tan KC, et al. Fulminant hepatic failure resulting from coexistent Wilson's disease and hepatitis E. Gut. 1994;35:849–53. *Acute liver failure in Wilson's disease triggered by viral hepatitis.*

Sallie R, Katsiyiannakis L, Baldwin D, et al. Failure of simple biochemical indexes to reliably differentiate fulminant Wilson's disease from other causes of fulminant liver failure. Hepatology. 1992;16:1206–11. *The difficulty in diagnosis of Wilson's disease in acute liver failure.*

Terada et al. Restoration of holocaeruloplasmin synthesis in LEC rat after infusion of recombinant adenovirus bearing WND cDNA. J Biol Chem. 1988;273: 1815–20. *First description of gene therapy in animal model of Wilson's disease.*

Walshe JM. Treatment of Wilson's disease: the historical background. Quart J Med. 1996;89:553–55. *Excellent historic review by the doyen of the disease.*

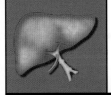

Chapter 22

Metabolic Diseases of the Liver

Richard G Quist, Alistair J Baker, Anil Dhawan and Nathan M Bass

INTRODUCTION

Metabolic disease of the liver is an arbitrary term that encompasses three distinct classes of disorders. Classically, the metabolic diseases of the liver are those that disrupt hepatic metabolic pathways and include specific congenital enzyme deficiencies in the pathways of carbohydrate, lipid, protein, and heme metabolism. These are typically discovered in infancy or early adulthood in which, due to the absence of a specific enzyme, substrate accumulation causes hepatotoxic and/or systemic toxic effects. Examples of these include:

- the glycogen storage diseases;
- disorders of tyrosine metabolism;
- galactosemia; and
- the hepatic porphyrias.

A second class of metabolic liver diseases are those that cause liver disease as a result of secondary systemic effects of the illness. Examples of this class include nonalcoholic steatosis and steatohepatitis (which are strongly associated with systemic disorders including obesity, diabetes, and hyperlipidemia), and genetic disorders such as α_1 antitrypsin deficiency, cystic fibrosis, Wilson's disease, and genetic hemochromatosis. Finally, a third category of metabolic liver diseases is comprised of those having direct effects on the liver through an infiltrative process. These include both primary and secondary forms of amyloidosis in which an abnormal matrix of extracellular material is deposited within the liver.

Patients who have metabolic conditions – previously largely restricted to the pediatric age group – are beginning to survive to adolescence and adulthood, and consequently are coming to the attention of adult gastroenterologists or hepatologists in significant numbers (Fig. 22.1). Care often continues in association with a specialist in metabolic medicine. By the time they are leaving pediatric services, patients with rare congenital conditions and their carers are likely to be well-versed in the nature, management, and problems of their disorder with knowledge gained from support groups, the internet, and personal experience. Among such patients are some with rare conditions that never or almost never present in the adult population, so are extremely unfamiliar to adult practitioners, but for whom continued treatment is essential. Examples include inborn errors of bile acid metabolism, classic galactosemia, hereditary fructosemia, and urea cycle disorders. Others may have undergone liver transplantation because of decompensating liver disease or because the liver is the seat of the inborn error. If well-controlled, such patients may be entire-

ly well and without clinical signs. Nevertheless, the ultimate prognosis with optimal modern treatment may be as yet unknown, and clinical supervision is required to ensure compliance and to monitor for possible complications.

This chapter broadly reviews common metabolic diseases of the liver as defined by these criteria, including fatty liver, nonalcoholic steatohepatitis (NASH), amyloidosis, α_1 antitrypsin deficiency, glycogen storage diseases, and the hepatic porphyrias. Other metabolic diseases of the liver including urea cycle defects, hemochromatosis, Wilson's disease, cystic fibrosis, and specific microvesicular fatty liver diseases are discussed elsewhere.

FATTY LIVER DISEASE

Fatty liver or hepatic steatosis is a common finding on liver biopsy and represents accumulation of lipid within hepatocytes. It is a common finding in liver biopsies and most cases are attributable to excessive alcohol intake. It may also occur in association with obesity, noninsulin-dependent diabetes mellitus (NIDDM),

Metabolic disorders in adults
With liver disease and specific treatments
Tyrosinemia Galactosemia Hereditary fructosemia Urea cycle disorders Inborn errors of bile acid nucleus synthesis
With extrahepatic manifestations for which liver transplantation may be required
Alpha$_1$-antitrypsin deficiency (PiZZ) Cystic fibrosis Hyperlipidemias Hereditary porphyrias Hyperbilirubinemias Propionic acidemia Primary oxaluria
Survivors of conditions usually having a poor prognosis in childhood
Mitochondrial respiratory chain disorders Niemann-Pick types A, B and C Gaucher's disease Wolman's disease

Figure 22.1 Metabolic disorders in adults. Increasingly metabolic disorders are becoming relevant to adult gastroenterologists because of improved survival and recognition.

hyperlipidemia, and drugs such as estrogens and corticosteroids. Fatty liver is, in general, benign. However, certain causes of liver fat accumulation are associated with a necroinflammatory process (i.e. NASH). This, in turn, carries a small risk of progression to chronic liver disease and cirrhosis. Since liver enzyme tests are included on routine chemistry panels, most patients with fatty liver are identified by findings of mild abnormalities of either serum aminotransferase or the cholestatic enzymes (γ-glutamyl transferase, alkaline phosphatase) activities in otherwise healthy individuals. Features consistent with fatty liver may also be found incidentally on an ultrasound or CT scans of the abdomen. Right upper quadrant pain may be a presenting symptom and has been reported in up to 20% of patients.

Pathogenesis

Fatty liver occurs as a result of accumulation of lipid products, predominantly triglycerides, within hepatocytes. Triglycerides are stored mainly in adipose tissue. Fatty acids are released from these stores into plasma by a hormone-sensitive lipase. Uptake of fatty acids by liver occurs via first-order kinetics as a function of blood concentration of fatty acids and may involve plasma membrane-associated carrier proteins. Fatty acids are also synthesized in the liver from acetate derived from glucose and amino acid metabolism. Disposition or metabolism of fatty acids occurs by two major routes in the hepatocyte (Fig. 22.2). Fatty acids may either be esterified to form triglycerides, phospholipids, and cholesteryl esters, and are subsequently exported to plasma with apoproteins as very low density lipoprotein (VLDL). Alternatively, they may be catabolized via fatty acid oxidation. Fatty acid oxidation occurs predominantly within the mitochondria (where fatty acid oxidation is coupled to ATP production for energy) and, to a lesser extent, in hepatic peroxisomes.

Peroxisomes contain oxidative enzymes and oxidize long-chain and very-long-chain fatty acids. Since the capacity of oxidative routes is limited, and since hepatic uptake of fatty acids is dependent on blood concentration, the liver is highly predisposed to fatty acid and hence triglycerides accumulation.

Causes

Fatty change in the liver may be categorized histologically as either microvesicular steatosis, where fat is present within numerous small vacuoles in the hepatocyte (small droplet); or macrovesicular steatosis with coalescence of fat vacuoles into large droplets, peripheral displacement of the hepatocyte nucleus, and alteration of hepatocyte morphology to the extent that it may resemble an adipocyte. These two morphologic types have specific causes (Fig. 22.3). Microvesicular steatosis occurs in the clinical setting of acute insults to hepatic metabolism. These include acute alcohol intoxication, acute fatty liver of pregnancy, and the effects of drugs and toxins such as aspirin and tetracycline. A common mechanism underlying microvesicular steatosis is acute impairment of fatty acid oxidation with subsequent rapid accumulation of fatty acids within hepatocytes.

Macrovesicular steatosis occurs in more chronic disease states such as chronic alcoholism, obesity (defined as greater than 10% of ideal body weight), adult onset diabetes, particularly if poorly controlled, chronic protein-calorie nutritional deficiency such as kwashiorkor, and chronic use of certain drugs including amiodarone, corticosteroids and, less commonly, estrogen therapy. Until recently, another common cause of macrovesicular steatosis was jejuno-ileal intestinal bypass surgery for morbid obesity. The 'J-I' bypass procedure was frequently performed until the mid-1970s. With this procedure, patients develop microvesicular fatty changes of the liver within weeks postoperatively, followed by steady pro-

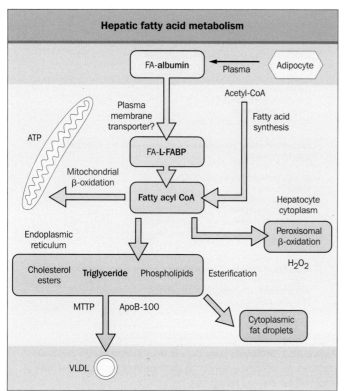

Hepatic fatty acid metabolism

Figure 22.2 Hepatic fatty acid metabolism. The accumulation of fat, predominantly triglyceride, in the liver reflects an imbalance between the rate of formation from fatty acids and the rate of secretion from the liver as very low density lipoprotein (VLDL). Fatty acids (FA) are activated to fatty acyl coenzyme A (CoA) on the surface of the mitochondria and endoplasmic reticulum. This intermediate, shown in the center of the diagram, is the activated form of fatty acid. Because of their limited solubility, long chain FA are transported in the plasma bound to albumin. Fatty acids enter the hepatocyte after dissociation from albumin and cross the plasma membrane possibly via a transporter facilitated mechanism. Once in the liver cell, the FA are bound to cytoplasmic liver FA binding protein (L-FABP). Under normal conditions of FA supply, FA are directed toward the mitochondria oxidation, which drives ATP synthesis, or to the endoplasmic reticulum for triglyceride, phospholipid, and cholesteryl ester biosynthesis. Under conditions of increased FA load or impaired mitochondrial β-oxidation, more FA is directed toward triglyceride biosynthesis, which may cause fatty liver, and towards extramitochondrial pathways of oxidation, mainly the β-oxidation pathway in the peroxisomes. The perioxomal pathway does not generate ATP, but hydrogen peroxide (H_2O_2). Triglyceride export from the liver occurs in the form of triglyceride-rich VLDL. VLDL assembly depends upon a supply of phospholipid, apolipoprotein B-100 (ApoB-100), and the microsomal triglyceride transfer protein (MTTP). Impairment of VLDL synthesis and secretion lead to fat accumulation in the hepatocyte. Examples include abetalipoproteinemia, which results from a gene defect in MTTP, and choline deficiency, which impairs phospholipid synthesis.

Causes of hepatic steatosis	
Microvesicular fat	**Macrovesicular fat**

Inborn errors:
  Mitochondrial β-oxidation
  Urea cycle enzyme deficiency
Acute fatty liver of pregnancy
Reye's syndrome
Drugs and toxins
  Salicylate
  Tetracycline
  Valproic acid
  Amiodarone*
  Perhexiline maleate
  Dideoxyinosine
Acute alcohol ingestion
	Chronic alcohol ingestion*
	Type II diabetes*
	Obesity*
	  Previous J-I bypass*
	Hyperalimentation*
	Protein-calorie malnutrition
	Limb lipodystrophy *
	Corticosteroids
	Abetalipoproteinemia *
	Wilson's disease
	Azitothymidine (AZT)

Figure 22.3 Clinical conditions that cause hepatic steatosis. These are subdivided into those predominantly causing microvesicular or macrovesicular steatosis. *Indicates conditions commonly associated with either steatosis or steatohepatitis.

gression to macrovesicular fatty change. If uncorrected, a substantial proportion of these patients may progress to steatohepatitis, cirrhosis, and end-stage liver disease. This is the main reason why the procedure has largely been abandoned.

Natural history

In most instances, fatty liver does not cause significant hepatic dysfunction, and is associated with a good prognosis. Exceptions to this rule include patients with ongoing toxic or metabolic insult to the liver, including those with chronic, excessive alcohol ingestion, treatment with drugs such as amiodarone, or the rare patient with an uncorrected J-I bypass. These circumstances carry a significant risk of progression to hepatic fibrosis and, ultimately, to end-stage liver disease. For those patients with fatty liver not associated with ongoing ingestion of alcohol or medications, a recent study of 26 patients followed for 10 years with repeat liver histology found that only one patient progressed to early fibrosis while no patient had developed cirrhosis or end-stage liver disease.

Treatment for fatty liver disease includes identification of the cause, removal of any toxic insult, and correction or control of the underlying metabolic abnormality. In patients with obesity, gradual, sustained weight loss has been shown to improve steatosis visualized on ultrasound with normalization of liver function tests. One small study of the effect of weight loss in obese patients also found histologic regression of steatosis.

NONALCOHOLIC STEATOHEPATITIS

Fatty liver with inflammation occurring in the absence of a history of significant alcohol use is termed nonalcoholic steatohepatitis (NASH). The term NASH was originally coined in 1980 as a histologic diagnosis described as macrovesicular fat with inflammatory changes including a polymorphonuclear infiltrate, usually with the presence of Mallory's hyalin. Histologically, it is identical to alcoholic hepatitis. A major clinical difference between NASH and simple fatty liver described in the previous

section is the potential for progression to hepatic fibrosis and cirrhosis in patients with NASH. Because NASH can progress to cirrhosis, it should be considered in the differential diagnosis of liver function test abnormalities or chronic liver disease in patients without other readily identifiable causes.

The prevalence of NASH in the general population has not been defined. However, studies of patients in Western countries undergoing diagnostic liver biopsy have reported NASH in 7–9% of total liver biopsies performed. In one autopsy series, NASH was found in 6% of 351 nonalcoholic patients. In Asia, and particularly Japan, the prevalence is very low, being seen in only 1–2% of liver biopsies performed. The average age at diagnosis is in the fifth and sixth decades. Nonalcoholic steatohepatitis has generally been considered to be more common in women. However, more recent autopsy data indicate that the condition may be more evenly distributed between the sexes. The diagnostic criteria for NASH are listed in Fig. 22.4.

Pathogenesis

The mechanisms of fat accumulation in the liver have been described in the previous section on fatty liver disease. The processes that stimulate inflammatory changes in the liver parenchyma in patients who have NASH have not been completely defined. There is evidence that steatosis alone is associated with lipid peroxidation, which may incite an inflammatory response. Malondialdehyde, an end-product of lipid peroxidation in the liver, has been shown to be proinflammatory in several ways. These include serving as a chemoattractant for neutrophils, inducing production of proinflammatory cytokines (including TNF-α and interleukin-8) and stimulation of stellate cells to produce collagen which leads to hepatic fibrosis. A second product of lipid peroxidation, hydrogen peroxide, has been shown to produce highly reactive oxygen free radicals in the liver in the presence of iron. Free radicals are known to be proinflammatory and are thought to play a role in stellate cell stimulation of collagen production. A role for iron accumulation in the liver has been suggested in the pathogenesis of NASH. An over-representation of the C282Y HFE gene mutation associated with hemochromatosis has been reported in some series of patients with NASH. This suggests a potential role for iron in the etiology of NASH and the basis for a genetic predisposition.

Diagnostic criteria for NASH	
History	Exclusion of significant alcohol use

Laboratory	Absence of viral markers for hepatitis B
	  and C viruses
	Negative markers for hemochromatosis,
	  autoimmune hepatitis, exclusion
	  of Wilson's Disease, primary biliary cirrhosis

Liver histopathology	Macrovesicular and/or microvesicular steatosis Mixed neutrophilic and mononuclear infiltrate Mallory's hyalin Focal hepatocellular necrosis +/– fibrosis

Figure 22.4 Diagnostic criteria for nonalcoholic steatohepatitis (NASH). The diagnosis of NASH is made on a combination of clinical, laboratory and histologic criteria. (Adapted from Neuschwander-Tetri BA, Bacon BR. Med Clin North Am. 1996;80:1147–64.)

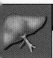

Clinical features

The clinical features of patients with NASH are outlined in Fig. 22.5. Patients who have NASH commonly do not present with specific symptoms. More than half of the patients are asymptomatic. Chronic right upper quadrant abdominal pain is a common complaint and occurs in about one-third. Less commonly, patients complain of generalized abdominal fullness and nausea. Physical findings are nonspecific and include hepatomegaly in about 30–40% of patients. Signs of portal hypertension are indicative of progression to cirrhosis. This contrasts with the portal hypertension that frequently occurs in alcoholic hepatitis, to which hepatocyte ballooning and secondary sinusoidal occlusion are important contributors, and portal hypertension in alcoholic hepatitis is often, at least partially, reversible.

The typical biochemical abnormalities in patients with NASH are shown in Fig. 22.5. Although considered to be insensitive indicators of the presence of NASH, aminotransferase activity tends to be mildly to moderately elevated. One autopsy series of patients with obesity revealed that nearly half of patients with histologic findings of NASH had normal aminotransferase activity. The pattern of the abnormality of the liver function tests tends to be milder than that in alcoholic hepatitis. Additionally, unlike alcoholic hepatitis, in NASH, alanine aminotransferase (ALT) is greater than aspartate aminotransferase (AST) activity with a ratio of 1.5:1. Evidence of cholestasis, including elevated serum bilirubin concentrations, is not common in patients with NASH unless they have advanced disease.

Associated clinical conditions

Clinical conditions that have been identified in association with hepatic steatosis are listed in Figure 22.3.

Obesity

Obesity is present in more than 70% of patients with NASH and is the greatest risk factor for the development of steatohepatitis.

In one study, 18.5% of patients with obesity had NASH, whereas only 2.5% of nonobese, nonalcoholic individuals had NASH at autopsy. When patients were categorized by grade of obesity (based on the percentage over ideal body weight), the prevalence of NASH was proportional to the grade of obesity. In childhood, NASH occurs almost exclusively in children with morbid obesity.

Noninsulin-dependent diabetes mellitus

Adult onset diabetes mellitus is a major risk factor for the development of NASH and is seen in 35–75% of patients. Diabetes is associated with a 2.6-fold increase in the prevalence of NASH over that of nondiabetics. Treatment with insulin is an independent risk factor for the development of NASH in diabetic patients. One study found that 20% of patients with NASH were insulin-requiring NIDDM (type II diabetic) patients, whereas 8.2% had diabetes treated with oral agents alone. Patients with insulin-dependent (type I) diabetes are not at increased risk for developing NASH. Hyperinsulinemia rather than hyperglycemia in NIDDM is thought to play a predominant role in the pathogenesis of NASH in this clinical situation.

Hyperlipidemia

Hyperlipidemia is present in 21–80% of patients who have NASH, but has not been shown to be an independent risk factor for its development. In certain types of lipodystrophy, chronic, abnormal mobilization of fat from peripheral stores causes a massively increased flux of fatty acids through the liver. These conditions are associated with NASH and progression to end-stage liver disease.

Jejuno-ileal bypass

The J-I (jejuno-ileal) bypass procedure was frequently performed for morbid obesity until the mid-1970s, when it became evident that it carried a substantial risk for the development of NASH with a greater potential for progression to cirrhosis. The precise cause of NASH in patients with previous J-I bypass procedures is unknown. Effective protein-calorie malnutrition and chronic, excessive mobilization of fatty acids from adipose tissue are thought to be contributory causes. However, mechanisms specific to the J–I bypass procedure must exist since other procedures inducing rapid weight loss, including rapid starvation diets and stomach stapling, have not been shown to cause NASH. Unlike other causes of steatosis, J-I bypass may result in rapidly progressive hepatic failure in 2–5% of patients.

Diagnosis

The diagnosis of NASH is based on the combination of histologic findings on biopsy and clinical history. Patients with abnormal liver function tests with suspected NASH should undergo a work-up to exclude other potential etiologies including viral hepatitis, chronic alcohol ingestion, metabolic diseases including hemochromatosis or Wilson's disease, autoimmune hepatitis, or drug-induced hepatitis. If biochemical signs of cholestasis are present, including elevated serum bilirubin levels, patients should undergo an ultrasound examination of the liver. Quantities of greater than 75–100g of alcohol on a weekly basis should raise concern that alcohol is the major contributing factor in patients with evidence of liver disease.

Right upper quadrant ultrasound of the liver should be performed as part of the work-up for abnormal liver function tests and is sensitive for detecting fat in the liver. Fatty change in the

Clinical and laboratory features of patients with NASH		
Age at diagnosis	Usually between 40–60 years Childhood subset 10–18 years	
Sex	Female to Male ratio 3:1	
Associated conditions	Obesity > 10% over IBW	70–100%
	Diabetes	35–75%
	Hyperlipidemia	20–80%
Symptoms	None	48–100%
	Right Upper quadrant pain	
	Generalized abdominal pain	
	Weakness and fatigue	
Laboratory features	Two- to threefold increase in plasma aminotransferase levels Normal or mildly elevated alkaline phosphatase levels Normal serum albumin, prothrombin time and bilirubin Possible elevation of serum ferritin	

Figure 22.5 Clinical and laboratory features of patients with NASH. The typical patient is a middle-aged, obese female, often asymptomatic and with coexisting diabetes mellitus or hyperlipidemia. IBW, ideal body weight. (Adapted from Sheth SG, et al. Ann Intern Med. 1997;126:137–45.)

liver characteristically appears as diffusely increased echogenicity throughout the liver parenchyma. Findings consistent with fatty liver by ultrasound are not specific and do not distinguish simple fatty change from NASH or even early cirrhosis. Computed tomography scanning reveals diffuse low-density changes in the liver in comparison to the spleen. Usually, this appears diffusely throughout the liver parenchyma. However, focal fatty change may be present in up to one-third of patients. The threshold for performing a liver biopsy in patients suspected of having NASH should be high, given the low risk of progression to cirrhosis and the fairly good diagnostic accuracy of combining a good clinical assessment with noninvasive tests. Typical histologic findings include varying degrees of hepatocellular steatosis, lobular inflammatory cell infiltrates, and often the presence of Mallory's hyalin or fibrosis (Figs 22.6 & 22.7).

Natural history and prognosis

Nonalcoholic steatohepatitis is considered to have a good prognosis in most patients, but data on the long-term natural history are lacking Most studies on the natural history of NASH have been retrospective analyses of small numbers of patients. Five- and 10-year probabilities of survival were reported at 67 and 59%, respectively, for 65 patients with NASH compared with 38 and 15%, respectively, for those with alcoholic hepatitis. Another

study of 49 patients with NASH found no significant changes in liver function over a 4-year period. In a follow-up study of 28 patients assessing histologic changes after a mean of 5 years after initial diagnosis of NASH, 3% showed improvement, 54% were unchanged, and 43% had histologic progression of liver disease. One patient developed liver failure secondary to NASH in this study. Previous studies of risk factors for NASH have shown that patients with greater than one risk factor for developing NASH have more severe histologic disease. This suggests that patients with more severe forms of obesity and diabetes are more likely to progress to cirrhosis.

Management

The management of NASH is dependent on both the severity and number of risk factors and on the severity of the histologic findings. In morbidly obese patients, weight loss and control of the underlying hyperlipidemia is advisable, particularly if there is evidence of fibrosis on liver biopsy. Weight loss should be gradual, as rapid weight loss may worsen steatohepatitis and could result in liver failure. In patients with diabetes, there is little evidence that tight glycemic control alters the course of disease. Nonetheless, patients with NASH and diabetes should maintain good glycemic control. Cessation of any potential drugs or toxins that may contribute to the development of NASH is clearly of importance.

Ursodeoxycholic acid may be beneficial for patients who have NASH but data are limited. One study of oral ursodeoxycholic acid with and without oral clofibrate for hyperlipidemic patients was performed. Patients underwent histologic and biochemical follow-up at 1 year. Interestingly, patients treated with ursodeoxycholic acid alone had significantly improved liver function tests as well as less hepatic steatosis on liver biopsy. However, no substantial improvement in the degree of inflammatory activity or fibrosis was noted.

ALPHA-1 ANTITRYPSIN DEFICIENCY

Alpha-1 antitrypsin deficiency is an autosomal recessively inherited disease, and is the most common genetic metabolic disease of the liver and is a common indication for liver transplantation in the pediatric population. Alpha-1 antitrypsin is synthesized and secreted by the liver and to a lesser extent in macrophages. It is present in tears, duodenal fluid, saliva, nasal secretions, cerebrospinal fluid, pulmonary secretions, and milk. It serves to inactivate a variety of proteases including trypsin, chymotrypsin, elastase, and proteases present in neutrophils. The homozygous form of the deficiency (PiZZ) is associated with the development of liver disease and cirrhosis in about 15–30% of both adult and pediatric patients. Recent evidence suggests that heterozygous forms such as PiZ, PiMZ, or PiSZ may also contribute to end-stage liver disease.

Epidemiology and pathogenesis

Alpha-1 antitrypsin deficiency occurs most commonly in Caucasians, particularly those of Northern European descent. In Scandinavians, the PiZZ phenotype is present in 1 in 1700 individuals. In the USA, data from eight separate studies suggest that the prevalence of α_1-antitrypsin deficiency is approximately 1 in 1800–2000 individuals. The disease is exceedingly rare in Hispanic, black, or Asian people.

Histologic findings in NASH	
Histologic findings	Percentage
Fatty change	100
Mild to moderate hepatocyte necrosis	96
Neutrophilic infiltrate	100
Mononuclear infiltrate	84
Mallory bodies	49
Fibrosis	65
Cirrhosis	16

Figure 22.6 Histologic findings in NASH. The mandatory fat and neutrophil infiltration are associated with a number of other features including fibrosis and cirrhosis. (Reproduced from Lee RG. Human Pathol. 1989;20:594–98.)

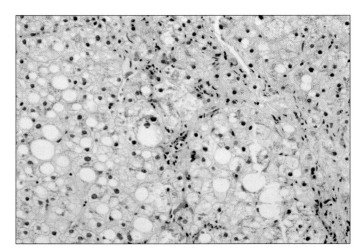

Figure 22.7 Liver histologic findings in NASH. Changes of both microvesicular and macrovesicular fatty change are present with a mild periportal neutrophilic infiltrate.

The gene for α_1-antitrypsin deficiency is 12.2kb long and is located on chromosome 14q31. It is polymorphic, encoding more than 75 allelic variants. Twenty of these alleles are associated with mild liver or lung disease, but only the Z and M (Malton) alleles are associated with end-stage liver disease.

Following synthesis of the protein, it is glycosylated in the endoplasmic reticulum prior to extracellular transport through the Golgi apparatus. In the genetic defect, the protein itself is normally produced in the endoplasmic reticulum, but abnormal glycosylation prevents transport of the enzyme to the extracellular matrix. The exact mechanism of liver injury is unknown. One theory proposes that liver damage occurs as a result of diminished serum α_1-antitrypsin levels and a proteolytic imbalance. A second theory suggests that liver damage occurs secondary to an abnormal immune response. Lymphocytes from infants with α_1-antitrypsin deficiency have been shown to produce a cytotoxic response to isolated hepatocytes. The third and more widely accepted theory proposes that over-accumulation of the protein within hepatocytes causes direct hepatocyte injury.

Clinical features

Neonatal jaundice and elevation of aminotransferase activity occur in 10% of homozygotes and a subset of these will progress to chronic liver disease and cirrhosis as adults. In infants presenting with neonatal cholestasis, α_1-antitrypsin deficiency is the second most frequent diagnosis after biliary atresia in populations of European descent. The mean age of onset of symptoms occurs at 2–3 weeks of age, but may occur anytime in the first 4 months. Jaundice usually lasts 2–3 months, but may last as long as 1 year. Physical findings include hepatosplenomegaly in up to 50% of symptomatic infants. The biochemical profile usually includes both signs of cholestasis and of hepatocellular damage. Once the cholestatic picture resolves, up to 70% of children with the deficiency will have persistently elevated aminotransferase activity. Liver disease may also be first discovered in late childhood or early adolescence. The affected child may present initially with signs of advanced liver disease, including portal hypertension with ascites or variceal hemorrhage.

The frequency with which adults develop liver disease secondary to α_1-antitrypsin deficiency is not clear. It is estimated that 10% of adults with homozygous deficiency will develop cirrhosis and end-stage liver disease. This is similar to the frequency, estimated at 5–10%, with which patients develop advanced pulmonary emphysema. Approximately two-thirds of adults who are homozygous for the disorder will be recognized medically at some point during their lifetime, while the remaining one-third of patients will remain completely asymptomatic. Adults may also present with cirrhosis and the rapid onset of portal hypertension, including ascites and variceal hemorrhage. Patients with cirrhosis secondary to α_1-antitrypsin deficiency have a very high incidence of hepatocellular carcinoma. In a cohort study of 94 autopsy cases of homozygous patients, the mean age of death from all causes was 58 years. Cirrhosis was present in 40% at the time of death, and 40% of cases with cirrhosis had primary liver cancer. Signs of chronic obstructive pulmonary disease were present in 50% of patients with cirrhosis.

Recent evidence suggests that the heterozygous phenotype may also play a role in the development of cirrhosis. A retrospective study of patients with end-stage liver disease referred for transplantation, reported a significantly greater frequency of phenotypes PiMZ and PiMS in patients with cirrhosis secondary to hepatitis C, alcoholic liver disease, hepatitis B, and hepatocellular carcinoma, suggesting a potential role for heterozygous forms of disease to predispose patients to cirrhosis and liver cancer in the setting of other causes of liver disease.

Diagnosis

Diagnostic tests for α_1-antitrypsin deficiency are listed in Fig. 22.8.

Serum levels of α_1-antitrypsin are useful in screening patients suspected of having the disease and provide evidence of deficiency when serum levels are 25% less than the lower limit of normal (usually 80mg/dL). However, the sensitivity of the serum protein level is low because α_1-antitrypsin is an acute phase reactant and elevated levels occur in various inflammatory states. Serum protein electrophoresis is useful in the setting of suspected disease since patients with the disorder have a marked reduction or absence of the α_1-globulin band. Percutaneous liver biopsy can be helpful in establishing the diagnosis in homozygotes. Histology reveals characteristic periodic acid–Schiff positive, diastase resistant globules in the endoplasmic reticulum of hepatocytes (Fig. 22.9). Alpha-1 antitrypsin phenotyping, by isoelectric focusing or immunofixation, should be performed in all cases of suspected disease and is the gold standard for establishing the diagnosis. Prenatal diagnosis may be made by genotype analysis via chorionic villous sampling, but this is rarely performed in practice. The phenotype of both parents should be established before genetic counseling.

Diagnostic tests for α_1-antitrypsin deficiency

Serum α_1-antitrypsin level <25% lower limit of normal

Serum protein electrophoresis with decreased α_1-globulin level

Immunofixation with phenotype analysis

Figure 22.8 Diagnostic tests for α_1-antitrypsin deficiency. Alpha-1 antitrypsin protein levels are used to screen for the disease, but the diagnosis is based on phenotypic analysis.

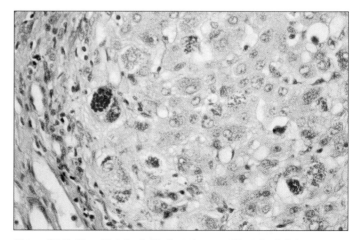

Figure 22.9 Liver histologic findings in α_1-antitrypsin deficiency. Abnormal α_1-antitrypsin deposits within the cytosol of hepatocytes shown by periodic acid–Schiff diastase stain.

Management

The management of patients with α_1-antitrypsin deficiency in the absence of chronic liver disease is largely supportive, including minimizing potential insults to the liver with avoidance of alcohol, maintaining adequate nutrition, and avoidance of smoking for the prevention of lung disease (Fig. 22.10). Some studies have suggested that breast-feeding neonates with the disease until the end of the first year of life is beneficial because it provides replacement of the enzyme in breast milk from maternal macrophages. Likewise, some benefit from ursodeoxycholic acid treatment in cholestatic neonates with the disorder has been suggested by small, nonrandomized trials. Liver transplant remains the only treatment for advanced disease. In the pediatric population, a study of 29 children transplanted for the disease showed an 80% 5-year survival, independent of the severity of disease before transplantation. Other experimental therapies include synthetic androgens, such as danazole, which can raise serum α_1-antitrypsin levels by 50%. Inhaled α_1-antitrypsin has been suggested to be safe for patients with pulmonary disease but does not normalize serum levels of the protein. This therapy has not been evaluated in patients with liver disease. Finally, gene replacement therapy using viral vectors has shown promise in short term correction of α_1-antitrypsin deficiency in animals, but this approach has not yet been tested in humans.

Management strategies for α_1-antitrypsin deficiency
Adequate nutrition
Oral supplementation with fat soluble vitamins
Abstinence from smoking and alcohol
+/- Ursodeoxycholic acid (neonatal cholestasis)
+/- Antioxidants - vitamin E
Orthotopic liver transplantation in end stage disease

Figure 22.10 Management of α_1-antitrypsin deficiency. The strategies range from nutritional manipulation to liver transplantation.

GLYCOGEN STORAGE DISEASE

Glycogen is the principle form of carbohydrate storage in the body and maintains glucose homeostasis during periods of fasting. In addition, during times of physiologic stress, glucagon and epinephrine (adrenaline) rapidly rise and cause glycogen breakdown to glucose for utilization. The formation and breakdown of glycogen is highly regulated by specific sets of enzymes predominantly in the liver, but also in muscle. In glycogen storage disease (GSD), enzymatic deficiencies at specific steps in the pathway of glycogen metabolism cause impaired glucose production and accumulation of abnormal glycogen in the liver. GSDs are rare, occurring in 1 in 100,000 births. Of the total of 12 recognized enzyme deficiencies associated with GSD, three (I, III, and IV) account for the majority of cases of clinical disease (Fig. 22.11). The mechanisms of the clinical and biochemical sequelae of GSD are outlined in Fig. 22.12.

Pathophysiology

Glycogen exists as a series of glucose molecules linked by hydroxyl groups at two specific locations on the glucose molecule: the 1,4 and 1,6 positions. The 1,4 linkage makes up 92–95% of the glycogen molecule. When the 1,4 position is hydrolyzed, a molecule of glucose-6-phosphate is released for further metabolism. The clinically important enzyme deficiencies that make up the GSDs include specific defects in glucose-6-phosphatase (types Ia and Ib), amylo-1,6-glucosidase also known as debranching enzyme (type III), and (-1,4-glucan-6-glycosyl transferase or branching enzyme (type IV). As a result of these defective steps in glycogen metabolism, abnormal forms of glycogen accumulate in the liver causing organ damage. Hepatocellular adenomas may develop in patients with GSD types I and III, and rarely progress to hepatocellular carcinoma. One study reported hepatic adenomas in 52% of patients with type I and III GSD. Although no patient developed hepatocellular carcinoma in this series over a 5-year duration, given the frequency of adenoma formation, the authors recommended that GSD patients receive routine follow-up with biannual ultrasound.

Clinicopathologic characteristics of hepatic glycogen storage diseases				
Type	Name	Deficient enzyme	Clinical manifestations	Treatment
I	Von Gierke's	Glucose-6-phosphatase	Hypoglycemia Lactic acidosis Hyperlipidemia Hyperuricemia	High carbohydrate diet Nocturnal enteral feedings Liver transplantation
III	Debrancher enzyme deficiency	Amylo-1,6 glucosidase	Mild hypoglycemia Hepatic fibrosis Muscle cramping Cardiac myopathy	High protein diet Liver transplantation
IV	Branching enzyme deficiency	β-1,4-glycosyl transferase	Early hepatic fibrosis Neuromuscular hypotonia Mild hypoglycemia	High protein diet Liver transplantation

Figure 22.11 Clinicopathologic characteristics of hepatic glycogen storage diseases (GSD). Summary of the clinicopathologic characteristics and treatment of GSD.

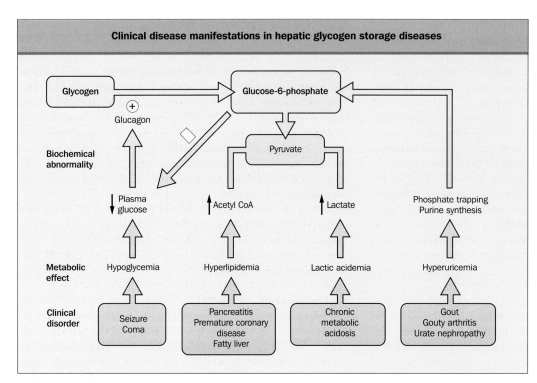

Figure 22.12 Clinical disease manifestations in hepatic glycogen storage diseases. Schematic illustration of the of the pathophysiologic mechanisms that lead to clinical disease manifestations in glycogen storage diseases.

Major types of glycogen storage disease

Glycogen storage disease types Ia and Ib

Type I GSD is caused by ineffective or absent glucose-6-phosphatase activity in the liver. It is divided into type Ia, which occurs due to genetic deficiency of glucose-6-phosphatase, and type Ib, which is due to deficiency of glucose-6-phosphate translocase that transports glucose-6-phosphate into the endoplasmic reticulum where it is metabolized by glucose-6-phosphatase. Patients with this disorder depend on dietary carbohydrate to maintain euglycemia. Presentation usually occurs within 3 weeks of birth, and is typically related to symptoms of hypoglycemia. These include lethargy, poor feeding tolerance, or in more advanced cases, seizures or coma. Blood glucose levels usually fall to about 850μmol/L (50mg/dL) after a 2–3 hour fast. During a prolonged fast, or development of infection, blood glucose may fall as low as 170–250μmol/L (10–15mg/dL). Findings on physical examination in children include marked hepatomegaly with variable splenomegaly. By ultrasound, the kidneys are typically enlarged secondary to abnormal glycogen deposition within renal parenchyma. Adults with the disorder may suffer complications of chronic renal disease. Type Ia GSD in children typically results in poor growth and delayed puberty. Nearly all adults are below the 50th centile for stature. Hyperuricemia develops secondary to chronic systemic carbohydrate deficiency and may cause complicated gouty disease or urate nephropathy. Hyperuricemia occurs due to the utilization of alternate pathways for the synthesis of ATP. This leads to chronically or acutely elevated levels of inosine, which then become metabolized to uric acid. The development of recurrent gout, gouty arthritis, and urate nephropathy have been described in adults with GSD I. Other causes of renal disease, particularly in older adult patients, include recurrent renal stones, pyelonephritis, and direct toxic effects of glycogen deposition.

Lipid abnormalities, including hypercholesterolemia and hypertriglyceridemia, occur frequently and are related to a relative increase in production of precursors of fatty acids from the glycolytic pathway and increased hepatic delivery of fatty acids. The latter stems from chronic adipose tissue triglyceride breakdown in response to a persistently elevated glucagon to insulin ratio. Serum triglyceride levels may be elevated to more than 6000mg/dL, causing episodes of acute pancreatitis. Total cholesterol typically remains in the 400–600mg/dL range, and premature coronary artery disease has occurred in young adults.

Hepatic adenomas are present in at least 75% of adults with GSD I and are often multiple in number. The cause is unknown but may be related to chronic hyperglucagonemia. Adenomas are typically 1–5cm in size; the mean age of development is 12–17 years of age. Of 27 patients with GSD I and hepatic adenomas, malignant transformation to hepatocellular carcinoma was observed in one patient.

A distinguishing feature of patients with GSD Ib is recurrent neutropenia and secondary bacterial infections. These may present as mild infections including otitis media, recurrent sinusitis, and stomatitis. Life-threatening infections including staphylococcal brain abscess and systemic fungemia have also been described. Treatment with granulocyte colony-stimulating factor (GCSF) may be required in these patients.

Diagnosis

The dramatic clinical features of GSD I often suggest the diagnosis in childhood. However, a percutaneous liver biopsy and direct measurement of glucose-6-phosphatase activity from hepatic tissue is necessary for definitive diagnosis. Carbohydrate challenge with oral galactose and fructose will demonstrate the absence of an increase in blood glucose levels.

Treatment

The goal of treatment in patients with GSD is prevention of adverse clinical effects of chronic disease by maintaining a normal blood glucose through adequate carbohydrate balance. Total par-

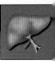

enteral nutrition is useful as treatment for metabolic derangements during decompensation and has been shown to improve growth rate in adolescents. However, this form of treatment is impractical for long-term feeding and carries risks of adverse events including catheter-related infection and sepsis. Additionally, chronic total parenteral nutrition may worsen underlying liver disease. In pediatric patients with early disease, successful treatment has been achieved by nocturnal feedings with high carbohydrate (cornstarch) enteric feeds via nasogastric feeding tube or gastrostomy during sleep. This, in conjunction with high carbohydrate meals consumed at frequent intervals (every 2–3 hours) during the day, have successfully prevented decompensation in pediatric patients and adults with severe forms of disease. Glucose requirements usually lessen as patients enter adulthood. Most adults are able to sustain carbohydrate balance with frequent daytime feedings alone.

Type III glycogen storage disease

In amylo-1,6-glucosidase (debrancher) deficiency, the glycogen molecule is a polymer of glucose subunits with 90% connected by 1,4 linkages with the remaining connected in the 1,6 position, creating branching points in the molecule. The debranching enzyme (amylo-1,6-glucosidase) moves the glucose subunits to the 1,4 position, and is deficient in GSD III disease. Type III GSD is characterized by accumulation of abnormal glycogen molecules in the liver. A distinguishing feature of this glycogenosis is the direct toxic effect of this abnormal form of glycogen in the liver, with the development of hepatic fibrosis and progression to end-stage liver disease.

Clinical presentation

The clinical manifestations of this disease are similar to those in patients with GSD I. However, metabolic manifestations related to carbohydrate deficiency are mild in comparison with GSD I. The usual presentation occurs in mid to late childhood or early adulthood. Symptomatic hypoglycemia is uncommon in adults with GSD III. Biochemical abnormalities including hyperuricemia and hyperlipidemia also tend to be milder. However, in GSD III disease, the development of glycogen deposit-related restrictive cardiomyopathy is common and has been described in up to a third of patients.

The diagnosis may be suggested by liver histology and confirmed by direct measurement of debranching enzyme activity using ^{14}C-labeled glucose. Hepatic fibrosis is common and occurs in 10–20% of patients with GSD III disease. However, progression to end-stage liver disease is uncommon. Treatment is similar to that in type I disease, including frequent, high carbohydrate meals and nocturnal feedings in more severe disease.

Type IV glycogen storage disease (amylopectinosis)

Type IV glycogenosis is a rare disorder caused by absence of the branching enzyme in glycogen synthesis. In this disorder, the glycogen molecule is markedly abnormal with long outer and inner chains of glucose units with formation of an amylopectin-like polysaccharide. Deposition of this form of glycogen in the liver leads to hepatic fibrosis and cirrhosis early in life with a median survival of 1 year following diagnosis. The natural history of this rare disease is adequately described in only 20–30 cases. Clinical symptoms typically begin during the first year of life and include failure to thrive, hepatosplenomegaly, abdominal distension, and signs of hepatic dysfunction and muscular hypotonia. Examination of the liver demonstrates pale, basophilic deposits within hepatocytes, and micronodular cirrhosis with broad bands of fibrous tissue. Treatment remains undefined, but clinical improvement has been seen with high protein, low carbohydrate feedings. Liver transplantation offers the only possibility of cure. Regression of amylopectin deposits in cardiac and peripheral muscles has been noted following liver transplantation.

HEPATIC PORPHYRIAS

The porphyrias are a group of metabolic disorders caused by genetic deficiencies of enzymes in the biosynthetic pathway of heme (Fig. 22.13). The heme molecule is a component of many proteins, including hemoglobin, myoglobin, cytochrome P450 enzymes, and electron transport cytochromes. Heme is synthesized mainly in the bone marrow (75–80%) and liver (15–20%). Current evidence favors the accumulation of heme precursors rather than a deficiency of heme as the cause of the clinical disease. The intermediates in the pathway of heme are known as porphyrins and normally have no known physiologic effects. There are a total of eight major enzymatic steps in the synthetic pathway of heme, and deficiency of any enzymatic step with exception of the first results in a specific form of porphyria. Fig. 22.13 outlines the enzymatic steps of heme biosynthesis, including the clinical porphyrias resulting from the known defects in these steps. Although the precise mechanisms of symptoms are unknown, elevated levels of porphyrins have toxic effects on neural and cutaneous tissue and are associated with a constellation of symptoms in these two organ systems.

Acute porphyrias are characterized by recurrent, severe attacks of neurovisceral symptoms including severe abdominal pain, nausea, vomiting, and neuropsychiatric disturbances. Cutaneous porphyrias, in which porphyrins are deposited in skin, are characterized by photosensitivity and characteristic vesiculobullous skin lesions.

Due to their unique and often dramatic presentations, the prophyrias have received popular attention in the past. Porphyrias have been proposed to have caused disease in such prominent figures as King George III and Vincent van Gogh, and have been fancifully speculated as the basis for mythologic creatures such as vampires and werewolves.

The most common forms of porphyria that are likely to be encountered by the primary care physician include:
- acute intermittent porphyria;
- porphyria cutanea tarda; and
- erythropoietic protoporphyria.

Acute porphyrias

The acute porphyrias include acute intermittent porphyria, hereditary coproporphyria, variegate coproporphyria, and δ-aminolevulinic acid (ALA) dehydratase deficiency. The symptoms are often severe and include recurrent and dramatic neurologic attacks with a wide variability and number of symptoms, including nausea, vomiting and abdominal pain, peripheral paresthesias and weakness, and even ascending paralysis or quadriplegia. Neuropsychiatric symptoms associated with acute porphyria are very common and include depression, acute psychoses, hallucinations, seizures or coma. The acute episodes may be precipitated by several factors that induce the hepatic P450

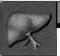

Heme biosynthesis pathway and the porphyrias

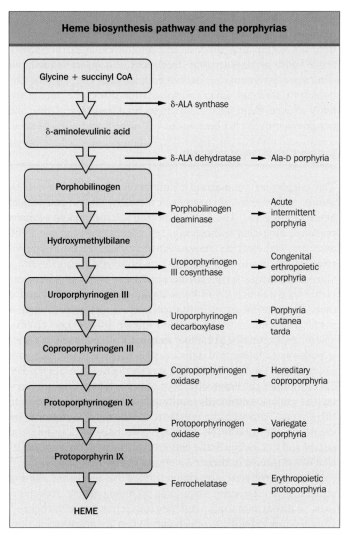

Figure 22.13 Heme biosynthesis pathway and the porphyrias. Heme biosynthesis pathway-specific enzyme deficiencies associated with the various types of porphyria.

Medications precipitating acute attacks of porphyria

Barbiturates	Griseofulvin
Estrogens	Imipramine
Phenytoin	Nifedipine
Sulfonamides	Progestogens
Chloramphenicol	Rifampin (rifampicin)
Chlordiazepoxide	Spironolactone
Diazepam	Theophylline
Ergot derivatives	Tolbutamide

Figure 22.14 Precipitants of porphyria. Medications associated with acute attacks of porphyria. (Reproduced from Scarlett YV, Brenner DA. J Clin Gastrol. 1998;27:192–8.)

extremities or even bulbar paralysis with respiratory involvement leading to death. Hyponatremia has been documented during acute attacks and may contribute to seizure activity. Medications that induce the cytochrome P450 enzymes, are common precipitants of acute attacks of AIP. Other factors that can contribute include premenstrual hormonal changes in females, prolonged fasting or rapid weight loss due to starvation diets.

The diagnosis of AIP is based on the identification of elevated urinary excretion of the porphyrin precursors δ-aminolevulinate (ALA) and porphobilinogen (PBG).

Prevention is the major goal in the management of acute attacks of porphyria. Individuals at risk should avoid excessive alcohol intake, drugs that induce the P450 enzyme system and prolonged periods of fasting. The treatment of AIP includes general supportive measures with intravenous fluids, narcotic analgesics for pain, and antiemetics if indicated. Intravenous dextrose solutions and intravenous heme therapy may be effective to diminish symptoms and duration of hospital stay if given early in the acute phase. These measures act by decreasing the activity of ALA synthase and reducing porphyrin precursor synthesis.

Hereditary coproporphyria and variegate porphyria
Hereditary coproporphyria (HCP) and variegate porphyria have clinical manifestations that include both neurologic and cutaneous symptoms. The former is autosomal dominant and is associated with the coproporphyrinogen oxidase deficiency. The neurologic symptoms of HCP tend to be more mild than acute intermittent porphyria. Clinical symptoms of HCP are identical to those of AIP, but also include photosensitivity, which does not occur with AIP. Photosensitivity is manifested as vesiculobullous lesions in sun-exposed areas and occurs in about 30% of patients with HCP. The biochemical picture of acute attacks of HCP is dominated by a dramatic increase in fecal excretion of coproporphyrin in addition to increased urinary PBG and ALA excretion. As with patients with AIP, treatment involves symptomatic relief with antiemetics, intravenous dextrose solutions, and intravenous heme. Identifying specific precipitants of acute attacks, most commonly medications that stimulate the cytochrome P450 enzymes, is key in the prevention of recurrent disease.

Variegate porphyria is a rare autosomal dominant disorder that occurs due to a heterozygous deficiency of protoporphyrinogen oxidase. The clinical symptoms are identical to those of other acute porphyrias, but variegate porphyria is characterized clinically by more severe photosensitive skin disease as well as a propensity to develop acute neurovisceral crises. Photosensitivity dominates the

enzyme system in the liver including alcohol, smoking, and specific medications including barbiturates, sulfonamides, corticosteroids, and sex steroid hormone replacement (Fig. 22.14). Attacks may also occur in the absence of specific stimuli.

Acute intermittent porphyria
Acute intermittent porphyria (AIP) is the most common of the acute porphyrias and is associated with porphobilinogen deaminase deficiency. It is transmitted genetically with autosomal dominance and incomplete penetrance. The typical age of onset is after puberty or in young adulthood, and it is more common in women than men. The incidence of AIP is higher in the psychiatric population where it has been reported to occur as frequently as 2.1 per 100,000.

The clinical syndrome is exclusively neurovisceral and neuropsychiatric without development of cutaneous lesions. Abdominal pain occurs in 85–95% of patients with AIP. Other common symptoms are secondary autonomic hyperactivity characterized by excessive sweating, nausea, vomiting, and tachycardia. Severe attacks may lead to life-threatening complications including refractory seizure, motor neuropathy with paresis of the

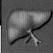

symptom complex in approximately 85% of patients.

Cutaneous porphyrias

The cutaneous porphyrias are caused by excess porphyrin deposition into the dermal basement membrane and capillaries. Light absorption in the 400–410nm range causes porphyrin excitation, generation of reactive oxygen species, and subsequent severe local inflammation. The typical lesions are vesicular or bullous and may be accompanied by hypertrichosis or pigment changes, which may be both increased or decreased, and white papules (milia).

Porphyria cutanea tarda

Porphyria cutanea tarda (PCT) is the most common of the porphyrias. Patients usually present in young adulthood. Lesions on the light-exposed skin, particularly the dorsa of the hands and the face, are the only consistent clinical feature of PCT. It may be inherited with an autosomal dominant pattern, but more commonly is acquired. Acquired forms of PCT are associated with alcoholism, iron overload, chronic renal failure, systemic lupus erythematosus, diabetes, human immunodeficiency virus, hepatitis C, and oral estrogens. Several forms of chronic liver disease are more common in patients with PCT, including infection with hepatitis B and C viruses, Wilson's disease, and hereditary hemochromatosis. A recent study of patients with PCT revealed that 73% of the patients carried a mutation of the HFE gene. About 42% of these patients were either heterozygous or homozygous specifically for the C282Y mutation of the HFE gene.

Liver disease is common in PCT. Most patients present with mild elevation of aminotransferase or alkaline phosphatase activities. Clinical evidence of liver disease at the time of diagnosis is rare. Histologically, most liver biopsies obtained in patients with PCT demonstrate evidence of iron deposition, mild fatty infiltration, and periportal inflammation. The frequency of cirrhosis is unclear but is seen in less than 15% of patients. Cirrhosis in association with PCT carries a higher risk of hepatocellular carcinoma than other causes of cirrhosis. Characteristic findings of PCT on histologic examination of the liver include increased concentrations of uroporphyrin, which often dramatically appear as crystals when examined with red fluorescence in long-wave ultraviolet light and are characteristic for PCT. The diagnosis is supported by the presence of up to greater than 100-fold increases in the urinary excretion of uroporphyrin.

Protoporphyria

Protoporphyria occurs as a result of deficiency of ferrochelatase, the last enzyme of the heme biosynthetic pathway. It is an autosomal dominant disorder. Clinical symptoms begin in early childhood and are characterized by photosensitivity with itching, painful erythema, and diffuse edema (Fig. 22.15). Vesicles and bullae, present in other forms of cutaneous porphyria, are absent in protoporphyria. Patients have a tendency to form protoporphyrin gallstones. Liver disease is common in protoporphyria and approximately 15–20% of patients will develop hepatic dysfunction, which may present as acute liver failure associated with marked accumulation of protoporphyrin in the liver. The diagnosis may be established by finding elevation of free erythrocyte protoporphyrin levels, but this is not a widely available assay. Protoporphyrin levels are elevated in both erythrocytes and feces. Urinary excretions of ALA and PBG are normal. The diagnosis is confirmed by measuring quantitative plasma, red blood cell, and fecal protoporphyrin. Treatment for this form of porphyria includes cholestyramine, which is thought to reduce photosensitivity by increasing protoporphyrin fecal excretion and interfering with the enterohepatic circulation of protoporphyrin. Oral β-carotene at doses of 120–180mg daily in adults is protective against photosensitivity reactions.

Patients with severe acute or advanced liver disease may be candidates for liver transplantation, although it is not considered curative since excessive porphyrin is produced mainly in the bone marrow, and may lead to recurrent disease.

Approach to the diagnosis of the porphyrias

The choice of screening tests depend upon the category of porphyria symptoms (Fig. 22.16). In the acute setting, particularly in patients with acute abdominal pain or other clinical features suggesting acute porphyria, establishing the diagnosis of porphyria is of more importance than determining the specific enzyme defect since the treatment is largely the same. For neurovisceral symptoms, the key rapid screening test is a qualitative test for PBG in the urine. If positive, the excretion of PBG and δ-ALA should be quantitated in a 24-hour urine collection. The majority of patients with acute porphyrias will markedly overexcrete PBG in urine. For symptoms of cutaneous porphyrias, a screening test for porphyrins in the urine is the most useful initial test. Protoporphyria is an exception in which elevated protoporphyrin levels are only measured in the stool.

INHERITED DISORDERS OF BILIRUBIN METABOLISM

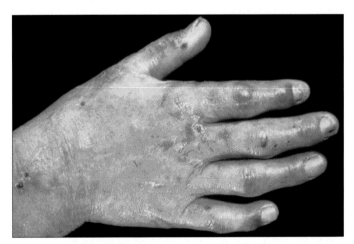

Figure 22.15 Porphyria. Hands of a patient with porphyria.

Laboratory diagnosis of porphyrias	
Type of porphyria	Diagnostic test
Acute intermittent porphyria	Urine PBG, ALA and porphyrins
Hereditary coproporphyria	Urine PBG, ALA and porphyrins Fecal coproporphyrin
Variegate porphyria	Urine PBG, ALA and porphyrins Fecal protoporphyrin
Porphyria cutanea tarda	Urine uroporphyrin
Erythropoietic porphyria	Red cell and fecal protoporphyrin

Figure 22.16 Porphyria. Diagnostic tests for porphyrias.

Bilirubin is mostly derived from breakdown of the heme moiety of hemoglobin. Unconjugated bilirubin is poorly water soluble but highly lipid soluble. Free unconjugated bilirubin in higher concentration is neurotoxic and may cause kernicterus at any age. In order to avoid the toxicity of bilirubin, it is carried to the liver bound with albumin for conjugation and subsequent excretion in bile. The conjugation of bilirubin with glucuronic acid is dependent on the microsomal enzymes, uridinediphosphoglucuronoside glucuronosyltransferases (UDPGs). Conjugated bilirubin is hydrophilic and is excreted across the biliary canaliculi into bile. Various inherited defects have been recognized as affecting either the conjugation or subsequent biliary excretion of bilirubin. The defects that affect the conjugation process lead to syndromes of unconjugated hyperbilirubinemias, while excretory defects cause conjugated hyperbilirubinemias.

Crigler–Najjar syndrome type I

Crigler–Najjar syndrome type I (Fig. 22.17) is a rare disorder that presents in the early neonatal period with severe unconjugated jaundice due to lack of the enzyme UDPG. The inheritance is autosomal recessive with worldwide occurrence. The clinical examination is essentially normal apart from the presence of deep jaundice. The standard tests of liver function are normal. The bile is usually pale due to absence of bile conjugates. The diagnosis is confirmed by documenting absence of UDPG in liver by enzyme assay. The mainstay of treatment in infants is phototherapy for up to 18 hours a day to avoid kernicterus. Phototherapy with ordinary fluorescent tube lights has helped a few patients to reach adulthood. Phototherapy imposes severe restrictions of lifestyle and also becomes less effective with increasing age. Liver transplantation has been performed to avoid kernicterus and reduce dependence on phototherapy with good effect. Auxiliary orthotopic liver transplantation appears more attractive and is equally effective in normalizing bilirubin levels, but with an added advantage of native liver acting as safety net in case of graft failure. Hepatocyte transplantation into the liver has also been attempted with partial success.

Tin protoporphyrin, a bilirubin-lowering agent, has also been used with variable success. The ultimate treatment is likely to be gene therapy in the native liver. Gene therapy has been successful in reducing bilirubin levels in Gunn rat, which is the animal model for this disorder. Its clinical application in human beings is eagerly awaited. Sudden increase in bilirubin should be managed with plasmapheresis or exchange blood transfusions as kernicterus can also occur in adults. Although there are no data available as to the safe level of unconjugated bilirubin in adults, levels of more than 400μmol/L (23.5mg/dL) may be toxic. Appropriate contraceptive advice should be given to sexually active females as high maternal unconjugated bilirubin can cross the placental barrier and cause kernicterus in the fetus. If contraception fails, termination of pregnancy is the only option as normal fetal development is not expected. Prenatal diagnosis is available in families with affected children.

Crigler–Najjar syndrome type II

Crigler–Najjar syndrome type II (see Fig. 22.17), first described in 1962 as chronic unconjugated hyperbilirubinemia in adults, is caused by partial deficiency of UDPG activity. Serum bilirubin is usually less than 300μmol/L (18mg/dL). The jaundice is usually present from infancy, but onset in adolescence is also reported. Unlike type I patients, neurologic complications are rare unless a sudden increase in bilirubin occurs secondary to infection or surgery. UDPG activity can be induced with phenobarbital or other microsomal enzyme inducers, leading to a decline in bilirubin levels. Recent insights in to the genetics of Crigler–Najjar syndrome have identified patients with type II disease who have a severe phenotype requiring phototherapy and who are at risk for kernicterus, but they are at least partly responsive to microsomal P450-inducing agents.

Gilbert syndrome

Augustin Gilbert, a French physician, described this disorder characterized by persistent mild unconjugated hyperbilirubinemia in 1901 (see Fig. 22.17). The incidence in the general population is between 2 and 7%. The serum bilirubin levels usually range between 20 and 80μmol/L (1.2–4.7mg/dL), increasing during periods of sleep deprivation, prolonged fasting, menstruation, and intercurrent infections. An increase in jaundice is often associated with nausea, malaise, and abdominal pain, but the incidence of these symptoms is similar to a normal control population. The diagnosis is usually suspected during routine medical examination or when blood tests are performed for other medical conditions. The clinical examination is unremarkable except for mild jaundice. Although the hepatic UGDP activity is low in Gilbert syndrome, the available enzyme activity appears to be sufficient to conjugate the daily turnover of bilirubin. The hepatic uptake of radiolabeled bilirubin is shown to be reduced. Hence, the precise mechanism of this disorder is unclear. Molecular studies have shown reduced expression of the UGDP 1 gene due to the addition of two nucleotides thymine adenine (TA) in the promoter region.

The diagnosis can be made by demonstrating an increase in serum bilirubin on a 300kcal diet for 48 hours, or after intravenous injection of nicotinic acid which increases the osmotic fragility of the red cells increasing the bilirubin production, or by demonstration of a reduction in bilirubin levels after administration of microsomal enzyme inducers such as phenobarbitone. However, in practice these tests are seldom required. Liver biopsy is not indicated. No treatment is required, life expectancy is

Clinical and laboratory features of inherited unconjugated hyperbilirubinemias			
Clinical laboratory parameter	**Crigler–Najjar syndrome**		**Gilbert's syndrome**
	Type I	**Type II**	
Inheritance	AR	AR/AD?	AD
Age of onset	Newborn	Newborn	Adolescence
Neurological complications	Common	Rare	Absent
Serum bilirubin μmol/L (mg/dL)	300–700 (18–41)	100–300 (6–18)	20–80 (1.2–4.7)
UGDP levels Reduction	Absent	Moderate reduction	Mild reduction
Response to enzyme inducers	Absent	Present	Present

Figure 22.17 Unconjugated hyperbilirubinemias. Clinical and laboratory features of Crigler–Najjar and Gilbert syndromes.

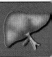

normal, and these individuals carry no extra risk for the purpose of assessment for life assurance.

Inherited disorders that cause predominant conjugated hyperbilirubinemia

Dubin–Johnson syndrome and Rotor syndrome are two inherited disorders that cause mild persistent conjugated hyperbilirubinemia. The clinical examination is essentially normal except for mild jaundice. Standard tests of liver function are also normal. There is defective functional excretion of bilirubin in Dubin–Johnson syndrome while hepatic storage of bilirubin is believed to be impaired in Rotor syndrome. The important features of these syndromes are shown in Fig. 22.18.

GALACTOSEMIA

The defect of galactose-1-phosphate uridyl transferase (GAL-1-PUT) is almost always revealed in the perinatal period when the infant is first exposed to milk feeding. Infants present with vomiting, hepatitis, liver failure, and disseminated intravascular coagulation, usually with sepsis. There may be a history of resolution of symptoms when feeding is discontinued. Hypoglycemia is seen in the majority if sought and when associated with Fanconi nephropathy explains the presence of galactose in the urine, giving the characteristic 'clinistix negative, clinitest positive' side-room test pattern when the infant is receiving feeds. Diagnosis is made from the level of GAL-1-PUT in the infant's red blood cells, remembering the false-negative effect of transfused blood, when a presumptive diagnosis can be made from the parents' heterozygote levels. Early management consists of removal of galactose from the diet and standard management of liver failure and sepsis. Despite the frequent presence of antenatally established liver disease, the prognosis is good except when the diagnosis has been repeatedly overlooked and liver failure or sepsis becomes overwhelming. Cataracts may be present from the neonatal period, and vitreous hemorrhage may have a poor prognosis.

The long-term prognosis with dietary management was once held to be good but it is clear that patients require long-term supervision. Monitoring of patients' understanding of the condition and knowledge of commercial dietary products containing galactose or lactose is required. Specialist cow's milk products, even when advertised lactose-free, may contain traces of lactose. Soymilk products are not contaminated, however. Urinary galactitol and plasma galactose-1-phosphate should be assessed regularly as an index of control and compliance. Poor control may be associated with risk of cataracts and Fanconi nephropathy. The majority of patients have mild neurodevelopmental or educational difficulties, not directly attributable to the quality of their dietary control, but due possibly to the perinatal insults or endogenous galactose production. The possibility of cataracts requires yearly opthalmology review.

Ovarian failure is well-recognized, and some degree of hypogonadism is almost universal for females. Patients without evidence of puberty by 14 years of age or with secondary amenorrhea but who are not pregnant should be referred to an endocrinologist. Pregnancy, although rare, requires particularly close supervision of diet and urine and plasma metabolites, as the fetus may be vulnerable to the toxic effects of galactitol. Transplantation of fertilized ova may be necessary to achieve

Conjugated hyperbilirubinemias		
Features	Dubin–Johnson syndrome	Rotor syndrome
Inheritance	Autosomal recessive	Autosomal recessive
Bilirubin levels	50–85μmol/L (3–5mg/dL) Rarely peaks to 300μmol/L (18mg/dL)	50–85μmol/L
Clinical examination and Liver function tests	Normal	Normal
BSP elimination	Secondary peak at 90 minutes	No secondary peak
Liver morphology	Jet black	Normal color
Liver histology normal	Dark pigment mainly in centrorilobular area	No pigment, normal histology
Oral cholecystography	Gallbladder not seen	Gallbladder seen
Prognosis	Benign condition	Benign condition
Treatment	None	None

Figure 22.18 Conjugated hyperbilirubinemias. Clinical and laboratory features of Dubin–Johnson and Rotor syndromes. BSP, bromsulphalein.

pregnancy. In late pregnancy and during lactation endogenous lactose production is increased resulting in deterioration in disease control with vomiting.

HEREDITARY FRUCTOSEMIA

Fructose aldolase deficiency is a rare cause of hepatomegaly, chronic hepatitis or steatohepatitis. Patients usually have a history of vomiting and failure to thrive from the time of weaning, but occasionally earlier due to the administration of honey as a 'tonic' in infancy in Mediterranean countries. The ubiquity of sucrose in manufactured foodstuffs may make it difficult to establish the relationship between foods and symptoms. Diagnosis is made from enzyme analysis of liver biopsy tissue. Treatment consists of removal of all fructose, sucrose, and maltose from the diet with the assistance of an expert dietitian. Water soluble vitamins, especially vitamin C, should be supplemented. Care should be taken that administered medications, including antibiotics for incidental infections, are sugar-free.

TYROSINEMIA TYPE I

The pathway of tyrosine catabolism is shown in Fig. 22.19. The autosomal recessive inherited fumaryl aceto-acetase deficiency may present early as neonatal jaundice with coagulopathy, often with hemorrhagic disease of the newborn. Infants may have a characteristic smell. There may be evidence of Fanconi nephropathy or hypertrophic cardiomyopathy. The pathognomonic feature is the presence of succinyl acetone, the major toxic metabolite of tyrosine in the urine. A second smaller group of patients presents in the early years of life or rarely early in the second decade. Features can include failure to thrive, metabolic bone disease, evidence of liver disease or hepatoma, or porphyria-like neurologic crises. Alpha-

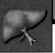

fetoprotein (AFP) is elevated with further increase indicating pre-malignant hepatocyte dysplasia or actual hepatoma. The introduction of 2-(2-nitro-4-trifluoromethylbenzoyl)-1,3-cyclohexanedione (NTBC)-blocking 4-OH phenylpyruvate reductase high in the catabolic pathway has transformed the previously unrewarding treatment. In effect tyrosinemia type 1 is converted to type 2. The latter is without the life-threatening complications, but still risks tyrosine crystal deposition in corneas and skin unless strict protein restriction and monitoring of serum tyrosine below 500µmol/L is maintained. Initiation of treatment is followed by rapid improvement in neurologic and liver features. Alpha-fetoprotein level falls to normal or near normal over weeks to months. The dose should be titrated to suppress succinyl acetone and δ-amino levulinic acid completely. In patients with acute liver failure, failure to clear jaundice is a poor prognostic marker indicating need for liver transplantation. Some may be left with well-compensated cirrhosis. After transplantation NTBC is discontinued, but low levels of renal derived abnormal metabolites may appear in the urine. Long-term follow-up is necessary to monitor control, the progress of any established liver disease, and the possible development of hepatoma. Of 220 patients treated, 90% responded, 5% died, and 5% underwent transplantation. Two cases of hepatoma have been seen in infants within 6 months of starting therapy.

UREA CYCLE DISORDERS

Ornithine transcarbamylase deficiency (OTCD) is the commonest and most characteristic of the conditions, except that its inheritance is X-linked codominant rather than autosomal recessive. Others include carbamyl phosphate synthetase 1 deficiency, argino-succinate synthetase deficiency, and arginase deficiency. Male patients with OTCD can present acutely in the perinatal period with respiratory distress and metabolic alkalosis on starting feeds. However, they may also present in the second decade of life following a large dietary protein load, with vomiting and encephalopathy sometimes mimicking a psychiatric condition. Acute presentation is associated with up to 50% mortality. There may have been previous behavior compatible with a psychiatric syndrome and learning difficulties. There is often a long-standing history of vomiting, particularly precipitated by high protein foods, or of self-restriction of diet perhaps interpreted as 'pickiness'. Hepatitis is frequently present and with coagulopathy may be mistaken for other causes of acute liver failure. Plasma ammonia is usually very high at presentation. Patients who have been managed with intravenous dextrose and fasted prior to admission to a specialist unit may have elevations of plasma ammonia that are not diagnostic, but fall in the range seen with acute liver failure. Plasma orotate is high and urea low. Liver ultrasound may show evidence of steatosis. Diagnosis is confirmed by enzyme analysis of liver biopsy tissue. The normal peak orotic acid level after an allopurinol challenge test is less than 13µmol/L creatinine compared with a range of 26–134µmol/L seen in six patients with urea cycle disorders. Females may be symptomatic to a milder degree with protein aversion, vomiting, and steatohepatitis.

Treatment consists of dietary protein restriction to 1g/kg per day

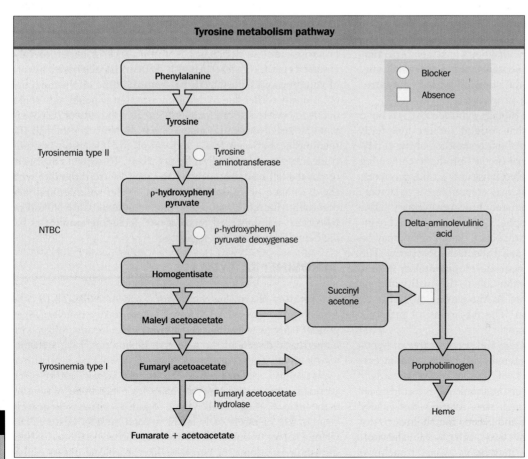

Figure 22.19 Tyrosine metabolism. The pathway of tyrosine metabolism is outlined. Filled rectangles represent blocked enzyme functions and filled circles represent absence of function due to inborn errors of metabolism. Porphyric crises in tyrosinemia result from succinyl acetone blocking heme synthesis with accumulation of δ-aminolevulinic acid which is a false neurotransmitter.

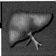

or less with additional vitamins and minerals to compensate for the absence of animal products. Higher protein intake may be permitted during periods of faster growth. Plasma amino acids are monitored to allow adjustment of protein intake. Sodium benzoate or phenylacetate is given to keep serum ammonia within the normal range. The prognosis is good, although severe developmental delay is usual in those with the neonatal presentation. Late presentation is associated with a poor prognosis and in one series only 41% survived and 28% had significant developmental delay, particularly when serum ammonia levels were over 350μmol/L. Persistent hyperammonemia is associated with cerebral atrophy, and neuronal loss. Liver transplantation resulted in good metabolic control in 14 survivors of 16 patients so treated, and although quality of life was good, the neurologic outcome was guarded.

INBORN ERRORS OF BILE ACID NUCLEUS SYNTHESIS

The complex pathways of synthesis of primary bile acids from cholesterol are summarized in Fig. 22.20. Defects are extremely rare and have yet to be precisely characterized. Two conditions 3β-hydroxy-C_{27}-steroid dehydrogenase/isomerase and Δ^4-3-oxosteroid 5β-reductase deficiencies, predominate, but with occasional even rarer or unclassifiable conditions. Patients may present with neonatal liver failure and hemochromatosis, neonatal cholestasis, or chronic cholestasis with metabolic bone disease. The characteristic features of low serum γ-glutamyl transpeptidase and absence of pruritus are not absolute. Diagnosis is made by analysis of plasma and urine bile acid profile on fast atom bombardment mass spectroscopy. Treatment is by downregulating the endogenous bile acid synthesis that results in hepatotoxic products using cholic and chenodeoxycholic acids orally. Ursodeoxycholic acid may also be given to promote resolution of the liver disease. Fat-soluble vitamins are also required initially. Patients treated before the onset of hepatocellular failure or portal hypertension have a good prognosis with full resolution of liver disease possible. Life-long follow-up and treatment are required. Regular plasma bile acid measurement is required to ensure anomalous production is fully suppressed.

PROPIONIC ACIDEMIA

Of patients with propionic acidemia 90% have a defect of mitochondrial propionyl coenzyme A carboxylase deficiency, implying an abnormality involving all tissues. Patients present typically soon after birth with vomiting and coma, with hypoglycemia and acidosis occurring spontaneously or precipitated by infection or protein ingestion. These crises are recurrent. Management is often problematic and is based on a high carbohydrate, low protein diet, and oral antibiotics to reduce gut-derived short-chain fatty acids, in addition to sodium benzoate to reduce hyperammonemia. The prognosis depends on the frequency and severity of crises, including associated neurologic insults. Liver transplantation, either complete or right lobe auxiliary, can abolish crises and allow an unrestricted diet. Patients still have sources of excess propionate such as the kidneys, so that organic aciduria is usual. They may continue to restrict their protein intake voluntarily, indicating continued intermittent nausea from organic acidemia.

PRIMARY OXALURIA TYPE I

In humans, oxalate is an obligate catabolite produced at a rate of about 1–3g/day by the liver. It is also a dietary component of leafy vegetables, rhubarb and strawberries. The enzyme for its catabolism, alanine glyoxylate aminotransferase (AGT), is normally found only in liver peroxisomes, and the deficiency leading to anomalous enzyme production is inherited in an autosomal recessive pattern. Oxalate is nephrotoxic, particularly if crystals are precipitated. The secondary means of its removal is via the kidneys where, since it is poorly water soluble, its rate of removal is dependent on glomerular filtration rate (GFR), rate of urine formation and urinary pH. The typical presentation of primary oxaluria (PO) is in the first or second decade with nephrolithiasis, but occasionally it is diagnosed in infancy. Plasma oxalate is elevated and diagnosis is made by enzyme measurement in liver biopsy material. Liver histology is normal or has minimal nonspecific changes. Early diagnosis can lead to preservation of renal function by maintaining a massive intake of water (up to 10L/day) combined with oral bicarbonate and depletion of oxalate from the diet. Patients with impaired GFR are likely to accumulate oxalate because clearance of oxalate is less efficient than that of creatinine, leading to further renal impairment. Retained calcium oxalate precipitates readily in bone and vascular endothelium so patients with end-stage renal disease may have large amounts of the mineral sequestered with associated arthritis and risk of pathologic fractures. There is debate as to whether calcium restriction is helpful. Low calcium diet can promote oxalate absorption so normal calcium intake is probably indicated. Hypertension is common.

About 20% of cases are pyridoxine sensitive, 50% resistant, and 30% show an intermediate response. High-dose pyridoxine has been associated with neuropathy. The role of transplantation has not yet been fully clarified. In late disease, renal transplantation liberates sequestered oxalate with consequent damage to the graft. Long-term high intensity hemodialysis (at least 50%

Primary bile acid synthesis	
Cholesterol	
Endoplasmic reticulum	Cholesterol 7 alpha hydroxylase **3-β hydroxy-C27 steroid dehydrogenase/isomerase** 12-α hydroxylase
Cytoplasm	**δ-4–3–oxosteroid 5-b reductase** 3-α-hydroxysteroid dehydrogenase
Mitochondria	Sterol C27 hydroxylase (CTX)
Cytoplasm	Alcohol dehydrogenase Acetaldehyde dehydrogenase
Endoplasmic reticulum	Bile acid CoA ligase
Peroxisome	Side chain oxidation **Zellwegger**
Primary bile acids	

Figure 22.20 Primary bile acid synthesis. Cholesterol is the substrate and there is extensive intracellular trafficking of products. Disease states are in bold. CTX, cerebrotendinous xanthomatosis.

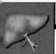
more than for control of serum creatinine) may reduce oxalate load before renal transplantation and protect the graft afterwards. Serum oxalate does not reflect the progress of this treatment in heavily oxalate-loaded patients, presumably because the serum contains only a small fraction of the total pool. Measurement of the dialysate oxalate indicates that 5–6g oxalate is removed per day. Liver transplantation is required as a means to remove oxalate and prevent further synthesis. There has been continued debate as to the relative immunologic benefit of synchronous same donor liver and kidney versus liver followed by kidney transplantation. The ideal management is liver transplantation before there is any evidence of renal damage and the GFR is still normal. The role of auxiliary transplantation appears limited as retained native liver is a source of endogenous oxalate that might contribute to further nephropathy. Patients with intermediate degrees of renal impairment should ideally receive a single donor liver and kidney, as immunosuppressive drugs are likely to cause further renal damage and precipitate renal failure. Patients with established end-stage renal disease are probably best managed by a two-stage procedure with initial liver transplantation followed by renal transplantation once the oxalate load has been reduced. In practice such patients tend to have vascular involvement and represent a very high risk.

MITCHONDRIAL RESPIRATORY CHAIN DISORDERS

This increasingly important cause of liver disease in children has not yet been described as a de-novo cause of liver disease in adults, but is a recognized cause of myopathy. The pediatric experience is brief and the manifestations protean, so it is possible that affected adults will be recognized in due course. Understanding of the condition is confused by the various historic nomenclatures of conditions now known to be of respiratory chain origin, and mitochondrial heteroplasmy so that tissues are affected unpredictably. In addition, the balance of normal to abnormal mitochondria may change in either direction with time. The nature of inheritance in that mitochondrial DNA is inherited mostly from the ova, that is, maternally. There is no 'gold standard' for diagnosing this condition.

Liver disease may be seen as the primary feature or additional to bone marrow, neurologic, endocrine, myopathic. or other manifestations. Prognosis is generally poor, but occasional long-term survivors are seen without severe central nervous system (CNS) or bone marrow disease. Primary liver disease may be as acute liver failure, steatohepatitis, or progressive liver disease including micronodular cirrhosis.

Acute liver failure in mitochondrial respiratory chain disorders (MRCDs) is characterized by a previous history of variable neurologic features including squint, speech or motor delay, or severe cerebral palsy. Epilepsy and the recent introduction of valproate are often background clinical features. Failure to thrive may be seen. Evidence of encephalopathy may be striking early in the course and, in association with mild jaundice, has been described as a 'Reye-like' presentation of this condition. Transaminase levels are initially very high, in the order of thousands or tens of thousands of units. Coagulopathy is rapidly progressive. Hypoglycemia may be present, particularly if there is a secondary defect of fatty acid oxidation. There may be evidence of other organ involvement with Fanconi nephropathy, cardiac, multiorgan or bone marrow failure.

Myoclonic jerks may be present. The above features may be known as 'Alper's syndrome', although the name was originally given to a condition characterized by neuropathologic features.

Serum lactate is elevated but not always in excess of that seen in liver failure of other cause. Elevated cerebrospinal fluid (CSF) lactate may indicate CNS involvement, which may be important diagnostically and prognostically, since it may herald a progressive encephalopathy. Direct measurement of CSF lactate may be prevented by coagulopathy, but indirect measurement of basal ganglion lactate by magnetic resonance spectroscopy may be valuable in deciding management strategies, particularly the exclusion of liver transplantation. Ultrasound of liver may show evidence of steatosis.

Features of chronic liver disease with MRCD are less specific but the above features and particularly bone marrow failure – so-called Pearson's syndrome – are suggestive of the condition. Respiratory chain enzyme analysis of liver and skeletal muscle, tissue, histology and histochemistry of skeletal muscle and analysis of mitochondrial DNA will yield the diagnosis in the majority of cases, but a proportion of patients with classic features of Alper's syndrome lack laboratory confirmation.

No effective specific treatments are available and liver disease should be managed conventionally. Antioxidants, N-acetyl cysteine and ursodeoxycholic acid may be beneficial. Respiratory chain enzyme preparations and cofactors have had anecdotal success, but have not been adopted universally. Avoiding excessive blood transfusion is important in Pearson's syndrome, as iron is a mitochondrial toxin. Often after a protracted course Alper's type of acute liver failure can recover, despite parameters that suggest a grave outcome in other types of liver failure. The patient may still die of the neurologic features or multiorgan failure, but occasional long-term survivors are known.

NIEMANN–PICK A, B AND C DISEASES

Although traditionally classified together because of clinical similarities, these rare conditions may be quite disparate in causation. Types A and B are associated with deficiency of sphingomyelinase in leukocytes or fibroblasts, and type C, of which there are two subtypes, have an enzymically undetermined defect of cholesterol esterification. The responsible genetic defect has been linked to a locus on chromosome 18. A functional defect of cholesterol esterification can be shown and is the confirmatory diagnostic test. All types present most often with neonatal hepatitis or neurologic features. Neurologic storage is absent in type B. Liver, reticuloendothelial, and, if present, CNS storage of lipid substances may have begun before birth. Type A may have storage in other tissues including lungs. In type C, two-thirds present with neonatal liver disease. Nine per cent died of early liver failure. Half of the remainder had persisting clinical liver disease and half had resolution of transaminase but with persisting splenomegaly in excess of other evidence of portal hypertension. The overall mortality is 67%. Progressive neurologic deterioration may be delayed for decades but the mean age of onset was 4.5 years with early features of ataxia, supranuclear opthalmoplegia or loss of cognitive skills, and is predicted by evidence of neuronal storage in ganglion cells of the myenteric plexus obtained by rectal biopsy. Neurologic features are independent of the severity of liver disease. Epilepsy typically occurs later. Adult patients may present with psychiatric features.

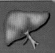

Diagnosis is made on bone marrow aspirate with periodic acid–Schiff-positive, diastase-resistant foamy blue material seen in macrophages (Fig. 22.21). Sphingomyelinase A and B levels in fibroblasts and leukocytes are normal in type C. In addition, the initial tendency to improvement of the liver disease may render the diagnosis of type C difficult until a later presentation with neurologic features. Management is entirely supportive. Bone marrow transplantation is unhelpful for progressive storage in the mouse model of Niemann–Pick disease type C. Liver transplantation has been recorded in a case of NPB. Combined liver and bone marrow transplantation has not been attempted, probably because of concerns that the neurologic disease will progress.

GAUCHER'S DISEASE

Gaucher's disease is the result of deficiency of lysosomal glucoceribrosidase and is the commonest of the lysosomal storage disorders. Types 2 and 3 present as neonatal hepatitis or hepatosplenomegaly, with evidence of storage in liver, and reticulo-endothelial and neurologic tissues. The massive organomegaly is often strikingly out of proportion to other evidence of liver disease, its duration or evidence of portal hypertension. Gaucher cells are sparse and may be difficult to recognize in the liver. Bone marrow aspiration shows the characteristic periodic acid–Schiff diastase-positive histiocytes containing striated material. Diagnosis is confirmed from enzyme levels in leukocytes or fibroblasts. The natural history is of variable neurodevelopmental deterioration with stable or slowly progressive liver disease, bone marrow infiltration with bone pain or fractures, and variable pancytopenia. Bone marrow transplantation has been performed for bone pain and pancytopenia. Treatment with regular infusions of the deficient enzyme has shown early promise in preventing progression of the disease and relieving symptoms.

Type 1 disease is more indolent and the neurologic features may be absent. Presentation may be as late as old age with hepatosplenomegaly, pancytopenia, or rarely features of portal hypertension or decompensation of liver function. Evidence of cardiac and pulmonary infiltration may be present. The serum ferritin may be raised. The liver histology typically shows sparse Gaucher cells, extramedullary hemopoiesis and pericentral fibrosis. Hypersplenism, abdominal discomfort, and pain from splenic infarction may justify splenectomy. Bone marrow and/or liver transplantation may be indicated in specific cases. The long-term benefit of enzyme replacement therapy is unknown.

CHOLESTEROL ESTER STORAGE DISEASE

Classic Wolman's disease presents before 6 months of age with diarrhea, vomiting, failure to thrive, and hepatosplenomegaly. There is no specific treatment and death occurs within months. The condition 'cholesterol ester storage disease' has the same deficiency of lysosomal acid lipase demonstrable (<10% activity) in fibroblasts or leukocytes. A more benign course with diagnosis occasionally delayed until adulthood is seen. Clinical features may be limited to hepatomegaly with splenomegaly of a mild degree in a minority of cases. Patients have hyperlipidemia with high free and esterified cholesterol. There is a predisposition to atheromatous vascular disease. Massive quantities of cholesterol esters and other lipid material are deposited in tissues including liver, reticuloendothelial system, and small intestinal mucosa. The liver biopsy is characteristically orange to the naked eye. Massive hepatocyte steatosis is seen histologically with fat-laden macrophages and septal fibrosis also present in some cases. Some patients have progressive liver disease and develop decompensation of liver function or portal hypertension. There is no specific treatment. Response to cholesterol-lowering agents is poor. Liver transplantation has been performed and may be indicated in cirrhosis when nonliver features are mild.

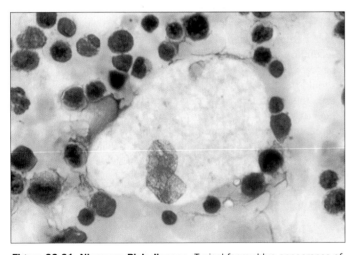

Figure 22.21 Niemann–Pick disease. Typical foamy blue appearance of macrophages or histiocytes.

PRACTICE POINTS

Illustrative case

A 15-year-old boy was suffering from splenomegaly and a 10-year history of a neurologic disorder that included mental retardation, vertical supranuclear gaze palsy, dysarthria, ataxia, and dystonia. Bone marrow aspirates revealed foamy cells with storage materials that were positive with filipin staining. Cultured skin fibroblasts derived from the patient showed moderate loss of sphingomyelinase activity and the impairment of cholesterol esterification.

Interpretation

The characteristic clinical presentations and typical histochemical findings of this patient met the diagnostic criteria of Niemann–Pick disease type C (NPC). In the fibroblasts from the patient, there was an accumulation of GM2 ganglioside around their cytoplasms. Increased levels of glycolipids including GM2 ganglioside are reported in the cerebral cortex of NPC, but not in the fibroblasts. The fibroblasts derived from NPC may reflect the abnormal metabolism of glycolipids in the central nervous system of NPC.

Illustrative case

A 58-year-old obese female with diabetes, hypercholesterolemia, and hypertension complains of intermittent right upper quadrant abdominal pain, and on routine physical examination is found to have an enlarged liver. There is no history of known liver disease, significant alcohol intake or hepatitis. Liver function tests reveal AST of 48 and ALT of 60. Bilirubin, alkaline phosphatase, complete blood count, albumin, and prothrombin time are normal. An abdominal sonogram reveals marked echogenic changes consistent with fatty liver, but otherwise normal liver contour, gallbladder, bile ducts, and spleen. Serologies for viral hepatitis, antimitochondrial antibody, and autoimmune markers are negative.

Interpretation

The management issues are about establishing the diagnosis and whether a liver biopsy should be considered. The patient presents with signs of NASH. She has no evidence of cirrhosis on physical examination and has normal hepatic synthetic function. In this situation there is little to be gained from a liver biopsy. She should be encouraged to gradually lose weight, control her cholesterol through diet and/or medication, and undergo clinical assessment with follow-up liver tests every 6 months.

Illustrative case

A 48-year-old female with moderate obesity and a long history of untreated hyperglycemia is admitted to the hospital after a single episode of coffee ground emesis. Six months earlier, the patient had lost 60lbs in a rapid weight loss program. An endoscopic examination reveals grade III esophageal varices that are not bleeding. Laboratory tests reveal an albumin of 2.6g/dL, a prothrombin time of 17 seconds but otherwise normal liver function tests. There is no history of alcohol abuse according to the patient and her spouse. The patient undergoes treatment for her varices and a percutaneous liver biopsy is performed, which reveals steatohepatitis with stage IV fibrosis.

Interpretation

This patient has signs of advanced liver disease, most likely secondary to NASH. Her disease was possibly aggravated by her rapid weight loss. Other potential causes of liver disease should be assessed by a careful history for significant alcohol use, measurement of markers of viral hepatitis including hepatitis B and C, serologic tests for autoimmune hepatitis, screening for hemochromatosis, and a right upper quadrant ultrasound with Doppler assessment of the hepatic vasculature. Given the patient's advanced liver disease, she should be referred for liver transplantation.

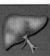

FURTHER READING

Ali M, Rellos P, Cox TM. Hereditary fructose intolerance. J Med Genet. 1998;35:353–65. *Significant genetic study.*

Bacon BR, Farashvash MJ, Janney CG, Neuschwander-Tetri BA. Nonalcoholic steatohepatitis: an expanded clinical entity. Gastroenterology. 1994;107:1103–1109. *Good clinical description of NASH.*

Beutler E. Enzyme replacement therapy for Gaucher's disease. Baillieres Clin Haematol. 1997;10:751–63. *Review of role of effective but expensive therapy for this condition.*

Bunchman TE, Majors H, Majors G, et al. The infant with primary hyper-oxaluria and oxalosis: from diagnosis to multiorgan transplantation. Adv Renal Replace Ther. 1996;3:315–25. *A modern view of the management of this condition.*

Butterworth RF. Effects of hyperammonaemia on brain function. J Inherit Metab Dis. 1998;21(Suppl 1):6–20. *Evidence for the need for close control of liver transplantation.*

Chowdhury JR, Chowdhury NR, Wolkoff AW, Arias IM. Heme and bile pigment metabolism. In: The liver: biology and pathobiology, 3rd edition. Arias IM, Boyer JL, Fausto N, et al., eds. New York: Raven Press; 1994. *Definitive review.*

George DK, Goldwurm S, MacDonald GA, et al. Increased hepatic iron concentration in non-alcoholic steatohepatitis is associated with increased fibrosis. Gastroenterology. 1998; 114:311–8. *Study implicating iron in the pathogenesis of NASH.*

Holme E, Lindstedt S. Tyrosinemia type 1 and NTBC (2-(2-nitro-4-tri-flouromethylbenzoyl)-1,3-cyclohexanedione). J Inherit Metab Dis. 1998;21:507–17. *Recent data on the efficacy of treatment that has transformed this condition.*

James OF, Day CP. Non-alcoholic steatohepatitis (NASH): a disease of emerging identity and importance. J Hepatol. 1998;29:495–501. *Extensive review of NASH.*

Labrune P, Trioche P, Duvaltier I, Chevalier P, Odievre M. Hepatocellular adenomas in glycogen storage disease type I and III. A series of 43 patients and review of the literature. J Pediatr Gastrol Nutr. 1996;24:276–79. *Good review of literature.*

McDonagh AF, Bissell DM. Porphyria and porphyrinology – The past fifteen years. Semin Liver Dis. 1998;18:3–13. *Good review of topic.*

Mowat AP. Alpha 1 antitrypsin deficiency (PiZZ): features of liver involvement in childhood. Acta Paediatr. 1994;393(Suppl):13–17. *Review of the spectrum of disease in childhood.*

Munnich A, Rotig A, Chretin D, Saudubray JM, Cormier V, Rustin P. Clinical presentations and laboratory investigations in respiratory chain deficiency. Eur J Paediatr. 1996;155:262–74. *Description of characteristic disease patterns.*

Rela M, Muiesan P, Andreani P, et al. Auxiliary liver transplantation for metabolic diseases. Transplant Proc. 1997;29:444–5. *Early experience of the application of auxiliary transplantation in metabolic disease.*

Talente GM, Coleman RA, et al. Glycogen storage disease in adults. Ann Intern Med. 1994;120:218–26. *Review of adult perspective of this condition.*

van der Veere CN, Sinaasappel M, McDonagh AF, et al. Current therapy of Crigler–Najjar syndrome type I: report of a world registry. Hepatology. 1996;24:311. *Defines neurologic prognosis in large cohort.*

Vanier MT. Lipid changes in Niemann–Pick disease type C brain: personal experience and review of the literature. Neurochem Res. 1999;24:481–9. *Current data from premier international authority.*

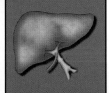

Section 3 Specific Diseases of the Liver

Chapter 23

Pediatric Liver Disease

Deirdre A Kelly

NEONATAL LIVER DISEASE

Jaundiced baby

Almost two thirds of children who have liver disease present in the neonatal period with persistent jaundice. Although physiologic jaundice is common in neonates (Fig. 23.1), infants who develop severe or persistent jaundice should be investigated to exclude hemolysis, sepsis or underlying liver disease. Neonatal jaundice that persists beyond 14 or 21 days should always be investigated, even in breast-fed babies.

Clinical features suggesting liver disease include pale stools and dark urine, dysmorphic features, bruising, petechiae or bleeding, hepatomegaly and/or splenomegaly, slow weight gain or failure to thrive, and previous family history or consanguinity. The differential diagnosis is between extrahepatic biliary disease, the neonatal hepatitis syndrome, and intrahepatic biliary hypoplasia.

Unconjugated hyperbilirubinemia

The commonest causes of unconjugated hyperbilirubinemia are physiologic jaundice or breast-milk jaundice (Figs 23.1 & 23.2), although systemic disease or hemolysis from any cause must be excluded. It is important to establish Coomb's positivity, and glucose-6-phosphate dehydrogenase deficiency, and to exclude red cell membrane defects such as spherocytosis. Systemic sepsis is an important cause of unconjugated hyperbilirubinemia in the early neonatal period and requires prompt treatment with antibiotics, fluids, phototherapy and/or exchange transfusion.

Inherited disorders: Crigler–Najjar type I and II

This autosomal recessive disease is secondary to a deficiency of the hepatic enzyme, bilirubin diglucuronide transferase, which causes high levels of unconjugated hyperbilirubinemia in the perinatal period. In Crigler–Najjar type I peak serum bilirubin levels vary between 15–50mg/dl (250–850µmol/L), whereas in Crigler–Najjar type II peak bilirubin levels are 12–18mg/dl (200–300µmol/L).

Diagnosis

The diagnosis of Crigler–Najaar type I is suspected by the high level of unconjugated hyperbilirubinemia in the absence of other clinical causes. Confirmation may be obtained by aspiration of bile from the duodenum as bilirubin diglucuronides are not present in Crigler–Najjar type I, but small amounts are detected in type II. Liver biopsy to measure enzyme levels is not necessary.

Management

Prompt treatment is required for Crigler–Najaar type I with exchange transfusion and phototherapy to prevent kernicterus. Infants do not respond to phenobarbital (phenobarbitone). Long-term phototherapy is essential, but becomes difficult when 12–16 hours per day are required for school-going children. Auxiliary liver transplantation is now the treatment of choice and effectively reduces bilirubin levels while retaining native liver for future gene therapy. Treatment for Crigler–Najaar type II is not required except for cosmetic reasons, but bilirubin levels reduce on phenobarbital 5–15mg/kg.

Extrahepatic biliary disease

Biliary atresia occurs in 1:14,000 live births worldwide. There is a slight female predominance. The etiology is unknown although the association of biliary atresia with other extrahepatic anomalies suggests an abnormality of the embryologic development of the biliary tree. There is no clear genetic basis despite the association of biliary atresia with trisomy 18 and human leukocyte antigen (HLA)-B12 subtype. Although isolated cases of biliary atresia are associated with proven viral infection (cytomegalovirus),

---

Physiologic neonatal jaundice
Peak 2–5 days after birth
Normal stools and urine
More severe in premature babies
Clears within 2 weeks
May persists for 4 weeks in breast-fed infants
Can rarely lead to kernicterus
Diagnosis: 80% total bilirubin is unconjugated
Treatment includes phototherapy, fluids, reassurance

Figure 23.1 Physiologic neonatal jaundice.

Causes of unconjugated hyperbilirubinemia
Physiologic/breast milk jaundice
Hemolysis
Immune
Red blood cell membrane abnormality
Metabolic disorders
Crigler–Najjar types I and II
Gilbert's syndrome
Galactosemia
Fructosemia
Hypothyroidism
Sepsis
Hypoxia

Figure 23.2 Causes of unconjugated hyperbilirubinemia.

numerous studies have not indicated an association with any hepatotropic RNA viruses such as reovirus or rotavirus.

Pathogenesis

Biliary atresia affects all parts of the biliary tree. There is gradual fibrosis and destruction of the extra- and intrahepatic biliary ducts with progressive cholestasis. The lumen of the extrahepatic duct may be obliterated at different levels leading to three main types: type I in which the common bile duct is obstructed; type II in which the common hepatic duct is obstructed; and type III in which there is fibrosis at the level of the porta hepatis – this occurs in 85% of cases.

Clinical features

Infants who have biliary atresia are usually born at term with a normal birth weight. Jaundice is apparent on the second day of life, but is mistaken for physiologic jaundice. Biliary obstruction, as evidenced by pale stools and yellow urine, gradually develops over the next 2–4 weeks, and is associated with a gradual increase in liver size and failure to gain weight adequately despite a good appetite. Approximately 25% of babies have associated anomalies: dextracardia, ventricular or atrial septal defects, polysplenia, and the hypovascular syndrome (HVS) (Fig. 23.3).

The spleen is not enlarged unless there is significant hepatic fibrosis. Ascites may occasionally be present.

Diagnosis

All children who have persistent neonatal jaundice need thorough investigation (Fig. 23.4).

A diagnosis of biliary atresia is dependent on:

- presence of conjugated hyperbilirubinemia
- liver biochemistry which indicates raised alkaline phosphatase (>600IU/L) and γ-glutamyltranspeptidase (γ-GT) (>100U/L), and moderate elevation of alanine and aspartate transaminases (100–200U/L);
- abdominal ultrasound performed after a 4-hour fast will either not demonstrate a gallbladder or indicate a small contracted gallbladder;
- radionuclide hepatobiliary imaging will not demonstrate biliary excretion from the liver into the gut after 24 hours (Fig. 23.5); and

histology that demonstrates the characteristic findings of expansion of portal tracts, proliferation of bile ducts and ductules with bile plugs, portal fibrosis, and portal edema – there may be an increase in inflammatory reaction at the porta hepatitis and variable giant cell transformation of hepatocytes (Fig. 23.6).

As none of these tests are pathognomonic for biliary atresia, the diagnosis should be confirmed by operative cholangiography with progression to a Kasai portoenterostomy if required. Endoscopic retrograde cholangiography (ERCP) in this age group is now pos-

Congenital abnormalities in biliary atresia	
Anomaly	**Comment**
Cardiac	
Dextrocardia	+/– situs inversus
VSD	
ASD	
Left atrial isomerism	With HVS
Vascular	
Preduodenal portal vein	}HVS
Absent interferior vena cava	}Azygous drainage
Splenic	
Polysplenia	+/– HVS
Double spleen	
Asplenia	
Malrotation	
Situs inversus	+/– HVS, NHP
Annular pancreas	
Immobile cilia syndrome	Bronchiectasis

Figure 23.3 Congenital anomalies in biliary atresia. ASD, atrial septal defect; HVS, hypovascular syndrome; VSD, ventricular septal defect; NHP, normal heart position.

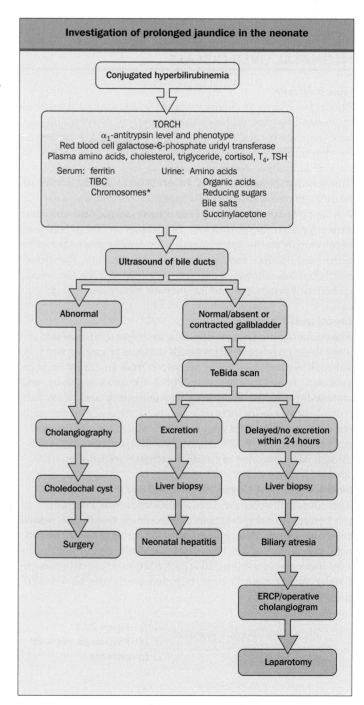

Figure 23.4 Investigation of prolonged jaundice in the neonate. T4, thyroxine; TIBC, total iron-binding capacity; TSH, thyroid-stimulating hormone; TORCH, serology for toxoplasma, other, rubella, cytomegalovirus, and herpes simplex viruses; TeBida, 99 technetium trimethyl-1-bromoimino diacetic acid. * Chromosomes for 18, 21, Alagille syndrome.

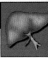

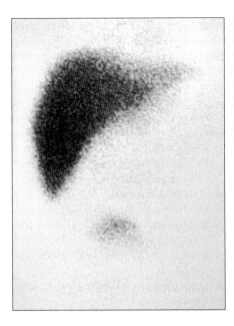

Figure 23.5 Radioisotope scanning demonstrating excellent uptake of radioisotope but no excretion at 24 hours. This represents either severe intrahepatic cholestasis, but more likely the diagnosis of extrahepatic biliary atresia.

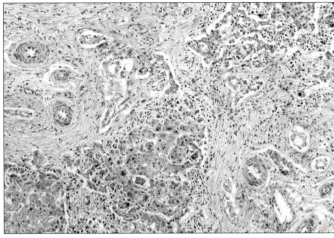

Figure 23.6 Biopsy showing features suggestive of biliary obstruction. These are portal fibrosis, biliary ductular proliferation with bile plugs, and portal edema. There may be considerable histologic overlap between biliary atresia and the neonatal hepatitis syndrome.

sible using prototype pediatric duodenoscopes. Biliary atresia can be confidently excluded if the biliary tree is visualized, but a failure to do so may either be due to technical failure or biliary atresia and progression to operative cholangiography and laparotomy is then required.

Management

The Kasai portoenterostomy involves resection of the obliterated biliary tract and formation of a Roux loop which is anastomosed to the porta hepatis. Between 50–60% of cases achieve biliary drainage which may be improved by administration of a short course of corticosteroids at the end of the first postoperative week. Revised Kasai operations are not indicated because of the poor success rate, and because of increased technical difficulties at subsequent liver transplantation.

The success of the Kasai portoenterostomy operation depends on a number of factors, which include the timing of the operation, the expertise of the surgeon, the degree of hepatic fibrosis at operation, and the presence or absence of other congenital abnormalities. Operations should be performed before 8 weeks of age, although there is no clear effect of age on survival unless the operation takes place after 100 days of age. Surgery is not recommended if there is evidence of advanced hepatic fibrosis with splenomegaly, ascites, or varices.

Cholangitis is most common in the immediate postoperative period. The incidence is reduced by prophylactic antibiotics, either intravenously for 10–14 days or orally for 3–6 months. The clinical signs include an increase in jaundice, pyrexia, acholic stools, and tenderness over the liver. Broad spectrum antibiotics (ceftazidime, amoxicillin, piperacillin or ciprofloxacin) are usually effective.

Malabsorption is usually associated with a partially successful Kasai portoenterostomy and is an important factor in the development of malnutrition in neonatal liver disease. The development of cirrhosis and portal hypertension is inevitable even in those children who have had a successful Kasai portoenterostomy, although the need for transplantation varies with the rate of progression of liver disease and complications. Unsuccessful Kasai portoenterostomy is an immediate indication for liver transplantation and these children should be referred early to specialized centers for follow-up.

Choledocal cyst

Choledocal cysts are localized cystic dilatation of all or part of the common bile duct. Cysts are more common in Japan (1:100,000 live births) and in females (4:1). Choledocal cysts may be congenital or acquired. There may be a structural weakness with subsequent dilatation in the wall of the biliary tree or alternatively the biliary dilatation may be secondary to pancreatitis associated with a common pancreaticobiliary channel or repeated cholangitis.

The cyst may present in infancy with prolonged jaundice and must be differentiated from biliary atresia or the neonatal hepatitis syndrome. In older children a history of abdominal pain, jaundice, and abdominal mass is classic, but is a rare presentation in childhood. Jaundice may be intermittent and associated with ascending cholangitis and recurrent pancreatitis.

Diagnosis

Choledocal cysts are diagnosed by abdominal ultrasound which may detect the cysts antenatally. Confirmation of the anatomy is obtained by radioisotope scan, percutaneous transhepatic cholangiogram, or endoscopically by an endoscopic retrograde cholangiopancreatography (Fig. 23.7). Histology of the liver usually indicates biliary fibrosis, cholestasis, and bile plugs in the portal tract. The histologic features are completely reversible following successful surgery.

Management

Surgical treatment includes excision of all the affected ducts and re-establishment of biliary drainage by forming a hepaticojejunostomy. Drainage of the cyst into adjacent duodenum or jejunum is now contraindicated, because of the potential malignant transformation. The results of surgery are excellent, cholangitis is an occasional complication, and there is a 2.5% risk of malignancy in the residual biliary tree in adult life.

Spontaneous perforation of the bile ducts

This is a rare complication in which perforation occurs at the junction of the cystic and common hepatic ducts, perhaps due to a congenital weakness, inspissated bile, or gallstones. Infants may present at any age from 2–24 weeks of age with abdominal distension, ascites, jaundice, and acholic stools. Biliary peritonitis, with bile in hydroceles, hernial sacs, and umbilicus may be obvious.

The diagnosis may be confirmed by abdominal ultrasound, which may show free intraperitoneal fluid and dilated intrahepatic ducts. Biochemical liver function tests may be abnormal, with conjugated hyperbilirubinemia and raised alkaline phosphatase and γ-GT. If the biliary leak is large, liver function tests may be virtually normal. Hepatobiliary scanning will demonstrate isotope into the peritoneal cavity. Treatment includes peritoneal drainage followed by repair of the perforation.

Inspissated bile syndrome and cholelithiasis

Bile duct obstruction secondary to inspissated bile syndrome may be secondary to total parenteral nutrition, prolonged hemolysis, and dehydration. It is more common in premature babies or those undergoing major surgery. The clinical picture is of biliary obstruction with pale stools, dark urine, and abnormal liver function tests. The diagnosis may be confirmed by ultrasound, which demonstrates a dilated intra- and extrahepatic duct system with biliary sludge. Percutaneous transhepatic cholangiography will outline the anatomy and may be therapeutic with lavage of the biliary tree, but laparatomy and decompression of the biliary tree may be required. The use of ursodeoxycholic acid (20mg/kg) and cholecystokinin may prevent the need for either surgical or radiologic intervention.

Cholecystitis may occur in infants in association with gallstones from hemolysis or total parenteral nutrition (TPN), while acalculus cholecystitis may occur as part of generalized sepsis. Operative cholecystectomy (rather than laparoscopic) is the treatment of choice in this young age group for symptomatic cholecystitis in association with gallstones.

Neonatal hepatitis syndrome

The neonatal hepatitis syndrome includes many different causes of neonatal liver disease (Fig. 23.8), which may have a similar presentation (see Fig. 23.4). The commonest causes are intrauterine infections or inherited metabolic diseases.

In contrast to children who have extrahepatic biliary disease, babies who have a neonatal hepatitis syndrome may have the following characteristics:
- they may be small for dates or have intrauterine growth retardation (Fig. 23.9);
- pigment is usually present in the stools although the urine will be yellow;
- dysmorphic features characteristic of Alagille syndrome or zellweger syndrome may be present; and
- hepatosplenomegaly is usually present.

Biochemical features include:
- conjugated bilirubin 6mg/L (>100mmol/L);

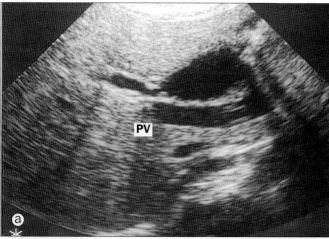

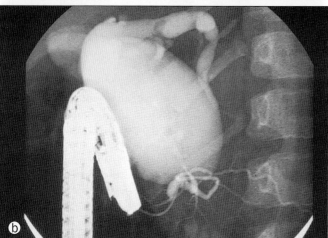

Figure 23.7 Abdominal ultrasound demonstrating a large cystic swelling. (a) Shows the cystic swelling, which was (b) confirmed to be a choledochal cyst on ERCP.

Neonatal hepatitis syndrome and diagnostic approach		
Disease	Diagnosis	Treatment
Intrauterine infection		
Cytomegalovirus	Urine for viral culture	Gancyclovir
Toxoplasmosis	IgM antibodies	Spiramycin
Rubella	IgM antibodies	Supportive
Herpes simplex	EM/viral culture of vesicle	Acyclovir
Syphilis	VDRL test	Penicillin
Metabolic		
AAT deficiency	AAT level and phenotype	Supportive
Cystic fibrosis	Sweat chloride, immunoreactive trypsin, ΔF08 mutation	Supportive
Galactosemia	Galactose-1-6-phosphate uridyltransferase	Galactose-free diet
Tyrosinemia	Urine succinylacetone, serum amino acids, α-fetoprotein	NTBC
Hereditary fructosemia	Enzymes in liver	Fructose-free diet
Niemann–Pick type A	Sphingomyelinase	Supportive
Niemann–Pick type C	Storage cells in bone marrow aspirate and liver biopsy; fibroblast culture	Supportive
Wolman disease	Abdominal radiograph of adrenal glands	Supportive
Primary disorders of bile acid synthesis	Urinary bile acids by FAB-MS	Bile acids
Zellweger syndrome	Very-long-chain fatty acids	Supportive
Endocrine		
Hypituitarism (septo-optic dysplasia)	Cortisol, TSH, T$_4$	Hormone replacement
Hypothyroidism	TSH, T$_4$, free T$_4$, T$_3$	Hormone replacement

Figure 23.8 Neonatal hepatitis syndrome and diagnostic approach.
AAT, α$_1$-antitrypsin; EM: electron microscopy; FAB-MS, fast atom bombardment ionization mass spectrometry; NTBC, 2(2-nitro-trifluoromethylbenzoyl)-1,3-cyclonescanedione; T3, triiodothyronine; T4, thyroxine; TSH, thyroid-stimulating hormone; VDRL, venereal disease research laboratory.

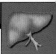
- alkaline phosphatase 600–800IU/L;
- aspartate aminotransferase (AST) and alanine aminotransferase (ALT) 200–300IU/L; and
- hypoglycemia (depending on etiology).

Liver histology is nonspecific and demonstrates a giant cell hepatitis with fibrosis of the portal tracts, extramedullary hemopoiesis, cholestasis, and biliary ductule proliferation. There may be histologic overlap with biliary atresia (Fig. 23.10).

Intrauterine infection

The commonest cause of intrauterine infection causing neonatal hepatitis is cytomegalovirus (CMV) infection. Infants are small for dates with hepatosplenomegaly and may have thrombocytopenia, choreoretinitis, or microcephaly. A diagnosis (see Fig. 23.8), is based on identification of immunoglobulin (Ig)M antibodies and virus culture. The outcome is variable. In most babies the hepatitis resolves completely within 3–6 months, but neurologic involvement with spasticity or sensorineural deafness and developmental delay may be present. Treatment with ganciclovir is rarely necessary.

Rubella hepatitis is almost unknown now following universal vaccination, but may present with neonatal hepatitis, cataracts, congenital heart disease, and deafness. Progressive liver disease has been reported.

Toxoplasmosis is prevalent in parts of France and Germany, but is unusual in the British Isles. It is associated with persistent neonatal jaundice, failure to thrive, hepatosplenomegaly, central nervous system involvement with choreoretinitis, hydrocephaly, microcephaly, and intracranial calcification. Treatment with spiramycin may be helpful for liver disease. The long-term outcome is related to the neurologic disease, as by the time of diagnosis many children are blind or severely handicapped.

Herpes simplex in the newborn usually causes a multisystem disorder with encephalitis and acute liver failure. Antiviral treatment with acyclovir is successful if started early enough.

Congenital syphilis is now rare, but may also cause a multisystem disease with intrauterine retardation, anemia, thrombocytopenia, nephrotic syndrome, skin rash, diffuse lymphadenopathy, and hepatomegaly. Diagnosis is based on serologic testing (see Fig. 23.8). Treatment with penicillin is usually curative.

Hepatitis A, B and C viruses and HIV are rare causes of persistent neonatal jaundice. Vertical transmission of hepatitis C virus (HBV) and hepatitis C virus (HCV) lead to an asymptomatic carrier state.

Endocrine disorders

The neonatal hepatitis syndrome is associated with pituitary or adrenal dysfunction in approximately 30% of patients. Hypopituitarism may be due to hypothalamic dysfunction and is associated with septo-optic dysplasia, which includes absence of the septum pelucidum or malformation of the forebrain and hypoplasia of one or both optic nerves.

Hypoglycemia is a prominent symptom that is not associated with the severity of liver disease. Other signs of hypopituitarism including microgenitalia in boys, midline facial abnormalities, or nystagmus. A number of children may have severe cholestasis with acholic stools and dark urine and differentiation from biliary atresia may be difficult.

The diagnosis is established by demonstrating abnormal thyroid function tests indicating hypothyroidism and a low random or 9.00am cortisol. A synacten test is rarely required for confir-

mation. Treatment is with hormone replacement with thyroxine, hydrocortisone, and growth hormone. If diagnosed early enough, liver disease will completely resolve, but hormone replacement is required lifelong.

Inborn errors of metabolism

The commonest inborn error of metabolism to present with persistent neonatal jaundice is α_1-antitrypsin deficiency, which is an autosomal recessive disorder with an incidence of 1:7000 live births worldwide. Infants may present with intrauterine growth retardation, cholestasis, failure to thrive, hepatomegaly, or a vitamin K responsive coagulopathy which is more likely in those infants who are not given prophylactic vitamin K at birth and who are being breast-fed. The coagulopathy may be obvious with bruising and bleeding from the umbilicus, but the initial symptom may be intraventricular hemorrhage which may result in neurologic disability.

Diagnosis

Liver biochemistry demonstrates a mixed hepatic/obstructive picture with elevated transaminases, alkaline phosphatase, and γ-GT. Radiologic investigations may indicate severe intrahepatic cholesta-

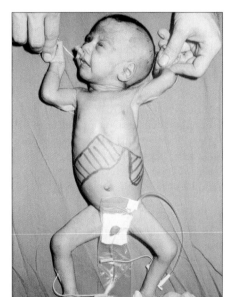

Figure 23.9 Neonatal hepatitis. This baby was born at 37 weeks' gestation, with obvious intrauterine retardation. He was jaundiced with hepatosplenomegaly, and malnourished with loss of fat and muscle stores. The most likely differential diagnosis is neonatal hepatitis secondary to a uterine infection or inborn error of metabolism.

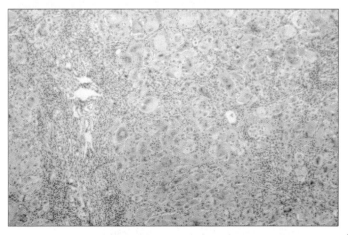

Figure 23.10 Most babies who have neonatal hepatitis have giant cell hepatitis with extramedullary hemopoiesis and a rosette formation of hepatocytes. This is a nonspecific finding and may represent many different causes of neonatal liver disease.

sis with a contracted gallbladder on a fasting ultrasound, and delayed or absent excretion of radioisotope on hepatobiliary scanning. In homozygotes the diagnosis is easily confirmed by detection of a low level of α_1-antitrypsin (<0.9g/L). Liver disease is usually associated with phenotype protease inhibitor PiZZ but may occur with PiMZ heterozygotes or other variants. Liver histology demonstrates a giant cell hepatitis with characteristic periodic acid–Schiff (PAS), diastase resistant, positive granules of α_1-antitrypsin in hepatocytes which may be detected by 6–8 weeks of age (Fig. 23.11).

Management

This consists of nutritional support, fat-soluble vitamin supplementation, and treatment of pruritus and cholestasis (Fig. 23.12).

The prognosis is varied. Jaundice disappears in most infants, of whom approximately one third regain normal function, one third develop an inactive fibrosis and/or cirrhosis, and one third develop chronic liver failure requiring transplantation. Respiratory disease is rare in childhood but long-term follow-up is essential to monitor growth, development, and the need for liver transplantation. Antenatal diagnosis by chorionic villus sampling is now available using synthetic oligonucleotide probes specific for the M and Z genes, or by restriction fragment length polymorphism.

Intrahepatic biliary hypoplasia

The term intrahepatic biliary hypoplasia refers to an absence or reduction of a number of interlobular bile ducts or ductules seen in portal tracts in association with normal-sized branches of the portal vein and hepatic arteries. Biliary hypoplasia may occur in a wide spectrum of liver diseases, such as α_1-antitrypsin deficiency, chromosomal abnormality such as Down syndrome, or intrauterine infection (CMV). However, this term is usually only associated with syndromic biliary hypoplasia or Alagille syndrome, or nonsyndromic biliary hypoplasia which includes Byler's disease and progressive familial intrahepatic cholestasis.

Alagille syndrome

This is an autosomal dominant condition with an incidence of 1:100,000 live births worldwide. It is a multisystem disorder which is associated with cardiac, facial, renal, occular, and skeletal abnormalities. The genetic abnormality has been identified as a deletion on chromosome 20p and has now been identified as Jag 1 gene. Infants may present with persistent cholestasis, severe pruritus, hepatomegaly, and failure to thrive. The characteristic facial features are very difficult to identify in infancy, but become more prominent later in childhood. They include a triangular face with high forehead and frontal bossing, deep widely spaced eyes, saddle-shaped nasal bridge, and pointed chin (Fig. 23.13).

Cardiac abnormalities include peripheral pulmonary stenosis, pulmonary and aortic valve stenosis, and Fallot's tetralogy.

Skeletal abnormalities are widespread and include abnormal thoracic vertebrae, 'butterfly' vertebrae, and curving of the proximal digits of the third and fourth finger. Posterior embryotoxin, which is detected on the inner aspects of the cornea near the junction of the iris, is demonstrated in 90% of patients by slit-lamp examination. Retinal pigmentation on fundoscopy and calcific deposits (optic drusen) in the optic nerve may be detected by ultrasound. Renal disease varies in severity from mild renal tubular acidosis to severe glomerular nephritis. One of the most difficult management problems is severe failure to thrive, which is complicated by gastrointestinal reflux and severe steatorrhea secondary to fat malabsorption or pancreatic insufficiency.

Diagnosis

Liver biochemistry indicates severe cholestasis with:
- conjugated bilirubin 6mg/dl (>100mg/dL);
- raised alkaline phosphatase >600IU/L;
- γ-GT >200IU/L;
- raised transaminases; and
- plasma cholesterol >6mmol/L with normal triglycerides 0.4–2mmol/L.

Tests of hepatic function such as albumin and coagulation are usually normal. Renal dysfunction may be identified by the presence of aminoaciduria or estimating urinary protein/creatinine ratio (normal <20).

The skeletal abnormalities are easily identified by radiologic examination of the chest and hands. Electrocardiography may demonstrate right bundle branch block or right ventricular hypertrophy in children who have peripheral pulmonary stenosis.

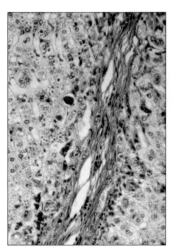 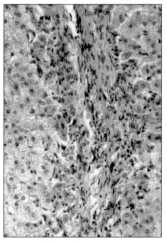

Figure 23.11 α_1-antitrypsin deficiency is the commonest inherited liver disease. The diagnosis is made on histology, demonstrating granules in hepatocytes either by a periodic acid–Schiff (PAS)-stain (a), or by immunoperoxidase staining (b), which may be detected as early as 6–8 weeks.

Management of neonatal liver disease	
Nutritional support	
Modular feed	Energy intake 150–200cal/kg
Carbohydrate	Glucose polymer (8–10g/kg/day)
Protein	Whey protein (2.5–3.5g/kg/day)
Fat	50/50 MCT/LCT (8g/kg/day)
Fat-soluble vitamins	
A: 5–10,000U/day E: 50–100mg/day K: 1–2mg/day D: 50ng/kg/day	
Pruritus/cholestasis	
Phenobarbital 5–15mg/kg Ursodeoxycholic acid 20mg/kg Rifampin (rifampicin) 3mg/kg Cholestyramine 1–2g/day Topical skin care	

Figure 23.12 Management of neonatal liver disease. MCT, medium chain triglyceride; LCT, long chain triglyceride.

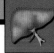

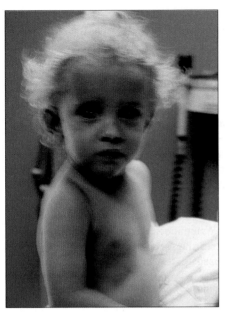

Figure 23.13 Alagille syndrome. This is an autosomal dominant disorder in which the typical facies may be less obvious in infants. This baby demonstrates hypertelorism, widely spaced eyes, depressed nasal bridge, and a pointed chin. He also has curving of the second metacarpal on his little finger, which is characteristic of this syndrome.

Echocardiography may be normal but if cardiac abnormalities are suggested clinically, then cardiac catheterization should be performed for confirmation.

Liver histology may be nonspecific. The reduction in interlobular bile ducts is often difficult to identify in the neonatal period, particularly if cholestasis and giant cell hepatitis are also present. The histologic appearance differs from extrahepatic biliary atresia because of the absence of portal fibrosis and biliary ductular proliferation.

Management

Intensive nutritional support is essential (see Fig. 23.12) and pancreatic supplements may be required. Pruritus may be intractable and an indication for liver transplantation. Prognosis is varied and depends on the extent of liver, cardiac, or renal disease. Approximately 50% of children may regain normal liver function by adolescence while others require liver transplantation in childhood. The indications for liver transplantation are the development of cirrhosis and portal hypertension, intractable pruritus or severe decompensated growth failure. Pretransplant cardiac surgery or balloon dilatation may be indicated for severe pulmonary stenosis.

Progressive intrahepatic cholestasis

Progressive intrahepatic cholestasis or progressive familial intrahepatic cholestasis (PFIC) is the term given to a number of poorly defined conditions in which there is persistent jaundice, cholestasis, hepatomegaly, pruritus, and failure to thrive. Many different variants and the genetic mutations underlying a number of these have been identified. (PFIC-1,2).

Byler's disease (PFIC-I)

This severe form of familial idiopathic cholestasis was first described in an Amish family. In contrast to children who have intrahepatic cholestasis of other causes, this group of children had a normal serum γ-GT. Low or normal serum cholesterol is also characteristic of this syndrome. The clinical presentation is with persistent conjugated hyperbilirubinemia, severe pruritus, and growth retardation. Histology shows a lack of hepatic inflammation but paucity of bile ducts and canalicular bile plugs. Cirrhosis develops in early childhood requiring liver transplantation.

The management consists of nutritional support (see Fig. 23.12) and treatment of pruritus which includes biliary diversion, an operative technique in which bile is diverted externally by an enterostomy. Most children have progressive fibrosis with the development of cirrhosis and portal hypertension requiring liver transplantation in childhood.

Inherited disorders of bile salt metabolism

The development of fast atom bombardment ionization mass spectrometry (FABMS) has allowed many defects in primary bile acid synthesis to be identified. A number of disorders have been identified (Fig. 23.14).

Infants present with cholestasis, hepatomegaly, and failure to thrive, with or without pruritus (Fig. 23.14). Biochemistry indicates nonspecific abnormalities of transaminases and elevated alkaline phosphatase and/or γ-GT. Liver histology indicates a giant cell transformation with cholestasis with rapid development of fibrosis and cirrhosis. The diagnosis is made by identifying the specific abnormal bile acid metabolites in urine. These diseases are fatal without liver transplantation, but treatment with a combination of cholic acid, chenodeoxycholic acid or ursodeoxycholic acid may prevent progression to cirrhosis and portal hypertension if started sufficiently early.

Zellweger syndrome (cerebrohepatorenal syndrome)

This is an autosomal recessive syndrome with multisystem disease. It is associated with absent or dysfunctional peroxisome biogenesis leading to secondary defects of bile acid synthesis and abnormal β-oxidation of fatty acids. The incidence is 1:100,000 live births. The initial presentation is with severe hypotonia, feeding difficulties, and failure to thrive. Jaundice is only present in 50% of babies, but dysmorphic features which include epicanthic folds, brush field spots, and a high forehead are common in association with psychomotor retardation. There is multisystem involvement involving the brain, heart, liver, and kidneys.

The diagnosis is confirmed by demonstrating abnormal bile salt metabolites using FABMS or the detection of very-long-chain fatty acids in serum. Initially hepatic pathology may appear normal, but there is excessive hepatic iron in the first few months with the subsequent development of fibrosis and micronodular cirrhosis. Ultra-electron microscopy may indicate abnormal mitochondria and the absence of peroxisomes.

Inherited disorders of bile acid synthesis		
Enzyme	**Features**	**Treatment**
3β-hydroxy-Δ^5-C$_{27}$-steroid dehydrogenase/isomerase	Neonatal hepatitis; normal γ-GT; low bile acid concentration; no pruritus	CDCA or UDCA
Δ^4-3-oxosteroid 5β-reductase	Jaundice, coagulopathy; elevated bile acid concentrations	UDCA + cholic acid
24,25-dihydroxy-cholanoic cleavage enzyme	Giant-cell hepatitis; normal γ-GT; elevated serum cholesterol; low bile acid concentrations	CDCA + cholic acid

Figure 23.14 Inherited disorders of bile acid synthesis. CDCA, chenodeoxycholic acid; γ-GT, γ-glutamyltranspeptidase; UDCA, ursodeoxycholic acid.

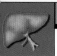

Treatment is supportive as death is inevitable. Liver transplantation is not indicated because of the progression of multisystem disease. Initial attempts to induce peroxisomes with hypolipemic drugs were unsuccessful. Primary bile acid therapy with cholic and chenodeoxycholic acid may produce some histologic improvement, but has no effect on survival.

Cystic fibrosis

Cystic fibrosis is an unusual cause of neonatal cholestasis accounting for <1% of children who have persistent jaundice. It is an autosomal recessive disorder with an incidence of 1:2000 live births. The genetic defect has been localized to the long arm of chromosome 7, and more than 300 mutations have been identified in the gene coding for the cystic fibrosis transmembrane conductance regulator (CFTR). The commonest mutation is Δ508, but no mutation is specific for liver disease. The prominent clinical symptoms include persistent cholestasis, meconium ileus, hepatomegaly, failure to thrive, and recurrent respiratory infections. If cholestasis is complete with acholic stools, differentiation from biliary atresia may be difficult.

Diagnosis

Biochemical liver function tests reveal raised transaminases, alkaline phosphatase, and γ-GT. Immunoreactive trypsin may be higher than normal for age [1300ng/dl (>130ng/mL)]. Serum cholesterol and triglycerides are usually normal. Although a sweat test is thought to be pathognomonic for this diagnosis, it is not usually worth doing this in babies under 4–6 weeks of age [values of 5mg/dl (<50mmol/L) for <5 years]. Liver histology is varied, but usually demonstrates diffuse cholestasis with bile duct proliferation, focal biliary cirrhosis, and portal fibrosis.

Management

The efficacy of ursodeoxycholic acid (20–50mg/kg/day) in the treatment of neonatal cholestasis secondary to cystic fibrosis is unknown. Preliminary data in older children suggest that there is a biochemical and perhaps histologic improvement with treatment. It is usual to treat children with cholestasis secondary to cystic fibrosis with ursodeoxycholic acid and fat soluble vitamin supplementation and appropriate nutritional support (see Fig. 23.12). In most children who have neonatal cystic fibrosis, liver disease with jaundice resolves, but persistent jaundice has been reported with the development of cirrhosis, portal hypertension, and liver failure. Ongoing malnutrition and respiratory disease may contribute to death in infancy.

Niemann–Pick disease type C

This is a rare autosomal recessive disorder in which there is a defect in cholesterol esterification that results in a neurovisceral lipid storage disorder with an extremely varied spectrum of clinical findings. About 60% of children will present with prolonged cholestasis and hepatosplenomegaly in infancy, some of whom may present with fetal ascites. A number of children present later (3–5 years of age) with isolated splenomegaly and/or neurologic signs and symptoms.

Diagnosis

Liver histology may indicate a giant cell hepatitis. The diagnosis is determined by detecting PAS diastase-resistant storage cells in Kupffer cells and hepatocytes. If there is an active hepatitis, it is

easier to detect these characteristic foamy storage cells in bone marrow aspirate. Neuronal storage indicating central nervous system involvement is present at birth and is best demonstrated in the ganglion cells of a suction rectal biopsy. Skin fibroblast cultures will define the enzyme defect and enable antenatal diagnosis.

Management

Jaundice subsides in most children although hepatosplenomegaly may persist with abnormal biochemical liver function tests. Hepatic fibrosis with progression to cirrhosis and portal hypertension is a rare occurrence. Sadly, all children develop neurologic complications at a median age of 5 years, which include ataxia, convulsions, developmental delay, and dementia. Supranuclear ophthalmoplegia is considered pathognomonic for this condition. Most children die in late childhood or early adolescence from respiratory infections. There is no specific treatment, although a low cholesterol diet has been suggested. Liver and bone marrow transplantation are not curative. Genetic counseling is essential, and antenatal diagnosis may be performed by chorionic villus biopsy.

LIVER DISEASE IN OLDER CHILDREN

Liver disease in children older than 6 months may be acute or chronic. As in infancy, there is a predominance of inherited disorders (Fig. 23.15) and multisystem involvement (Fig. 23.16).

Acute liver disease
Acute viral hepatitis

All forms of acute viral hepatitis may occur in children and include hepatitis A virus (HAV), HBV, post-transfusion HCV, epidemic hepatitis E virus (HEV), Epstein–Barr virus (EBV), and CMV. In contrast to many adults, most children are asymptomatic and anicteric, and many episodes of hepatitis are subclinical. In symptomatic cases a prodromal illness with vomiting, abdominal pain, lethargy, and jaundice are common, as in adults. The diagnosis is confirmed by elevations of serum aminotransferases (ALT and AST 10–100 × normal) and specific viral serology. Liver biopsy is not required for diagnosis unless the clinical course is complicated. Centrilobular necrosis and inflammation are typical histologic changes of acute viral hepatitis.

Management

Uncomplicated acute hepatitis is managed at home. Hospital admission is required only if the child has severe vomiting leading to dehydration, abdominal pain or lethargy, if coagulation parameters are prolonged or transaminase activity remains high. Fulminant hepatitis is a complication in less than 5% of pediatric cases. The main differential diagnoses are metabolic liver disease (e.g. Wilson's disease) or drug-induced liver disease.

Chronic hepatitis

Hepatitis B virus and HCV are the commonest of viral hepatitis in childhood, but are unlikely to lead to serious liver disease until later in adolescence or adult life.

Hepatitis B virus infection

Children are infected in childhood by vertical transmission from a carrier mother; horizontal transmission from parents and other family members; by infected blood products; sexual abuse; or, in adolescents, drug abuse. There is an increased risk of environmen-

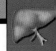

ing fulminant liver failure. In the order of 70% of infants infected perinatally will become chronic carriers unless immunized at birth.

The natural history of chronic HBV infection in childhood is not yet established. Children are usually asymptomatic without signs of chronic liver disease. Biochemical parameters indicate mild elevation of transaminases (80–150U/L) with normal albumin, coagulation, and alkaline phosphatase. Liver histology indicates a chronic hepatitis in over 90% of the carriers, which may be mild or nonspecific in 40% of children. Progression to cirrhosis is likely and has been reported in Mediterranean populations, although the exact incidence is unknown.

Children who have chronic HBV not only provide a continuing source of infection, but are at risk of developing cirrhosis and/or primary hepatocellular carcinoma. Chronic carriers should, therefore, remain under medical supervision so that the family may be supported and educated, as well as to screen and immunize family members. In addition, the patient should be monitored for evidence of seroconversion or progressive liver disease and/or hepatocellular carcinoma.

Annual review should include HBV serology and viral markers of HBV DNA, standard liver function tests, α-fetoprotein, and abdominal ultrasound.

Management

The indications for treatment in childhood are persistently raised serum aminotransferases, presence of HBe antigen with detectable HBV DNA in serum, and features of chronic hepatitis on liver biopsy. Interferon-α (5–10mu/m^2 thrice weekly) by subcutaneous injection for 6 months has a sustained clearance rate of 40–50% of those treated. Children who have active histology, low HBV DNA levels (<1000pg/mL), high serum aminotransferase enzymes, and horizontal transmission are more likely to respond to interferon. Pretreatment with corticosteroids remains unproven in the short term, but may have a long-term effect on seroconversion over 3–4 years. The antiviral agent lamivudine has not yet been evaluated in children.

The most important strategy to prevent HBV transmission in childhood includes routine antenatal screening of all women during pregnancy, with immunization of at-risk infants, or universal immunization of all infants. The implementation of universal immunization continues to be controversial, although a number of countries in Europe and North America have adopted this policy.

Hepatitis C virus infection

The importance of hepatitis C virus infection in children lies in its propensity to develop chronic liver disease. Children infected with HCV form three main groups: those who were parenterally infected prior to blood product and donor organ screening in 1990; children who have been vertically infected; and a group of children who have been sporadically infected but the route of acquisition remains obscure. In contrast to HBV infection, vertical transmission of HCV is unusual, ranging from 2–10% of offspring born to HCV-RNA-positive mothers. The risk of transmission is increased up to 48% by coexisting maternal HIV infection and in those who have high HCV RNA titers. Breast feeding is not contraindicated.

Diagnosis

Diagnosis is made by screening children at risk. Serum aminotransferases are typically normal or very slightly elevated, HCV serology will indicate anti-HCV antibodies and the presence of

Liver diseases in older children	
Disease	**Diagnostic investigations**
Chronic hepatitis	
Chronic hepatitis	Portal inflammatory hepatitis infiltrate on biopsy
Hepatitis B, C, D, EBV, CMV	Serology
Autoimmune hepatitis	IgG >2g/dl (>20g/L)
	C3, C4, LKM, ANA, SMA
Wilson's disease	Serum Cu, ceruloplasmin, urinary Cu
α₁-antitrypsin deficiency	α₁-antitrypsin level and phenotype
Cystic fibrosis	Sweat test, liver biopsy
Cryptogenic cirrhosis	Liver biopsy
Primary sclerosing cholangitis	ERCP and liver biopsy
Tyrosinemia type I	Urinary succinylacetone
Hereditary fructose intolerance	Fructose 1-6-phosphate aldolase in liver

Figure 23.15 Liver diseases in older children. ANA, antinuclear antibodies; C3, C4, complement; ERCP, endoscopic retrograde cholangiopancreatography; LKM, liver, kidney microsomal antibodies; SMA, smooth muscle antibodies.

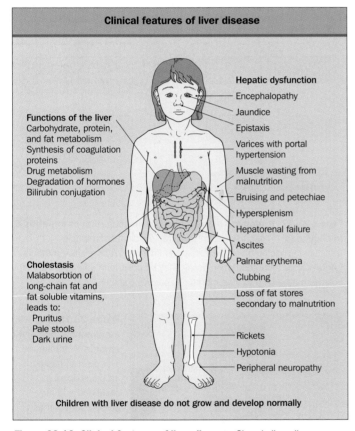

Clinical features of liver disease

Hepatic dysfunction
- Encephalopathy
- Jaundice
- Epistaxis
- Varices with portal hypertension
- Muscle wasting from malnutrition
- Bruising and petechiae
- Hypersplenism
- Hepatorenal failure
- Ascites
- Palmar erythema
- Clubbing
- Loss of fat stores secondary to malnutrition
- Rickets
- Hypotonia
- Peripheral neuropathy

Functions of the liver
Carbohydrate, protein, and fat metabolism
Synthesis of coagulation proteins
Drug metabolism
Degradation of hormones
Bilirubin conjugation

Cholestasis
Malabsorbtion of long-chain fat and fat soluble vitamins, leads to:
Pruritus
Pale stools
Dark urine

Children with liver disease do not grow and develop normally

Figure 23.16 Clinical features of liver disease. Chronic liver disease affects every organ in the growing child and leads to significant growth failure and psychosocial delay, which are indications for liver transplantation.

tal transmission in residential institutions and hemodialysis centers. Perinatal transmission occurs mainly through placental tears, trauma during delivery, or contact of the infant mucous membrane with infected maternal fluid. Intrauterine transmission has been reported, but is not a major route of transmission. Hepatitis B virus carrier mothers, who are HBe antigen positive, have the highest infectivity with a 70–90% risk of transmission. Those mothers who are HBe antigen negative, but HBe antibody positive may also transmit infection, and their infants are particularly at risk of develop-

HCV RNA by reverse transcriptase polymerate chain reaction (RTPCR). Histology reveals classic features of chronic hepatitis C, which include mild portal tract inflammation, lymphoid aggregates, and mild periportal piecemeal necrosis with steatosis and apoptosis. A giant cell hepatitis in association with HCV infection has been described in neonates.

Management
The first step is to establish the diagnosis by measuring not only anti-HCV antibody, but confirming that active infection is present by detecting HCV RNA by RTPCR (Fig. 23.17).

The range of genotypes identified in childhood resemble those in adult populations and does not help in diagnosis, but may provide long-term data on epidemiology and prognosis. The natural history of chronic HCV in childhood is not known. The natural seroconversion rate appears to be approximately 20% in children who have received blood products. No long-term data are available on vertically infected infants, as yet.

Children who have persistent positivity of HCV RNA and evidence of liver disease should be selected for therapy. Meta-analysis of interferon-α therapy in adults has indicated that monotherapy with interferon is unlikely to produce sustained clearance of HCV RNA or biochemical remission in more than 25% of patients. Although long-term controlled trials in childhood have not yet been performed, preliminary studies indicate that the response to interferon is no different in children. Evaluation of interferon and ribavirin in childhood has not yet been performed. Future treatment strategies that are under consideration are daily interferon (3 mu/m^2), pegylated (PEG) interferon, and combination therapy with ribavirin and interferon.

Autoimmune hepatitis
Autoimmune hepatitis is a chronic inflammatory disorder affecting the liver, which is usually responsive to immunosuppressives. It may affect children of any age from 6 months onwards, although there is a 3:1 female preponderance. Both forms of autoimmune hepatitis type I [antinuclear antibodies (ANAs), and smooth muscle antibodies (SMAs)] and type II [liver, kidney microsomal antibodies (LKMs)] present in childhood.

Clinical features
In type I autoimmune hepatitis, the median age of onset is 10 years and the clinical presentation varies from acute hepatitis with autoimmune features to the insidious development of cirrhosis, portal hypertension, and malnutrition. The association of multiorgan disease is higher in type I hepatitis with autoimmune thyroiditis, celiac disease, inflammatory bowel disease, hemolytic anemia, and glomerulonephritis being the most common (Fig. 23.18).

In type II autoimmune hepatitis, the age of onset is younger (median age 7.4 years); the clinical presentation is more likely to be acute with fulminant hepatic failure in 11%; and multiorgan disease is less common. The form LKM II may develop in association with hepatitis C or secondary to drugs such as antiepileptic drugs.

The diagnosis is made in the same way as in adults by the identification of:
- elevated serum aminotransferases;
- increased total globulin or IgG concentrations greater than 1.5 times above the normal limit;
- nonspecific autoantibodies – seropositivity for ANA, SMA or LKM I antibodies – titers greater than 1:40 (up to 25% of chil-

dren may not have detectable autoantibodies on presentation);
- characteristic histologic features of chronic hepatitis (Fig. 23.19); and
- exclusion of hepatitis C and Wilson's disease.

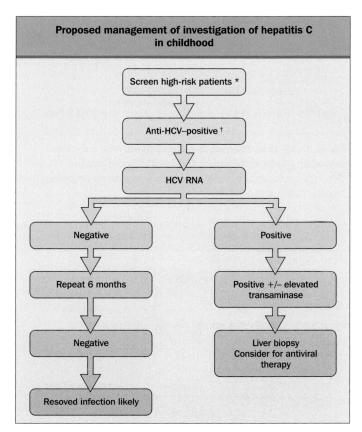

Proposed management of investigation of hepatitis C in childhood

Screen high-risk patients *

↓

Anti-HCV–positive †

↓

HCV RNA

↓ ↓

Negative | Positive

↓ ↓

Repeat 6 months | Positive +/– elevated transaminase

↓ ↓

Negative | Liver biopsy Consider for antiviral therapy

↓

Resoved infection likely

Figure 23.17 Prolonged management of investigation of hepatitis C in childhood. * High risk patients include recipients of multiple transfusions/pooled blood products, and infants of HCV positive mothers. † Anti-HCV by third generation assay. May be positive in infants of HCV positive mothers up to nine months by passive transfer.

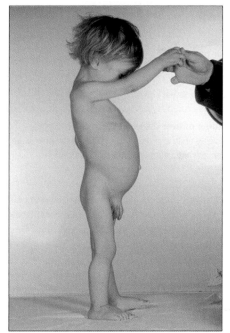

Figure 23.18 Boy with autoimmune hemolytic anemia. Autoimmune liver disease has an insidious onset in childhood and may present with cirrhosis and portal hypertension. Type I autoimmune hepatitis may also present with multisystem involvement, as in this patient.

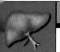

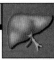

Management

Both forms of autoimmune hepatitis respond to immunosuppression with prednisolone 2mg/kg/day (maximum 60mg) in association with azathioprine 0.5–2mg/kg/day. About 90% of children will respond to the above regimen, but cyclosporine (2–4mg/kg/day) may be helpful in inducing or maintaining remission. There has been no established optimal duration of treatment. Discontinuation of corticosteroids and/or azathioprine may be considered if liver function tests have been normal for at least 1 year, but up to 80% of children will relapse following discontinuation of treatment.

Despite a biochemical response to immunosuppression, histologic progression may develop over many years. Failure of medical treatment is more likely in patients presenting at an early age, those who have type II autoimmune hepatitis, coagulopathy, high bilirubin, and established cirrhosis at presentation. Indications for liver transplantation include a presentation with fulminant hepatic failure, progression to end-stage liver failure, or intolerable side effects or failure of medical treatment. Transplantation may not provide a complete cure as the recurrence rate is approximately 25%, although this is relatively easy to control with corticosteroids.

Sclerosing cholangitis

The spectrum of sclerosing cholangitis in childhood includes neonatal sclerosing cholangitis and autoimmune sclerosing cholangitis in association with type I autoimmune hepatitis or immunodeficiency (Fig. 23.20).

Clinical features include abdominal pain, weight loss, intermittent jaundice resembling autoimmune hepatitis; and cholestasis with cholangitis and pruritis or cirrhosis with portal hypertension. Laboratory investigation will indicate elevated alkaline phosphatase (>16 × normal) and γ-GT (50–100 × normal). Bilirubin levels may be normal or intermittently elevated in at least 50% of patients; serum transaminases are moderately elevated (× 50 normal); and prothrombin times and albumin levels are usually normal early in the disease. Elevated prothrombin time may be due to fat-soluble vitamin deficiency and is responsive to vitamin K. The diagnosis is confirmed by cholangiography [either operative, percutaneous, transhepatic, endoscopic, or magnetic resinance imaging (MRI)], which reveals typical lesions of irregular intrahepatic ducts, focal saccular dilatations, short anular strictures, an abnormally large gallbladder, or extrahepatic ductular irregularities. Histology may demonstrate pathognomonic fibrous obliterative cholangitis with periductular fibrosis, but more often indicates features of chronic hepatitis with cholestasis.

Management

Immunosuppression is only of benefit in sclerosing cholangitis associated with autoimmune hepatitis. Treatment of inflammatory bowel disease does not prevent progression of sclerosing cholangitis. Medical therapy is directed towards treatment of cholestasis with fat-soluble vitamin supplementation, nutritional support, and management of pruritis. Treatment with ursodeoxycholic acid (20mg/kg/day) may be of benefit, but there are no control data available in children. Although isolated biliary strictures may

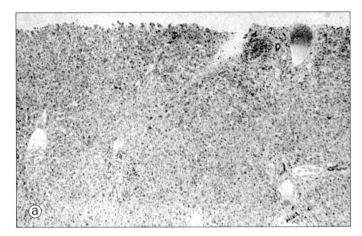

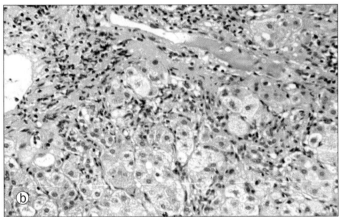

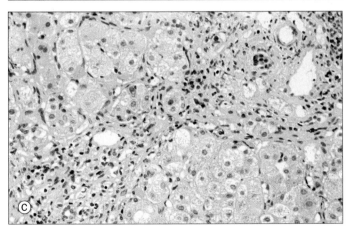

Figure 23.19 Histology of chronic hepatitis. The features of chronic hepatitis in childhood are very similar to those in adults, with an increase in inflammatory infiltrate in the portal tracts (a). This may extend beyond the limiting plate [piecemeal necrosis (b)] leading to bridging fibrosis (c). Differential diagnosis is between an autoimmune hepatitis, chronic viral hepatitis, or Wilson's disease.

Diseases associated with sclerosing cholangitis in childhood	
Disease	**(%)**
Autoimmune hepatitis I	? 50
Inflammatory bowel disease	33
Histocytosis X	19
Immunodeficiency	12
Other	3
Neonatal onset	18
No associated disease	22

Figure 23.20 Diseases associated with sclerosing cholangitis in childhood.

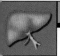

require radiologic or surgical intervention, surgical drainage procedures are not generally indicated and may increase the risk of ascending cholangitis and progression of liver disease.

The majority of children will progress to liver failure and develop the complications of portal hypertension. Median survival or time to transplantation is 10 years from the onset of disease.

Indications for liver transplantation include progressive cholestasis and intractable pruritis or the development of cirrhosis and portal hypertension. Extrahepatic disease, such as colitis may become more severe following liver transplantation.

Drug-induced liver disease

The mechanisms leading to drug-induced liver damage are similar in adults and children, although there is less risk of adverse drug reactions in younger children compared with adults, which may reflect polypharmacy or concurrent disease. However, in childhood there is a specific increased risk of valproate hepatotoxicity in children less than 3 years of age (see page 23.18).

Acetaminophen (paracetamol) poisoning

Acetaminophen toxicity is the most common cause of drug-induced fulminant liver failure. It leads to a direct dose-dependent hepatotoxic effect. In childhood, acetaminophen toxicity may develop in children aged under 3 years of age, either by deliberate acetaminophen poisoning by carers, long-term chronic ingestion of acetaminophen, or deliberate overdose in adolescents. Children have a lower incidence of liver failure with acetaminophen overdose than adults (unless taken with alcohol), perhaps because the rate of glutathione resynthesis is higher.

Aspirin

Aspirin gives rise to dose-dependent hepatotoxicity that is mild, asymptomatic, and reversible. Adverse effects are associated with levels exceeding 15mg/dL in 90%, which may occur in children treated for juvenile chronic arthritis. Hepatic features include an asymptomatic elevation in transaminases with a normal bilirubin level, which usually occurs 6 days after initiation of treatment. In less than 5% of children, severe hepatocellular injury may ensue with prompt recovery on withdrawal of treatment.

Reye's syndrome may be defined as an acute, noninflammatory encephalopathy with hepatic injury occurring without a recognized cause. It has been associated in children with ingestion of aspirin in 90% of cases, especially in children who have intercurrent illnesses such as chickenpox or influenza. The pathogenesis is multifactorial and may reflect a genetic predisposition with a mitochondrial enzyme abnormality in which the viral infection or aspirin ingestion may have induced the hepatocellular insult. There is no relationship between salicylate level and severity of hepatic dysfunction. Reye's syndrome in association with aspirin ingestion is now almost unknown due to the recommendation that aspirin should not be prescribed in children under the age of 12 years.

Metabolic disease in older children

Metabolic disease in older children presents with hepatomegaly often without jaundice, with or without splenomegaly or neurologic involvement. The main causes of metabolic liver disease in older children include α_1-antitrypsin deficiency, cystic fibrosis, Gaucher's disease, tyrosinemia type I, glycogen storage diseases, hereditary fructose intolerance, and Wilson's disease.

Glycogen storage disease

The hepatic glycogen storage disorders (GSDs) are a group of inherited disorders affecting the metabolism of glycogen to glucose. Characteristic findings include hepatomegaly, growth failure, and hypoglycemia. The diagnosis is based on demonstrating the respective enzyme deficiency. All are autosomal recessive, except for phosphorylase kinase deficiency which is X-linked.

Glycogen storage disease type Ia

Glucose-6-phosphatase is a microsomal enzyme found in hepatocytes, renal tubular epithelium, pancreatic and intestinal mucosa, and is essential for hepatic glucose export. Deficiency of the enzyme results in complete dependency on exogenous carbohydrate. The clinical and biochemical effects of the disease result from hypoglycemia and the body's response to hypoglycemia.

Infants usually present with hypoglycemic seizures, hepatomegaly, and failure to thrive. Biochemical investigations reveal fasting hypoglycemia (<1.5g/L) with lactic acidosis (>5mmol/L), hyperlipidemia (cholestcrol >6mmol/L and triglycerides >3mmol/L), and hyperuricemia. Hepatic transaminases are usually normal or mildly elevated. Liver histology reveals steatosis and glycogen storage with no fibrosis. Histochemical stains for glucose-6-phosphatase are negative and the enzyme will not be detected in liver.

The initial aim of dietary treatment is to provide a continuous supply of exogenous glucose in order to maintain normal blood sugars and suppress counter-regulatory responses. This is best achieved in infants by frequent day-time feeding, use of oral uncooked corn starch which is hydrolysed in the gut to release glucose slowly over hours, and continuous nocturnal enteral glucose feeds. If dietary control is strict in infancy, normal growth and development will take place, although hepatomegaly and hyperlipidemia persist. Long-term complications include osteoporosis, renal dysfunction and calculi, and hepatic adenomata which have the potential for malignant transformation. Liver transplantation will correct the hepatic metabolic defect, but is not indicated for metabolic control. The gene for glucose-6-phosphatase has been isolated and many mutations described and antenatal diagnosis by chorionic villus sampling is possible if a known mutation has been identified within the family.

Glycogen storage disease types 1b and 1c

In these disorders glucose-6-phophatase is normal, but dysfunctional. Type 1b is due to a defect in glucose-6-phosphate transport into the microsome, while type 1c is due to abnormalities of phosphate transport out of the microsome. The clinical and biochemical features are similar to GSD type 1a. In GSD type 1b, neutropenia with recurrent infections from oral ulcers and inflammatory bowel disease has been reported. As the gene defect in GSD 1b and 1c has not yet been characterized, antenatal diagnosis is not possible.

Glycogen storage disease type 3

In this disorder there is deficiency in the debrancher enzyme or amylo-1-6-glucosidase deficiency. The metabolic defect is mild as other routes of gluconeogenesis are intact and there is no renal involvement. The defect is expressed in muscle in 85% of cases (type 3a). The clinical presentation is similar to GSD type 1, without renal involvement. In time a peripheral myopathy and cardiomyopathy may develop. As the abnormally structured residual glycogen is fibrogenic, hepatic fibrosis and cirrhosis are complicating features. Diagnosis is by identifying the deficient enzyme in leukocytes or liver tissue.

Dietary treatment is similar to that of GSD type I, but a higher protein intake is recommended due to the demand of gluconeogenic amino acids. Most metabolic abnormalities diminish at puberty and long-term outcome is determined by the development of myopathy, cardiomyopathy, or cirrhosis. Antenatal diagnosis is possible by enzyme measurement or mutation analysis on chorionic villi samples.

Glycogen storage disease type 4

This rare disease is due to a deficiency of the branching enzyme. It usually presents with evidence of severe liver disease in late infancy but there may be cardiac, muscle, and neurologic involvement. Hepatic histology demonstrates cirrhosis and accumulation of abnormally shaped glycogen that is diastase resistant. Dietary treatment is as for other forms of GSD. There is rapid development of cirrhosis necessitating liver transplantation in the first 5 years of life. Progression of extrahepatic disease has been reported post-transplantation.

Glycogen storage disease types 6 and 9

These variants are due to defects in hepatic phosphorylase and phosphorylase kinase, respectively. The phenotype of both GSD types 6 and 9 is milder than in other forms of GSD. Children present with hepatomegaly and growth failure, but hypoglycemia is rare. Hyperlipidemia and ketosis may occur. Hepatic transaminases are often slightly raised, but progression to cirrhosis is unusual. Dietary treatment other than nocturnal corn starch is rarely necessary and spontaneous catch-up growth occurs before puberty. Neither cardiomyopathy nor myopathy have been recognized, and the long-term outlook is excellent.

Hereditary fructose intolerance

This autosomal recessive disorder is due to the absence or reduction of fructose-1-phosphate aldolase B in liver, kidneys, and small intestine. The incidence has been estimated at 1:20,000 live births. The genetic mutation has been identified and is on chromosome 9. Clinical presentation is related to the introduction of fructose or sucrose in the diet. Vomiting is a prominent feature with failure to thrive, hepatomegaly, and coagulopathy. Occasionally infants may present with acute liver failure with jaundice, encephalopathy, and renal failure. Renal tubular acidosis and hypophosphatemic rickets occur (Fig. 23.21).

Older children demonstrate aversion to fructose-containing food.

Biochemical liver function tests indicate raised hepatic transaminases, hypoalbuminemia, and hyperbilirubinemia. Plasma amino acids may be elevated secondary to liver dysfunction and there may be hyperuricacidemia and hypoglycemia. Hematologic abnormalities such as anemia, acanthocytosis, and thrombocytosis are associated. Urinary investigations will indicate frutosuria, proteinuria, amino aciduria, and organic aciduria in association with a reduction in the tubular reabsorption of phosphate.

Diagnosis is suggested by reducing substances in the urine and confirmed by a reduction or absence of enzymatic activity in liver or intestinal mucosal biopsy or by mutation analysis.

Hepatic pathology varies from complete hepatic necrosis to diffuse steatosis and periportal intralobular fibrosis which may progress to cirrhosis if fructose is continued. Fructose elimination reverses hepatic and renal dysfunction. Antenatal diagnosis is possible by chorionic villus sampling.

Gaucher's disease

This autosomal recessive disorder is secondary to a deficiency of glucosyl-ceramide-β- glucosidase which is deficient in leukocytes, hepatocytes and amniocytes. It may present in infancy with acute liver failure, but is more usual in late childhood with hepatosplenomegaly, and respiratory, neurologic, and bone disease. The diagnosis is suggested by the identification of large multinucleated Gaucher cells in bone marrow aspirate and liver, confirmed by enzyme assay. Hepatic fibrosis may be severe leading to cirrhosis. Recent therapy for Gaucher's disease includes enzyme replacement, bone marrow, or liver transplantation.

Wilson's disease

Wilson's disease is an autosomal recessive disorder with an incidence of 1:30,000 live births. The Wilson's disease gene is on chromosome 13 and encodes a copper-binding ATPase.

Clinical features

Clinical features in childhood include hepatic dysfunction (40%) and psychiatric symptoms (35%). Children under the age of 10 years usually present with hepatic symptoms. The hepatic presentation of Wilson's disease resembles that of adults who have hepatomegaly: vague gastrointestinal symptoms; subacute or fulminant hepatitis; and chronic hepatitis or cirrhosis. Neurologic symptoms are nonspecific. Children may present with deteriorating school performance, abnormal behavior, lack of coordination, and dysarthria. Renal tubular abnormalities, renal calculii, and acute hemolytic anemia are associated features. The characteristic Kayser–Fleischer rings are not usually detected before the age of 7 years and may be absent in up to 80% of older children.

Diagnosis

Biochemical liver function tests indicate chronic liver disease with low albumin [<3.5g/dl (<35g/L)], minimal transaminitis, and a low alkaline phosphastase (<200U/L). There may be evi-

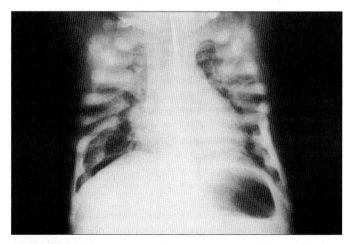

Figure 23.21 This chest radiograph demonstrates an enlarged heart secondary to fluid overload, and severe rickets secondary to renal tubular acidosis. The most likely diagnosis is between tyrosinemia type I and hereditary fructosemia.

dence of hemolysis on blood film. The diagnosis is established by detecting a low serum copper [<1μmol/dl (<10μmol/L)], a low serum ceurolplasmin [<20mg/dl (<200mg/L)], excess urine copper (>1μmol/24h), particularly after penicillamine treatment (20mg/kg/day), and an elevated hepatic copper (>250mg/g dry weight of liver). Approximately 25% of children may have a normal or borderline ceruloplasmin as it is an acute phase protein. Radioactive copper studies are only indicated in children who have equivocal copper and/or ceruloplasmin values in whom liver biopsy is contraindicated.

Histologic features of Wilson's disease depend on the clinical presentation. There may be microvesicular fatty infiltration of hepatocytes, chronic hepatitis (see Fig. 23.19), hepatocellular necrosis, multinucleated hepatocytes and Mallory's hyaline, hepatic fibrosis, and cirrhosis. In children who have fulminant hepatitis the histologic features are those of severe hepatocellular necrosis with an underlying cirrhosis.

Management
Current management includes a low copper diet and penicallimine (20mg/kg/day), which is effective if started before the development of significant hepatic fibrosis. If penicillamine toxicity is unacceptable, alternative therapy includes trientine (trietheline tetramine) 25mg/kg/day, in addition to oral zinc. In asymptomatic children or in those who have minimal hepatic dysfunction, the outlook is excellent, although fulminant hepatic failure with hemolysis may occur if treatment is discontinued. Liver transplantation is essential therapy for children who present with subacute or fulminant hepatitis and in those children who have advanced cirrhosis and portal hypertension.

It is essential for the family to be screened in order to treat asymptomatic patients and to detect heterozygotes. The development of mutation analysis may be more reliable than measurement of serum copper and ceruloplasmin.

Cystic fibrosis liver disease
The incidence of liver disease in children who have cystic fibrosis varies from 4.5 to 20%, depending on age and the definition of significant liver disease.

Pathophysiology
The etiology of cystic fibrosis liver disease has only been partially explained. Despite major advances in the understanding of the genetic defects in cystic fibrosis, no definite genetic mutation has been associated with the development of liver disease. A low familial concordance of the development of liver disease within siblings suggests that environmental factors may be important. There is an increased frequency of the HLA antigens A2, C7, DR2 (DRW15), and DQW6, suggesting that genetic factors controlling the lymphocyte-mediated immune response might be implicated. The recent discovery of the cystic fibrosis transmembrane receptor (CFTR) in the apical membrane of biliary epithelial cells may be a major step in the understanding of the etiology.

Bile acid malabsorption is a constant finding in untreated children who have cystic fibrosis. In the duodenum the total concentration of bile salts is decreased, but increases in the glycine/taurine ratio, and the percentage of potentially toxic dihydroxy bile salts have been noted. The abnormally low duodenal pH secondary to pancreatic insufficiency further exacer-

bates bile acid malabsorption and impairs micellar formation. Supplementation with taurine improves the glycine/taurine ratio of bile salts in the serum but not in the duodenum. It is possible that the abnormalities in bile salt concentration and the increase in hydrophobic and toxic bile acids may play an important role in the production of viscous bile and or biliary sludge, which may lead to partial biliary obstruction and focal biliary fibrosis.

Clinical features
Most children who have cystic fibrosis and liver disease are asymptomatic in the early stages. In infants, cholestatic neonatal hepatitis may be a presenting feature (see above), but more commonly the presentation is associated with asymptomatic hepatosplenomegaly or the complications of portal hypertension. Biliary disease includes asymptomatic gallstones in 20% and microgallbladder on ultrasound in 10–40%, but biliary strictures are now considered uncommon.

Diagnosis
Early detection of liver disease using serum liver function tests is unsatisfactory. In general, however, there will be transient abnormalities of alkaline phosphatase in up to 50% of patients; increases in γ-GT in 30% of males and 60% of females occur; and serum bilirubin levels and coagulation times remain normal until late in the disease. Ultrasonography may detect increased echogenicity in 41% of patients, but does not differentiate fatty infiltration from fibrosis. Microgallbladder with or without gallstones is found in 25% of patients. Hepatobiliary scanning demonstrates pooling in intrahepatic bile ducts, which may be a normal finding, or the presence of biliary strictures.

Liver histology may indicate fatty infiltration, focal biliary cirrhosis, and multilobular cirrhosis. Steatosis is the commonest finding at biopsy and includes a mixture of micro- and macrovesicular fatty infiltration. Nonspecific mild inflammation around the portal tracts is commonly found in association with chemical cholangitis (granular eosinophilic secretions in bile ducts in association with ductal proliferation of bile ducts). Fibrosis develops initially around the portal tracts and gradually extends between portal tracts until cirrhosis has developed. Cholestasis and bile plugs are rarely identified. Liver biopsy should be performed to establish the extent and severity of liver disease and is indicated when there is persistent transaminitis, hepatic echogenicity on ultrasound, hepatomegaly and/or splenomegaly, or evidence of hepatic dysfunction.

Management
Treatment consists of nutritional support and the prevention and management of hepatic complications. Nutritional support is critically important in children who have cystic fibrosis, regardless of whether they have liver disease. If cystic fibrosis is complicated by clinically significant liver disease, then the following is recommended:
- increasing energy intake to 150% of average requirements by carbohydrate supplements, such as glucose polymer, or by increasing the percentage of fat;
- increasing the proportion of medium chain triglyercides to 50% of the fat content; and
- supplementation with fat soluble vitamins, including vitamin A (5–15,000IU/day), vitamin E (100–500mg/day), vitamin D (50ng/kg), and vitamin K (1–10mg/day).

The use of ursodeoxycholic acid in the management of cystic

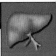

fibrosis liver disease remains controversial. There is clear evidence that treatment with ursodeoxycholic acid improves the biochemical indices of liver function, but is unlikely to affect the natural history of the disease unless prescribed before the stage at which it becomes significant.

The main hepatic complication of cystic fibrosis liver disease is the development of portal hypertension and the development of esophageal varices, which should be diagnosed by endoscopy. Prophylactic sclerotherapy is not recommended, but injection sclerotherapy or banding is usually effective once variceal hemorrhage develops. In order to avoid repeated anesthetics for sclerotherapy or banding, inserting a transjugular intrahepatic portal systemic shunt (TIPSS), which can be performed in quite young children, may be preferable.

Current data indicate that cystic fibrosis liver disease is a progressive disease leading eventually to cirrhosis and portal hypertension in all cases. Indications for liver transplantation include the development of end-stage liver failure with jaundice, ascites, and coagulopathy, which are late features in this disease. Liver transplantation is indicated in children who have cystic fibrosis liver disease before the development of significant pulmonary complication (<70% of normal function) in order to prevent the necessity for heart, lung, and liver transplantation. The use of pulmonary DNAs preoperatively is recommended. Perioperative antibiotics should be based on the sensitivity of colonized pulmonary bacteria. The outcome following liver transplantation is similar to that in children transplanted for other causes of liver disease. Lung function may improve after transplantation.

Hepatic tumors

Liver tumors are relatively rare in childhood and occur in the region of 0.5–2.5 per million population. Hepatocellular carcinoma in childhood occurs at an older age than hepatoblastoma in association with underlying cirrhosis secondary to hepatitis B, hepatitis C, or α_1-antitrypsin deficiency. A rare fibrolamellar hepatocellular tumor is occasionally seen in childhood and occurs in noncirrhotic livers. Hepatoblastoma is most commonly seen in children under the age of 18 months and is rare after the age of 5 years. There is a male predominance of 3 to 2. The commonest presenting feature is of an abdominal mass and distension, and rarely anorexia, weight loss, pain, vomiting, and jaundice. Hepatoblastoma is sometimes associated with sexual precoscities due to the release of human chorionic gonadotropic hormones (β-HCG). Osteoporosis may occur in up to 20% of cases leading to bone fractures and vertebral compression. Hepatoblastoma occurs with certain well-recognized associations, in particular hereditary polyposis coli.

Diagnosis

Laboratory investigations will demonstrate:
- a normocytic normochromic anemia in 50% of children;
- thrombocytosis (greater than $1000 \times 10^9/L$) in 30% of children;
- normal liver function tests in hepatoblastoma, but may be abnormal in hepatocellular carcinoma due to underlying cirrhosis;
- α-fetoprotein may be a useful diagnostic and prognostic marker and is elevated in 90% of hepatoblastoma patients and 60% of hepatocellular carcinoma patients; and
- transcobalamin-1 may be a useful marker in fibrolamellar hepatocellular carcinoma.

Abdominal ultrasound, computed tomography (CT) scanning or MRI imaging will determine the site and extent of the lesion, and establish the presence of any metastases while providing information as regards suitability for surgical resection. Vascular structures are best identified on angiography or MRI imaging and are an essential investigation before surgery. Chest radiograph and CT scanning are important baseline investigations to define the presence of pulmonary metastases. Liver biopsy is necessary for histologic confirmation and selection of chemotherapy, despite the risks of disseminating tumor.

Hepatoblastoma may be classified into four groups; fetal, embryonal, macrotrabecular, and small-cell undifferentiated tumors. Microscopic features distinguishing hepatocellular carcinoma from hepatoblastoma are the presence of tumor cells that are larger than normal hepatocytes with frequent tumor giant cells, broad cellular trabeculi, nuclear neomorphism, and the absence of hematopoiesis. The fibrolamellar variant of hepatocellular carcinoma consists of plump tumor cells with deeply eosinophilic cytoplasm and a marked fibrous stroma separating epithelial cells into trabeculi.

It is important to differentiate a hepatoblastoma and hepatocellular carcinoma from other undifferentiated embryonal sarcoma and this is only possible on histologic criteria. Benign vascular tumors such as hemangioma or hemangioendotheliomas are usually differentiated by the radiologic appearance on CT scanning and histology. Focal nodular hyperplasia is a rare benign tumor of childhood which may be single or multiple.

The malignant tumors must also be differentiated from hepatic adenomas which present with a pattern similar to that seen in adults. They may occur at any age, including in neonates and have even been reported in the fetus *in utero*. There is no link between maternal contraceptive use and childhood adenoma. Adenomas have been reported in patients receiving anabolic steroids, GSD type I, familial diabetes mellitus, hemosiderosis, and galactosemia. Histologically, the tumors may be partially encapsulated, and consist of thick cords of benign hepatocytes lacking portal structures and bile duct. It may be particularly difficult to distinguish between adenoma and well-differentiated hepatocellular carcinoma.

Management

About 90% of hepatoblastomas will respond to chemotherapy and surgery. At minority will require liver transplantation for unresectable tumors. Current chemotherapy includes a combination of cisplatinum and doxorubicin (PLADO), which will reduce the tumor in the majority of patients. Of the total, 71% will be amenable to surgical resection with an 82% 5-year survival rate. Most tumors, which are multifocal, central in situation or involving the portal vein, are not amenable to resection and these children should be considered for liver replacement. An increasing number of patients have been successfully transplanted with a 5-year survival rate of 80%.

Hepatocellular carcinomas are less responsive to treatment and only 50% will respond to PLADO chemotherapy. Surgical resection is less successful. The recent addition of carboplatim to PLADO may improve the response rate in these tumors. Response to therapy may be monitored by serial measurement of α-fetoprotein levels. Patients who have good responses to chemotherapy will have a rapid fall of serum α-fetoprotein, while those children with persistent elevation of α-fetoprotein are likely to have residual disease or metastases.

ACUTE LIVER FAILURE IN INFANCY AND CHILDHOOD

The definition of acute liver failure or fulminant hepatic failure (FHF) is the development of hepatic necrosis with coagulopathy and encephalopathy occurring within 8 weeks of the onset of liver disease. This definition is hard to apply in pediatric practice, as many infants present with acute liver failure from an inborn error of metabolism implying pre-existing disease. Secondly, encephalopathy may be difficult to detect in infants and small children and be less severe than coagulopathy in the early stages. Thus, caution is required when defining fulminant hepatitis or acute liver failure in infancy. The etiology of acute liver failure may include many causes common in adult practice, the main difference being the high incidence of acute liver failure associated with metabolic liver disease (Fig. 23.22).

Acute liver failure in infancy

Acute liver failure in infancy usually presents with multisystem involvement. The diagnosis may initially be difficult as jaundice may be a late feature. Infants are usually small for gestational dates, with hypotonia, severe coagulopathy, and encephalopathy. Neurologic problems such as nystagmus and convulsions may be secondary to cerebral disease or encephalopathy. Renal tubular acidosis is common. Investigations include a search for multiorgan disease.

Galactosemia

This rare autosomal disorder is secondary to a deficiency of galactose-1-phosphase uridyltransferase. Acute illness results from the accumulation of the substrate galactose-1-phosphate (gal-1-P) following the introduction of milk feeds. Infants present with collapse with sepsis, hypoglycemia, and encephalopathy in the first few days of life or with progressive jaundice and liver failure. Cataracts are present. The disease may be complicated by Gram-negative sepsis, which stimulates a life-threatening severe bleeding diathesis.

The diagnosis is established by the detection of urinary reducing substances in the absence of glycosuria, and confirmed by reduced enzyme activity in erythrocytes. Hepatic pathology demonstrates fatty change, periportal bile duct proliferation, and

Acute liver failure in children	
Etiology	**Diagnostic investigations**
Infection Viral hepatitis A, B, C, undefined, EBV, CMV	Viral serology
Poison/drugs Acetaminophen (paracetamol) Isoniazid, halothane Animata phalloides	Acetaminophen levels Halothane antibodies
Autoimmune hepatitis	Autoimmune screen
Metabolic Wilson's disease Tyrosinemia	Cu, ceruloplasmin Urinary succinylacetone
Reye's syndrome	Microvesicular fat in liver Urinary dicarboxylic acids

Figure 23.22 Acute liver failure in children.

iron deposition with extra medullary hematopoiesis. If galactose ingestion persists, hepatic fibrosis and cirrhosis may develop or be present at birth.

Liver function improves following exclusion of galactose from the diet unless liver failure or cirrhosis has developed. Galactose elimination is life-long, but efficacy may be limited by endogenous synthesis of gal-1-P. The long-term outcome is disappointing. Learning difficulties and growth disturbance are described and are more common in girls, 75% of whom also develop ovarian failure. Detection of galactosemia in a neonatal screening program will lead to early detection, except for infants who present with fulminant hepatitis. Antenatal diagnosis is possible by chorionic villi sampling.

Neonatal hemochromatosis

This presumed autosomal recessive disorder is the commonest cause of acute liver failure in the neonate. It is characterized by the prenatal accumulation of intrahepatic iron, due either to a primary disorder of fetoplacental iron handling, or a secondary manifestation of fetal liver disease. Intrauterine growth retardation and premature delivery is common. Clinical features include hypoglycemia, jaundice, and coagulopathy within the first 2 weeks, with a fatal outcome without treatment.

Biochemical liver function tests demonstrate an elevated bilirubin, and reduced transaminases and albumin. Serum iron binding capacity is low and hypersaturated (90–100%), with a grossly elevated ferritin level [100ng/dl (>1000ng/L)]. Diagnostic liver biopsy is not feasible because of the coagulopathy, but extrahepatic siderosis is found in minor salivary glands obtained by lip biopsy. Magnetic resonance imaging may confirm excess hepatic or extrahepatic iron. Liver histology at autopsy demonstrates pericellular fibrosis, giant cell transformation, ductular proliferation, and regenerative nodules. The distribution of siderosis is similar to adult hereditary hemochromatosis, with hepatocellular and extrahepatic parenchymal deposition, and sparing of the reticuloendothelial systems.

Medical management includes supportive therapy for acute liver failure and an 'antioxidant cocktail', which combines N-acetylcysteine (150mg/kg/day), vitamin E (25mg/kg/day), selenium (2–3μg/kg/day), prostaglandin E_1 (0.4–0.6μg/kg/h), and desferrioxamine (30μg/kg/day). Some children have responded to this regimen, but the majority require liver transplantation. Extrahepatic iron is mobilized following successful liver transplantation.

Currently early antenatal diagnosis is not possible, but the diagnosis may be suspected by the detection of nonspecific abnormalities such as hydrops fetalis or intrauterine growth retardation. Prenatal iron accumulation may be detected by MRI, but the sensitivity is unknown. A recent report of maternal autoimmune disease preceding this syndrome (presence of anti-RO and anti-LA antibodies) may be relevant to etiology.

Disorders of mitochondrial energy metabolism

This group of disorders include a wide range of clinical phenotypes with any mode of inheritance: autosomal recessive; autosomal dominant; or transmission through maternal DNA. A number of different defects involving the electron transport chain have been described. The clinical feaures develop secondary to electron transport chain dysfunction, which results in cellular ATP deficiency and the generation of toxic-free radicals. Clinical symptoms vary, depending on the nature

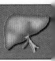

of the primary defect, the tissue or organ distribution and abundance, and the importance of aerobic metabolism in the affected tissue. The constituent proteins of the electron transport chain are encoded in two genomes, either nuclear DNA or mitochondrial DNA (mDNA) which is maternally inherited. In the context of liver failure, two entities are relevant: isolated deficiencies of the electron chain enzymes and mDNA depletion syndromes.

Deficiencies of the electron transport chain enzyme

The most common isolated defects are complexes 4 and 1, although multiple deficiencies have been reported. Infants present with multisystem involvement with hypotonia, cardiomyopathy, and proximal renal tubulopathy and a severe metabolic acidosis. Relevant diagnostic investigations include elevated blood lactate, lactate/pyruvate ratio >20, increased 3-OH-butyrate/acetoacetate ratio >2, or an increase in lactate, possible ketone bodies and, following a glucose load (2g/kg × 50g), the detection of specific organic acids such as urinary 3-methyl-glutaconic acid or other Krebs cycle intermediates. Coagulopathy is usually extreme, and may prevent liver or muscle biopsy, or cerebrospinal fluid (CSF) examination. The definitive diagnosis is based on demonstrating biochemical dysfunction of electron chain function in liver or muscle by histochemistry or enzyme analysis in fresh tissue. Demonstration of an elevated CSF lactate compared with plasma lactate indicates neurologic involvement.

Supportive management is usually the only option. Liver transplantation is only successful if the defect is confined to the liver, but is contraindicated if multisystem involvement is obvious as neurologic deterioration persists or may develop post-transplant.

Antenatal diagnosis is rarely possible as the underlying gene defects are unknown.

Mitochondrial DNA depletion syndromes

Mitochondria normally contain more than one copy of mDNA and replication is regulated by a number of factors encoded by nuclear genes. Mutations in these nuclear genes lead to a reduction in copy numbers of mDNA resulting in mitochondrial depletion. The clinical presentation and biochemical findings are similar to those of infants presenting with isolated electron transport chain deficiencies. In most patients tissue measurement of electron chain activities show deficiencies in complexes 1, 3, and 4, although activity may be within the normal range. The diagnosis is confirmed by demonstrating an abnormally low ratio for mDNA/nuclear DNA in affected tissue. Treatment is supportive as liver transplantation is contraindicated. Antenatal diagnosis is not currently possible.

Tyrosinemia type I

Tyrosinemia type I is an autosomal recessive disorder due to a defect of fumaryl acetoacetase (FAA), which is the terminal enzyme in tyrosine degradation. The gene for FAA is on the short arm of chromosome 15 and many mutations have been described. Intermediate metabolites such as maleyl- and fumarylacetoacetate are highly reactive compounds that are locally toxic within the liver, whereas the secondary metabolite succinylacetone has local and systemic effects, including inhibition of porphobilinogen synthase, and is thought to be responsible for cardiac, renal, and neurologic disease.

Clinical features

This is heterogeneous, even within the same family. Acute liver failure is a common presentation in infants between 1 and 6 months of age who present with mild jaundice, coagulopathy, encephalopathy, and ascites. Hypoglycemia is common, either due to liver dysfunction or hyperinsulinism from pancreatic islet cell hyperplasia. In older infants, failure to thrive, coagulopathy, hepatosplenomegaly, hypotonia, and rickets are common (see Fig. 23.21). Older children may present with chronic liver disease, a hypertrophic cardiomyopathy, renal failure or a porphyria-like syndrome with self-mutilation. Renal tubular dysfunction and hypophosphatemic rickets may occur at any age. There is a high risk of hepatocellular carcinoma.

Diagnosis

Biochemical liver function tests reveal an elevated bilirubin, transaminases, alkaline phosphatase, and a reduced albumin. Plasma amino acids indicate a three-fold increase in plasma tyrosine, phenylalanine, and methionine with grossly elevated α-fetoprotein levels. Urinary succinyl acetone is a pathognomonic but not an invariable finding. The diagnosis is confirmed by measuring FAA activity in fibroblasts or lymphocytes. Proximal tubular dysfunction may be suspected if there is phosphaturia and aminoaciduria, and confirmed by a reduction in renal tubular absorption of phosphate (<80%).

Echocardiography may reveal a hypertrophic cardiomyopathy, while radiologic examination may indicate severe hypophosphatemic rickets. Hepatic histology is nonspecific with steatosis, siderosis, and cirrhosis, which may be present in infancy (Fig 23.23). Hepatocyte dysplasia is common and is associated with a risk of hepatocellular carcinoma.

Management

Initial management is with a phenylalanine and tyrosine-restricted diet which may improve overall nutritional status and renal tubular function, but does not effect progression of liver disease. The recent discovery of 2(2-nitro-trifluoromethylbenzoyl)-1,3-cyclohexenedione (NTBC), which prevents the formation of toxic metabolites, has altered the natural history of this disease in childhood. Worldwide more than 100 children have been treated with NTBC. There is rapid reduction of toxic metabolites, normalization of tubular function, prevention of porphyria-like crises, and improvement in both nutritional status and liver function, particularly in those who have acute liver failure.

The long-term outcome of children who have tyrosinemia type I treated with NTBC is unknown. These children require long-term monitoring and follow-up with 6-monthly abdominal ultrasounds and CT scans, or MRI and α-fetoprotein estimation for early detection of hepatocellular carcinoma (Fig 23.24). The current indications for liver transplantation for this condition include the development of acute or chronic liver failure unresponsive to NTBC, or suspicion of development of hepatocellular carcinoma. Antenatal diagnosis is possible either by chorionic villus sampling which measures FAA directly, or from mutation analysis, or by measurement of succinyl acetone in the amniotic fluid. Prospective affected siblings may benefit from early NTBC therapy.

Familial hemophagocytic lymphohistocytosis

This rare disorder may be inherited as an autosomal recessive condition, or be secondary to a viral illness. There is progressive vis-

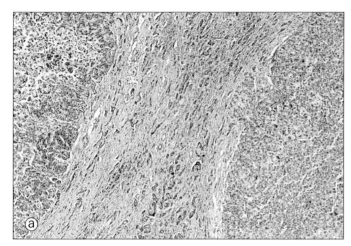

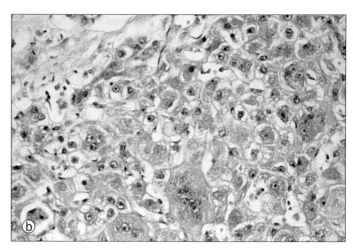

Figure 23.23 Histology of a liver biopsy. (a) Indicating non-specific steatosis and fibrosis. (b) There is early hepatic dysplasia, which is a frequent finding in tyrosinemia type I. A focus of hepatocellular carcinoma was found elsewhere in the liver at transplantation.

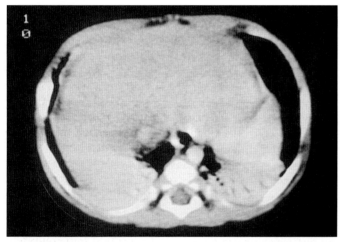

Figure 23.24 CT scan indicating multiple nodules in a patient who has tyrosinemia type I. These nodules may represent regenerative nodules or foci of hepatocellular carcinoma.

ceral, neurologic, and bone marrow infiltration with lymphocytes and large erythrophagocytic histioctyes. Children present with fever, hepatosplenomegaly, jaundice, skin rash, edema, and encephalopathy in the first year of life. There is a pancytopenia, coagulopathy, and biochemical features of acute liver failure, hypofibroginemia, and hypotriglyceridemia. Diagnosis is established by identifying the characteristic erythrophagocytic histiocytes in bone marrow, liver, and CSF. The disease is usually fatal, although treatment with antimetabolites and corticosteroids, or bone marrow transplantation may be helpful. Liver transplantation is contraindicated if there is extensive bone marrow or neurologic involvement.

Acute liver failure in older children
Fulminant viral hepatitis
All forms of acute viral hepatitis may present in childhood and the presentation will be similar to that of FHF in adults, except where specified below.

In infants, infection with herpes simplex virus (HSV-1, HSV-2, HSV-6, varicella-zoster virus, or CMV) may cause par-

ticularly severe forms of hepatic failure, often in immuno-compromised hosts.

In older children, hepatitis A is the commonest cause of fulminant hepatitis with an incidence ranging from 1.5 to 31%. Hepatitis B infection from vertical transmission from an HBsAg-positive mother, with anti-HBe antibody, has been documented to produce fulminant hepatitis in infants aged 3 months. The pathogenesis of this disease is unknown, but may be related to the lack of protection of anti-E antibody in the neonate. The commonest cause of fulminant hepatitis, as in adults, is sporadic non-A–G hepatitis (NA–G), which accounts for almost two thirds of children who have FHF. As in adults, this carries a particularly poor prognosis.

Drugs and toxins
Liver injury due to drugs and toxins is the second most common cause of acute liver failure in older children. Sodium valproate has been associated with more than 150 cases of fatal hepatotoxicity worldwide, although the mechanism is unclear. Valproate has a complex metabolic fate undergoing partial mitochondrial β oxidation, forming acyl compounds with coenzyme A and carnitine and inhibiting cellular carnitine uptake. Hepatotoxicity has occurred in patients who have abnormalities of fatty acid oxidation, mitochondrial energy metabolism, the urea cycle, and those who have presumed metabolic disorders such as Alpers' syndrome, suggesting that the normal response to valproate may precipitate hepatotoxicity in those who have abnormal intermediary metabolism.

Hepatotoxicity may occur at any age, but is more likely in children aged <2 years, those on multiple epileptic therapy, and those who have previous neurologic abnormalities or developmental delay. Clinical features include nausea, vomiting, increasing seizure frequency, jaundice, edema, and hypoglycemia leading to drowsiness and coma usually within the first 6 months of treatment. Biochemical investigations reveal moderate increases in hepatic transaminases and bilirubin, hypoaminemia, and severe coagulopathy. Hepatic histology demonstrates is severe microvesicular fatty change with hepatocellular necrosis and occasionally cirrhosis.

Once liver disease is established, the outlook is poor unless valproate has been promptly discontinued. Carnitine is not effective in preventing or treating hepatotoxicity, but *N*-acetylcysteine may have a hepatoprotective role. Liver transplantation is contraindicated as neurologic disease may progress.

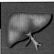
Progressive neuronal degeneration of childhood (Alpers' syndrome)

The etiology of this familial disorder is unknown. It is thought to be autosomal recessive, and in some cases an electron chain transport defect has been identified. Despite a normal neonatal period, there may be both physical and developmental delay followed by the sudden onset of intractable seizures between the ages of 1 and 3 years. Although biochemical evidence of liver dysfunction is often present at this stage, clinical liver involvement is a preterminal event. Hepatic disease presents as jaundice, hepatomegaly, and coagulopathy with rapidly progressive liver failure.

There are no specific biochemical features. Electroencephalogram demonstrates high amplitude polyspikes; CT or MRI scans show low density areas in the occipital and posterior temporal areas. There are gradual extinction of visual evoked responses. Liver histology characteristically shows microvesicular fatty change, bile duct proliferation, focal necrosis leading to bridging fibrosis and cirrhosis. Neuropathology reveals cortical involvement with neuronal cell loss and astrocyte replacement.

The condition is uniformly fatal, with most children dying before 3 years within a few months of developing overt liver disease. It is important to avoid the use of valproate as it is likely to accelerate the development of liver disease. Liver transplantation is contraindicated, as neurologic progression continues after transplant. Antenatal diagnosis is currently impossible.

Immune and metabolic mechanisms

Autoimmune hepatitis type II [associated with liver, kidney and microsomal antibodies (LKMs)] is a common cause of acute liver failure in childhood. The diagnosis is established by identifying elevated serum immunoglobulins and LKM antibodies (see Fig 23.15). A minority of patients will respond to immunosuppressant therapy in this situation and most will require liver transplantation. Acute liver failure has also been recorded with juvenile rheumatoid arthritis, although therapy with immunosuppressive agents is more effective.

Although most inborn errors of metabolism present early in infancy, Wilson's disease, tyrosinemia type I, or Alpers' disease present in older children.

Clinical manifestations of acute liver failure

The onset of liver disease varies according to etiology. There may be a prodromal illness with lethargy, fatigue, malaise, vomiting, diarrhea, and jaundice with the subsequent development of coagulopathy and encephalopathy. Encephalopathy is difficult to detect in infants and may present with drowsiness, irritability or day/night reversal of sleep rhythm. Older children become aggressive, which is misinterpreted as antisocial behavior. The later stages of encephalopathy and hepatic coma are similar in older children and adults. A poor prognosis is indicated if any of the following features are present:

- rise in bilirubin [>18mg/dl (>300mmol/L)];
- a fall in transaminases without clinical improvement and increasing coagulopathy;
- prothrombin time >60s;
- metabolic acidosis (pH <7.3);
- hypoglycaemia (glucose less than 4mmol/L);
- a decrease in liver size (not usual in metabolic liver disease); and
- increasing hepatic coma grade II or III.

Supportive management for acute liver failure in childhood includes:

- maintaining blood glucose levels greater than 4mmol/L with 10–50% dextrose;
- fluid restriction (50–75% of standard maintenance) using colloid to maintain circulating volume;
- prevention of gastrointestinal hemorrhage from stress erosions using H_2 receptor antagonists (ranitidine 3mg/kg q8h) and sucralfate (2–4g/day);
- prevention of sepsis with broad-spectrum antibiotics (amoxicillin, cefuroxime, and metronidazole);
- prophylactic antifungal therapy (fluconazole);
- treatment of coagulopathy if required with fresh frozen plasma and intravenous vitamin K (2–10 mg);
- management of hepatic encephalopathy. In the early stages reduction of protein intake to 1–2g/kg and provision of high calorie feeds using glucose polymer (8–10g/kg) and oral lactulose may be sufficient. Increasing encephalopathy unresponsive to conservative management requires elective ventilation; and
- the development of cerebral edema by clinical signs, such as deepening coma which may be detectable on CT scan, is an ominous sign. Conservative management includes fluid restriction (<50% of maintenance), mannitol (0.5g/kg q6h–q8h), and elective hyperventilation. The role of intracranial pressure monitoring is controversial. Electrodes may be difficult to insert in children who have severe coagulopathy, particularly as the blood product replacement may exacerbate cerebral edema. Intracranial pressure monitoring may improve selection for transplantation but does not affect overall survival.

Liver transplantation should be carefully considered in all children who have acute liver failure, but difficulties arise in the selection of infants who have inborn errors of metabolism, because of the difficulty in excluding multisystem disease. Liver transplantation is indicated in those children who have poor prognostic factors, namely NA–G hepatitis, rapid onset of coma grade III or IV, or severe coagulopathy (may be more severe than encephalopathy in metabolic disease). There should be no evidence of irreversible brain damage on CT scans or evidence of multisystem disease (normal muscle biopsy, normal electrocardiogram, etc).

The mortality rate is greater than 70% for children who are in grade III or IV coma, or who have persistently abnormal coagulation (prothrombin time >60s). Prognosis may be better in children who have hepatitis A or who have taken an acetaminophen overdose. The causes of death in children not transplanted were sepsis (15%), hemorrhage (50%), renal failure (30%), and cerebral edema (56%). There is between 50 and 70% 1-year survival rate following liver transplantation, which is less than transplantation for children who have other indications. Survivors with liver transplantation face the psychologic sequelae of such a procedure and the long-term complications of this operation.

Of the range of hepatic support, only exchange blood transfusion and plasmaphoresis have had any value in pediatric practice in reducing coagulopathy and prolonging life until a donor liver was obtained. Artificial liver support using either porcine hepatocytes or a liver cell line have not been evaluated in children.

LIVER TRANSPLANTATION

The success of pediatric liver transplantation has revolutionized the prognosis for many infants and children who would otherwise die of liver failure. The main factors in improving survival in this age group include advances in preoperative management such as the treatment of hepatic complications, nutritional support, and selection for transplantation. The rapid development in innovative surgical techniques to expand the donor pool have extended liver transplantation to the neonatal age group, while improvements in postoperative management including immunosuppression have led not only to increased survival, but also improved quality of life. The range of indications for liver transplantation in children now include semi-elective liver replacement and transplantation for inborn errors of metabolism with extrahepatic disease and unresectable hepatic tumors.

Indications

As in adults, most children are transplanted for chronic liver failure. Biliary atresia is the commonest indication for children transplanted under the age of 2 years (Fig. 23.25).

As many children who have cirrhosis and portal hypertension have well-compensated hepatic function, the timing of liver transplantation may be difficult to decide. In general, the most useful guide is a serial estimation of hepatic function, such as:
- a persistent rise in total bilirubin [6mg/dl (>100μmol/L)];
- prolongation of prothrombin time (international normalized ratio [INR] >1.4);
- progressive fall in serum albumin [<3.5g/dl (<35g/L)];
- the development of protein energy malnutrition resistant to nutritional management (deterioration in measurements of triceps skin-folds, midarm muscle area, negative growth velocity); and
- hepatic complications such as chronic hepatic encephalopathy, refractory ascites, intractable pruritus, or recurrent variceal bleeding nonresponsive to optimal medical management.

Children who have chronic liver disease have a significant reduction in developmental motor skills which may be reversed following liver transplantation; thus these children should be transplanted before the complications of their liver disease impairs the quality of their lives and before growth and development are irreversibly delayed.

Acute liver failure

The indications for liver transplantation for children who have acute liver failure depend on the etiology and the extent of the multisystem disease. In general children who have fulminant hepatitis should be referred early to a specialist unit in the field of transplantation in order to provide time for stabilization and consideration for liver transplantation.

Children who have a poor prognosis and, therefore should have early listing for liver transplantation, include those who have:
- NA–G hepatitis;
- rapid onset of coma with progression to grade III or IV hepatic coma;
- diminishing liver size; and
- a fall in serum transaminases associated with increasing bilirubin [>18mg/dl (>300μmol/L)] and persistent coagulopathy (>50s).

Liver transplantation is contraindicated for children who have evidence of multisystem involvement (e.g. mitochondrial disease) or irreversible brain damage from cerebral edema or hypoglycemia.

Inborn errors of metabolism

Liver transplantation is indicated for inborn errors of metabolism if the hepatic enzyme deficiency leads to irreversible liver disease or liver failure and/or hepatoma (e.g. tyrosinemia type I, Wilson's disease) or severe extrahepatic disease. Selection of patients who have severe extrahepatic disease is difficult, as it is necessary to evaluate the quality of life of the child on medical management and to compare the potential mortality and morbidity of their original disease with the risk of complications following liver transplantation. The timing of transplantation in these disorders depends on the rate of progression of the disease, the quality of life of the affected child on conservative management, and the development of severe reversible extrahepatic disease.

Indications for transplantation for liver tumors includes either unresectable benign tumors causing hepatic dysfunction or unresectable malignant tumors refractory to chemotherapy without evidence of extrahepatic metastases.

Evaluation

The aim of the evaluation process is to:
- assess the severity of liver disease and the extent of hepatic complications;
- consider the technical aspects of the operation with regard to vascular anatomy and size;
- exclude any significant contraindications to successful transplantation; and
- prepare the child and family psychologically.

The histologic diagnosis of the original disease should be reviewed and the severity and extent of hepatic function determined by evaluating:
- albumin [3.5g/dl (< 35g/L)];
- coagulation time (INR>1.4);
- bilirubin – rise in bilirubin [9mg/dl (>150μmol/L)] is usual is cholestatic patients, but may be a late feature in other diseases such as cystic fibrosis; and
- the extent of portal hypertension – this should be estimated by visualizing esophageal and gastric varices by gastrointestinal endoscopy.

It is normal to establish baseline renal function, hematologic parameters, and background serology, which includes CMV status. The most important technical information required is the

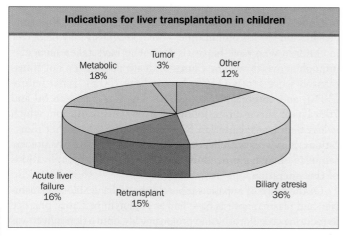

Indications for liver transplantation in children

Tumor 3%
Other 12%
Metabolic 18%
Acute liver failure 16%
Retransplant 15%
Biliary atresia 36%

Figure 23.25 Indications for liver transplantation in children. Birmingham Program, 1988 – 1998.

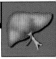

vascular anatomy and patency of the hepatic vessels. Most of this information may be obtained by color-fluid doppler ultrasound, and examination of the liver and spleen, although occasionally MRI or angiography may be required to clarify abnormal anatomy in the hypovascular syndrome or to determine the extent of portal vein thrombosis. Liver transplantation causes important hemodynamic changes during the operative and anhepatic phases, and thus baseline information on cardiac and respiratory function is essential and may be obtained from an electrocardiogram, echocardiogram, or oxygen saturation study.

One of the main aims of liver transplantation is to improve quality of life post-transplant, and thus it is essential to exclude any neurologic or psychologic defects that may be irreversible after transplantation. The psychologic and developmental assessment of children may be performed using the standard tests, such as the Griffith's developmental scale (children under the age of 5 years), the Bailey developmental scales, or Stanford B and A intelligence scales for children of all ages.

Chronic liver disease has an adverse effect on the dentitian of young children, which include hypoplasia, staining of the teeth, and gingival hyperplasia. As gingival hyperplasia may be a significant problem post-transplant, good methods of dental hygiene should be established before transplantation.

Contraindications to transplantation

As medical and surgical expertise is improved, there are fewer contraindications to pediatric liver transplanted based on technical restrictions of age and size. Increased experience has indicated that certain medical conditions are not curable by transplantation and these include:

- the presence of severe systemic sepsis, particularly fungal sepsis;
- HIV-positive children whose long-term prognosis is still unknown;
- malignant hepatic tumors with extrahepatic spread;
- severe extrahepatic disease which is not reversible post-transplant, including severe cardiopulmonary disease, not amenable to corrective surgery; or severe structural brain damage; and
- mitochrondial disease with multisystem involvement.

Preparation for transplantation

Most live vaccines are contraindicated post-transplant, and thus it is essential to ensure that routine immunizations are complete, namely diphtheria, pertussis, tetanus and polio, pneumovax as protection from streptococcal pneumonia, and haemophilius infuenzae b vaccine. In children older than 6–9 months, measles, mumps, rubella, and varicella vaccination should be offered. Hepatitis A and B vaccinations may also be prescribed pretransplant.

The treatment of specific hepatic complications is an important part of preoperative management. Acute variceal bleeding should be managed in a standard way with resuscitation, endoscopic sclerotherapy or esophageal banding, vasopressin or octreotide infusions. Esophageal banding is preferable to injection of sclerotherapy, if technically possible, as the inevitable development of postsclerotherapy variceal ulcers may be further adversely affected by post-transplant immunosuppression. In children who have uncontrolled variceal bleeding, the insertion of a transjugular intrahepatic portal systemic shunt has proved an effective management strategy, even in quite small children. Sepsis, particularly cholangitis and spontaneous bacterial peritonitis, should be appropriately treated with broad-spectrum

antibiotics (cefuroxime 20mg/kg/q8h, amoxicillin 25mg/kg/q8h, metronidazole 8mg/kg/day, are useful first-line antibiotics). In children who have acute liver failure, antifungal therapy should be started while awaiting liver transplantation with either fluconazole or liposomal amphotericin.

Fluid retention leading to ascites and cardiac failure is inevitable in most children who have liver failure. It is managed with a combination of salt and fluid restriction (to 2/3 of maintenance fluids), diuretics [spironolactone 3mg/kg/day or furosemide (frusemide) 0.5–2mg/kg/day], albumin infusions (either 4.5 or 20%). Hemodialysis or hemofiltration are rarely required for children who have chronic liver failure, but may be essential in managing fluid retention and cerebral edema in children who have acute liver failure.

The development of effective nutritional strategies has been an important advance in the preoperative management of children who have chronic liver failure which may have improved morbidity and mortality post-transplant. A high calorie protein feed should provide between 150–200% of average energy requirements. Problems arise providing these high energy feeds in fluid-restricted patients and therefore modular feeds provided by a nocturnal nasogastric enteral feeding or continuous feeding may be useful. Parenteral nutrition may be required if enteral feeding is not tolerated due to ascites and variceal bleeding.

Psychologic preparation

One of the most important aspects of the transplant assessment is the psychologic counseling and preparation of both child and family. A skilled multidisciplinary team, which includes a play therapist and psychologist, is essential to the success of this preparation and may be successfully achieved through innovative play therapy and toys and books suitable for children. Particularly careful counseling is required for parents of children referred for liver transplantation because of an inborn error of metabolism, which has not led to liver failure. These parents may find it more difficult to accept the risks and complications of the operation, the potential mortality, and the necessity for long-term immunosuppression. Parents of children who require transplantation for fulminant hepatitis may be too distressed to appreciate fully the significance and implications of liver transplantation and may require ongoing counseling and education postoperatively.

Innovative surgical techniques

The traditional form of operation, orthotopic liver transplantation, is now a rare occurrence in pediatric liver transplantation due to the shortage of size-matched organs for young children. This scarcity of size-matched donors lead to a high waiting list mortality and the view that liver transplantation was contraindicated in infants who weighed less than 10kg.

The development of reduction hepatectomy, in which left lateral segments of a larger liver are cut down to fit a child, have reduced the waiting list deaths from 15% to less than 5%, and extended the range of liver transplantation to young infants under the age of 1 year. Although morbidity may be higher in children receiving reduction hepatectomy, there is no long-term difference in outcome or survival compared with orthotopic liver transplantation. The continuing problem of donor shortages has lead to the development of split-liver transplantation in which a single donor liver is offered to two recipients. Recent results, which involve *in situ* liver splitting with cooperation between transplant centers, has improved both graft and patient survival. Of particular relevance for pediatric liver transplantation is the development of living related transplantation, which originated in Japan when this was the only form of transplantation permissible in that country. There are a number of ethical problems associated with this procedure which are related to the donor morbidity and potential mortality. The main advantages are related to the ability to electively transplant children who have end-stage failure before they have significant hepatic and nutritional deterioration, the use of 'good quality grafts', and the reduction in pressure on the organ donor pool.

Recent results demonstrate that there is a 91% survival in children receiving living related grafts transplanted electively, but survival in children who have FHF is only 57%, which is comparable with the results using cadaver donors. The choice of living related transplantation in the management of children who have FHF remains controversial, as not only is graft survival less likely, but it is difficult for parents to make clear decisions in this emotional situation.

Auxiliary liver transplantation is a particularly attractive technique in which part of the donor liver is inserted beside or in continuity with the native liver, which is retained in case of graft failure or for future gene therapy. It is particularly appropriate for children who have metabolic liver disease who have a functionally normal liver but severe extrahepatic disease. Auxiliary liver transplantation is now the operation of choice for children who have Crigler–Najjar type I and has proved successful in reducing the levels of unconjugated bilirubin and improving quality of life. Its role in other metabolic diseases, such as organic acidemias, has yet to be established.

Postoperative management

The immediate postoperative period is concerned with monitoring graft function, initiating immunosuppression, and preventing or managing complications. The majority of children remain in the intensive therapy unit for 24–48 hours, unless there are complications of graft function or cardiac difficulties. Graft function is evaluated in the standard way by measuring acid-base status, blood glucose levels, coagulation times, serum bilirubin, transaminases and alkaline phosphatase. Immunosuppression is initiated with corticosteroids (intravenous hydrocortisone or methylprednisolone transferring to enteric coated prednisolone once oral feeds are resumed), cyclosporine (Neoral) 5mg/kg, and azathioprine 2mg/kg. Alternative first-line immunosuppression, including tacrolimus (0.15mg/kg) with corticosteroids, is currently being evaluated in children.

Prophylactic antibiotics may be prescribed for 48 hours unless there is continuing infection. The incidence of stress ulcers and excess gastric acid secretion is particularly high in children recovering from liver transplantation, which may be prevented with ranitidine 3mg/kg q8h, sucralfate 2–4 q6h, and/or omeprazole 10–20mg q12h. Antiplatelet drugs, such as aspirin and dipyridamole, are prescribed to prevent vascular thrombosis which is particularly high in children, but these are discontinued at 3 months.

Early complications after liver transplantation

- Primary graft failure is a rare occurrence now with improved medical and surgical management, but may occur secondary to nonfunction (within 48 hours), hyperacute rejection (up to 4 days), or hepatic artery thrombosis (0–10 days). The only successful treatment is retransplantation, but the mortality

for retransplantation in this setting is up to 50%.
- Hepatic artery thrombosis is more common in children than in adults because of the small size of the vessels and occurs in 10% of children. The incidence has fallen following the introduction of reduction hepatectomy with the use of larger donor blood vessels
- Oliguria may develop in association with poor graft function, hypovolemia, or immunosuppressive therapy. Most children improve with conservative management and less than 10% require dialysis for renal failure unless transplanted for acute liver failure.
- Hypertension from cyclosporine or tacrolimus or prednisolone therapy is common and responds to fluid restriction and standard therapy with nifedipine (5–10mg/PRN) and/or atenolol (25–50mg/q12h).
- Acute cellular rejection responsive to increased immunosuppression occurs in 50–80% of children between 7 and 10 days. It is less common in infants (20%), which may be related to immune tolerance in this group. Most acute rejection episodes respond to prednisolone (20–40mg/kg/day) intravenously over 2 or 3 days. Conversion to a more potent immunosuppressive drug such as tacrolimus may be required in a minority of children.
- Chronic rejection is less common, but may occur at any time post-transplant. There may be a response to an increase in immunosuppression or a change to tacrolimus immunosuppression, but many children require retransplantation.
- Biliary complications occur in 18–20% of children and are more common in those receiving reduction hepatectomies than in those receiving full liver grafts. Biliary strictures may be secondary to anastomotic stricture, edema of the bile ducts or hepatic artery ischemia, whereas biliary leaks may be secondary to leakage from the cut surface of the liver in reduction hepatectomy or more commonly from hepatic artery ischemia. Most biliary leaks will settle with conservative management, but large leaks leading to biliary peritonitis, biliary abscess or sepsis will require surgical drainage and reconstruction. Many biliary strictures may now be managed medically with ursodeoxycholic acid (20mg/kg/day) or radiologically using percutaneous transhepatic cholangiography and dilatation of the stricture, and placement of a biliary stent.
- Bacterial sepsis remains the commonest complication following liver transplantation and may be related to central line insertion.
- Fungal infections (*Candida albicans* or aspergillosis) have been documented in up to 20% of patients, particularly those receiving liver transplantation for acute liver failure.

Late complications after liver transplant

Late complications may occur at any time after transplantation and they include the following.

Cytomegalovirus and Epstein–Barr virus infections

Cytomegalovirus and EBV infections are common as the majority of children undergoing liver transplantation are negative for both CMV or EBV. Pretransplant infection with CMV is a particular problem after transplantation in pediatric practice, because the majority of donor livers (particularly reduction hepatectomies from adults) are likely to be CMV-positive. Infection with CMV is inevitable between 4 and 6 weeks post-transplant, despite prophylaxis with acyclovir or ganciclovir. The risk of CMV disease is directly related to receiving a CMV-positive donor, but may be treated effectively with high dose ganciclovir (5mg/kg) and hyperimmune CMV globulin.

The development of primary EBV infections is a significant long-term problem. As many as 65% of children undergoing liver transplantation will be EBV-negative, and 75% of this group will have a primary degree of infection within 6 months of transplantation. It is important to diagnose primary EBV infection as early as possible (EBV early capsid antigen and polymerase chain reaction [PCR]), so that immunosuppression may be reduced to prevent further progression to lymphoproliferative disease.

Lymphoproliferative disease

There is a close relationship between primary EBV infection and the development of lymphoproliferative disease, which ranges from benign hyperplasia to malignant lymphomas. In the majority of children the clinical features represent infectious mononucleosis, with a minority developing isolated lymphoid involvement or malignant lymphoma. The diagnosis is based on identifying the characteristic histology from the affected tissue, which may also demonstrate polymorphic B-cell proliferation or lymphomatous features. It may be necessary to differentiate monoclonal from polyclonal infiltrates using immunofluorescence staining for heavy and light chain immunoglobulins. Although almost every organ in the body may be affected, the liver and gut are most usually involved. It is clear that lymphoproliferative disease is more likely in the presence of intense immunosuppression, particularly with more than one agent (OKT3 antilymphocyte globulin). Treatment includes reduction of immunosuppression and acyclovir (3mg/m^2), which is effective in the majority. If the lymphoproliferative disease becomes overtly malignant, chemotherapy with standard lymphoma treatment is required.

Side effects of immunosuppression

These are numerous and are mostly similar in children as those in adults. The major difference in pediatric practice is the effect of corticosteroids on growth and ultimate height. Hirsuitism and gingival hyperplasia, which are well-known side effects of cyclosporine, have an important effect on quality of life, particularly in adolescents. The prevention of nephrotoxicity, which is common to both cyclosporine and tacrolimus, needs careful monitoring of immunosuppressive levels to minimize this long-term effect.

Late technical problems

These include biliary strictures and hepatic artery or portal vein thrombosis; management is the same as in adult patients.

Growth failure

Growth failure affects approximately 20% of children after liver transplantation. The most important factors related to growth failure are:
- excessive corticosteroid dosage;
- recurrent hepatic complications and cholestasis;
- intercurrent illnesses, such as EBV and CMV; and
- behavioral problems with interfere with calorie intake.

Successful management of growth failure involves a skilled multidisciplinary team, including dietitian and psychologist, ensuring adequate calorie intake (by nasogastric tube, if necessary) and early reduction or discontinuation of corticosteroid therapy.

Recurrence of disease

This is an increasingly important problem. As with adults, hepatitis B and C can recur, but the scale of the problem is much shorter. Recent data indicates that up to 25% of children transplanted for autoimmune hepatitis will have a recurrence, both immunologically and histologically. Giant cell hepatitis with autoimmune hemolytic anemia is a rare disorder that has been shown to recur post-transplant and is now considered a contraindication to transplantation. The outcome for children transplanted for malignant hepatic tumors is related to the rate of recurrence, which is low if there are no extrahepatic metastases present at the time of surgery.

Survival

Current results from international units indicate that 1-year survival after pediatric liver transplantation may be as high as 90%, while long-term survival rates (5–8 years) ranges from 60 to 80%. Patients receiving elective living related transplantation may have a higher 1-year survival (94%) compared with those receiving cadaveric grafts (78%). Nutritional status pretransplant is a significant risk factor for morbidity and mortality, as data indicating that children who had malnutrition had a 60% chance of surviving the first year compared with 95% in better nourished children, highlighting the necessity for intensive preoperative nutritional support. It is clear that short-term survival is better in children transplanted electively compared with those transplanted for acute liver failure or fulminant hepatitis who continue to have survival rates of 60–70% 1-year survival compared with 80–90%, which is related not only to the severity of the liver disease, but is also due to multiorgan failure.

Outcome after metabolic liver transplantation

In α_1-antitrypsin deficiency, Byler's disease and Wilson's disease, there are both phenotypic and functional cures of the original disease. In tyrosinemia type I, liver transplantation corrects hepatic enzyme deficiency and prevents the development of liver cancer, although the kidney continues to produce toxic metabolites. Long-term nephrotoxicity from immunosuppressive agents is, therefore, a problem in this group of children. In Crigler–Najjar type I, urea cycle defects and primary oxalosis, the metabolic defect is completely corrected, and rehabilitation depends on the extent of extrahepatic disease pretransplant.

In organic acidemia, such as proprionic acidemia and methalmonomic acidemia, the metabolic defect is widespread throughout body tissue, but liver replacement provides sufficient hepatic enzyme to prevent metabolic acidosis, under normal conditions. The majority of these children are able to take a normal protein intake, but will be at risk of mild metabolic acidosis during intercurrent infections.

Quality of life after transplantation

Children who survive the initial 3-month post-transplant period without major complications should achieve a normal lifestyle, despite the necessity for continuous immunosuppressive monitoring. Prospective studies have indicated a rapid return to normal nutritional status in over 80% of children within 1 year post-transplant. Linear growth may be delayed between 6 and 24 months post-transplant, which is directly related to corticosteroid dosage and to malnutrition and preoperative stunting.

Early studies of neuropsychologic development pre- and post-transplant demonstrated that the rate of improvement post-transplant is related to the extent of motor or psychologic developmental delay pretransplant, thus highlighting the necessity for early transplantation, particularly for infants who have chronic liver disease. Prospective studies have shown that there is an initial deterioration in psychosocial development post-transplant, which is maybe related to the prolonged hospitalization, and to stress of the transplant operation. Following the resumption of normal life there is a return to pretransplant psychosocial scores within 1–2 years. Most children return to nursery or normal school within 3 months of transplantation.

Long-term studies have shown that children surviving liver transplantation enter puberty normally, girls will develop menarche, and both boys and girls will have pubertal growth spurts. Successful pregnancies have been reported.

PRACTICE POINT

Case I

A 3-week-old male infant was referred for investigation because of prolonged neonatal jaundice. He had been born at term, following a normal pregnancy and delivery, weighing 3.5kg. He was fully breast-fed and feeding well, but had been jaundiced since the second day of life. His stools were described as pale and his urine as yellow. On examination he was found to be gaining weight satisfactorily, but to be mildly jaundiced with a firm enlarged liver.

Investigations indicated a bilirubin of 100μmol/L, AST 80U/L, ALT 120U/L, alkaline phosphatase 600IU/L, albumin 38g/L, and γ-GT 200U/L. Prothrombin time, hematology, and renal function were normal. Stools contained some pigment and urine was moderately yellow. Screen for congenital infection and inborn errors of metabolism were negative. Abdominal ultrasound, after a 4-hour fast, revealed a small contracted gallbladder (Fig. 23.26). Hepatobiliary scanning revealed no excretion of isotope after 24 hours. Liver histology demonstrated a giant cell hepatitis with minimal fibrosis and mild biliary ductular proliferation (Fig. 23.27).

Interpretation

The clinical features and presentation (namely normal birth weight, progressive jaundice since birth, enlarged firm liver) all suggested a diagnosis of biliary atresia. Liver histology performed at 4 weeks of age showed no evidence of portal fibrosis, or biliary ductular proliferation suggestive of biliary atresia. The options were either to perform an endoscopic retrograde angiography, or an operative cholangiogram to confirm the diagnosis of biliary atresia. An endoscopic retrograde cholangiography and pancreatography (ERCP) was attempted, and although the ampulla was identified, no bile was detected before or after cholecystokinin injection, and cannulation of the biliary tree was unsuccessful. The therapeutic options were either to treat medically with ursodeoxycholic acid and phenobarbital to improve bile flow and re-evaluate in 1–2 weeks, or to proceed to an operative cholangiogram and a Kasai portoenterostomy if biliary atresia was established. Although the diagnosis to establish biliary atresia is not usually difficult, between 3 and 4 weeks there is considerable overlap with the neonatal hepatitis syndrome, and a high degree of suspicion is required to ensure that early diagnosis and palliative surgery is performed.

Case 2

An 11-year-old girl presented to her general practitioner with a history of jaundice for 6 weeks, weight loss (2 stones), anorexia, and lack of energy. She gave a previous history of a similar illness 2 years ago, after the family returned from a Mediterranean holiday. No investigations had been performed at that time and she had apparently made a good recovery. On examination she was found to be mildly jaundiced, and to

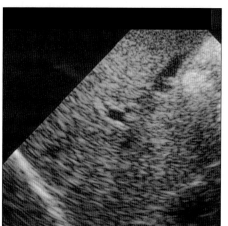

Figure 23.26 Abdominal ultrasound of gallbladder. The gallbladder is usually enlarged after a 4-hour fast. The gallbladder may be small or absent in babies with severe intrahepatic cholestasis or biliary atresia.

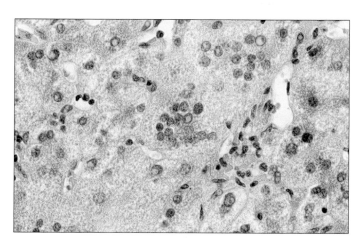

Figure 23.27 The histology of the liver demonstrates typical giant cell hepatitis. There is considerable histologic overlap between biliary atresia and neonatal hepatitis. The histologic findings of biliary atresia may not be obvious if the biopsy is performed before 4 weeks of age (see Fig. 23.10).

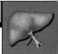

have a tremor in both hands, hepatosplenomegaly, palmar erythema, and eight spider nevi. She was referred for further investigation. There was no history of drug ingestion or any family history of autoimmune disease. The parents were not related. On examination her blood pressure was normal, her height was on the 50th centile and her weight on the 10th centile (indicating recent weight loss). Neurologic examination was grossly normal, apart from a fine tremor of both hands. Laboratory investigations showed that hemoglobin was 10g/L (normal >12g/L), white cell count 2.0×10^9/L, and platelet count 60×109/L; there were no reticulocytes or any evidence of hemolysis. Liver function tests showed that bilirubin was 150µmol/L, AST was 450U/L, ALT was 700U/L, alkaline phosphatase was 500U/L, albumin was 30g/L (normal >35g/L), and prothrombin time was 19/13s. Other investigations indicated: immunoglobulins, IgG 25g/L (normal 8–15g/L); ANA 1:100; SMA negative; and LKM negative. Serum copper was 12µmol/L (normal >10). Ceruloplasmin was 220mg/L (normal >200). Urinary copper was 2µmol/L in 24 hours (normal <1µmol/L in 24 hours). Urine copper increased following treatment with penicillamine to 3µmol/24 hours. Serology for hepatitis A, B, and C viruses, EBV, and CMV was negative.

A liver biopsy was performed that demonstrated increased portal inflammatory infiltrate of mainly lymphocytes with a variable number of plasma cells. There was piecemeal necrosis and some early bridging necrosis (see Fig. 23.19).

Interpretation

The differential diagnosis lay between an autoimmune liver disease and Wilson's disease. Autoimmune liver disease type I is commoner in girls than in boys (3:1) and often presents with an insidious course over 1–2 years. Thus, at clinical presentation, the elevated immunoglobulins and positive ANA with supportive histology would suggest autoimmune liver disease. On the other hand, Wilson's disease in childhood often presents with a very similar clinical picture with nonspecific symptoms and chronic hepatitis. Serum copper and ceruloplasmin levels may not be reduced in children presenting with the hepatic form of the disease, and the diagnosis is often most reliably made on the basis of an elevated urinary copper, particularly if there is a significant increase following oral penicillamine. In addition, other features of Wilson's disease such as Kayser–Fleischer rings and neurologic involvement may be absent in up to 50% of cases and 75% of children. Histologic findings may be identical in autoimmune hepatitis and Wilson's disease. Differentiation may be necessary using radioactive copper studies.

The treatment for autoimmune hepatitis is with prednisolone and/or azathioprine, while treatment for early Wilson's disease is penicillamine. In this case, diagnostic features in favor of autoimmune hepatitis were the immunoglobulin level, the positive ANA, and the histologic features. Factors that made Wilson's disease less likely, despite the equivocal copper and ceruloplasmin levels and the excess urinary copper excretion, were the absence of hemolysis and a relatively normal alkaline phosphatase. The patient was treated with prednisolone 2mg/kg for 4 weeks with complete res-

olution of biochemical findings, and was maintained in remission on alternate day prednisolone and azathioprine. The tremor resolved with improved nutrition.

Case 3

A 4-month-old male infant presented with vomiting, diarrhea, failure to thrive, and the recent onset of drowsiness and irritability. He was born to nonconsanguinous parents following a normal pregnancy and had had a normal delivery with a birth weight of 3kg (normal). He had made good developmental progress in the first 4 months of the year, and his parents had no concerns until the recent illness.

He was found to be mildly jaundiced, had evidence of recent weight loss, was generally hypotonic, but eye movements were normal and he made appropriate eye contact. Central nervous system examination was essentially normal. He was found to have a firm liver without splenomegaly or ascites. Hematology and renal function were normal, liver function tests indicated a bilirubin of 130µmol/L, AST 400U/L, ALT 350U/L, prothrombin time 40/13s, and serum ammonia 100 (elevated µmol/L); plasma amino acids were nonspecifically elevated consistent with acute hepatic dysfunction. Investigations for known inborn errors of metabolism were negative, including tyrosinemia type I, galactosemia, and hereditary fructose intolerance. Serum ferritin was mildly elevated.

A diagnosis of acute liver failure, probably secondary to an inborn error of metabolism was made. The infant was treated conservatively with acute liver failure support: nutrition, lactulose, and coagulation support. His condition deteriorated over the next 2–3 weeks, with an increase in coagulation time (prothrombin <60s) and further drowsiness.

Interpretation

The diagnostic dilemma revolves on whether transplantation is indicated for an infant who has acute liver failure secondary to a probable (but undiagnosed) metabolic disease. Under these circumstances it is important to establish whether the inborn error of metabolism is confined to the liver and thus liver transplantation may be curative, or whether there is disease of other organs (muscle, brain, kidney, or heart), which would preclude successful transplantation. Severe coagulopathy prevented liver biopsy and CSF analysis, and the infant was too small for successful transjugular liver biopsy.

A electroencephalogram indicated nonspecific hepatic encephalopathy, a CT scan was essentially normal, cardiac examination revealed a structurally normal heart, and tests of renal function were normal. A muscle biopsy demonstrated ragged red fibers secondary to cytochrome enzyme deficiency (secondary to a mitochondrial disorder) which was confirmed biochemically (Fig. 23.28).

The parents were counseled that the child had a mitochondrial disorder involving the liver and muscle and probably the brain, and that liver transplantation would not be curative. The child died 4 months later, following development of obvious neurologic deterioration with recurrent convulsions and respiratory failure. Liver biopsy at autopsy showed the microvesicular fatty infiltration which is common in this disorder (Fig. 23.29).

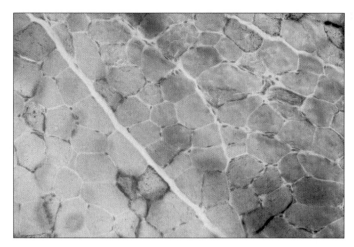

Figure 23.28 Muscle biopsy. Most mitochondrial disorders affect muscles secondary to defects of the respiratory chain enzymes. The classic finding of ragged red fibers (Gomori's 1-step trichrome stain) usually indicates a respiratory chain defect that must be confirmed enzymatically.

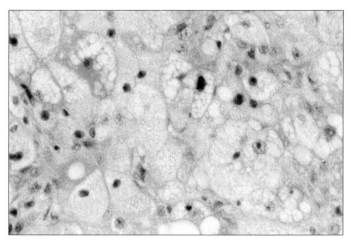

Figure 23.29 Histology of liver biopsy taken at autopsy. It indicates microvesicular fatty infiltration in hepatocytes, which is characteristic of Reye's syndrome, Alpers' disease, or mitochondrial disorders.

FURTHER READING

Balistreri WF. Bile acid therapy in pediatric hepatobiliary disease: the role of urseodeoxycholic acid. J Pediatr Gastroenterol Nutr. 1997;24:573–89. *Comprehensive summary of this partially proven therapy.*

Beath SV, Boxall EH, Watson RM, Tarlow MJ, Kelly DA. Fulminant hepatitis B in infants born to anti-HBe hepatitis B carrier mothers. Br Med J. 1992;304:1169–70. *Important lesson for management of hepatitis B mothers and children.*

Beath SV, Brook GD, Kelly DA, et al. Successful liver transplantation in babies under 1 year. Br Med J. 1993;307:825–8. *Pioneering work in transplantation.*

Bhaduri BR, Mieli-Vergani G. Fulminant hepatic failure: pediatric aspects. Semin Liver Dis. 1996;16:349–55. *Good summary of this rare disease.*

Bortolotti F, Jara P, Diaz C, et al. Post-transfusion and community-acquired hepatitis C in childhood. J Ped Gastroenterology and Nutrition. 1994;18(3):279–83. *Useful information on hepatitis C in childhood.*

Bull LN, Carlton VE, Stricker NL, et al. Genetic and morphological findings in progressive familial intrahepatic cholestasis (Byler disease [PFIC-1] and Byler syndrome): evidence for heterogeneity. Hepatology. 1997;26:155–64. *Outstanding description of genetic disorders.*

Devictor D, Tahiri C, Rousset A, Massenavette B, Russo M, Huault G. Management of fulminant hepatic failure in children – an analysis of 56 cases. Crit Care Med. 1993;21(9 Suppl):348–9. *Comprehensive summary of French practice in this disease.*

De Ville de Goyet J, Hausleithner V, Reding R, et al. Impact of innovative techniques on the waiting list and results in paediatric liver transplantation. Transplantation. 1993;56:1130–6. *Highlights new developments in transplantation.*

Gregorio GV, Portmann B, Reid F, et al. Autoimmune hepatitis in childhood: a 20-year experience. Hepatology. 1997;25:541–7. *A good paper on outcome of rare disease.*

Li L, Krantz ID, Deng Y, et al. Alagille syndrome is caused by mutations in the human *Jagged 1*, which encodes a ligand for Notch 1. Nature Genet. 1997;16:243–51. *New important research.*

Lindstedt S, Holme E, Lock E, et al. Treatment of hereditary tyrosinaemia type I by inhibition of 4-hydroxphenyl pyruvate dioxygenase. Lancet. 1992;340:813–17. *Pioneering paper on the new therapy for this disease.*

McClement JW, Hard ER, Mowat AP. Results of surgical treatment for extrahepatic biliary atresia in the United Kingdom. Br Med J. 1985;290:345–7. *Important summary of surgical experience.*

Mieli-VerganiG, Howard ER, Portman B, Mowat AP. Late referral for biliary atresia – Missed opportunities for effective surgery. Lancet. 1989;1:421–3. *Highlights the difficulty in educating medical professionals.*

Moukarzel AA, Najm I, Vargas J, McDiarmid SV, Busuttil RW, Ament ME. Effect of nutritional status on outcome of orthotopic liver transplantation in paediatric patients. Transplant Proc. 1990;22:1560–3. *Important work indicating prognostic effect of nutrition on liver transplantation.*

Rivera-Penera T, Gugig R, et al. Outcome of acetaminophen overdose in pediatric patients and factors contributing to hepatotoxicity. J Pediatr. 1997;130:300–4. *Important in understanding the incidence and outcome of acetaminophen overdose.*

Sira JK, Boxall E, Sleight E, Ballard A, Yoong AK, Kelly DA. Long-term treatment of chronic hepatitis B carrier children in the UK (abstract). Hepatology. 1997;26:427A. *Indicates the value of prednisolone priming in the treatment of hepatitis B.*

Thomson M, McKiernan P, Buckels J, Mayer D, Kelly D. Generalised mitochondrial cytopathy is an absolute contraindication to orthotopic liver transplantation in childhood. Liver Transplant Surg. 1995;1:428. *Important paper relating to selection for transplantation.*

Yandza T, Gauthier F, Valayer J. Lessons from the first 1000 liver transplantation in children at Bicetre Hospital. J Pediatr Surg. 1994;29:905–11. *Good summary of evolution of pediatric transplantation.*

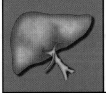

Chapter 24
Benign Tumors and Cystic Diseases of the Liver

John Karani

INTRODUCTION

There are very few issues in clinical hepatology that invoke as much debate as the pathogenesis, diagnosis, and management of benign liver tumors. Advances in radiologic techniques have led to an improvement in lesion conspicuity that allows the demonstration of small liver tumors that would not have been detected a decade ago. The number of pathologic entities that are now diagnosed, both independently or in association with chronic liver diseases or multisystem disorders, continues to increase. Although didactic algorithms defining lines of investigation and management are of value, there will always be a variance in observation and expertise in radiologic and pathologic interpretation that may adversely affect or advance the diagnostic pathway. In addition, the natural history of many of these tumors, particularly the rarer types, is not yet clearly established and therefore predictions of prognosis may be erroneous. However, any individual clinical practice should establish the basic principles of management and audit their outcome.

General principles of investigation and management

A common clinical scenario is that a focal lesion has been detected on imaging. Often this will be an incidental finding that is unrelated to the patient's symptoms. There is a differential diagnosis that will include tumors of a wide pathologic spectrum. Each of these tumors will require different treatment and carry a different prognosis. The role of clinical and radiologic investigations is to predict the pathology of these tumors and reserve surgical or image-guided biopsy for lesions that demonstrate indeterminate characteristics. It is important in the clinical assessment to ascertain whether the tumor has arisen within normal parenchyma or if there is clinical and biochemical evidence of diffuse parenchymal liver disease. There is an association of certain benign lesions in patients who have multisystem disorders and therefore this possibility should be sought in the clinical history. Liver function tests will be normal in the majority of patients with benign tumors. As a general rule any asymptomatic lesion in a patient who has normal liver function that exhibits the pathognomonic radiologic characteristics of an individual benign tumor should be managed conservatively. Repeat imaging can be used to confirm that the size and morphology of the lesion does not change.

The indications for surgery are difficult to define and are often not dependent upon the type of tumor. Hepatic resection and embolization carry a significant morbidity, but are indicated and may be life saving in those patients presenting with severe spontaneous hemorrhage. If pain is the presenting feature and is attributable to the tumor and also cannot be controlled by medical

management, then surgery is indicated. This has to be preceded by a thorough risk versus benefit analysis for each individual patient.

Histologic classification

Benign tumors can arise from all of the cellular components of the liver. Hepatocytes can give rise to hepatocellular adenomas; cystadenomas can arise from biliary epithelium and hemangiomas from mesenchymal tissue and a combination of cells may be found in the tumor-like lesions such as focal nodular hyperplasia. Figure 24.1 represents an abbreviated version of the pathologic classification that is now accepted worldwide.

The specific pathologic characteristics of the more important of these lesions are described in the following text.

Radiologic techniques and objectives

There are now a number of techniques to detect and characterize benign liver lesions, including ultrasound (US), computed tomography (CT), magnetic resonance imaging (MRI), nuclear scintigraphy, and arteriography. Each of these has its own merit, but in practice none is pre-eminent. The correct diagnosis is usually made by a correlative imaging strategy that is interpreted by

Histologic classification of tumors
Benign epithelial tumors
Liver cell adenoma
Bile duct adenoma
Bile duct cystadenoma
Biliary papillomatosis
Benign nonepithelial tumors
Hemangioma
Infantile hemangioendothelioma
Lymphangioma
Angiomyolipoma
Pseudolipoma
Fibroma (fibrous mesiothelioma)
Leiomyoma
Tumor like lesions
Cysts
Fibropolycystic disease
Focal nodular hyperplasia
Nodular regenerative hyperplasia
Mesenchymal hamartoma
Biliary hamartoma (von Meyenberg complex)
Inflammatory pseudotumor

Figure 24.1 Histologic classification of tumors.

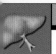
an experienced radiologist who has knowledge of the clinical spectrum and associations of these lesions. The following text outlines the simple questions that these techniques have to answer, either singularly or in combination.

- Is the lesion cystic or solid, or a combination of both these features? This question is reliably answered by US, supplemented by CT or MRI to determine the relative proportion of the cystic and solid elements.
- Is this a single lesion or are other tumors present and do they have similar characteristics indicating the same pathology? It is important to remember that lesions of less than 5mm are detected by all of these techniques.
- Is the lesion vascular or avascular? This can be determined by contrast enhanced CT, US or MRI, and the pattern of enhancement through the arterial, portal venous, and delayed phases of these studies will be a differentiating characteristic between lesions. For example, centripetal enhancement with delayed 'filling in' is characteristic, but not pathognomonic, of a cavernous hemangioma. Arteriography can confirm the pattern of vascularity and the arterial pattern may be characteristic of an individual tumor. Focal nodular hyperplasia and cavernous hemangioma are examples of this situation.
- Are Kupffer cells present in the lesion? Technetium-99m sulfur colloid scintigraphy or MRI with intravenous superparamagnetic iron oxide (SPIO) particles will define the distribution of Kupffer cells in the lesion.
- Are hepatocytes present in the lesion? Technetium-99m-iminodiacetic acid (IDA) derivative scintigraphy or MRI with the paramagnetic chelate manganese dipyridoxyl diphosphonate (Mn-DPDP) will define the distribution of hepatocytes in the lesion.
- Is there another specific tissue characteristic present by which the tumor can reliably be diagnosed? The presence of a capsule, calcification, or hemorrhage is a recognized diagnostic feature of certain types of tumors.
- Is there evidence of chronic parenchymal liver disease or portal hypertension?
- Is the lesion resectable? The segmental anatomy and vascular relationships of the lesion have to be accurately assessed by CT or MRI.
- At what stage can the investigations be terminated? It may be possible to stop the radiologic pathway after a single investigation. For example, cavernous hemangiomas of less than 3cm generally have pathognomonic features on US. They are echogenic with posterior acoustic enhancement, and lie peripherally but close to a major hepatic vein. If these features are observed in an asymptomatic patient the investigative sequence should be terminated.
- Is a biopsy required and can this be performed with safety? As a general rule, all lesions that have indeterminate radiologic characteristics should be biopsied. If the lesion is large and symptomatic and will be resected independent of its pathologic characteristics, then preoperative image-guided biopsy is not necessary.

LIVER CELL (HEPATOCELLULAR) ADENOMA

This is the most intensively studied benign tumor of the liver with the spectrum of lesions now defined. 'Spontaneous' liver cell adenoma do occur in adults and children of both genders,

but are rare, and the majority of cases are associated with hormone therapy. The commonest cause of liver cell adenomas is the use of the oral contraceptive pill, or it may be a sequel to therapy with androgenic anabolic steroid therapy for impotence, or to enhance muscle development in body builders and athletes. Children of either sex treated with the same drugs for Fanconi's syndrome, refractory anemia, and bone marrow aplasia carry an equivalent risk of liver cell adenoma development. All the compounds incriminated have been 17-alkyl (α-ethinyl) substituted derivatives of the basic steroid structure with methyltesterone, oxymethalone, and norethandrolone being the most frequently incriminated drugs. Rarer etiologic factors are glycogen storage disease type 1a, familial diabetes mellitus, and Kleinfelter syndrome and therapy with clomiphene, danazol, and norethisterone.

Incidence

The estimated annual incidence has been put at 3.4 per 100,000 contraceptive users, which is equivalent to approximately 300 cases per year in the USA. Case–control studies and epidemiologic evidence have shown that the development of liver cell adenoma in a woman relates to the dose, duration of usage, and increasing age. Low-dose oral contraceptives in current use carry little or no risk of tumor development.

Clinical features

Symptomatic patients present with episodic or acute abdominal pain. The latter is invariably secondary to hemorrhage within the tumor. This may be further complicated by rupture into the peritoneum (Fig. 24.2).

If not recognized and appropriately treated, this sequel carries a mortality of approximately 10%. The factors that adversely influence the risk of spontaneous rupture are the size of the tumor, pregnancy, and menstruation.

The simultaneous occurrence of liver cell adenoma and focal nodular hyperplasia has been observed, but this is uncommon. Peliosis hepatis is often present and may be extensive if the tumor is due to anabolic androgenic steroids. Reports of spontaneous regression after drug withdrawal and progression or malignant change are rare. Most gonadal steroid-related liver tumors do not produce α-fetoprotein and do not metastasize, even though the histologic appearance may be equivocal and difficult to differentiate from hepatocellular carcinoma.

Diagnosis
Pathology
Macroscopically the tumors arise in an otherwise normal liver and are typically large, often measuring up to 10cm at presentation (Fig. 24.3).

Pedunculation is present in approximately 10% of cases. The majority of these lesions are solitary and well demarcated, but are seldom encapsulated on sectioning. The color varies from yellow to tan and they are highly vascular with areas of hemorrhage, and infarction is a characteristic feature. Rarer instances of multiple tumors occur. This disorder is termed liver cell adenomatosis and probably represents a distinct pathologic entity of differing etiology.

Microscopically the tumor is composed of liver cells arranged in plates that are two or three cells thick, separated by compressed

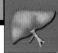
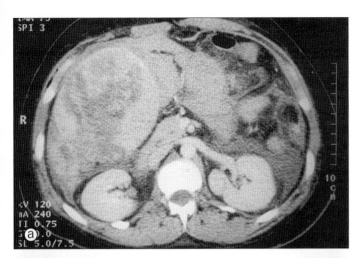

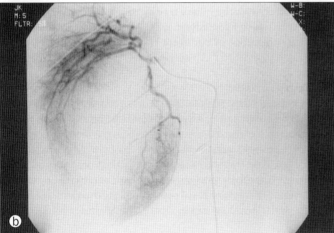

Figure 24.2 Ruptured liver cell adenoma. (a) CT demonstrating a hypervascular adenoma that has undergone spontaneous rupture with development of a hemoperitoneum. (b) Selective hepatic arteriography demonstrates the abnormal vessels on the periphery of the lesion with the central avascular area representing the line of rupture with contained hemorrhage.

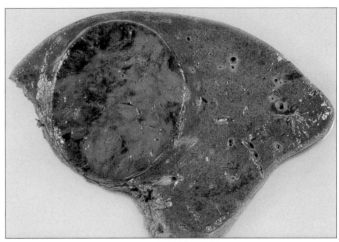

Figure 24.3 Liver cell adenoma. Liver cell adenoma in a 38-year-old woman. Bisected right hepatectomy specimen showing an encapsulated tumor mass with foci of hemorrhage. (Courtesy of Professor B. Portmann.)

sinusoidal spaces lined by endothelium. Enzymatically active Kupffer cells may be present and these are demonstrated by periodic acid-Schiff (PAS) diastase or Perle's stains. Mitoses are absent or few in number and the cell nuclei are uniform in appearance. Excess glycogen or fat may be present in larger than normal hepatocytes producing pale and eosinophilic cytoplasm. Bile ducts are absent but bile may be present as droplets within the cytoplasm or as plugs in distended canaliculi.

Radiology

Irrespective of the imaging technique being used, the characteristics of a liver cell adenoma depend upon its size, the degree of hemorrhage or infarction complicating the tumor, or the amount of fat or glycogen present. Supportive diagnostic features may be present such as diffuse fatty replacement of the liver supporting a pre-existing storage disorder or the presence of free intraperitoneal hemorrhage.

Sonography typically demonstrates a large hyperechoic mass with central anechoic areas corresponding to zones of internal hemorrhage. Severe necrosis may develop following infarction resulting in a complex cystic sonographic appearance. Color flow and spectral scanning demonstrate the enhanced peripheral vascularity of the tumor.

Unenhanced CT usually demonstrates a hypodense or isodense lesion, but in the presence of severe fatty replacement the tumor may appear to be of higher density than the surrounding abnormal hypodense parenchyma. Hyperdense areas of fresh hemorrhage may be present. Typically, the non-necrotic and nonhemorrhagic regions of the lesion will show transient enhancement during the arterial phase with a centripetal pattern of enhancement developing through the portal and late venous phases (Fig. 24.4).

Unlike hemangiomas, this pattern of peripheral enhancement does not persist and the lesion becomes isodense or hypodense by the portal venous phase as a consequence of arteriovenous shunting.

On MRI studies, variable characteristics are present, but adenomas may show increased signal intensity on T1-weighted images resulting from the presence of fat or glycogen. The presence of an increased signal on T2-weighted images and enhancement following gadolinium are suggestive as diagnostic features. No adenomas have been reported showing uptake of ferrite, reflecting the lack of Kupffer cells in the nodule.

Characteristic angiographic features are of a hypervascular mass with centripetal flow and abnormal peripheral arteries. A more generalized abnormality of the liver may be present with an abnormal hepatogram phase that is characteristic of peliosis.

Management

Current opinion is that adenomas that are greater than 10cm in diameter carry a sufficiently high risk of hemorrhage to warrant surgical excision. In a patient presenting with acute abdominal pain, severe active hemorrhage or shock, emergency radiologic intervention with arterial embolization is indicated as a prelude to resection. The most commonly encountered clinical scenario is the patient on oral contraceptives in whom the tumor has been detected as an incidental finding on imaging. In this situation, a conservative approach can be followed, as the natural history is not so well defined that the prognosis can predicted with accuracy. Complete resolution, as well as progression, on

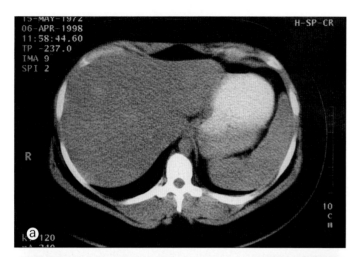

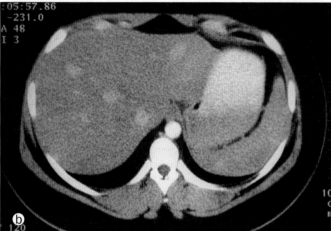

Figure 24.4 Liver cell adenoma. (a) CT demonstrating multiple liver cell adenoma appearing as hyperdense nodules within a fatty liver on the unenhanced scan. (b) Following intravenous contrast the lesions become more conspicuous by their enhancement in the arterial phase of the scan.

withdrawal of estrogen have been documented. A policy of close observation by imaging can be adopted. If the tumor enlarges, or the patient develops symptoms attributable to the lesion, surgical intervention should be considered. Following successful surgical resection, the long-term prognosis is good.

An elective radiologic approach using selective arterial embolization with coils and particulate material to ablate the vascularity of the tumor can provide a therapeutic alternative, particularly if the lesions are multiple or the anatomy mitigates against risk hepatic resection carrying the minimal operative risk. As with many uncommon liver tumors with variable presentation, management options, and biologic activity, establishing and recruiting patients to a long-term case–control study to establish the role of radiologic intervention as alternatives to surgery and conservative management is difficult. However, individual experience and reports indicate that this approach merits consideration.

BILE DUCT CYSTADENOMA

This is a rare tumor that is not unique to the liver and tumors of similar characteristics reported in the pancreas and ovary. They constitute less than 5% of cysts of biliary origin, with 85% aris-

ing from the intrahepatic biliary tree and the remainder arising from the extrahepatic bile ducts or gallbladder. The similarity to pancreatic neoplasms is explained by the derivation of the pancreas and biliary system from the endodermal diverticula of the gut. The primordial germ cells normally migrate from the posterior wall of the yolk sac along the wall of the hindgut through the yolk stalk, a structure that is intimately related with the gut from which the primordia of the hepatobiliary system and pancreas arise. This embryologic association may also explain the ovarian-like stroma visible in these tumors, which is reported as a feature carrying a better prognosis.

Clinical features
The majority of these tumors occur in women, with a peak incidence in the fifth decade. Patients present with pain or discomfort and a palpable mass. Biliary cystadenomas do not communicate with the biliary tree although compression or projection into major bile ducts may occur and result in features of obstructive jaundice or recurrent cholangitis.

Diagnosis
Pathology
They are usually large multiloculated cystic tumors lined by columnar, mucin-producing epithelium. Categorization of the tumor into benign or a malignant cystadenocarcinoma is largely dependent upon the histologic assessment of the epithelium, which may show internal papillary structures or cystic invaginations. Foci of cellular atypia, particularly nuclear enlargement and hyperchromasia, multilayering or solid epithelial masses indicate 'borderline' change, while capsular invasion is an indicator of malignant change.

Radiology
The tumors are slow growing and by the time of presentation usually measure over 10cm in diameter. They are therefore easily detected by imaging (Fig. 24.5).

Specific radiologic features are the complex cystic appearance of the tumor with multiple loculi containing mucinous fluid that may be detected by any of the available techniques. The tumors are characteristically avascular on angiography. There are no specific radiologic criteria to differentiate cystadenocarcinoma and cystadenoma, but an increased mural nodularity favors malignant change. Therefore, the role of imaging is three-fold: first, to give an indication as to the potential diagnosis; second, to define the segmental anatomy and vascular relationships before liver resection; and finally to exclude a pancreatic or ovarian primary cystadenocarcinoma metastasizing to the liver.

Management
If anatomically possible, surgical resection is the treatment of choice and carries a good prognosis even if there is histologic evidence of malignant transformation. Occasional cystadenocarcinomas have been managed by liver transplantation with excellent results.

BILE DUCT ADENOMAS AND MICROHAMARTOMAS

Bile duct adenomas are rare tumors, with hamartomatous features that are formed by numerous small non-malignant ducts separated by mature connective tissue. They are usually an inci-

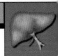

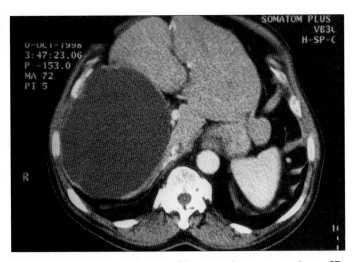

Figure 24.5 Biliary cystadenoma. Biliary cystadenoma appearing on CT as a large hypodense lesion with mural nodularity. There is atrophy of the posterior segments of the right lobe of the liver.

dental finding at laparotomy or autopsy appearing as single, pale, well circumscribed nodules. Over 90% are subcapsular in position and therefore easily resected.

Microhamartomas or von Meyenburg complexes represent a not uncommon finding in wedge biopsies from the liver or at autopsy. They are tiny, usually multiple lesions composed of small dilated, angulated bile ducts in a stroma of fibrous tissue. They lie within or adjacent to portal tracts. They are usually asymptomatic but have been reported in association with portal hypertension similar to congenital hepatic fibrosis. The development of cholangiocarcinoma within these complexes has been reported.

HEMANGIOMA

This is the most common benign tumor of the liver, with a reported incidence of 1–20% of the population. This latter figure is a result of a prospective autopsy-based study in which a dedicated search for this lesion was performed. Most reports suggest a predominant prevalence in women. Although this tumor may occur in any age group, it is most commonly found in the third, fourth and fifth decades. Serial longitudinal growth studies have shown that most hemangiomas remain stable, although they may occasionally increase or decrease in size. Hormonal influences in growth have also been documented with enlargement of some tumors during pregnancy and regression of others after steroid therapy.

Clinical features
The vast majority of hemangiomas will remain asymptomatic and are discovered as an incidental finding on imaging investigations performed for an unrelated condition. In most instances knowledge of the characteristic features should allow a definitive diagnosis to be made and obviate the need for any further investigations. Abdominal pain may occur with larger lesions with hemorrhage, infarction or compression of adjacent viscera complicating the tumor. Thrombocytopenia from platelet sequestration, hypofibrinogenemia from deposition of intravascular fibrin clot, and spontaneous rupture are all rare complications.

Diagnosis
Pathology
Hemangiomas may be single or multiple, intraparenchymal, or pedunculated, with a diameter varying from a few millimeters to greater than 20cm. However, the vast majority of hemangiomas are solitary, of less than 5cm in size, and are most commonly found in a subcapsular site in the right lobe adjacent to peripheral divisions of the hepatic vein. They are derived from mesodermal elements and are composed of cavernous vascular spaces lined by a single layer of flat epithelium and filled with blood. Thin fibrous septae separate the vascular channels. They have a predisposition to thrombosis with subsequent development of fibrosis, dystrophic calcification, or ossification. Larger hemangiomas have a propensity to involute, developing a central fibrocollagenous scar as vascular occlusion and organization of central thrombi occurs. Central necrosis is a potential sequel. Rarely, vascular occlusion may lead to total sclerosis of the hemangioma and formation of a fibrous nodule.

Radiology
Each radiologic technique has characteristic features by which hemangiomas may be reliably diagnosed, but there is a significant minority that are atypical. The latter require a combination of radiologic techniques to establish the diagnosis. The appearances will reflect the varying representation of the histologic elements within the tumor. Larger tumors often have mixed or atypical features and the differentiation from other benign or malignant tumors may be difficult. None of these techniques is pre-eminent and it is often a correlative imaging analysis by an experienced hepatobiliary radiologist that allows the diagnosis to be made with confidence.

Characteristic appearances on ultrasound are of a well-circumscribed hyperechoic lesion of less than 3cm, exhibiting posterior acoustic enhancement. These lie in a subcapsular position adjacent to an hepatic vein. If fatty infiltration of the liver is present, the tumors may be hypoechoic. Demonstration of bloodflow on color Doppler flow imaging is a variable feature occurring in between 10 and 50% of hemangiomas in published series. Large (greater than 3cm) or giant (greater than 10cm) hemangiomas will have varying degrees of hemorrhage, calcification, or fibrosis, modifying the ultrasound appearances.

On CT, hemangiomas are characteristically of low density, although in the presence of fatty infiltration they may appear hyperdense relative to the surrounding hepatic parenchyma. After intravenous contrast agent administration, there is nodular peripheral enhancement of the tumor by the large feeding vascular nidus of the tumor. Centripetal enhancement then occurs with 'filling in' of the tumor (Fig. 24.6).

Although small lesions 'fill in' completely, large hemangiomas may show central avascular zones corresponding to the central fibrotic scar (Fig. 24.7).

The rate of 'filling in' of the tumor is variable and is dependent on the flow dynamics of the hemangioma and on the timing of the acquisition of the scan relative to the bolus of contrast, but may be delayed for up to 20 minutes after the injection. It is important to emphasize that only approximately 54% of large hemangiomas have this characteristic perfusion pattern. However, only 2% of other primary, benign and malignant tumors exhibit these features so their presence typically should allow a confident diagnosis of a hemangioma to be made. The converse argument is that up to 46% of hemangiomas exhibit atypical features of either absent, mixed or central enhancement or incomplete 'filling in' on delayed scans so that clear differentiation from malignant tumors may not be possible in these cases. Therefore, it is an important rule that in the CT evaluation of a patient who has a documented extrahepatic malignancy, strict adherence to these criteria is essential to ensure a metastasis is not misinterpreted as an atypical hemangioma.

With MRI, hemangiomas characteristically demonstrate marked hyperintensity on T2-weighted images that may contain low intensity areas correlating with the pathologic zones of fibrosis. After administration of the vascular phase contrast agent gadolinium diethylenetriaminepentaacetic acid (Gd-DTPA) there is early peripheral nodular enhancement with 'filling in' on delayed scans paralleling the characteristics of CT. Smaller hemangiomas more often demonstrate uniform enhancement, potentially indistinguishable from the appearances of hypervascular metastases or hepatocellular carcinomas (Fig. 24.8).

Increasing the T2-weighting of the acquisition may improve the discrimination, with hemangiomas usually being of higher signal intensity than malignant nodules. As hemangiomas do not contain Kupffer cells or normal hepatocytes they do not enhance with either SPIO particles or manganese-DPDP.

Hemangiomas cause a focal defect on both hepatobiliary excretion and sulfur colloid scintigraphy that is accompanied by normal uptake in the surrounding liver. Tagged red blood cell scans may be diagnostic, again showing the features of centripetal uptake with 'filling in' on delayed scans.

Angiography is usually reserved for the atypical tumors when assessment by noninvasive techniques singularly or in combination has not resulted in a definitive diagnosis. The appearances are pathognomonic with small pools of contrast, which persist beyond the late venous phase without evidence of tumor neovascularity or arteriovenous shunting (Fig. 24.9).

Management

It is the severity of the clinical presentation rather than any specific morphologic characteristic of the hemangioma that direct management. Rupture and hemorrhage are at the extreme of the clinical spectrum, and the requirement for surgical intervention is without question. In the patients who have abdominal pain, the clinical analysis is frequently more

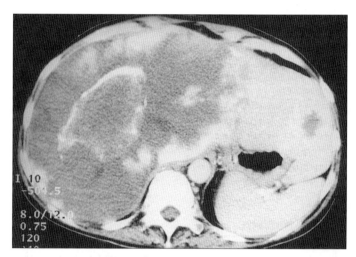

Figure 24.7 Hemangioma. CT demonstrates a central scar within a cavernous hemangioma of the right lobe of the liver. There is a small hemangioma in the left lobe that also exhibits centripetal enhancement.

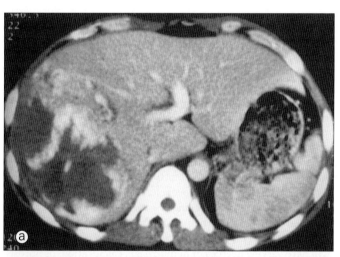

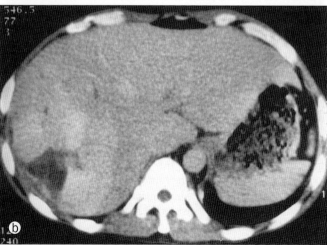

Figure 24.6 Hemangioma. CT demonstrating a giant cavernous hemangioma with (a) centripetal enhancement in the early vascular phase and (b) 'filling in' in the delayed phase.

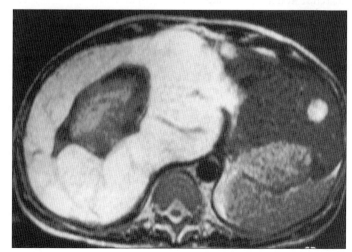

Figure 24.8 Hemangioma. T2-weighted MRI scans of same case as Fig. 24.5 demonstrate the characteristic hyperintensity of the hemangioma with the central hypointense scar. The smaller lesion in the left lobe appears uniformly hyperintense.

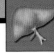

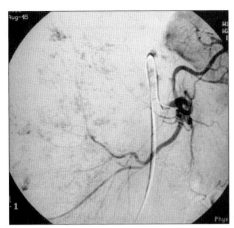

Figure 24.9 Hemangioma. Selective hepatic arteriography demonstrates the characteristic features of a hemangioma with pools of contrast and absent venous shunting.

difficult. If it is clear that the patient's symptoms are attributable to a large hemangioma, and if radiologic assessment confirms that the lesion is resectable, surgery is indicated. Radiologic intervention with particulate embolization of the arterial supply is a therapeutic alternative but as yet there is no controlled trial to confirm its efficacy. Neither of these interventions, with their inherent morbidity, should be undertaken unless an objective risk–benefit analysis of the patient's symptoms has been undertaken.

INFANTILE HEMANGIOENDOTHELIOMA

Clinical features

This is the commonest mesenchymal tumor of the liver and may represent part of a generalized mesenchymal disorder with cutaneous hemangiomata present in over 50% of cases. Less commonly there are accompanying lesions in the gastrointestinal tract, trachea, pulmonary parenchyma, or central nervous system. More than 80% are diagnosed in the first 6 months of life and there is an approximately equal sex incidence. Complications include congestive cardiac failure secondary to arteriovenous shunting, rupture, and consumptive coagulopathy. Anemia, thrombocytopenia and hemolytic jaundice are other presenting features. Occasionally these lesions present as an asymptomatic mass that resolves spontaneously without complication.

Diagnosis
Pathology

The tumors can be solitary or multicentric, varying in size from a few millimeters to more than 15cm in diameter. They are well demarcated but nonencapsulated. The cut surface exhibits a reddish-brown appearance with a spongy consistency that may show central areas of focal hemorrhage, scarring or calcification. Histologically the tumor is composed of anastomosing vascular channels lined by a solitary (type 1) or multiple layers (type 2) of plump endothelial cells. The infiltrative growth pattern between the liver cell plates is the feature that distinguishes the tumors from cavernous hemangiomas. The tumor cells are benign and mitoses are rare. Extramedullary hemopoiesis is a frequent finding. Low-grade angiosarcomas may also present in infancy and, as these carry different management and prognostic implications, are the most important histologic diagnostic differential of the type 2 lesions.

Radiology

The radiologic features reflect the degree of arterialization and arteriovenous shunting within the tumor. High volume shunts are associated with a hyperdynamic arterial flow, dilatation of the draining hepatic veins, and features of cardiac failure with cardiomegaly and pulmonary plethora on chest radiograph. The infants who present within the first few days of life with these features are often misdiagnosed as having congenital heart disease with an intracardiac shunt. The role of radiology is to examine the extent of replacement of the normal liver parenchyma by the hemangioendothelioma, assess the degree of vascularity and pathologic shunting, and to determine whether any other organs are involved.

The US features of these tumors vary. Many of the tumors are well circumscribed, but their internal structure may differ in characteristics. Diffuse alteration in the parenchymal pattern with complete replacement of the normal liver pattern may be present, even in the presence of normal liver function as assessed by synthetic capability. Doppler US characteristics are diagnostic in the majority of infants with a high volume systolic and end diastolic arterial flow and dilatation of anatomically normal main hepatic veins.

Computed tomography demonstrates the focal vascular spaces as enhancing masses on both the arterial and portal venous phases of contrast enhancement. The degree of persistence of tumor enhancement on the delayed phase will be dependent on the degree of arteriovenous shunting. The tumors with high volume shunts will be characterized by a rapid clearance of contrast and dilated hepatic veins (Fig. 24.10).

Those who do not have a major arteriovenous shunt will show persistent and increasing enhancement with 'filling in' resembling adult cavernous hemangiomata (Fig. 24.11).

Magnetic resonance imaging will demonstrate the tumors as hyperintense vascular spaces on T2-weighted images. The enlarged hepatic arteries and decompressing hepatic veins are demonstrable on conventional multiplanar imaging or dedicated vascular image acquisition techniques (magnetic resonance angiography). Areas of focal calcification, hemorrhage, and necrosis, which have variable representation within the tumors, will all have their characteristic appearances with the individual techniques.

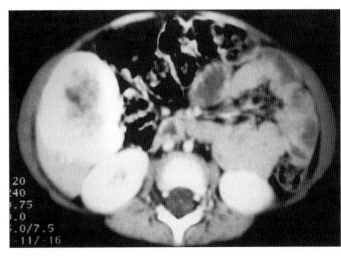

Figure 24.10 Hemangioendothelioma. Segmental hemangioendothelioma presenting in an infant appearing as a hypervascular mass on CT.

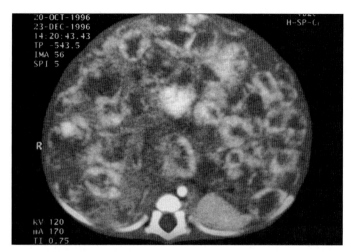

Figure 24.11 Hemangioendothelioma. Diffuse hepatic hemangioendothelioma of infancy with multiple enhancing nodules within an enlarged liver.

Angiography provides a conclusive diagnosis, detailed anatomy of the tumor, and its feeding arteries. Hypervascular tumor vessels are present with varying degrees of arteriovenous shunting and enlargement of the hepatic veins and hepatic artery. There is often diminution in the size of the abdominal aorta distal to the origin of the enlarged hepatic artery, as a consequence of the steal of blood through the liver.

Management
The management of these tumors is dependent on the severity of the clinical presentation. This is a rare benign tumor and yet there are many treatments advocated in published series and individual case reports. Mild degrees of cardiac failure may be treated with digoxin and diuretics, but the response to steroids and interferon seems to vary from center to center. Radiotherapy has been used, but all of these nonsurgical management lines have to be judged by the natural history of these tumors that may undergo spontaneous regression and involution in the first few months of life without any intervention. Surgery is mandatory for intraperitoneal hemorrhage, but surgery in the presence of severe cardiac failure, unresponsive to medical treatment, is more contentious. Hepatic resection, hepatic artery ligation, or embolization and transplantation all have a potential role.

Hepatic artery ligation is a well established technique with numerous published reports attesting to its efficacy. It remains to be seen whether it can be totally superseded by embolization as a method of occluding the arterial inflow to the hemangioendothelioma. Occluding the arterial supply with a metallic spring embolus delivered following percutaneous catheterization of the hepatic artery should result in the same alteration in hemodynamics as with surgical ligation, but without the operative morbidity. Resection is a surgical option when the tumor is confined to a lobe or segment, but is feasible in only a minority of cases. The greatest risk from resection lies in intraoperative hemorrhage. Liver transplantation may be the only option if arterial ligation fails with development of early arterial collateralization of the tumor and recurrence of severe cardiac failure.

LYMPHANGIOMA

Hepatic lymphangiomas commonly occur as multiple masses of dilated lymphatic channels containing proteinaceous fluid or blood. Multiple organ involvement, including the spleen, peritoneum, kidneys, lungs, gastrointestinal tract, and skeleton may be present, especially in children.

LIPOMATOUS TUMORS

Hepatic lipomas are uncommon benign tumors that are generally asymptomatic incidental findings on imaging. They may be composed solely of fat cells, or may contain varying proportions of adenomatous, angiomatous, and myomatous tissue, resulting in adenolipomas, myelolipomas, and angiomyolipomas.

Clinical features
Approximately 10% of patients who have tuberous sclerosis and renal angiomyolipomas will have hepatic fatty tumors, either lipoma or angiomyolipoma. There is no sex predilection and they have been reported in a broad adult age range of 24–70 years.

Diagnosis
Pathology
The tumors are composed of vessels, smooth muscle, fat, and hemopoietic tissues in various combinations. The unusual histologic appearances may cause diagnostic difficulty, especially with the leiomyomatous element, which may be either spindle or epithelioid in nature. Electron microscopy and immunocytochemistry readily identify the various components of the tumor.

Radiology
The radiologic appearance of these fatty lesions is dependent on their internal composition. Fat has specific tissue characteristics. On US it is of increased echogenicity with acoustic enhancement posterior to the lesion. It has a specific density on CT of –20 to –115 Hounsfield units (HUs) and on MRI it is hyperintense on both T1 and T2-weighted acquisitions. The presence of angiomatous or myomatous tissue will necessarily alter the homogeneity of these characteristic features. Although pure lipomas do not enhance after vascular phase contrast agents, fatty hepatic tumors with angiomatous or adenomatous elements may show variable enhancement and make diagnosis by imaging more difficult. In these cases, a tissue diagnosis by image-guided biopsy may be necessary.

Management
No treatment is indicated if a definitive histologic or radiologic diagnosis has been made in an asymptomatic patient. The tumors that are characterized by the presence of angiomatous features may present with hemorrhage and abdominal pain. In these rare instances surgical resection or embolization will have to be considered.

FOCAL NODULAR HYPERPLASIA

Clinical features
Even though the overall incidence is low, focal nodular hyperplasia (FNH) is the second most common tumor and constitutes approximately 8% of primary hepatic tumors found at autopsy.

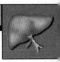
It is found most commonly in females during their reproductive years. Fewer than 20% are found in children and these account for 2% of the childhood tumors. The etiology of the lesion is unknown. The preponderance in women, as with adenomas, suggests an association with estrogens, but the prevalence of oral contraceptive use in these cases is similar to that of a matched control population. The majority of lesions are discovered incidentally and only approximately 15% result in symptoms, usually non-specific abdominal discomfort. Rupture and hemoperitoneum are rare. Patients who have focal nodular hyperplasia frequently have other vascular and neuroendocrine anomalies including cavernous hemangiomas, glioblastomas, astrocytomas, phaeochromocytomas, and multiple endocrine neoplasias. Lesions in children have been described in association with glycogen storage disease type 1, sickle cell disease, and cyanotic congenital heart disease.

Pathogenesis

The pathogenesis of FNH has been related to neoplastic change, hamartomatous malformation, or focal liver injury. The current view is that it represents a hyperplastic response to an abnormal blood flow caused by a pre-existing vascular malformation within the liver or abnormal or absent portal venous flow. It has been suggested that increased and turbulent bloodflow results in platelet disruption with arterial thrombosis and release of platelet-derived growth factors that may then stimulate liver cell hyperplasia.

Diagnosis
Pathology

This lesion is typically solitary and forms a well circumscribed fibrous lobular mass (Fig. 24.12).

The majority of tumors are smaller than 5cm, with a mean diameter of 3cm at the time of diagnosis. They are rarely encapsulated and 20% are pedunculated. The typical lesion tends to bulge on its cut surface and displays multiple yellow–brown nodules of liver parenchyma separated by fibrous septa. Histologically it resembles cirrhosis, but is focal and surrounded by normal liver parenchyma. A central stellate scar is often seen and it may contain thick-walled vessels. The frequent finding of bile duct

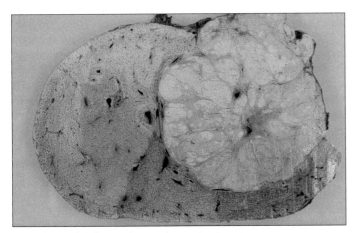

Figure 24.12 Focal nodular hyperplasia. Right hepatectomy specimen with a well circumscribed tumor measuring 8×8×6cm in the inferior aspect of the specimen. The lesion bears a central fibrous scar with radiating septa and appears lobulated and paler than the adjacent parenchyma. (Courtesy of Professor B. Portmann.)

proliferation around the liver cell nodules may be a response to cholestasis. The nodules consist of normal liver cells arranged in plates two or three cells thick and contain increased amounts of glycogen or fat. Focal nodular hyperplasia is distinguished from liver cell adenoma by its multinodularity, and the presence of septa and proliferating bile ductules.

Radiology

Up to 60% of FNH lesions contain Kupffer cells with reticuloendothelial cellular function, and these lesions may therefore demonstrate normal or increased uptake on sulfur colloid scintigraphy. The remainder may be seen as a photon defect. If uptake is present this may provide a differentiating feature from an adenoma. Hepatobiliary excretion scans show tracer uptake in the majority of cases, and isotope excretion can be observed in 50% of delayed scans. In practice, nuclear scintigraphy has a very limited role both in the detection and tissue characterization of focal liver lesions such as FNH with greater reliance placed upon other imaging techniques.

Sonographically, FNH may have a variable appearance, but the majority of these lesions are well demarcated lesions that are hyperechoic or isoechoic relative to the surrounding liver. Although a central scar is a common feature, it is not specific to FNH and it may not be visible on US. The color flow Doppler characteristics mimic the angiographic and macroscopic feature of increased bloodflow with a pattern of blood vessels that radiates peripherally from a central feeding artery.

On unenhanced CT studies, FNH is typically hypodense or isodense to the liver parenchyma. Its presence can often be inferred by an alteration in the surface contour of the liver and a hypodense central scar. The degree of enhancement following iodinated contrast medium is variable, but they generally rapidly enhance in the arterial and early portal venous phase, becoming isodense in the late portal phase (Fig. 24.13).

Apart from a possible central scar, which will maintain its hypodensity, enhancement of the tumor is uniform throughout these phases. It is this feature and the rapidity at which they occur that may distinguish FNH from cavernous hemangioma where the centripetal pattern of enhancement and 'filling in' is considerably slower to develop. Spontaneous intratumoral hemorrhage and a capsule are not features of FNH and if present favor the diagnosis of an adenoma.

On MRI most lesions are isointense or hypointense on T1-weighted images and show increased signal on T2. However, some lesions are isointense on both sequences and, as with the isodense tumors on CT, may only be detected by the expansion of the liver surface they create by their mass effect and a central scar when present. Following intravenous gadolinium, a rapid intense blush may occur that rapidly fades leaving the tumor close to isointensity in the equilibrium delayed phase of the examination. Delayed and increasing enhancement of the central scar on delayed scans is a characteristic of FNH. It is proposed that this feature is due to the presence of vascularized myxoid tissue in the scar. Fibrolamellar hepatocellular carcinomas and malignant cholangiocellular tumors also contain scars but do not demonstrate this radiologic sign.

Angiographically, FNH is a hypervascular tumor with a centrifugal arterial supply creating a 'spoke-wheel' pattern in the majority of lesions. During the capillary hepatogram phase an intense blush develops and large draining veins are visible (Fig. 24.14).

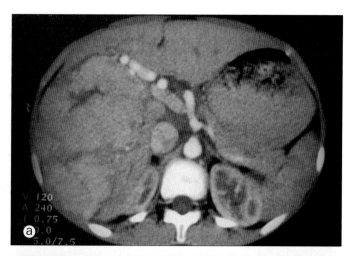

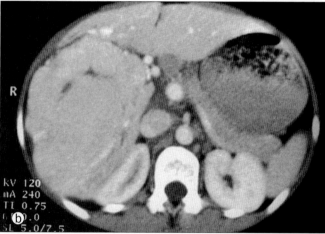

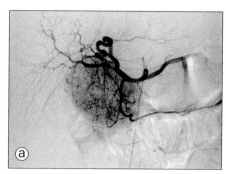

Figure 24.14 Focal nodular hyperplasia. Arteriography demonstrates the characteristic signs of focal nodular hyperplasia with (a) a centrifugal 'spoke-wheel' arterial pattern and (b) an intense blush with draining veins.

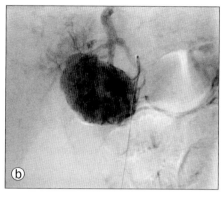

Figure 24.13 Focal nodular hyperplasia. (a) Focal nodular hyperplasia exhibiting characteristic features of increased density, with enlarged peripheral arteries and stellate scars in the arterial phase CT. (b) The lesion becomes isodense in the portal venous phase.

Management

In the asymptomatic patient it is important to establish the diagnosis by confirming the presence of characteristic features on imaging. Image-guided biopsy for a histologic diagnosis is reserved for lesions that demonstrate atypical or indeterminate radiologic features. In those rare patients presenting with spontaneous hemorrhage, surgical resection or embolization is indicated. In the patients who have nonspecific abdominal pain the decision to intervene is far more difficult. It must be clear that the patient's symptoms are attributable to this lesion by excluding any other cause and conducting a careful analysis of the risks of morbidity from surgery versus the potential symptomatic benefit in each individual patient.

NODULAR REGENERATIVE HYPERPLASIA

This is a rare entity that has been known by numerous synonyms, including nodular transformation of the liver, noncirrhotic nodulation, miliary hepatocellular adenomatosis, and adenomatous liver. However, the term of nodular regenerative hyperplasia (NRH) is now universally accepted. This condition need not involve the whole liver, but may be accentuated near the porta

hepatis and in this situation the term partial nodular transformation has been used. Autopsy series have shown a prevalence as high as 0.6%, but only one third of these cases had clinical features in life potentially attributable to this diagnosis.

Clinical features

It has been reported in all age groups with equal sex incidence. In the western world, NRH is the major cause of noncirrhotic portal hypertension. Clinical manifestations may be nonspecific, including malaise, fatigue, and abdominal pain, particularly if it has developed in association with a multisystem disorder. Alternatively it may be related to complications of portal hypertension with ascites and variceal hemorrhage. Synthetic liver function is usually preserved with minimal elevation of the serum transaminases, bilirubin, and prothrombin time.

Various systemic diseases are associated with NRH including rheumatoid arthritis, Felty's syndrome, polyarteritis nodosa, CREST (calcinosis cutis, Raynaud phenomenon, esophageal hypomobility, sclerodactyly, telangiectasia) syndrome, subacute bacterial endocarditis, tuberculosis, diabetes, myeloproliferative disorders, lymphomas, and after steroid or cytotoxic therapy. It also occurs in recipients of bone marrow, renal, and liver transplants, and in this setting therapy with azathioprine has been implicated in the causation. Common to all these disorders is a circulatory or vascular disorder and it has been postulated that NRH is a secondary and nonspecific adaptation of the liver parenchyma to an alteration in total liver bloodflow.

Diagnosis
Pathology
Confirming the diagnosis by liver biopsy is difficult and many cases are only diagnosed at surgery or autopsy. The liver is divided into nodules that vary in size between 0.1cm and 1cm, although rarely nodules measuring up to 10cm in diameter have been reported. Histologically the nodules are composed of cyto-

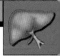
logically normal hepatocytes arranged in abnormal cell plates that are two or more cells thick. The features are of pure liver cell nodularity, enlarging and distorting acini or lobules but not replacing them. Histologically, this disorder can be distinguished from micronodular cirrhosis by the absence of fibrous septa between the nodules. Obliterative vascular changes may also be present.

Radiology

The radiologic features are those of portal hypertension with splenomegaly, varices, ascites, and variable degrees of alteration in the hepatic parenchyma. Nodules may be present on all imaging techniques, but the liver parenchyma may remain uniform. Differentiation from cirrhotic portal hypertension may be difficult on imaging appearances alone, but hepatic and portal vein venous pressure studies confirm the hemodynamic profile of presinusoidal portal hypertension in association with a patent portal vein. These are important diagnostic criteria that support the diagnosis of NRH.

Management

The management is dependent on the degree and manifestations of portal hypertension. It commences with medical therapy to reduce portal pressure and ablation of varices once they have bled. Some cases proceed to shunting and portal decompression when recurrent variceal hemorrhage is resistant to the first-line therapeutic measures.

MESENCHYMAL HAMARTOMA

This lesion probably represents a failure of normal development *in utero* of the ductal plate.

Clinical features

These lesions are benign and account for approximately 6% of primary liver tumors in children. The majority will present in childhood with two thirds of patients presenting in the first year of life. Almost all patients present before the age of 5 years but, rarely, this may be delayed until adolescence or early adult life. There is a slight male preponderance. The commonest presentation is with symptoms of progressive abdominal enlargement. Less commonly, infants may present with respiratory depression or peripheral edema from the mass effect of the lesion.

Diagnosis
Histology

There is a mixture of mesodermal and endodermal structures in a loose connective tissue stroma and fluid-filled spaces without an endothelial lining. Bile duct, liver cell, and angiomatous elements are present, and the appearance is of well differentiated ductal structures surrounded by loose mesenchyme containing fibroblasts. The prominent mesenchymal and cystic components that are visible on histology and radiologic investigations, will allow differentiation from FNH and liver cell adenoma.

Radiology

Ultrasound and CT assessment will demonstrate a well circumscribed complex cystic lesion with internal septation (Fig. 24.15).

With contrast enhancement or angiography, the lesion is predominantly avascular, but neovascularity is seen in the more solid elements. The MRI appearances depend on whether an individual lesion is predominantly stromal or cystic. The lesions with a fibrotic stroma predominating will appear hypointense relative to the surrounding liver on T1-weighted images. Alternatively, if the lesion is mainly cystic its major feature will be its hyperintensity on the T2-weighted images. The fibrous stroma and internal septation are the features that will distinguish this tumor from a simple cyst.

Management

The characteristic natural history is of progressive enlargement of the lesion secondary to degeneration and fluid accumulation within the cystic component. Treatment is removal by a combination of resection and enucleation. Marsupialization into the peritoneal cavity or transplantation are alternative treatments for unresectable lesions.

INFLAMMATORY PSEUDOTUMOR

Synonyms for this very rare lesion include 'pseudolymphoma', 'histiocytoma', and 'plasma cell granuloma'. Only about 50 cases have been reported to arise within the liver, and they are known to occur at other sites including the lung and orbits.

Clinical features

Most patients are young with a significant male preponderance. The clinical presentation is of an acute infection with relapsing fever, abdominal pain, vomiting, diarrhea, and jaundice. No causative organism or definite predisposing factor has been confirmed. Leukocytosis, a raised erythrocyte sedimentation rate, and polyclonal hyperglobulinemia are present in about 50% of cases.

Diagnosis

Macroscopically, the lesion is tumor-like. It may be either solitary or multiple, and measure up to 25cm in diameter. Microscopically, the lesion contains chronic inflammatory cells in which polyclonal plasma cells predominate. There is a lamellar pattern of sclerosis. The lesions commonly resolve slowly with involution, but biliary strictures and sepsis are rare sequelae of those arising and involving the porta hepatis (Fig. 24.16).

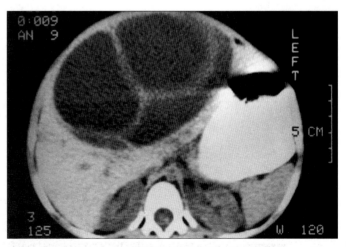

Figure 24.15 Mesenchymal hamartoma. This scan demonstrates the characteristic CT features of a mesenchymal hamartoma. This tumor presented in infancy with the appearances of a multiseptate cyst.

MISCELLANEOUS TUMOR-LIKE LESIONS

This group of conditions is of marginal importance in clinical practice but include infections that may produce a solitary necrotic nodule, including hydatid disease, tuberculosis, and larval infection. Pseudolipoma represents the attachment of omental or pericolic fat lobules to the liver. Focal fat deposition occurs with obesity, alcoholic liver disease, diabetes, and hyperlipidemia. This produces a characteristic radiologic pattern on US and CT of 'geographic liver', where fat replaces normal liver parenchyma but without distortion of the portal vasculature.

Compensatory lobar hyperplasia may follow segmental intrahepatic or extrahepatic portal vein or bile duct occlusion. Endometriosis of the liver site is recorded, arising in either a subcapsular or intrahepatic site. Adrenal nest tumors that arise from ectopic adrenal tissue that are identical to that in adrenocortical tumors and ectopic pancreas are both documented causes of tumor-like lesions of the liver.

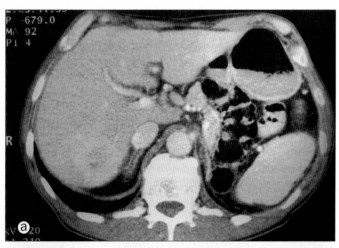

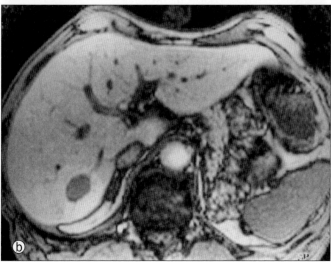

Figure 24.16 Inflammatory pseudotumor. (a) The CT demonstrates a lesion in the right lobe posteriorly with peripheral enhancement and central low density. (b) T2-weighted MRI scan following Mn-DPDP demonstrates the tumor as a hypointense lesion with manganese enhancement of the periphery of the lesion.

SIMPLE HEPATIC CYST

This is defined as a single unilocular cyst lined by a single layer of cuboidal, bile duct epithelium. The wall is a thin layer of fibrous tissue of less than 1mm in thickness. They may be single or multiple and typically arise in a subcapsular site. The adjacent hepatic parenchyma is normal, distinguishing these cysts from the simple cysts occurring in polycystic disease in which the parenchyma shows regions of fibrosis with von Meyenberg complexes.

Clinical features

These cysts vary in size from less than 1cm to over 20cm. They are much more common in females, with a ratio of females to males of 4–5:1. They have an overall incidence of 2.5% in the general population, but are generally found in less than 1% of patients less than 60 years of age but rising to approximately 7% in those patients who are older than 80 years of age. Autopsy series have reported an incidence as high as 14%. Patients are usually asymptomatic, but symptoms can develop secondary to their mass effect with abdominal pain, rupture, infection, or intracystic hemorrhage as presenting features.

Diagnosis

With US imaging, the cysts appear as well defined, echo-free lesions that transmit sound with posterior acoustic enhancement. Thin septations can be present but thicker septa or eccentric mural thickening of the cyst are indications of a complicated cyst or neoplasm. With CT, simple cysts appear as homogeneous, well-circumscribed, hypodense lesions with HU measurements in the range of simple fluid (<20HU). Small lesions may show artificially high density because of partial volume averaging of the adjacent hepatic parenchyma. They do not enhance following intravenous contrast. On MRI they characteristically show uniform low signal on T1-weighted images, and high signal on T2-weighted images. Small central cysts may be indistinguishable from both vessels and small cavernous hemangiomas on T2-weighted acquisitions. Postintravenous contrast studies with gadolinium may allow differentiation by demonstrating enhancement of both the hepatic vessels and hemangiomas.

Management

The most effective treatment for symptomatic cysts is wide excision and drainage. Guided percutaneous drainage is an option, particularly to assess whether this cures the pain that is being attributed to the lesion. However, there is a high recurrence with reaccumulation of fluid within the cyst. Sclerosing the cyst with alcohol following percutaneous decompression reduces the rate of recurrence.

POLYCYSTIC LIVER DISEASE AND CONGENITAL HEPATIC FIBROSIS

Polycystic disease is characterized by multiple hepatic cysts. The cysts are lined by bile duct epithelium but do not communicate with the biliary tree. Approximately 50–75% of patients who have adult polycystic kidney disease will have liver cysts (Fig. 24.17).

There is no correlation between the severity of the renal disease and the extent of liver involvement. Polycystic liver dis-

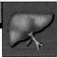
ease can occur in the absence of renal involvement. The parenchyma surrounding the cysts is abnormal, frequently containing von Meyenburg's complexes and increased fibrosis. Synthetic liver function is usually normal but the severity of the mass effect may prompt surgical intervention with cyst excision and drainage, lobar resection or transplantation, representing the spectrum of surgical options. Occasionally, the cysts impair hepatic venous outflow causing ascites and these cases usually require liver transplantation.

Congenital hepatic fibrosis is part of the spectrum of hepatic cystic disease. It is characterized by aberrant bile duct proliferation and periductal fibrosis. Clinically the majority of patients present in childhood with features of portal hypertension with variceal hemorrhage, splenomegaly, and ascites. The cysts are not grossly visible and the radiologic features are those of portal hypertension.

CAROLI'S DISEASE

Caroli's disease is a rare cystic developmental malformation of the intrahepatic bile ducts with intervening relatively normal bile ducts. The relationship to the more classic choledochal cyst is unclear. The whole of the biliary system may be involved or just a single segment or lobe. It is usually associated with hepatic fibrosis and cystic renal disease. The condition may be complicated by recurrent cholangitis and may present with fever without jaundice. Caroli classified two types of malformation. The rarer type 1, which presents with recurrent cholangitis and type 11 associated with hepatic fibrosis, portal hypertension, and renal cystic disease (Fig. 24.18).

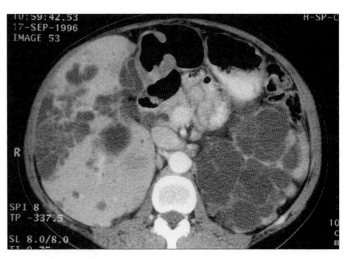

Figure 24.17 Polycystic disease. Multiple cysts demonstrated with CT as hypodense lesions in the liver and left kidney.

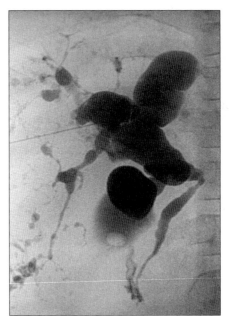

Figure 24.18 Caroli's disease. Caroli malformation of the bile duct with dilatation of the common hepatic, main right, and left ducts, with peripheral communicating bile duct cysts demonstrated by percutaneous cholangiography.

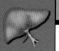

PRACTICE POINT

Illustrative case

A 34-year-old woman presented with high upper quadrant pain associated with nausea and vomiting. The pain was not colicky in nature and persisted after the nausea and vomiting had subsided. There were no clear precipitating factors or other associated symptoms. She had otherwise been well. She had used the oral contraceptive pill for 6 years and afterwards had two uneventful pregnancies. The physical examination was entirely normal apart from mild tenderness in the epigastrium.

All laboratory investigations were within normal limits. A US of the liver revealed a 5cm mass lesion in segment 4 of the liver. There was no evidence of gallstones or bile duct dilatation. The remainder of the examination was normal. A CT scan confirmed the presence of a mass in segment 4 of the liver with a central scar. A liver biopsy was performed which was compatible with a diagnosis of FNH. Endoscopic examination of the upper gastrointestinal tract was normal.

The nausea and vomiting resolved quickly with symptomatic treatment, but the discomfort in the right upper quadrant persisted. This started to interfere with work and sleep patterns, and she began using increasing amounts of analgesia, eventually progressing to regular use of narcotics. The imaging was repeated and there was no change in the size or nature of the lesion. The lesion was embolized with coils and particulate matter on two occasions, but there was only a marginal reduction in the size of the lesion, and there was no change in the symptoms. Surgical excision of the lesion was not considered to be feasible with an acceptable degree of risk. After protracted counseling she accepted that the lesion was benign and should be asymptomatic. All analgesia was withdrawn over a 6-week period and the symptoms resolved.

Interpretation

This case is typical of the problems that can be encountered when interpreting the significance of unexpected findings during the investigation of common symptoms. The US was intended to screen for gallstones and bile duct dilatation but detected a benign liver tumor. The diagnosis of FNH was not problematic and this finding did not credibly explain the patient's symptoms. Nevertheless, by the time these findings were explained to the patient she was convinced that there was a relationship between her symptoms and the liver tumor. It only became clear later that she also was convinced that the tumor was malignant despite the explanation to the contrary. The pressure to treat the lesion was patient driven and surgery would probably have been performed if the lesion had been more accessible. The management of incidental benign tumors requires careful and circumspect investigation and treatment.

FURTHER READING

Bartolozzi C, Lencioni R, Paolicchi A, et al. Differentiation of hepatocellular adenoma and focal nodular hyperplasia of the liver: comparison of power Doppler imaging and conventional color Doppler sonography. Eur Radiol. 1997;7:1410–5. *Comparison of sonographic techniques in the investigation of benign tumors.*

Baum JK, Holtz F, Bookstein JJ, et al. Possible association between benign hepatomas and oral contraceptives. Lancet. 1973;2:926–9. *One of the first descriptions of the association between adenoma and the contraceptive pill.*

Choi CS, Freeny PC. Triphasic helical scanning of hepatic focal nodular hyperplasia: incidence of atypical findings. Am J Radiol. 1998;170:391–5. *Diagnostic approach to atypical lesions.*

De-Carlis L, Pirotta V, Rondinara GF, et al. Hepatic adenoma and nodular hyperplasia: diagnosis and criteria for treatment. Liver Transplant Surg. 1997;3:160–5. *Series which illustrates the key issues in both diagnosis and management.*

Freeny PC, Vimant TR, Barnett TC. Cavernous hemangioma of the liver: ultrasonography, arteriography, and computed tomography. Radiology. 1979;132:143–8. *Comparison of different techniques in the assessment of hemangiomas.*

Holcomb GW, O'Neill JA, Mahboubi S, et al. Experience with hepatic hemangioendothelioma in infancy and childhood. J Pediatr Surg. 1988;23:661–6. *Outline of treatment options in infantile hemangioendothelioma.*

Homer LW, White HJ, Read RC. Neoplastic transformation of von Meyenburg complexes. J Pathol Bacteriol. 1968;96:499–502. *Description of cholangiocarcinoma arising in these normally innocuous lesions.*

Ishak KG, Willis GW, Cummins SD, et al. Biliary cystadenoma and biliary cystadenocarcinoma. Cancer. 1977;39:322–8. *Authoritative review of these rare biliary lesions.*

Klatskin G. Hepatic tumors: possible relation to use of oral contraceptives. Gastroenterology. 1977;73:386–94. *Good review of this topic.*

Mergo PJ, Ros PR. Benign tumors of the liver. Radiol Clin North Am. 1998;36:319–31. *Good review.*

Ribiero A, Burgart LJ, Nagorney DM, Gores GJ. Management of liver adenomatosis: results with a conservative surgical approach. Liver Transplant Surg. 1998;4:388–98. *Review of eight cases.*

Srouji MN, Chatten J, Schulman WM, et al. Mesenchymal hamartoma of the liver in infants. Cancer. 1988;42:2483–9. *Description of a rare lesion.*

Vana J, Murphy GP, Aronoff BL, et al. Primary liver tumors and oral contraceptive. JAMA. 1977;238:2154–8. *Large review of primary liver tumors in US including 212 benign tumors.*

Weimann A, Ringe B, Klempnauer J, et al. Benign liver tumors: differential diagnosis and indications for surgery. World J Surg. 1997;21:983–91. *Series of 437 patients, 173 of whom underwent surgery.*

Williams RA, Ferrell LD. Pediatric liver tumors. Pathology. 1993;2:23–42. *Review of pathologic findings in pediatric tumors.*

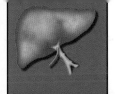

Chapter 25

Malignant Tumors of the Liver

Philip J Johnson

INTRODUCTION

Tumors of the liver enter into the differential diagnosis of many patients presenting to the hepatologist, and tend to be managed by hepatologists and hepatobiliary surgeons rather than by oncologists. A sound knowledge of these tumors is therefore required by all involved in the practice of clinical hepatology. In many parts of the world hepatocellular carcinoma (HCC) is one of the most common malignant tumors and represents a major public health problem. The liver is also the most frequent, and often the clinically predominant, organ site of metastatic malignant disease. This chapter deals firstly with the most common primary malignant tumor of the liver, HCC, then other primary liver tumors, and finally secondary liver tumors.

HEPATOCELLULAR CARCINOMA

Introduction

Hepatocellular carcinoma is the sixth most common cancer in the world, and 540,000 new cases were diagnosed in 1996, accounting for 5.2% of all new cancers. It tends to present late in its natural history, because small tumors cause few symptoms and the large size of the liver precludes easy palpation of the tumor until it has gained considerable dimensions. The large functional reserve of the liver also delays symptomatic presentation with disturbances such as jaundice or ascites. Patients who are carriers of the hepatitis B virus (HBV), hepatitis C virus (HCV), or those who have cirrhosis of any other etiology, are at a very high risk of HCC development. Physicians managing such patients need to maintain a high index of suspicion (Fig. 25.1).

Epidemiology and pathogenesis

Elucidation of the epidemiology of HCC is one of the medical success stories of the 20th century. Not only have the most important risk factors been identified and their impact quantified, but also preventive measures based on these results are now being implemented.

Age-adjusted incidence rates vary from less than 2/100,000 in Northern Europe, the USA, and Australia up to more than 100/100,000 in parts of sub-Saharan Africa and the Far East (Fig. 25.2). These data may hide important information. For example, within the USA, where the overall incidence rate is low, there is marked variation in relation to ethnicity with rates per 100,000 of 18, 4, and 2 for Chinese, black Americans, and white Americans respectively. Furthermore, within individual countries there may be very striking geographic differences in incidence, even among ethnically homogenous peoples (Fig. 25.3).

Key features of hepatocellular carcinoma and secondary liver tumors	
HCC	Secondary liver tumours
HCC usually presents late, when the tumor is already large	Liver metastases are present in 40% of patients who have extrahepatic malignancy who come to autopsy
The nontumorous liver is usually cirrhotic	Survival is directly related to the size of the tumor
Resection offers the only hope of long term survival, but is only an option for a minority of patients because: the tumour has already metastasized, or liver function is too poor, or the tumor is too large	All solitary lesions should be investigated for the possibility of surgical resection
Recurrence after resection or transplantation is common particularly when the tumor is large or there is histologic evidence of vascular invasion	In patients who have good performance status cytotoxic chemotherapy should be considered, either given as standard intravenous regimen or as a chronic infusion
HBV vaccination should ultimately decrease the incidence of HCC in many high incidence areas	Postoperative adjuvant treatment improves survival and decreases the risk of hepatic metastases in patients who have Duke stage C colorectal cancer

Figure 25.1 Key features of hepatocellular carcinoma (HCC) and secondary liver tumors.

Age-adjusted incidence rates of HCC			
	Country	Male	Female
Low incidence areas	UK	1.6	0.8
	USA (white)	2	1
	Australia	1.1	0.5
	Germany	4	1.2
	Denmark	3.6	2.3
Intermediate incidence areas	Italy	7.5	3.5
	Spain	7.5	4
	Romania	11.8	7.9
	Argentina	8	5
High incidence areas	Japan	20	5
	Hong Kong	32	7
	Mozambique	113	31
	Zimbabwe	65	25
	Senegal	25	9
	Taiwan	85	–

Figure 25.2 Age-adjusted incidence rates of HCC (per 100,000 of population) in various countries. Where figures for different areas of the same country are available, typical values have been given. Most registries do not distinguish between HCC and other primary tumors, so the figures should, at best, be considered as a rough guide.

Rates are consistently higher for men than for women. The incidence of HCC rises with age in all areas of the world (Fig. 25.4).

In 70–90% of cases of HCC there is an associated hepatic cirrhosis. The overall rate of tumor development in cirrhotic subjects is in the order of 2–5% per annum. All factors linked to the development of HCC, including HBV, HCV, and alcohol, also cause cirrhosis. If the factor causing cirrhosis, for example alcohol in alcoholic cirrhosis, or iron in the case of hemochromatosis, is removed, the high risk of HCC does not decrease.

Hepatitis B virus infection

Areas of the world with the highest HCC incidence have carriage rates for hepatitis B surface antigen (HBsAg) of greater than 10% (Fig. 25.5). A landmark study of 22,707 HBsAg seropositive male Chinese civil servants for HCC development, showed conclusively that chronic HBV infection precedes HCC development and the relative risk for a male HBsAg carrier for HCC was about 100. Other cancers did not develop with undue frequency among HBV carriers.

The association of HBV and HCC is confined to chronic HBV infection, particularly when acquired at birth or during childhood. The period from acquisition of the virus to tumor development can be as short as 4 years and as long as 80 years. Although the weight of epidemiologic evidence linking chronic HBV infection to the subsequent development of HCC is now overwhelming, elucidation of the mechanism has proved elusive. Hepatitis B virus DNA, integrated in to the host genome, can be detected in most cases, even in the absence of serologic evidence of HBV infection. However, there does not appear to be a consistent integration site and HBV does not contain recognized oncogenes.

It is hoped that vaccination against HBV will dramatically decrease the incidence of this tumor. Preliminary evidence from Taiwan where mass vaccination was introduced in 1984 for children of mothers who were HBsAg carriers, and universally in 1986, shows that this a realistic aim. A steady decrease in the number of children who have HCC, aged 6–14 years, is already evident. The incidence rate has fallen from 0.7/100,000 (1981–1986) to 0.57 (1986–1990) and to 0.36 (1990–1994).

Hepatitis C virus infection

With the development of tests for antibodies to the HCV in 1989 it became apparent, at least in Europe and Japan, that HCV was at least as important as HBV in the pathogenesis of HCC. In Europe, HCV positivity in patients who have HCC ranges from 20 to 76%, with a tendency to increase from north to south (Fig. 25.6). There appears to be a very long incubation period as assessed by following up patients who have hemophilia in whom the time of acquisition could be accurately documented. Since HCV has no reverse transcriptase activity and is not a retrovirus, it should, in theory, have no direct oncogenic potential. Most authors have attributed the association with HCC to the chronic liver disease that HCV may cause. Hepatitis C virus-related HCC is starting to become a major clinical problem in the West, perhaps following intravenous drug abuse in the1960s.

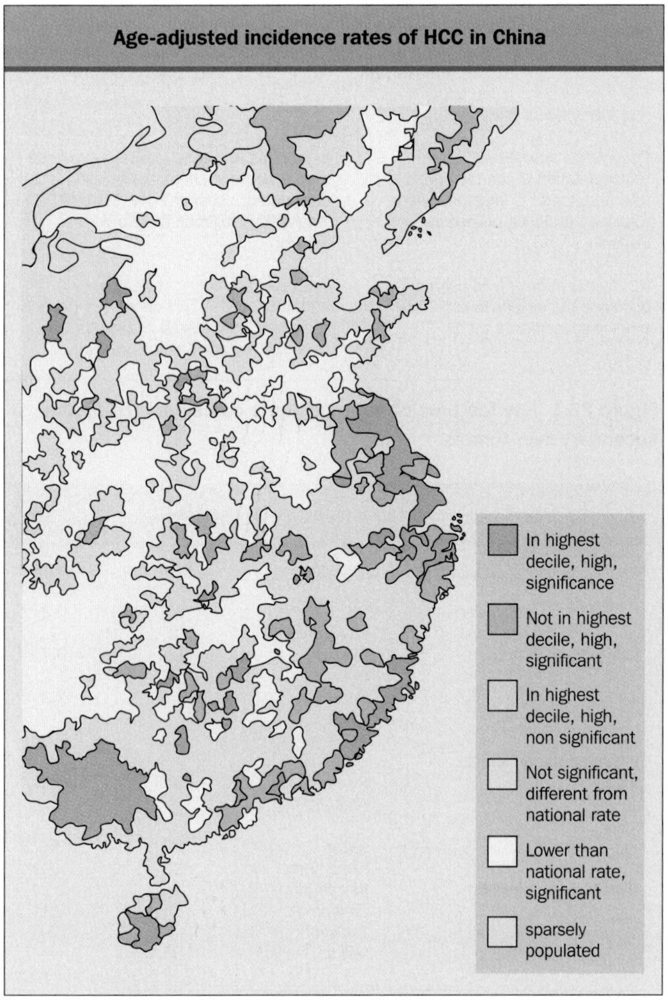

Age-adjusted incidence rates of HCC in China

In highest decile, high, significance

Not in highest decile, high, significant

In highest decile, high, non significant

Not significant, different from national rate

Lower than national rate, significant

sparsely populated

Figure 25.3 Age-adjusted incidence rates of HCC in China in relation to the national average. Note that, although the prevalence of hepatitis B carriage is fairly constant throughout China, there is a great deal of geographic variation, with cases tending to cluster (red and purple areas) strongly around the coastal strip.

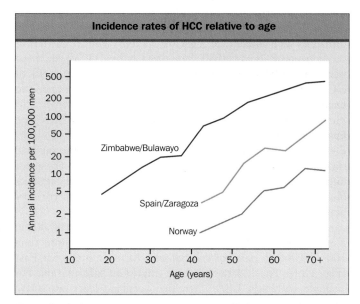

Figure 25.4 The change in incidence rates of HCC according to age in three different geographic areas. (Munoz and Bosch. In: Okuda and Ishak, eds. Neoplasms of the liver. Tokyo: Springer Verlag, 1987.)

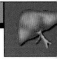

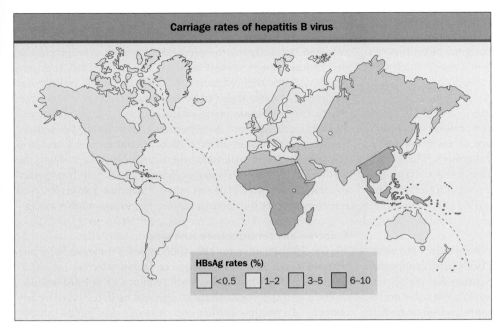

Figure 25.5 Worldwide carriage rate of the hepatitis B virus. Note that the areas with the highest carriage rates coincide with the areas that have the highest incidence of HCC.

With the prospect of effective treatment of both hepatitis B and C, the question of whether this will decrease the likelihood of the development of HCC arises. The relevant trials are currently underway. Initial experience with interferon treatment of HCV is encouraging (Fig. 25.7).

Aflatoxin exposure and other possible etiologic factors

Aflatoxins are mycotoxins generated by the fungi *Aspergillus flavus* and *Aspergillus parasiticus*. These mycotoxins are the most potent naturally occurring carcinogens known. Humans are exposed following ingestion of nuts and meal that are stored under hot humid conditions where these molds grow. The relative risk of HCC for individuals exposed to aflatoxin is very high, similar to that for HBV carriage, but for individuals who have both risk factors the relative risk is increased in a multiplicative manner. These are likely to be major etiologic factors in humid parts of China and Africa.

There now seems little doubt that there is true association between contraceptive preparations and benign hepatic adenomas, although the risk is extremely small and the risk that such lesions will lead to significant symptoms is even smaller. The current consensus is that while there may possibly be a significantly increased risk of the development of HCC after prolonged (>8 years) usage, the absolute risk remains extremely small.

Clinical features and disease associations

The most common mode of presentation is with the triad of abdominal pain in the right upper quadrant, weight loss, and hepatomegaly. Patients who present in this manner usually have a tumor larger than 6cm in diameter and diameters of 15cm are not uncommon. The pain is usually a dull ache, sometimes referred to the shoulder. Sudden attacks of more severe pain may be caused by spontaneous bleeding into the tumor. Hepatomegaly, often massive, is an invariable feature of symptomatic malignant liver tumors. The liver feels firm or stony hard. The combination of a vascular bruit, which can be heard in about 25% of cases, and a rub on auscultation over the liver are said to be diagnostic of HCC. Usually the symptoms will have

Anti-HCV positivity in hepatocellular carcinoma		
Country	% of HCC patients	% of control population
Italy	76	<1
France	58	<1
Spain	75	7.5
Greece	40	6
UK	10	<1
USA	20	1
Japan	68	7

Figure 25.6 Rate of positivity for anti-HCV among patients who have HCC in various countries compared with a control population from the same country. There is considerable variation within country and figures may even depend on the particular assay used. Figures should therefore only be taken as rough estimates.

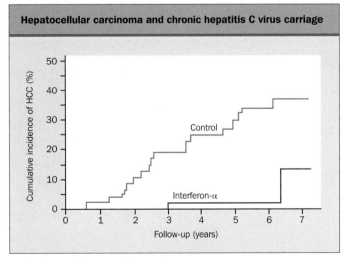

Figure 25.7 Cumulative incidence of HCC in chronic carriers of the HCV who receive interferon-α. Note that tumors start to be detected in the control group well within the first year, implying that they were already present on entry into the study, although at a preclinical stage. (Nishiguchi et al. Lancet. 1995;346:1051–5.)

been present for a only a few weeks in high incidence areas, or for a few months in lower incidence areas. Delay in seeking medical advice is seldom a reason for late diagnosis or a factor that can be held responsible for delayed intervention. Less common presentations are listed below.

Hepatic decompensation

In a male who has previously well-controlled cirrhosis who develops ascites, recurrent variceal hemorrhage or encephalopathy, HCC must always enter the differential diagnosis. The ascites becomes difficult to control with standard diuretic therapy and may be bloodstained. Jaundice of the hepatocellular type becomes steadily progressive.

Gastrointestinal hemorrhage

About 10% of cases will present with gastrointestinal bleeding. In 40% of the cases the bleed will have been from esophageal varices; this is much more frequent if the patient has portal vein invasion by the tumor, which presumably increases the portal pressure. Bleeding from duodenal ulceration and other benign causes accounts for the remaining 60% of cases. A rare event is bleeding from direct invasion of the gastrointestinal tract, stomach, or duodenum, by the tumor.

In both the above-mentioned presentations, the patient may have cutaneous stigmata of chronic liver disease, but this is by no means always the case. The majority of patients who present with HCC, as well as having no history of chronic liver disease, have no clinical signs thereof. The failure to detect clinical signs of chronic liver disease does not imply its absence.

Tumor rupture – 'hemoperitoneum'

Spontaneous rupture is a particularly dramatic presentation of the tumor (Fig. 25.8). There is a sudden onset of abdominal pain and swelling. Although hemoperitoneum is a frequent event late in the course of the disease, it is a presenting feature in less than 5% of cases. The patient presents with shock and a rigid, silent abdomen. The diagnosis is established by paracentesis, which reveals bloodstained fluid.

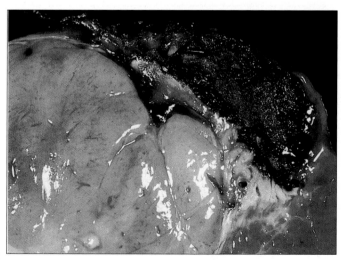

Figure 25.8 Macroscopic picture of ruptured HCC. Note the large blood clot on the surface of the liver. The vessels responsible for the hemorrhage are visible. (Courtesy of Dr CT Liew.)

Asymptomatic presentation

Increasingly, because of screening programs, tumors are being detected before any symptoms develop. With current imaging procedures, tumors as small as 0.5cm can be detected. It is even being suggested that, using tumor marker screening, tumors may be detected before they can be seen on ultrasound imaging (i.e. during the preclinical phase of the disease). The frequency of asymptomatic diagnosis is entirely dependent on the intensity of the screening program. In most countries those cases detected at this stage remain a small fortunate minority. Not surprisingly, the natural history of these very early lesions is different from symptomatic tumors and apparent survival is much better. Surgical resection or liver transplantation may be curative in this group.

Endocrine and paraneoplastic syndromes

Hepatocellular carcinoma has a reputation for paraneoplastic presentations, but this is largely due to highly selective reporting. Overall less than 1% of all cases will present with any of these syndromes, although asymptomatic cases will be detected more frequently if sought assiduously. Among the paraneoplastic syndromes, a high red cell count (erythrocytosis) is well recognized, and is presumed to be related to ectopic production of erythropoietin or an erythropoietin-like substance. Two types of hypoglycemia are recognized. The first ('type A'), occurs during the terminal stage of a rapidly growing tumor and is seldom symptomatic. A much greater clinical problem is type B disease, in which severe symptomatic hypoglycemia occurs relatively early in the disease course. The hypoglycemia does not respond consistently to any therapeutic approach and the physician usually resorts to long-term enteral glucose administration. Other even rarer presentations include gynecomastia, hypercalcemia, and hyperthyroidism.

Other rare modes of presentation

Spread to involve the hepatic vein is a cause of the Budd–Chiari syndrome with massive tense ascites. Obstructive jaundice may be due to compression of the bile ducts by tumor rather than hepatocellular failure. In approximately half the cases the site of obstruction is extrahepatic. Other rare causes of jaundice include direct growth of the tumor into the bile duct or bleeding from the tumor into the biliary system (hematobilia). Hepatocellular carcinoma has occasionally been reported as a cause of 'pyrexia of unknown origin' (PUO). The PUO occurs late in the disease and leads to diagnostic difficulties during management. With established cases of HCC it may be difficult to differentiate between a pyrexia of malignant disease from a sepsis-related fever in patients who are neutropenic following chemotherapy.

Clinical features of specific histologic subtypes

Three rare, histologically defined, primary liver cancers deserve special consideration since they have specific clinical correlates. The fibrolamellar variant of HCC has several distinctive clinical features, including a young age at presentation (median age 20 years), normal α-fetoprotein (AFP) levels, and a lack of any association with cirrhosis. Patients are invariably HBV-negative. The histologic picture is one of central dense fibrotic bands and eosinophilic tumor cells. The tumor, which is very rare in high incidence areas, carries a better prognosis than the normal type of HCC. Another histologic variant with which fibrolamellar carcinoma may be confused has very marked sclerosis, but does not carry a better prognosis. It is often associated with hypercalcemia and is easily mistakenly classified as a cholangiocarcinoma. The unusual vascular tumor, now termed 'epithelioid hemangioendothelioma', may occasionally arise in the liver. Its distinction from HCC is important as the prognosis is distinctly better.

Hepatocellular carcinoma in the noncirrhotic liver

In all areas of the world 10–20% of HCC cases arise within a histologically normal liver. This type has distinctive clinical features. Compared with HCC complicating cirrhosis, the incidence in females is higher, the typical age of presentation is lower, the tumor is less often AFP-positive, and survival is slightly better. The characteristic clinical features are detailed in Figure 25.9,

Features of cirrhotic and noncirrhotic hepatocellular carcinoma		
	No cirrhosis	Cirrhosis
Demographics		
Age (years)	36±14	56±13*
Male	56	98
Female	44	2*
Presentation		
Abdominal pain	50	44
Awareness of a mass	36	7*
Weight loss	32	36
Hemoperitoneum	2	2
Hepatic decompensation		
jaundice	10	24*
fluid retention	8	28*
upper gastrointestinal hemorrhage	0	11*
encephalopathy	0	3*
Laboratory features		
Elevated SAP	90	96
Elevated AST	58	93*
elevated bilirubin	34	65*
Low serum albumin	40	73*
Prolonged PT	30	50*
AFP positive	87	46*
Median log AFP (ng/ml)	7000	7000

Figure 25.9 Clinical and laboratory features of a group of 50 patients who have noncirrhotic HCC compared with 100 patients with cirrhotic HCC. All figures quoted are percentages except where stated otherwise. AST: aspartate aminotransferase activity; PT, prothrombin time; SAP, serum alkaline phosphatase activity. The series was predominantly based on a series from a low-incidence Western area. *Indicates that the difference is statistically significant at $P>0.05$ level. (Adapted from Melia et al., 1984.)

where they are compared with those of HCC associated with cirrhosis. The distinction is important since, as the regenerative capacity of the normal liver is greater than that of the cirrhotic liver, the options for more aggressive surgical management are greater. However, these tumors have longer presymptomatic stages than HCC complicating cirrhosis, and consequently tend to present with greater tumor size and bulk.

Diagnosis

One of the symptom complexes described above will raise the suspicion of HCC. The initial investigations comprise three processes:
- imaging procedures (including plain chest radiograph);
- laboratory investigations (AFP estimation, routine liver function tests, and serology for chronic viral hepatitis); and
- the histologic confirmation of the diagnosis.

However, the natural desire to confirm the diagnosis histologically, particularly in view of the gravity of the prognosis, needs to be tempered with a consideration of benefit to risk ratio for the patient. For example, in a patient who has severely decompensated cirrhosis, and in whom liver transplantation is not an option, it is unlikely that establishing the diagnosis will have any impact on further management and will certainly risk hemorrhage, which may lead to further decompensation.

Imaging

The approach to documentation of the presence of a space occupying lesion within the liver will depend on local availability and expertise. Ultrasound examination, which is usually the initial procedure, shows the tumor as hypoechoic while small, becoming progressively hyperechoic with ill-defined margins as it enlarges. This investigative approach is particularly appropriate for regular screening of cirrhotic patients for the development of HCC, since lesions as small as 0.5cm can be detected. Ultrasound scanning can also assess the patency of the portal and hepatic veins, particularly when Doppler flow studies are undertaken (Fig. 25.10). It permits differentiation between solid and cystic space occupying lesions, and can allow accurate measurement of the main tumor size and daughter nodules, if present. Tumor and cirrhotic nodules can often be differentiated, but the entire examination is very operator-dependent. Computed tomography (CT) scanning is equally sensitive but, in addition, a detailed search for primary or secondary lesions outside the abdomen is possible,

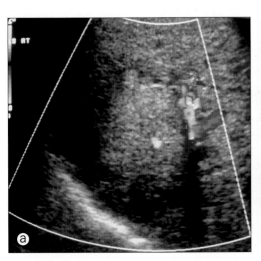
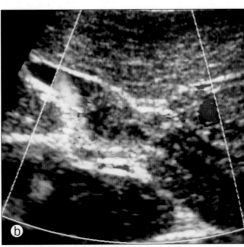

Figure 25.10 Color Doppler studies. (a) Large right HCC compressing the portal veins and (b) portal vein thrombosis secondary to HCC. (Courtesy of Dr Wei Tse Yang.)

although examination time and expense may limit applicability. Hepatocellular carcinoma is seen as a hypodense lesion that does not enhance after contrast administration. The plain chest radiograph should not be forgotten and occasionally lung metastases are seen at presentation; this clearly has implications for the extent to which further investigation would be appropriate. In addition, it may be possible to see a bulge on the left diaphragm, which is a finding that is very characteristic of HCC.

Frequently, the radiologist will report a suspicious lesion, and AFP levels are only minimally raised. Hepatic angiography with or without CT scanning after lipiodol injection into the hepatic artery may be helpful in such cases. Distinction between hemangiomas and HCC is a frequent problem, particularly when screening the asymptomatic patient, and dynamic CT scanning is the most widely used approach (Fig. 25.11). In cases of doubt, hepatic angiography is used to differentiate the blush that is characteristic of tumor neovascularization from the venous phase filling of an hemangiomatous lesion. Arteriography the most sensitive radiologic technique for the detection of HCC. It is useful for the detection of lesions below the diagnostic threshold of scanning in patients who have elevated APF levels and for the most accurate possible preoperative definition of tumor distribution.

Laboratory investigations

At the time of presentation, serum AFP levels are elevated above the reference range of 0–10 ng/mL in 50–80% of patients who have HCC (Fig. 25.12). The median value is in the order of 3000ng/mL in low incidence areas and 10,000ng/mL in high incidence areas, where levels may reach 10,000,000ng/mL (10g/L). The test is primarily of value in the diagnosis of HCC developing in patients who have cirrhosis where a level above 500 ng/mL is, in the presence of a liver mass, virtually diagnostic. Levels above 100 should raise the possibility of HCC, but levels as high as 1000ng/mL may occur in other nonmalignant liver diseases, particularly severe untreated chronic hepatitis and acute liver failure. However, trends are as important as absolute values and a steadily rising value over a 1–2 month period is very strongly suggestive of HCC. Levels of

APF correlate with changes in tumor bulk in individual patients, but isolated values are not reliable general indicators of the extent of the tumor. Recently, 'hepatoma-specific' isoforms of AFP have been described and may help distinguish AFP derived from HCC from that derived from benign liver disease.

α-Fetoprotein is less useful in distinguishing between primary and secondary tumors in the noncirrhotic liver. Only 50% of such cases of HCC arising in normal livers have elevated levels, and up to 10% of patients who have hepatic metastases will have elevated levels. Other primary tumors such as nonseminomatous germ cell tumors and hepatoblastomas also consistently express a high concentration of AFP, but there is seldom any clinical difficulty in differentiating such tumors from HCC. Other tumor markers are of value in the diagnosis of the fibrolamellar variant of HCC, and these include the vitamin B_{12}-binding protein and neurotensin.

The standard liver function tests are not of diagnostic significance for HCC, but form part of the initial assessment because, if grossly deranged, they may influence the degree to which the physician goes to establish the diagnosis. The significance of the viral serology depends on local conditions. In low incidence areas its detection would be counted in favor of the diagnosis of HCC, whereas in high incidence areas, such as sub-Saharan Africa and the Far East, where the great majority of patients are carriers, its absence would indicate that biopsy for histologic confirmation would be important.

Histologic confirmation of the diagnosis

Two distinct aims need to be distinguished. The first is to decide whether the lesion detected by an imaging procedure is malignant, and the second is to determine the histiogenesis of the lesion, or at least to distinguish between a primary and a secondary tumor. The first aim is usually relatively easy, although to distinguish between a very well-differentiated HCC and a benign adenoma may, on occasion, prove difficult. However, the pathologist will often have more difficulty in confidently distinguishing between primary and secondary tumors when the tumor is poorly

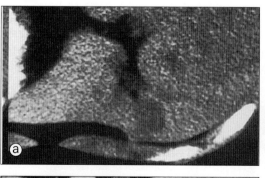
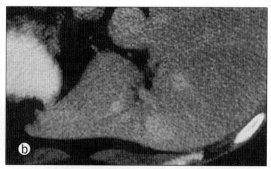
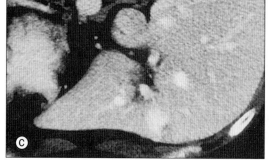
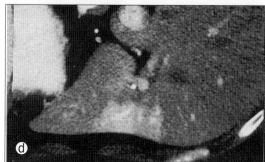

Figure 25.11 CT scans of hemangioma in the left lobe of the liver. The progressive filling in of the lesion on a dynamic contrast CT scan (a>b>c>d) is characteristic of a hemangioma rather than HCC. (Courtesy of Dr Wei Tse Yang.)

differentiated. This distinction may be important in clinical management when, for example, deciding whether to proceed to further investigation with a view to resection. Under these circumstances the serum AFP may be helpful, a grossly raised value supporting the diagnosis of HCC. An alternative strategy is to biopsy the nontumorous part of the liver. If this is cirrhotic, then a primary lesion becomes the more likely diagnosis.

The stage at which biopsy should be undertaken requires careful consideration because of the small risk of tumor dissemination along the needle track. Provided that normal criteria for safe liver biopsy are met, the conventional percutaneous approaches using Menghini, Trucut, or fine-needle (the latter depending on the availability of expert cytology) are appropriate. The frequency with which tumor tissue can be obtained can be increased by using ultrasound to guide the operator or by combining biopsy with laparoscopy. The former approach is now routine practice in most institutions. When there is reason to believe that the lesion

may be resectable, many surgeons prefer to avoid preoperative biopsy, and the possible risks of tumor dissemination, and await frozen section confirmation at the time of operation.

Following careful physical examination, and with the above investigations to hand, the physician is in a position to make an initial assessment. In many instances a confident diagnosis can be established at this stage, particularly in high incidence areas. In the presence of an hepatic mass that is radiologically consistent with HCC, a known history of chronic liver disease or a positive test for chronic HBV or HCV infection, and an AFP level of greater than 500ng/mL, the diagnosis of HCC is almost certain, even in the absence of histologic confirmation. Under other circumstances the diagnosis should be confirmed histologically either by percutaneous biopsy or at laparotomy.

Natural history and prognosis

In high incidence areas the median survival from the time of diagnosis is, in the absence of resection, measured in weeks. In low incidence areas the figure is in terms of 6–12 months. Those with large tumors, vascular invasion, poor liver function, or evidence of metastases do very poorly. On the other hand those with small tumors (<3cm), which develop in a patient with good liver function (Child's grade A cirrhosis), may survive up to 3 years without treatment (Fig. 25.13). The Okuda staging system is most widely used and it should be noted that the underlying liver function is the primary determinant of survival (Figs 25.13 & 25.14).

Physicians searching the literature for effective treatment of HCC should be aware that clinical trials are often undertaken on patients who have characteristics that suggest a better prognosis within this spectrum. The results are then compared (usually favorably) with figures for the overall group, leading to an overstatement of the therapeutic potential in an unselected population of patients who have HCC (Fig. 25.15).

Management

At the time of writing the only potentially curative treatment is surgical resection including transplantation. Unfortunately, however, most cases will fall within the category of being unresectable. The major reasons why patients cannot undergo

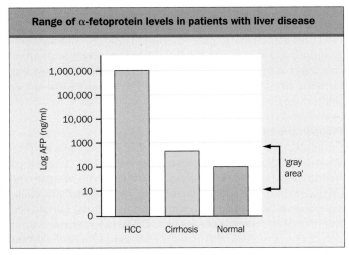

Figure 25.12 Range of α-fetoprotein (AFP) levels in patients with liver disease. Note the wide range of levels that can be seen in HCC patients, and the 'gray area' of overlap between patients who have chronic liver disease (but no HCC) and those who have HCC. AFP levels will be raised in 75% of HCC patients, but only about 5% of those who have chronic liver disease.

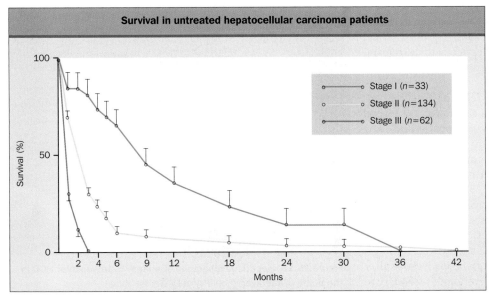

Figure 25.13 Survival in untreated patients who have HCC, in relation to disease stage. The stage classification is shown in Figure 25.14. (From Okuda et al. Cancer. 1985;56:918–28.)

Staging of hepatocellular carcinoma		
Clinical feature		Points
Tumour size (on anterior projection of liver scan)	>50%	1
	<50%	0
Ascites	Present	1
	Absent	0
Serum albumin (g/l)	<30	1
	>30	0
Serum bilirubin (μmol/l)	>35	1
	<35	0
Total score	Stage	Median survival (months)
0	1	28
1,2	2	8
3,4	3	1

Figure 25.14 Staging of HCC. (Adapted from Okuda, 1985.)

Some prognostic factors in hepatocellular carcinoma		
Poorer (less than 1 month)	Median (3–6 months)	Better (up to 3 years)
Larger tumor (>8cm)		Small tumors
Vascular invasion		No vascular invasion (macro- or microscopic)
Poor liver function bilirubin >2N PT> 2sec. prolonged albumin <25g/L		Normal liver function
Hepatic decomposition		No ascites or encephalopathy
Metastases extra-hepatic intra-hepatic		No metastases

Figure 25.15 Some prognostic factors in HCC.

conventional resectional surgery with a view to cure are the extent of the tumor, the implications of the associated cirrhosis, extrahepatic metastases, or unrelated co-morbidity. The presence of cirrhosis does not preclude resection, but the results are best in patients who have Child's A disease. Liver transplantation is feasible in patients who have small tumors, irrespective of the Child's category. Extensive, bilobar disease and/or invasion of the major vessels including the inferior vena cava, main portal vein, and common hepatic artery commonly preclude surgical resection.

Surgical approaches

Liver resection is a major operation that carries an operative mortality of about 5% in noncirrhotic, and 10–15% in cirrhotic patients. No single liver function test can predict the survival of an individual patient undergoing liver resection, but once the liver disease decompensates patients almost always develop liver failure after resection. Child's grade C cirrhosis is therefore usually considered to be a contraindication to surgery, but liver failure can still occur after resection in those who have Child's grades A or B. It has been proposed that the presence of portal hypertension, as judged by a hepatic venous pressure gradient of >10mmHg, is the best single test predicting postoperative liver failure. The amount of intraoperative blood loss, the duration and degree of hypotension, and the extent of ischemia to the remaining liver remnant due to hilar clamping or injury to its blood supply all also influence survival.

Although cirrhosis is no longer considered an absolute contraindication, the operative mortality is significant for several reasons. Many cirrhotic patients have a coagulopathy and a low platelet count because of hypersplenism. Portal hypertension increases the risks of bleeding because of the opening up of portosystemic collaterals in the retroperitoneum. The cirrhotic liver is firm, difficult to manipulate, and does not readily take suture material. Most of these problems are now surmountable with technical advances, but surgical successes are often negated by postoperative complications. Estimates of the functional capacity of the residual tissue are difficult to determine preoperatively and this may prove to be inadequate after surgery. Initial adequate function may deteriorate secondary to

infection and cirrhotic patients are intrinsically immunocompromised and at high risk of sepsis. A patient who has a normal liver can tolerate resection of about 75% of the liver, but in a cirrhotic liver a right lobectomy (55% resection) is the upper limit of surgical resectability.

Preoperative investigations

Computed tomography and selective hepatic angiography (Fig. 25.16) are the usual preoperative investigations. Computed tomography shows the site and extent of the disease, but may miss up to one third of nodules detected at surgery. Angiography delineates the vascular anatomy, confirms patency of the portal vein, and may detect tumor not seen on CT. The most reliable way of detecting macroscopic abdominal spread and assessing the extent of liver involvement is during laparotomy. Intraoperative ultrasound locates otherwise undetected small primary and secondary lesions and tumor thrombus in portal and hepatic veins. It also helps to determine the resection margins and the plane of liver transection in relation to the hepatic vasculature, thereby helping to preserve as much functioning liver tissue as possible.

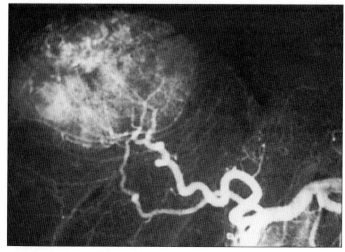

Figure 25.16 Hepatic angiography of a large hypervascular HCC in the dome of the liver. (Courtesy of Dr Wei Tse Yang.)

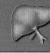

Resection

The liver can be divided into eight segments, each receiving its hepatic arterial, portal venous, and biliary duct branches (Fig. 25.17). The hepatic venous branches are distributed between, rather than within, the individual segments. Accurate delineation of the segments to be excised has been facilitated by intraoperative ultrasound, and by the injection of dyes into the portal or arterial blood supply. The five commonly used lobar and/or segmental resections are shown in Fig. 25.18. In a right trisegmentectomy, the right lobe of the liver and medial segment of the left lobe are removed. In a left trisegmentectomy,

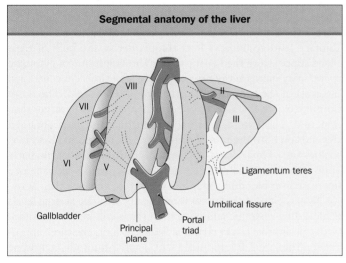

Figure 25.17 The segmental anatomy of the liver which forms the basis for the standard surgical resections.

the left lobe of the liver and the anterior segment of the right lobe are removed. An extended right hepatectomy usually refers to a right trisegmentectomy, but may also refer to a slight modification of right lobectomy in which the hepatic parenchyma is transected well to the right of the falciform ligament rather than at this ligament, thus sparing most of the medial segment. An extended left lobectomy should not be confused with the left trisegmentectomy, since it does not result in removal of the full anterior segment of the right lobe. Nonanatomic resection refers to resection of the liver along nonanatomic planes. In general, this results in more bleeding and can leave behind parts of the liver remnants deprived of their blood supply and subject to necrosis.

About 10–15% of patients who have HCC will come to operation and the 5-year survival rate is about one third to one half. Postoperative disease recurrence, usually intrahepatic, is the main cause of death. Pre- and postoperative adjuvant treatment are often given but are not, as yet, of proven benefit.

Orthotopic liver transplantation

Orthotopic liver transplantation potentially overcomes the problems of tumor distribution and/or hepatic insufficiency that limits the application of conventional resection. Many of the first patients to achieve long-term survival after transplantation had malignant liver disease. They tolerated the operation well and recovered rapidly but, despite careful preoperative assessment that attempted to exclude those who had extrahepatic spread, tumor recurrence was common. Presumably this stemmed from undetectable micrometastases, and was perhaps promoted by the requisite immunosuppression. This led many groups to abandon transplantation for malignant disease other

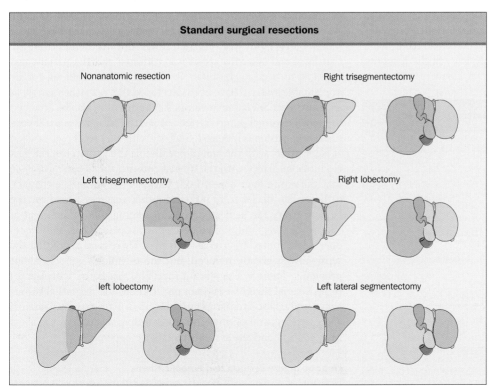

Figure 25.18 Standard surgical resections.

than when the tumor was found incidentally in a patient undergoing transplantation for advanced cirrhosis. Indeed, evidence is now emerging that tumor size, number and/or the degree of vascular invasion are the major factors influencing recurrence rates. Small tumors of up to 4cm in diameter and not numbering more than two may have a prognosis similar to those cirrhotic patients without HCC who undergo liver transplantation. Transplantation recurrence is the rule with tumors greater than 8cm diameter or in those that are multifocal (Fig. 25.19). The results in the intermediate group are currently considered to be too low to warrant transplantation, but this may improve with preoperative therapy, for example chemoembolization.

The question whether, in a particular patient, resection or transplantation is to be preferred is controversial. When the patient has decompensated liver disease the answer is clearly transplantation, but in other circumstances, and while the results with liver transplantation are still improving, referral for an opinion to a center where both options can be considered should be undertaken. In addition to the surgical considerations, the potential for further *de novo* malignant change in the cirrhotic tissue left *in situ* can influence the decision.

Management of the patient who has inoperable disease

The physician must clearly define the aims and limitations of any proposed treatment. These aims should be set out before the patient in a manner that, while realistic, avoids destroying all hope. There are now so many options for the management of patients who have inoperable disease that it is easy to lose sight of certain basic principles. For the vast majority of cases the aim is good palliation; no treatment has yet been convincingly and consistently proven to increase survival.

Systemic therapy

Effective systemic therapy, with a role similar to that used so effectively in childhood liver cancer (hepatoblastoma), remains elusive. Doxorubicin the most active single cytotoxic agent, has a response rate of only 15–20%, and in only 5% will the response be complete. The responses are usually brief and do not significantly improve overall survival. Combination therapy has not been shown to be superior to single agent treatment, although recently combinations of conventional cytotoxic drugs and α-interferon have been reported to produce some dramatic remissions including complete pathological responses.

There have been some controlled studies reporting that tamoxifen, an antiestrogenic agent, may improve survival. Although the most recent, and best designed study, could not confirm the earlier optimistic reports, several physicians have started to use tamoxifen as a safe and nontoxic treatment of last resort, and one that has some, albeit limited, documented evidence of efficacy from randomized clinical trials.

Intra-arterial treatment and locoregional therapy

Primary (and secondary) liver tumors derive the bulk of their blood supply from the hepatic artery. Direct infusion of cytotoxic agents may increase the drug exposure (the time/concentration interval) of the tumor to the drug by up to 400-fold. The dose-limiting toxicity then becomes regional (i.e. hepatic), rather than systemic. The extent to which regional advantage is obtained depends on both the rate of drug elimination and the blood perfusion rate. Thus, drugs with a short half-life are particularly appropriate for this route of administration and measures to decrease liver bloodflow may be expected to enhance their activity. Nonetheless, if the tumor is maximally sensitive at drug levels achieved by systemic administration there will be no advantage with this approach. On pharmacologic grounds, the most appropriate drugs are 5-fluorouracil (5-FU) and 5-fluorodeoxyuridine (FUDR), both of which have half-lives of only a few minutes. Unfortunately, 5-FU, at least as a single agent, falls into the category of ineffective therapy for patients who have HCC.

Successful arterial infusion therapy also depends on adequate perfusion of the entire liver and a safe delivery system. In early studies, a catheter was inserted percutaneously via the brachial or femoral artery, but this approach suffered from the disadvantage that local and systemic sepsis was common and the patient was confined to bed and hospital. To overcome this problem, totally implantable systems have been developed that act either simply as an access port or contain a pump. The former can also be attached to a small external pump carried around the patient's waist if continuous perfusion is required. Such systems are usually introduced at laparotomy with the aim of positioning the catheter in the gastroduodenal artery with the tip just entering the hepatic artery so that the entire liver is perfused. This has the advantage that the catheter can be securely tethered; other vessels coming off the hepatic artery can be ligated; the surgeon can assess the extent of disease directly; and, unlike percutaneous placement, the procedure is less limited by arterial anomalies. There is no doubt that the sepsis rate is greatly reduced, but the technique is not without problems. There is a significant mortality associated with laparotomy, arterial thrombosis is not uncommon, and migration to various extrahepatic sites has occurred in up to 10% of cases. Gastritis and gastric ulceration may still occur despite ligation of the short gastric artery and the systems tend to be expensive.

Hepatic artery ligation and embolization

Ligation of one or both hepatic arteries at laparotomy, as a treatment for liver tumors, has been practised for many years. Nowadays injecting emboli under fluoroscopic control, at the

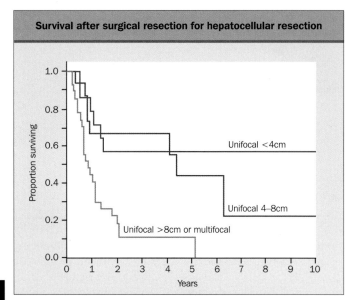

Survival after surgical resection for hepatocellular resection

Unifocal <4cm

Unifocal 4–8cm

Unifocal >8cm or multifocal

Proportion surviving / Years

Figure 25.19 Survival of patients who have HCC after surgical resection in relation to tumor size and number. (McPeake et al. 1995.)

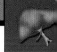

time of diagnostic hepatic arteriography, is more widely used. It is preferable to surgical ligation because anesthesia and laparotomy are avoided, and subsequent growth of collateral circulation is delayed, as occlusion is induced at the periphery. The procedure can be repeated on several occasions. The main indication is pain relief, which is effected in about 65% of cases and, although more than half the patients show evidence of tumor regression, there is little evidence that survival is prolonged. Particular caution is required in older patients and those in whom there is evidence of hepatic decompensation.

Use of lipiodol to target intra-arterial chemotherapy

When lipiodol, an oily based contrast medium, is injected into the hepatic artery, sequential CT scanning shows that it is cleared from normal hepatic tissues but accumulates in malignant tumors. This is probably because of the increased permeability of the neovascular tissue, coupled with the lack of lymphatic clearance from tumor tissue. These observations made lipiodol an ideal vehicle for chemotherapy delivery. Most commonly doxorubicin is thoroughly mixed with 15ml of lipiodol and injected into the tumor-feeding arteries. This is followed by embolization with 0.5–1mm of gelatin cubes [so called 'transcatheter oily chemoembolization' (TOCE)]. It is important to confirm, before the procedure, that the portal vein is patent and, after the procedure, that the appropriate arteries have been embolized.

Effective embolization is usually associated with fever, pain, and vomiting for up to 3–5 days, after which these symptoms settle. Liver failure may be precipitated by TOCE. Antibiotic prophylaxis is required, starting on the day before the procedure, together with adequate analgesia and control of nausea. Other side effects are uncommon, but include accidental embolization of other organs including the gallbladder and spleen. Portal vein thrombosis is usually a contraindication to TOCE since the cirrhotic liver is crucially dependent on the hepatic artery in this situation and any further interruption thereof may precipitate liver failure. The presence of Child's grade C cirrhosis is also a relative contraindication.

Until recently TOCE was widely regarded as standard treatment for inoperable HCC. However, two recent controlled trials that have shown no survival benefit and a high incidence of complications have tempered the initial optimism. While there is little doubt that the procedure causes tumor volume reduction, even uncontrolled studies have suggested that long-term survival for which other factors such as tumor type, degree of spread and the serum AFP level value were more significant than the treatment. Indeed it is not inconceivable that most of the effect seen is due to the embolization – there being no proof that the lipiodol targeting adds significant benefit.

Percutaneous ethanol injection

The injection of alcohol, directly into liver tumors, leads to extensive coagulative necrosis. Under real-time ultrasonic or CT guidance about 5ml of sterile 95% ethanol is injected through a 20cm long, 21 or 22 gauge needle. The procedure is repeated depending on the size of the tumor and extent of necrosis obtained. The advantage of this approach is its simplicity, lack of side effects, and cheapness. On the other hand, while small tumors (<2cm) only require 3–4 sessions, larger tumors require up to 20. Many workers have found it difficult to gain a homogenous distribution of alcohol throughout the lesion. The patient often

complains of mild pain, and some fever. If the alcohol escapes into the peritoneal cavity, severe pain ensues. This can be avoided by very slow infiltration of the alcohol.

Survival at 1, 3, and 5 years has been reported to be 96, 72, and 51% for Child's A cirrhosis; 90, 72, and 48% for Child's B cirrhosis; and 94, 25, and 0% for Child's C cirrhosis. It has also been reported that results, at least over the first 3 years after treatment, are not dissimilar to those obtained by surgical resection. Other injection agents, such as hot water and saline, are currently being assessed.

Radiotherapy

The application of external beam irradiation for the treatment of liver tumors has been limited by the radiosensitivity of normal hepatocytes. Maximum tolerance of normal liver to radiation is between 2500 and 3000cGy. Above this the risk of radiation hepatitis (veno-occlusive disease with perivenular congestion and fibrosis) increases rapidly. External irradiation to treat HCC has therefore received little attention, although recently encouraging results have been obtained using conformal radiotherapy and intrahepatic arterial 5-FUDR as a radiosensitizer.

Internal irradiation with intra-arterial radioisotopes

Lipiodol-[131]iodine emits mainly γ-radiation with an energy of 364KeV and has a physical half-life of 8.04 days. This treatment is at least as effective (in small tumors) as TOCE and has far fewer side effects. The prescribed dose of lipiodol-^{131}I ranges from 555 to 2220MBq. [90]Yttrium, a pure β emitter, is more powerful than [131]I. It has a physical half-life of 64 hours and a mean energy of 936KeV. The yttrium can be tagged to resin microspheres and introduced into the hepatic artery. With such an approach a therapeutic dose of radiation can be delivered without causing radiation hepatitis. Optimal tumor regression and a reduction in the serum AFP level are seen when the average radiation dose to the tumor is above 12,000cGy.

Leakage of microspheres into the right gastric artery or gastroduodenal artery may occasionally cause radiation gastritis or duodenitis. Systemic leakage of the microspheres to involve the lungs, which are sensitive to radiation, may occur if there is extensive arteriovenous shunting within the tumor. For this reason, the degree of lung shunting must be determined before administration of the radioisotope. Technetium-99m macroaggregated albumin (^{99m}Tc-MAA) with γ camera scanning is used to predict the percentage of lung shunting and the relative tumor to nontumor uptake ratio (T/N ratio). Those who have high lung shunting (>15%) and poor T/N ratio are not suitable for [90]yttrium microsphere treatment (Fig. 25.20).

Guidelines for the approach to the patient who has 'inoperable' disease

Several other locoregional approaches, including cryotherapy, focused ultrasound, and microwaves, have been described. All are effective in reducing tumor bulk, but there is no conclusive evidence of improved survival. Faced with a multiplicity of options, none of which have conclusively been shown to alter the natural history, the practitioner is left with difficult decisions in many cases. In the face of liver failure, with overt jaundice, ascites or encephalopathy, it is reasonable to offer no active treatment. When there is extrahepatic spread, local therapy is also not worthwhile. It may be reasonable to give a couple of courses of systemic

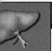

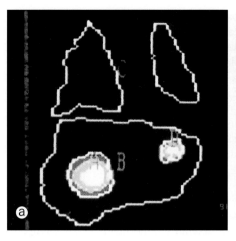
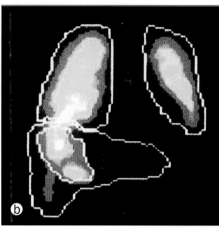

Figure 25.20 Gamma scan of the liver after injection of technetium-labeled macroaggregated albumin. This serves as a simulation to examine the distribution of yttrium-labeled microspheres that will occur when these are given as treatment for HCC. In (a) the activity is concentrated in the two liver tumors, indicating a high tumor to normal ratio and no shunting to the lungs. In (b) there is massive lung shunting. If this latter patient were given yttrium treatment, radiation pneumonitis would be very likely to occur. (Courtesy of Dr Stephen Ho.)

treatment with either adriamycin (doxorubicin) or the more recently described regimen of interferon and cytotoxic drugs to patients who have very extensive intrahepatic disease. It is important not to continue treatment if there is no response after two courses or if the side effects outweigh any potential benefit. Those patients who have a solitary tumor, or a small number of well-defined nodules, should be considered for one of the locoregional treatments described above. In the absence of proven benefit the one that offers least in the way of side effects and compilation should be chosen. Ethanol injection where feasible is simple, cheap, and with minimal morbidity; where facilities are available yttrium is highly effective and almost devoid of side effects.

Recurrent disease after surgical resection or transplantation

Tumor will recur after apparently curative resection in more than 50% of patients. A few of these 'recurrences' may represent new primary tumors, but in the majority of cases they reflect growth of tumor that was presumably present, but microscopic at the time of surgery. Of recurrences, 90% will be clinically apparent within 3 years of the operation. Certain characteristics of the original tumor predict an increased likelihood of recurrence and these include tumor size greater than 5cm in diameter, histologic evidence of vascular invasion, and lack of encapsulation. The AFP status of the original tumor and the recurrence do not change, so that if the original tumor secreted AFP then the recurrence will, and vice versa. It should be noted that normalization of AFP after resection does not necessarily imply complete tumor removal, and should not decrease the physician's index of suspicion for recurrence. The site of relapse is usually intrahepatic after conventional surgical resection and will be readily screened for, and detected by, ultrasound examination. After transplantation the sites of recurrence are more widespread and the commonest sites are the liver graft, adrenal bed, lungs, and bones. Computed tomography scanning of areas suggested on the basis of clinical examination and symptoms will need to be undertaken. In those who had raised AFP levels preoperatively, a rising AFP in the postoperative period invariably means impending clinical recurrence, which it may precede by several months. Tumor growth is considerably accelerated after liver transplantation because of immunosuppression, and as a consequence the response to chemotherapy is poor and most patients die within 6 months of detection of recurrent disease.

Currently there is no proven effective adjuvant therapy, but postoperative intra-arterial lipiodol-I[131] has, in a small prospective randomized controlled trial, been shown to decrease the rate of tumor recurrence. The acyclic retinoid polyprenoic acid, which inhibits hepatocarcinogenesis, and induces apoptosis and differentiation in human-derived cell lines, has been shown, in a recent controlled trial, to prevent the development of second primary tumors after resection. These therapeutic approaches need to be validated in extended studies.

Screening programs for hepatocellular carcinoma

Whole population screening is not an option, but there are well defined high risk groups – patients who have chronic liver disease and those who carry the HBV or HCV – who may benefit from HCC surveillance programs. The lifetime risk of HCC development for a male who has cirrhosis in any of these groups is in the range 10–40%. In such an individual, who has access to the necessary resources, it seems likely that a 3–6 monthly AFP estimation and ultrasound examination will detect tumor development before it becomes clinically apparent. If liver transplantation is available a case can be made for screening all those at risk, as this is the only effective way of diagnosing the disease while it is still curable with transplantation. Surveillance programs are commonly promoted in the West, but it should be stressed that, at the time of writing, this practice is not supported by evidence showing that it is either cost effective or leads to improved survival. It should also be remembered that the patient undergoing resection or transplantation faces a 5–15% perioperative mortality, whereas without operation the survival with an asymptotically detected tumor may be up to 3 years. In the absence of an available transplant program, it is reasonable not to screen patients who have Child's grade C cirrhosis.

OTHER PRIMARY LIVER TUMORS

The ratio of HCC : cholangiocarcinoma : other primary malignant liver tumors is in the order of 100:10:1 (cholangiocarcinomas are dealt with in Chapter 26). It follows that in most units physicians and pathologists will have only a very limited experience of 'other' primary liver tumors. It is, however, important that such diagnoses are established accurately since some of the tumors described below have a significantly better prognosis than HCC and are more often cured by surgery. Histologic review by a pathologist who has a special interest in liver tumors is always rec-

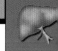
ommended if there is any doubt whatsoever about the diagnosis. Fibrolamellar carcinoma is considered a 'variant' of HCC and has been described above.

Sarcomas – angiosarcomas and malignant hemangioendotheliomas

Angiosarcomas

Angiosarcomas present in a manner similar to those of other malignant tumors of the liver, usually with hepatomegaly, pain, and weight loss, or hemoperitoneum. In about 25% of cases a history of occupational exposure to vinyl chloride (VC), thorotrast, or arsenic can be obtained. Precursor features are well-recognized and include periportal and subcapsular fibrosis and evidence of activation of hepatocytes in the sinusoid lining cells. The inhalation of the VC monomer appears to be responsible for the liver damage. Exposure to VC is now strictly controlled during the production of polyvinyl chloride so that cases are likely to decrease significantly. A similar situation exists with thorotrast, a radiologic contrast medium containing a colloidal suspension of thorium dioxide (a powerful emitter of α particles), which was first used in the 1920s but has been withdrawn since 1950. The minimum period between exposure and tumor development is 15 years, but cases are still being encountered more than 40 years after the agent was withdrawn from use. The radioactive emission of the thorotrast can be readily detected by autoradiography and the particles of thorotrast can be seen by electron microscopy.

Epithelioid hemangioendotheliomas

Epithelioid hemangioendotheliomas represent the malignant end of a spectrum starting with the typical hemangioma. There are no specific presenting features and are most often seen in young and middle-aged females. The tumors are usually multiple at presentation and metastases are detectable in about half of all cases. Although the tumor may appear epithelioid on routine histologic examination, its endothelial origins can be confirmed by staining for factor-VIII-related antigen, and the malignant cells have characteristic ultrastructural features. The prognosis is very variable. Most patients will die from the tumor, but prolonged survival periods of up to 10 years, even without treatment, have been reported. The standard surgical approaches of resection where this is possible, or liver transplantation, are still recommended.

Biliary cystadenocarcinoma

This is a rare cystic tumor that represents the malignant end of the adenoma–carcinoma spectrum and is analogous to similar tumors found in the pancreas. They are usually multilocular and intrahepatic with only a small minority presenting in the biliary tract. Symptoms are nonspecific, and although imaging with CT may suggest the diagnosis, differentiation between the malignant and benign counterparts can only be made confidently after complete resection. Complete resection should be undertaken wherever possible, after which the prognosis is good with a very high chance of cure.

Primary hepatic lymphomas

Such tumors are even rarer than those mentioned above. Their diagnosis remains controversial since it is often difficult to establish that they are truly primary. Occasionally cases can be cured by resection or palliated with chemotherapy, but the prognosis is very poor in the majority of cases.

Malignant liver tumors in childhood – hepatoblastoma

Malignant liver tumors are rare in children, but when present are usually hepatoblastomas. Of hepatoblastomas, 90% occur within the first 5 years of life and they outnumber HCC in this age group by a ratio of 2:1. The usual presentation is with an enlarging upper abdominal mass together with pain, weight loss, and anorexia. Association with congenital abnormalities is well-described as are cases of precocious puberty related to β-human chorionic gonadotropin (HCG) production by the tumor cells. Serum AFP is consistently elevated, often to very high levels. It accurately reflects tumor mass and is useful in monitoring treatment. On imaging the tumor is hypervascular, usually solitary, and often exhibits calcification.

Primary liver tumors in childhood are uniformly fatal without resection. As with adult HCC, the main hope of cure is complete surgical resection. About 50% will be suitable for resection and half of these will survive long term. However, the tumor is highly sensitive to chemotherapy (usually adriamycin and *cis*-platinum) and postoperative adjuvant therapy, even in the presence of incomplete resection, has been found to improve survival rates. Currently, in several centers, preoperative chemotherapy is given to all patients irrespective of the perceived degree of operability. Long-term survival rates in the order of 80% are being achieved. All children who have hepatoblastoma should be managed in centers conversant with a multimodality approach to treatment.

SECONDARY LIVER TUMORS

Introduction

Until recently the approach to the patient who have hepatic metastases has been largely nihilistic. The detection of metastases immediately heralded withdrawal of all active therapy. However, it is now recognized that, with careful selection, a small percentage of patients may be cured by surgery, a significant proportion may have their survival prolonged, and others can be offered a significant improvement in quality of life by cytotoxic chemotherapy. Equally, however, administration of cytotoxic therapy to patients who have poor performance status and widely disseminated disease may dramatically decrease the quality of life for their few remaining months. A carefully balanced approach is therefore needed. Hepatic metastases are often only one site of metastatic disease and the overall management of such cases is the purview of the oncologist. The following section is confined mainly to those cases in which the liver is the sole or predominant site of disease.

Epidemiology and pathogenesis

Liver metastases are found at 1% of all autopsies. After lymph nodes, the liver is the most common site of metastatic disease, being involved in 40% of adult patients who have primary extrahepatic malignancy who come to autopsy. The tumors may be solitary or multiple, but unlike HCC they tend to be umbilicated and infiltrate the normal liver tissue (Fig. 25.21). Up to 75% of primary tumors drained by the portal venous system (pancreas, large bowel, and stomach) will have metastatic involvement. About 10% of these will have solitary liver metastases; this figure is much lower for other tumors such as those of breast and lung.

Clinical features and disease associations

Patients who have hepatic metastases present with pain, weight loss, anorexia, and hard hepatomegaly in which discrete masses

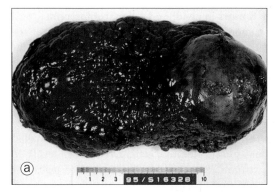
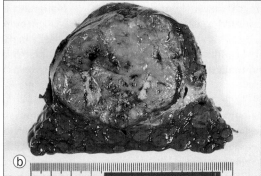
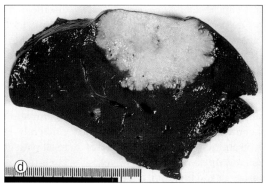
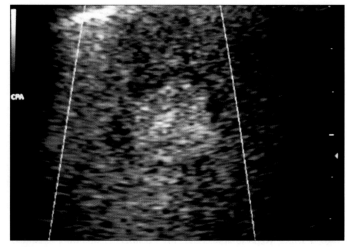

Figure 25.21 A comparison of the macroscopic appearances of primary and secondary liver tumors. Note that the primary tumor (HCC) arises as a well-circumscribed, solitary nodule in an extensively macrocirrhotic liver and bulges from the surface of the liver (a & b). In marked contrast the secondary tumor arises in a noncirrhotic liver, is infiltrating in nature, and umbilicated (c & d). (Courtesy of Dr CT Liew.)

can often be palpated. The abdomen may be distended with ascites and there may be other, extrahepatic, signs of malignancy. These are all clear signs of advanced disease. Patients who have hepatic metastases who may be candidates for surgical resection often have their tumors detected before symptoms develop. As a very broad generalization, it is not cost-effective to screen all patients who have primary tumors for liver deposits. Rather, it is better to confine investigation to those who have clinical signs or symptoms, or biochemical evidence of liver dysfunction. Certain metastatic tumors, particularly carcinoid and other 'apudomas' including islet cell carcinomas, appear to involve the liver with relatively little disruption of hepatic function.

Diagnosis

Routine liver function tests are not very helpful in diagnosing liver metastases, although metastases are unlikely if all routine liver function tests are entirely within their reference ranges. As noted above any abnormality, particularly a raised activity of hepatic alkaline phosphatase, is an indication for further imaging of the liver.

Imaging

In terms of sensitivity, there is little to choose between conventional ultrasound (US) scanning and contrast-enhanced CT, if the aim is to detect the presence or absence of metastases. With both techniques the sensitivity is in the order of 85%. For 'lesion by lesion' detection CT is rather more accurate. The sensitivity may be increased to 95% by employing CT with arterial portography, which is usually used when surgical resection is contemplated and the number and exact location of each lesion are required to be known. Both techniques can miss lesions on the surface of the liver. With intraoperative US scanning the sensitivity reaches 100% (by definition, as this is the gold standard by which other techniques are judged). It should be stressed that the figures quoted above refer to the detection of metastases when the reporting radiologist has been specifically requested to examine the liver with a view to

detecting tumors. Similar figures will not be obtained with routine scanning when the operator is not focused on the search for tumors.

On CT scans metastases show lower attenuation than the surrounding liver, both before, and after, contrast. Both CT and ultrasound will often show peripheral ring enhancement (Fig. 25.22). In contrast to primary liver tumors, metastases tend to be umbilicated and do not expand and distort the liver surface to the same extent (see Fig. 25.21). About 20% of patients who have hepatic metastases from colorectal cancer will show calcification on CT or US. Interestingly these patients seem to have a significantly better prognosis. All too frequently patients present with malignant liver disease (usually adenocarcinoma on biopsy), but no obvious primary extrahepatic site can be detected after full physical examination. Extensive radiologic investigations such as barium meal, barium enema, and intravenous pyelography are not indicated as

Figure 25.22 Characteristic liver secondary seen on ultrasound examination as a 'target' lesion with a hypoechoic rim and a hyperechoic center. (Courtesy of Dr Wei Tse Yang.)

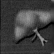

the occult tumor is seldom situated in the gut or kidney and both false-positive and false-negative results are frequent. Computed tomography scanning is also the most rewarding investigation, but in a proportion of these patients the primary is never identified.

Serologic tests
Estimation of the serum concentration of carcinoembryonic antigen (CEA) is the only tumor marker widely applied. It is used mainly to detect recurrence after resection of the primary colorectal tumor. A rising level in this situation usually heralds metastases, most often in the liver. It is not clear whether this early diagnosis of recurrence leads to improved survival.

Histology
In the presence of widespread metastatic disease, particularly when active treatment is not contemplated, histologic confirmation of suspected hepatic metastases is not indicated. However, when the lesion is solitary, biopsy is indicated unless resection is to be undertaken. The presence of metastases obviously has major implications for the patient, but this diagnosis should not be presumed if a solitary lesion is detected as this may be an unrelated benign lesion. When the primary tumor from which an hepatic metastasis has originated is not apparent, histologic examination may provide a clue to the site of the primary (Fig. 25.23).

Adenocarcinomas are usually of colorectal or pancreatic origin, but intrahepatic cholangiocarcinomas also have a similar appearance. Anaplastic tumors are usually of bronchial origin. Recently developed histologic methods involving special stains, immunocytochemistry, and electron microscopy often permit distinction of the origin of these highly anaplastic tumors. This means that the surgeon must collaborate very closely with the pathologist so that biopsy specimens can be placed in the appropriate medium. Detection of a lymphoma on the basis of positive B-cell or T-cell surface markers may lead to specific therapy.

Natural history and prognosis
There is a linear relation between percentage survival and log survival time (from diagnosis) with secondary liver tumors (Fig. 25.24). About 50% of patients are alive at 3 months and less than 10% at 1 year, although individual cases may show wide variations. Patients who have multiple metastases have a significantly worse prognosis than those who have solitary metastases, as do those who have any evidence of other, extrahepatic, metastases. Among those who have solitary lesions receiving no active treatment, a 20% 3-year survival rate has been quoted. This observation should not be forgotten when assessing the efficacy of surgical resection of solitary metastases in uncontrolled studies. Metastases from primary carcinoid tumors are the only secondary tumors to exhibit a significantly better prognosis, survival periods of up to 10 years not being uncommon. With the wide use of more sophisticated radiologic techniques the diagnosis is being established earlier, often while the patient is asymptomatic, and this makes for an apparent increase in survival.

Management
As with primary tumors, the aim of investigation is to identify that small subgroup that might benefit from surgical resection.

Surgical resection
Currently surgical resection offers the only hope of cure, but it is only in cases of metastatic colorectal cancer that sufficient numbers of cases have been accrued to draw any general conclusions. Overall, between 2.5 and 5% of all patients who have hepatic metastases will be candidates for surgical resection with curative intent. A review of the literature shows that survival at 1, 3, 5, and 10 years is of the order of 85, 50, 35, and 20% respectively. Although the complication rate can be high, the perioperative mortality should now be below 5%.

The precise indications vary from unit to unit. Some consider that any case in which all obvious tumors can be removed should be candidates. Others confine surgical resection to those who have solitary lesions, or at most, three small lesions confined to one lobe. Such decisions remain a matter of philosophy and resource. Resection is less likely to be successful as the tumor size and the number of nodules decreases, and as the time between resection of the primary and detection of the recurrence increases. An

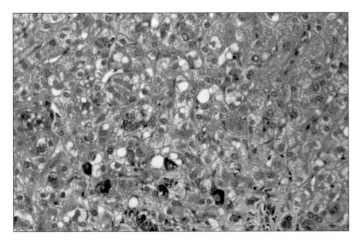

Figure 25.23 Hepatic metastasis for a primary melanoma. The site of a secondary tumor can seldom be confidently made on routine histologic examination. Here the presence of melanin confirms metastasis from a primary melanoma. (Courtesy of Dr Bernard Portmann.)

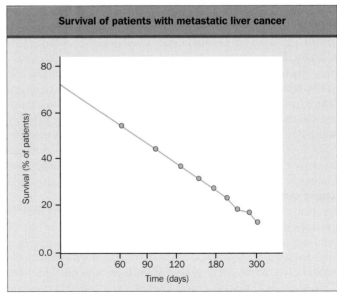

Figure 25.24 Overall survival of patients with metastatic liver cancer. Note that the time axis is logarithmic. (Data from Jaffe, Surg Gynaecol Obstet 1969 127:1–11).

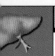

involved margin after resection is always a harbinger of subsequent recurrences.

Management of inoperable hepatic metastases

5-Fluorouracil remains the commonest treatment for metastatic HCC. Using the standard regimens 10–15% of patients will obtain objective responses. These responses are short-lived (<6 months) and only very occasionally complete. There is no overall improvement in survival. The response rate can be improved by increasing the dose intensity or by administering the drug as a prolonged infusion. Nonetheless, there is little effect on overall survival, and any small improvement in response rate is counterbalanced by increased cost, toxicity, and patient inconvenience.

The combination of 5-FU and folinic acid is superior to 5-FU alone. There is an increased response rate, some of the remissions are prolonged and complete, and there is a trend towards an increase in survival. It may also be effective in patients who have previously failed on other regimens. Complications include stomatitis, bone marrow depression, and diarrhea, particularly when 'high dose' leukovorin is used. The most appropriate regimen at the time of writing is probably the so-called low-dose regimen. Leukovorin is given at a dose of 20mg/m², immediately followed by 5-FU at a dose of 370mg/m². Both drugs are given by rapid intravenous injection for 5 consecutive days with courses repeated every 4 weeks. Although it seems likely that the combination of 5-FU and leukovorin is a significant advance and offers the prospect of palliation and the possibility of improved survival at an acceptable cost in terms of complications, it must be recognized that the benefits remain modest, and not all investigators concur with these sentiments.

Intra-arterial infusion chemotherapy for metastatic liver cancer

There is a high response rate when FUDR is infused chronically into the hepatic artery. The time to tumor progression in the liver is significantly prolonged, but there is no improvement in overall survival. The toxicity is quite distinct from that seen with systemic administration of 5-FU. Nausea, vomiting, diarrhea, and myelosuppression are all uncommon. The toxicity relates to ulcer disease and hepatic toxicity. The former is presumed to be due to gastric and duodenal perfusion from small branches of the hepatic artery. The most common lesion is a sclerosing cholangitis, probably due to primary damage of the blood vessels feeding the bile ducts, which also derive their blood supply from the hepatic artery. The overall cost, inconvenience, and side effects of chronic intra-arterial chemotherapy still limit this approach. However, in highly motivated patients, with good performance status and modest disease burden, controlled studies have shown that significant improvement in quality of life can be obtained (Fig. 25.25).

Use of chemotherapy in an adjuvant setting

Because of the high recurrence rate, particularly to the liver in patients who have Dukes' grade C colorectal cancer, the role of adjuvant chemotherapy has been extensively investigated. In a trial involving 1296 patients, 1 year of treatment with the combination of systemic 5-FU plus levamisole in patients who have Dukes' grade C disease gave a marked reduction in recurrence and death rates. The disease-free survival in those receiving adjuvant therapy at 3 years was 66% compared with 47% in the control group – a very highly significant difference. It should be noted that the role of levamisole is unknown, there being little evidence

that it is of any value alone either as active treatment or as adjuvant, and a combination of 5-FU and folinic acid is becoming more widely used. A recent US National Institutes of Health consensus conference has recommended that chemotherapy should be given to all patients with Dukes' grade C colorectal cancer. It should be noted, however, that meta-analyses show only more modest benefit, with improvement in 5-year survival being no more than 5%.

Hepatic metastases from other primary sites

Early trials employing the 'FAM' regimen (5-FU, adriamycin, and mitomycin C) in metastatic disease originating from stomach, pancreas or bile duct were encouraging, but more recent reports fail to confirm any increased activity over the single agents. Metastases from breast cancer are more sensitive to chemotherapy with response rates of over 50%, particularly with doxorubicin or taxol-based regimens. Other tumors, such as small cell carcinoma of the lung, germ cell tumors, and lymphomas that are sensitive to chemotherapy, may also involve the liver. Isolated hepatic metastases from those primaries that may be surgically resected are most unusual as the liver involvement is usually part of widespread metastatic disease.

CARCINOID SYNDROME

The development of the carcinoid syndrome invariably implies metastatic spread from a primary lesion in the small bowel to the liver. The syndrome comprises facial flushing, diarrhea, and, less often, wheezing, and cardiac complications. Abdominal pain may be due to obstruction by the primary small bowel tumor. Diagnosis is based on an elevated level of urinary 5-hydroxyindoleacetic acid (5HIAA) and the characteristic histologic pattern of a neuroendocrine tumor involving the liver. It is highly characteristic that the patient's general clinical state can be remarkably good, even in the presence of massive liver involvement.

In the absence of symptoms, there no indication for active treatment of hepatic carcinoid metastases unless complete surgical resection is feasible. Symptoms of the carcinoid syndrome

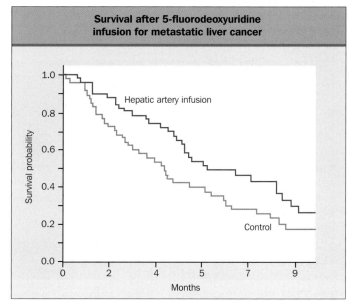

Figure 25.25 Improvement in survival, with a normal quality of life after chronic infusion with 5-fluorodeoxyuridine (FUDR). (Allen-Marsh TG et al., Lancet. 1994;344:1255–60.)

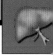

may be controlled by reduction of tumor mass (by surgery, arterial embolization, or cytotoxic chemotherapy) or pharmacologic interference with production or action of the tumor products. These approaches may have unpleasant side effects and should be employed only when symptoms become severe.

By the time the carcinoid syndrome has developed, the tumor is usually too widespread for curative resection to be attempted, but it may be successful in occasional patients and the approach to assessment is, as with other tumors, outlined above. Liver transplantation has been employed in carefully selected cases. Control by 'shelling out' individual deposits has now been superseded by hepatic artery embolization. About 80% of patients achieve complete resolution of symptoms, which may last for 1 month to 3 years. The procedure can be repeated and some patients have had multiple embolizations over several years.

Streptozotocin is the most active cytotoxic agent to have been used but it leads to a reduction in tumor mass in only 30% of cases. The addition of other agents, such as adriamycin and 5-FU, may give rather higher response rates but at the cost of considerably greater toxicity. All these approaches to decreasing tumor bulk may be associated with the massive release of vasoactive peptides from the tumor tissue. To prevent the resultant complications, patients are treated with blocking agents for 2 days before the procedure and 3 days after: parachlorophenylalanine 500mg four times daily and cyproheptadine 4mg three times daily. Cytotoxic chemotherapy should be the treatment of last resort and only used after embolization and pharmacologic approaches have failed.

Pharmacologic control

α-Methyl-dopa and parachlorophenylalanine, which inhibits key enzymes in the biosynthesis of serotonin from tryptophan, has now been largely superseded by the long-acting somatostatin analog octreotide. Octreotide is usually dramatically effective against diarrhea and frequently against flushing too. The disadvantage is that it needs to be administered subcutaneously two or three times per day. Most patients, however, learn to administer the drug themselves, and effective slow release intramuscular formulations are becoming available that will only require weekly or even monthly administration. A dose of 50mg three times per day is used initially and increased until symptoms are controlled. The drug is also very effective in managing carcinoid crises during surgery. The aim of therapy is symptom control and early reports of tumor shrinkage have not been substantiated. When octreotide becomes ineffective, the addition of interferon-α may further control symptoms. Control of diarrhea with codeine phosphate or loperamide and careful avoidance of precipitating factors such as alcohol, stress and certain foods may also be effective. The effect of the latter is mediated by various kinins and phenoxybenzamine and chlorpromazine are occasionally effective.

PRACTICE POINT

Illustrative case

A 38-year-old man has been found to be a chronic carrier of HBV during a routine health check. The only positive physical finding was mild hepatomegaly. All routine liver tests fell within the reference range. His physician recommended 6-monthly estimations of the serum AFP level and US examination. Two years after presentation serum AFP level was reported to be 65ng/mL (reference range <10ng/mL) and this had risen to 125ng/mL within a month. As the US examination remained unchanged from previous examinations a decision was taken to re-evaluate the patient after 2 months. This time, however, the AFP level has increased to 469ng/mL. Ultrasound examination, CT scan with lipiodol, and angiography all failed to show any evidence of tumor. Within a further 2 months the AFP level had reached 1200ng/mL. Although ultrasound remained normal, a further angiogram revealed a 1×1.5cm lesion in the caudate lobe. However, the surgeon noted advanced macronodular cirrhosis. In view of the extensive cirrhosis and young age, 3-monthly AFP and US examination together with 6-monthly CT scans were recommended. One year later a 1.2cm lesion was detected by US examination and confirmed on CT scan. α-fetoprotein was negative. On this occasion liver transplantation was recommended. The procedure was uneventful with no evidence of recurrence at 6 months postoperation.

Interpretation

Chronic carriers of HBV have a greatly increased risk of developing HCC. There is as yet no evidence that routine screening will, overall, increase survival, but undoubtedly some lucky individuals will have their tumor detected in time for effective therapeutic intervention. Despite the extreme nodularity of the patient's liver, note that liver function tests were still within the reference range, and that there were no cutaneous features of chronic liver disease. Once patients have significant dysfunction, even if a tumor is detected by screening, it will seldom be amenable to surgical resection. A steadily rising AFP level should be taken seriously. Note that the failure to detect a lesion should not lead the physician to assume that this is a 'false positive' result – levels of AFP often rise before there is any evidence of tumor on conventional imaging techniques. The second tumor was AFP-negative and this suggests that a new malignant clone had developed. Although the second tumor was technically resectable, the path of liver transplantation was chosen. Firstly, it is clear that the liver is highly unstable and further new or metastatic tumor was likely. Secondly, with future resections, liver failure was only a matter of time. Thirdly, further operation may make the subsequent transplantation more hazardous. Transplantation while the patient was fit would avoid subsequent decompensation and abolish the risk of further HCC. With the small size of the tumor, the risk of developing recurrence in the transplanted liver is small and the patient can look forward to a better than 75% chance of being alive and well at 5 years. It is likely that treatment of 'screened' HCC patients will become an important indication for liver transplantation.

FURTHER READING

Allen-Marsh TG, Earlam S, Fordy C, Abrams K, Houghton J. Quality of life and survival with continuous hepatic-artery floxuridine infusion for colorectal liver metastases. Lancet. 1994;344:1255–60. *One of the very few studies that has seriously addressed quality of life issues in a controlled trial. The authors showed that not only was survival prolonged in patients who had colorectal metastases (405 versus 226 days), but also that survival was with a normal quality of life.*

Atlas of Cancer Mortality in the People's Republic of China. The Editorial Committee for the Atlas of Cancer Mortality in the People's Republic of China. China Map Press. *This volume is not widely known in the West, but it represents a fascinating summary of a mammoth undertaking to plot out the geographic variation in the incidence of tumors, including HCC, throughout China. The results imply that chronic HBV infection cannot account for all the geographic variation in the incidence of HCC.*

Beasley RP. Hepatitis B virus the major etiology of hepatocellular carcinoma. Cancer. 1988;60:1942. *The definitive summation of the data implicating, and in the case of Taiwan, quantifying the risk of HCC in chronic carriers of the hepatitis B virus.*

Chang MH, Chen CJ, Lai MS, et al. Universal hepatitis B vaccination in Taiwan and the incidence of hepatocellular carcinoma in children. N Engl J Med. 1997;336:1855–9. *The first evidence that universal vaccination against the HBV may decrease the incidence of HCC. A landmark paper.*

Colombo M, Kuo G, Choo QI, et al. Prevalence of antibodies to hepatitis C virus in Italian patients with hepatocellular carcinoma. Lancet. 1989;2:1006–8. *One of the earliest studies to demonstrate the association between chronic HCV infection and the subsequent development of HCC. Although the specificity of the assay used was in some doubt, later application of more specific assays has confirmed the strong association.*

Dube S, Heyen F, Jenicek M. Adjuvant chemotherapy in colorectal carcinoma. Results of a meta-analysis. Dis Colon Rectum. 1997;40:35–41. *This paper is a detailed analysis of the impact of adjuvant treatment following resection of Dukes' C colorectal cancer. The incidence of metastatic disease, particularly to the liver, is significantly decreased, but the absolute improvement in terms of survival benefit is not impressive.*

Group d'Etude et de Traitement du Carcinome Hepatocellulaire. A comparison of lipiodol chemoembolization and conservative treatment for unresectable hepatocellular carcinoma. N Engl J Med. 1995;332:1256–61. *A controlled trial that found no survival benefit of TOCE. Although open to several criticisms another recent trial has also arrived at the same conclusion. While subgroups of patients may, in the long run benefit from TOCE, it seems unlikely that this procedure will have major impact on survival.*

Lau WY, Ho SKW, Leung TWT, et al. Selective internal radiation therapy for inoperable hepatocellular carcinoma with intraarterial infusion of yttrium[90] microspheres. Int J Rad Oncol Biol Phys. 1998;40:583–92. *Describes a new loco-regional therapy for HCC and the emerging concept of preoperative treatment aiming at increasing the resectablity rate of large tumors.*

Lau WY, Leung TWT, Ho SKW, et al. Adjuvant intra-arterial lipiodol-iodine-131-labelled lipiodol for resectable hepatocellular carcinoma – a prospective randomised trial. Lancet. 1999;353:797–801.

Leung TWT, Patt YZ, Lau WY, et al. Complete pathological remission is possible with systemic combination chemotherapy for inoperable hepatocellular carcinoma. Clinical Cancer Research. 1999;5:1676–81.

McPeake JR, Portmann B. Hepatic malignancy, Budd–Chiari syndrome and space-occupying conditions. In: Williams R, Portmann B, Tan KC, eds. The practice of liver transplantation. London: Churchill Livingstone; 1995:57–71. *A review of the indications and results of liver transplantation for malignant disease.*

Muto Y, Moriwaki H, Ninomiya M, et al. Prevention of second primary tumors by an acyclic retinoid, polyprenoic acid, in patients with hepatocellular carcinoma. N Engl J Med. 1996;334:1561–7. *The first evidence that 'differentiation' agents may prevent hepatic cancer. In this case, the agent was administered after surgical resection or percutaneous ethanol injection.*

Nishiguchi S, Kuroki T, Nakatani S, et al. Randomised trial of effects of interferon-α on the incidence of hepatocellular carcinoma in chronic active hepatitis C with cirrhosis. Lancet. 1995;346:1051–5. *Evidence that treating chronic hepatitis C with interferon not only improves liver function but also decreases the incidence of cancer development.*

Paradinas FJ, Melia WM, Wilkinson ML, et al. High serum vitamin B_{12} binding capacity as a marker of the fibrolamellar variant of hepatocellular carcinoma. Br Med J. 1982;285:840–42. *An early description of fibrolamellar carcinoma and a novel tumor marker.*

Ross RK, Yuan JM , Yu MC, et al. Urinary aflatoxin biomarkers and risk of hepatocellular carcinoma. Lancet. 1992;339:943–6. *This study strongly suggests that the combined risks of HBV carriage and aflatoxin exposure are much more than additive, although the number of cases developing HCC are still very small.*

Tranberg K, Bengmark S. Metastatic tumours of the liver. In: Blumgart LH, ed. Surgery of the liver and biliary tract. London: Churchill Livingstone; 1994:1385–97. *Covers diagnosis and surgical treatment of secondary liver cancers. This book also covers all aspects of surgical management of liver tumors.*

Schuster MJ, Wu GY. Gene therapy for hepatocellular carcinoma: progress but many stones yet unturned. Gastroenterology. 1997;112:656–9. *A glimpse into the future, but with a realistic appreciation of the problems that remain.*

Van Kaick G, Muth H, Kaul A, et al. Results of the German thorotrast study. In: Boice JD Jr, Fraumeni JF Jr, eds. Radiation carcinogenesis epidemiology and biological significance. New York: Raven Press; 1984:253–62. *A meticulous study of the consequences of the 'thorotrast tragedy' from which cases are still being seen to this day. The relation of radiation to subsequent development of malignancy in terms of dose and latency and tumor site are particularly well-documented.*

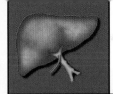

Chapter 26   Biliary and Cholestatic Diseases

Gregory T Everson

INTRODUCTION

This chapter describes a group of miscellaneous disorders of the biliary tract: cholelithiasis, cholecystitis, fibrocystic diseases, simple hepatic cysts, and cholangiocarcinoma. The specific aims are to describe the epidemiology and pathogenesis of these disorders, define the key clinical syndromes, provide methods for diagnosis, and elucidate the natural history and impact of therapy.

CHOLELITHIASIS

Epidemiology and risk factors

Epidemiologic studies suggest that more than 20,000,000 Americans have gallstones and that nearly 750,000 cholecystectomies are performed annually in the USA, at an estimated total cost of over 7 billion dollars per year. The majority of gallstones are composed predominantly of cholesterol, and risk factors for gallstones include: age, female gender, use of exogenous estrogen or contraceptive steroids, pregnancy, obesity, and rapid weight loss in obese subjects. Gallstones are highly prevalent in Hispanic populations and in native American populations of the southwestern USA. Additional risk factors for gallstones include: use of fibric acid derivatives (clofibrate), prolonged total parenteral nutrition, ileal resection or jejunoileal bypass, ileal disease (e.g. Crohn's disease), celiac disease, vagotomy, spinal cord injury, diabetes mellitus, chronic hemolytic disease, and cirrhosis.

An integral feature of the Third National Health and Nutrition Examination Survey (NHANES III) was the inclusion of gallbladder ultrasonography to define the prevalence and risk factors for gallbladder disease in adults (age range 20–74years) in the USA. Screening ultrasonography was performed in over 14,000 participants in NHANES III and gallbladder disease was defined by either the presence of cholelithiasis or prior gallbladder surgery. The overall prevalence of gallbladder disease was 20.5 million, and 8.7 million had had prior cholecystectomy. As demonstrated in nearly every population study previously conducted in other parts of the world, the prevalence of gallbladder disease in the USA was greater in women and increased with age in both men and women (Fig. 26.1). The difference in prevalence between men and women was greatest in younger age groups. Alcohol consumption was associated with lower risk and diabetes mellitus and obesity were associated with higher risk of gallbladder disease in both sexes. In women, risk of gallbladder disease correlated with number of completed pregnancies, use of cigarettes, and reduced physical activity. The design of NHANES III allowed comparison of differences in prevalence of gallbladder disease between ethnic groups. Nonhispanic black men had a lower prevalence of gallbladder disease than

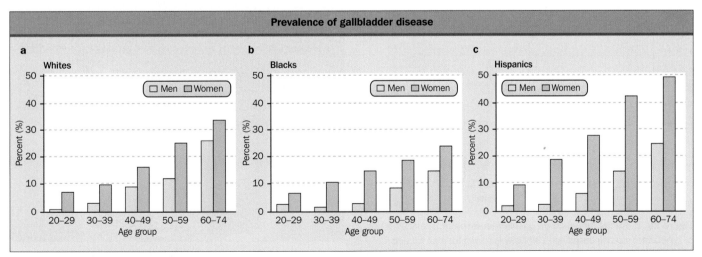

Figure 26.1 Prevalence of gallbladder disease. (a) Non-Hispanic whites; (b) non-Hispanic blacks; (c) Hispanics. The prevalence of gallbladder disease (gallstones on screening ultrasonography or prior cholecystectomy verified by absence of gallbladder on screening ultrasonography) in the United States for men and women as determined from the Third National Health and Nutrition Examination Survey (NHANES III) is shown. In all age groups, women have a greater prevalence of gallbladder disease than men; the difference is most dramatic at younger ages.

either nonhispanic white men or hispanic men (Fig. 26.2a). The latter two groups had similar prevalences. Hispanic women had the highest prevalence of gallbladder disease, which persisted even after controlling for comorbid conditions and other risk factors. In addition, nonhispanic black women had a lower risk for gallbladder disease than either hispanic or nonhispanic white women (Fig. 26.2b), which was particularly pronounced at older age and with increasing body mass index (BMI). Pathophysiologic mechanisms to explain these differences have not been defined.

Pathogenesis

Gallstones are typically classified by their chemical composition: cholesterol, black pigment, and brown pigment. Cholesterol gallstones are defined as gallstones that are more than 50% cholesterol by weight. Cholesterol gallstones are not made of pure cholesterol; salts of calcium, pigments, and glycoprotein may be found in the center, in radiating spikes, or in concentric rings within the stone. Pigment gallstones are poor in cholesterol and contain carbonate, phosphate, calcium salts of bilirubin, and palmitate distributed throughout the stone material. Black pigment stones are composed almost entirely of salts of bilirubin, occur in the setting of chronic hemolytic disease, and are formed in the gallbladder under sterile conditions. Brown pigment stones are soft, amorphous, and contain bilirubin salts plus a number of other components. They are the main type of primary bile duct stones, and tend to form in the setting of infection.

Current understanding of the pathogenesis of cholesterol gallstones suggests that three processes may be required: secretion of 'lithogenic' bile by the liver, nucleation of molecules to initiate crystal formation, and stasis of bile in the gallbladder to allow crystals to elongate and agglomerate to form 'sludge' and stones.

The secretion of bile that is supersaturated with cholesterol is a prerequisite for cholesterol gallstone formation. Supersaturation may result from either enhanced cholesterol secretion (obesity, pregnancy, contraceptive steroids, estrogens) or reduced bile acid

secretion (fasting, ileal disease or resection, rapid weight loss). The initial secretion of cholesterol by hepatocytes into bile is tightly coupled to phospholipid secretion in the form of unilamellar vesicles. When bile is unsaturated bile acid enhances the disappearance of vesicles as cholesterol is transferred to cholesterol/bile acid/phospholipid micelles. When bile is saturated, the unilamellar vesicles aggregate into large, cholesterol-rich, multilamellar vesicles, which favors nucleation of cholesterol molecules to form crystals and, ultimately, gallstones.

Gallbladder mucin and other glycoproteins secreted by the liver and, possibly, gallbladder mucosa have been proposed as pronucleation factors. These glycoproteins have been shown to promote the formation of cholesterol crystals from saturated biles and often are found in the core matrix of both cholesterol and pigment gallstones. In contrast, antinucleation factors (apoproteins A-1 and A-2) found in nonlithogenic bile may prevent the formation of cholesterol crystals from vesicular aggregates.

The healthy gallbladder prevents formation of gallstones by acidifying and concentrating bile, and by vigorously expelling crystals and sludge during contractions. Cholesterol nucleation takes place over days, if the gallbladder empties vigorously several times daily, removing mucus as well as bile from the gallbladder, then crystal formation and development of gallstones may not occur. Gallbladder hypomotility may be a factor in the formation of gallstones during total parenteral nutrition, rapid weight loss, prolonged fasting, pregnancy, celiac disease, massive small bowel resection, and biliopancreatic bypass procedure for treatment of obesity.

Clinical manifestations of gallstones
Asymptomatic gallstones

Most patients with gallstones are asymptomatic and will remain asymptomatic for several years. Such patients are regularly detected on routine ultrasonography (Fig. 26.3). One study of the natural history of truly asymptomatic gallstones indicated that only 20% of these patients will develop symptoms when fol-

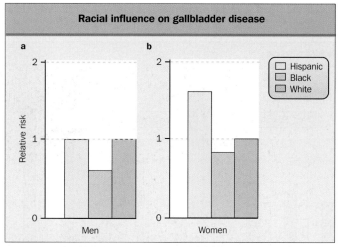

Figure 26. 2 Racial influence on gallbladder disease. The relative risk of gallbladder disease based upon ethnicity is shown for men (a) and women (b). Non-Hispanic black men had a lower risk of gallbladder disease compared with both non-Hispanic white men and Hispanic men. Compared with non-Hispanic white women, Hispanic women had a higher risk and non-Hispanic black women had a lower risk of gallbladder disease. Relative risk was adjusted for age and BMI, body mass index.

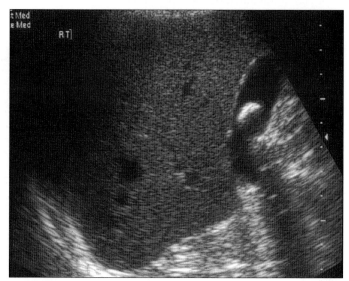

Figure 26.3 Ultrasound detection of gallstones. This ultrasonograph demonstrates a gallstone within the gallbladder lumen. Criteria for diagnosis include: echogenic concretions in the lumen, shadowing of the ultrasonographic beam, and mobility of the concretions with positioning of the patient. (By kind permission of Dr. H. Irving.)

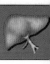

lowed up to 25 years. It has been suggested that the asymptomatic gallstone population is really comprised of two populations: those that ultimately become symptomatic (usually within the first 5 years of follow-up) and those that never develop symptoms. The risk of developing symptoms is 1–3% per year for the first 5–10 years, but then drops to 0.1–0.3% with prolonged observation. The risk of developing serious complications from gallstones (acute cholecystitis, cholangitis, pancreatitis, sepsis, gangrenous gallbladder) is low, only about 0.1% per year. In the most comprehensive long-term study of natural history, biliary colic always preceded any serious complication by several months. Given the costs associated with cholecystectomy, the relatively benign natural history, and the fact that biliary colic nearly always precedes more serious complications, prophylactive cholecystectomy is not recommended for asymptomatic patients. However, prophylactic cholecystectomy may be considered in the following circumstances: patients with large ileal resections, patients with known gallstones who will be traveling or working in remote regions of the world, and certain populations or medical conditions that are associated with high rates of complications or cancer (Pima Indians, calcified gallbladder, porcelain gallbladder, gallstones associated with sickle cell disease). One decision analysis suggested that patients with diabetes mellitus do not benefit from prophylactic cholecystectomy.

In general, most gallstones do not spontaneously dissolve or exit the gallbladder asymptomatically. In the National Cooperative Gallstone Study 1% of patients experienced spontaneous clearance of gallbladder stones over a period of 2 years while taking placebo. Even this low rate of clearance was questioned as the technique used to detect gallstones was oral cholecystography, which is much less sensitive than the currently recommended method of real-time ultrasonography (98% sensitivity and specificity). In contrast, two recent ultrasonographic studies suggested that one-third of cholesterol gallstones that develop during pregnancy may dissolve. Small stones (<0.5cm diameter) that are composed predominantly of cholesterol are more likely to dissolve during the postpartum period. In general, calcified stones, pigment stones, and stones that have persisted over several years are not likely to dissolve spontaneously. Gallstones that are symptomatic are not likely to disappear spontaneously.

Symptomatic gallstones

Biliary colic is the most specific symptom of cholelithiasis and is defined as pain that is localized to either the right upper quadrant of the abdomen or epigastrium. It is characterized by a short crescendo period of increasing pain (5–15 minutes), a plateau of steady pain (15 minutes to several hours), and a decrescendo period of decreasing pain and resolution of pain (15 minutes to 2 hours). Patients are asymptomatic between attacks of colic. Nonspecific symptoms that do not correlate well with gallstones include the following: nausea, vomiting, dyspepsia, diarrhea, weight loss or gain, and heartburn. Elderly, diabetic, and immunocompromised patients may present with serious complications of gallbladder disease (gangrenous gallbladder, empyema of the gallbladder, perforation of the gallbladder, suppurative cholangitis) and may exhibit few or no localizing abdominal complaints or findings on physical examination. In these patients gallbladder disease may present as fever, altered mental status, loss of appetite and weight loss, or sepsis.

The best data that address the natural history after an episode of biliary colic are from the National Cooperative Gallstone Study.

Patients entering the trial had a preceding history of biliary colic and were then randomized to receive one of two doses of chenodeoxycholate or placebo. A total of 305 patients were enroled in the placebo arm and were followed clinically. Patients with frequent attacks of biliary-type pain 12 months before entry into the trial continued to experience frequent attacks of pain, some developed complicated biliary disease, and many required cholecystectomy. In contrast, those who had infrequent attacks of pain continued to have few attacks, experienced a lower complication rate, and had lower rates of cholecystectomy. In general, patients with biliary colic can be expected to continue to experience biliary colic during follow-up. The severity of the attacks is highly variable but may be relatively consistent within a given individual. Patients with frequent, severe episodes may be at greatest risk for complicated gallbladder disease.

Rarely, a large gallstone in the gallbladder will erode through the gallbladder wall into an adjacent viscus (usually duodenum), traverse the bowel, impact at a point of narrowing (usually terminal ileum), and cause bowel obstruction or gastric outlet obstruction (Bouveret's syndrome).

Therapeutic options

A conservative noninterventional approach is only warranted for patients with asymptomatic gallstones. Once gallstones become symptomatic the gallbladder should be removed. Chronic use of analgesics in the treatment of biliary pain is discouraged as it merely masks symptoms and may increase the likelihood that the patient will only present later with more serious biliary complications of the disease. Most clinicians recommend therapy for symptomatic disease based upon the high likelihood of recurrent symptoms and the risk of developing serious complications once biliary colic has occurred. Diabetic patients may be at particularly high risk for complications compared with nondiabetics. Complications include either severe cholecystitis, gangrenous gallbladder, empyema of the gallbladder, or perforated gallbladder. The operative mortality with emergency surgery for acute complications of gallstones in diabetic patients has been reported to be as high as 15–20%, or four to five times higher than that for matched groups of nondiabetic patients.

Oral bile acid therapy

Two dihydroxy bile acids, chenodeoxycholic acid (CDCA) and ursodeoxycholic acid (UDCA), have proven effective in dissolving gallstones in randomized controlled trials. Criteria for use of these agents are: radiolucent gallstones on plain film of the abdomen (or CT scan), functioning gallbladder by oral cholecystography or HIDA-scintigraphy, and an intact enterohepatic circulation. Calcified stones are a contraindication to use of bile acid therapy because they are insoluble and will not dissolve. Patients who lack a functioning gallbladder should not be treated with oral bile acids because the bile acids will not enter or concentrate within the gallbladder, a requirement for effective therapy. Patients with ileal disease or resection may not absorb the orally administered bile acids. Because CDCA and UDCA reduce biliary cholesterol by different but complementary mechanisms, most investigators in the field recommend use of both agents simultaneously (CDCA 8mg/kg per day + UDCA 8mg/kg per day). One meta-analysis of 23 trials of gallstone dissolution involving 1949 patients described the range of dissolution rates to be 0–63%. Highest rates of dissolution were observed with combination therapy (versus monotherapy with either CDCA or UDCA), higher doses, longer duration of treatment, and smaller diameter gallstones (<1cm). The success rate of treating small stones (1–3mm) that float within gallbladder bile is as high as 80%. Ursodeoxycholic acid is highly effective in preventing cholesterol stones from forming during rapid weight loss induced by very-low-calorie diets. Disadvantages of oral bile acid therapy include: slow rates of dissolution, the fact that it is most effective in a minority of patients (nonobese patient, <5mm solitary stone, radiolucent), and high recurrence rates even with effective dissolution (10% per year for first 5 years). Patients with multiple stones before dissolution have a higher risk of recurrence than those with single stones.

Extracorporeal shock-wave lithotripsy

This is effective in fragmenting gallstones within both the gallbladder and common bile duct. Extracorporeal shock-wave lithotripsy (ESWL) of gallstones is always done with concomitant use of oral bile acids and is restricted to use in patients with a functioning gallbladder. It reduces larger stones to smaller stones, increasing total surface area of stones, which then increases the success rate of oral bile acids to dissolve the stones. The combination of lithotripsy and bile acid therapy is 40–50% effective (stone and fragment-free at 6 months) when used on single gallstones of less than 30mm diameter. The advantages of lithotripsy are: low morbidity, lack of general anesthesia, outpatient setting, and minimal interruption of lifestyle. The main disadvantages of ESWL are the lack of efficacy in patients with multiple stones and the high recurrence rate once oral bile acid therapy is stopped (10% per year for at least 5 years).

Methyl-tert-butyl-ether (MTBE)

Methyl-tert-butyl-ether (MTBE) is 50-fold more potent than oral bile acids in dissolving cholesterol. Like oral bile acids, it is only effective against radiolucent gallstones. Treatment with MTBE requires percutaneous puncture of the gallbladder, placement of an indwelling gallbladder catheter, continuous infusion and aspiration of MTBE into and out of the gallbladder, and careful close monitoring of the patient by the treating physician. The majority of cholesterol gallstones may be dissolved by one or two treatment sessions with MTBE. Despite the effectiveness of MTBE to dissolve the cholesterol component of the stone, a pigmented or calcified shell or collection of debris often persists. This material serves as a nidus for future stone formation. Indeed, as predict-

ed, stone recurrence rates are high. Criteria for use of MTBE are: radiolucent gallstone, functioning gallbladder or patent cystic duct, and the patient must be able to tolerate percutaneous transhepatic puncture of the gallbladder. Disadvantages of MTBE include: spillage of MTBE into the duodenum which can cause severe duodenitis, systemic absorption which may result in anesthesia of the patient, and risks associated with percutaneous puncture of the gallbladder. In general, MTBE treatment is only performed in specialized centers. Treatment with MTBE is currently done only for patients with a prohibitive operative risk.

The great success and high patient acceptance of laparoscopic cholecystectomy have virtually eliminated the widespread clinical application of oral bile acid dissolution therapy, shock-wave lithotripsy, and percutaneous puncture of the gallbladder for MTBE treatment.

Endoscopic sphincterotomy

This is recommended in the treatment of choledocholithiasis and its complications of obstructive jaundice, cholangitis, or pancreatitis. Numerous studies of endoscopic sphincterotomy for choledocholithiasis have verified its efficacy at nearly eliminating the risk of subsequent complications of passage of additional bile duct stones. Patients who are reasonable surgical candidates should undergo cholecystectomy once stabilized after endoscopic retrograde cholangiopancreatography (ERCP) and sphincterotomy. The risk of acute cholecystitis in patients who have had endoscopic sphincterotomy but whose gallbladder has been left in place is 5–20% during a 3–5 year follow-up.

Surgery for symptomatic gallstones

Elective cholecystectomy is the preferred treatment for symptomatic cholelithiasis. There are two basic techniques: open laparotomy or laparoscopic. Until the late 1980s, open laparotomy and cholecystectomy were the standard surgical methods against which all other therapies were judged. In 1988, it was shown that the gallbladder could be safely and effectively removed by the laparoscopic technique. Since this initial experience most surgeons performing cholecystectomy have switched from the open to the laparoscopic technique and several studies have compared results from the two methods. A significant advantage for laparoscopic cholesystectomy in terms of complication rate, duration of hospital stay, and hospital costs has been demonstrated (Fig. 26.4). Advantages of laparoscopic cholecystectomy include: short duration of hospital stay, early return to home and job, high patient

Surgical series of laparoscopic cholecystectomy					
Year of study	Patients	% to open	Mortality	Major comps	Bile duct injury
1992	1963	4.5	0.1	2.1	0.3
1991	1518	4.7	0.07	1.5	0.5
1991	1236	3.6	0.0	1.6	0.3
1992	618	2.9	0.0	1.6	0.2
1991	500	1.8	0.0	1.0	0.0
1992	400	4.0	0.0	5.0	0.5
1991	381	3.0	0.9	3.4	0.0

Figure 26.4 Surgical series of laparoscopic cholecystectomy. Large series confirm low complication rates after laparoscopic cholecystectomy with conversion rates to open cholecystectomy under 5%.

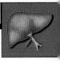

acceptance, and low rate of complications. Disadvantages include: higher risk of major morbidity when the surgery is done by technically inexperienced surgeons, potential need to convert an elective cholecystectomy to an urgent cholecystectomy if complications occur, and higher rate of serious bile duct injuries. Open cholecystectomy may still be the preferred approach to patients with complex gallbladder disease [empyema, infarction, perforation causing generalized peritonitis or subphrenic abscess, biliary–enteric fistula leading to bowel obstruction (gallstone ileus) and bacterial cholangitis].

Reported operative mortality rates for diabetics and nondiabetics are shown in (Fig. 26.5). Stable diabetics who undergo elective cholecystectomy have no major increase in expected operative mortality. In contrast, diabetics who are poorly controlled and who undergo cholecystectomy for complicated biliary tract disease do experience increased morbidity and mortality. For these reasons, the development of biliary colic in a diabetic patient with gallstones is an indication for early elective cholecystectomy.

Postcholecystectomy syndrome

Approximately 5% of patients will have persistence or recurrence of nonspecific symptoms after cholecystectomy. Most commonly, patients complain of dyspepsia or upper abdominal pain. The differential diagnosis is extensive and includes recurrent or retained calculi in cystic or common bile duct, pancreatitis, cholangitis, papillary stenosis, or operative injury to the biliary tree. Once anatomic or mechanical factors have been eliminated one needs to consider the possibility of disordered biliary motility, biliary dyskinesia, as the basis for pain. Biliary dyskinesia implies a disorder of the normal contraction of the gallbladder or altered function of the sphincter of Oddi. After removal of the gallbladder, the source of biliary dyskinesia is limited to the sphincter of Oddi. The latter may be responsible for postchole-

cystectomy syndrome in 5–15% of patients. The diagnosis of sphincter of Oddi dysfunction is dependent upon accurate measurement of the basal pressure of the sphincter via biliary manometry at ERCP. Patients with basal sphincter pressures greater than 40mmHg experience relief of their pain after endoscopic sphincterotomy (Fig. 26.6). Additional features that support the diagnosis and a response to sphincterotomy are: dilated common bile duct (CBD), abnormal liver tests, and prolonged retention of contrast in the biliary system at the time of ERCP. Some patients have postcholecystectomy pain but lack any objective evidence for biliary disease ('type III' sphincter of Oddi dysfunction). In general, these patients do not respond to sphincterotomy, suggesting that sphincter function is not related to their symptoms. One group examined these patients for underlying visceral hyperalgesia in response to balloon distension of rectum and duodenum and selectively reproduced symptoms with duodenal distension. They also found that these patients were characterized by somatization, depression, obsessive–compulsive behavior, and anxiety.

CHOLECYSTITIS

Cholecystitis may or may not be associated with the presence of gallstones. Calculous cholecystitis implies gallbladder inflammation in the presence of gallstones. Clinical features of calculous cholecystitis include fever, right upper quadrant abdominal pain with tenderness to palpation, leukocytosis, and ultrasonographic images that demonstrate cholelithiasis. Additional ultrasonographic features of cholecystitis may include thickening of the wall of the gallbladder and pericholecystic fluid.

Gallbladder sludge refers to gallbladder mucin with entrapment of particulate matter nucleated from bile (Fig. 26.7). Sludge formation occurs within the gallbladder when gallbladder emptying is slow and incomplete. It is often associated with

Mortality rates from acute complications of biliary tract disease: effect of diabetes mellitus						
	Mortality rates (%)					
	Diabetes mellitus			No diabetes		
Period	Surgery	No surgery	Total	Surgery	No surgery	Total
1953–1958	31	13	20	10	3	4
1960–1981	7	0	7	2	8	3

Figure 26.5 Mortality rates from acute complications of biliary tract disease: effect of diabetes mellitus. Mortality rates from biliary tract disease are consistently higher in patients with diabetes mellitus.

Effectiveness of endoscopic sphincterotomy for sphincter of Oddi dysfunction								
	SO pressure <40mmHg				SO pressure >40mmHg			
Patient group	Outcome (%)							
	n	Good	Fair	Poor	n	Good	Fair	Poor
Sham ES	12	31	18	67	12	15	10	75
ES	12	7	12	58	11	80	11	9
	(P = NS)				(P <0.05)*			

Figure 26.6 Effectiveness of endoscopic sphincterotomy for sphincter of Oddi dysfunction. Sphincter of Oddi (SO) pressures >40mmHg identify the patients most likely to benefit from endoscopic (ES) sphincterotomy.

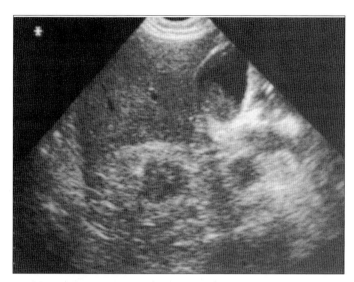

Figure 26.7 Biliary sludge. This ultrasonograph demonstrates 'sludge' within the gallbladder lumen. In contrast to the features of cholelithiasis, sludge is echogenic and mobile but fails to cast an ultrasonographic shadow. (By kind permission of Dr. H. Irving.)

prolonged fasting or lack of stimulation of intestinal release of cholecystokinin. Although sludge is a reversible stage in gallstone pathogenesis, gallstones may develop in a large percentage of patients, leading to symptomatic biliary tract disease. Sludge is a risk factor for gallstones, but it may be evacuated from the gallbladder and gallstone formation may be prevented.

Acalculous cholecystitis is inflammation of the gallbladder in the absence of gallstones and represents 2–5% of cases of proven acute cholecystitis. The pathogenesis is unknown. Risk factors for acute acalculous cholecystitis include: prior surgical procedure (nonbiliary), severe trauma, burns, total parenteral nutrition (TPN), multiorgan failure, immunocompromised host (AIDS, cancer chemotherapy, leukemia/lymphoma, uremia), and elderly age.

Diagnosis

Murphy's sign, which is also known as 'inspiratory arrest', is a valuable sign of acute cholecystitis. The patient is asked to take a deep inspiration while the examining fingers are held under the liver border, usually around the tip of ninth rib where the gallbladder may descend upon them. Inspiration is arrested in midcycle by painful contact with the fingers. Carcinoma of the gallbladder may produce a similar sign when it has invaded through the gallbladder wall involving the serosa or visceral peritoneum overlying the gallbladder.

One may be nearly certain of the diagnosis in the appropriate clinical situation when the following are present: leukocytosis, fever, and right upper quadrant tenderness to palpation. In the absence of the latter findings one must rely upon imperfect confirmatory radiologic studies (ultrasonography, HIDA-scintigraphy). Findings on ultrasonography that support the diagnosis of cholecystitis are: a thickened edematous gallbladder wall and a pericholecystic fluid collection. Although patients with acalculous cholecystitis may have sludge within the gallbladder lumen, sludge alone may not be pathologic. Sludge may be present in the absence of cholecystitis and absent in the presence of cholecystitis. A positive scan by HIDA-scintigraphy for acute

cholecystitis is characterized by normal uptake and clearance of HIDA by the liver, rapid excretion into the biliary system, visualization of the extrahepatic bile ducts, and appearance of HIDA in the intestine, but no visualization of the gallbladder. False-positive scans may occur in patients on TPN, alcoholics, or those who have had a prolonged fast or who have just eaten. In addition, in acalculous cholecystitis the cystic duct may be patent and allow entry of radionuclide into the gallbladder lumen, resulting in a false-negative scan. Positive findings on ultrasonography or HIDA-scintigraphy need to be assessed carefully before proceeding to cholecystectomy.

Mirizzi's syndrome is a clinical syndrome of cholecystitis and jaundice that develops when a stone impacts in the cystic duct. The resulting inflammation compresses and obstructs the common hepatic duct or CBD. Obstruction of the bile duct further promotes the development of cholangitis. The stenosis of the bile duct can mimic a malignant stricture. Acute cholecystitis is often associated with mildly abnormal liver tests, but a serum bilirubin greater than 85µmol/L (5mg/dL) strongly suggests CBD obstruction. If untreated, the stone may erode into CBD and create a biliobiliary fistula. Management involves drainage of the biliary system, antibiotic therapy, intravenous fluids, and cholecystectomy.

ACUTE CHOLANGITIS

Acute cholangitis results from impaction of a gallstone in the bile duct and ascending infection behind the obstruction. Biliary pain, jaundice, and fever (with chills and rigors) occurring together constitute Charcot's triad, which indicates acute cholangitis. The triad occurs in 70% of cases of acute cholangitis and is the most common complication of choledocholithiasis. Refractory sepsis manifested by hypotension and mental confusion in a patient with Charcot's triad constitutes Raynold's pentad. Only 10% of patients with acute suppurative cholangitis present with all five of these features.

Therapy for cholangitis should be individualized because of the wide spectrum of severity of illness. Antibiotic therapy and intravenous hydration should be initiated promptly on an empiric basis. Antibiotics are tailored to the types of organisms associated with acute cholangitis: *Escherichia coli*, *Klebsiella pneumoniae*, *Streptococcus faecalis*, *Pseudomonas aeruginosa*, and *Bacteroides fragilis*. In the elderly or immunocompromised patient anaerobic coverage is necessary since these patients are at increased risk for developing suppurative cholangitis. Effective antibiotic regimens include: ampicillin (or amoxicillin) plus an aminoglycoside, piperacillin alone, or fluoroquinolones. In cases where bacteroides are suspected, the addition of metronidazole is recommended. Sulfonamides and cephalosporins are not recommended for acute cholangitis. It is important to remember that antibiotics are viewed as adjuncts to the primary therapy: duct drainage.

The majority of patients with cholelithiasis are cured by cholecystectomy, although a few may have residual stones within the bile duct. The incidence of bile duct stones increases with increasing age and is more likely to occur in patients with multiple gallstones. The diagnosis of retained CBD stone is suggested by recurrence of biliary colic, abnormal liver tests, pale stools, dark urine, and dilatation of the bile duct on ultrasonography. However, retained stones may be present without dilatation of the CBD or abnormal liver tests. The diagnosis is

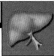

established by cholangiography. The preferred diagnostic test is ERCP, because the retained stone may also be easily treated with this modality.

About 70% of patients will respond with stabilization of their clinical course. Patients failing to respond to empiric therapy within 24 hours should be considered for immediate biliary decompression. The latter may be accomplished by endoscopic sphincterotomy and removal of the impacted stone, endoscopic placement of nasobiliary drainage tube, percutaneous transhepatic drainage (radiology), or cholecystectomy plus CBD exploration or placement of T-tube. The choice of each of these modalities depends upon the expertise of the available specialists, the condition of the patient, and estimated operative risk. In general, either endoscopic or surgical treatment is recommended. Radiologic placement of drainage catheters is usually restricted to the circumstance when endoscopy is unsuccessful. Several trials have examined the role of urgent endoscopy versus early surgery and have demonstrated that ERCP done early in the course of acute cholangitis is safe and effective in controlling biliary tract sepsis (Figs 26.8 & 26.9). It is not yet determined whether outcome is superior with the combination of early ERCP, sphincterotomy, CBD stone extraction, and drainage of the biliary system followed by elective laparoscopic cholecystectomy compared with urgent cholecystectomy, CBD exploration, and T-tube placement. There have been no critical evaluations of costs associated with these two approaches.

GALLSTONE PANCREATITIS

Although alcohol is the commonest cause of pancreatitis, gallstones are responsible for 25–40% of cases. Impaction of a gallstone at the ampulla of Vater causes hypertension in the pancreatic duct, which initiates the inflammation. Impaction may be more frequent in patients with high basal pressures in the sphincter of Oddi or in patients whose sphincter fails to relax in response to physiologic stimuli. Clinical clues that suggest gallstones as the etiology include: significant abnormalities in liver tests, cholelithiasis on ultrasonography, an amylase greater than 1500IU/L, or a rapid rise and fall in amylase. However, clinical features of gallstone pancreatitis may be indistinguishable from other forms of pancreatitis.

Recurrence rates of either cholangitis or gallstone pancreatitis differ depending upon whether the patient has a retained bile duct stone. In most cases of cholangitis the bile duct stone is too large to pass spontaneously and recurrence of cholangitis is predicted if the stone is not removed. In contrast, as many as 90% of bile duct stones may pass into the intestine in the setting of gallstone pancreatitis. Nonetheless, the existence of residual stones in the bile duct or gallbladder is sufficient to ensure recurrence. As many as 60% of patients will experience recurrent pancreatitis within 6 months of the initial episode. Endoscopic retrograde cholangiopancreatography with sphincterotomy is recommended early for severe biliary pancreatitis, which will allow removal of impacted CBD stones.

GALLBLADDER CARCINOMA

There is an association between chronic cholecystitis and gallbladder malignancy. The incidence of carcinoma increases with

Severe acute cholangitis: mortality		
Cause	Surgery group (n = 41)	Endoscopic drainage group (n = 41)
Heart failure (n)	2	0
Bronchopneumonia (n)	2	2
Renal failure (n)	1	0
Multiorgan failure (n)	4	2
Sepsis (n)	3	0
Cerebellar hemorrhage (n)	1	0
Total	13	4 P <0.03

Figure 26.8 Severe acute cholangitis: mortality. Mortality in patients with severe acute cholangitis: a randomized trial comparing urgent biliary tract surgery to endoscopic cholangiography and drainage. This randomized study confirmed lower mortality rates with endoscopic therapy.

Severe acute cholangitis: morbidity		
Complication	Surgery group (n = 41)	Endoscopic drainage group (n = 41)
Heart failure (n)	1	3
Bronchopneumonia (n)	15	7
Wound dehiscence (n)	1	0
Wound infection (n)	7	1
Gastrointestinal bleeding (n)	2	0
Renal dysfunction (n)	11	7
Bleeding after papillotomy (n)	0	1
Disseminated intravascular coagulopathy (n)	2	0
Total	39	19 P <0.05

Figure 26.9 Severe acute cholangitis: morbidity. Morbid complications in patients with severe acute cholangitis: a randomized trial comparing urgent biliary tract surgery to endoscopic cholangiography and drainage. This randomized study confirmed lower complication rates with endoscopic therapy.

age and with gallstones greater than 3cm in diameter. Approximately 0.1–3% of gallbladders removed for symptomatic cholelithiasis or cholecystitis, especially in the elderly, contain adenocarcinoma. Pima Indians, who have an extremely high prevalence of gallstones, also have the highest rate of gallbladder cancer and mortality in the USA. Calcified (porcelain) gallbladders pose an extreme risk for development of carcinoma, as high as 25%. Most tumors are adenocarcinomas and they are locally very aggressive. Tumor that extends beyond the gallbladder wall has a poor prognosis.

Courvoisier's sign is represented by the demonstration of a palpable, distended, nontender gallbladder. The etiology is usually a malignant obstruction of the bile duct. It is uncommon with choledocholithiasis. One reason for the lack of distension of the gallbladder with common duct stones is that the gallbladder, which is the source of the gallstone, is also likely to be a victim of chronic cholecystitis. Fibrosis and scarring render the organ nondistensible.

FIBROCYSTIC DISEASES OF THE LIVER

The diseases included in fibrocystic diseases of the liver are: autosomal-dominant polycystic disease, solitary hepatic cysts, congenital hepatic fibrosis, choledochal cysts, and Caroli's disease. Histopathologically they are characterized by ectasia of intrahepatic bile ducts, cysts of biliary epithelial cell origin, portal fibrosis, and persistence or lack of remodeling of the embryonic ductal plate (ductal plate malformation). The clinical spectrum ranges from an asymptomatic state to cholangitis or manifestations of liver failure. Polycystic liver disease is highlighted since there have been many recent advances in its natural history, genetics, and treatment.

Polycystic liver disease

Autosomal-dominant polycystic kidney disease (ADPKD) is one of the most common inherited disorders (10 times more common than sickle cell disease and 15 times more common than cystic fibrosis), and is second only to hemochromatosis in inherited disorders involving the liver. As polycystic patients survive for longer periods of time, due to improvements in the management of renal cystic disease, i.e. dialysis and transplantation, complications arising in hepatic cysts are recognized with increasing frequency. Many patients may be completely asymptomatic, with normal renal function, and unaware of their underlying disease. Others develop abdominal complaints, infections in cysts, cyst hemorrhage, or rarely, hepatic decompensation.

Natural history

The natural history of hepatic cysts that occur in the setting of polycystic kidney disease has been extensively described. Hepatic cysts occur uncommonly before puberty, but prevalence of hepatic cysts increases dramatically from the onset of puberty through the early, child-bearing years of adult life (Fig. 26.10). Most patients are asymptomatic without clinical consequences; they possess only a few hepatic cysts or have hepatic cysts whose diameters range from a few millimeters to one or two centimeters. Some patients develop massive hepatic cystic disease (almost exclusively restricted to women) during early adult life and many of these patients will become symptomatic, usually with abdominal pain or discomfort, early postprandial fullness, or shortness of breath. Rarely, patients may experience complications of advanced liver disease such as portal hypertension with variceal hemorrhage. As patients live into late adult life, there is a risk of renal failure due to renal cystic disease and need for either hemodialysis or renal transplantation. Complications that arise in hepatic cysts may occur more frequently in this population. In series of hemodialysis patients, 10–15% experienced complications in hepatic cysts, usually hemorrhage or infection, and, rarely, cyst carcinoma.

Pathogenesis

Increasing age, female gender, severity of renal cystic disease and severity of renal dysfunction are the four major risk factors

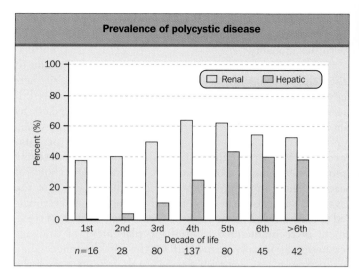

Figure 26.10 Prevalence of polycystic disease. The frequency of renal and hepatic cysts is displayed by age in a population at risk for ADPKD. Cysts were detected by real-time ultrasonography. The population at risk included 239 patients with ADPKD and 189 unaffected family members. The number of subjects in each decade is indicated at the bottom.

for development of hepatic cysts in ADPKD. Hepatic cysts are rarely detected before puberty, but the prevalence increases dramatically during the child-bearing years of adult life. By age 60 years nearly 50% of patients with ADPKD may have hepatic cysts (see Fig. 26.10). Although the age-related prevalence of hepatic cysts is similar in men and women, women experience greater numbers and larger sizes of hepatic cysts. This female tendency to develop extensive hepatic cystic disease correlates with both pregnancy and the use of exogenous female steroid hormones (Fig. 26.11).

The severity of hepatic cystic disease also correlates independently with both the severity of renal cystic disease and the degree of renal dysfunction. The correlation with renal cystic disease likely represents the parallel organ expression of the underlying genetic defect. However, the correlation with renal dysfunction suggests that the progression of liver cystic disease may be modified by toxic or metabolic factors that accumulate due to renal failure.

The autosomal-dominant inheritance of *ADPKD1* was established in 1957 in a study of 284 patients and their family members. Subsequent reports confirmed this pattern of inheritance and indicated that spontaneous mutations accounted for only a minority of cases, fewer than 10%. However, it was not until nearly 30 years later, that the first gene for ADPKD, *ADPKD1*, was localized to the short arm of chromosome 16 by linkage techniques. Eight years later, the *ADPKD1* gene was identified, cloned and sequenced. The protein encoded by this gene is designated as polycystin-1. The amino acid sequence for polycystin-1 has been determined from knowledge of the nucleotide sequence of the *ADPKD1* gene and the protein structure has been inferred from the amino acid sequence. This analysis has suggested that polycystin-1 is an ubiquitous protein, found in nearly all tissues in the body, and that it is likely to be an integral membrane protein involved with calcium flux and cell signaling.

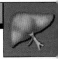

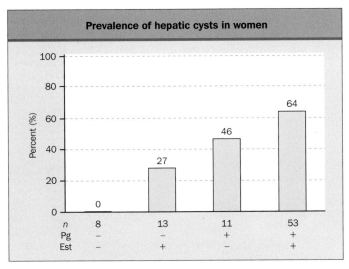

Figure 26.11 Prevalence of hepatic cysts in women. The prevalence of hepatic cystic disease as detected by screening ultrasonography is shown for women stratified by history of prior pregnancy (Pg) or prior use of female steroid hormones (Est). The number above each bar is the percent prevalence and n = number of subjects in each group.

In 1988, 3 years after the discovery of the chromosomal localization of *ADPKD1*, two publications described polycystic families that did not exhibit linkage to markers on the short arm of chromosome 16. Five years later, the location of the *ADPKD2* gene was assigned to chromosome 4q and a further 3 years later the *ADPKD2* gene was identified, sequenced, and cloned. The protein encoded by the *ADPKD2* gene is called polycystin-2. Polycystin-2 shares little sequence homology with polycystin-1, but is ubiquitous and also thought to be a membrane embedded protein that works in concert with polycystin-1 to regulate calcium flux and cell signaling.

It was long suspected that some families had a form of polycystic disease that was uniquely restricted to the liver. Affected family members had extensive hepatic cystic disease with either no or only a few renal cysts. Proof of a liver-restricted form of autosomal-dominant polycystic disease was provided by a Dutch family with isolated polycystic liver disease that was transmitted through three generations. None of the affected family members exhibited linkage to the genetic markers for either *ADPKD1* or *ADPKD2*. The chromosomal location, gene, and encoded protein have not yet been identified.

Symptoms

Most patients with polycystic liver disease are asymptomatic or may note only a protuberant abdomen. Patients with polycystic liver disease have been arbitrarily divided into two groups, massive or minimal, based upon a definition for massive of a total liver cyst: parenchymal volume ratio greater than 1. Using this definition, most symptomatic cases were restricted to patients with massive hepatic cystic disease. Both abdominal pain or discomfort and shortness of breath correlate with severity of hepatic cystic disease. Pain related to hepatic cystic disease is dull and aching and may be positional. Patients commonly describe abdominal fullness and often resort to ingestion of frequent small meals, since they experience early post-prandial fullness when they eat larger meals.

The majority of patients rarely exhibit any features of hepatic decompensation. Likewise, biliary complications are rare. The major consequence of growth of hepatic cysts is the development of abdominal symptoms without any major clinical manifestations of hepatic failure (Fig. 26.12). Rarely, a patient with polycystic liver disease will experience hepatic decompensation and variceal hemorrhage, ascites, or encephalopathy. Quantitative tests of hepatic function have indicated that nearly all polycystic patients, including those with massive hepatic cystic disease, have preserved hepatic metabolic capacity as judged from the clearance of caffeine and antipyrine. In contrast, there is a slight but significant increase in portosystemic shunting in those with massive hepatic cystic disease (Fig. 26.13). The increase in portosystemic shunting is modest and not usually associated with either variceal bleeding or other features of portal hypertension.

The most common, clinically relevant complications that arise in hepatic cysts are intracystic hemorrhage, infection, or post-traumatic rupture. Rare reports of cyst adenocarcinoma, biliary obstruction, Budd–Chiari syndrome, or hepatic failure exist. Figure 26.12 lists the complications, the preferred method of diagnosis, and options for medical or surgical management. In addition to these complications, patients with polycystic disease may have a variety of other associated conditions including: mitral valve prolapse, diverticulosis, inguinal hernias, and berry aneurysms of the cerebral circulation.

Laboratory investigation

Blood count and standard biochemical tests of liver disease are usually normal. Some patients with hepatic cystic disease exhibit elevations in γ-glutamyl transferase (GGT), and there

Clinical complications in polycystic liver disease		
Complication	**Diagnosis**	**Treatment**
Cyst infection	CT, MRI, In-WBC scan	Antibiotics (fluoroquinolones); drainage, if not responding
Cyst hemorrhage	CT, MRI	Medical management, pain control
Cyst adenocarcinoma	CT, MRI, aspiration cytology	Surgical resection
Portal hypertension	Endoscopy, hepatic angiography	EST/EVL, P-S shunt, OLTx
Hepatic failure	Clinical diagnosis	Medical management or OLT
Budd–Chiari	Hepatic venography	Cyst decompression, if unsuccessful then resection or OLTx
Rupture of cyst	Clinical suspicion	Medical management, pain control
Biliary obstruction	ERCP	Stent placement, cyst decompression

Figure 26.12 Complications in polycystic liver disease. The range of potential complications and the appropriate investigation and management. In-WBC scan, indium-labeled white blood cell scan; EST, endoscopic sclerotherapy; EVL, endoscopic variceal ligation; P-S shunt, portosystemic shunt; OLTx, orthotopic liver transplantation; ERCP, endoscopic retrograde cholangiopancreatography.

Portosystemic shunts

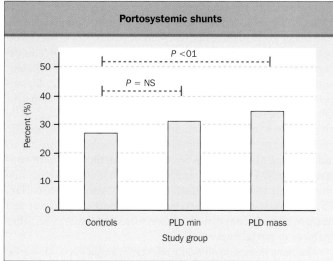

Figure 26.13 Portosystemic shunts. Portosystemic shunting is slightly increased in patients with polycystic liver disease (PLD) who have the most severe hepatic cystic disease. Min, minimal; mass, massive.

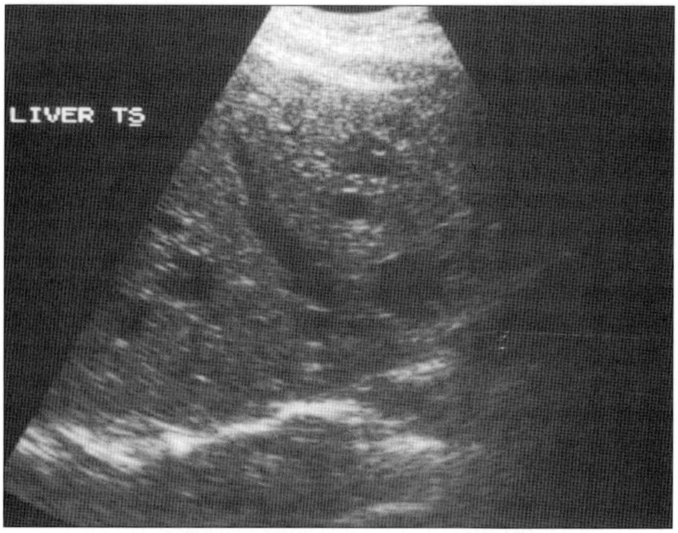

Figure 26.14 Cysts on ultrasonography. Multiple cysts are seen throughout the liver in a patient with polycystic liver disease. (By kind permission of Dr. H. Irving.).

is a weak, but significant, correlation of GGT with severity of hepatic cystic disease. Plain radiographs of chest and abdomen are usually normal, except for elevation of the right hemidiaphragm in those with massive disease. Barium studies are unremarkable except for liver enlargement and mass effect of the enlarged liver and kidneys extrinsically to compress the column of barium in the colon. Polycystic patients may have extensive diverticular disease that is expressed at a relatively early age.

Modern imaging methods (ultrasonography, CT, nuclear scans, and MRI) easily demonstrate hepatic cysts. Ultrasonography is preferred as the initial screening test, and other scans are reserved for specific indications or research applications. Hepatic cysts appear as thin-walled cavities without intraluminal echogenicity on ultrasonography (Fig. 26.14). Computed tomography scans reveal similar findings with minor differences in Hounsfield units between cysts. However, CT scans may exhibit significant heterogeneity between uncomplicated cysts. Standard radio-isotope scans are of little diagnostic value; HIDA scans are normal; and indium-labeled white blood cells scans may be useful in diagnosing hepatic cyst infection.

Cyst fluid

There have been several analyses of hepatic cyst fluid and all demonstrate that the composition is consistent with a biliary origin for hepatic cysts. Electrolytes reflect plasma levels, glucose is low to nondetectable, secretory immunoglobulin A is present, and cyst fluid is relatively enriched in GGT. *In vivo*, cyst secretion studies suggest that hepatic cysts may secrete fluid in response to intravenously administered secretin. Under ultrasound guidance, catheters were placed in hepatic cysts and cyst fluid labeled with [99m]technetium-HIDA. After measurement of basal excretion water secretion, secretin was administered intravenously and stimulated secretion was assessed. Analysis of isotopic dilatation suggested that these cysts secreted fluid in response to secretin. *In vitro* studies have further confirmed the biliary origin and nature of hepatic cystic epithelium.

Treatment
medical
There are no medical therapies for polycystic liver disease that are effective in causing cyst involution or that prevent cyst formation. The finding of secretin-induced secretion by hepatic cysts prompted clinicians to attempt to reduce cyst volume using long-acting somatostatin analog. This anecdotal experience failed to demonstrate any significant effect on hepatic cyst growth or size. One of the more intriguing observations is the finding that hepatic cystic disease may be influenced by female gender, pregnancy, or use of exogenous female steroid hormones. A recent prospective study quantitated liver (cyst and parenchymal) and kidney volumes at baseline and after 1 year of follow-up in ADPKD women on and off estrogen replacement therapy. Exogenous estrogen did not influence renal cyst growth but the growth of hepatic cysts was significantly greater in women on estrogen therapy (Fig. 26.15). The clinician must individualize the case for estrogen treatment by weighing this potentially deleterious effect against the potential for other benefits (bone metabolism, amelioration of estrogen-withdrawal symptoms, lipid metabolism) or risks (thromboembolism, uterine, or breast cancer).

Radiologic cyst aspiration and sclerosis
Symptomatic patients with polycystic disease are often referred to interventional radiologists for cyst aspiration and cyst sclerotherapy (alcohol, doxycycline). This approach should be restricted to patients with one, or a few dominant cysts. Most patients with polycystic disease have too many cysts or the cysts that they have are of insufficient size to warrant percutaneous aspiration and sclerotherapy. Cyst sclerotherapy requires ultrasound- or CT-guided percutaneous puncture of the targeted cyst and placement of an intracystic drainage catheter. Fluid is aspirated from the cyst and then a sclerosant, usually ethanol or a tetracycline derivative (doxycycline), is infused. The patient is moved to ensure contact of the sclerosant with the entire epithelial lining of the cyst cavity. The goal of treatment is destruction

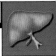
of the epithelial surface. The sclerosant is then aspirated and the catheter is either removed or placed to gravity drainage or low intermittent suction. For large cysts (>100mL or diameter of >6cm) we prefer to leave the catheter to drain for 24 hours and perform a second treatment the next day, before removing the catheter. Success in obliterating individual cysts in polycystic patients is approximately 90%.

Cyst fenestration

Cyst fenestration is the most commonly-applied surgical treatment in the management of symptomatic massive hepatic cystic disease (Fig. 26.16). Two approaches have been used: open laparotomy and, more recently, laparoscopy. Several series of open laparotomy, encompassing large numbers of patients, indicate that this approach results in satisfactory resolution of symptoms. However, open laparotomy is associated with prolonged hospitalization and the morbidity of major abdominal surgery. Operative mortality is low (<1%) and reported rates of postoperative complications (bleeding, infection, bile leak, ascites) range from 0 to 50%. Because of its less invasive nature, laparoscopic cyst fenestration is gaining increasing acceptance as an alternative surgical technique. Advantages of laparoscopic surgery include: less morbidity, reduced duration of hospital stay, and the potential for outpatient surgical management. Individual center experience with laparoscopic cyst decompression is rather limited but the sum of the results in the reported literature suggests that this approach is effective and associated with low mortality (<1%) and morbidity (0–25%).

Liver resection

One center recently reported their experience with partial liver resection in the management of 31 patients with highly symptomatic, massive hepatic cystic disease. Their ages ranged from 34 to 69, the gender ratio (male:female) was 3:28, and renal function varied from normal to dialysis-dependency.

Nearly all patients experienced significant relief from symptoms and long-term sustained reduction in symptoms was common (>95%). However, over 50% experienced significant perioperative morbidity and there was one perioperative death (due to rupture of an intracranial aneurysm). Although resection is promising for some patients, we would currently reserve hepatic resection for those cases that fail to respond to or are refractory to cyst decompression.

Liver transplantation

Polycystic patients with hepatic failure may be considered for hepatic transplantation using the standard criteria that are applied to all patients with end-stage liver disease. However, as noted above, the vast majority of patients with polycystic liver disease have preserved hepatic function, and hepatic failure sufficient to warrant transplantation is rarely encountered. The patient with massive hepatic cystic disease should only be considered for hepatic transplantation when other options are unavailable or have failed. Isolated liver transplantation is considered for those patients with preserved renal function, but who have massive hepatic cystic disease with symptoms or complications not amenable to other interventions. Combined liver and kidney transplantation should be considered in those patients with end-stage renal disease (ESRD), on or near dialysis, with symptomatic massive hepatic cystic disease that is not amenable to radiologic, laparoscopic or alternative surgical interventions. Cyst infection, hemorrhage, and adenocarcinoma are not indications for hepatic transplantation. Cyst reduction procedures (fenestration, resection, sclerosis) are preferred in the initial management of Budd–Chiari syndrome or biliary obstruction due to hepatic cysts.

Solitary hepatic cyst

Solitary hepatic cysts are relatively common, usually asymptomatic, and most often discovered incidentally during the

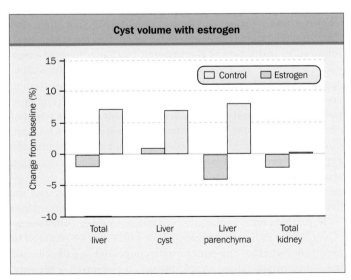

Figure 26.15 Cyst volume: postmenopausal estrogen increases liver volume. Percentage of volume change in liver and kidney at the end of 1 year of follow-up is shown. Estrogen-treated patients are depicted by green bar and non-treated controls as orange bar.

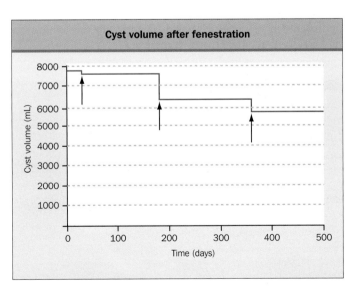

Figure 26. 16 Cyst volume after fenestration. The reduction in liver volume achieved by sequential laparoscopic cyst fenestration in a single patient is shown. Initial liver volume was 7710mL and final, after 3 procedures (arrows indicates the days of laparoscopic cyst decompression), was 5677mL.

evaluation of a wide variety of abdominal symptoms or disorders. Exact prevalence of solitary hepatic cysts for the US population is unknown, but the female:male ratio is approximately 4:1. A recent Taiwanese study used ultrasonography in a large-scale community-based screening programme for simple hepatic cysts to explore the age- and sex-specific prevalence, and in a hospital-based study to record the size of simple hepatic cysts. A total of 3600 subjects in eight communities underwent screening ultrasonography, and 156 simple hepatic cysts in 132 study subjects were detected. The overall prevalence was, therefore, 3.60%. Prevalence increased with age, ranging from 0.83% below age 40 to 7.81% in subjects over 60 years of age. The sizes of 219 hepatic cysts in 167 hospitalized patients were measured; 53% had diameters between 1 and 3cm, and only 7% were larger than 5cm. Cysts occurred more commonly in the right lobe and were twice as prevalent in women. All of these cysts were asymptomatic and none of the patients suffered clinical consequences (Fig. 26.17).

Clinical features

Solitary cysts that become symptomatic typically have diameters greater than 5cm and they present with localized pain in the right upper quadrant of the abdomen. Rarely, solitary hepatic cysts may develop intracystic hemorrhage, infection, or neoplasia. The latter complications may be diagnosed by radiologic imaging studies or cyst aspiration, culture, or cytologic and chemical analysis of cyst fluid.

Treatment

Asymptomatic solitary hepatic cysts are best managed conservatively. The preferred treatment of symptomatic cysts is ultrasound- or CT-guided percutaneous cyst aspiration followed by alcohol (or doxycycline) sclerotherapy. This approach is more than 90% effective in controlling symptoms and ablating the cyst cavity. The recurrence rate after successful ablation is only 5–15%. If the radiologically guided, percutaneous approach is ineffective or unavailable, treatment may include either laparoscopic or open surgical cyst fenestration. The laparoscopic approach is increasingly utilized for anatomically accessible cysts and greater than 90% efficacy is reported.

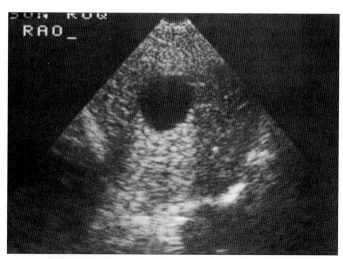

Figure 26.17 Solitary hepatic cyst. Ultrasonography of a large cyst in the right lobe of the liver. (By kind permission of Dr. H. Irving.).

CONGENITAL HEPATIC FIBROSIS

Congenital hepatic fibrosis is a rare, inherited, autosomal-recessive disorder that is most often associated with autosomal recessive polycystic kidney disease. Other clinical associations include adult ADPKD, renal dysplasia, nephronophthisis, Meckel–Gruber syndrome, Ivemark syndrome, Jeune syndrome, vaginal atresia, and tuberous sclerosis. Congenital hepatic fibrosis can coexist with other fibrocystic liver diseases such as Caroli's disease and choledochal cyst. The histopathologic features may vary, but in nearly all cases there is fibrous enlargement of the portal tracts, which contain abnormally shaped bile ducts. Congenital hepatic fibrosis typically involves all lobes of the liver equally, but on occasion one lobe of the liver may be preferentially affected. Von Meyenburg complexes (VMCs), also referred to as bile duct microhamartomas, are dilated, ectatic, intra- and interlobular bile ducts embedded in a fibrous stroma, and occur in nearly all patients with congenital hepatic fibrosis (VMCs are also commonly found in both ADPKD and Caroli's disease).

Clinical features

Congenital hepatic fibrosis presents in three clinical forms: portal hypertension, recurrent cholangitis, and asymptomatic or latent disease. The first two forms are usually diagnosed in early childhood in patients who present with variceal hemorrhage or unexplained biliary sepsis, respectively. In contrast, some patients will be detected later, during their adult years, when they are evaluated for unexplained hepatomegaly or portal hypertension. Rarely, patients present with evidence of both portal hypertension and cholestasis, the latter due to either associated biliary anomalies (Caroli's disease) or to intrinsic destructive cholangiopathy. In general, hepatic function is well preserved, despite portal hypertension or bouts of cholangitis, although some patients experience progressive hepatic failure in long-term follow-up.

Treatment

The first-line treatment of variceal hemorrhage is endoscopic variceal eradication (either sclerotherapy or ligation treatment), followed by institution of β-adrenergic blockade. In most cases, varices may be successfully obliterated by the endoscopic approach, thereby controlling this potentially life-threatening complication. Surgical shunts or transjugular intrahepatic portosystemic shunt (TIPS) are reserved for patients who fail endoscopic therapy, bleed from gastric varices or who have portal hypertensive gastropathy. Occasionally patients will experience progressive hepatic fibrosis and hepatic dysfunction after long-standing portosystemic shunt surgery, and development of this complication may necessitate consideration for liver transplantation.

In patients with cholangitis, radiologic imaging (ultrasonography, biliary radioscintigraphy, CT, or MRI) may be required to determine whether the patient with congenital hepatic fibrosis has concomitant biliary cystic disease. If the latter is present, the treatment of cholangitis is centered around provision of adequate biliary drainage, relief of obstruction (papillotomy with stone extraction or stricture dilatation), and control of infection with antibiotics. In the absence of biliary cystic disease or cholangiocarcinoma (said to occur in as many as 6% of cases

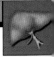

of congenital hepatic fibrosis), cholestasis may be related to idiopathic inflammatory destructive cholangiopathy and respond to UDCA therapy.

In general, patients with congenital hepatic fibrosis lack evidence of significant hepatic dysfunction or hepatic failure and they respond to the management of complications as noted above. Indications for hepatic transplantation include:

- variceal hemorrhage or hemorrhage from portal hypertensive gastropathy that is not responsive to endoscopic treatment or amenable to portosystemic shunt surgery or TIPS;
- recurrent cholangitis that is not amenable to medical, endoscopic, radiologic or surgical therapy; and
- hepatic failure (development of coagulopathy, biochemical deterioration, ascites, or portosystemic encephalopathy).

Since patients with congenital hepatic fibrosis often have autosomal-recessive polycystic kidney disease, one may need to consider combined liver–kidney transplantation in suitable candidates.

CHOLEDOCHAL CYST

Choledochal cysts are cystic dilatations that may occur throughout the macroscopic intra- and extrahepatic biliary tree. Although the term choledochal cyst has been used for any cystic dilatation of the biliary tree, isolated choledochal cysts are usually restricted to only the common hepatic or bile duct. Despite the uncommon occurrence of choledochal cysts, there are hundreds of reports in the literature encompassing over 3000 cases.

Choledochal cyst is a rare condition in the Western hemisphere, but, it is relatively more common among Japanese and other Oriental populations. Several classifications of choledochal cysts have been proposed but the most commonly cited in the medical literature is outlined in Fig. 26.18. The pattern of inheritance is unclear and there have been no definitive studies of either the genetic markers or molecular biology of choledochal cysts.

The pathogenesis of choledochal cyst is unknown. Several theories have been proposed. The most favored theory is that congenital weakness of the common bile duct and relative distal obstruction, due to congenital pancreatobiliary malformation, facilitate ascending infection of the bile duct (cholangitis) or chronic reflux of pancreatic enzymes. Support for this theory is found in experimental models in which choledochal cysts have been produced by removing epithelium, ligating the distal portion of the bile duct, and anastomosing the pancreatic duct directly to the biliary system. Histologically, the cyst walls are made up of fibrous tissue representing a chronic inflammatory process and the epithelial lining is either partially or completely absent.

Clinical features

The most common clinical presentation of choledochal cyst is a relatively young patient (child or adolescent) with pain, mass in the right upper quadrant or epigastrium, and jaundice. In one series of 740 cases jaundice was the most common and consistent presenting feature. In infants, jaundice is often the only sign and the disorder may be difficult to distinguish from biliary atresia. The majority of the patients have been diagnosed before age 30 years and the male:female ratio in most series is about 1:4.

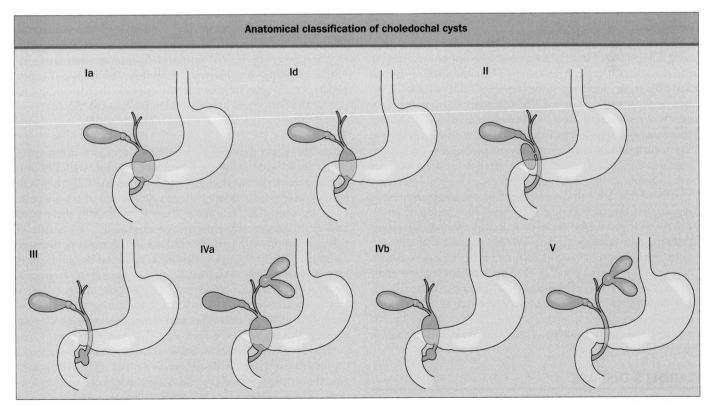

Figure 26.18 Anatomical classification of choledochal cysts. The various anatomic types of choledochal cysts are shown. Type Ia, choledochal cyst; type Ib, segmental choledochal dilatation; type Ic, diffuse or cylindrical duct dilatation; type II, extrahepatic duct diverticulum; type III, choledochocele; type IVa, multiple intra- and extrahepatic duct cyst; type IVb, multiple extrahepatic duct cyst; type V, intrahepatic duct cyst (Caroli's disease). (Reprinted with permission. Todani et al, AMJ. 1977;134:263–9.)

Reported complications include spontaneous and traumatic rupture, rupture during pregnancy, liver abscess, cirrhosis, and complications related to portal hypertension including gastroesophageal varices and development of cholangiocarcinoma. The incidence of cholangiocarcinoma ranges from 2.5 to 17.5%, which is 5–35 times greater than the population at-large. The incidence of carcinoma increases throughout life and approaches 50% by age 50 years. Internal drainage procedures without cyst excision appear to accelerate the development of cholangiocarcinoma. Bacterial overgrowth and increased levels of secondary bile acids may contribute to cyst metaplasia and carcinoma. The tumors may originate in different parts of the pancreatobiliary system, including liver, gallbladder, intrahepatic ducts, pancreatic ducts, and pancreas.

Diagnosis

The diagnosis of a choledochal cyst should always be suspected in a child presenting with recurrent abdominal pain, jaundice, and raised serum amylase. Initial imaging of the biliary tree by ultrasonography or radioscintigraphy (HIDA scans) is usually diagnostic. Confirmation and anatomic definition may require CT, ERCP, or percutaneous transhepatic cholangiogram (PTC). Patients with extrahepatic choledochal cysts have an increased incidence of anomalous pancreaticobiliary junction, which requires ERCP when planning for excision of the cyst. In recent years endoscopic ultrasonography has been a useful imaging method for patients with suspected anomalous pancreaticobiliary junction. Prenatal ultrasonography can detect choledochal cysts *in utero*, which may help antenatal counseling since early neonatal cyst excision and duct revision may be required.

Treatment

It is generally agreed that choledochal cysts require surgical treatment. The preferred surgical treatment is complete cyst excision with Roux-en-Y hepaticojejunostomy. This eliminates any opportunity for stasis, infection, stone formation, and possible development of cholangiocarcinoma. The procedure provides excellent long-term results with low morbidity and mortality, but life-long follow-up may be necessary to avoid potential problems, such as biliary cirrhosis. Internal cyst drainage procedures (cystoduodenostomy, cystojejunostomy) have often been unsatisfactory with a complication rate as high as 50%, and this procedure may actually accelerate the development of cholangiocarcinoma. Unilobar intrahepatic cystic disease is usually treated by resection of the affected lobe of the liver. Radiologic and endoscopic drainage procedures are used to stabilize patients with acute or recurrent cholangitis. However, recurrent symptoms are common and the risk of development of cholangiocarcinoma is not eliminated. When features of end-stage liver disease develop, due to long-standing, progressive biliary obstruction, or when endoscopic, radiologic or surgical therapy have failed to resolve the biliary infectious complications, orthotopic liver transplantation may be considered.

CAROLI'S DISEASE

In 1958, Caroli described a syndrome of congenital malformation of intrahepatic bile ducts characterized by segmental cystic dilatation of the intrahepatic ducts, increased incidence of biliary lithiasis, cholangitis and liver abscesses, absence of cirrhosis and portal hypertension, and association of renal cystic disease. Subsequent to Caroli's initial reports two distinct disease entities associated with Caroli's disease have been recognized: the simple type, which is associated with medullary sponge kidney in 60–80% of cases; and the periportal fibrosis type, which is associated with congenital hepatic fibrosis, cirrhosis, portal hypertension, and esophageal varices.

Clinical features

The most common presenting symptoms of Caroli's disease are recurrent episodes of fever, chills, and abdominal pain due to cholangitis, with peak incidence in early adult life. Males and females are equally affected, in contrast to the female predominance of polycystic disease, simple hepatic cysts, and choledochal cysts. More than 80% present with symptoms before the age of 30 years. Rarely, the disease presents later in life with evidence of portal hypertension and its complications, most commonly bleeding esophageal varices. The risk of development of cholangiocarcinoma in Caroli's disease is about 7%. Biliary lithiasis is found in one-third and predisposes patients to recurrent episodes of cholangitis due to obstruction and ascending infections. Occasional patients also experience multiple liver abscesses. The genetics are unclear, with both autosomal-dominant and autosomal-recessive patterns of inheritance proposed. There have been no molecular biologic studies of Caroli's disease.

Diagnosis

Caroli's disease is typically discovered by ultrasonography performed during evaluation of biliary obstruction or cholangitis. Communication of the intrahepatic cysts with the biliary tree is usually confirmed by scintigraphy, CT scan after biliary contrast, ERCP or PTC. Some studies have suggested that CT is superior to ultrasonography in the initial evaluation of adult patients. Ultrasonography is preferred in children. Percutaneous transhepatic cholangiography and ERCP provide detailed examination of the biliary tree and may aid in therapy (fig. 26.19).

Treatment

Adequate biliary drainage is the primary approach in the management of Caroli's disease. Endoscopic therapy with ERCP is effective in removing sludge or stones from the CBD but is of limited utility in providing adequate drainage of intrahepatic cysts. In contrast, PTC is more effective in draining these cysts and avoids recurrent episodes of cholangitis, especially if patients comply with periodic flushing and changing of drainage catheters. Rarely the cystic disease is confined to one hepatic lobe, and, in this circumstance, hepatic lobectomy is often curative. Although some have advocated hepaticojejunostomy after partial hepatectomy as primary therapy, the long-term efficacy of this procedure is uncertain, and the extensive surgery could compromise the outcome from hepatic transplantation.

There are two main indications for hepatic transplantation in Caroli's disease: hepatic decompensation and recurrent cholangitis that is unresponsive to endoscopic or radiologic interventions. Most patients with Caroli's disease have preserved hepatic function but some have associated congenital hepatic fibrosis and portal hypertension. Bleeding from esophageal varices is usually controlled by endoscopic therapy (sclerotherapy or ligation). Transjugular intrahepatic portosystemic

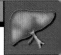

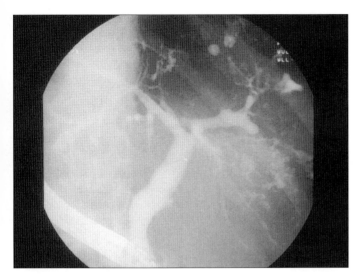

Figure 26.19 Caroli's disease. This ERCP demonstrates the typical intrahepatic biliary cysts of Caroli's disease. (By kind permission of Dr. H. Irving.)

shunt placement to decompress portal hypertension is relatively contraindicated due to the extensive cystic disease, similar to polycystic liver disease. If, however, variceal bleeding recurs despite the maximum endoscopic therapy or if the patient develops cirrhosis (biliary type), and experiences decompensation with the development of ascites or encephalopathy, then transplantation is preferred. The most common indication for transplantation is recurrent cholangitis despite prior interventions. Transplantation should be considered if patients experience two or more bouts of cholangitis despite maximum radiologic or endoscopic therapy.

CHOLANGIOCARCINOMA

Cholangiocarcinoma is defined as primary malignancy of the biliary ductular epithelium or the periductular biliary glands. The tumor may develop anywhere along the course of the large ductular biliary system and it is commonly defined by either anatomic location (intrahepatic, extrahepatic, or intraductular) or histology (cholangiocarcinoma versus hepatocholangiocarcinoma). Tumors that arise at the hilum of the liver, near the bifurcation of the left and right ducts, are commonly referred to as Klatskin's tumors. Risk factors for development of cholangiocarcinoma include: choledochal cysts, primary sclerosing cholangitis, chronic choledocholithiasis, exposure to thorium dioxide, and oriental cholangiohepatitis due to *Clonorchis sinensis*. In Western countries the most common association is with primary sclerosing cholangitis (PSC). Most patients with PSC who develop cholangiocarcinoma have had PSC for many years (>10 years) and have had a clinical course characterized by obstructive jaundice and repeated bouts of bacterial cholangitis. However, cholangiocarcinoma may develop in the absence of these features. In published series, cholangiocarcinoma complicated PSC in 10–20% of all cases and was an incidental finding in up to 9% of patients undergoing liver transplantation for PSC. One case–control study suggested that smoking was a risk factor for development of cholangiocarcinoma in PSC. Development of thrombophlebitis in a patient with PSC may also be a harbinger of underlying cholangiocarcinoma.

Diagnosis

The most common presenting symptom is jaundice, which is usually painless or associated with mild discomfort in the right upper quadrant of the abdomen. Pruritus is common, especially in those with underlying PSC. Late features of the disease include anorexia, weight loss, weakness, and fatigue. The biochemical profile reflects extrahepatic obstruction with elevations primarily in conjugated bilirubin, alkaline phosphatase, and GGT. There is no sensitive and specific serologic marker for cholangiocarcinoma, although CA 19-9 is elevated in most cases and some reports suggest that this test can be useful in detecting the development of cholangiocarcinoma in the setting of PSC. One recent study suggested that positron emission tomography may be sensitive and specific in diagnosing cholangiocarcinoma. Until these initially promising results can be verified in larger studies, the diagnosis is dependent upon demonstration of intraductal tumor by cholangiography (Fig. 26.20), positive biliary cytology (on repeated testing), or tissue biopsy.

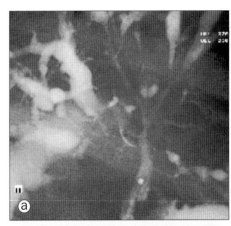

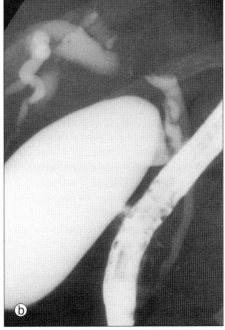

Figure 26.20 Cholangiocarcinoma. (a) Cholangiocarcinoma of the common hepatic duct with proximal dilatation of intrahepatic ducts. (b) Cholangiocarcinoma of the common hepatic duct in another patient. The stricture causes accumulation of dye distally in the gallbladder at ERCP. (By kind permission of Dr. H. Irving.)

Treatment

Standard oncologic regimens, employing external-beam irradiation and systemic chemotherapy, have been ineffective. Surgery is indicated for patients with locally confined, resectable tumors who lack metastatic disease. However, few patients meet these criteria and advanced liver disease related to PSC precludes extensive hepatobiliary surgery. The results with liver transplantation have also been disappointing: the 5-year patient survival after liver transplantation for cholangiocarcinoma is only 17% (Fig. 26.21). This poor result has prompted many to suggest that the diagnosis of cholangiocarcinoma is an absolute contraindication to hepatic transplantation.

A number of new approaches are currently under evaluation: high-dose, external beam irradiation, endoscopic-guided photodynamic therapy, combination treatment with iridium implants and systemic chemotherapy, and combination therapies before and after hepatic transplantation. Multivisceral transplantation (liver, stomach, duodenum, pancreas) has also been proposed as therapy for cholangiocarcinoma. The benefits and outcomes from these approaches remain to be defined.

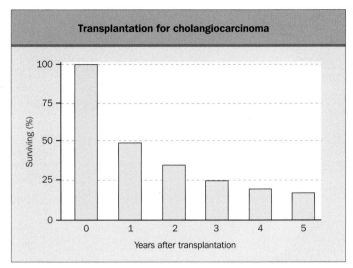

Figure 26.21 Liver transplantation for cholangiocarcinoma. Survival of patients with cholangiocarcinoma after hepatic transplantation is shown. Five-year outcome is poor with only 17% surviving. Innovative strategies employing peri- and postoperative chemotherapy and radiation offer promise in the treatment of this difficult clinical problem.

PRACTICE POINT

Illustrative case

A 35-year-old woman presented with upper abdominal discomfort. Her mother had died 1 year previously after an unsuccessful liver and kidney transplant for polycystic disease. Two of her three siblings were known to have polycystic disease. She had three children but they had not been screened for polycystic disease. She was taking the oral contraceptive pill but no other medication. The remainder of her medical history was uneventful. On physical examination the noted abnormalities were a blood pressure of 155/102mmHg and a palpable liver 2cm below the costal margin. Ultrasound examination confirmed the presence of cysts in the liver and a small number of renal cysts. The patient requested information on her future.

Interpretation

The confirmation of the diagnosis came as no surprise to the patient, although she had hoped that her symptoms were a psychological reaction to her mother's death. The use of the oral contraceptive pill was considered as a factor that might change the rate of expansion of the cystic disease and she was advised to use alternative means of contraception. The indications for transplantation in her mother were discussed and it was concluded that the venous outflow obstruction that led to the liver transplant was unlikely to occur, but that the need for a renal transplant was much more likely. She was advised of the importance of maintaining good control of the hypertension because of the association between polycystic disease and Berry aneurysm. Finally, she was advised to have her children screened for polycystic disease.

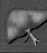
FURTHER READING

DeSautels SG, Slivka A, Hutson WR, et al. Postcholecystectomy pain syndrome: pathophysiology of abdominal pain in sphincter of Oddi type III. Gastroenterology. 1999; 116:900–905. *Good clinical study of the features of disordered tone of the sphincter of Oddi.*

Diehl AK. Epidemiology and natural history of gallstone disease. Gastroenterol Clin North Am. 1991;20:1–20. *Good review of the epidemiology and natural history of gallstones.*

Everhart J, Khare M, Hill M, Maurer KR. Prevalence and ethnic differences in gallbladder disease in the United States. Gastroenterology. 1999;117:632–9. *Results of over 14,000 ultrasound assessments for cholelithiasis.*

Fick GM, Gabow PA. Natural history of autosomal dominant polycystic kidney disease. Ann Rev Med. 1994; 45:23–9. *Clinical review of topic.*

Gabow PA. Autosomal dominant polycystic kidney disease. N Engl J MEd. 1993; 329:332–42. *First description of the gene responsible for ADPKD2.*

Huang JF, Chen SC, Lu SN, et al. Prevalence and size of simple hepatic cysts in Taiwan: community- and hospital-based sonographic surveys. Kao-Hsiung i Hsueh Ko Hsueh Tsa Chih [Kaohsiung J Med Sci]. 1995; 11:564–7. *Study of prevalence of simple cysts in 3600 subjects.*

Ko CW, Sekijima JH, Lee SP. Biliary sludge. Ann Intern Med. 1999;130:301–11. *Recent review of biliary sludge.*

Lai ECS, Mok FPT, Tan ESY, et al. Endoscopic biliary drainage for severe acute cholangitis. N Engl J Med. 1992;326:1582–6. *Randomized comparison of endoscopic and surgical management of cholangitis.*

May GR, Sutherland LR, Shaffer EA. Efficacy of bile acid therapy for gallstone dissolution: a meta-analysis of randomized trials. Aliment Pharmacol Ther. 1993;7:139–48. *Good analysis of the efficacy of efficacy of bile acid therapy for gallstones involving 23 trials and 1949 patients.*

Parfrey PS, Bear JC, Morgan J, et al. The diagnosis and prognosis of autosomal dominant polycystic kidney disease. N Eng J Med. 1990;323:1085–90. *First description of the gene responsible for ADPKD1.*

Que F, Nagorney DM, Gross JB Jr, Torres VE. Liver resection and cyst fenestration in the treatment of severe polycystic liver disease. Gastroenterology. 1995;108(2):487–94. *Description of surgical management of 31 cases with severe disease.*

Rha SY, Stovroff MC, Glick PL, Allen JE, Ricketts RR. Choledochal cysts: a ten year experience. Am Surg. 1996;62(1):30–4. *Description of extensive clinical experience of choledochal cysts.*

Shiffman ML, Kaplan GD, Brinkman-Kaplan V, Vickers FF. Prophylaxis against gallstone formation with ursodeoxycholic acid in patients participating in a very low calorie diet program. Ann Intern Med. 1995; 122:899–905. *Role of bile acids preventing gallstone recurrence.*

Steiner CA, Bass EB, Talamini MA, Pitt HA, Steinberg EP. Surgical rates and operative mortality for open and laparoscopic cholecystectomy in Maryland. N Engl J Med. 1994; 330:403–8. *Study demonstrating the advantages of laporoscopic therapy.*

Thistle, JL, Cleary, PA, Lachin, MJ, et al. The natural history of cholelithiasis: The National Cooperative Gallstone Study. Ann Intern Med. 1984;101:171–5. *Study of the natural history of biliary colic.*

Tikkakoski T, Makela JT, Leinonen S, et al. Treatment of symptomatic congenital hepatic cysts with single-session percutaneous drainage and ethanol sclerosis: technique and outcome. J Vasc Intervent Radiol. 1996; 7(2):235–9. *Good results obtained with aspiration and sclerosis of cysts.*

Todani T, Watanabe Y, Narusue M, Tobuchi K, Okajima K. Congenital bile duct cysts: classification, operative procedures and review of 37 cases including cancer arising from choledochal cyst. Am J Surg. 1977;134:263–9.

Ward CJ, Turley H, Ong ACM, et al. Polycystin, the polycystic kidney disease 1 protein, is expressed by epithelial cells in fetal, adult, and polycystic kidney. Proc Natl Acad Sci USA. 1996; 93(4):1524–8. *Characterization of the protein coded for by the gene associated with ADPKD1.*

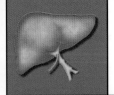

Chapter 27

Vascular Diseases of the Liver

Peter Clive Hayes and Syed Hasnain Ali Shah

INTRODUCTION

The vasculature of the liver is unusual in that it has both an arterial and a venous blood supply. Blood from the high pressure, highly oxygenated arterial side mixes with the low pressure, poorly oxygenated blood from the portal venous system in the hepatic sinusoids. These porous blood channels drain into central veins which in turn drain into hepatic veins before entering the inferior vena cava close to the right atrium. The hepatic artery supplies 35% of the blood flow and 50% of the oxygen to the liver. There is a little understood mechanism between the hepatic artery and portal vein which maintains a constant blood flow to the liver.

In this chapter diseases that affect the vascular structures will be considered (Fig. 27.1) with the exception of hyalinization of the space of Disse (a common and important pathologic process in the development, for example, of alcoholic cirrhosis) and hepatoportal sclerosis ('idiopathic portal hypertension'). Vascular disorders that occur secondary to systemic circulatory disturbances such as cardiac failure or cardiogenic shock likewise will not be discussed further (see Chapter 32).

HEPATIC ARTERIAL DISEASE

Hepatic artery occlusion
Hepatic artery occlusion is relatively uncommon and may give rise to a variety of clinical sequelae ranging from that which is asymptomatic to hepatic infarction and death. The consequences of hepatic artery occlusion depend upon the site of occlusion, the extent of the collateral circulation, and the speed of occlusion. If, for example, a thrombosis forms slowly in the hepatic artery, a collateral circulation from the gastric and gastroduodenal arteries may provide sufficient arterial flow with the whole process being asymptomatic and found incidentally at autopsy. Sudden occlusion, particularly if the portal venous in-flow is compromised, is likely to be fatal. In certain circumstances hepatic infarction may occur without occlusion of the hepatic artery, for example in cardiogenic shock.

Etiology and pathogenesis
Occlusion of the hepatic artery may be due to atheromatous disease, polyarteritis nodosa, giant cell arteritis or embolism in patients who have bacterial endocarditis. Thrombosis of the hepatic artery after liver transplantation is more common in those 20% of donor livers who have anomalous hepatic arterial anatomy. Occlusion may also be secondary to arterial dissection after hepatic arteriography or trauma. Where hepatic arterial occlusion gives rise to infarction this is usually segmental with the central area being pale, surrounded by a hemorrhagic region. As mentioned above, the size and extent of infarction is related to the adequacy of the collateral circulation.

Clinical features
The classic features of hepatic infarction are severe right upper quadrant abdominal pain accompanied by tachycardia, hypotension, fever and leukocytosis. If the liver damage is severe, then features of fulminant hepatic failure will develop. Liver function tests show a parenchymal injury pattern with marked increases in serum transaminases. Hepatic artery occlusion is well-recognized in the postoperative phase following liver transplantation, where a dramatic deterioration of the patient's condition occurs with the development of acute liver failure. Urgent retransplantation is then required. In transplant patients who have more gradual thrombosis, biliary strictures secondary to ischemia are common.

Sites and causes of hepatic vascular disease

Hepatic veins:
thrombosis
tumor

Inferior vena cava:
thrombosis
web
tumor

Venules:
veno-occlusive
disease

Portal vein:
thrombosis
tumor

Sinusoids

Splenic vein

Hepatic artery:
thrombosis
aneurysm

Superior mesentric
vein

Figure 27.1 Sites and causes of hepatic vascular disease.

Diagnosis

The diagnosis will usually be suggested by Doppler ultrasonography and confirmed by hepatic arteriography. Computed tomography (CT) and magnetic resonance imaging (MRI) may be useful in determining the extent of ischemic damage.

Natural history and prognosis

The outcome for patients who have hepatic artery occlusion, as mentioned above, depends to a great extent on the anatomic position of the occlusion, the rate of occlusion, and the state of the portal circulation. If, for example, the occlusion occurs proximal to branching of the gastric and gastroduodenal arteries, the collateral circulation cannot develop and the extent of infarction is consequently considerably greater. Sudden occlusion is more likely to give rise to hepatic infarction than slow thrombosis. If there is portal vein occlusion or a simultaneous occlusion of the hepatic artery and portal vein, the prognosis is extremely poor. If hepatic artery occlusion follows soon after liver transplantation, similarly the outcome is poor without urgent retransplantation.

Management

The management of patients who have hepatic artery occlusion depends upon the clinical sequelae. If acute liver failure develops then management should be instituted as described in Chapter 30. In patients who have less severe complications, management may be expectant and antibiotics should be used to prevent secondary infection in infarcted liver tissue.

Hepatic artery aneurysms

Aneurysm of the hepatic artery is a rare condition, the cause of which may be atheroma, polyarteritis nodosa, systemic infections (e.g. endocarditis, tuberculosis, and syphillis), and intra-abdominal sepsis; or it may be traumatic, for example following liver biopsy, or congenital. The aneurysm can be either intra- or extrahepatic and may show considerable variation in size. The aneurysm may thrombose, causing infarction or rupture giving rise to a hemorrhage. Hepatic artery aneurysms are commonest in middle-aged men and are often asymptomatic for long periods. The most common symptom is abdominal pain which can be severe particularly if there is arterial dissection. Rupture, which occurs in up to 80% of cases, may give rise to intraperitoneal hemorrhage or hemobilia. The triad of abdominal pain, jaundice, and gastrointestinal hemorrhage is said to be suggestive of hepatic artery aneurysms, but only occurs in approximately 30% of cases. Occasionally the aneurysm may compress the biliary tree giving rise to obstructive jaundice. The prognosis for hepatic artery aneurysm is poor if treatment has to be undertaken after rupture and urgent surgery is required. There is 80% mortality. However, in asymptomatic patients an aneurysm of the common hepatic artery proximal to the gastroduodenal artery can be ligated, but more peripheral aneurysms, including those involving the gastroduodenal artery, require reconstructive surgery. Intrahepatic arterial aneurysms may be treated by hepatic resection, segmental arterial ligation, or by embolization (Fig. 27.2).

Arterioportal fistulae

An arterioportal fistula is a rare but potentially treatable cause of portal hypertension. Fistulae within the liver are generally secondary to liver biopsy, blunt trauma, hepatocellular tumors or hereditary hemorrhagic telangiectasia. Extrahepatic fistulae usually follow rupture of an hepatic arterial aneurysm into the portal vein, or rupture between the splenic artery or vein.

Arterioportal fistulae give rise to portal hypertension associated with gastrointestinal bleeding and ascites and may also cause abdominal pain and intestinal ischemia. The diagnosis is usually made by either Doppler ultrasonography or by CT scanning. A hepatic bruit is usually present. Treatment of arterioportal fistulae depends on their size and position. Extrahepatic fistulae tend to increase in size and should be treated by surgery or embolization. Small intrahepatic fistulae may require no treatment.

PORTAL VEIN THROMBOSIS

Thombosis may occur in any part of the portal vascular system between the mesenteric veins and the portal radicals in the liver. Thrombosis can occur in an otherwise normal venous system, particularly in association with thrombophilic disorders. It may be associated with intra-abdominal inflammation or malignancy, or may be secondary to portal hypertension.

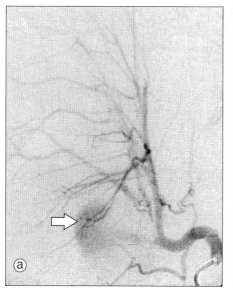
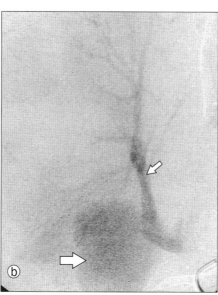

Figure 27.2 Hepatic arterial aneurysm.
(a) Traumatic hepatic arterial aneurysm filling with radiographic contrast (arrow). (b) The same aneurysm now filled (arrow). Early filling of a portal vein branch has occurred via an arteriovenous fistula (small arrow).

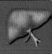
Etiology and pathogenesis

Thrombosis in the main portal vein accounts for approximately 10% of cases of portal hypertension in Western countries, and in approximately 50% of these cases no cause for the thrombosis is identified. In children, umbilical infections in particular are believed to be the commonest cause predisposing to portal vein thrombosis, but systemic infection leading to dehydration and hemoconcentration may also be important. Umbilical catheterization is believed to predispose to portal vein thrombosis, but evidence to support this is limited. In the majority of cases the thrombosis is discovered many years later rather than at the time of infection. Deficiency of protein C, protein S, or antithrombin III are common in children who have portal vein thrombosis, but this is probably secondary rather than causal. Predisposing factors to portal vein thrombosis in adults include intra-abdominal inflammation and malignancy, thrombophilia, and abdominal trauma (Fig. 27.3).

The frequency with which portal vein thrombosis complicates cirrhosis is probably less than was originally estimated from autopsy studies. For example, in a large cohort of Japanese patients who had cirrhosis, portal vein thrombosis was identified in less than 1%. Portal vein thrombosis complicating cirrhosis is probably commoner in those who have more advanced liver disease. The flow of blood within the portal vein may be reduced or reversed or even be stationary in cirrhosis. Overestimation may occur in studies using Doppler ultrasonography. Portal vein thrombosis may also occur in cases of portal hypertension not associated with cirrhosis, such as idiopathic portal hypertension and in partial nodular transformation of the liver. Thombosis in an otherwise normal portal vascular system is unusual and may be associated with thrombophilia. In these situations hepatic vein thrombosis may also be present. Thrombophilic disorders include protein C and protein S deficiency and the factor V Leiden mutation (see later).

Clinical features

Acute thrombosis

Acute thrombosis in the portal venous system presents with acute abdominal pain with or without diarrhea. Patients in whom portal vein thrombosis complicates intra-abdominal inflammation or malignancy may obviously present with features of the underlying disorder such as a perforated viscus or necrotizing pancreatitis. In patients who have intra-abdominal malignancy, the development of ascites may be due to portal vein thrombosis. In liver transplant recipients, portal vein thrombosis is generally less serious than hepatic artery thrombosis and loss of the graft is unusual.

Chronic portal vein thrombosis

This disorder is frequently asymptomatic and presents with splenomegaly or with complications of portal hypertension or is identified incidentally.

Children

Neonatal umbilical infection or childhood intra-abdominal inflammation may cause portal vein thrombosis. The presentation is often delayed for years and presenting features include gastrointestinal bleeding, hypersplenism, and splenomegaly. Presentation with ascites or encephalopathy is rare. Bleeding from gastroesophageal varices usually presents in adolescents and is unusual before the age of 3 years. In those who remain asymptomatic, evidence of hepatic dysfunction may develop in adulthood with mildly abnormal liver function tests.

Adults

The commonest presenting feature in adults who have portal vein thrombosis is gastrointestinal bleeding from gastroesophageal varices. In those who have associated cirrhosis, ascites may develop and encephalopathy is not unusual, particularly after variceal hemorrhage. Portal vein thrombosis is a relative contraindication to transplantation for liver disease especially if the thrombosis is extensive.

Investigations

Investigations used in the identification of portal hypertension are described in Chapter 6. They include abdominal ultrasound with Doppler studies to identify blood flow within the portal venous system and angiography which is used to define more accurately the extent of thrombosis. Wedged hepatic venous pressure in portal hypertension due to portal vein thrombosis is normal, but where the thrombosis is secondary to hepatic disease wedged hepatic venous pressure may be elevated. Gastrointestinal endoscopy is invaluable in identifying esophageal and gastric varices and in their treatment. Computed tomography may show the thrombosis within the vein lumen and MRI may also be valuable. The venous phase of angiography shows a filling defect, but the presence of extensive collaterals may make this investigation less reliable than expected (Figs 27.4 & 27.5).

Causes of portal vein occlusion
Sepsis, (e.g. systemic infection or portal pyemia)
Umbilical vein catheterization
Thrombophilia including myeloproliferative disorders:
paroxysmal noctural hemoglobinuria
Pregnancy and the oral contraceptive drugs
Surgery or abdominal trauma
Cirrhosis or hepatic venous occlusion
Neoplasia including liver tumors and tumors of structures
around the portal vein
Pancreatitis
Congenital
Idiopathic

Figure 27.3 Causes of portal vein occlusion.

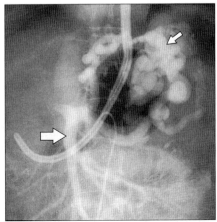

Figure 27.4 Venous phase of a mesenteric angiogram. Showing portal vein occlusion (large arrow). There is an extensive collateral circulation with varices (small arrow).

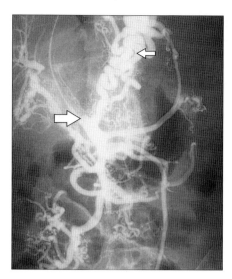

**Figure 27.5
Transhepatic
venogram showing
thrombosis in the
portal vein (arrow).**
There is a widespread
collateral circulation
(small arrow).

Liver function tests are generally normal in patients who have portal vein thrombosis not secondary to parenchymal liver disease, although mild abnormalities may be present in adults who have portal vein thrombosis. In such patients liver biopsy may show portal tract fibrosis with chronic inflammatory cell infiltration and with regular atrophy. Full blood count may show thrombocytopenia and leukopenia with or without anemia related to hypersplenism.

Prognosis

In patients who have acute thrombosis of the portal vein, there may be extensive thrombosis extending into the mesenteric veins in whom early surgical intervention for bowel infarction is essential. The prognosis of patients who have chronic portal vein thrombosis is to a large degree dependent upon any associated underlying disorder, such as cirrhosis. In those patients in whom no associated condition is identified, the outlook is good. Tolerance, for example, to gastrointestinal bleeding is better than in patients who have cirrhosis because of the preserved liver function. In children who present with variceal bleeding secondary to portal vein thrombosis, the risk of hemorrhage decreases after adolescence and hepatic dysfunction may occur years later associated with atrophy and portal tract fibrosis.

Management

The identification of portal vein thrombosis alone does not require intervention, but its complications do. If there is a reversible underlying cause this should be treated. In the majority of patients, portal vein thrombosis presents with variceal hemorrhage and control for this bleeding is the same as that used for other causes of variceal hemorrhage. Prevention of rebleeding is also generally the same as for other causes of variceal hemorrhage, although surgical intervention, especially splenorenal shunt surgery, is more often considered because of the preserved hepatic function and reduced risk of subsequent encephalopathy. Other surgical treatments such as esophageal transection or ligation of varices with splenectomy are less often useful, because of the high incidence of gastric varices. In children under the age of 10 years, because of technical difficulties related to portosystemic shunt surgery, endoscopic sclerotherapy is usually preferred. Currently band ligation of varices is technically difficult in small children. In occasional cases portal venous angioplasty may be

successfully undertaken. Successful thrombolysis for acute portal vein thrombosis has also been reported. Transjugular intrahepatic portal systemic stent shunts (TIPSS) are not normally indicated in this situation and would usually be impossible to establish.

Regional portal hypertension

Thrombosis of either splenic vein or mesenteric veins may give rise to regional portal hypertension. Thrombosis restricted to mesenteric veins is rare (Fig. 27.6), but may present with gastrointestinal bleeding in patients who do not have splenomegaly or esophageal varices.

Splenic vein thrombosis
Pathogenesis

The commonest causes for splenic vein thrombosis are pancreatitis with or without pancreatic pseudocysts and pancreatic tumors. Retroperitoneal infections or fibrosis, liver cirrhosis, and upper abdominal surgery are unusual causes. Thrombosis of the splenic vein gives rise to the development of collateral vessels between the spleen and the portal vein, namely portoportal shunts, or between the spleen and the vena cava or azygos vein, namely portosystemic shunts. In particular a collateral circulation develops via the short gastric veins into the gastric fundus, and then to the left gastric vein and portal vein. The result is prominent gastric varices but few in the lower esophagus.

Clinical features

The majority of patients who have splenic vein thrombosis present with gastrointestinal bleeding usually from gastric varices since esophageal varices are less common. Other patients may present with features related to the associated underlying disorder such as pancreatic neoplasia. The classic clinical feature is splenomegaly.

Diagnosis

The diagnosis of splenic vein thrombosis should be considered in patients who have splenomegaly and endoscopic findings of gastric varices. The diagnosis would generally be confirmed by Doppler ultrasonography, but venous phase mesenteric angiography may be required. Occasionally the slow retrograde flow in the splenic vein in patients who have cirrhosis may erroneously be interpreted as thrombosis. Hematologic investigations may reveal evidence of hypersplenism.

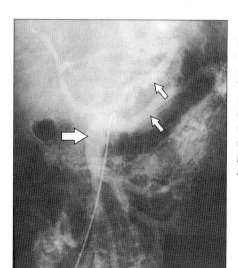

**Figure 27.6 Venous
phase of a superior
mesenteric artery
angiogram.** Showing a
thrombus in the superior
mesenteric vein (large
arrow). There is
retrograde filling of the
splenic vein and left
gastric vein (small
arrows).

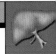
Prognosis
Prognosis depends to a large extent on the underlying predisposing cause. In those without serious underlying pathology the prognosis is good.

Management
In patients in whom thrombosis is confined to the splenic vein, splenectomy is the definitive treatment and curative. Endoscopic treatment, which is less effective in the management of gastric than in esophageal varices, is not usually helpful. Patients in whom splenic vein thrombosis is identified before variceal bleeding should be considered for prophylactic splenectomy, although they will need to understand fully the risks and benefits of such a procedure.

HEPATIC VENOUS OUTLET OBSTRUCTION

Many disorders give rise to obstruction of the hepatic veins. The obstruction can arise at a variety of sites between the acinar central veins and the inferior vena cava. For this reason the all-inclusive term of hepatic venous outlet obstruction is used rather than the more restricted terms of Budd–Chiari syndrome and veno-occlusive disease. These latter terms are used to describe disorders of the main hepatic veins and hepatic venules, respectively. Hepatic venous outlet obstruction will be discussed below under three main headings:
- disorders of the main hepatic veins;
- disorders affecting the inferior vena cava; and
- disorders of the hepatic venules.

Main hepatic vein disease
The clinical problem that arises from disorders that affect the main hepatic veins is commonly referred to as Budd–Chiari syndrome, named after Budd who described the disorder in 1845, and Chiari who reported a series of cases in 1899. The clinical syndrome produced varies considerably depending upon the cause, speed, and completeness of the hepatic vein occlusion.

Etiology and pathogenesis
The cause of obstruction of the main hepatic veins is most commonly due to thrombosis, but other causes such as tumor invasion are occasionally responsible. In the majority of patients in whom thrombosis in hepatic veins occurs, there is an underlying thrombogenic propensity, but in a significant minority no cause can be found. A list of the predisposing thrombogenic disorders is outlined in Figure 27.7.

The most important cause (a primary myeloproliferative disorder, which is associated with 60% of cases) may be readily identified by traditional hematologic investigations, but in some patients the culture of bone marrow cells is necessary to identify increased spontaneous formation of erythroid colonies. This abnormality may not be confined to just erythropoietin-independent growth of erythroid colonies, but defects may also affect the megakaryocyte and granulocyte–macrophage hemopoietic cell lines. This type of latent myeloproliferative disorder is responsible for a significant proportion of cases of thrombosis of the main hepatic veins classified as idiopathic in early series.

Recently a genetic disorder due to mutation of a single base pair in the factor V gene (factor V Leiden) has been identified which gives rise to thrombophilia, as a result of a defect in the

anticoagulant response to activated protein C (APC). This is now believed to be the cause of Budd–Chiari syndrome in around 25% of cases.

Another important predisposing risk factor is the use of the oral contraceptive pill, although in certain cases this drug probably has an additive effect to an underlying thrombophilia. Other disorders such as paroxysmal nocturnal hemoglobinuria, connective tissue disorders, and deficiencies in the thrombolysis system are uncommon, but can be screened for easily.

Obstruction of a single main hepatic vein is usually without clinical sequelae and it is only when obstruction of two of the three main hepatic veins occurs that symptoms arise (Fig. 27.8).

The obstruction to hepatic venous drainage gives rise to increased sinusoidal pressure with sinusoidal dilatation and congestion, particularly around the central vein of the hepatic lobules, and thus to portal hypertension. The increase in sinusoidal

---

Causes of hepatic venous flow obstruction

Myeloproliferative disorders: latent or overt
Coagulopathy: lupus anticoagulant and anticardiolipin antibodies, deficiency of antithrombin III, protein C or protein S, factor V Leiden mutation, Behçet's disease
Paroxysmal nocturnal haemoglobinuria
Drugs: oral contraceptives, dacarbazine
Pregnancy
Blunt abdominal trauma
Malignancy: hepatocellular carcinoma, renal cell or adrenal carcinoma, leiomyosarcoma of the IVC
IVC web
Infections: amoeibic abscess, schistosomiasis, hydatid disease
Idiopathic

Figure 27.7 Causes of hepatic venous outflow obstruction.

Drainage of the hepatic veins into the inferior vena cava

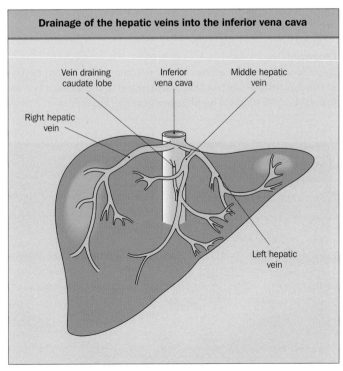

Figure 27.8 Schematic representation of the drainage of the hepatic veins into the inferior vena cava. A separate vein drains the caudate lobe which results in sparing of this lobe when the other veins are blocked.

pressure enhances filtration of interstitial fluid increasing hepatic lymphatic flow which may overflow through the liver capsule causing ascites. The reduced flow within the sinusoids also causes hepatocellular ischemia and necrosis, and where the thrombosis occurs rapidly acute liver failure may result. Where the occlusion is more gradual collateral vessels develop and nodular regeneration takes place within the liver, along with centrilobular fibrosis leading, sometimes within months, to cirrhosis. Because the caudate lobe drains independently into the inferior vena cava (see Fig. 27.8) it may be spared in the thrombotic process, and caudate lobe hypertrophy takes place. This may be marked and in fact may compress the inferior vena cava, but is only present in around 50% of cases.

Clinical features

These can vary from the development of fulminant hepatic failure within a few days (rarely), or within a few weeks, to a chronic form which develops over many months. The classical triad is abdominal pain, ascites, and hepatomegaly. In the acute form ascites develops rapidly, along with hepatomegaly, abdominal pain, and jaundice. Fulminant liver failure, with rapid progression to coma and death may occur. In the more common subacute or chronic form ascites is the classic feature. This may be resistant to medical management and be associated with functional renal failure, or it may respond, at least initially, to medical management. Those patients in whom ascites is readily controlled medically have a better prognosis. Abdominal pain and anorexia are common while jaundice, vomiting, diarrhea, and fever are variable. Gastrointestinal hemorrhage is also a recognized complication. Splenomegaly occurs as portal hypertension develops and a palpable caudate lobe may be found on examination. A negative hepatojugular reflex (i.e. absence of filling of the jugular vein with pressure exerted over the liver) may be observed. Differentiation of the Budd–Chiari syndrome from cardiac failure is important.

Diagnosis

In patients who have ascites and hepatomegaly in whom hepatic venous outflow obstruction is suspected, the diagnosis is confirmed in 75% of cases by ultrasonography (Fig. 27.9).

This is suggested by the presence of echogenic material in the lumen of the main hepatic veins, or stenosis of the veins with proximal dilatation. Ultrasonography will also allow assessment of the patency of the portal and superior mesenteric veins and the inferior vena cava. Computed tomography is useful, particularly in patients in whom the ultrasonographic diagnosis is not diagnostic. Contrast tomography may provide additional information. Magnetic resonance imaging may also be valuable in acute Budd–Chiari syndrome, the caudate lobe may have shorter T2 relaxation values with a lower water content than the remainder of the liver.

Venography can be valuable in confirming the diagnosis and is important in decision making for treatment, particularly in defining patency of the inferior vena cava. Pressure measurements within the inferior vena cava may help in deciding on the site of obstruction. Venography can be undertaken by retrograde cannulation of the hepatic veins or by a transhepatic route using a thin needle to puncture an hepatic venous radical.

Liver biopsy is in many cases unnecessary in the diagnostic work-up of patients who have occlusion of the main hepatic veins. Classic features of centrilobular congestion are present (Fig. 27.10), but may not be apparent in patients who have chronic venous outflow obstruction if they have developed cirrhosis.

Analysis of the ascitic fluid is of limited value since, although it is commonly exudative with a high protein content, particularly in the acute presentation, it can be variable from 5–50g/L.

Laboratory investigations are not usually helpful in establishing a diagnosis, although they are valuable in identifying predisposing disorders (see Fig. 27.7). In patients who have the acute form of hepatic venous outflow obstruction the transaminase levels are more elevated than in those who have more long-standing disease. A marked coagulopathy is characteristic of those who have an acute presentation, but is less marked in those who have a more gradual onset. Hypoproteinemia may be present due to a protein losing enteropathy.

Prognosis

The prognosis following hepatic venous outflow obstruction is highly variable and depends upon the extent of hepatic venous outflow obstruction and the speed with which it develops. In the

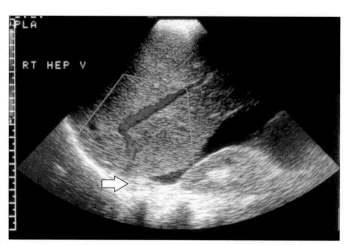

Figure 27.9 Doppler ultrasound scan showing blockage of an hepatic vein (arrow) with no filling of the inferior vena cava.

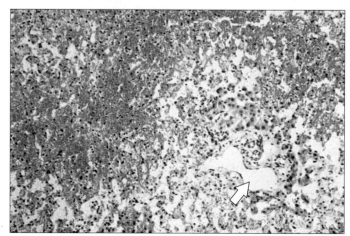

Figure 27.10 Histology of the liver in a patient with Budd–Chiari syndrome. There is loss of hepatocytes in zone 3 around the central vein (arrow) and extensive surrounding hemorrhage.

most acute form fulminant hepatic failure may develop and result in death over a few days without liver transplantation. In the more chronic forms the severity of liver decompensation is variable and overall the prognosis at 3 years is approximately 50%.

Management

As mentioned above, treatment varies depending upon severity of the underlying hepatocellular dysfunction. In those in whom fulminant hepatic failure supervenes urgent transplantation may be required. In the commoner presentation of the chronic variant ascites is the major therapeutic target but response is highly variable. In approximately 30% the ascites is diuretic resistant from the outset, while in the remainder diuretic therapy controls the ascites, at least initially. In a recent series comparing venous decompression versus transplantation, the latter was associated with better survival. Venous decompression, usually by side-to-side portacaval shunting, should probably be reserved for those who have acute and potentially reversible portal hypertension and good liver function. Splenorenal and mesocaval H-graft shunts are more prone to thrombosis. Insertion of a TIPSS may be useful in selected cases, but its precise role is at present unclear. Anticoagulant therapy is widely used to reduce the risk of thrombosis or recurrence after transplantation. Thrombolytic treatment has been proposed in some cases and can be effective up to several weeks. Recombinant tissue plasminogen activator is probably the agent of choice. For that minority of patients in whom occlusion of the main hepatic veins is secondary to malignant invasion, the prognosis is poor and acute liver failure may develop. Metastatic spread to the right side of the heart and lung is common.

Inferior vena caval disease

Primary disorders of the inferior vena cava (IVC) include thrombosis and membranous obstruction (vena caval web). Rarely cardiac disorders can lead to diagnostic difficulties or cause secondary IVC thrombosis, such as congestive cardiac failure, constrictive pericarditis or right atrial tumors (myxoma). In membranous obstruction of the inferior vena cava, which has been reported principally in South Africa and Japan, the level of the obstruction is generally at or superior to the ostia of the main hepatic veins. The severity of the disorder is dependent upon the number of hepatic veins obstructed, although in general one vein remains patent, allowing blood to return to the heart via dilated lumbar and azygos collateral veins.

Epidemiology and pathogenesis

Membranous obstruction of the IVC is the major cause of Budd–Chiari syndrome in South Africa and Japan. The obstruction may vary from a web or membrane to an occlusion several centimeters thick, containing fibrous and elastic tissue, and smooth muscle. Although congenital formation of inferior vena caval webs has been proposed, there is increasing evidence that in many cases it is acquired, and in some cases can be attributed to an underlying thrombogenic disorder similar to those described in patients who have main hepatic vein outlet obstruction (see Fig. 27.7).

Clinical features

The main difference between membranous obstruction of the inferior vena cava and primary disorders of the hepatic veins is

that clinical manifestations develop more slowly. Patients may present with obvious abdominal, lumbar, and thoracic lateral veins, and in many ascites is absent. Probably for this reason hepatic fibrosis and cirrhosis at the time of presentation is more common. Edema of the lower limbs is common unlike Budd–Chiari syndrome without IVC involvement. In a significant proportion of patients, hepatitis B viral infection coexists, and hepatocellular carcinoma may develop in a significant minority of patients.

Diagnosis

The imaging techniques described above in the investigation of patients who have hepatic venous outlet obstruction are also those employed in the diagnosis of primary obstruction of the inferior vena cava. Ultrasonography, for example, may show echogenic material in the lumen of the inferior vena cava; venography is important in determining the patency of the inferior vena cava and has important implications in treatment (Fig. 27.11).

Hemodynamic pressure studies may be valuable in identifying the pressure gradient across an IVC web.

Management

In patients who have membranous obstruction of the inferior vena cava transcardiac membranotomy or percutaneous vascular angioplasty may be undertaken in situations where at least one main hepatic vein remains patent. In patients who have occlusion of the main hepatic veins portoatrial or mesoatrial shunts using prosthetic grafts have been attempted, although the results are poor because of thrombosis of the prosthetic graft.

Disorders of the hepatic venules

Involvement of the hepatic venules in various disease processes is well recognized. For example, in acute alcoholic hepatitis sclerosing hyaline necrosis affecting the central hepatic vein is characteristic, but the major disorder that primarily affects the hepatic venules is veno-occlusive disease. As with disorders that affect the main hepatic veins, presentation in patients who have veno-occlusive disease can be acute and cause acute liver failure, or may be subacute or chronic where hepatic fibrosis and cirrhosis may supervene.

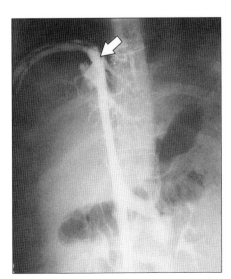

Figure 27.11 A venogram of the vena cava showing total occlusion of the inferior vena cava above the level of the liver (arrow).

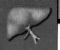

Epidemiology and pathogenesis

There are three major causes of veno-occlusive disease, namely:
- poisoning with pyrrolizidine alkaloids;
- hepatic irradiation; and
- antineoplastic drug therapy.

The pathologic feature of veno-occlusive disease is concentric narrowing of the central venule or sublobular veins by loose connective tissue which does not affect larger hepatic veins. This is associated with hemorrhagic congestion and hepatocellular death affecting zone 3 of the hepatic lobule. Progression of the disorder leads to perivenular fibrosis with fibrotic scar formation replacing the central veins, leading eventually to cirrhosis. The earliest form of the condition can be recognized as subendothelial edema with extravasation of red blood cells into the space of Disse.

The underlying pathogenic mechanisms behind veno-occlusive disease will vary with the cause. In the variety due to ingestion of pyrrolizidine alkaloids, first recognized in Jamaica, poisoning is usually due to ingestion of 'bush teas', but may follow eating contaminated flour or taking herbal medicine. Ingestion of large quantities produces acute disease, whereas long-term low dose ingestion causes the chronic variant. The most common plant genera involved in this disorder are *Heliotropium*, *Crotolaria*, and *Senecio*. These plants are a common cause of liver failure in grazing animals.

In veno-occlusive disease secondary to hepatic irradiation, the injury is dose-dependent. The disorder is unusual with radiation doses less than 3000 rads. Clinical features present between 2 and 5 weeks after the radiation administration.

The development of veno-occlusive disease has been strongly associated with high dose combinations of cytoreductive therapy including cyclophosphamide, busulphan, carmustine, and etoposide. The drug most commonly implicated is azathioprine (and related 6-mercaptopurine). The combination of cyclophosphamide, alkylating agents, and whole-body irradiation as used for conditioning for bone marrow transplantation commonly causes veno-occlusive disease.

Rarely veno-occlusive disease may be due to oral contraceptives, systemic lupus erythematosis or familial immunodeficiency. Alcohol can produce a veno-occlusive disease syndrome in those who have severe central hyaline sclerosis.

Clinical features

The clinical features of veno-occlusive disease can be highly variable and dependent upon the underlying cause. In the acute form, which most commonly follows ingestion of a large amount of pyrrolizidine alkaloid, there is the rapid development of hepatomegaly or abdominal pain and ascites which may be preceded by a 1–2 week febrile illness. This may progress to fulminant hepatic failure, although complete recovery can take place. The subacute variant follows incomplete recovery of the acute form. Chronic veno-occlusive disease may occur after long term ingestion of small amounts of pyrrolizidine alkaloids or after antineoplastic drug administration. The clinical features are the same as those of cirrhosis, although ascites is especially common. Cirrhosis may develop within a few months of the acute presentation. The veno-occlusive disease that follows azathioprine administration occurs any time after 6 months of continuous administration and presents with jaundice and hepatomegaly.

Diagnosis

In veno-occlusive disease liver biopsy is usually required for diagnosis. Ultrasonography is valuable in demonstrating patency of the main hepatic veins whilst histology shows abnormalities of small hepatic veins. In some cases coagulopathy or thrombocytopenia may be a contraindication to percutaneous liver biopsy and in these cases transjugular liver biopsies may be valuable. A wedged hepatic venous pressure gradient greater than 10mmHg is highly suggestive of veno-occlusive disease in the setting of bone marrow transplantation (see above).

Natural history and prognosis

The natural history of veno-occlusive disease is to a large degree dependent upon the underlying cause and the presentation. In those in whom it presents acutely, fulminant hepatic failure and death can occur, but recovery can be complete. Those who have a subacute or chronic presentation will have incomplete recovery, particularly where cirrhosis has developed. In a recent study of bone marrow transplantation patients, veno-occlusive disease developed in 54% of patients and was severe in a quarter of these. Mortality rate was extremely high in those with severe disease, but less than 10% in mild cases. Pre-existing liver disease manifested by abnormal aminotransferases before transplantation increases the risk.

Management

This will depend on the underlying cause and presentation. For those people presenting with acute liver failure, intensive supportive treatment will be required which might include liver transplantation. In those who have more chronic disease management of the complications of cirrhosis, particularly ascites, will be required. Obviously where possible the causal factor should be discontinued, such as ingestion of plant alkaloids and use of drugs such as azathioprine. Transjugular intrahepatic portosystemic stent shunts have recently been used with some promise as a method of portal decompression in patients who have veno-occlusive disease after bone marrow transplantation.

Peliosis hepatis

This disorder is characterized by blood-filled spaces within the liver which are not lined by sinusoidal cells. Although rare, it is increasingly recognized, particularly in immunocompromised individuals.

Etiology and pathogenesis

Peliosis hepatis may develop secondary to drug treatment with estrogens or anabolic steroids and immunosuppressive agents such as azathioprine, and in patients who have chronic infections. This latter cause has recently assumed increasing importance because of the frequency of peliosis in patients who have acquired immune deficiency syndrome (AIDS). In such patients chronic bacillary infection by two species from the genus *Bartonella*, namely *B. quintana* and *B. henselae*, may cause peliosis hepatis as well as bacillary angiomatosis and bacteremia. It is seen most commonly following transplantation, particularly in renal transplants patients, when there is a prevalence of approximately 3%.

Clinical features

Peliosis hepatis may be asymptomatic or cause such problems as hepatomegaly, portal hypertension, ascites or liver failure. Rupture of the vascular lesions may cause intraperitoneal hemorrhage.

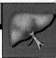

Diagnosis

At laparoscopy peliosis hepatis can be recognized as dark blebs on the surface of the liver. Imaging by means of ultrasound, CT, and MRI may suggest the diagnosis, but it is usually made histologically.

Prognosis

The prognosis of peliosis hepatis is highly variable and in many patients depends on the underlying predisposing condition, for example post-transplantation or human immunodeficiency virus infection.

Management

Where possible the cause should be removed. In patients who have AIDS the bacillary form may be treated with erythromycin, and in cases where drug therapy is suspected withdrawal may lead to disease regression. For patients who present with hemorrhage or problems with portal hypertension, surgical intervention such as a hepatic dearterialization may be effective.

PRACTICE POINT

Illustrative case

A 26-year-old male was admitted with a 4-week history of increasing abdominal distension. He had previously been well and there was no relevant past medical history. His mother had a history of two femoral vein thromboses during pregnancy and was maintained on long-term anticoagulants.

On examination he looked well and had a normal mental state. There were no signs of chronic liver disease, he had no signs of cardiorespiratory disease, but abdominal distension was marked and was due to ascites.

Preliminary laboratory investigations showed: a normal full blood count; normal electrolytes, urea and creatinine; prothrombin time was prolonged at 18s (control 12); alanine transferase 120IU/L; alkaline phosphatase 520IU/L; serum bilirubin 30mmol/L (1.8mg/dL); and serum albumin 35g/L. An ultrasound examination confirmed ascites, the spleen was at the upper limit of normal, the liver was uniformly enlarged but of normal texture. The portal venous system was normal, but there was thrombosis in all hepatic veins with normal flow in the inferior vena cava. A diagnosis of subacute Budd–Chiari syndrome was made.

Further investigation revealed that the patient and his mother had factor V Leiden.

It was decided to manage the situation with a shunting procedure and a TIPSS was successfully performed. Three days later the patient became confused and disoriented and jaundice was clinically obvious. Investigation showed: alanine transferase 560IU/L; alkaline phosphatase 540IU/L; serum bilirubin 65mmol/L (3.8mg/dL); and prothrombin time 36s. Ultrasound showed that the TIPSS was patent.

Hepatic decompensation was diagnosed with deteriorating hepatic function, and the patient was listed for emergency hepatic transplantation.

Interpretation

The case illustrates the dilemma in treating the Budd–Chiari syndrome between a venous decompression procedure and hepatic transplantation. In patients who have preserved liver function and no evidence of chronic liver disease, the preferred option is usually some form of shunt. Hence TIPSS was performed in this case; there was, however, mild hepatic dysfunction. The shunt procedure precipitated encephalopathy and jaundice, and there was continuing deterioration of liver function, also probably related to extensive hepatic venous thrombosis. The prolonged prothrombin time was an indication of this, despite the underlying thrombotic tendency due to the factor V mutation. Hepatic transplantation was probably the optimal treatment and would also correct the factor V Leiden defect.

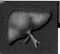

FURTHER READING

Bertina RM, Koeleman BPC, Koster T, et al. Mutation in blood coagulation factor V associated with resistance to activated protein C. Nature. 1994;369:64–7. *A landmark paper describing the single point mutation in the factor V gene which codes for Factor V Leiden.*

Gupta S, Blumgart LH, Hodgson HJ. Budd–Chiari syndrome: long term survival and factors affecting mortality. Quart J Med. 1986;60:781–91. *A description of long-term survival in 18 patients with Budd–Chiari syndrome. Those who survive the initial years of illness, particularly variceal hemorrhage, have a better prognosis than previously believed.*

Junker P, Egeblad M, Nielsen O, Kamper J. Umbilical vein catheterisation and portal hypertension. Acta Paediatr Scand. 1976;65:499–504. *Portal hypertension is a rare complication of umbilical vein catheterization. There is an increased risk of thrombosis with catheterization longer than 2 days. Thirty-eight cases are reviewed.*

MacDonald GB, Hinds MS, Fisher LD, et al. Veno-occlusive disease of the liver and multiorgan failure after bone marrow transplantation. A cohort study of 355 patients. Ann Intern Med. 1993;118:255–67. *A comprehensive review of this topic. Veno-occlusive disease developed in 54% of bone marrow transplant recipients. It is frequently associated with renal and cardiopulmonary failure.*

Okuda K, Ohnishi K, Kimura K, et al. Incidence of portal vein thrombosis in liver cirrhosis. An angiographic study in 708 patients. Gastroenterology. 1985;89:279–86. *A detailed angiographic study showing that thrombosis of the portal vein occurred secondary to cirrhosis in only 0.6% of cases, far fewer than previously suggested.*

Ringe B, Lang H, Oedhafer K-J, et al. Which is the best surgery for Budd–Chiari syndrome: venous decompression or liver transplantation? A single multicentre experience with 50 patients. Hepatology. 1995;21:1337–44. *A useful summary of the role of surgery in Budd–Chiari cases.*

Simpson IW. Membranous obstruction of the inferior vena cava and hepatocellular carcinoma in South Africa. Gastroenterology. 1982;82:171–8. *A comprehensive review of this syndrome, confirming the high incidence of membranous obstruction of the IVC in South Africa. There is a strong association with hepatocellular carcinoma.*

Tavill AS, Wood EJ, Creel L, Jones EA, Gregory M, Sherlock S. The Budd–Chiari syndrome: correlation between hepatic scintigraphy and the clinical, radiological, and pathological findings in 19 cases of hepatic venous outflow obstruction. Gastroenterology. 1975;68:509–18. *An important paper documenting the importance of a thrombotic tendency in the etiology of the Budd–Chiari syndrome. An excellent description of the enlargement of the caudate lobe as it is preserved from injury due to its separate venous drainage.*

Thompson EN, Williams R, Sherlock S. Liver function in extrahepatic portal hypertension. Lancet. 1964;2:1352–6. *An important early clinical paper describing follow up of patients who had extrahepatic portal hypertension due to portal vein thrombosis. Liver function deteriorates over time.*

Tygstrup N, Winkler K, Mellengaard K, Andreassen M. Determination of the hepatic arterial blood flow and oxygen supply in man by clamping the hepatic artery during surgery. J Clin Invest. 1962;41:447–54. *An important paper describing the application of physiologic techniques in clinical investigation.*

Warren WD, Henderson JM, Millikan WJ, Galambos JT, Bryan FC. Management of variceal bleeding in patients with non-cirrhotic portal vein thrombosis. Ann Surg. 1988;207:623–34. *An important paper describing the use of the distal splenorenal shunt in patients who have extrahepatic portal vein thrombosis. A good result in the medium term was reported in 83% of patients.*

Webb LJ, Sherlock S. The aetiology, presentation and natural history of extrahepatic portal venous obstruction. Quart J Med 1979;48:627–39. *A comprehensive description of a 16-year experience of 97 patients who have portal vein obstruction. Fifty-seven per cent present in childhood but 43% presented in adult life.*

Zamboni P, Pisano L, Mari C, Galeotti R, Feo C, Liboni A. Membranous obstruction of the inferior vena cava and Budd–Chiari syndrome. J Cardiovasc Surg 1996;37:583–7. *A paper stressing the importance of membranous obstruction in the development of thrombosis in hepatic venous drainage.*

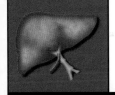

Section 3 Specific Diseases of the Liver

Chapter 28 Pregnancy and the Liver

Michael A Heneghan

INTRODUCTION

Alteration in aspects of liver function is normal during pregnancy. Severe liver dysfunction is rare, but when it occurs it may do so in a catastrophic fashion for both mother and infant. It is appropriate therefore to consider the liver in relation to pregnancy in three separate categories:

- liver dysfunction specific to the pregnant state (i.e. conditions occurring only in the setting of pregnancy);
- management of the pre-existing disorders that may be aggravated by the pregnant state (i.e. pre-existing liver disease that must cope with the extra physiologic demands of pregnancy); and
- liver disease coincident with pregnancy (i.e. apparent concurrent liver conditions occurring in a pregnant individual, most of which do not effect either the pregnancy or the natural history of the disease state). A classification of these conditions is given in Fig. 28.1.

Classification of liver disease in pregnancy

Liver disease specific to pregnancy

Hyperemesis gravidarum
Acute fatty liver of pregnancy
Intrahepatic cholestasis of pregnancy
Hypertension-associated liver disease of pregnancy:
   Pre-eclampsia and eclampsia
   Hepatic infarction, hematoma and rupture
   HELLP syndrome

Pre-existing liver disease

Cirrhosis with portal hypertension
Autoimmune hepatitis
Congenital hyperbilirubinemias
Primary biliary cirrhosis
Primary sclerosing cholangitis
Liver tumors in pregnancy
Wilson's disease

Liver disease coincident with pregnancy

Acute viral hepatitis:
   Hepatitis A-E
   Herpes simplex hepatitis
Drug toxicity
Acetaminophen toxicity
Biliary disease
Budd–Chiari syndrome
Liver transplant recipients

Figure 28.1 Classification of liver disease in pregnancy. These include diseases specific to pregnancy, pre-existing, and coincident liver diseases.

NORMAL PREGNANCY

Some of the normal physiologic changes of pregnancy mimic signs associated with chronic liver disease. The presence of palmar erythema and spider nevi on the neck, face, and back may arise in 60% of pregnant women. These signs are due to an increase in blood volume and cardiac output that occurs predominantly in the second and third trimesters. The spider nevi do not always resolve after completion of the pregnancy.

Bloodflow to the liver remains within the normal range so that the fractional bloodflow to the liver decreases from approximately 35 to 28% of the cardiac output. The liver itself may be impalpable during pregnancy due to upward pressure from the gravid uterus. Small esophageal varices have been identified in approximately 50% of pregnant women due to compression of the inferior vena cava and increased flow in the azygous system. Gallbladder motility decreases and the lithogenicity of bile increases, in part due to increased hepatic cholesterol synthesis.

Laboratory tests can be misleading during pregnancy unless they are interpreted in the context of stage of gestation. The aminotransferases, asparate (AST) and alanine aminotransferase (ALT) remain normal throughout pregnancy as does the level of γ-glutamyl transpeptidase, 5′-nucleotidase, total bile acids, bilirubin, γ-globulins, and prothrombin time. The serum alkaline phosphatase activity increases steadily to the seventh month and then rises more rapidly to a peak at full-term. It rarely exceeds twice the upper limit of normal and returns to the normal range within 2 weeks of delivery in most cases. Increases in the measured levels of alkaline phosphatase activity reflects production in the placental syncytiotrophoblast, but it also parallels skeletal maturation of the fetus. Serum albumin falls by one fifth due to hemodilutional effects of increased plasma volume. Reductions are also seen in levels of α- and β-globulins, packed cell volume, urea, urate, and total protein levels. All lipids increase progressively during pregnancy except for lysolecithin. Triglycerides levels show a three-fold increase, whereas cholesterol increases two-fold. The serum bilirubin may rise by 2–6%, but will not usually be reflected in alterations to the profile of liver function tests. In approximately 20% of pregnancies the levels of conjugated bilirubin will be increased, and this reflects impaired bilirubin excreting capacity, which characteristically decreases after mid-pregnancy. Alpha-fetoprotein (AFP) is synthesized in fetal embryonal liver cells and levels peak at 30 weeks of gestation, with a rapid fall towards full term. Levels of AFP are usually undetectable in normal pregnancy unless fetal anencephaly, open spina bifida, or maternal hepatocellular carcinoma is present. Laboratory findings are summarized in Fig. 28.2.

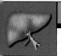
Laboratory assessment	
Parameter	**Alteration from nonpregnant state**
Packed cell volume	Decreased
Urea	Decreased
Uric acid	Decreased
Total protein	Decreased
Albumin	Decreased
α-globulins	Increased
β-globulins	Increased
γ-globulins	No alteration
Alkaline phosphatase	Increased (placental and bone production)
Prothrombin time/INR	No alteration
Fibrinogen	Increased
Cholesterol	Increased
Triglycerides	Increased
Bilirubin	Increased
Total bile acids	No alteration
Aminotransferases (AST/ALT)	No alteration
γ-glutamyl transpeptidase	No alteration
5'-nucleotidase	No alteration
α-fetoprotein	No alteration unless spina bifida, fetal anencephaly, or maternal HCC present

Figure 28.2 Laboratory assessment. Pregnancy causes a range of deviations from standard values in the nonpregnant state.

Liver biopsy findings show normal hepatic architecture with occasional reactive Kupffer cells and a variation in nuclear size and shape, including an increase in binucleate hepatocytes. Electron microscopy shows proliferation of smooth endoplasmic reticulum, and giant mitochondria with an increase in paracrystalline inclusions reflecting increased protein synthesis and energy requirements.

INVESTIGATION OF LIVER DISEASE DURING PREGNANCY

The approach to the investigation of liver dysfunction in pregnancy is modified to take account of the physiologic changes and the desire to minimize exposure to radiation. Liver function tests should be interpreted in the light of the physiologic changes described above and summarized in Fig. 28.2. The risks of liver biopsy are similar to those in the nonpregnant state, and contraindications to liver biopsy are as in any patient. The necessity for a histologic diagnosis prepartum should, however, be balanced against the clinical need, and many biopsies can safely be delayed until the postpartum period. Ultrasound carries no risk to the fetus and is the radiologic examination of choice. Computed tomography examination should be carried out based on the clinical need prepartum, with shielding to the fetus. Endoscopic retrograde pancreatography (ERCP) with sphincterotomy for the treatment of choledocholithiasis has been performed safely in the second trimester of pregnancy without adverse outcomes.

LIVER DISEASES SPECIFIC TO PREGNANCY

Hyperemesis gravidarum

Nausea and vomiting occur so commonly within the first trimester that it is considered to be a normal complaint of pregnancy. Hyperemesis gravidarum is vomiting that is protracted, resulting in dehydration, ketosis, weight loss (>5% of total body weight), and excessive salivation. Hyperthyroidism has been described in association with hyperemesis gravidarum. Jaundice is rare and bilirubin levels rarely exceed four times normal levels. Elevations in AST or ALT are seen in 50% of patients but seldom exceed 200IU/L. The differential diagnosis includes other conditions that cause vomiting, including pancreatitis, acute hepatitis, and diabetic ketoacidosis.

The syndrome is commonly associated with obese, nonsmoking mothers in their first pregnancy. Patients have a lower rate of fetal loss than unaffected women and there is an association with babies of low birth weight. An increased prevalence of the condition is seen in patients with pregnancy complicated by hydatidiform moles.

Epidemiologic risk factors suggest that high levels of circulating estrogens are important in the pathogenesis of the condition. High levels of gonadotropins have been detected in the first trimester. Liver dysfunction is thought to be a secondary event and not the cause of vomiting.

Management is largely supportive, and following hydration with intravenous fluids and initial restriction of oral intake most patients improve with resolution of the abnormal transaminases. Most patients will be discharged within 3–7 days of admission following hydration therapy, but relapse is common. Recently, ondansetron has been used with success in this condition. In very severe cases, thiamine deficiency can occur and in these circumstances it is appropriate to supplement the vitamin, especially in patients who have not eaten for some time. Usually, however, this condition resolves as the patient enters the second half of the gestational period.

Acute fatty liver of pregnancy

Although this condition has been recognized since the mid-nineteenth century, it was not until 1940 that Sheehan described 'obstetric yellow atrophy' as a specific cause of jaundice in pregnancy. The absence of liver necrosis in the presence of microvesicular fat within swollen hepatocytes with centrally located nuclei, differentiated it from 'acute yellow atrophy' of fulminant hepatitis. Many of the original cases described the condition in the setting of intravenous tetracycline administration and initially the drug was thought to be responsible. Despite changes in obstetric practice including the discontinuation of tetracycline usage in pregnant women, acute fatty liver has persisted. Its incidence in the USA is 1 in 14,000 pregnancies, but is probably underestimated as cases with mild or subclinical disease will not come to attention.

Pathogenesis

Acute fatty liver of pregnancy is regarded as one of the family of diseases that are characterized by a mitochondrial cytopathy, which also includes conditions such as Reye's syndrome, drug-related liver disease (including tetracycline, sodium valproate, and fialuridine), and other genetic defects in mitochondrial function. Experimentally, tetracycline causes microvesicular change similar to that with acute fatty liver of pregnancy that is known to localize in the mitochondria. These conditions are characterized by vomiting, hypoglycemia, lactic acidosis, hyperammonemia, and microvesicular fat in organs. Acidosis occurs as a result in defective energy supply within the mitochondria during oxida-

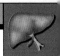
tive phosphorylation. Hypoglycemia in these disorders may relate to failure of mitochondrial tricarboxylic acid cycle enzymes.

The understanding of the pathogenesis of the condition has been greatly enhanced by the description of a full-term infant born to a mother with acute fatty liver of pregnancy in whom hypoglycemia, hepatic encephalopathy, and steatosis developed. The infant was found to have a defect in fatty acid oxidation and specifically was deficient in long-chain 3-hydroxyacyl coenzyme A dehydrogenase (LCHAD). The mother was found to be heterozygous for deficiency of this enzyme. This pattern has also been noted in 11 patients whose pregnancies were complicated by acute fatty liver with features of hemolysis, elevated liver enzymes, low platelets (HELLP) syndrome. Six babies from this series were found to have LCHAD deficiency. Heterozygosity for LCHAD in the mother appears to be responsible at least in part for the development of disease in the infant. The molecular basis has been identified as the substitution of guanosine to cytosine in the α-subunit that catalyses the last three steps of β-oxidation. Consistent with these findings is the fact that in murine models, pregnancy decreases fatty oxidation with the effect mediated by estrogens and progesterones

An alternative hypothesis relates to medium-chain acyl coenzyme A dehydrogenase deficiency resulting in secondary carnitine deficiency in mitochondria. This results in the absence of an essential cofactor in fatty acid transport into mitochondria. Pregnancy causes relative deficiency in carnitine and in genetically susceptible individuals can precipitate symptoms. Despite these clues, the initiating factors in the development of acute fatty liver of pregnancy and other mitochondrial cytopathies remain unknown.

Presentation and diagnosis

Patients present in the second half of pregnancy, usually between the 30th and 38th weeks. Commonly the patient presents with lethargy and malaise followed by nausea and vomiting. Jaundice follows but is usually mild. Persistent vomiting is the predominant symptom and hematemesis may occur as a consequence of esophageal and gastric inflammation. Other symptoms include ankle swelling, headache, polydipsia, polyuria, abdominal pain, and tenderness. Ascites and fever are rarely present. Pre-eclampsia has been reported in approximately 50% of patients with acute fatty liver of pregnancy. It is also more likely to occur in primagravid women or in twin pregnancies. Patients with this condition may also present with hyperacute liver failure and the associated complications of bleeding, hypoglycemia, jaundice and encephalopathy. In severe cases renal failure may also occur.

Laboratory findings depend on the severity of the underlying disease. A raised white cell count in association with toxic granulation is common. Thrombocytopenia is common and associated with impaired coagulation and disseminated intravascular coagulation (DIC) in approximately 10%. This is reflected in decreased fibrinogen and increased fibrin degradation products (FDPs) or D-dimers in severe cases. The presence of low platelets may be due to disseminated intravascular coagulation or may suggest the presence of HELLP syndrome. Figure 28.3 illustrates

Characteristics of liver disease in pregnancy						
Disease	Trimester	Symptoms	Jaundice	Laboratory findings	Incidence	Adverse events
Hyperemesis gravidarum	1/2	Nausea and vomiting	Mild	↑ Bilirubin (× 4) ↑ AST/ALT (× 2–4)	0.3–1.0 %	Low birth weight
Acute fatty liver of pregnancy	3	Abdominal pain Nausea and vomiting Confusion (late)	Common	↑ Bilirubin (late x 6–8) ↑ AST/ALT (× 5–10) ↑ FDPs (common) ↓ Platelets	0.008%	↑ Maternal mortality LCHAD in fetus ↑ Fetal mortality
Pre-eclampsia and eclampsia	2/3	Abdominal pain Hypertension Edema Confusion (late)	Late (10%)	↑ Bilirubin (late × 2–5) ↑ AST/ALT (× 10–50) ↑ FDPs (<10%) ↓ Platelets (<10%) Proteinuria	5–10%	↑ Maternal mortality
Hepatic infarction and rupture	3 Postpartum	Abdominal pain Hypotension Nausea and vomiting	Common	↑ AST/ALT (× 100) ↑ FDPs (common) ↓ Platelets (common)	Unknown	↑ Maternal mortality
Cholestasis of pregnancy	1/2/3	Itch	Common (20–60%)	↑ Bilirubin (× 6) ↑ AST/ALT (× 6) ↑ Bile acids	0.1–0.2% in USA	Stillbirth Prematurity Fetal mortality (3%)
HELLP syndrome	3	Abdominal pain Nausea and vomiting Confusion (late)	Late (10%)	↑ AST/ALT (× 10–20) ↑ LDH ↑ Urate ↓ Platelets ↑ FDPs (20–40%)	0.1% 4–12% of women with pre-eclampsia Twin pregnancy	↑ Maternal mortality ↑ Fetal mortality (30%)

Figure 28.3 Characteristics of liver disease in pregnancy. Clinical and laboratory parameters of the range of pregnancy-specific diseases. FDP, fibrin degradation products.

the differences between the various liver conditions specific to pregnancy. Elevations in AST and ALT are rarely above 10 times the upper limit of normal and tend to fall after delivery. Uric acid, urea, and creatinine levels also increase and may continue to do so until delivery. Uric acid levels may rise before the development of symptoms. In severe cases, especially those with signs of liver failure, the differential diagnosis will include severe pre-eclampsia, HELLP syndrome, acute hepatitis, hemolytic uremic syndrome, pancreatitis, and thrombotic thrombocytopenic purpura.

Radiologic evaluation includes ultrasound, which should be performed to define liver echogenicity and to exclude the presence of biliary disease. Usually this will show increased reflectivity (Fig. 28.4). However, as the ultrasound examination may be normal it will be important to perform CT evaluation of the liver in patients with evidence of more severe disease. Computed tomography findings may illustrate decreased attenuation within the liver when compared with the attenuation of the spleen (Fig. 28.5). Serial evaluation will show reversal of this pattern, with the attenuation of the liver returning to a higher attenuation than the spleen when normality resumes. Computed tomography evaluation will also reveal patients with intrahepatic or subcapsular hemorrhage and liver rupture.

Histology

The variation in the clinical presentation is also reflected in that seen in liver biopsy specimens. Fatty infiltration rapidly resolves after delivery. Histologic evaluation typically shows microvesicular fatty infiltration that does not displace the nucleus. In early cases this is manifest as ballooning of the hepatocyte. This pattern is most prominent around the central veins, although it can be found throughout the liver lobule (Fig. 28.6). In severe cases the fat infiltration may be macrovesicular with hepatocyte necrosis seen as cells drop out. Although bridging necrosis is not seen, lobular inflammation may occur and be confused with viral hepatitis. Cholestasis and bile plugging is common. Microvesicular fat may be seen also in cases of toxemia-related liver disease and in HELLP syndrome. Although intrasinusoidal fibrin deposition and hemorrhage has been described in patients with fatty liver of

pregnancy it is rare and more characteristic of toxemia-related liver disease. Other organs may have fat infiltration, including the heart, kidney, and pancreas. Follow-up biopsy shows a return to complete morphologic normality.

Electron microscopy shows the presence of fat that is non-membrane bound, and dilated smooth endoplasm reticulum. Mitochondrial pleomorphism with paracrystalline deposits have also been described.

Management

The key to management of severe cases is multidisciplinary care involving both the obstetrician and the hepatologist. Immediate delivery is the primary treatment and a liver biopsy can usually be safely postponed until after delivery. Alternatively, biopsy via the transjugular route can be performed if a significant coagulopathy exists. Resolution of the syndrome can only begin after delivery. As acute fatty liver of pregnancy is a disease of the 3rd trimester, the fetus is mature and delivery of the baby is usually undertaken. In mild cases, careful fetal monitoring can be undertaken and gestation prolonged, but the disadvantage of this is that change may occur quickly and the progression of liver disease may be rapid.

Vaginal delivery is the preferred route in most cases. In more severe disease, cesarean section may be performed under spinal or epidural anesthesia if coagulation studies are normal. If signs or symptoms of acute liver failure are present, emergency cesarean section should be performed under general anesthesia. Obstetric complications frequently reflect the severity of liver dysfunction, but in all instances close observation is necessary in the immediate postpartum period. Postpartum bleeding is common and may be out of proportion to the degree of abnormality reflected in laboratory tests of coagulation. Transfusion with fresh frozen plasma, cryoprecipitate, and platelets is recommended. Deficiency in antithrombin III has been reported and this may be supplemented. In severe cases, when inability to control bleeding has occurred, hysterectomy has been performed.

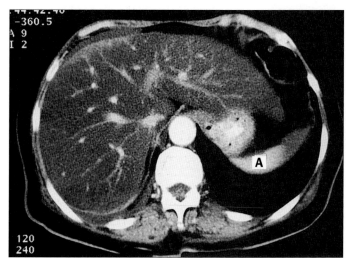

Figure 28.5 Computed tomography evaluation. Contrast enhanced abdominal CT scan showing a hypodense parenchyma within the liver consistent with fat infiltration. The attenuation of liver in this setting is several houndsfield units lower than that of the spleen, which is white (A). A thin rim of ascites is seen anterior to the liver. (Courtesy of Drs Pauline Kane and Sarah Kirwin.)

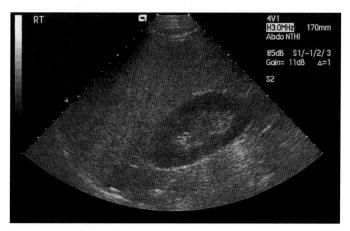

Figure 28.4 Ultrasound evaluation. Ultrasound of the liver and right kidney showing normal echo pattern within the kidney with the liver showing increased echogenicity from fat infiltration. (Courtesy of Dr Paul Sidhu.)

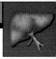
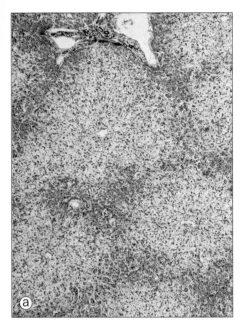
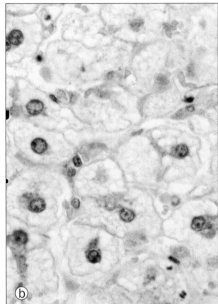
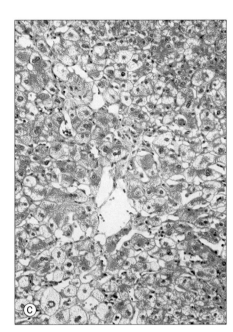

Figure 28.6 Histology of acute fatty liver. Light microscopy of a liver biopsy specimen from a patient with acute fatty liver of pregnancy. (a) Extensive fatty change involving zones 2 and 3, with relative sparing of zone 1. (Hematoxylin and eosin). (b) Hepatocytes are enlarged and ballooned with a microvesicular fatty infiltration of the cytoplasm without nuclear displacement. (Hematoxylin and eosin). (c) Resolving acute fatty liver of pregnancy showing patchy residual fatty change maximal in the perivenular areas. Although this pattern may be seen in patients recovering from acute hepatitis, the degree of parenchymal collapse is considerably less in this case. (Hematoxylin and eosin.) (Courtesy of Professor Bernard Portmann.)

Management of acute liver failure should follow standard practice outlined in Chapter 30. Renal dysfunction is an early feature and renal replacement therapy should be instituted as required. Orthotopic liver transplantation is not frequently indicated and is reserved for those patients who fail to respond to conventional treatment. Expeditious delivery and adequate attention to other aspects of care usually obviates the need for this intervention. As a consequence of heightened awareness of the condition, coupled with better intensive care monitoring and management, mortality for this condition is now substantially less than 10% for the affected mother and less than 20% for the fetus.

Although several series report many successful pregnancies without subsequent recurrence, the condition has also been described as recurring in other case reports. This reiterates the importance of close observation of these patients in subsequent pregnancies.

HYPERTENSION-RELATED LIVER DISEASE OF PREGNANCY

Pre-eclampsia is a common condition affecting between 7 and 10% of all pregnancies, and even in developed countries it is still the major cause of maternal death. The term 'toxemia' has fallen out of favor and it is more appropriate to consider a spectrum of disease that relates to the presence of hypertension in pregnancy, with the severity of liver disease reflecting the severity of the (pre-)eclamptic process. This incorporates pre-eclampsia, eclampsia, hepatic infarction, and rupture. Included in this continuum is a condition defined in 1982 by Weinstein by the presence of hemolysis, elevated liver enzymes and low platelets, called the HELLP syndrome.

Pre-eclampsia and eclampsia
Pre-eclampsia is characterized by a triad of hypertension, proteinuria, and edema. Hypertension is defined as an elevation in blood pressure of 30mmHg (systolic) or 15mmHg (diastolic) above the value recorded in the first trimester, or any value greater than 140/90mmHg. It occurs predominantly late in the second trimester or in the third trimester. Risk factors include pre-existing hypertension, extremes of child-bearing age, first pregnancy, and multiple gestation. Eclampsia is marked by seizures or coma in addition to the signs of pre-eclampsia.

Pathogenesis
Two hypotheses have been proposed to explain the changes seen in hypertension-related liver disease. The first includes the deposition of fibrin secondary to the presence of disseminated intravascular coagulation. The second and more plausible hypothesis is that segmental vasospasm results in the vasculopathy and secondary damage. A summary of this mechanism is illustrated in Fig. 28.7.

Presentation and diagnosis
The major symptoms of pre-eclampsia are epigastric or right upper abdominal pain, which may mimic an acute abdomen. The liver is usually normal in size and tender on palpation. Other symptoms include visual change including blurred vision and the presence of scotomota, headache, nausea, and vomiting. In rare instances patients may be asymptomatic. Others may present with seizures before the development of the more usual presenting symptoms. The principal physical signs include edema, which may be nondependant, hyper-reflexia, and fundoscopic changes. The disorder is a multisystem one involving the central nervous system, kidneys, liver, and hematologic

Hypertension-related disease

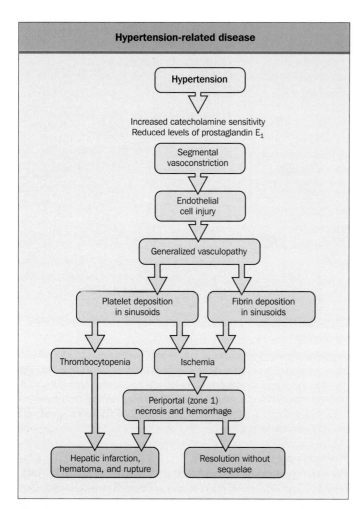

Figure 28.7 Hypertension-related disease. A schema illustrating the pathogenetic mechanisms.

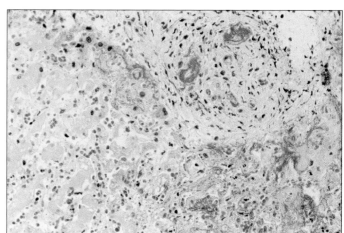

Figure 28.8 Histology in eclampsia-related liver disease. Severe eclamptic liver disease showing characteristic periportal fibrin deposition. The degree of staining correlates with the increase in AST values. Periportal bleeding occurs in severe cases. (Hematoxylin and eosin.) (Courtesy of Professor Bernard Portmann.)

system. Severe cases will have renal failure. Over 80% of maternal deaths are due to the central nervous system complications, but the hepatic complications are responsible for most of the remaining mortality.

The degree of abnormality of liver function tests reflects the severity of the hypertension. About 24% of patients with mild hypertension have abnormal liver function tests, but this rises to over 80% in the setting of severe hypertension. The cardinal abnormality is an elevation in the AST and ALT, and in severe cases the levels may be as high as those seen in acute hepatitis. The bilirubin is rarely elevated unless hemolysis or hepatic rupture has occurred. Levels of antithrombin III have been found to correlate inversely with the outcome in severe disease. Thrombocytopenia may be present and is known to occur before the development of hypertension.

Histology

Histologic examination of the liver is generally normal in mild disease, although focal necrosis may be seen. In more advanced disease the lesion typically is one of fibrinogen deposition within the space of Disse with hemorrhage leading to hepatocyte necrosis. In one report in which liver histology was available in 102 patients with eclampsia-related liver disease (97 autopsies and five liver biopsies), periportal fibrin deposition involving most portal tracts

was the dominant abnormality (Fig. 28.8). Immunostaining shows fibrinogen within sinusoids in approximately one third of cases. The degree of staining has been shown to correlate with the level of transaminases in serum. Capillary thrombi, and more rarely hepatic arterial and intrahepatic portal vein thrombosis, were noted. The progression of this condition is to hepatic infarction, the development of hematoma, and liver rupture. For this reason, it is important to screen these patients serially with ultrasound evaluation or CT scanning. The presence of liver infarction is usually reflected by very high aminotransferase values.

Management

The disorder follows an unpredictable course with some patients remaining stable for days to weeks, while in other patients a rapid deterioration either from a neurologic or hepatologic standpoint is seen. The management of the liver abnormalities reflects the general management of the condition with early delivery remaining the key to successful outcome. The normalization of liver function tests is similar to that observed following ischemic damage to the liver, with abnormalities in AST/ALT and bilirubin resolving within days of delivery. The γ-glutamyl transpeptidase rises until 7–10 days after delivery of the baby and resolves approximately 2 months later.

Hepatic infarction, hematoma, and rupture

Hepatic infarction, the development of hematomas (Fig. 28.9), and liver rupture are associated with severe pre-eclampsia, eclampsia, and HELLP spectrum of disease in over 80% of cases. It has been seen occasionally in patients with acute fatty liver of pregnancy, and other conditions that predispose to liver rupture in pregnant patients include adenoma, hemangioma, hepatocellular carcinoma (HCC) and liver abscess.

Patients typically present in the third trimester, or early after delivery, with severe right upper quadrant pain and fever. When liver rupture occurs, the patient progresses to abdominal swelling in association with a falling hematocrit and circulatory collapse. Diagnostic paracentesis reveals blood in the peritoneum. The

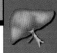

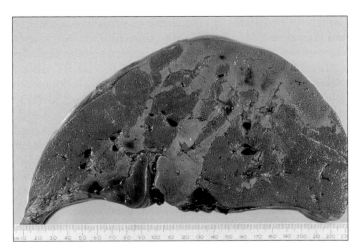

Figure 28.9 Hepatic infarction in eclampsia. Gross appearance of liver infarction occurring in the setting of severe eclampsia-related liver disease. Liver cut surface shows extensive pale areas of infarction. (Courtesy of Professor Bernard Portmann.)

differential diagnosis includes perforation of any intra-abdominal viscus. A high level of suspicion of liver rupture should be entertained in any patient postpartum with right upper quadrant pain with or without a history of pre-eclampsia. Maternal mortality has been reported as high as 59%, while that of the offspring has been reported as up to 62%.

Laboratory testing will usually show a raised white cell count, anemia and elevations in transaminases, frequently in excess of 3000IU/L. Abnormalities in clotting tests may be present early in the clinical course. If the hematoma is large, abnormalities in fibrinolysis may occur and DIC ensues. This process may be aggravated by infection within the infarcted areas. Infarcts may involve either lobe, although hematomas are most commonly found in the anterior or superior aspect of the right lobe. Rupture usually involves the inferior margin of the liver. Reports exist of

the diaphragm being penetrated with ensuing hemothorax. In some patients the rupture may be contained within the hepatic capsule and subcapsular hematoma is detected on CT scanning (Figs 28.10 & 28.11).

Conservative management is the treatment of choice for infarction and hematomas. Careful radiologic evaluation is essential. In cases with isolated infarction or hematoma without liver rupture, serial CT examinations will display resolution. In cases that are actively bleeding, hepatic angiography followed by embolization of the appropriate segmental arterial branches will be appropriate before surgical intervention. The principal advantage of this approach is that the segmental anatomy of the injured liver can be defined. At laparotomy, the surgeon may be faced with a liver oozing from multiple tears in the liver capsule that are not amenable to suturing. Control of bleeding can usually be gained by packing the liver followed by re-exploration and removal of packs when appropriate. Liver transplantation has been successfully performed in a small number of cases.

Hemolysis, elevated liver enzymes, low platelets syndrome
A combination of hemolysis, elevated liver enzymes, and low platelets occurring in pregnancy was recognized by Pritchard in 1954, but the acronym 'HELLP syndrome' was popularized by Weinstein in 1982. The pathophysiology of HELLP syndrome is similar to that of pre-eclampsia-related liver injury described in Fig. 28.7. The hemolysis, however, is due to the passage of red blood cells through damaged vascular intima, with liver necrosis occurring due to fibrin deposition in the sinusoids.

The typical patient is Caucasian, older than 25 years, is at less than 36 weeks of gestation, and has a past history of poor outcome in pregnancy. Criteria have been proposed for the diagnosis of HELLP syndrome. Hemolysis is documented if there is an abnormal blood film in combination with a bilirubin of greater than 1.1mg/dL (18.8μmol/L) and an elevation of lactate dehydrogenase greater than 600IU/L. Liver enzymes are considered elevated if the AST is greater than 70IU/L (approximately 1.5 times the upper limit of normal levels). A

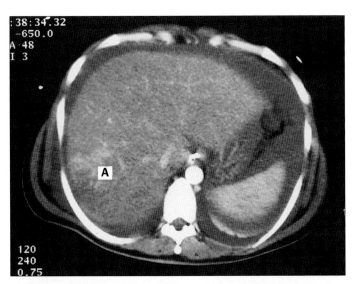

Figure 28.10 Intrahepatic hemorrhage. Contrast-enhanced abdominal CT scan showing ascites and intrahepatic bleeding (A) within the right lobe, without evidence of liver rupture in a patient with eclampsia. (Courtesy of Drs Pauline Kane and Sarah Kirwin.)

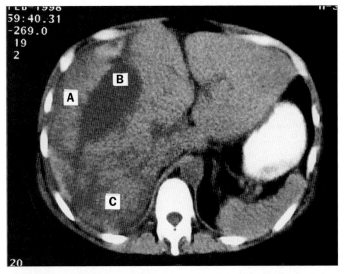

Figure 28.11 Subcapsular hematoma. Nonenhanced CT scan showing a large right subcapsular hematoma (A) compressing the right lobe of liver. There is an area of infarction (B), and contusion (C) within the right lobe of liver. (Courtesy of Drs Pauline Kane and Sarah Kirwin.)

platelet count of less than 100×10^9/L is considered thrombocytopenic. This combination of findings is present in between 3 and 5% of patients with pre-eclampsia, and in one series of 112 patients the syndrome occurred between 26 weeks of gestation and at the time of delivery in 69% of cases. The remaining 31% occurred after delivery and in only 80% of these cases was there evidence of pre-eclampsia. Patients typically present with a history of malaise. This is in association with right upper quadrant pain in over 90% of cases. Nausea and vomiting are also common. There may be associated DIC in up to 38% of cases. On clinical examination over 80% of patients will have right upper quadrant tenderness and 60% report rapid weight gain. One-fifth of patients will not have hypertension and proteinuria is absent in 15%. Additional laboratory studies may reveal a prolonged activated partial thromboplastin time (APTT), as well as reduced creatinine clearance.

The differential diagnosis is broad and includes viral gastroenteritis, appendicitis, acute fatty liver of pregnancy, viral hepatitis, pyelonephritis, and other causes of thrombocytopenia. Complications relating to HELLP syndrome are most severe when DIC is present. In one series of 112 women with HELLP syndrome, placental abruption occurred in 20%, DIC in 38%, acute renal failure in 8%, pleural effusions in 7%, and pulmonary edema in 5%. Ruptured liver hematoma (Fig. 28.12) occurred in 2% and there were two maternal deaths. The same series reported a 33.3% perinatal mortality including a 19.3% incidence of stillbirths.

Patients with confirmed HELLP syndrome are for the most part treated as severe eclamptics. Urgent delivery is usually planned if the gestation is over 34 weeks. A strategy of low-dose aspirin in association with corticosteroids prolonged the gestational period for an average of 5.5 weeks in five patients with a perinatal mortality rate of 28%. Other alternatives have included the use of plasma expansion and plasmapheresis with or without prostacyclin, but none of these therapeutic modalities have been subjected to rigorous evaluation in the form of controlled clinical trials. A novel approach to the treatment of HELLP is the use of 5-nitrosoglutathione, a nitric oxide donor with a profound inhibitory effect on platelet activation. The basis for this treatment is the hypothesis that the disease may represent a systemic disorder of nitric oxide deficiency. Current obstetric practice recommends that vaginal delivery be attempted if the patient is in labor and where gestation has gone beyond 32 weeks. However, when the gestation is less than 32 weeks and there are other obstetric indications to terminate the pregnancy, delivery should be performed using cesarean section.

An evaluation of 158 patients with HELLP syndrome found that thrombocytopenia and elevation in transaminases peaked at between 24 and 48 hours postpartum, with abnormalities resolving over 3–4 days in most instances. However, abnormalities may persist for up to 2 weeks postpartum. Recurrence of HELLP syndrome in subsequent pregnancies has been recorded at levels as low as 3.4%.

Acute fatty liver of pregnancy and pre-eclamptic liver disease overlap

Frequently, patients present with disease that does not fit neatly into the categories of liver disease outlined above. This is supported by the finding of hypertension and signs of pre-eclampsia in patients with acute fatty liver of pregnancy. The converse is also true in that a series exists of 41 patients with pre-eclampsia-related liver dysfunction who had microvesicular fat on liver biopsy when oil red stains were performed. This fat was visible in only 28% of cases on conventional hematoxylin and eosin staining. Moreover, the density of oil red staining correlated well with serum urate concentration and correlated inversely with platelet count. From a practical standpoint, the priority in all instances will be expeditious delivery when appropriate, with close monitoring and detailed peripartum clinical care.

Intrahepatic cholestasis of pregnancy

Approximately 20% of cases of jaundice that occur in pregnancy result from intrahepatic cholestasis. Its prevalence is between 0.5 and 1% of pregnancies. There is an increased prevalence of the condition in Scandinavia (1–1.5%), where a seasonal variation in prevalence has been described, and in Araucanian Indians in Chile (4.7–10%). In twin pregnancies in Chile, the prevalence has been reported to be 20.9%. Familial cases have been noted sug-

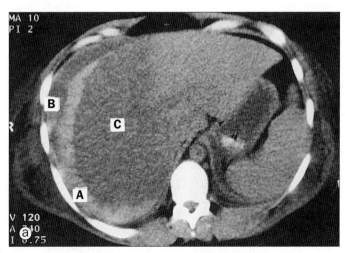
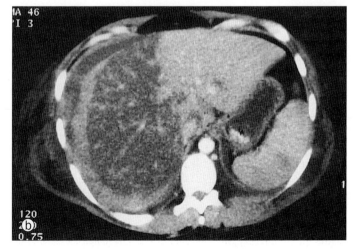

Figure 28.12 Severe eclampsia and HELLP syndrome. These are complicated by liver rupture. (a) Nonenhanced CT scan showing subcapsular hematoma (A), with free blood within the abdominal cavity (B). Segmental hypoperfusion is seen within the right lobe (C). (b) Contrast enhancement confirmed hypoperfusion of the right lobe and liver infarction with free blood still visible as before. (Courtesy of Drs Pauline Kane and Sarah Kirwin.)

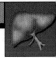

gesting a genetic predisposition to the disease. It has been described in oriental populations, but only rarely in blacks. The syndrome has been associated with other forms of cholestasis. Specifically, 50% of women who develop cholestasis while taking oral contraceptives will develop intrahepatic cholestasis of pregnancy, although this is less common nowadays with the use of low estrogen preparations.

Pathogenesis

Possible pathogenic mechanisms have been proposed for this condition, including an increased sensitivity of the bile excretory system to both endogenous or exogenous estrogen. Progesterone has also been suggested as a triggering factor in some studies. Associations have been described between intrahepatic cholestasis of pregnancy and twin pregnancy, *in vitro* fertilization, prematurity, and hypertension.

Recently, homozygous nonsense mutation in the human multidrug resistance 3 (MDR3) gene has been identified as being responsible for a subtype of progressive familial intrahepatic cholestasis (PFIC) with high γ-glutamyltranspeptidase. MDR3 P-glycoprotein is a canalicular phospholipid translocator that is involved in the biliary secretion of phospholipids. Heterozygosity for this mutation has been identified as being potentially responsible for intrahepatic cholestasis of pregnancy. Evidence for this comes from a single family in whom six women had at least one episode of intrahepatic cholestasis of pregnancy, resulting in fetal deaths in three women, and spontaneous and progressive disappearance of cholestasis after delivery. Genomic DNA was available for four of the women and they were found to be heterozygous for the 1712delT nonsense mutation, which results in the production of a truncated protein. Although the precise effects of this truncated protein is unclear, the coexistence of nongenetic factors such as female sex hormones and their metabolites could modify heterozygous MDR3 expressivity directly by decreasing normal allele expression or indirectly by impairing the function of the transport systems involved in bile secretion.

Presentation and diagnosis

Patients can present at any time from late in the first trimester onwards. The condition is, however, commoner in the second and third trimesters. Itch is the predominant symptom and may be present without jaundice. Jaundice usually follows the onset of pruritus by 2 weeks and is associated with pale stools and dark urine. The presence of right upper quadrant pain is rare and should suggest another diagnosis. Itch may be severe and lead to lack of sleep, anorexia, and weight loss. Physical examination usually is noncontributory and the only finding may be excoriation. Symptoms usually continue for the duration of the pregnancy and resolves within 2 weeks of delivery. The differential diagnosis includes acute viral hepatitis or gallstone disease.

Although total serum alkaline phosphatase is increased in pregnancy, in intrahepatic cholestasis of pregnancy the levels are usually 5–10 times normal. Fractionation of the enzyme shows it to be of hepatic origin rather than placental. Serum 5′-nucleotidase levels and bile acids (chenodeoxycholic acid, deoxycholic acid, and cholic acid) are also increased. These acids are deposited in the skin and may be up to 10 times normal concentration. Serum bilirubin is also elevated, but usually not more than six times normal, and is predominantly conjugated. With disease progression there may be a decreased production of the vitamin K-dependent clotting factors that are synthesized in the liver (II, VII, IX, X) with prolongation of the prothrombin time. Serum transaminases are usually in the normal range, but when elevated are rarely more than 5–10 times normal and never in the range that is associated with acute hepatitis. A further association with intrahepatic cholestasis of pregnancy is the finding of disturbed carbohydrate metabolism, with higher postprandial glucose levels in these patients compared with age-matched controls. Ultrasound of the liver should be performed to exclude extrahepatic biliary obstruction.

Although liver biopsy is not necessary to diagnose the condition. The periportal areas show no changes and significant necrosis or inflammation are unusual. The bile canaliculi may be dilated with bile plugging (Fig. 28.13). Electron microscopy shows destruction of villi in the bile canaliculi. After delivery, the changes regress.

Management

Itching is treated with antihistamines or with cholestyramine (8–16g/day in three to four divided doses), with greatest success noted when treatment is started soon after the onset of symptoms. Cholestyramine, despite its effectiveness, has the disadvantage of exacerbating vitamin K deficiency. Towards the end of the pregnancy, it is important to supplement vitamin K parenterally. Ursodeoxycholic acid (UDCA) 14mg/kg/day has been used as an alternative to cholestyramine with good effect, returning bile acid profiles towards normal in the mother without influencing the presence of major bile acids in meconium including the toxic metabolite lithocholic acid. These results suggest that UDCA is beneficial for the mother and not harmful to the fetus. Other agents which have been used with varied success include phenobarbitone 90mg taken at night and dexamethasone 12mg/day for 1 week followed by a 3-day tapered withdrawal. Another approach to the condition is the use of S-adenosyl-L-methionine, 800mg once daily in 500mL of saline intravenously. Its method of action appears to occur through alteration in membrane fluidity through an increase in the methylation of the mem-

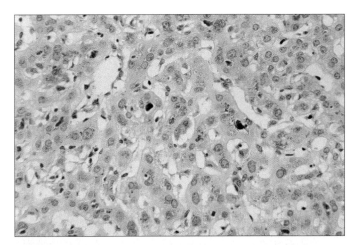

Figure 28.13 Cholestasis of pregnancy. Light microscopy shows pure cholestasis with occasional bile plugs in hepatocytes and canaliculi. These findings are predominantly located in zone 3. Inflammation and necrosis are usually not observed. (Hematoxylin and eosin.) (Courtesy of Professor Bernard Portmann.)

brane phospholipids. Alternatively, an increase in the methylation of 2-hydroxylated estrogens may cause a reduction in the microsomal membrane binding of these compounds.

The risk of premature birth and fetal death may be increased in patients with this condition. The premature birth rate has been reported to be as high as 50%, although some studies have failed to detect an increase in fetal loss. In one series of 83 pregnancies (yielding 86 neonates) complicated by intrahepatic cholestasis, the incidence of prematurity was 44% and intrapartum fetal distress was 22%. The perinatal mortality rate has been reported to be as high as 35%. It is recommended that the onset of labor in these patients should not proceed beyond term. There is a substantial risk of recurrence in subsequent pregnancies.

PRE-EXISTING LIVER DISEASE AND PREGNANCY

Amenorrhea is common in women with cirrhosis of child-bearing age, affecting up to 50%. Although primary amenorrhea occurs, secondary amenorrhea is the most common presentation. Other menstrual abnormalities in women with established cirrhosis include menorrhagia, oligomenorrhea, and menstrual cycle irregularity. The endocrinologic effects of menstrual disturbance in patients with cirrhosis include central effects involving the hypothalamic–pituitary axis, peripheral effects secondary to portosystemic shunting, and systemic effects based on patient's nutritional condition. Figure 28.14 illustrates the interaction of several proposed mechanisms in the development of infertility of these patients.

Alcohol alone can have a significant effect on the hypothalamic–pituitary axis. Up to 60% of women with a history of alcohol abuse have a history of menstrual disturbance that is reversible with abstinence. A number of abnormalities have been described in these women, including fewer than expected developing follicles and absent corpora lutea. Premature ovarian failure has been suggested in other instances. However, many cases of amenorrhea are reversible after orthotopic liver transplantation. Resumption of normal menstrual function was noted in 28 of 34 patients, and in 90% of these menstruation returned within 10 months of the transplant.

Cirrhosis with portal hypertension
Controversy exists regarding the risk of bleeding from varices

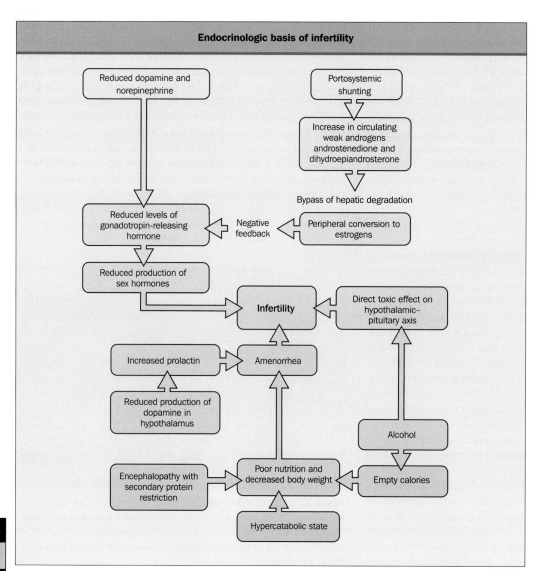

Figure 28.14 Endocrinologic basis of infertility. The complex interactions in the pathogenesis of infertility in patients with cirrhosis.

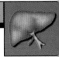
during pregnancy in patients with cirrhosis. The increase in circulating blood volume, cardiac output, azygous vein flow, and the pressure of the gravid uterus should in combination theoretically increase the risk of bleeding. However, this may be counterbalanced by the vasodilatation associated with pregnancy. Bleeding should be treated in the same fashion as in the nonpregnant patient with particular care given to effective resuscitation and the prevention of hypotension.

The situation is more complex in patients who have large varices that have not previously bled. A review of 53 patients with cirrhosis and portal hypertension concluded that pregnancy did not predispose to fatal hemorrhage in patients with pre-existing varices. In addition, the risk of bleeding could not be predicted from a past history of bleeding in earlier pregnancies. Vaginal delivery was not associated with an increased risk of bleeding. Prophylactic shunt surgery had been advocated by some authors, but this practice is no longer considered necessary, even though in one series the risk of bleeding was calculated to be 24.3% in nonshunted patients compared with 3.3% in those that had undergone shunting. Some of the cases described in that series date from 1923 and are not relevant to current practice.

The optimal hepatologic practice in patients with cirrhosis who conceive is an endoscopic evaluation of the upper gastrointestinal tract to screen for the presence of varices. If the varices are large, or if mucosal stigmata indicating an increased risk of bleeding are present, propranolol should be commenced in doses similar to those used in the nonpregnant patient. Currently, there is no good evidence to suggest that prophylactic sclerotherapy or endoscopic banding ligation of esophageal varices is superior to adequate nonselective β blockade in the primary prevention of variceal bleeding in patients with portal hypertension. The paradigm, however, should be close monitoring of hepatic function during the pregnancy and clear communication with the patient regarding the natural history of their disease.

Autoimmune hepatitis

An early observation in patients with autoimmune hepatitis (AIH) was an association between other endocrine disorders and the presence of reduced fertility. However, in these patients, menstruation can commence or resume once disease activity lessens and pregnancy has been described in some patients. A high incidence of obstetric complications was reported in early series, including toxemia of pregnancy and premature delivery in 30% of cases, low birth weight in 35%, and a cesarean section rate of 26%. A more recent study described 32 live births including one twin pregnancy resulting from 33 pregnancies in 18 women with AIH. This series included six women with cirrhosis and 12 women who were noncirrhotic. *In vitro* fertilization was used to achieve pregnancy in two instances. In 24% of pregnancies patients received prednisolone alone, in 9% azathioprine alone, and in 46% combination therapy with steroids and azathioprine. Azathioprine was withdrawn before conception in two cases, and during the first trimester in a further two patients who were subsequently maintained on steroids throughout the pregnancies. Median doses of prednisolone and azathioprine were 10mg/day (range 5–30mg/day) and 75mg/day (range 50–125 mg/day), respectively. Seven pregnancies were managed without any pharmacologic intervention either before or after delivery. Fetal loss after 20 weeks of gestation occurred in two instances, one associated with a maternal death from pulmonary hyper-

tension. Flares in disease activity requiring increased immunosuppression occurred during 9% of pregnancies and within 3 months of delivery in a further 12%. No drug-related side effects were described among the 32 live births after a median follow up of 9 years.

Controversy exists with regard to the appropriateness of azathioprine in pregnant patients with AIH. There is scanty evidence suggesting that this drug or its metabolite is toxic in human pregnancy. However, since many side effects of the drug are described as occurring within the first few months of commencing therapy, it may be prudent to attain remission of the disease using steroid monotherapy when it presents during pregnancy. In patients who become pregnant while taking azathioprine, there is no evidence to suggest that there should be either a dose reduction or drug withdrawal.

Congenital hyperbilirubinemias

Dubin–Johnson syndrome may present *de novo* in pregnancy due to a decrease in the maximal bilirubin secretory capacity during pregnancy. Jaundice and conjugated hyperbilirubinemia manifest themselves in the third trimester, with resolution to prepregnancy levels after delivery. The maternal course during pregnancy is usually uncomplicated. Other familial hyperbilirubinemias such as Gilbert's and Rotor syndromes are unaffected by pregnancy.

Primary biliary cirrhosis and primary sclerosing cholangitis

Successful pregnancy has occurred in patients with both primary biliary cirrhosis (PBC) and primary sclerosing cholangitis (PSC). For both conditions, the diagnosis is usually established before pregnancy. However, pregnancy may unmask previously undiagnosed PBC or trigger a deterioration of the disease. Previously, cholestyramine was used in PBC to ameliorate itch but recent reports suggest the use of UDCA in pregnant patients with PBC is safe. Moreover, it has the added benefits of reducing symptoms and normalizing liver function tests. The effects of pregnancy on PSC are less well known. One child born to a mother with PSC had high bile acid levels in the fetal circulation and subsequent fetal compromise, but the significance of this anecdotal observation is unclear.

Liver tumors in pregnancy

Hepatocellular carcinoma, cholangiocarcinoma, adenomas, cavernous hemangiomas, and focal nodular hyperplasia have all been reported. In general, their clinical presentation does not differ from that in the non pregnant state. Median survival of pregnant women with HCC is shorter than that in nonpregnant controls. As with adenomas, HCC may rupture with catastrophic consequences.

In women without pre-existing liver disease, hepatic adenoma is the most likely tumor to be encountered. It is associated with a past history of use of the oral contraceptive, and these tumors appear to be particularly susceptible to rupture during pregnancy. Although it has been suggested that pregnancy is contraindicated in patients with unresected adenomas, many patients will proceed through pregnancy oblivious to the presence of the benign tumor. Ultrasound surveillance of adenomas has been used to screen for size alterations. Cavernous hemangiomas tend to present with abdominal pain due to rapid enlargement of the tumor. The presence of high levels of estrogen in pregnancy are likely to account for the enhanced growth of these benign tumors.

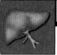
Wilson's disease

Successful pregnancy has been reported in patients with Wilson's disease when disease activity is presymptomatic and in patients stabilized on penicillamine. Pregnancy is rare in patients with cirrhosis. Improvement in the manifestations of Wilson's disease in pregnancy has been described, reflecting increased fetal demand for copper and a four-fold increase in maternal circulating ceruloplasmin. Penicillamine and trientene therapy is safe during pregnancy and should be continued throughout. Worsening of liver function tests and hemolysis has been seen in patients in whom therapy was discontinued.

LIVER DISEASE COINCIDENT WITH PREGNANCY

Acute viral hepatitis

Acute hepatitis is the commonest cause of jaundice in pregnant women. The presentation of hepatitis in pregnancy and its management in similar to that in the nonpregnant state, except that pharmacotherapy should be avoided where possible. There is a slightly increased prevalence of prematurity, but no increased risk of malformation. In the developed world, mortality for acute viral hepatitis is similar in pregnant and nonpregnant patients, whereas in developing countries acute hepatitis ranks third as a cause of maternal mortality. Obstetric practice should follow standard protocol.

Hepatitis A

The clinical course resembles that in the nonpregnant state. The risk to the fetus is minimal. Antibodies to hepatitis A virus cross the placenta and maternal passive prophylaxis with immunoglobulin appears to protect the infant against infection.

Hepatitis B and D

Hepatitis B (HBV) virus infection is the major cause of liver disease worldwide, and increased screening of pregnant women for the presence of the virus has led to a focus on the appropriate management strategies during pregnancy and the purperium. Infection is not transmitted transplacentally, but occurs at the time of delivery. Transmission of the virus occurs in 50% of infants born to mothers with acute hepatitis B, with the greatest risk occurring when infection occurs during the third trimester. Transmission rates are approximately 5% in patients who are chronic carriers of HBV. Risk of transmission of disease is greatest in Chinese populations where the prevalence of hepatitis B e antigen (HBeAg) is high. Over 80% of children born to HBeAg-positive mothers from this population will become hepatitis B surface antigen (HBsAg) chronic carriers, with most remaining asymptomatic until adult life.

All infants born to mothers who are HBsAg-positive should receive immunoprophylaxis. The risk of infection is significantly decreased by a schedule of 0.5mL of intramuscular hepatitis B immunoglobulin (HBIg) administered at birth, followed by hepatitis B vaccine administered within the first week of life, at 1 month and at 6 months of age. An alternative schedule suggests vaccination at birth, 1 month, 2 months, and 12 months, but there are no data comparing the efficacy of the two dosing schedules. Close contacts of the pregnant HBV carrier should be tested for the presence of HBsAg and vaccinated if negative. Unlike HBV infection, hepatitis D has rarely been transmitted to the new-born as antibodies are transferred via the placenta. Immunoprophylaxis against hepatitis B will also protect against transmission of hepatitis D virus. Postexposure prophylaxis can be given without risk. A strategy of universal screening of mothers at 14 weeks of gestation has been advocated, and this could in time result in a dramatic reduction in the incidence of HBV infection worldwide.

Hepatitis C

Risk of transmission of hepatitis C virus (HCV) infection from mother to infant is estimated at 0–2%. This risk is increased in infants born to mothers coinfected with HIV. Chronic HCV infection is not adversely effected by pregnancy. In infants born to HCV-infected mothers, antibodies to HCV are detectable in sera for approximately 6 months, as the antibodies are transmitted transplacentally.

Hepatitis E

This waterborne, epidemic form of viral hepatitis has been recognized as having both an increased prevalence and a poor prognosis in pregnancy. Hepatitis E virus (HEV) has been recognized as the principal cause of high mortality associated with viral hepatitis in pregnancy. In one series from India, mortality was 17.3% in pregnant women, 2.1% in nonpregnant women, and 2.8% in men. Similar patterns of mortality have been noted in other developing countries. Transmission to the fetus has not been recognized. Administration of intramuscular immunoglobulin at birth to the infants of infected mothers has been recommended by some authors.

Herpes simplex hepatitis

Infection with herpes simplex is rare but may be associated with either an acute or subacute course. The condition usually presents in the third trimester with vague symptoms and vesicular lesions on the skin, perineum, or cervix. Laboratory findings are usually typical of acute hepatitis with aminotransferases greater than 10–20 times normal. Pneumonitis or encephalitis may be present in addition to the liver and skin disease. Histology shows hemorrhagic and necrotic areas with associated eosinophilic inclusion bodies. Serology and culture may help confirm the diagnosis. Treatment includes supportive care in addition to aciclovir.

Acetaminophen toxicity

Acetaminophen (paracetamol) is frequently recommended as an analgesic in pregnancy, and overdoses may be encountered either accidentally or in a premeditated fashion in the context of unwanted pregnancy. N-acetylcysteine has been utilized in the treatment of acetaminophen toxicity even in early pregnancy. Fetal losses occur when disturbance of coagulation is severe. A pregnancy test should be performed on all young women presenting with hyperacute liver failure, as concealment of pregnancy is not unusual.

Biliary disease

Several factors contribute to the development of gallstone disease during pregnancy. In addition to risk factors such as the presence of choledochal anomalies (Fig. 28.15), other factors include a reduction in gallbladder motility, an increase in the lithogenicity of bile, increased cholesterol synthesis, increased delivery of cholesterol to the liver, and impairment of the catabolism of cho-

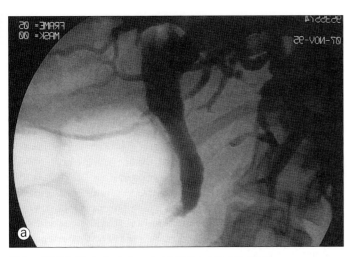

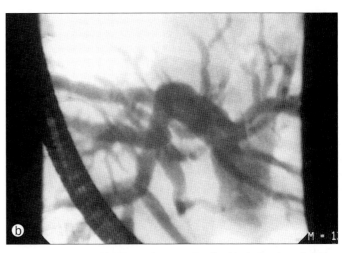

Figure 28.15 Choledochal cyst. (a) Endoscopic retrograde cholangiopancreatography showing a fusiform choledochal cyst with dilatation of intrahepatic bile ducts in a patient presenting at 20 weeks of gestation with ascending cholangitis. (b) Filling defects are visualized in the intrahepatic bile ducts. Despite intravenous antibiotics and surgical excision of the cyst, fetal death occurred. (Courtesy of Drs Pauline Kane and Sarah Kirwin.)

lesterol to bile acids. These factors result in prevalences of 31 and 9% for the presence of gallbladder sludge and gallstones respectively. Moreover, patients who have had oral contraceptives prior to pregnancy have an increased prevalence of gallstone disease. Obstruction to the biliary tree should be managed conventionally. Endoscopic retrograde cholangiopancreatography and sphincterotomy have been performed uneventfully in pregnancy. Surgery involves a higher risk of fetal loss.

Budd–Chiari syndrome

Rarely the Budd–Chiari syndrome occurs in pregnancy or in the early postpartum period (Fig. 28.16). The clinical features, investigations, and management of such patients is similar to that in the nonpregnant state. The increased prevalence of the syndrome in pregnancy relates to the presence of a hypercoagulable state and reduced levels of antithrombin III. Maternal mortality has been reported to be high. Repeat pregnancy has been reported in some patients despite the presence of the syndrome.

Liver transplant recipients

A successful liver transplant allows for the return of normal menstrual patterns in the majority of patients of child-bearing age. Although pregnancies in liver graft recipients are less common than renal transplant recipients, several centers have reported a number of successful deliveries. In one series of 37 patients treated largely with cyclosporine-based immunosuppression regimens, drug-induced hypertension was reported in 46%, eclampsia/pre-eclampsia in 21%, allograft rejection in 17%, and graft loss in 5.7%. In addition there was a high rate of prematurity and low birth weight. A similar study of tacrolimus-based immunosuppression regimens reported 35 deliveries from 27 women with a cesarean section rate of 49% and a perinatal survival rate of 94%. The infants who did not survive were born

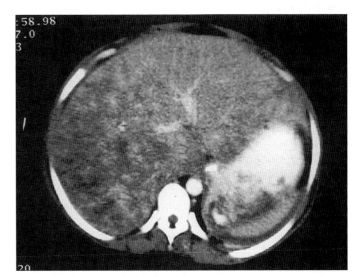

Figure 28.16 Segmental Budd–Chiari syndrome. Contrast-enhanced abdominal CT scan showing hepatomegaly and a segmental arterioportal geographic perfusion pattern involving the right lobe. These findings were found in a 30-year-old primagravida with venous outflow block involving the right hepatic vein secondary to factor V Leiden deficiency. (Courtesy of Drs Pauline Kane and Sarah Kirwin.)

to mothers who conceived early post-transplant. Rejection occurred in 22% of women during pregnancy and 11% postpartum. The incidence of hypertension was 11%. Tacrolimus may cause transient renal impairment in the newborn due to transplacental transfer of the drug. Liver transplantation has been performed successfully in pregnant patients presenting with acute liver failure.

PRACTICE POINT

Illustrative case

A 27-year-old woman, para[1+0] presented at 33 weeks of gestation with a 2-day history of abdominal pain and ankle edema. There was no significant past medical history and her pregnancy had been uncomplicated. Blood pressure was 160/90mmHg and clinical examination revealed mild tenderness in the right upper quadrant with a gravid uterus correct for dates. There was no encephalopathy. Testing of the urine showed proteinuria. Liver function tests were appropriate for pregnancy. Renal function, clotting and hematologic profiles were within the normal range. An expectant approach to management was undertaken and the patient was admitted for bed rest and monitoring of presumed pre-eclampsia. Dexamethasone was administered in order to facilitate maturation of the fetal lung.

Two days later, the abdominal pain returned and in association with this, the following were noted: blood pressure 140/85mmHg; white cell count 16.9×10^9/L [normal range (NR) 4.5–11 $\times 10^9$/L]; platelets 63×10^9/L (NR 160–440 $\times 10^9$/L). Serum alkaline phosphatase was 167IU/L (NR 30–115IU/L); bilirubin 3.2mg/dL (NR 0.3–1.5mg/dL); AST 654IU/L (NR 0–45IU/L); and albumin 17g/L (NR 35–50g/L). Urea was 27mg/dL (NR 8–25mg/dL) and creatinine 2.0mg/dL (0.6–1.5mg/dL). International normalized ratio (INR) was 2.25 (NR 0.9–1.2). Clotting abnormalities were corrected by administration of fresh frozen plasma and platelets, and cesarean section performed. After delivery of a 2050g male infant, the patient was transferred to the intensive treatment unit.

On admission, her abdominal scar was edematous with a hematoma present within it. Ultrasound showed increased echogenicity within the liver with patent vessels. Computed tomography scanning showed no alteration in density between the liver and spleen, but bilateral pleural effusions were present and a large hematoma was noted within the uterine cavity. The patient remained hypoxic despite being intubated, was oligoanuric and hypertensive, (blood pressure 200/120mmHg). Hyper-reflexia was present on examination in association with ankle clonus. The differential diagnosis was hypertension-related liver disease complicated by either HELLP syndrome or acute fatty liver of pregnancy given the sonographic findings.

Further treatment included fluid resuscitation, support of coagulopathy, institution of N-acetylcysteine, intravenous antibiotics for sepsis, magnesium sulfate and hydralazine for hypertension, and continuous venovenous hemofiltration for renal failure. Ventilatory support was required for 5 days. Peak in serum creatinine occurred on day 3 postpartum (7.5mg/dL), whereas the hypertension remained problematic for 3 weeks while the patient was on antihypertensive agents. She was discharged from hospital 3 weeks postpartum with normal liver function tests and labetelol for hypertension.

Interpretation

Cases such as this illustrate the difficulty in identifying a unifying hypothesis in patients with pregnancy-related liver disease. What is clear is that features of the three common liver diseases of the third trimester may be present to a variable extent. Extensive radiologic investigation may not elucidate the exact cause of hepatic and other end organ dysfunction. Liver biopsy may be appropriate in the recovery phase, but should not alter or impede management decisions.

In this case, hypertension-related liver disease was the predominant pathology, although features of HELLP syndrome and acute fatty liver were also present. What is also apparent from cases such as this, is that significant end organ damage may occur long into the postpartum course and may peak as long as 7 days postpartum. Attention to all organ systems should be the paradigm, and intensive care management will be appropriate in many instances. Clotting disorders should be supported aggressively and a search for DIC performed on a daily basis.

FURTHER READING

Depue RH, Bernstein L, Ross RK, et al. Hyperemesis gravidarum in relation to estradiol levels, pregnancy outcome, and other maternal factors: A seroepidemiologic study. Am J Obstet Gynecol. 1987;156:1137–41. *This series reviews vomiting in pregnancy in 1250 women and outlines the associations with young age, first pregnancy, and low fetal loss, as well as hormonal changes.*

Heneghan MA, Norris SM, O'Grady JG, Harrison PM, McFarlane IG. Autoimmune hepatitis: optimal management in pregnancy and review of maternal and fetal outcomes. Hepatology. 1998;28:393A. *This series describes 32 live births from 18 women with AIH, six of whom had cirrhosis. Relapse rates of AIH during pregnancy were 9% and 12% in the first 3 months postpartum.*

Jacquemin E, Cresteil D, Manouvrier S, Boute O, Hadchouel M. Heterozygous non-sense mutation of the MDR3 gene in familial intrahepatic cholestasis of pregnancy. Lancet. 1999;353:210–11. *Report in which the association between intrahepatic cholestasis of pregnancy and heterozygosity in the MDR3 gene was described.*

Martin JN Jr, Blake PG, Perry KG, et al. The natural history of HELLP syndrome. Patterns of disease progression and regression. Am J Obstet Gynecol. 1991;164:1500–3. *A total of 158 patients with HELLP syndrome have been evaluated, showing peak abnormalities in liver function at 48 hours postpartum.*

Molmenti EP, Jain AB, Marino N, Rishi NK, Dvorchik I, Marsh JW. Liver transplantation and pregnancy. Clin Liv Dis. 1999;3:163–74. *This paper reviews the complete literature on pregnancy in liver transplant recipients with particular reference to 35 deliveries in 27 women on tacrolimus immunosuppression at the University of Pittsburgh. Details of tacrolimus concentrations in maternal, placental, and infant serum are given.*

Riely CA, Latham PS, Romero R, Duffy TP. Acute fatty liver of pregnancy. A reassessment based on observations in nine patients. Ann Intern Med. 1987;106:703–706. *The clinical characteristics of acute fatty liver of pregnancy are reported in nine patients. All had pre-eclampsia and one had HELLP syndrome.*

Rolfes DB, Ishak KG. Liver disease in toxemia of pregnancy. Am J Gastroenterol. 1986;81:1138–44. *This report reviews the pathologic findings of hypertension-related liver disease of pregnancy in 103 women.*

Sibai BM, Taslimi NM, El-Nazer A. Maternal-perinatal outcome associated with the syndrome of hemolysis, elevated liver enzymes, and low platelets in severe pre-eclampsia–eclampsia. Am J Obstet Gynaecol. 1986;155:501–9. *This report is of 112 patients with HELLP syndrome from a series of 1153 women with pre-eclampsia in pregnancy. Maternal mortality was 2% and perinatal mortality 33%.*

Treem WR, Rinaldo P, Hale DE, et al. Acute fatty liver of pregnancy and long-chain 3 hydroxyacyl-coenzyme A dehydrogenase deficiency. Hepatology. 1994;19:339–45. *This report describes the mechanism and association between acute fatty liver of pregnancy and LCHAD.*

Weinstein L. Syndrome of hemolysis, elevated liver enzymes, and low platelet count: A severe consequence of hypertension in pregnancy. Am J Obstet Gynecol. 1982;142:159–67. *This is the original report which coined the term 'HELLP syndrome'. The characteristics of 29 patients with HELLP are reviewed.*

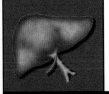

Section 3 Specific Diseases of the Liver

Chapter 29 Drug- and Toxin-Induced Liver Disease

Suzanne Norris

INTRODUCTION

Drug-induced liver diseases are clinicopathologic syndromes in which hepatotoxicity is caused by drugs and other foreign chemicals. Such syndromes are a potential complication of nearly every medication that is prescribed, as the liver is central to the metabolic disposition of virtually all drugs and toxins. The severity varies from minor nonspecific injury to hepatic necrosis resulting in acute liver failure, chronic hepatitis, cirrhosis, and liver tumors. While removal of the offending drug will usually ameliorate the injury, its continuation may lead to liver failure or chronic liver disease. Early recognition of hepatic drug reactions is therefore a major concern for clinicians. Some types of drug-induced liver disease result from dose-dependent toxic mechanisms. Most, however, are adverse hepatic drug reactions, and unintentional side effects occurring at conventional doses used for prophylaxis and therapy. Such drug-induced hepatic reactions are rare and unpredictable complications of commonly used drugs. The clinical syndromes and histopathology they produce mimic all known hepatobiliary diseases and one drug may damage the liver through a variety of mechanisms, leading to different histologic appearances in different patients. Methyldopa, for instance, can cause acute or chronic hepatitis, granulomas, or cholestasis. It is therefore likely that multiple pathogenetic mechanisms operate or that the response of the liver to injury may vary between individuals, thereby resulting in diverse clinicopathologic features.

EPIDEMIOLOGY

Drug-induced liver injury is rarely encountered in general practice, but accounts for between 2–5% of hospital admissions for jaundice in the USA, and between 2–3% of all hospital admissions due to adverse drug reactions. For more serious forms of liver disease that result in fatal outcome, drugs are disproportionately represented. In the USA, drugs account for up to 30% of cases of fulminant hepatic failure. Suspected drug-induced liver injury accounts for 4–7% of all reports of adverse drug effects voluntarily reported to central registries. While between 600 and 1000 drugs have been implicated in the etiology of a wide variety of liver diseases, only a few agents produce clinically significant liver injury in more than 0.1% of individuals exposed. For most drugs, the risk of liver injury is in the range of 1–10 per 100,000 individuals exposed, although there are some notable exceptions (Fig. 29.1).

Frequencies of drug-induced liver diseases	
Drug	Frequency (cases per 100,000 exposed)
Isoniazid	1000–2500
Chlorpromazine	500–1000
Dantrolene	1000
Valproic acid	3–200
Ketoconazole	7–9
Phenytoin	<10
Diclofenac	1–5
Amoxicillin and clavulinic acid	0.1–0.5

Figure 29.1 Frequencies of drug-induced liver diseases. (Adapted from Farrell GC. Drug-induced liver disease. Churchill Livingstone;1994:1–673.)

BASIC PRINCIPLES OF DRUG METABOLISM

The vulnerability of the liver to damage by drugs and toxins is a consequence of its central role in metabolism. The position of the liver between the gastrointestinal tract and peripheral organs results in its constant exposure to ingested foreign substances, the metabolism of which may result in noxious intermediates that can cause or augment liver injury.

Many drugs and toxins are lipophilic, entering the body through the gastrointestinal tract, and require conversion from water-insoluble (nonpolar) to water-soluble (polar) metabolites for their elimination in urine and bile. The liver is uniquely suited to metabolize lipophilic drugs due to the fenestrations in the endothelium lining the sinusoidal spaces (Fig. 29.2). These fenestrations allow the passive diffusion of most blood-borne proteins from the sinusoid to the space of Disse (Fig. 29.2) where protein-bound drugs come into contact with the hepatocyte plasma membrane. From here, the proteins can be actively transported or diffuse passively into the hepatocyte where the drugs are metabolized and then excreted into the space of Disse, sinusoids, and ultimately the systemic circulation to be excreted by the kidney. Alternatively, the metabolites may be excreted in bile.

Biotransformation is the process by which therapeutic agents are rendered more hydrophilic. The enzyme systems responsible

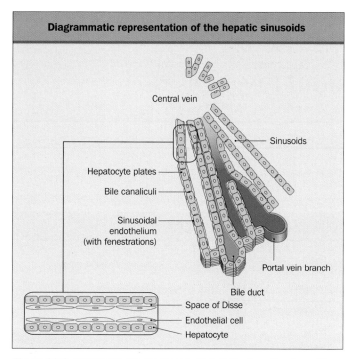

Diagrammatic representation of the hepatic sinusoids

Central vein

Sinusoids

Hepatocyte plates

Bile canaliculi

Sinusoidal endothelium (with fenestrations)

Portal vein branch

Bile duct

Space of Disse

Endothelial cell

Hepatocyte

Figure 29.2 Diagrammatic representation of the hepatic sinusoids.

Drug biotransformation

Lipid-soluble drug

Phase I: Mixed function oxidase/P450

Products of: oxidation reduction hydrolysis

Phase II: Conjugation

Water-soluble compound

Urine   Bile

Figure 29.3 Schematic representation of drug biotransformation.

for biotransformation are located in the smooth endoplasmic reticulum of the hepatocyte and include mixed function oxidase or mono-oxygenase (MFO), cytochrome c-reductase and cytochrome P450. Biotransformation consists of two phases (Fig. 29.3).

Phase I prepares the compound for conjugation by providing polar groups through hydroxylation or oxidation, thereby modifying the primary structure of the drug. In phase II, the resulting metabolite is conjugated with glutathione (GSH), glucuronate, sulfate, glycine, or water, which enhance its water solubility. The conjugate can then be excreted. Differences between the phase I and II pathways of metabolism are demonstrated in Figure 29.4.

The key enzyme in phase I reactions is cytochrome P450, a large multigene family of enzymes with nearly 300 members. P450 enzymes are composed of an apoprotein and a heme group which binds oxygen after electron-transfer reactions from nicotinamide adenine dinucleotide phosphate, reduced form (NADPH), resulting in hydroxylation, dealkylation, or dehalogenation. Each group of genes composes a family whose isoenzymes function in a similar fashion, and three distinct P450 gene families (termed CYP1, CYP2, and CYP3) account for the majority of phase I metabolism. Each family contains members that are more than 40% homologous in terms of amino acid sequence. These families are subdivided into subfamilies which share greater than 55% amino acid sequence homology. Each isoenzyme has specific substrates on which it can act; for example, CYP2E1 is the major isoenzyme responsible for the production of metabolites of acetaminophen (paracetamol), while CYP3A is concerned with the metabolism of cyclosporine. There are marked differences between patients in their ability to perform phase I liver metabolism of some drugs, and genetic differences in the catalytic activity of P450 isoenzymes may determine idiosyncratic reactions to drugs. One example is the poor metabolism of the antihypertensive agent, debrisoquin

Differences between phase I and phase II pathways of drug metabolism		
	Phase I Oxidation	**Phase II Conjugation**
Enzyme system	Cytochrome P450	Acetyltransferases Glucuronyltransferases Sulfotransferases
Location in liver	Centrilobular	Periportal
Location within cell	Microsomal	Can be nonmicrosomal
Location within microsomal membrane	Surface	Interior
Endoplasmic reticulum	Smooth	Rough

Figure 29.4 Differences between phase I and phase II pathways of drug metabolism.

(debrisoquine), which occurs in approximately 5% of the Caucasian population. The debrisoquin 'poor metabolizer' phenotype is inherited as an autosomal recessive trait and results from genetic defects in several alleles for a single P450 enzyme, CYP2D6, leading to its deficiency. This enzyme system also metabolizes most neuroleptics and β blockers. More recently, it has been reported that approximately 2% of Caucasians are 'rapid extensive metabolizers' of debrisoquin and these patients demonstrate rapid metabolism of other drugs that are CYP2D6 substrates. The rate of hepatic drug metabolism may also be affected by compounds that, through induction of the cytochrome P450 system, accelerates the metabolism of certain drugs (Fig. 29.5).

It is generally accepted that women should not rely on the oral contraceptive pill alone if they are also taking rifampin (rifampicin) or antiepileptic medication, both of which cause

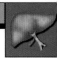

induction of CYP3A4 with subsequent accelerated metabolism of sex hormones. P450 induction also leads to accelerated production of toxic metabolites, as demonstrated by ethanol which induces CYP2E1, thereby enhancing the toxicity of acetaminophen (paracetamol). Cigarette smoke is also a potent inducer of certain P450 enzyme species.

RISK FACTORS FOR DRUG-INDUCED HEPATOTOXICITY

Individual susceptibility to drug- and toxin-induced liver injury may be affected by a variety of host factors such as age, sex, genetic make up, pregnancy, nutritional status, and coexisting disease (Fig. 29.6).

The increased susceptibility of the elderly to hepatotoxicity from drugs such as nonsteroidal anti-inflammatory drugs (NSAIDs) and isoniazid may result from age-related changes including reduced hepatic bloodflow, decreased activity of the hepatic cytochrome P450 enzyme system, and reduced renal clearance. Women are particularly predisposed to drug-induced hepatitis, for example chronic hepatitis due to nitrofurantoin or diclofenac, while cholestatic drug reactions are equally found in both sexes. However, male renal transplant recipients are more predisposed to azathioprine-induced liver disease than females.

Obesity may increase the risk of hepatotoxicity through prolonged hepatic exposure to fat-soluble drugs released from stores in adipose tissues. Impairment of GSH synthesis and its depletion in the hepatocyte in patients with malnutrition and chronic alcoholism may be responsible for their increased susceptibility to acetaminophen toxicity. Glutathione depletion in patients with acquired immune deficiency syndrome may also be associated with the increased susceptibility of this patient group to drug toxicity from oxacillin and sulfa drugs. The association between hypoalbuminemia and hepatotoxicity from aspirin may reflect the reduced binding of aspirin to plasma proteins and subsequent increased tissue levels. Inborn errors of metabolism, such as defects in mitochondrial β-oxidation, have been associated with microvesicular fat infiltration in children exposed to aspirin or valproic acid. Deficient uridine diphosphate (UDP) glucuronosyl transferase activity in patients with Gilbert's syndrome may be associated with increased sensitivity to acetaminophen.

PATHOGENESIS OF DRUG-INDUCED HEPATOTOXICITY

Drugs with the potential for hepatotoxicity can be divided into intrinsic or predictable hepatotoxins and unpredictable or idiosyncratic hepatotoxins (Fig. 29.7).

Characteristics of human liver P450		
P450	Drug substrates	Probable inducers
CYP1A2	Caffeine Acetaminophen Theophylline Cimetidine	Cigarette smoke Omeprazole
CYP2C	Omeprazole Diazepam Tolbutamide Phenylbutazone Tienilic acid	
CYP2D6	Debrisoquin Codeine Fluoxetine Quinidine Most β blockers Many neuroleptics	
CYP2E1	Acetaminophen Ethanol	Ethanol Isoniazid
CYP3A4	Cyclosporine A Erythromycin Ketoconazole Estrogens Nifedipine Acetaminophen Midazolam/triazolam Tamoxifen Lovastatin	Rifampin Glucocorticoids Antiepileptic medication

Figure 29.5 Characteristics of human liver P450.

Host variables for individual susceptibility to drug-induced liver injury		
Host factor		Increased susceptibility
Age	Infancy Old age	Valproic acid, salicylates NSAIDs, isoniazid, nitrofurantoin
Sex	Male Female	Amoxicillin–clavulinic acid, azathioprine Isoniazid, zidovudine, halothane, methyldopa
Racial background Asian/African		Isoniazid
Pre-existing disease	Liver Renal AIDS	Acetaminophen, isoniazid NSAIDs Oxacillin, trimethoprim–sulfamethoxazole
Nutrition	Obesity Fasting	Halothane, methotrexate Acetaminophen
Pregnancy		Acetaminophen
Other drugs	Alcohol Isoniazid Antiepileptics	Acetaminophen Acetaminophen Acetaminophen
Genetic polymorphism/defect	Slow acetylators Urea cycle Mitochondrial β-oxidation UDP glucuronosyl transferase HLA phenotypes	Isoniazid Valproic acid Valproic acid Acetaminophen See text

Figure 29.6 Host variables for individual susceptibility to drug-induced liver injury.

The former produce liver injury in a predictable, dose-dependent manner that can be reproduced in experimental animals. Characteristically, these toxins cause liver necrosis that affects predominantly one area of the liver lobule, for example acetaminophen which causes centrilobular or zone 3 necrosis. In contrast, the latter group produce liver injury in an unpredictable manner (while administered within an acceptable therapeutic range), are not dose-dependent, are not reproducible in animal models, and produce a more diffuse form of liver injury. An example here is isoniazid.

Most intrinsic hepatotoxins produce injury through the toxic effects of their reactive metabolites after phase I biotransformation. These reactive metabolites, which include electrophilic radicals, free radicals, or reactive oxygen, can form covalent bonds with cellular molecules such as proteins, lipids, and nucleic acids, with subsequent disruption of their function. This cellular distortion produces liver injury by inactivating key enzymes or by forming protein–drug complexes that are potential targets for immune-mediated liver injury (Fig. 29.8).

In the past, covalent binding has been considered to be a key mechanism of drug-induced liver injury; it appears to be the main mechanism by which acetaminophen causes necrosis and by which electrophilic metabolites of carcinogens distort DNA. However, the extent of covalent binding of drug intermediates to cellular proteins does not correlate with the level of hepatic necrosis in experimental models, questioning the importance of this mechanism. Nevertheless, the specificity of the proteins covalently bound by metabolites may be more important than the extent of covalent modification.

Oxidative processes are also important to the development of cell damage through the generation of oxidative stress, an imbalance between pro-oxidants and antioxidants. Electrophilic metabolites of acetaminophen metabolism can act as cellular oxidants resulting in oxidation of thiol groups in proteins. Oxidative stress is also an important mechanism for activating apoptosis. Glutathione, a major intracellular antioxidant that protects against the toxic effects of covalent binding, is important for the conjugation of several metabolites (such as acetaminophen) and facilitates their excretion in the bile. Depletion of GSH can therefore potentiate or augment hepatic injury. Lipid peroxidation is another major mechanism by which free radicals and active oxygen cause cellular injury. Peroxidative injury may also result from the generation of superoxide anions.

Most of the intrinsic hepatotoxins (such as acetaminophen) produce cellular injury as an indirect consequence of depletion of essential molecules or interference with biochemical pathways essential for cell integrity, which subsequently results in secondary structural damage. However, some intrinsic hepatotoxins produce a direct destructive effect on hepatocyte structure through the effects of peroxidation [such as carbon tetrachloride (CCl_4)] (Fig. 29.7). This structural alteration leads to secondary metabolic defects. Irrespective of whether the initial insult is metabolic or structural, ultimately it results in cell death. It is uncertain whether a final common pathway exists for drug-induced liver injury. Disruption of cellular calcium homeostasis, impairment of energy production and depletion of ATP have all been postulated to be key determinants of cell death (Fig. 29.9).

In addition to these biochemical mechanisms of liver injury, other factors play a role. Activated hepatic macrophages release proteases, nitrogen radicals, superoxide, and cytokines, which also recruit lymphocytes and neutrophils from the systemic circulation to the hepatic inflammatory response. Cytokines produced by activated macrophages can be hepatotoxins in their own right, for example tumor necrosis factor-α (TNF-α) which is thought to exert its hepatotoxic effect by producing intramitochondrial oxidative stress. Studies have reported that anti-TNF-α antibodies protect against CCl_4-induced hepatotoxicity in rats.

Immunologic mechanisms may also be involved in idiosyncratic drug-induced hepatotoxicity. The term immunologic idiosyncrasy assumes an allergic basis for drug-induced liver injury. However, the mechanism of the immune response is still not fully understood. The basis of the injury is thought to be hypersensitivity which

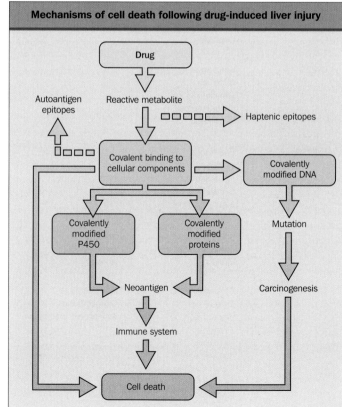

Mechanisms of cell death following drug-induced liver injury

Figure 29.8 Mechanisms of cell death following drug-induced liver injury.

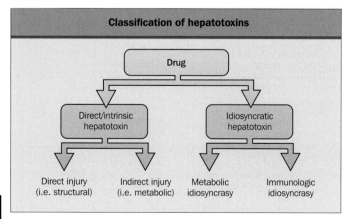

Classification of hepatotoxins

Figure 29.7 Classification of hepatotoxins.

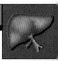

Effect of disruption of cellular calcium homeostasis

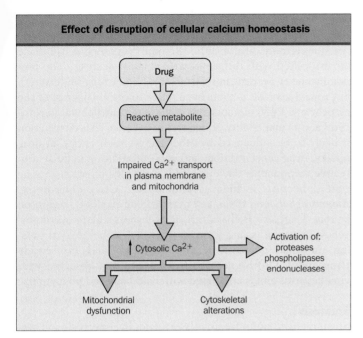

Figure 29.9 Effect of disruption of cellular calcium homeostasis.

Drug-induced liver disease and autoantibody expression

Drug	Autoantibody
Nitrofurantoin	ANA, SMA
Methyldopa	ANA, SMA
Chlorpromazine	ANA (AMA negative)
Tienilic acid	LKM_2
Diclofenac	ANA
Sulphonamides	ANA
Iproniazid	AMA (E6 moiety)
Halothane	PDG (E2 moiety)
Nimesulide	ANA
Alverine	ANA

Figure 29.10 Drug-induced liver disease and autoantibody expression. ANA, antinuclear antibody; SMA, smooth muscle antibody; AMA, antimitochondrial antibody; LKM_2, liver kidney microsomal type 2; PDG, pyruvate dehydrogenase.

develops after a period of 1–5 weeks, recurs quickly on readministration of the drug, and is accompanied by fever, rash, eosinophilia, lymphocytosis, and an inflammatory infiltration of the liver. In some cases, the liver is involved as part of a systemic hypersensitivity reaction. For drugs to induce an immune response, it is generally assumed that they covalently alter an endogenous macromolecule forming a carrier hapten-conjugate, which then acts as an immunogen and elicits a humoral and/or a cellular immune response directed against the liver. The immune response may be directed against three types of antigenic determinants (epitopes) of the altered macromolecule: epitopes that include the bound drug metabolite (haptenic epitopes); novel epitopes of the carrier molecule, namely neoantigens that result from the covalent modification; and native or autoantigen epitopes normally seen as self molecules but rendered immunogenic by covalent modifications (Fig. 29.8).

Autoantibodies have been documented in the sera of patients taking the antihypertensive diuretic, tienilic acid (Fig. 29.10). These patients developed a high incidence of anti-liver-kidney microsomal type 2 (anti-LKM_2) autoantibodies that recognize epitopes specific to CYP2C9, the major cytochrome P450 involved in the biotransformation of tienilic acid. Anti-LKM_2 autoantibodies are highly specific for drug-induced autoimmune-like chronic hepatitis and have a different pattern of immunofluorescence staining from the anti-LKM_1 autoantibodies found in type 2 autoimmune hepatitis. Another example of autoantibodies associated with drug-induced liver injury is the recognition of the E2 subunit of pyruvate dehydrogenase (PDC) by sera of patients with a history of halothane hepatitis. E2, the major autoantigen recognized by antimitochondrial antibodies in primary biliary cirrhosis, mimics the epitope common to several trifluoroacetylated proteins produced as a result of halothane exposure, representing an example of molecular mimicry. Non-tissue-specific autoantibodies, such as antinuclear and anti-smooth muscle antibodies, may occur in drug hepatitis caused by nitrofurantoin, methyldopa, and minocycline. Major histocompatibility antigens (MHC) class I and class II molecules present antigenic peptides to T lymphocytes, and as human

leukocyte antigen (HLA) molecule expression is genetically polymorphic it is possible that certain haplotypes may modulate the immune response. Weak associations have been reported with the MHC complex HLA-A11 for halothane-induced and diclofenac-induced hepatotoxicity, and HLA-DR6 for nitrofurantoin-induced liver injury. Other drugs that are thought to mediate immunologic-mediated liver damage include phenytoin, dapsone, sulfonamides, and diclofenac. Idiosyncratic hepatotoxicity not associated with hypersensitivity is thought to depend on metabolic idiosyncrasy and examples include isoniazid and valproic acid. Figure 29.11 compares the features that suggest immunoallergy or metabolic idiosyncrasy (see also Fig. 29.7).

Hepatotoxicity is normally prevented or limited by a number of protective mechanisms. Cytochrome P450 can be inactivated by the reactive metabolites themselves when they covalently bind to the apoprotein of cytochrome P450. Reactive epoxides undergo transformation by epoxide hydrolases to stable compounds. Other enzymes such as glutathione peroxidase and catalase protect against lipid peroxidation. Failure of these protective mechanisms therefore contributes to drug-induced liver injury.

PATTERNS OF DRUG-INDUCED HEPATOTOXICITY

Although the mechanisms by which drugs can interfere with bilirubin metabolism and produce jaundice are many and the spectrum of histologic change they induce is varied, two broad categories of liver injury are commonly found, cholestasis and hepatocellular (or cytolytic) damage. The former is characterized by a predominantly elevated alkaline phosphatase (Alk.P.) and γ-glutamyltransferase (γ-GT), while in the latter the aminotransferases [alanine (ALT) and aspartate (AST)] are significantly elevated, although mixed patterns of abnormalities are common. While some drugs can produce a characteristic lesion, others are associated with a broader spectrum of pathologic change. A variety of chronic lesions related to vascular damage, neoplastic change or fibrosis has also been described. These patterns of hepatotoxicity are summarized in Figures 29.12 & 29.13.

HEPATOCELLULAR INJURY

Hepatocellular injury can be acute or chronic and includes necrosis, steatosis, and hepatitis in various combinations.

Necrosis

Many drugs can cause necrosis but differ in the extent and severity of this injury. Necrosis induced by intrinsic hepatotoxins is often zonal (centrilobular or zone 3, midzonal or zone 2, and periportal or zone 1), whereas that produced by idiosyncratic reactions is more diffuse, although some drugs such as halothane are associated with diffuse as well as zonal necrosis. The predominance of necrosis in selected areas is not fully understood, but zone 3 necrosis is thought to relate to the abundance of the cytochrome P450 metabolizing systems in centrilobular hepatocytes and a vulnerability of this area to hypoxia. This distribution is likely to be influenced by other factors such as rate of drug uptake, drug concentration, and concentrations of cellular protective components such as GSH. Examples of drugs causing zone 3 necrosis include acetaminophen, CCl_4, chloroform, *Amanita phalloides* toxin, and pyrrolizidine alkaloids. Periportal or zone 1 necrosis is characteristic of ferrous sulfate overdoses, yellow phosphorus, and toxins such as allylalcohol. Agents causing midzonal necrosis include beryllium and furosemide (frusemide). Diffuse necrosis is similar to that observed with viral hepatitis and is associated with halothane and phenytoin.

Steatosis

Steatotic liver injury frequently precedes liver necrosis and two types are described according to their pathologic patterns.

Comparison of drug-induced immunologic and metabolic idiosyncrasy		
Feature	Immunologic type	Metabolic type
Frequency	0.01% exposed	0.1–2% exposed
Gender	More common in women	Slightly more common in women
Latent period	Relatively constant	Highly variable
Response to rechallenge	Invariable fever in 12–72 hours	Usual, abnormal liver function tests after 3–30 days
Fever	Common	Less striking
Rash, arthralgia	Common	Rare
Eosinophilia	20–70% cases	Less than 10% cases
Granulomas	Common	Rare
Autoantigens	Common	Rare
Examples	Diclofenac Methyldopa	Isoniazid Ketoconazole

Figure 29.11 Comparison of drug-induced immunologic and metabolic idiosyncrasy. (Adapted from Farrell GC. Drug-induced liver disease. Churchill Livingstone;1994:1–673.)

Morphologic classification of drug-induced acute liver injury	
Type of injury	Examples
Hepatocellular (cytolytic) Zonal necrosis Steatosis: macrovesicular microvesicular Hepatitis	Acetaminophen, CCl_4, halothane Ethanol, methotrexate Tetracycline, valproic acid, methotrexate Methyl dopa, isomiazid
Cholestatic Hepatocanalicular (pericholangitis) Canalicular (noninflammatory)	Amoxicillin–clavulinic acid, chlorpromazine Estrogens, 17α-substituted steroids (anabolic)
Vascular Hepatic vein occlusion Venohocclusive disease Peliosis hepatitis	Estrogens Antineoplastic agents, pyrrolizidine alkaloids Anabolic steroids

Figure 29.12 Morphologic classification of drug-induced acute liver injury.

Morphologic classification of drug-related chronic liver injury	
Type of injury	Examples
Chronic hepatitis Autoimmune-like	Methyldopa, dantrolene, sulfonamides, diclofenac
Viral hepatitis-like	Amiodarone, isoniazid, halothane, aspirin
Chronic cholestasis Ductal (sclerosing cholangitis) Ductopenia Hepatocanalicular	Floxuridine (FUDR) Flucloxacillin, tricyclic antidepressants Chlorpromazine, barbituates, cimetidine, phenytoin, tolbutamide, amitriptyline
Granulomas (more than 50 drugs implicated)	Sulpha drugs, allopurinol, carbamazepine, chlorpromazine, diazepam, diltiazem, gold, phenytoin, penicillin, nitrofurantoin tolbutamide, quinidine, isoniazid
Chronic steatosis	Ethanol, methotrexate, antineoplastic agents
Phospholipidosis	Amiodarone, perhexilene maleate, thioridazine
Vascular Nodular regenerative hyperplasia Noncirrhotic portal hypertension Hepatic vein occlusion Veno-occlusive disease Peliosis hepatitis	Azathioprine, 6-thioguanine Vinyl chloride, azathioprine, 6-thioguanine Estrogens Antineoplastic agents, pyrrolizidine alkaloids Anabolic steroids
Neoplasms Adenoma Hepatocellular carcinoma Angiosarcoma	Estrogens Estrogens, anabolic steroids, vinyl chloride Vinyl chloride, thorotrast
Fibrosis	Methotrexate, vitamin A, vinyl chloride

Figure 29.13 Morphologic classification of drug-induced chronic liver injury.

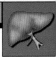
Steatosis may predominate in either the centrilobular or periportal region. Occasionally, the fat cells may coalesce to form fatty cysts or become surrounded by histiocytes to form lipogranulomas. Triglyceride is the predominant lipid that accumulates and this occurs when the rate of formation exceeds that of disposition into lipoproteins or hydrolysis to fatty acids. In macrovesicular steatosis, the hepatocyte contains a single large droplet of fat which displaces the nucleus to the periphery of the cell, giving it the appearance of an adipocyte (Fig. 29.14a). This pattern of fat deposition is seen with obesity, diabetes, ethanol, malnutrition, and jejunoilial bypass.

With microvesicular steatosis, the hepatocyte is occupied by numerous small droplets of fat leaving the nucleus centrally placed so that the cell retains its hepatocyte-like appearance (Fig. 29.14b). The pathogenesis appears related to inhibition of the mitochondrial oxidation of fatty acids and several drugs demonstrate this entity including valproic acid and tetracycline. Another form of lipid accumulation is phospholipidosis, which occurs when amphiphilic drugs accumulate within lysosomes forming a stable complex with phospholipids. Phospholipidosis can histologically resemble alcoholic hepatitis. The liver injury induced is usually mild but can be associated with Mallory's hyaline, and can progress to overt disease. Cirrhosis has been observed in patients taking amiodarone and perhexilene maleate. Alcohol-like liver injury without phospholipidosis has also been reported in patients taking nifedipine and diltiazem.

Hepatitis

Nonspecific hepatitis is typical of many types of drug-induced hepatotoxicity. It lacks the typical appearance of autoimmune hepatitis and is associated with scattered foci of necrosis and a variable inflammatory infiltrate. It is usually not associated with progressive liver disease. Granulomatous hepatitis is characterized by aggregates of epitheloid histiocytes and accompanying inflammatory cells. Drug-induced granulomas are usually noncaseating and their presence suggests an immunologic idiosyncrasy (see Fig. 29.11). Chronic hepatitis that resembles autoimmune hepatitis in its histologic and clinical features has been described for a number of drugs (see Fig. 29.13). Pathologic changes include portal and periportal inflammatory infiltration by lymphocytes and plasma cells, often associated with degeneration of surrounding cells (piecemeal necrosis). Autoantibodies are frequently present in the sera.

CHOLESTASIS

Intrahepatic cholestasis is a common manifestation of hepatotoxicity. It is predominantly noted as centrilobular bile staining of hepatocytes and as bile casts in the canaliculi. If the cholestasis is severe, the periportal area is also involved and bile plugs occur. Several forms of cholestatic liver disease have been described (see Figs 29.12 & 29.13).

Bland, pure or canicular cholestasis

Bland, pure or canalicular cholestasis as exemplified by anabolic and contraceptive steroids, is characterized by a bland accumulation of bile in canaliculi and cells, and necrosis and inflammatory features are minor or absent (Fig. 29.15).

Hepatocanicular cholestasis

In hepatocanalicular cholestasis, cholestasis is accompanied by a portal and lobular inflammatory infiltrate. Necrosis may also occur. This type of liver injury is observed with chlorpromazine and erythromycin.

Ductopenic cholestasis

The inflammatory cholestasis may also be accompanied by destruction of the small bile ducts resulting in ductopenic cholestasis or 'vanishing bile duct syndrome'. Drugs implicated in this form of liver injury include: chlorpromazine, tricyclic antidepressants, flucloxacillin, haloperidol, thiabendazole, tolbutamide, and carbamazepine. In some cases, the bile duct destruction occurs without an inflammatory infiltration, but frank cholangitis with neutrophilic infiltration of bile ducts is more common. This form of liver injury can persist for months and even years before resolving, but may progress to secondary biliary cirrhosis.

Ductular or cholangiolar cholestasis

Another form of cholestasis associated with bile casts in the cholangiocytes is known as ductular or cholangiolar cholestasis and is exemplified by benoxaprofen.

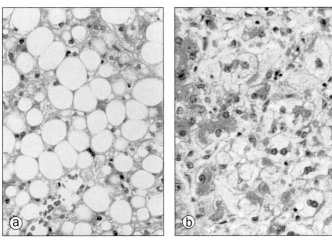

Figure 29.14 Steatosis. (a) Macrovesicular steatosis;
(b) Microvesicular steatosis.

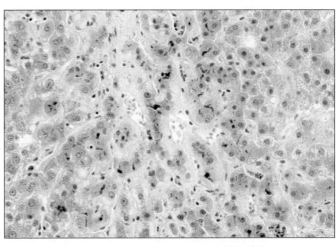

Figure 29.15 Bland, or pure, cholestasis following anabolic steroid use.

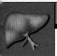
Ductal cholestasis

Ductal cholestasis associated with intra- and extrahepatic sclerosing cholangitis has been described following intra-arterial administration of floxuridine and fluorouracil for treatment of metastatic liver carcinoma.

OTHER CHRONIC LESIONS

Chronic forms of liver disease almost always depend on continued exposure to the drug rather than a self-perpetuating process instigated by the initial insult. However, in a few cases cirrhosis may develop despite discontinuation of the drug; this may occur with amiodarone and perhexiline maleate treatment as they can persist for many months in the liver. Portal hypertension has also been described following drug-induced liver injury due to the development of portal fibrosis. This noncirrhotic portal hypertension, or hepatoportal sclerosis, has been described with vitamin A intoxication, chronic exposure to arsenicals, vinyl chloride, and copper sulfate. Periportal fibrosis has also been reported following methotrexate administration. Portal hypertension due to vascular lesions may also result from drug administration such as oral contraceptive-induced hepatic vein occlusion and antimetabolite-induced veno-occlusive disease (see Fig. 29.13).

Drug administration has been linked to tumor development, both benign and malignant disease. Oral contraceptives have been implicated in the growth of hepatic adenomas and hepatocellular carcinoma, while the use of anabolic steroids has also been associated with the development of these lesions. Angiosarcomas have been reported in those exposed to vinyl chloride and arsenic, while cholangiocarcinoma has been reported in those using anabolic and contraceptive steroids. However, the causal relationship between these agents and cholangiocarcinoma remains to be proven.

DRUG-INDUCED LIVER INJURY ACCORDING TO DRUG CLASS

Steroids: anabolic and contraceptive drugs

Natural and synthetic steroids have a number of effects on the liver:

- pure cholestasis;
- development of tumors, hepatic adenoma, and hepatocellular carcinoma;
- architectural disturbance with the development of focal nodular hyperplasia (FNH);
- increased incidence of gallstones;
- hepatic vein occlusion; and
- peliosis hepatis.

Many of these effects have been reported for both oral contraceptive steroids (OCSs) and anabolic steroids. Both groups of drugs are intrinsic hepatotoxins and the presence of an alkyl or ethinyl group on carbon 17 appears to be essential for the development of cholestatic liver disease. However, there are some differences in the type of liver injury they produce. Anabolic and androgenic steroids have been more frequently associated with malignant tumors, while contraceptive steroids are more commonly associated with benign liver tumors. Hepatic vein occlusion may relate to thrombogenic effects of the estrogenic component of contraceptive steroids. Anabolic steroids more commonly produce peliosis hepatis.

Oral contraceptive steroids are associated with pure cholestasis in approximately 10 per 100,000 women exposed in Western Europe and 25 per 100,000 in Chile and Scandinavia, and it occurs within 2–3 months of commencing therapy (see Fig. 29.15). The estrogenic component is probably responsible for the cholestasis as pure estrogens also cause cholestasis. The injury is dose-dependent and is less common with low-dose preparations. Oral contraceptive steroid-induced cholestasis occurs in women with a history of cholestasis of pregnancy, and has also been observed in sisters, suggesting a genetic component. The mechanism by which estrogens and related steroids produce cholestasis is uncertain, but it appears to result from interference with bile excretion. Decreased bile flow, biliary secretion of bile acids, plasma membrane fluidity, and Na^+ and K^+-ATPase activity have all been reported in experimental animals. Biliary excretion of sulfobromophthalein (BSP) is also impaired. Estrogens may also alter the membrane lipid composition. Following cessation of OCS, the cholestasis resolves and the prognosis is excellent. Pure cholestasis may also complicate the use of stanozolol, a C-17 substituted testosterone, and danazol, a C-17 substituted androgen used in endometriosis.

The risk of developing hepatic adenomas and hepatocellular carcinoma appears to be increased by OCS and anabolic/androgenic use (Fig. 29.16), and most cases are associated with 17-α-alkylated steroids.

Adenomas have also been reported with norethisterone, a progestin, and clomiphene. The true incidence of OCS-related adenomas is unknown but the risk seems to be time-dependent, that is, the relative risk is unchanged for administrations of less than 1 year, but increases 116-fold at 5 years. Adenomas may regress after cessation of the drug, but can recur with readministration of OCS or with pregnancy. Estrogen-associated adenomas are highly vascular and have a tendency to hemorrhage into the tumor or into the peritoneal cavity. Whether adenomas progress to hepatocellular carcinoma (HCC) is controversial. Foci of dysplasia or malignancy have been described in resected adenomas, and the incidence of HCC is increased when OCS have been used for greater than 5 years, but not with use for less than 5 years. However, other cofactors may be important in the pathogenesis of HCC in OCS users and anabolic steroid users, such as hepatitis B and alcohol excess. Like adenomas, steroid-induced HCC may regress after cessation of the drugs. Oral contraceptive steroid use has also been linked to the development of epithelioid hemangioendothelioma, and the enlargement of existing hemangiomas. Angiosarcomas have been reported with anabolic steroid use.

The risk of hepatic vein occlusion, or Budd–Chiari syndrome, is increased 2.5-fold in OCS users, consistent with their perceived thromboembolic potential. This thrombogenic trait is ascribed to the estrogenic component of the drug which may exacerbate an underlying thromgenic disorder. Peliosis hepatis is characterized by blood-filled cavities within the hepatic parenchyma which may be lined by sinusoidal endothelium, and numerous cases have been reported in association with anabolic/androgenic steroids.

Anticonvulsant and psychoactive drugs
Anticonvulsant drugs
Phenytoin

Phenytoin-induced acute and chronic hepatotoxicity have been well described. While most patients are adults, hepatoxic effects have been reported in patients as young as 8 months. Clinical

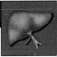

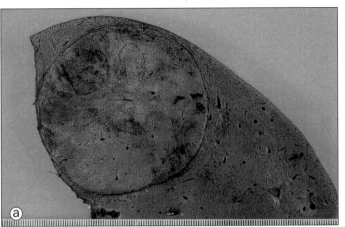

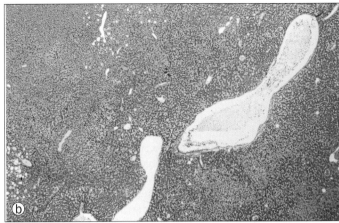

Figure 29.16 Hepatic adenoma secondary to long-term oral contraceptive steroids (OCS) usage. (a) Macropathology (b) Micropathology.

symptoms and signs occur within 6 weeks of administration and include rash, fever, lymphoadenopathy, and eosinophilia, suggesting a hypersensitivity or immunologic basis to the injury. This is supported by the occasional occurrence of a pseudomononucleosis syndrome of lymphoadenopathy, lymphocytosis, and serum sickness-like features. Some patients exhibit manifestations of Stevens–Johnson syndrome. Histologically, the lesion resembles acute viral hepatitis with diffuse hepatocellular degeneration, foci of necrosis, and an inflammatory infiltrate. Granulomas have also been described. However, phenytoin-induced liver injury may also result from the adverse effects of toxic intermediates, as it is metabolized by the cytochrome P450 system with the production of reactive arene oxide metabolites, which may subsequently bind covalently to tissue macromolecules, producing liver injury (Fig. 29.17).

Differences in individual susceptibilities to phenytoin-induced liver damage may be due to genetic differences in rates of biotransformation, as deficiencies in epoxide hydrolase activity (required for detoxification) have been reported in those affected and their family members.

Carbamazepine

Carbamazepine is similar to phenytoin in its structure and also utilizes epoxide hydrolase in its biotransformation. Minor liver dysfunction is seen in approximately 5–10% of asymptomatic subjects using the drug. Liver damage begins within 1 month of commencing therapy and hepatocellular, cholestatic, and granulomatous reactions (Fig. 29.18) have been described.

Carbamazepine may also cause cholangiolitis and has been reported as a cause of ductopenia.

Valproic acid

Valproic acid-induced liver injury has a particular predilection for children, especially for those less than 2 years of age. Symptoms occur between 10 and 12 weeks of therapy and seem to be dose-related in some cases. The pathologic lesions include submassive necrosis with microvesicular steatosis, and bile duct injury. The mechanism of injury is not certain. A branched medium-chain fatty acid itself, valproic acid inhibits mitochondrial oxidation of long-chain fatty acids, with reduction in hepatocellular acetyl-coenzyme-A and impairment of urea cycle enzymes. Patients with inborn errors in the urea cycle are susceptibile to valproate hepatotoxicity. Polypharmacy, through enzyme induction or competitive inhibition of metabolizing enzyme systems, may also be a factor in valproate-induced liver injury.

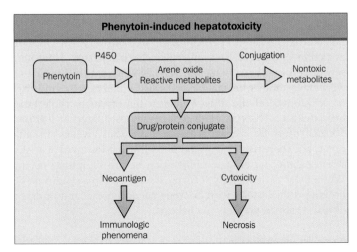

Figure 29.17 Phenytoin-induced hepatotoxicity.

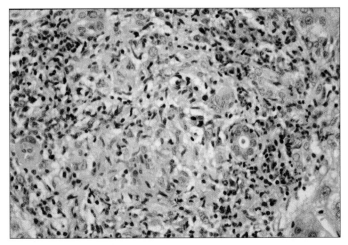

Figure 29.18 Carbamezepine-induced hepatic granulomatous liver disease.

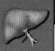
Psychoactive drugs
Chlorpromazine
Chlorpromazine is a cause of cholestatic jaundice in 1% of those that take the drug, but subclinical liver dysfunction may occur in as many as 40–50% of chronic users. It occurs within 5 weeks of therapy and is heralded by a prodrome of flu-like symptoms, followed by a rash and fever in up to 60% of cases. The histologic pattern includes cholestasis in zone 3 and portal inflammation with eosinophils in 20–50% of cases, and granulomas have been described. The prognosis is generally good, but a small number of patients develop a prolonged cholestatic syndrome with hypercholesterolemia and xanthelasmata. In these patients, the histology can resemble primary biliary cirrhosis, but antimitochondrial antibodies are negative, although some patients have antinuclear antibodies in their sera. The clinical features suggests a hypersensitivity basis for chlorpromazine-induced liver damage, but chlorpromazine and its metabolites do directly interfere with the mechanisms necessary for bile secretion. Altered membrane fluidity, impaired membrane Na$^+$ and K$^+$-ATPase activity and impaired solute transport are changes that contribute to the development of chlorpromazine-induced cholestasis. Furthermore, chlorpromazine affects the cytoskeleton, causing dilatation and diverticuli in the canaliculi.

Antidepressants: tricyclic antidepressants
Many members of this class of psychotropic drugs (imipramine, amineptine, amitriptyline, desipramine) are hepatotoxic and asymptomatic liver dysfunction may occur in approximately 10% of users. The injury can be either cholestatic or hepatocellular, although amitriptyline has caused a prolonged cholestatic lesion with portal fibrosis and inflammation. The mechanism of hepatotoxicity is thought to be due to reactive arylating intermediates.

Antidepressants: monoamine oxidase inhibitors
Hepatotoxicity is commonly seen in this group with jaundice reported in 1–2% of patients. Iproniazid, an amine oxidase inhibitor, was originally used to treat tuberculosis, but occasionally resulted in fatal liver necrosis with a mortality of 20% in those who developed jaundice. Clinical features occur within 4–5 weeks of treatment. Histology reveals diffuse hepatocellular necrosis that can progress to massive necrosis in some patients, resembling that associated with acute viral hepatitis. Iproniazid hepatitis is usually associated with anti-M6 antimitochondrial antibody. Angiosarcomas have been reported in experimental animals following administration of phenylhydrazine.

Cocaine
Cocaine use may result in severe liver damage with associated systemic failure, rhabdomyolysis, and renal failure. Pathologic examination reveals zone 3 centrilobular necrosis but also microvesciular steatosis, suggesting impaired fatty acid oxidation. It is metabolized by the cytochrome P450 enzyme system to the active hepatotoxic metabolite norcocaine nitroxide. The mechanism of toxicity is due to these free radicals, but hepatotoxicity may also be due to hepatic ischemia as cocaine increases the systemic levels of norepinephrine and epinephrine (noradrenaline and adrenaline), and these agents reduce hepatic artery bloodflow.

Ecstasy (3,4-methylenedioxymethamphetamine)
Several case reports have described an acute hepatotoxic syndrome similar to that seen with cocaine, that is, hyperthermia, rhabdomyolysis, and hepatic necrosis. Chronic ecstasy ingestion has been associated with recurrent episodes of acute hepatitis.

Antibiotics
Antibacterial agents
Tetracyclines
Tetracyclines can rarely cause severe acute liver injury. The majority of cases have been in pregnant women where tetracycline was used to treat urinary tract infections. However, males and nonpregnant women are also susceptible to tetracycline-induced liver damage, especially at higher doses of more than 1.5g per day. Within 2–3 days of intravenous administration of tetracycline, jaundice occurs with nonspecific symptoms such as malaise, anorexia, and vomiting. Histologically, the main lesion is microvesicular fat (see Fig. 29.14b) resembling that seen in fatty liver of pregnancy, Reye's syndrome, and valproic acid hepatotoxicity, and tetracycline in high doses impairs hepatic mitochondrial oxidation. The mechanism of injury appears to be a toxic effect of the drug or its metabolites rather than an immunologic effect, and suggested methods of injury include failure of ATP synthesis and inhibition of protein synthesis. Similar toxic effects can be seen with oxytetracycline and chlortetracycline, but minocycline has been reported to cause liver injury with predominantly allergic features.

Erythromycin
Administration of erythromycin estolate can cause a cholestatic jaundice in approximately 1–2% of recipients. The risk of cholestatic jaundice for all erythromycin preparations is 3.6 per 100,000 users, and jaundice secondary to erythromycin stearate and propionate has been recorded. Symptoms occur between 1 and 3 weeks after commencing treatment and rash, fever, and eosinophilia in tissue and blood have suggested an allergic mechanism of injury. However, erythromycin estolate can impair bile flow and interfere with canalicular membrane Na$^+$and K$^+$-ATPases, which indicates a direct hepatotoxic effect. Erythromycin toxicity may also present as an acute cholangitis or cholecystitis. Liver biopsy reveals centrilobular cholestasis and a portal infiltration rich with eosinophils.

Flucloxacillin
Hepatotoxicity due to penicillins is rare, and very few cases of penicillin-G-induced liver injury have been reported. However, several semisynthetic penicillin derivatives have been associated with cholestatic or hepatocellular injury which rapidly improves on withdrawal of the drug. Flucloxacillin produces cholestatic liver disease. The risk of liver injury is estimated at 7.6 per 100,000 users. Symptoms usually occur within 3 weeks of treatment, but there can be a period of well-being for up to 3 weeks after cessation of drug administration before symptoms occur. While most patients fully recover, some develop a syndrome of prolonged cholestasis with ductopenia, and portal and bridging fibrosis that can progress to cirrhosis.

Ampicillin and amoxicillin
These semisynthetic penicillins have little hepatotoxicity when used alone. However, when amoxicillin is used in combination

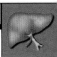

with clavulinic acid, the risk of cholestasis is 1 per 100,000 users. Symptoms occur between 1 and 2 weeks of treatment but can be delayed for up to 6 weeks following withdrawal of the drug. Histology reveals cholestasis with minimal inflammation or necrosis. Granulomas may be present. The mechanism of injury probably relates to immunologic idiosyncrasy.

Sulfonamides

Sulfa drugs are associated with a wide spectrum of pathologic changes in the liver. The precise risk of injury following administration of these drugs is unknown, but the incidence of hepatic injury appears to be less than 5%. The clinical pattern of sulfonamide hepatotoxicity is usually cholestatic or mixed hepatocellular–cholestatic and the clinical course can resemble viral hepatitis. Hypersensitivity phenomenon such as a rash, fever, arthralgia, and eosinophilia are not uncommon. Sulfonamides in combination with other drugs also cause liver injury. Sulfasalazine induces an allergic-type hepatitis with low levels of serum complement and circulating immune complexes, mimicking serum sickness. Although the sulfpyridine is believed to be responsible for the liver injury, the 5-aminosalicylate moiety may also play a part (see below). Pyrimethamine-sulfadoxine, used as antimalaria prophylaxis, causes hepatic necrosis and fatalities have been described from massive necrosis. Granulomatous hepatitis has also been described. Trimethoprim-sulfamethoxazole can lead to cholestatic hepatotoxicity, and fatalities due to fulminant liver failure have been recorded. However, the majority of patients fully recover when the drug is withdrawn.

Nitrofurantoin

This antibiotic is associated with a wide variety of adverse effects such as peripheral neuropathy, pulmonary infiltration, and skin reactions, and it can also lead to a cholestatic hepatitis with hypersensitivity features suggesting an underlying immunoallergic mechanism as the basis for the injury. However, it has been associated with chronic hepatitis and cirrhosis, particularly in women over the age of 40 years who have taken the drug for longer than 4–6 months. The chronic hepatitis is associated with a number of autoimmune features such as hyperglobulinemia and positive antinuclear and anti-smooth muscle autoantibodies. Associations with HLA-DR6, HLA-DR2, and HLA-B8 have been reported.

Antifungal agents

Ketoconazole

Ketoconazole has been well-documented as a hepatotoxic drug, with an estimated risk of injury of 1 per 15,000 cases. Asymptomatic liver dysfunction occurs in 5–10% of users. Symptoms occur within 1–6 months of treatment and are commoner in women. Liver biopsy reveals a diffuse hepatocellular necrosis, occasionally with bridging necrosis, but fatalities are rare.

Griseofulvin

This antifungal agent produces hepatocellular carcinoma and a porphyria-like syndrome in experimental animal models. Humans taking this drug may develop porphyrinuria and those with acute intermittent porphyria may relapse. Cholestatic injury has also been documented in humans, and alcohol-like lesions in mice.

Antituberculous agents

Most of the antituberculous drugs can cause hepatic damage in susceptible individuals, but as these drugs are administered in combination to prevent resistant bacterial strains emerging, it may be difficult to attribute liver dysfunction to a particular agent. Furthermore, drug interactions can potentiate hepatotoxicity.

Isoniazid

Isoniazid is one of the most important causes of drug-induced liver injury, and two types of injury are observed. Mild hepatotoxicity is the commoner lesion seen in approximately 10–20% of users and occurs in the first few months of treatment. It produces a mild nonspecific focal hepatitis (Fig. 29.19) that is clinically inapparent and that resolves despite continuation of the drug.

The less common isoniazid-induced hepatitis occurs in approximately 1% of all users, but in 2% of those over 50 years of age. It appears to be more common in women and alcoholics. For two thirds of patients, symptoms begin within the first 3 months of treatment, but this can be delayed for up to 12 months. Clinically, the symptoms and signs are those of an acute viral illness. There is a rising serum transaminase level and histologic findings include acute hepatitis, bridging necrosis, submassive necrosis, and chronic hepatitis. The drug must be stopped. The mortality for clinically jaundiced patients is 10%. The mechanism of injury involves the production of toxic metabolites. Isoniazid first undergoes biotransformation in the liver by acetylation, producing the harmless acetylisoniazid which then undergoes hydrolysis to monoacetylhydrazine. This product is oxidized by the cytochrome P450 system to form reactive metabolites that covalently bind to tissue macromolecules. It has been suggested that the rate of acetylation of isoniazid to subsequent toxic metabolites may be important for individual susceptibility to hepatotoxicity and studies reported that rapid acetylators were at greatest risk of injury. Subsequent studies have not confirmed this claim and have even suggested that slow acetylation status may be more important as a risk factor for hepatic injury.

Rifampin

Rifampin-induced liver injury occurs in approximately 1–4% of users and occurs within 3 weeks of therapy. However, it is usually given in combination with isomiazid. Clinically, it produces an acute hepatitis similar to that seen with isoniazid. The histology reveals hepatocellular injury and necrosis is common.

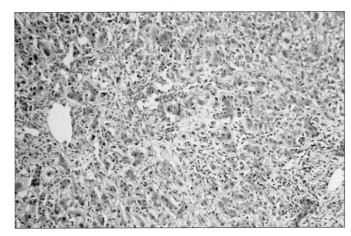

Figure 29.19 Mild hepatitis secondary to isoniazid administration.

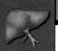
Rifampicin impairs the hepatic uptake of bile acids and bilirubin in a dose-dependent manner, and impaired BSP excretion is observed in experimental animals. It induces drug-metabolizing systems in the endoplasmic reticulum and this may explain the higher incidence of hepatotoxicity in recipients of combination therapy compared with those using monotherapy.

Analgesic and anti-inflammatory drugs
Acetaminophen
Acetaminophen (paracetamol) is a popular and, when taken at the recommended doses (0.5–3g daily), relatively safe analgesic and antipyretic drug. At higher doses, however, it can lead to liver damage. This may occur in two ways: first, intentional overdoses; and second, high therapeutic doses (4–8g daily), where other factors may influence the individual susceptible to acetaminophen-induced liver damage such as chronic alcohol ingestion, co-ingestion of drugs that induce the cytochrome P450 metabolizing system, pre-existing liver disease, and conditions that are associated with low glutathione stores such as malnutrition. Individuals with Gilbert's syndrome may also have an increased susceptibility to acetaminophen-related liver injury due to their deficiency of hepatic UDP-glucuronyltransferase. In the UK, it is one of the most popular means of attempting suicide, and is the most common cause of fulminant hepatic failure. In the USA, it has become the commonest drug involved in deliberate overdose. Acetaminophen is an intrinsic hepatotoxin; the effect on the liver is predictable and dose-dependent.

Clinically, there are three phases:
- phase 1 (1–24 hours) when the patient complains of nausea vomiting and diaphoresis;
- phase 2 (24–48 hours) during which time there may be no symptoms or clinical evidence of liver disease – this may be the latent period during which there is progressive formation of reactive metabolites; and
- phase 3 (2–10 days) with the onset of overt liver disease, which may recover completely with no sequelae or progress to liver failure, cerebral edema, and multiorgan failure (see Chapter 30).

The characteristic histologic lesion is centrilobular or zone 3 necrosis which may develop into submassive or massive hepatic necrosis (Fig. 29.20).

The zone 3 location of the initial histologic change is a consequence of the location in this area of the cytochrome P450 enzyme that is involved in metabolizing the drug (CYP2E1). At low doses, acetaminophen is largely conjugated with sulfate or glucuronic acid (Fig. 29.21) and these conjugates are then excreted in the urine.

A small proportion of drug (approximately 5%) is metabolized by the CYP2E1 isoenzyme resulting in the formation of the highly toxic and reactive electrophile N-acetyl-p-benzoquinone imine (NAPQI). This is rendered harmless by conjugation with GSH and, after further conversion to acetylcysteine derivatives, is excreted in the urine as a mercapturic acid (Fig. 29.21). Glutathione, therefore, normally provides protection against the toxic intermediate at low levels of acetaminophen ingestion. However, with larger doses of acetaminophen, the sulfate and glucuronide pathways are saturated and therefore a larger amount of drug is available for biotransformation via the P450 enzyme system. Subsequent detoxification depends on conjugation with GSH and therefore tissue levels of GSH are critical to the development of hepatic necrosis. When doses of acetaminophen are large enough to deplete GSH stores by more than 70%, detoxification of NAPQI cannot be sustained; it can then covalently bind to tissue macromolecules which are essential for cellular homeostasis, resulting in structural and functional disruption of key cellular components by oxidation of protein and nonprotein thiols. Lipid peroxidation is a late event

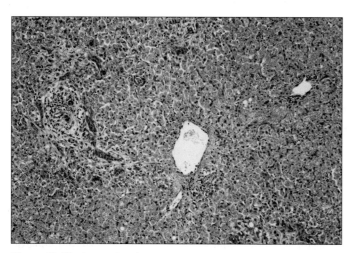

Figure 29.20 Acetaminophen-induced submassive hepatic necrosis.

Figure 29.21 Schematic representation of acetaminophen biotransformation.

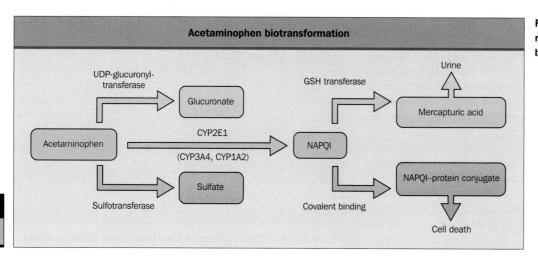

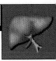

and may be the result rather than the cause of tissue necrosis. Through the covalent modification of plasma membrane and mitochondrial proteins, intracellular calcium homeostasis is destroyed, resulting in a cascade of endonuclease-, phospholipase-, and protease-induced cellular damage that ends in cell death. *N*-acetylcysteine and methionine increase hepatic GSH stores by promoting GSH synthesis. Other agents that inhibit the CYP2E1 isoenyzme, such as cimetidine, offer protection against liver injury in experimental animals, but do not appear to be of benefit in humans.

Salicylates

Aspirin is another intrinsic hepatotoxin with a dose-dependent and reversible form of liver injury. Hepatic injury may occur with high therapeutic doses in children and adults with chronic rheumatologic or collagen vascular diseases, or following a deliberate overdose. The injury is usually associated with serum salicylate levels of greater than 2.5μmol/L (25mg/dL) but can occur at lower serum drug levels. Hypoalbuminemia may predispose to aspirin-induced hepatotoxicity by increasing the unbound fraction of the drug. The hepatotoxic effects of aspirin may be involved in the development of Reye's syndrome. In most cases, it presents as an asymptomatic dysfunction in liver function and jaundice occurs in less than 5% of cases. Liver biopsy is compatible with a nonspecific focal hepatitis with minimal inflammatory changes in the portal areas. Recovery is complete on cessation of drug ingestion.

Nonsteroidal anti-inflammatory drugs

The hepatotoxicity induced by this group of drugs is not uniform. Most cause hepatocellular damage but several lead to cholestasis. Likewise, the frequency of liver damage that they produce is variable; for example, mefanamic acid rarely causes liver injury unlike ibufenac, which caused fatal liver damage and was ultimately withdrawn from the market. Although the mechanism of injury appears to be idiosyncrasy, for some drugs it is immunologically mediated with accompanying hypersensitivity phenomena. Others appear to have a metabolic basis for their injury. The risk of hepatotoxicity for the group as a whole is estimated to be approximately 3.7 per 100,000 users. Associated risk factors for liver injury include old age, renal disease, and alcohol excess.

Diclofenac

Women and patients with osteoarthritis appear to be more susceptible than others to diclofenac-induced hepatotoxicity which causes asymptomatic liver dysfunction in 15% of users. Duration of administration before the onset of liver dysfunction is widely variable, ranging from 1 to 14 months. Allergic features are rare. Liver biopsy demonstrates a nonspecific acute hepatitis with zonal necrosis. Recovery is usual but fatalities have been recorded. Diclofenac has also been associated with an autoimmune-like chronic hepatitis.

Phenylbutazone

This drug has been associated with clinically apparent liver injury in 0.25% of users. Symptoms usually begin within 6 weeks of treatment and are similar to a viral hepatitis. Rash, fever, and arthralgia are common. The histology may vary from hepatocellular necrosis to bridging necrosis to granulomatous hepatitis.

Less commonly, cholestasis with minimal hepatocellular features can be seen.

Sulindac

As with diclofenac, the mechanism of injury with sulindac appears to be hypersensitivity-based. The illness begins within 6 weeks of drug administration. The liver biopsy reveals a cholestatic injury in most patients, although hepatocellular features have been recorded in some patients. Approximately, 5% of jaundiced cases are fatal. Recovery may take months.

Ibuprofen

This drug appears to be one of the least commonly implicated NSAIDs in the generation of liver injury despite its frequent use. It is associated with hepatocellular injury that has many of the clinical hallmarks of the hypersensitivity syndrome.

Nimesulide

This agent is a new NSAID of the sulfonanilide class and is a more selective cyclo-oxygenase type 2 (cox-2) inhibitor than cox-1 inhibitor. A recent report of nimesulide-induced hepatotoxicity described six patients who presented with jaundice following administration of this agent. Histology revealed hepatocellular necrosis in four of the patients, although two had pure cholestasis. Autoantibodies were present in the sera and some showed hypersensitivity features.

Cardiovascular drugs
Antihypertensive agents
Methyldopa

Both acute and chronic liver disease has been described in patients taking methyldopa, although the incidence has fallen as it has been replaced by newer antihypertensive agents. Asymptomatic liver dysfunction occurs in 5–30% of users within 1–6 weeks, and may resolve despite continued use of the drug. Overt hepatic disease occurs in 1% of users. The commonest histologic lesion resembles acute viral hepatitis with hepatocellular necrosis. Portal and periportal inflammation is prominent. More importantly, methyldopa can cause an autoimmune-like chronic hepatitis that has been reported to progress to fibrosis and macronodular cirrhosis in some patients.

The mechanism of injury appears to be both an immunologic and metabolic idiosyncrasy. Methyldopa undergoes biotransformation via the cytochrome P450 system by oxidation to a reactive metabolite thought to be a quinone or semiquinone. These intermediates may covalently bind to cellular macromolecules, resulting in a conjugate that can act as a neoantigen becoming a target for immune recognition. Evidence for immunologic disturbance is suggested by a positive Coombs' test, positive autoantibodies, and inhibition of cytotoxic T cell function. Despite these findings, clinical evidence of hypersensitivity is rare. The mortality is similar to that for other causes of drug-induced hepatocellular injury, with a rate of 10% in those who develop clinically apparent jaundice.

Angiotensin-converting enzyme inhibitors

This class of drugs occasionally produces liver damage. Acute hepatocellular injury occurs over a widely variable period of time. The mechanism of injury is unknown although hypersensitivity phenomena have been described with captopril. Cross-reactivity of hepatotoxicity can occur between captopril and enalapril.

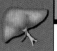

Thiazide diuretics

Despite widespread use, thiazide diuretics rarely cause liver injury. Cholestatic hepatitis has rarely been reported with chlorthiazide. In mice, furosemide causes zone 3 necrosis.

Hydralazine

This vasodilator can cause a variety of liver injuries including hepatocellular hepatitis and granulomatous hepatitis, particularly on a background of a lupus-like syndrome. The drug can also produce an effect mimicking acute cholangitis. Non specific organ antibodies are found in the serum and anti liver microsomal antibodies directed against CYP1A2 have been reported.

Antiarrhythmic agents
Amiodarone

Amiodarone is an amphophilic drug with a lipophilic ring complex and a hydrophilic side chain, a structure that results in its accumulation in lysosomes. Within the lysosomes, it binds to phospholipids and prevents their degradation by phospholipases, thereby producing secondary phospholipid storage. This results in increased density on computed tomography (CT) scanning due to the iodine content of the stored drug. Toxicity is not confined to the liver and lysosomal inclusions are also found in other tissues. The range of liver injury sustained with amiodarone is diverse, and both acute and chronic liver disease has been reported. Approximately 15–50% of users develop an asymptomatic rise in liver function tests, while clinically apparent disease occurs in less than 3% of patients. Jaundice is rare. Acute hepatitis in those taking the drug for a few weeks usually resolves upon cessation of therapy. Chronic injury can be insidious and patients may present with complications of cirrhosis. Histologic appearances include granulomas, cholangitis, and micronodular cirrhosis, but the typical appearance is that of alcoholic hepatitis with steatosis, focal necrosis, centrilobular fibrosis, Mallory's hyaline, and polymorphonuclear infiltration (Figs 29.22 & 29.23).

Interference with mitochondrial fatty acid oxidation by amiodarone in animal models may be a factor in the pathogenesis of this pseudoalcoholic liver injury.

Quinidine

Quinidine administration may result in liver injury within 6–12 days of treatment. The clinical symptoms are similar to those of acute viral hepatitis and liver biopsy confirms hepatocellular necrosis. Granulomas have also been described.

Calcium channel blockers

Verapamil has been reported to have hepatotoxic effects within 2–3 weeks of commencing therapy, producing a mixed cholestatic and hepatocellular pattern. Nifedepine can cause steatosis and zone 3 necrosis. It has also been implicated in pseudoalcoholic liver disease. Diltiazem may rarely cause fatal hepatotoxicity.

Anti-anginal agents
β-Adrenergic blocking drugs

Most of the drugs in this group rarely induce liver disease. Labetolol can cause hepatocellular necrosis within 2 months of treatment, and fatalities have been recorded. Metoprolol is metabolized by the CYP2D6 isoenyzme, which is also responsible for debrisoquin metabolism. It induces an acute hepatitis.

Perhexilene maleate

A lipophilic drug that accumulates in lysosomes, this agent produces pseudoalcoholic liver disease similar to that described for amiodarone, which can also progress to cirrhosis despite cessation of drug ingestion. Deficiency of the CYP2D6 metabolizing isoenzyme, which is responsible for perhexilene hydroxylation, may be a predisposing factor for perhexilene-induced liver damage. Susceptibility to perhexilene hepatotoxicity has been associated with HLA-B8 phenotype.

Antihyperlipidemic agents
3-Hydroxy-3-methylglutaryl coenzyme A reductase inhibitors

Asymptomatic elevation in transaminases occurs in 1–5% of users in the first few weeks of treatment and this abnormality is usually dose-related. The mechanism of liver function abnormality may be the accumulation of metabolites whose conversion to cholesterol has been blocked by inhibiting the 3-hydroxy-3-methylglutaryl coenzyme A reductase enzyme.

Clofibrate

Clofibrate may also produce asymptomatic elevation in aminotransferases. Cholestasis, granulomatous inflammation, and an increased incidence of gallstones have been reported following clofibrate administration. In animal models they cause an increase

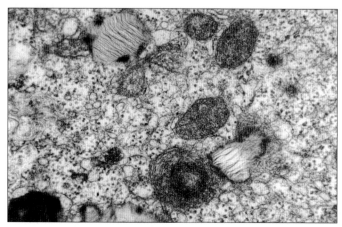

Figure 29.22 Amiodarone-induced phospholipidosis. Electron microscopy reveals phospholipidic inclusions.

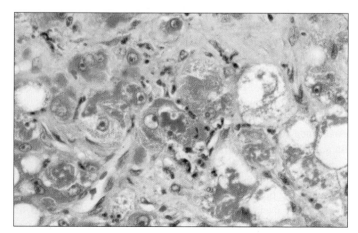

Figure 29.23 Amiodarone-induced liver disease demonstrating Mallory bodies and hepatic fibrosis.

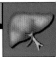

in hepatocyte peroxisomes which may be related to the development of hepatic neoplasms in these animals.

Immunomodulatory drugs

Immunomodulatory drugs, a group of drugs that includes antineoplastic drugs, antimetabolites, immunosuppressant agents, and antiviral drugs, produce a wide spectrum of hepatotoxicity ranging from mild hepatocellular hepatitis to cirrhosis. However, it can be difficult to identify the cause of the injury due to the multiple potential causes of liver dysfunction in patients receiving these drugs. The differential diagnosis may include the underlying disease itself, metastatic disease, opportunistic infection, sepsis, and polypharmacy with multiple drug interactions.

Antimetabolites
Methotrexate
The potential for hepatotoxicity with long-term use of methotrexate is well-known. The risk of liver injury seems related to the duration of therapy but other contributing factors may include obesity, diabetes, alcohol excess, underlying liver disease, and renal impairment. Because the progression of methotrexate-induced liver injury to fibrosis and cirrhosis is usually subclinical, it has become accepted practice to recommend liver biopsy after cumulative doses in excess of 1.5g, although this is controversial as patients with rheumatoid arthritis treated with methotrexate have a low incidence of significant liver damage. In addition, progression to fibrosis has been reported despite normal liver function tests. However, monitoring of liver function is advisable as methotrexate has been associated with hepatocellular and fulminant liver failure. Histololgic abnormalities include steatosis, necrosis, a mixed portal inflammatory infiltration, and ultimately cirrhosis. The mechanism of liver injury is unclear.

Antipurines
Azathioprine, frequently used to treat chronic liver disease, is metabolized in the liver to produce 6-mercaptopurine. Liver injury induced by this drug ranges from portal inflammation with cholestasis to peliosis hepatis, nodular regenerative hyperplasia, veno-occlusive disease, and hepatoportal sclerosis (or idiopathic portal hypertension), suggesting a susceptibility of the vascular endothelium to injury by azathioprine. There is a strong association between male renal transplant recipients and azathioprine-induced veno-occlusive disease. 6-Mercaptopurine, used to treat leukemia, is also hepatotoxic. It can produce jaundice in 5–40% of users, although hepatocellular injury is more common than cholestatic injury. 6-Thioguanine produces histologic hepatotoxicity similar to that described for azathioprine, in particular veno-occlusive disease, nodular regenerative hyperplasia, and hepatoportal sclerosis. Cytosine arabinoside produces a mild cholestatic injury.

Antipyrimidines
One of the most important drugs that causes hepatotoxicity in this group is 5-fluorouracil, which produces little liver damage when administered orally as a single agent. However, the coadministration of a pyrimidine synthesis inhibitor (phosphono-acetyl-l-asparate), used to enhance the efficacy of 5-fluorouracil, results in cholestatic injury. A derivative of 5-fluorouracil, floxuridine, has been reported to cause irreversible sclerosing cholangitis and cholecystitis when infused into the hepatic artery as

treatment for metastatic liver disease.

Alkylating agents
Many drugs in this group are capable of hepatic injury. Cyclophosphamide, used in high dosage or in combination with other agents for bone marrow pre-conditioning, can lead to veno-occlusive disease (Fig. 29.24).

Busulfan (UK: busulphan), at high doses used in bone marrow pre-conditioning, produces a similar lesion but may also induce a cholestatic hepatitis. The nitrogen mustards are rarely hepatotoxic. Chlorambucil can produce hepatocellular injury which has been reported to progress to cirrhosis.

Antiviral agents
Nucleoside analogs
Zidovudine (AZT) hepatotoxicity has been well-established in patients positive for HIV. The typical histologic abnormality is a severe macrovesicular steatosis with minimal necrosis or inflammation. However, fulminant liver failure has been reported following its use. The mechanism of injury is uncertain, but seems to relate to a toxic effect on mitochondrial function with subsequent fat accumulation, lactic acidosis, and multiorgan failure.

Naturally occurring immunomodulatory agents
L-asparaginase
This agent usually induces a mild steatosis that resolves with cessation of the drug. Large doses can cause hepatic necrosis. Toxicity may result from impaired hepatic protein synthesis as deamination of asparagine is facilitated by asparaginase, resulting in depletion of asparagine stores.

Alkaloids
These agents rarely cause liver injury, but when used in combination with irradiation, vincristine, and vinblastine can lead to a severe hepatitis. Pyrrolizidine alkaloids induce veno-occlusive disease. Etoposide and other podophylline alkaloids in high doses can cause hepatic necrosis.

Adriamycin (doxorubicin hydrochloride)
This agent and the related minomycin have been implicated in the development of veno-occlusive disease. Bleomycin can induce steatosis.

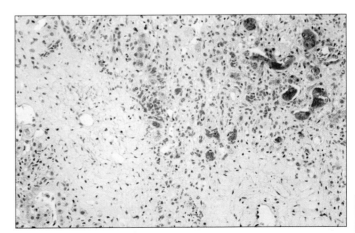

Figure 29.24 Cyclophosphamide-induced veno-occlusive disease.

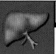

Cyclosporine
Cyclosporine has been reported to cause cholestasis. In experimental models, it impairs bile flow, suggesting a direct effect on bile secretion.

Anesthetic agents
Halothane
Halothane is the prototype for anesthetic-induced hepatotoxicity. The risk of liver injury ranges from 1 per 35,000 to 1 per 10,000 anesthetics administered. Risk factors for developing halothane-induced hepatotoxicity include obesity, female sex, advancing age, and repeated exposure to the agent, which implies a sensitization process. The risk of injury has been reported to be 7 per 10,000 in those who had previously experienced this anesthetic agent. Asymptomatic liver dysfunction occurs in approximately 20–25% of those exposed. Nonspecific symptoms appear within 2 weeks of exposure (but may occur as quickly as 2–3 days in those previously exposed) and resemble those of acute viral hepatitis. Histologic features include zone 3 necrosis which can progress to massive necrosis. Other less severe lesions include spotty necrosis, diffuse hepatitis, and bridging necrosis. The mechanism of injury appears to be toxic metabolites produced by biotransformation. In humans, 20% of halothane is metabolized, producing bromide ion and trifluoroacetic acid (TFA) which are not hepatotoxic. In animal studies, reactive metabolites of halothane covalently bound to tissue macromolecules and induced liver injury only in the presence of tissue hypoxemia. Trifluoroacetic acid–protein conjugates have been demonstrated in the sera of patients who have been exposed to halothane anesthesia and seem to act as neoantigens, producing antibodies in patients with severe liver injury. These antibodies may cross-react with endogenous proteins; antibodies to the E2 component of PDC have been reported. This may explain the hypersensitivity phenomena such as fever, rash, eosinophilia, and increased frequency of toxicity with repeated exposure.

Other anesthetic agents
Enflurane-induced liver injury is less common than that due to halothane but produces a similar clinical and histologic picture. Isoflurane is metabolized less extensively than halothane and therefore is less commonly implicated as a cause of anesthesia-related liver dysfunction.

Industrial and naturally occurring toxins
Carbon tetrachloride
Carbon tetrachloride, an intrinsic hepatotoxin, is a well-recognized cause of liver injury. Occupational exposure may occur in those in contact with dry-cleaning, grain fumigants, or working with fire-fighting equipment, and inhalation and ingestion are the commonest forms of exposure. Starvation and alcohol excess appear to enhance the toxicity of CCl_4, possibly by inducing the microsomal metabolizing enzyme system, in particular the CYP2E1 isoenzyme. Hypoxia enhances the conversion of CCl_4 to the reactive metabolite CCl_3. Symptoms occur within 24 hours of exposure, and jaundice appears after 2–4 days. Renal impairment is also apparent. Histology shows zone 3 necrosis and fatty change is not uncommon.

Yellow phosphorous
Yellow phosphorous-induced hepatic injury occurs by inhalation or ingestion of rat poison, and produces a clinical syndrome similar to that described for CCl_4. It is characterized by rapidly deteriorating liver and renal function, and can lead to fulminant liver failure within 3–4 days following exposure. The breath, vomitus, and feces typically have a garlic odor and are phosphorescent. The pathologic findings are zone 1 necrosis with macrosteatosis.

Selenium
At low concentrations this is an essential trace element for human growth and it contributes to cellular mechanisms that protect against lipid peroxidation. However, in higher concentrations selenium is hepatotoxic and inhibits protein synthesis with subsequent deficiency of methionine and cysteine. Acute toxicity results in microvascular steatosis. Like phosphorous toxicity, the breath and excreta have a garlic odor.

Vinyl chloride
Vinyl chloride has been associated with a range of liver pathologies, but principally angiosarcoma, fibrosis, and hepatoportal sclerosis. Liver injury appears to be related to duration of exposure, but other factors may include smoking and alcohol. The most characteristic histologic lesion is capsular and subcapsular fibrosis. Angiosarcomas are often peripherally placed and associated with terminal retroperitoneal hemorrhage. Vinyl chloride at low concentration can be metabolized by alcohol dehygrogenase, but at higher levels, metabolism is performed by the microsomal enzyme systems. Extrahepatic manifestations of vinyl chloride toxicity include Raynaud's phenomenon and scleroderma-like skin changes.

Pesticides (insecticides, herbicides, fungicides)
Pesticides have rarely produced significant liver injury in humans despite experimental evidence of perivenular necrosis in rodents. However, their potential for hepatotoxicity and hepatocarcinogenesis is a concern as, after exposure, they are stored for a long time in body fat and in the liver. The pesticide dichlorodipenthyltrichloroethane (DDT) is listed by the World Health Organization as a carcinogenic agent. Cholestasis with bile duct degeneration and necrosis has been reported following paraquat ingestion, but its clinical importance is superseded by the more toxic effects of this agent on the pulmonary and gastrointestinal systems.

Arsenic
This poison produces acute and chronic liver injury and usually results from accidental ingestion. Following acute poisoning, features of hypersensitivity are prominent. Histologic abnormalities include hepatocellular necrosis and severe steatosis. Alternatively, patients may present with a cholestatic syndrome, reflected histologically by cholestasis and portal infiltration, which may progress to a primary biliary cirrhosis-like entity. Chronic arsenic exposure is associated with hepatosclerosis, cirrhosis, hepatocellular carcinoma and angiosarcoma.

Mushroom poisoning
Ingestion of *Amanita phalloides* (death cap) and *Amanita verna* (destroying angel) is associated with severe liver injury, especially in children. *Amanita phalloides* is recognized by its green–brown cap, white gills, and stem. Toxicity is due to the amatoxins, which bind to RNA polymerase and inhibit the formation of messenger RNA, and phallotoxins, which impair cell membrane function by interfering with the polymerization–depolymerization cycle. As little as three mushrooms can be fatal as they

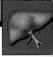

contain approximately 7mg of amatoxins. Symptoms occur within 8–12 hours of ingestion followed by a period of apparent improvement before clinically overt liver dysfunction occurs. Histology reveals zone 3 hemorrhagic necrosis with severe steatosis. In those that survive, a minority can progress to have a histologic picture of chronic autoimmune-like hepatitis with autoantibodies, hyperglogulinemia, and circulating immune complexes in the serum.

Aflatoxins

Aflatoxins are derived from the *Aspergillus* species and have been identified as a contaminant of nuts, corn, wheat, barley, soy beans, and rice. There are 12 naturally occurring parent forms, and they have been classified into two major groups: aflatoxin B and aflatoxin G. The former toxin is the most common aflatoxin contaminant found in food. Hepatotoxicity is due to impairment of RNA synthesis, possibly due to inhibition of RNA polymerase or interaction with nuclear chromatin. Ingestion of aflatoxin-contaminated food results in acute hepatotoxicity heralded by nausea, vomiting, and jaundice with subsequent development of portal hypertension. Liver biopsy demonstrates cholestasis with periductal fibrosis. Chronic ingestion in animals results in veno-occlusive disease and hepatocellular carcinoma; aflatoxins are also carcinogenic in humans. They have been postulated as cocarcinogens with hepatitis B virus.

Herbal medicines

The increasing use and growing popularity of alternative medicines has resulted in an increasing awareness of their potential toxicities. Hepatotoxicity due to herbal remedies can be difficult to diagnose, as frequently patients will not remember to include these self-prescribed remedies in a drug history. Some of the more commonly used remedies include germander, which is used to treat obesity. However, seven cases of acute hepatitis associated with germander ingestion at the recommended dose have been reported in France. Symptoms of abdominal pain and jaundice developed within 3–18 weeks of germander administration in capsular form or as tea. Histology revealed nonspecific hepatocellular necrosis. Symptoms resolved quickly on withdrawal of the agent, but rapidly reappeared upon germander readministration. Fatal fulminant liver failure has been reported following germander administration. Animal studies have reported depletion of GSH and protein thiols due to germander-derived reactive metabolites, activated by the cytochrome P450 enzyme system. Chinese herbal remedies have also been associated with acute hepatitis, in particular xiao-chai-hu-tang, used as an antidote to the common cold, but also used to treat liver diseases in Japan. Acute hepatitis may also follow administration of mistletoe (*Viscus album*) used to treat asthma, skullcap (*Scutellaria*) and valerian (*Valeriana officinalis*) used to treat stress, and chaparral leaf.

CLINICAL FEATURES OF DRUG-INDUCED LIVER INJURY

There are few, if any, clinical features associated with drug-induced hepatotoxicity that are pathognomonic for drug-induced injury to the liver. Many drugs cause a nonspecific viral hepatitis-type picture with an initial prodrome of nausea, anorexia and vomiting followed by abdominal pain and jaundice (Fig. 29.25).

Fever, rash, and arthralgia are hallmarks of hypersensitivity which may indicate an immunologic idiosyncrasy to drugs, but these signs also occur with viral hepatitis. Classical indicators of toxin-induced liver injury, such as the garlic odor of breath, vomitus, and feces of yellow phosphorous hepatotoxicity, are rare. Syndromes of acute liver disease occur in three phases as characterized by injury due to acetaminophen, hepatotoxic mushrooms, and CCl$_4$: early severe gastrointestinal and neurologic symptoms; a period of apparent improvement; and finally overt liver injury with subsequent multiorgan involvement. Some drugs mimic clinical entities such as cholecystitis (erythromycin) and cholangitis (chlorpromazine), pseudomononucleosis, lymphadenopathy and serum sickness-like syndromes (phenytoin, sulfonamides, sulindac, dapsone), bone marrow suppression (immunomodulatory drugs), and systemic vasculitis (allopurinol, sulfonamides). Hepatic adenomas may present as a painless abdominal mass or hemoperitoneum following rupture of the tumor.

DIAGNOSIS OF DRUG-INDUCED LIVER INJURY

Because the majority of clinical manifestations of drug-induced liver injury are nonspecific, making the correct diagnosis at an early stage is extremely difficult. Furthermore, liver deterioration may represent progression of the underlying disease, a complication of the underlying disease, or an unrelated clinical episode such as sepsis. In addition, the administration of mul-

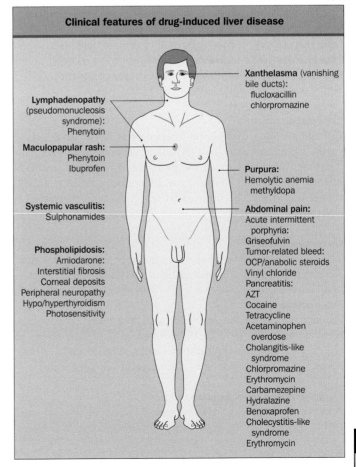

Clinical features of drug-induced liver disease

Xanthelasma (vanishing bile ducts): fluicloxacillin chlorpromazine

Lymphadenopathy (pseudomonucleosis syndrome): Phenytoin

Maculopapular rash: Phenytoin Ibuprofen

Systemic vasculitis: Sulphonamides

Phospholipidosis: Amiodarone: Interstitial fibrosis Corneal deposits Peripheral neuropathy Hypo/hyperthyroidism Photosensitivity

Purpura: Hemolytic anemia methyldopa

Abdominal pain: Acute intermittent porphyria: Griseofulvin Tumor-related bleed: OCP/anabolic steroids Vinyl chloride Pancreatitis: AZT Cocaine Tetracycline Acetaminophen overdose Cholangitis-like syndrome Chlorpromazine Erythromycin Carbamezepine Hydralazine Benoxaprofen Cholecystitis-like syndrome Erythromycin

Figure 29.25 Clinical associations of drug-induced liver disease.

tiple drugs in seriously ill patients further complicates the process of drug-induced liver damage. A low threshold of suspicion is therefore necessary to make the correct diagnosis at an early stage in the illness when withdrawal of the offending agent should result in complete recovery. Central to the diagnosis is a thorough history including recent and past drug exposure (including herbal remedies, vitamins, and homeopathic medicines), and occupational hazards with exposure to potential toxins. Ideally, the diagnosis should be based on a history of illness subsequent to drug ingestion and improvement on cessation of therapy. Confirmation of the diagnosis by a drug rechallenge is rarely justifiable. In recent years, a clinical scale for the diagnosis of drug-induced hepatitis has been developed and validated (Fig. 29.26).

Investigations

Liver function tests

It has been suggested that drug-induced liver injury is diagnosed as hepatocellular when the ALT and AST are greater than twice above the upper limit of normal or when the ALT/alkaline phosphatase (Alk) ratio is equal to or greater than 5. The injury is cholestatic where the Alk is twice the upper limit of normal or where the ALT/Alk ratio is less than or equal to 2. However, many drug reactions frequently cause a mixed pattern of liver function abnormality. Hypoalbumenemia is particularly associated with salicylate toxicity, but this may just reflect the severity of the underlying liver disease, if present.

Full blood count

Lymphocytosis and eosinophilia are associated with immunologic phenomena. Leukopenia and thrombocytopenia may reflect bone marrow suppression as a result of drug toxicity or as a secondary toxic event following liver failure. A low platelet count may also indicate disseminated intravascular coagulation (DIC) which may follow acute toxic injury to the liver.

Coagulation screen

A prolonged international normalized ratio (INR) or activated partial thromboplastin time (APTT) reflects deteriorating liver function. These indices are the most useful prognostic markers of acute liver failure following acetaminophen overdose. A DIC screen (fibrinogen, fibrin degradation products or D-dimers) is also useful.

C-reactive protein

This is an acute phase protein which can be elevated as a nonspecific response to a hypersensitivity reaction.

Autoimmune screen

Autoantibodies found in association with drug-related liver impairment are listed in Figure 29.10. Elevated IgG levels are observed with autoimmune-like syndromes. Increased IgE levels have been described following gold and carbamazepine administration.

Electrolytes and renal function

A markedly elevated K^+ may indicate rhabdomyolysis associated with acute liver failure, in particular, cocaine-induced liver injury.

Toxicology screen

This can be useful to aid the diagnosis of suspected drug overdose.

Others

Amylase, creatine phosphokinase (CPK) and lactate may indicate muscle necrosis secondary to rhabdomyolysis. A rapidly rising lactate accompanies impaired mitochondrial fatty acid oxidation.

Radiology

Ultrasound and CT examination can be useful to rule out nondrug-related causes of liver dysfunction. Hepatic adenomas and carcinomas can be diagnosed and subsequently confirmed by

Drug-induced liver injury diagnostic scale	Score
Temporal relationship between drug intake and the onset of clinical picture	
Time from drug intake until the onset of first clinical or laboratory manifestations:	
4 days to 8 weeks (or less than 4 days in cases of re-exposure)	3
Less than 4 days or more than 8 weeks	1
Time from withdrawal of the drug until the onset of manifestations:	
0 – 7 days	3
8 – 15 days	0
More than 15 days*	–3
Time from withdrawal of the drug until normalization of laboratory values **:	
Less than 6 months (cholestatic or mixed patterns) or 2 months (hepatocellular)	3
More than 6 months (cholestatic or mixed) or 2 months hepatocellular)	0
Exclusion of alternative causes*	
Viral hepatitis	
Alcoholic liver disease	
Biliary tree obstruction	
Other (pregnancy, acute hypotension):	
Complete exclusion	3
Partial exclusion	0
Possible alternative cause detected	–1
Probable alternative detected	–3
Extrahepatic manifestations	
Rash, fever, arthralgia, eosinophilia (>6%), cytopenia:	3
4 or more	2
2 or 3	1
1	0
None	
Intentional or accidental re-exposure to the drug	
Positive rechallenge test	3
Negative or absent rechallenge test	0
Previous report in the literature of cases of DILI associated with the drug:	
Yes	2
No (drugs marketed for up to 5 years)	0
No (drugs marketed for more than 5 years)	–3
Total score	

Figure 29.26 Drug-induced liver injury diagnostic scale. Description of the component elements and scores attributed. *Except cases of prolonged persistence of the drug in the body after drug withdrawal (e.g. amiodarone). **Normalization: decrease to values below 2× the upper limit of normal values. ***Use the exclusion criteria considered appropriate in each case. Definite drug associated injury >17, probable 14–17, possible 10–13, unlikely 6–9, excluded <6. (Adapted with permission from Maria VAJ. Hepatology. 1997;26:664 .)

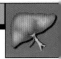

angiography. Fatty infiltration of the liver may be first suggested by ultrasound screening. Amiodarone produces a classical CT appearance with increased liver density due to the iodine content of the retained drug stored within the lysosomes. Examination of hepatic vein patency by CT and Doppler studies may aid the diagnosis of drug-related Budd–Chiari and veno-occlusive disease.

Liver biopsy

Histologic features suggestive of drug-related liver disease are listed in Figure 29.27.

MANAGEMENT

The main treatment for drug-induced hepatotoxicity is withdrawal of the offending agent. While the majority of patients will recover completely, for some the adverse effects continue to deteriorate, despite cessation of therapy. The basic principles of management involve supportive care and alleviation of symptoms such as pruritis. Cholestyramine, antihistamines, opiate antagonists, and odansatron may alleviate pruritis, but some patients may require plasmaphoresis. Rifampin has also been used to treat pruritis. Corticosteroids have no established role in the treatment of drug-related liver injury, but may be used in the setting of immunologic idiosyncrasy to suppress features of

Histologic features that implicate a drug-induced etiology	
Zonal necrosis	Pure cholestasis
Microvesicular steatosis	Peliosis hepatis
Granulomas	Veno-occlusive disease
Eosinophilic inflammatory infiltration	

Figure 29.27 Histologic features that implicate a drug-induced etiology.

hypersensitivity or in autoimmune-like syndromes. Specific antidotes exist for overdose of some drugs such as acetaminophen, where *N*-acetylcysteine can replenish hepatic GSH stores. Carnithine has been suggested in cases where defects in mitochondrial fatty acid defects are prominent, but there is little evidence to indicate that this is of major benefit. Hyperbaric oxygen has been suggested as an adjunct to therapy in cases of CCl_4 toxicity as hypoxemia potentiates the hepatotoxic effects. Liver transplantation may ultimately be necessary if clinical and biochemical parameters continue to deteriorate (see Chapter 34).

PRACTICE POINT

Illustrative case

A 21-year-old female was admitted to hospital with a 24-hour history of left upper and lower limb weakness and a 2-month history of right-sided frontoparietal headache. Examination revealed a left-sided hemiparesis and a CT brain scan confirmed a right parietal hemorrhage. Biochemical parameters of liver, renal, and hematologic function were normal. She was prescribed phenytoin at a standard dose as prophylaxis against seizure activity and referred to a stroke rehabilitation unit.

Nineteen days later she complained of right thoracolumbar pain and pain in the right upper quadrant. This was associated with a high fever of 39–40°C. Initial investigations were as follows: white cell count 3.7×10^9/L, erythrocyte sedimentation rate 76mm/h, and eosiniphilia 0.6×10^9/L. Urea and electrolytes were normal, but urine microscopy revealed significant proteinuria. A presumptive diagnosis of urinary tract infection was made and she was commenced on appropriate antibiotic therapy. However, the high pyrexia continued intermittently over the next few days and she underwent investigation for pyrexia of unknown origin (PUO). This included blood and urine cultures, echocardiography, CT abdomen and thorax, intravenous urography, immunoglobulin, and autoantibody screen (which included

lupus anticoagulant, double-stranded DNA, anticardiolipin antibodies) and HIV testing – all investigations were negative. Despite antibiotics, the fevers continued. Liver function tests became abnormal at this time: alkaline phosphatase (ALP) 182 IU/L, γ-GT 173 IU/L, and AST 277 IU/L. Bilirubin remained normal at 4μmol/L (0.2mg/dL). Over the next 7 days she became jaundiced and liver biochemistry progressively deteriorated: bilirubin 160μmol/L (8mg/dL), ALP 408 IU/L, AST 3033 IU/L, prothrombin time (PT) 24s, APTT 54s, INR2.1. Her clinical condition deteriorated with the development of tender hepatomegaly, posterior cervical lymphadenopathy, and a widespread desquamating pruritic erythematous maculopapular rash. Phenytoin was withdrawn at this time. Viral serology for hepatitis A, hepatitis B, and Epstein–Barr virus was negative. In view of deteriorating liver function, she was transferred to a specialist unit for subsequent management.

At the specialist unit, initial assessment revealed jaundice without stigmata of chronic liver disease. Cervical and axillary lymphadenopathy were noted. She had a resolving mobiliform erythematous rash and tender hepatomegaly without ascites or splenomegaly. A presumptive diagnosis of phenytoin-induced hepatitis was made. This was confirmed by liver biopsy, which revealed florid hepatitis with severe

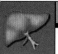

perivenular necrosis. The portal and periportal areas were heavily infiltrated by inflammatory cells including plasma cells, eosinophils, and lymphocytes. In addition, there was marked cholestasis. She was commenced on supportive therapy, including intravenous n-acetylcysteine, and antibiotics.

However, liver function continued to deteriorate: bilirubin 702µmol/L (33mg/dL), ALP 245 IU/L, γ-GT 163 IU/L, AST1391 IU/L, INR5.9. She subsequently developed grade 3 encephalopathy, requiring incubation and ventilation, and, in view of progressive liver failure, was listed for liver transplantation.

Interpretation

This case illustrates two points about drug-induced liver injury. First, making the correct diagnosis at an early stage is extremely difficult as the majority of clinical manifestations of drug-induced liver injury are nonspecific. In this case, the diagnosis was not made until 3 weeks after the onset of symptoms and until other cases of a PUO had been excluded. The combination of symptoms such as rash, fever, and lymphadenopathy has been reported for many diseases, and therefore the diagnosis of drug-induced injury may only occur when clinical suspicion is high. Secondly, while most cases of drug hepatotoxicity run a benign course with no chronic sequelae, liver failure may occasionally develop, as in this case. With the development of rash, fever, and lymphadenopathy (indicating a hypersensitivity or immunologic bases to the disease process), corticosteroids were used to try and suppress these features. Unfortunately, the patient's clinical condition continued to deteriorate and she fulfilled criteria for liver transplantation for acute liver failure.

FURTHER READING

Beaune PH, Lecoeur S. Immunotoxicology of the liver: adverse reactions to drugs. J Hepatol. 1997;26(suppl. 2):37–42. *An excellent review of the mechanisms of liver injury following drug administration.*

Berson A, Freneaux D, Larrey D, et al. Possible role of HLA in hepatotoxicity. An exploratory study in 71 patients with drug-induced idiosyncratic hepatitis. J Hepatol. 1994;20:336–42. *A key study of HLA associations and drug-induced liver injury.*

Ellis AJ, Wendon JA, Portmann B, Williams R. Acute liver damage and ecstasy ingestion. Gut. 1996;38:454–58. *An excellent review of ecstasy-induced liver failure.*

Farrell GC. Drug-induced liver disease. Edinburgh: Churchill Livingstone; 1994:1–673. *A very comprehensive textbook of drug-induced liver disease covering classification, mechanisms of liver injury, diagnosis, and management.*

Fromenty B, Pessayre D. Impaired mitochondrial function in microvesicular steatosis. Effects of drugs, ethanol, hormones and cytokines. J Hepatol. 1997;26 (suppl. 2):43–53. *This is a superb review of drug-induced steatosis, covering normal mitochondrial function, inborn errors of metabolism, and acquired impairment of β-oxidation.*

Gitlin N. Clinical aspects of liver disease caused by industrial and environmental toxins. In: Schiff L, Schiff ER, eds. Diseases of the liver. Philadelphia: Lippincott; 1993:1018–50. *A superb text covering occupational and industrial toxins and their effect on liver function.*

Gut J, Christen U, Huwyler J, et al. Molecular mimicry of trifluoroacetylated human liver protein adducts by constitutive proteins and immunochemical evidence for its impairment in halothane hepatitis. Eur J Biochem. 1992;210:569–76. *This paper presents a mechanism for drug-induced liver injury, suggesting molecular mimicry as a principal mechanism in halothane hepatitis.*

Larrey D. Hepatotoxicity of herbal remedies. In: Arroyo V, Bosch J, Bruguera M, Rodes J. Therapy in liver diseases. Barcelona: Masson; 1997:233–8. *This text offers a concise review of the most popular herbal medicines and their toxic effects on the liver.*

Larrey D, Vial T, Pauwels A, et al. Hepatitis after germander (*Teucrium chamaedrys*) administration: another instance of herbal medicine hepatotoxicity. Ann Intern Med. 1992;117:129–32. *This paper offers a review of seven cases of hepatitis following germander ingestion, their presentation, and subsequent follow-up.*

Larrey D, Pageaux GP. Genetic predisposition to drug-induced hepatotoxicity. J Hepatol. 1997;26(suppl. 2):12–21. *This is a fascinating and in-depth review of the detoxification mechanisms of the liver and the genetic predisposition to variation in these systems.*

Lee WM. Drug-induced hepatotoxicity. N Engl J Med. 1995;333:1118–27. *A quality review of the clinical presentation of drug-induced liver disease.*

Maria VAJ, Victorino RMM. Development and validation of a clinical scale for the diagnosis of drug-induced hepatitis. Hepatology. 1997;26:664–9. *A useful guide for determining the likelihood of drug-induced liver injury when the diagnosis is uncertain.*

Makin AJ, Wendon J, Williams R. A 7-year experience of severe acetaminophen-induced hepatotoxicity (1987–1993). Gastroenterology. 1995;109:1907. *A comprehensive study of the clinical and biochemical parameters of acetaminophen-induced liver failure from a single center.*

Pohl LR. Drug-induced allergic hepatitis. Semin Liver Dis. 1990;10:305–15. *A solid review of the mechanisms of drug-related hypersensitivity phenomena.*

Smilkstein MJ, Douglas DR, Daya MR, et al. Acetaminophen poisoning and liver function. N Engl J Med. 1994;331:1310–12. *An interesting exchange of letters concerning the management of acute acetaminophen poisoning.*

Steenbergen WV, Peeters P, De Bondt J, et al. Nimesulide-induced acute hepatitis: evidence from six cases. J Hepatol. 1998;29:135–41. *A review of the selective cox-2 inhibitory NSAIDs and liver injury.*

Watkins PB. Role of cytochromes P450 in drug metabolism and hepatotoxicity. Semin Liver Dis. 1990;10:235–50. *A very comprehensive review of the genetics and molecular basis of P450 induction.*

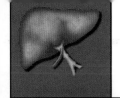

Section 3 Specific Diseases of the Liver

Chapter 30

Acute Liver Failure

John G O'Grady

INTRODUCTION

Acute liver failure is a complex medical emergency that evolves after a catastrophic insult to the liver. The liver damage is sufficiently severe to cause encephalopathy, and this develops within a matter of days or weeks of the insult to the liver. Acute liver failure is a heterogeneous condition that incorporates a range of clinical syndromes. The dominant factors that give rise to this heterogeneity include the underlying etiology, the age of the patient and the duration of time over which the disease evolves. The natural history of the condition is very variable within this spectrum and survival rates without recourse to transplantation range from 10 to 90% for different cohorts. The treatment involves an integrated, multidisciplinary strategy with the hepatologist, intensivist, and transplant surgeon playing pivotal roles. The key components of the management strategy are the assessment of the severity of the disease and the associated prognosis, prevention or treatment of the complications that may arise, and the use of transplantation when spontaneous survival is considered unlikely. Consequently, this condition should ideally be managed in specialist centers where the management protocols are achieving considerably improved survival rates in the range from 40% to in excess of 90%, depending on the underlying etiology.

DEFINITIONS

The term fulminant hepatic failure was first used in the late 1960s, and was defined as the development of encephalopathy within 8 weeks of the onset of symptoms in patients who had no previous history of liver disease. Late-onset hepatic failure was later used to describe a group of similar patients in whom this interval ranged between 9 and 26 weeks. A French nomenclature from the 1980s defined fulminant hepatic failure as the onset of encephalopathy within 2 weeks of the onset of jaundice (rather than symptoms), and subfulminant hepatic failure was used to describe the cases who were jaundiced for 3–12 weeks before the development of encephalopathy.

The most recent proposal for the classification of the condition attempted to achieve a closer alignment between the categories and differences in the associated natural history and clinical features (Fig. 30.1). This uses the core term acute liver failure to describe the development of encephalopathy within 12 weeks of the onset of jaundice, and prefixes the terms 'hyper' and 'sub' to describe subgroups with distinct clinical characteristics in whom this interval is up to 7 days and 5–12 weeks, respectively. This definition excludes patients who have previous symptomatic liver disease, but allows the inclusion of subclinical chronic liver disease

characteristic of Wilson's disease and some patients who have hepatitis B-related liver failure.

Hyperacute liver failure is defined as the development of encephalopathy within 7 days of the onset of jaundice. This group has the highest likelihood of recovery with medical management, despite the characteristic rapid deterioration, high incidence of cerebral edema, and the severe prolongations of prothrombin time that are observed. In acute liver failure the encephalopathy develops between 8 and 28 days after the onset of jaundice. This group has a high mortality, a high incidence of cerebral edema, and prolongations of prothrombin time that are as severe as in hyperacute liver failure. The interval between the onset of jaundice and the development of encephalopathy in subacute liver failure ranges from 5 to 12 weeks. This group also have a high mortality rate, despite a very low incidence of cerebral edema and much less severe prolongations of prothrombin time.

Young children who have acute liver failure may not develop classic encephalopathy until late in the disease process. Increasingly in this group the diagnosis of acute liver failure is made on the basis of a coagulopathy. It has also been argued that, in adults who have severe liver damage, drugs like benzodiazepines may mimic encephalopathy, and that a coagulopathy is a more reliable parameter to differentiate severe hepatitis or liver injury from acute liver failure.

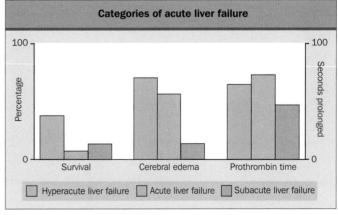

Figure 30.1 Categories of acute liver failure. Hyperacute liver failure has the best prognosis despite the high incidence of cerebral edema and marked prolongation of prothrombin time. Acute liver failure shares the same characteristics but has a much poorer prognosis. The outcome in subacute liver failure is poor despite the low incidence of cerebral edema and less marked prolongation of prothrombin time. The survival figures relate to the period 1973–85 before liver transplantation confused natural history studies, and the survival rate for the hyperacute group is now considerably higher.

ETIOLOGY AND PATHOGENESIS

There is considerable variation worldwide in the etiology of acute liver failure (Fig. 30.2).

Viruses and drugs account for the majority of cases. However, a significant number of patients have no definable viral cause and have no history of exposure to drugs or toxins. This condition is referred to as seronegative hepatitis in this chapter, but is also known as non-A–E hepatitis and acute liver failure of indeterminate etiology. The overall incidence of acute liver failure complicating acute hepatitis in the USA is 0.9%, and this equates to about 2000 deaths annually. Most of the drug-induced cases are rare idiosyncratic reactions, but some such as acetaminophen (paracetamol) are in part dose-related toxic events.

Viral

Acute liver failure is a very uncommon complication of hepatitis A infection, occurring in 0.14–0.35% of hospitalized cases, and in 0.4% of all cases seen in the USA. As hospitalized and notified cases represent only a proportion of all cases of acute hepatitis A, the real prevalence is probably considerably lower. Exposure to hepatitis A in childhood is becoming less common and the risk of death increases with age at the time of infection. Consequently, hepatitis A has emerged as the commonest defined viral cause of acute liver failure in the UK. This trend may be reversed by the appropriate targeting of populations at risk for vaccination against hepatitis A. The diagnosis of acute hepatitis A is made by the detection of the IgM antibody in serum and this is present in 95% of cases at the time of presentation. The remaining 5% become positive on repeat testing.

The incidence of acute liver failure following hepatitis B is 1–4% of hospitalized patients, and the risk increased when there was associated hepatitis D or δ virus co-infection. Hepatitis D was found in 34–43% of patients who had acute liver failure due to hepatitis B, compared with 4–19% of less severe cases. The majority (58–79%) were due to superinfection in chronic hepatitis B virus carriers and the remainder were a consequence of acute co-infection. The presence of the IgM antibody to hepatitis B virus (HBV) core-antigen in serum is the most accurate way of diagnosing acute liver failure due to hepatitis B, as hepatitis B surface antigen (HBsAg) was undetectable in 12–55% of cases at the time of presentation. Viral replication had ceased in most cases as evidenced by the detection of HBeAg in serum in 12–37% and HBV DNA in only 9% of patients. The detection of HBsAg does not necessarily implicate hepatitis B in the pathogenesis of the acute liver failure. In one series, 15% of HBsAg-positive cases were attributed to non-A, non-B hepatitis on the basis of the absence of IgM antibodies to hepatitis A virus (HAV), core-antigen, and hepatitis D. However, it is now recognized that acute liver failure may also occur during spontaneous reactivation of chronic hepatitis B infection (HBV DNA levels markedly elevated), seroconversion from hepatitis B 'e' antigen

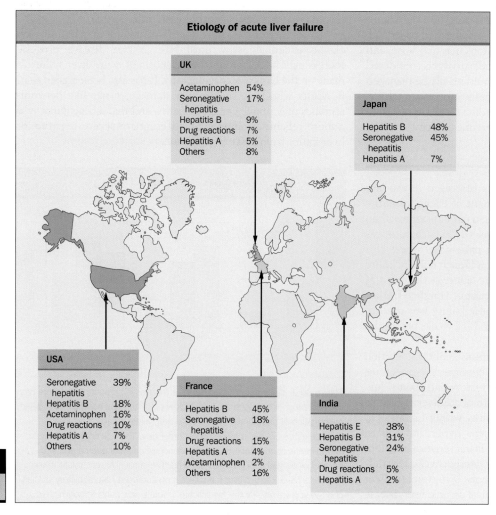

Etiology of acute liver failure

UK

Acetaminophen	54%
Seronegative hepatitis	17%
Hepatitis B	9%
Drug reactions	7%
Hepatitis A	5%
Others	8%

Japan

Hepatitis B	48%
Seronegative hepatitis	45%
Hepatitis A	7%

USA

Seronegative hepatitis	39%
Hepatitis B	18%
Acetaminophen	16%
Drug reactions	10%
Hepatitis A	7%
Others	10%

France

Hepatitis B	45%
Seronegative hepatitis	18%
Drug reactions	15%
Hepatitis A	4%
Acetaminophen	2%
Others	16%

India

Hepatitis E	38%
Hepatitis B	31%
Seronegative hepatitis	24%
Drug reactions	5%
Hepatitis A	2%

Figure 30.2 Etiology of acute liver failure. There are considerable geographic variations in the etiology of acute liver failure. Acetaminophen is especially common in the UK, while hepatitis B and hepatitis E are particularly prominent in France and India, respectively.

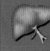

(HBeAg) to hepatitis B 'e' antibody (HBeAb), and following the cessation of immunosuppressive drugs, including cytotoxic drugs, in chronic hepatitis B carriers. Studies of the role of mutants, especially the pre-core mutants that are unable to secrete HBeAg, have failed to link them conclusively to the pathogenesis of hepatitis B-related acute liver failure. Women appear to have a higher risk of developing acute liver failure following infection with HBV. A number of interesting cases have been described where sequential female sexual partners of hepatitis B carriers have developed acute liver failure.

The risk of developing acute liver failure after exposure to hepatitis C appears to be very low, and in a number of studies of patients with acute liver failure the overall hepatitis C positivity rate was only 2%. Contrary reports have emerged from series of Japanese and Hispanic Californian patients, but these populations have relatively high carrier rates for hepatitis C and the association is probably not causal. Post-transfusion hepatitis, which is usually due to hepatitis C, rarely leads to acute liver failure. It has been suggested that chronic hepatitis C virus infection may be a co-factor with acute HBV infection in increasing the risk of developing acute liver failure. A report describing hepatitis F as a viral cause of acute liver failure has not been confirmed, and no evidence has emerged to link hepatitis G to acute liver failure.

Seronegative or non-A–E hepatitis is the commonest presumed viral cause in some parts of the Western world. In the UK it accounts for 56% of such cases. Middle-aged females are most frequently effected and the risk of developing acute liver failure with seronegative hepatitis was calculated at 2.3–4.7% of hospitalized cases. The diagnosis remains one of exclusion. However, there must be considerable doubt as to whether many or all of the cases in this category are due to a viral infection. Cases are usually sporadic and unidentified toxins or autoimmune processes may contribute to the causation of acute liver failure in this cohort.

Hepatitis E is common in parts of Asia and Africa and the risk of developing acute liver failure ranges from 0.6 to 2.8% in men and nonpregnant women to over 20% in pregnant women, being particularly high during the third trimester. Hepatitis E is also encountered in Europe and the USA, and may account for up to 8% of cases that would previously have been described as seronegative hepatitis. A history of travel to a high endemic area was not always present in these cases. Unusual causes of viral acute liver failure include herpes simplex 1 and 2, herpesvirus-6, varicella-zoster virus, Epstein–Barr virus, and cytomegalovirus. The cases due to herpes simplex may have external manifestations of herpetic infection and are important to detect as they usually respond to acyclovir. Herpes simplex was implicated in 3% of adult cases of acute liver failure in France.

Drugs

Acetaminophen overdose is the commonest cause of acute liver failure in the UK. It appears to be increasing in the USA and other English-speaking countries, but is unusual in continental Europe and the rest of the world. In the UK it is usually taken with suicidal or parasuicidal intent, but up to 8% of cases follow the therapeutic use of acetaminophen. This is either because of unintentional overdosing or in people who have liver enzyme induction as a consequence of antiepileptic therapy or regular alcohol usage. The patients developing acute liver failure represent only about 2–5% of those presenting after overdosing with acetaminophen. The median dose of acetaminophen causing acute liver failure in the UK is 40g (range 5–210g), and the mortality was highest at doses exceeding 48g. The pattern in the USA may be somewhat different, as one small urban study suggested that 70% of cases were suicidal and 30% were accidental in undernourished or alcoholic subjects. Although the latter took an estimated average of 12g of acetaminophen, compared with 20g in the suicidal group, they had higher rates of coma (33 versus 6%) and death (19 versus 2%).

Halothane hepatitis was one of the more frequently encountered idiosyncratic drug reactions, accounting for up to 5% of cases of acute liver failure in the UK between 1973 and 1985, but the incidence has dramatically decreased since repeated exposure to halothane was discouraged. Acute liver failure occurs in sensitized individuals and develops within 5–15 days of the second or subsequent exposure to halothane. It has a predilection for obese, atopic, middle-aged females. Although a specific halothane-antibody test has been described, most diagnoses are made on clinical grounds. Acute liver failure has also been described after enflurane and isoflurane anesthesia.

Most cases of acute liver failure attributed to idiosyncratic drug reactions develop during the first exposure to the drug and some of the offending agents are listed in Figure 30.3. Estimates of the risk of developing acute liver failure as a result of an idiosyncratic reaction range from 0.001% for nonsteroidal anti-inflammatory drugs to 1% for the isoniazid/rifampin (rifampicin) combination. Ecstacy (methylenedioxymethamphetamine – a synthetic amphetamine) is a recent addition to this list and it has been associated with a number of clinical syndromes ranging from rapidly progressive acute liver failure associated with malignant hyperpyrexia to subacute liver failure. The diagnosis is made on the basis of a temporal relationship between exposure to the drug and the development of acute liver failure.

Other etiologies

Acute liver failure associated with pregnancy tends to occur during the third trimester. Typically there is a constellation of features, including liver failure with encephalopathy, sepsis, impaired renal function, and disseminated intravascular coagulation. Acute fatty liver of pregnancy usually occurs in primagravids carrying a male fetus, and is characterized by severe microvesicular steatosis which

Drugs that cause acute liver failure	
Category 1	Category 2
Acetaminophen	Benoxyprofen
Halothane	Phenytoin
Isoniazid/rifampicin	Isoflurane
Nonsteroidal anti-inflammatory drugs (NSAIDs)	Enflurane
Sulphonamides	Tetracycline
Flutamide	Allopurinol
Sodium valproate	Ketoconazole
Carbamazepine	Monoamine oxidase inhibitors (MAOIs)
Ecstacy	Disulphiram
	Methyldopa
	Amiodarone
	Tricyclic antidepressants
	Propylthiouracil
	Gold
	2,3-Dideoxyinosine (ddl)

Figure 30.3 Drug causes of acute liver failure. The drugs that cause acute liver failure are divided into two categories; category 1 is the frequently recurring causes and category 2 the occasional causes.

is often detectable by ultrasound. Serum uric acid levels are markedly elevated in these patients. The HELLP syndrome (hemolysis, elevated liver enzymes, low platelets) may be similar clinically. Acute liver failure complicating pre-eclampsia or eclampsia may also present with a similar syndrome, or may exhibit very high serum transaminase levels and abnormal tissue perfusion patterns on CT scanning that reflect the microvascular infarction that is characteristic of this condition.

Wilson's disease may present as acute liver failure, usually during the second decade of life. It is characterized clinically by a Coombs' negative hemolytic anemia and demonstrable Kayser–Fleischer rings in the majority of cases. The serum ceruloplasmin levels are usually, but not invariably, low and the serum and urinary copper levels are increased. Although the latter is the most specific feature of Wilson's disease, increases of lesser magnitude can occur in other causes of acute liver failure. A serum alkaline phosphatase-total bilirubin ratio of <2.0 had been suggested as an accurate discriminator of Wilson's disease from other causes of acute liver failure.

Poisoning with *Amanita phalloides* (mushrooms) is most commonly seen in central Europe, South Africa, and the west coast of the USA. Severe diarrhea, often with vomiting, is a typical feature and commences 5 or more hours after ingestion of the mushrooms. Liver failure develops 4–5 days later. Autoimmune chronic hepatitis may present as acute liver failure but it is usually no longer amenable to rescue with corticosteroid therapy. Anti-liver-kidney-microsomal antibodies are often the only detectable autoantibody in these cases. The diagnosis may be difficult to establish as autoantibodies in low titers are found in a proportion of patients who have seronegative hepatitis. The Budd–Chiari syndrome may present with acute liver failure and the diagnosis is suggested by hepatomegaly and confirmed by the demonstration of hepatic vein thrombosis. Malignant infiltration, especially with lymphoma, is another rare cause of acute liver failure that is typically associated with hepatomegaly. Ischemic hepatitis is being increasingly recognized as a cause of acute liver failure, especially in older patients. Other unusual causes of acute liver failure include heat-stroke and sepsis.

Pediatric cases

Children are at risk of developing most of the causes of acute liver failure discussed above, but also have some unique underlying causes, especially in the category of metabolic disease. Neonatal hemochromatosis presents within the first few weeks of life and has been treated by liver transplantation as early as 5 days of age. Acute liver failure due to mitochondrial disorders may be triggered by bacterial infections and they are characterized by high lactate levels in the blood. Other metabolic causes include tyrosinemia, galactosemia, and fructose intolerance. Young infants can develop acute liver failure with viral infections such as adenovirus, coxsackievirus, and cytomegalovirus.

CLINICAL SYNDROME

Acute liver failure causes a syndrome of multisystem failure potentially involving all the major body systems and these will be described in turn. Jaundice is present in most patients, but some cases of hyperacute liver failure develop encephalopathy before jaundice becomes clinically apparent. Most of the other signs of liver failure are notable by their absence. Fetor and flapping

tremor are not prominent features associated with the encephalopathy of acute liver failure, but are more likely to be seen with subacute liver failure than with the more rapidly progressive subtypes. Ascites is also unusual in Western patients except in subacute liver failure, Wilson's disease, and in the recovery period from acute liver failure when there is coexisting persistent renal failure. In India, however, ascites is a prominent feature and may be the indication of a poor prognosis in the absence of clinical encephalopathy. Other signs of portal hypertension are also unusual, but bleeding from esophageal varices has been documented especially in subacute liver failure.

Encephalopathy

All patients who have acute liver failure have some degree of encephalopathy. Patients who have grades 1 or 2 encephalopathy exhibit degrees of drowsiness or disorientation, but they can be roused and they respond appropriately to verbal stimuli. Progression to grade 3 encephalopathy is often heralded by a short period of extreme agitation before the patient becomes very confused and at best obeys simple commands. Grade 4 encephalopathy signifies deep coma with the patient being responsive only to painful stimuli or totally unresponsive. In acetaminophen-induced acute liver failure, the encephalopathy develops on the third or fourth day after drug ingestion, but in other etiologies the onset and rate of progression of the encephalopathy is variable.

The pathogenesis of the encephalopathy is incompletely understood and is probably multifactorial. Ammonia, phenols, fatty acids, middle-molecular weight substances, and mercaptans have all been proposed as possible causative agents. These toxins interfere with neuronal energy metabolism, and may also contribute to alterations in blood–brain barrier permeability by direct toxicity. The inhibitory neurotransmitter γ-aminobutyric acid (GABA) is increased in acute liver failure and this may act independently or in synergy with the benzodiazepine receptor which forms a supramolecular complex with the GABA receptor on neuronal plasma membranes. Other possible mechanisms include the development of false neurotransmitters (e.g. octopamine) and imbalances in the ratios of plasma and intracerebral amino acids.

Intracranial hypertension

This complicates grade 4 encephalopathy and develops in up to 70% of patients who have hyperacute liver failure, in up to 55% of patients who have acute liver failure and in less than 15% of patients who have subacute liver failure. It is a major cause of death and frequently disqualifies patients from transplantation when it is severe. The term intracranial hypertension covers a range of events including bloodflow-related episodic increases in intracranial pressure, followed by more sustained increases in intracranial pressure secondary to cerebral edema, and finally sustained impairment of cerebral perfusion pressure (Fig. 30.4).

In the early phase, sudden surges in intracranial pressure occur either spontaneously or in response to tactile or auditory stimuli. There is an associated increase in mean arterial pressure so that cerebral perfusion pressure is maintained and neuronal oxygenation is satisfactory. The risk to life at this stage is by means of classical brainstem herniation if the peak intracranial pressure is severe. As the complication progresses, the baseline intracranial pressure increases and sudden surges may continue to increase the

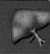

Main changes seen with intracranial hypertension			
Baseline intracranial pressure	Normal	Increased	Increased
Surges in intracranial pressure	Yes	Possible	May occur
Mean arterial pressure	Normal or increased	Normal or low	Low
Cerebral perfusion pressure	Normal	Normal or low	Low
Cerebral oxygen metabolism	Normal or increased	Normal or reduced	Reduced
Cerebral autoregulation	Maintained	Lost	Lost
Potential cause of death	Brain stem herniation		Hypoxic brain

Figure 30.4 Intracranial hypertension. This is a breakdown of the main changes in the key parameters as intracranial hypertension progresses through a spectrum of increasing severity from early to late stages.

pressure to dangerous levels. The arterial pressure no longer increases so that cerebral perfusion is variably reduced and there is some reduction in oxygen delivery to the brain. In the later stages, the intracranial pressure is so high, or the main arterial pressure is so low, that adequate cerebral perfusion is no longer exists. The main cause of death at this stage is hypoxic brain damage.

The clinical features of cerebral edema include systemic hypertension, 'decerebrate' posturing, hyperventilation, abnormal pupillary reflexes, and ultimately impairment of brainstem reflexes and functions. Papilledema, however, is rarely seen. Neurologic death can occur as a consequence of classic brainstem herniation or hypoxic brain damage, and consequently therapeutic approaches focus on the reduction of intracranial pressure or the optimization of neuronal oxygen metabolism. Most cases managed medically make full recoveries or succumb to this complication. A few exceptions were described in whom residual neurologic deficits occurred with medical management, but this was most often observed following liver transplantation. In the absence of direct intracranial pressure monitoring, systemic hypertension is a useful surrogate marker of paroxysms of increased intracranial pressure in the early stages, but this effect is lost as the severity of the complication increases. There is no evidence to support the use of CT scanning of the brain to diagnose or monitor cerebral edema in these patients, and the movement involved in bringing these patients to and through the scanner may be harmful.

Renal failure
Renal failure occurs in 75% of patients who develop grade 4 encephalopathy following an acetaminophen overdose and in 30% of other etiologies of acute liver failure. Renal failure after an acetaminophen overdose is a consequence of direct renal toxicity and usually develops early in the course of the illness. Patients with most other etiologies develop renal impairment when the encephalopathy is advanced, and it progresses through a stage of 'functional' renal failure [urinary sodium <10mmol/L (10mEq/L), urine/plasma osmolarity ratio >1.1] before demonstrating the characteristics of tubular damage. Urea synthesis is impaired in acute liver failure and it is not an accurate guide to the severity of renal dysfunction. Serum creatinine levels are therefore preferred for the monitoring of renal function.

Metabolic disorders
Hypoglycemia is common and can lead to impairment of consciousness before the onset of the encephalopathy characteristic of acute liver failure. The classic signs and symptoms of hypoglycemia are often masked and regular blood glucose monitoring is required. Metabolic acidosis is present in 30% of patients developing acute liver failure after an acetaminophen overdose and is associated with a particularly high mortality (>90% if the pH of arterial blood is <7.30 on the second or subsequent days after the overdose). This acidosis precedes the onset of encephalopathy and is independent of renal function. In contrast, a metabolic acidosis is found in 5% of patients who have other etiologies of acute liver failure, occurring later in the disease process and also associated with a poor outcome. Increased serum lactate levels have been documented in patients who have a metabolic acidosis, and these correlate inversely with mean arterial pressure, systemic vascular resistance and oxygen extraction ratios. The hyperlactatemia possibly reflects tissue hypoxia resulting from impaired oxygen extraction as a result of microvascular shunting of blood away from actively respiring tissues. In most etiologies of acute liver failure, alkalosis is the dominant acid–base abnormality and it may be associated with hypokalemia. Hyponatremia may reflect sodium depletion in patients who are vomiting or it may be dilutional due to excessive antidiuretic hormone secretion or intracellular sodium shifts. Hypophosphatemia is most frequently encountered in acetaminophen-induced acute liver failure when renal function is preserved.

Hemodynamics
The hemodynamic changes in acute liver failure are very similar to those observed in the systemic inflammatory response syndrome (SIRS). The early hemodynamic profile reflects a hyperdynamic circulation with increased cardiac output and reduced systemic peripheral vascular resistance. Profound vasodilatation may cause relative hypovolemia, and monitoring of pulmonary artery and left end-diastolic pressures is used to determine appropriate fluid regimens and adequate intravascular volumes. Progressive disease leads to circulatory failure either as a result of a falling cardiac output or an inability to maintain an adequate mean arterial pressure. This is a common cause of death in acute liver failure. Cardiac arrythmias may occur and are usually caused by a definable precipitating event (e.g. hypo- or hyperkalemia, acidosis, hypoxia, or cardiac irritation by a catheter, especially Swan–Ganz catheters).

Pulmonary complications
Pulmonary complications occur in approximately 50% of cases. Hyperventilation may be due to intracranial hypertension or may be due to a coexisting metabolic acidosis. Intracranial hypertension may also suppress respiratory function by compromising the brainstem, but most patients are mechanically ventilated before this occurs. Aspiration of gastric contents is an early risk to pulmonary status in patients who have encephalopathy who are also vomiting. Airway protection is critical in these patients, especially when they are being transported within or between institutions. Radiologic evidence of infection was found in 24% of patients, while pathogens were cultured from sputum in up to 46% of patients. Pulmonary edema occurred in 37% of patients, including almost half of those who had radiologic evidence of pneumonia. The pulmonary edema is largely noncardiogenic in origin

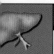

(pulmonary capillary wedge pressure corrected for serum albumin <18mmHg), and is especially frequent in cases resulting from an acetaminophen overdose. The relative contributions of increased endothelial permeability and neurogenic factors to the noncardiogenic pulmonary edema is unclear. Intrapulmonary hemorrhage and basal atelectasis are other pulmonary complications that are encountered in patients who have acute liver failure.

Hematology

The liver is responsible for the synthesis of most of the coagulation factors (except factor VIII, which is produced by endothelial cells) and some of the inhibitors of coagulation and fibrinolysis. In acute liver failure circulating levels of fibrinogen, prothrombin, and factors V, VII, IX, and X are reduced, and the prothrombin time is widely used as an indicator of the severity of liver damage. In addition to decreased synthesis of coagulation factors by the liver, there is evidence of increased peripheral consumption. While overt disseminated intravascular coagulation is unusual, sensitive techniques point to the presence of a low-grade process in most patients. Both quantitative and qualitative defects in platelet function are well described in acute liver failure and platelet counts of $<100 \times 10^9/L$ are seen in up to 70% of patients. Platelet aggregation is impaired, but there is an increase in platelet adhesiveness, a pattern that may be due to increased levels of circulating von Willebrand factor in acute liver failure.

Hemorrhage was documented in 73% of patients who had acute liver failure and was described as severe in 30%. The clinical coagulopathy is managed by the appropriate use of fresh frozen plasma, cryoprecipitate, and platelet concentrates. However, there is a tendency for the clinical coagulopathy to be much less profound than coagulation parameters would suggest, unless there is an associated thrombocytopenia or a frank disseminated intravascular coagulation syndrome. Gastrointestinal hemorrhage was common and was attributed to gastric erosions, but the incidence and severity have been decreased by gastric mucosal protection regimens. The other main sites include nasopharynx, lungs, kidneys, retroperitoneum, and skin puncture sites. Anemia not related to bleeding may be due to hemolysis or bone marrow disease. A Coombs' negative hemolytic anemia is a characteristic of Wilson's disease and a Coombs' positive hemolytic anemia may be seen in acute liver failure secondary to autoimmune hepatitis. Aplastic anemia is associated with seronegative hepatitis, especially in younger patients, and has been seen in up to one third of cases in pediatric series. This may be related to parvovirus B19 infection, although this is not necessarily the cause of the associated acute liver failure. Erythrohemophagocytosis is an increasingly recognized occurrence in acute liver failure.

Infection

Patients who have acute liver failure are at increased risk of infections and this has been calculated as twice the expected rate for similarly ill patients without liver disease. It is another of the common causes of death playing an integral role in the evolving cycle of hemodynamic instability and multisystem failure. It also frequently disqualifies potential candidates for emergency liver transplantation. Infection may be difficult to detect with confidence as there is a poor correlation between the presence of infection and body temperature or white cell counts. Patients who

have at least grade 2 encephalopathy had bacterial infection in up to 80% of cases and fungal infection in 32% of cases. The source of positive cultures included blood, urine, sputum, and vascular cannulae. The predominant bacteria were *Staphylococcus aureus*, streptococci, and coliform bacteria, while *Candida* spp. accounted for most of the fungal infections. The fungal infections were particularly difficult to diagnose and were detected antemortem in only 50% of cases. The risk factors for both bacterial and fungal sepsis include coexisting renal failure, cholestasis, treatment with thiopentone, and liver transplantation. Surveillance cultures are required on a daily basis.

Underlying etiology of acute liver failure		
Etiology	**Investigation**	**Comment**
Hepatitis A virus (HAV)	IgM anti-HAV	95% positive initially – 100% on repeat testing
Hepatitis B virus (HBV) acute infection seroconversion	IgM anti-core	Always positive but HBsAg often undetectable
	Full HBV profile	HbsAg positive, HBeAg negative, HBeAb initially negative, HBV DNA negative
increased replication	Full HBV screen	HBsAg positive, HBeAg positive, HBV DNA markedly elevated
Hepatitis D virus (HDV)	IgM anti-HDV	IgM anti-core may be positive (co-infection) or negative (superinfection)
Hepatitis E virus (HEV)	Anti-HEV	IgM antibody test not routinely available
Seronegative hepatitis	All tests	Diagnosis of exclusion
Acetaminophen	Drug levels in blood	May be negative on third or subsequent days after overdose
Halothane	Antibody test	Diagnosis usually made on clinical grounds
Idiosyncratic drug reactions	Eosinophil count	Most diagnoses based on temporal relationship
Ecstacy	Blood, urine, hair analysis	Medium-term exposure can be mapped from analysis of hair
Autoimmune	Autoantibodies, IgGs	High titers or anti-KLM suggest diagnosis
Pregnancy-related syndromes: fatty liver	Ultrasound, uric acid, histology	First pregnancy
HELLP syndrome	Platelet count	Disseminated intravascular coagulation a prominent feature
toxemia	Serum transaminases	Very high transaminase, appropriate obstetric history
Wilson's disease	Urinary copper, ceruloplasmin	Deeply jaundiced, anemic, second x obstetric history interruption in drug compliance
Amanita phalloides		History of ingestion of mushrooms, diarrhea
Budd–Chiari syndrome	Ultrasound or venography	Ascites, prominent caudate lobe on imaging
Malignancy	Imaging and histology	Imaging may be interpreted as normal
Ischemic hepatitis	Transaminases	Transaminases very high
Heatstroke	Myoglobinuria	Rhabdomyolysis a prominent feature

Figure 30.5 Underlying etiology of acute liver failure. The investigations required to establish the underlying cause of acute liver failure.

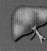

DIAGNOSIS

The diagnosis of acute liver failure is a clinical one based on the detection of evidence of encephalopathy in patients who have acute liver disease. Formal psychometric testing may be useful in patients who have subacute liver failure to detect subtle changes to the mental state, but in most patients the diagnosis of encephalopathy is made on overt clinical criteria. Commonly hypoglycemia and unusually uremia may mimic hepatic encephalopathy in patients who have acute liver failure, and these need to be excluded before the diagnosis is confirmed.

The etiology of acute liver failure must be accurately identified and the appropriate investigations are outlined in Figure 30.5. The investigation of the complications of acute liver failure is dealt with in Figure 30.6.

Histologic assessment of liver tissue may aid the diagnosis of the cause of acute liver failure, but this is often only available after death or transplantation. Confluent necrosis is the commonest histologic finding and this may be zonal or involve all of the parenchyma. Necrosis that is zonal within the acinus, and that which is coagulative or eosinophilic is more likely to be secondary to a toxic insult or ischemia (Fig. 30.7). The features of necrosis and parenchymal collapse may he interspersed with evidence of regeneration (Fig. 30.8). The regeneration may either occur in a diffuse pattern of small areas throughout the liver or in randomly occurring larger nodules that give the 'map-like pattern' that has been described in this condition (Figs 30.9 & 30.10). The

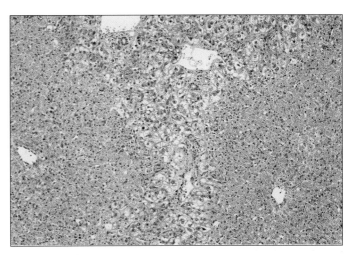

Figure 30.7 Liver histology. Submassive eosinophilic necrosis following an acetaminophen overdose showing few viable hepatocytes. This appearance can underestimate the capacity for regeneration to occur and the likelihood of spontaneous recovery. (Courtesy of Professor B. Portmann.)

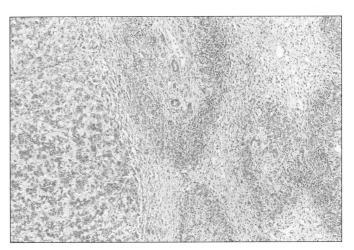

Figure 30.8 Liver histology. Adjacent regeneration (right) and severe collapse (left) occurring in a patient who has subacute liver failure. This appearance can overestimate the likelihood of spontaneous recovery. (Courtesy of Professor B. Portmann.)

Interpretation of laboratory parameters in acute liver failure	
Investigation	**Interpretation**
Hemoglobin	Hemorrhage, hemolytic or nonhemolytic anemia, aids fluid replacement
White cell count	Partial indicator of presence of sepsis
Platelet count	Important risk factor for bleeding, DIC syndrome, erythrohemophagocytosis, may be very low in acetaminophen cases
Serum bilirubin	Very variable, levels >700μmol/L (41g/dL) indicate hemolysis
Transaminases	Very variable and of no prognostic value
Serum albumin	Normal early but falls with disease progression, very low in hyperthermia
Prothrombin time	Very variable but of strong prognostic value
Serum sodium	Often low and may reflect sodium deficiency or dilution
Serum potassium	Low initially but rising with onset of renal failure
Serum phosphate	Low in acetaminophen cases with preserved renal function
Blood glucose	Regular estimations the only reliable screen for hypoglycemia
Acid–base status	Alkalosis common but acidosis associated with a poor prognosis
Arterial oxygen	Best screen for pulmonary disease even when chest X-ray is normal
Serum creatinine	Best indicator of renal dysfunction
Serum amylase	Essential to screen for co-existing pancreatitis

Figure 30.6 Interpretation of laboratory parameters. Abnormalities in investigations are interpreted in the context of acute liver failure. DIC, disseminated intravascular coagulation.

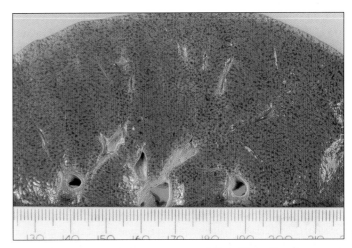

Figure 30.9 Macroscopic appearance of liver. The uniformly shrunken liver is characteristic of hyperacute liver failure. (Courtesy of Professor B. Portmann.)

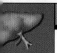

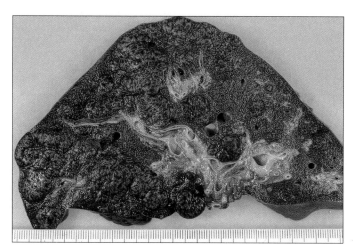

Figure 30.10 Macroscopic appearance of liver. The areas of regeneration randomly interspersed with collapse gives the 'map-like' pattern. The areas of regeneration may achieve significant volumes without improving the clinical condition. (Courtesy of Professor B. Portmann.)

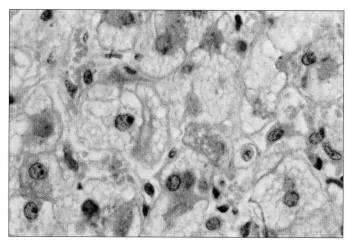

Figure 30.11 Diagnostic biopsy. This biopsy from a pregnant woman who has acute liver failure shows extensive fatty infiltration and is an example of the minority of biopsies that establish a specific diagnosis. (Courtesy of Professor B. Portmann.)

latter pattern is most commonly seen in patients who have subacute liver failure. The defined viral causes of acute liver failure have similar histologic appearances, and in true acute HBV infection there are usually no tissue markers detectable to implicate hepatitis B as the cause. The detection of hepatitis B markers suggests seroconversion to HBeAb positivity, a surge in hepatitis B replication or superinfection with δ viruses or viruses unrelated to HBV as the cause of the acute liver failure.

Histologic features may suggest specific diagnoses including sodium valproate toxicity, malignant infiltration, Wilson's disease, pregnancy-related syndromes, and Budd–Chiari syndrome. Sodium valproate toxicity is characterized by microvesicular steatosis. Screening for malignant infiltration as the cause of acute liver failure is one of the stronger indications for performing a liver biopsy in this condition. The benefit from a histologic diagnosis is strongest when lymphoma is the underlying diagnosis, as this may be responsive to chemotherapy. Patients who have Wilson's disease presenting as acute liver failure usually have established cirrhosis, commonly associated with interface hepatitis resembling autoimmune disease, hepatocyte ballooning, and steatosis. Liver histology may be very useful in making a precise diagnosis within the spectrum of pregnancy-related liver diseases, ranging from the fatty infiltration characteristic of acute fatty liver of pregnancy (Fig. 30.11), to the fibrin microthrombi and associated necrosis that is a feature of liver dysfunction secondary to pre-eclampsia or eclampsia. The histologic features of Budd–Chiari syndrome are extreme sinusoidal dilatation, congestion, and coagulative necrosis.

PROGNOSIS

The range of parameters that correlate with prognosis in acute liver failure is great. The skill is not in identifying these parameters, but adapting them so that they are universally useful in the decision-making process. The grade of encephalopathy, not unsurprisingly, correlates strongly with outcome and this is true for both the maximum grade attained and the grade of encephalopathy at the time of presentation to a specialist unit. The prognosis deteriorates further when grade 4 encephalopathy is

complicated by cerebral edema, and even further when the latter coexists with renal failure. Reliance on the development of these clinical complications to determine prognosis is not helpful when defining the scope and application of liver transplantation in this condition. Furthermore, subsets of patients have very poor prognoses without the development of cerebral or renal failure. The use of transplantation intensified the need for early indicators of prognosis so that those in need of this intervention could be identified as quickly as possible.

The prognosis of acute liver failure varies greatly with the underlying etiology (Fig. 30.12), as well as a number of other factors. Determination of prognosis drives two key management issues when assessing patients who have acute liver failure, namely, the need for referral to specialist centers and the indications for transplantation. Indications for referral to specialist units have been suggested for acetaminophen and other etiologies of acute liver failure (Figs 30.13 & 30.14).

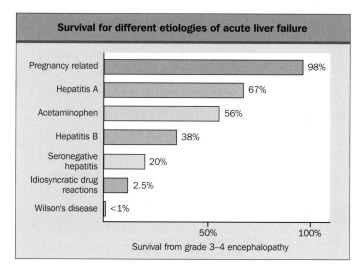

Figure 30.12 Impact of etiology on prognosis. The survival rates attained at King's College Hospital with medical management of patients progressing to acute liver failure is given for the underlying etiology. Similar results have been reported from Japan.

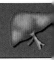

Referral to specialist units following acetaminophen ingestion		
Any of these criteria should prompt referral		
Day 2	**Day 3**	**Day 4**
Arterial pH <7.30	Arterial pH <7.30	INR >6 or PT >100s
INR >3.0 or PT >50s	INR >4.5 or PT >75s	Progressive rise in PT to any level
Oliguria	Oliguria	Oliguria
Creatinine >200μmol/L (1.5mg/dL)	Creatinine >200μmol/L (1.5mg/dL)	Creatinine >300μmol/L (2.3mg/dL)
Hypoglycemia	Encephalopathy	Encephalopathy
	Severe thrombocytopenia	Severe thrombocytopenia

Figure 30.13 Referral to specialist units. Criteria are suggested to select patients with acetaminophen-induced liver damage for referral to a specialist center. INR, international normalized ratio; PT, prothrombin time.

Referral to specialist units in non-acetaminophen etiologies		
The presence of any of the following criteria should prompt referral		
Hyperacute	**Acute**	**Subacute**
Encephalopathy	Encephalopathy	Encephalopathy
Hypoglycemia	Hypoglycemia	Hypoglycemia (less common)
PT >30s	PT >30s	PT >20s
INR >2.0	INR >2.0	INR >1.5
Renal failure	Renal failure	Renal failure
Hyperpyrexia		Serum sodium <130mmol/L (130mEq/L)
		Shrinking liver volume

Figure 30.14 Referral to specialist units. Criteria are suggested to select patients with non-acetaminophen-induced liver damage for referral to a specialist center. INR, international normalized ratio; PT, prothrombin time.

Separate criteria have been identified for use within specialist centers to identify the cohort most in need of liver transplantation, and the King's College criteria, which are widely used, are given in Figures 30.15 & 30.16.

One of the problems with there criteria is the difficulty applying the coagulation parameters outside the UK. The scale on which prothrombin times is reported in the USA is dramatically shorter than that in the UK, reflecting differences in technique and the reagents used. The use of the International Normalized Ratio (INR) did not solve this problem because of inaccuracies at higher readings. In France, the factor V levels are used in preference to either the prothrombin time or INR. Factor V levels less than 20% in patients under the age of 30 years, and less than 30% in older patients are indicative of a poor prognosis once encephalopathy develops. Factor V levels have not been used extensively in clinical practice outside France. A study from the UK assessed the prognostic value of factor V levels and validated their use in nonacetaminophen causes of acute liver failure, but found that they were not discriminatory in cases secondary to acetaminophen.

The King's College criteria, which are early indicators of prognosis, have a major advantage in that largely they can be applied quickly and before the patient progresses to the advanced stages of encephalopathy. In nonacetaminophen cases, etiology, the age of the patient, and the interval between the onset of jaundice and the development of encephalopathy are the static variables used to assess prognosis (see Fig. 30.16). These are combined with two commonly used dynamic parameters, serum bilirubin and prothrombin time, to complete the model. In acetaminophen cases, the pH of arterial blood has the strongest predictive value, and a pH <7.30 suggests a very poor prognosis. In patients who did not develop an acidosis the coexistence of a prothrombin time >100s (INR 6.7), serum creatinine >300μmol/L (2.3mg/dL), and grade 3 encephalopathy was necessary to be reasonably certain of a poor prognosis. However, despite the prompt identification of patients who have a poor prognosis after an acetaminophen overdose, liver transplantation could only be achieved in a minority of cases because of very rapid progression of the dis-

Indicators of a poor prognosis in acetaminophen-induced acute liver failure			
Parameter	**Sensitivity**	**Specificity**	**Positive predictive**
Arterial pH <7.30	49%	99%	81%
All 3 of the following concomitantly: Prothrombin time >100s or INR >6.5, Creatinine >300μmol/l (2.3mg/dL) and Grade 3–4 encephalopathy	45%	94%	67%

Figure 30.15 Indicators of a poor prognosis. The King's College criteria indicating a poor prognosis in acetaminophen-induced acute liver failure. INR, international normalized ratio.

Indicators of a poor prognosis in nonacetaminophen etiologies of acute liver failure			
Parameter	**Sensitivity**	**Specificity**	**Positive predictive**
Prothrombin time >100s or INR >6.7	34%	100%	46%
Any 3 of the following: Unfavorable etiology (seronegative hepatitis or drug reaction), age <10 or >40 years, acute or subacute categories, serum bilirubin >300μmol/l (2.3mg/dL), PT >50s or INR >3.5	93%	90%	92%

Figure 30.16 Indicators of a poor prognosis. The King's College criteria indicating a poor prognosis in causes of acute liver failure other than acetaminophen. INR, international normalized ratio; PT, prothrombin time.

ease. The criteria are still used as originally described with a few exceptions. In the original analysis the discriminatory power of a metabolic acidosis with an arterial pH <7.30 on the second or subsequent day after an acetaminophen overdose was very strong (95% mortality), but the more liberal use of N-acetylcysteine and aggressive early rehydration appear to have improved the outcome in these patients. As a result the interpretation of a transient acidosis in isolation from other prognostic indicators is more cautious. The criteria were not validated in a number of rarer etiologies, particularly pregnancy-related syndromes, Wilson's disease, and *Amanita phalloides* poisoning.

Assessment of the volume of viable hepatocytes by histologic examination is considered by some to be of prognostic value. The critical mass that suggests a good prognosis has been calculated at between 25 and 40%. This parameter has been used in isolation and in combination with other criteria to select patients for liver transplantation, but the potential for sampling error is considerable. A biopsy taken from an area of total collapse will show few viable hepatocytes even though the adjacent tissue may be regenerating. In addition, the poor prognosis in patients who have subacute liver failure may not be apparent from the relative healthy appearance of a biopsy taken from a regenerative nodule (see Fig. 30.8).

A small liver on clinical or radiologic assessment, or more particularly a liver that is found to be shrinking rapidly, is an indicator of a poor prognosis. This feature is especially useful in subacute liver failure when the degree of encephalopathy and the severity of the derangement of coagulation may not be particularly marked. In Japan, CT scanning has been used to assess both the size of the liver and the functional reserve, and this was useful in determining prognosis. Serial ultrasonic assessments of liver size are commonly used to detect changes in liver size, but the ease with which this can be done has to be weighed against the relatively subjective assessment of liver volume with this technique.

A number of parameters have been shown to have prognostic value in certain circumstances. Patients who have acute hepatitis B who have cleared HBsAg from serum are more likely to survive than those who have persistent HBsAg in blood. Serum α-fetoprotein levels are higher in patients who have acute liver failure due to hepatitis B who survive. Serial arterial ketone body ratios have also been shown to identify likely survivors in a number of studies. Although these parameters are of academic interest they are not routinely used to guide decision making in clinical practice.

MANAGEMENT

Overall strategy

Each patient who has acute liver failure needs an overall management strategy plan that starts with identification of etiology and an initial assessment of prognosis. Appropriate patients should then be referred to specialist centers where a decision on the need for liver transplantation is made. Patients are then monitored for the complications that may develop and these are treated as they emerge to the point of recovery, death or transplantation. Patients not initially considered for transplantation may change status on the basis of prognostic indicators or the pattern of clinical complications that emerges. Likewise, patients listed for transplantation may develop complications that preclude this intervention or occasionally may show unexpected signs of recovery before a donor organ becomes available. The final decision on transplantation is made when an organ is available. The potential to develop 'bridges to transplantation' using hepatectomy and/or extracorporeal liver support devices is likely to be increasingly tested in the forthcoming decade.

General measures

There has been scant reward from 30 years of research activity seeking the panacea for acute liver failure. Efforts have focused on reducing tissue injury, removing accumulated toxins, and promoting hepatocyte regeneration (Fig. 30.17).

Initial promising reports of efficacy followed by disappointing negative trials have been a recurring theme. There is no role for corticosteroid therapy and controlled studies suggest that in general they are contraindicated. Occasional patients who have late-onset hepatic failure are steroid responsive, but they are not yet readily identifiable on the basis of serologic markers. Insulin and glucagon infusions have been used to promote hepatic regeneration without convincing evidence of efficacy. Circulating interferon levels were found to be markedly reduced in one study of patients who had acute liver failure of viral etiology, and improved survival rates were reported for patients treated with interferon for 3 or more days. However, this observation has also been refuted in a larger study. Similarly, an initial enthusiastic report of the benefits of prostaglandins could not be reproduced within the construct of a controlled trial.

There are a few drugs with well-defined roles in specific etiologies of acute liver failure. Penicillin, and possibly silamyrin, should be added at the earliest opportunity to the standard supportive measures in patients who have *Amanita phalloides* toxicity. *N*-acetylcysteine is well-proven in the management of acetaminophen-induced acute liver failure. It was initially used to prevent liver damage when administered orally within 8 hours and intravenously within 15 hours of acetaminophen ingestion. The drug is given on the basis of the level of acetaminophen in the blood by time after the ingestion of the drug. Standard curves have been developed in the UK and the USA to indicate when *N*-acetylcysteine is indicated, and a third line has recently been proposed for high-risk patients (Fig. 30.18). The latter include patients taking enzyme

General management measures in acute liver failure		
Measure	**Controlled trials**	**Comment**
Corticosteroids	Yes	Old study but no benefit seen
Interferon	No	Initial positive report but no benefit seen in larger study
Insulin and glucagon	Yes	Early anecdotal suggestion of benefit but not confirmed in controlled study
Prostaglandin E₁	Yes	No survival benefit when controlled trial was performed
N-acetylcysteine	Yes	Beneficial in paracetamol cases, broader use not confirmed in clinical studies
Bowel decontamination	Yes	Inconclusive results
Charcoal hemoperfusion	Yes	No survival benefit, re-emerging as component of some extracorporeal circuits incorporating hepatocytes
Resin hemoperfusion	No	Preliminary studies only, inconclusive
Extracorporeal circuits	Yes	Early studies are either uncontrolled or are small – results of definitive trials awaited

Figure 30.17 General management measures. Almost all specific treatments applied to acute liver failure have been found to be ineffective.

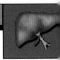

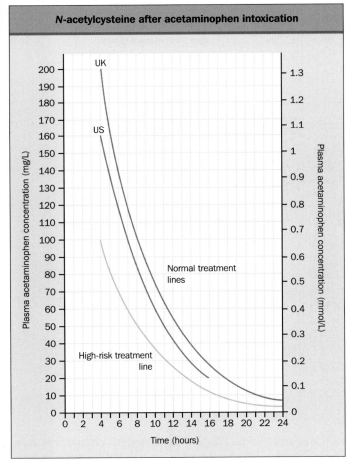

Figure 30.18 *N*-acetylcysteine after acetaminophen intoxication. The nomogram shows the blood levels that indicate a high risk of hepatotoxicity after acetaminophen ingestion in the UK and the USA. The lowest line is used in high-risk patients including the malnourished, chronic alcohol consumers, and patients taking enzyme inducing drugs (e.g. anti-epileptics).

inducing drugs (e.g. antiepileptic therapy), regular alcohol consumers, and malnourished patients. An extended role for this drug in acetaminophen-induced acute liver failure was first suggested by a retrospective study of 100 patients showing that *N*-acetylcysteine given 10–36 hours after drug ingestion was associated with a significant decrease in mortality (37 versus 58%), despite the development of comparable prolongations in prothrombin time. These observations were confirmed in a prospective controlled trial of 50 patients, in which patients in the active treatment limb were commenced on *N*-acetylcysteine 36–80 hours after drug ingestion. Although adequate studies of the overall effect of *N*-acetylcysteine on survival have not been performed for other etiologies of acute liver failure, it is increasingly used for ischemic and toxic insults, as well as a modulator of cellular oxygen metabolism.

Charcoal hemoperfusion was extensively assessed as a system to reduce circulating toxins. A study of 76 patients suggested a significant increase in survival with hemoperfusion when it was commenced while the patient was in grade 3 rather than grade 4 encephalopathy. Subsequently, controlled trials to assess the efficacy and optimal duration of hemoperfusion were carried out in 137 patients. Seventy-five patients with grade 3 encephalopathy were randomized to receive 5 or 10 hours of hemoperfusion daily, and there was no difference in survival between the two groups

(51.3 versus 50.0%). Sixty-two patients with grade 4 encephalopathy were randomized to receive either no hemoperfusion or 10 hours of hemoperfusion daily, and survival rates were also similar in the two groups (39.3 versus 34.5%). Even though these studies included 137 patients it has been argued that the numbers may have been inadequate to detect a significant clinical effect, and this illustrates graphically the difficulty of constructing meaningful controlled studies in acute liver failure. Plasmapheresis and exchange transfusions have also been used, and although temporary improvement in encephalopathy may be observed no sustained benefits have been established using these techniques. Interest in high-flux plasma exchange has recently been revived.

Two extracorporeal bioartificial liver support systems have been developed for clinical assessment in recent years. The hybrid bioartificial liver (BAL) intermittently exposes separated plasma to a cartridge containing porcine liver cells attached to collagen-coated microcarriers after the plasma has been passed through a charcoal column designed to remove substances toxic to the hepatocytes. This has been assessed as a bridge to transplantation in uncontrolled pilot studies and some neurologic benefits have been attributed to it. The extracorporeal liver assist device (ELAD) continuously exposed whole blood to cartridges containing approximately 200g of well-differentiated human hepatoblastoma cells that retain contact inhibition. The pilot studies performed so far include small controlled studies of the device, both as a bridge to transplantation and as an aid to spontaneous survival. These did not demonstrate any clinical benefit, but modest biochemical changes were observed. These systems, and any future improved versions, warrant assessment in properly constructed trials that take cognizance of the heterogeneity of acute liver failure. These systems need to be assessed both as potential bridges to liver transplantation as well as devices that may support some patients to a full recovery without surgery. *Ex-vivo* perfusion using pig or human livers that are unsuitable for transplantation has also been described as a bridge to transplantation in a small number of patients. Similar extracorporeal circuits using xenografts are likely to be assessed in pilot studies in the near future. Hepatocyte transfusions are also attracting some interest as a method of augmenting liver function, but as yet no significant clinical outcomes have been reported with this approach.

Liver transplantation

Orthotopic liver transplantation has revolutionized the management of acute liver failure by offering a lifeline to those cases that have a poor prognosis despite all the advances that have occurred in supportive care. It is now an integral part of the management of acute liver failure.

Grafts and graft allocation

Acute liver failure now accounts for 5% of all liver transplant activity in the USA and 11% in Europe. Most donor organ allocation systems prioritize acute liver failure; in the United Network for Organ Sharing (UNOS) system it is classified as category 1 and in the UK it is the only primary diagnosis on the 'super-urgent' registration list. Series from specialized centers in the USA, continental Europe, and the UK are remarkably consistent in showing that 45–51% of patients admitted with acute liver failure underwent liver transplantation (Fig. 30.19). In 13–27% of cases liver transplantation was considered to be contraindicated at the time of admission, and between 6 and 18% of patients were removed from the waiting list

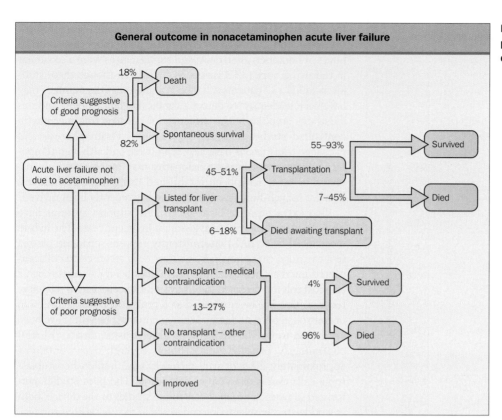

Figure 30.19 The general outcome for patients who have acute liver failure not due to acetaminophen.

or died before an organ became available (see Fig. 30.19). The UK figures exclude cases due to acetaminophen which accounts for 56–57% of the population with acute liver failure, but of these only 7–9% underwent transplantation (Fig. 30.20).

The waiting times for donor organs are pivotal in determining the policy on liver transplantation in the management of acute liver failure. The UNOS allocation system was changed to try to reduce the median waiting time of 5.5 days, while the UK system allows the majority of patients to be transplanted within 48 hours of registration. The waiting times also influence the attitude to the use of ABO mismatched grafts, fatty liver, and other suboptimal potential grafts. ABO incompatible grafts were used in 11% of adult transplants and 18% of pediatric transplants in the USA. A French group achieved a 93% transplantation rate by adopting a policy of using the first available organ irrespective of quality or blood group and achieved 1-year and 5-year survival rates of 68 and 61%, respectively. However, the European data show that the graft survival rate for ABO incompatible liver grafts used for emergency transplantation was only 32% at 1 year, compared with 54 and 49% for matched and unmatched but compatible grafts, respectively. A policy of accepting any organ increases the retransplantation rate and puts even more pressure on the restricted donor resource.

Patient selection

The optimization of the results requires the identification of suitable candidates as soon as possible in the disease process. The development of encephalopathy in association with a progressive coagulopathy is the most commonly used selection criterion. However, survival rates of 39–67% are being achieved with medical management in some etiologies; in these categories there is considerable scope for performing unnecessary transplants based

on this approach. The King's College Hospital criteria indicating a poor prognosis have been used as a method of selecting patients for liver transplantation. This model is sensitive to the urgency with which patients who have a poor prognosis need to be identified, is considered user-friendly, does not rely on the development of advanced disease before transplantation is indicated, and maximizes the time available to obtain a suitable donor organ. In addition to recognizing the heterogeneity within the syndromes of acute liver failure, this prognostic model is also sensitive to the paradox that young people who have rapidly progressive disease (hyperacute liver failure) have the best chance of survival without transplantation. Criticisms of this model include its apparent rigidity, nonuniversal applicability, and disservice to marginal cases in the light of the dramatic improvements seen in survival rates after liver transplantation for acute liver failure.

Alternatively, it has been suggested that all patients who have acute liver failure should be listed for transplantation and the decision to proceed made in the light of the clinical situation when an organ becomes available. This approach has the attraction of maximizing the delivery of transplantation to this patient population, but it increases the risk of unnecessary transplantation and may result in too much of a valuable resource being diverted to the management of this condition. Other approaches use factor V levels, liver histology, computed liver volume, and unbound plasma Gc levels. A review of the sensitivity and specificity indices for the systems currently in use indicates that the perfect model remains elusive.

The deselection of patients, whose clinical condition has deteriorated to the extent that proceeding to transplantation is futile, is difficult but important so as not to waste a valuable resource. No definite role has yet been confirmed for intracranial pressure monitoring or cerebral metabolic rates for oxygen in deciding

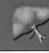

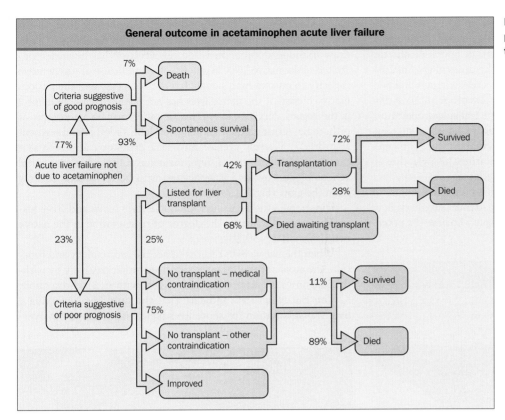

General outcome in acetaminophen acute liver failure

Figure 30.20 The general outcome for patients who have acute liver failure due to acetaminophen in the UK.

the vexed question of when potentially irreversible brain damage should preclude the use of liver transplantation in these patients. Deselecting patients who have cerebral perfusion pressures <40mmHg for 2 or more hours has been advocated and has resulted in a reduced incidence of failure of neurologic recovery after transplantation. However, two studies have documented survival both with and without transplantation in such patients. Accelerating inotrope requirements, uncontrolled sepsis, and severe respiratory failure are other imprecise contraindications to transplantation. These contraindications to transplantation are age-sensitive as younger patients are more resilient and more likely to reverse these complications after liver transplantation.

Transplant operation

The surgical aspects of standard liver transplantation are not as challenging as theoretic considerations might suggest. The repletion of coagulation factors, and platelets where necessary, before surgery adequately reverses the clinical coagulopathy in most cases, and intraoperative blood losses are remarkably low. This is in part a reflection of the poor correlation between studies of coagulation factors and the risk of surgical bleeding, but also the absence of portal hypertension. The liver is usually pale and shrunken but the presence of regenerative nodules protruding from the surface of the liver should not persuade the surgeon to abandon transplantation (Figs 30.21 & 30.22).

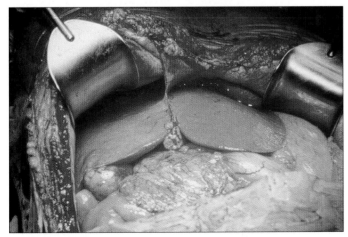

Figure 30.21 Transplant operation. The appearance of a liver in a patient undergoing liver transplantation for acute liver failure 5 days after an acetaminophen overdose. The liver is very pale.

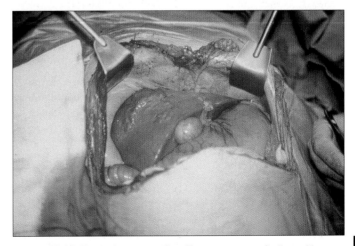

Figure 30.22 Transplant operation. The appearance of a liver with regeneration nodules in a patient undergoing liver transplantation for subacute liver failure following seronegative hepatitis.

Cerebral edema persists during and for up to 12 hours after a technically successful transplant and presents one of the major management issues. The dissection phase of the operation and the period immediately after reperfusion are the times of greatest risk for increases in intracranial pressure and decreases in cerebral perfusion pressure. In contrast, these parameters often improve dramatically during the anhepatic phase of the transplant operation. Cerebral autoregulation is restored within 48 hours of successful transplantation. Monitoring of intracerebral pressure and cerebral perfusion pressure should continue during this period in all patients who are susceptible to cerebral edema.

The relative ease of transplant surgery has permitted the use of innovative surgical techniques in these patients. Auxiliary liver transplantation has been pioneered for patients who have the poten-

tial to recover normal liver function and morphology. In theory, it combines the advantages of transplantation with the ability to withdraw immunosuppression when regeneration has been demonstrated in the native liver. In practice, the prediction of regenerative capacity to normal morphology has not been easy and the perioperative biopsy of the native liver has not been particularly helpful in this regard. Auxiliary liver transplantation may be heterotopic or orthotopic, replacing the right lobe, left lobe, or left lateral segment (Fig. 30.23). Current opinion favors the orthotopic approach as it preserves anatomic relationships, maintains autoregulation of portal venous blood flow, and is associated with better venous outflow from the graft (Fig. 30.24).

Functional studies using radionucleotide scans and liver histology are used to assess the degree of regeneration in the native liver (Figs 30.25–30.28).

When the native liver returns to normal morphology and function, the auxiliary transplant is sacrificed either passively by withdrawing immunosuppression or actively with surgical resection.

The European data indicate that the outcome of auxiliary liver transplantation for acute liver failure is similar to the over-

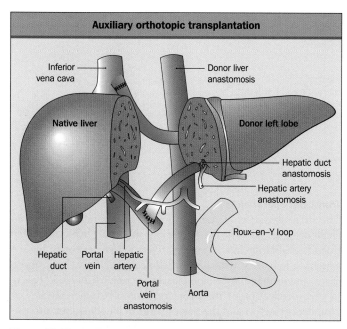

Figure 30.23 Auxiliary orthotopic transplantation. The liver can be subdivided to allow transplantation of the right lobe, left lobe, or left lateral segment. Most auxiliary transplants use either the right or left lobe.

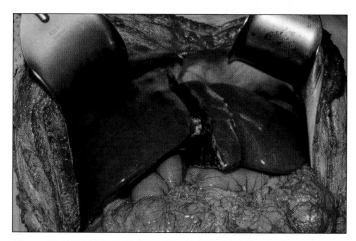

Figure 30.24 Auxiliary transplant. The appearance at the end of the operation with a perfused right auxiliary graft in a patient who has acetaminophen-induced acute liver failure.

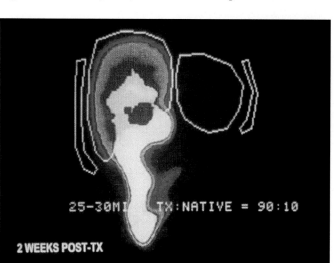

Figure 30.25 Auxiliary transplant. Radionucleotide scan showing 90% of function in the right lobe auxiliary transplant 2 weeks after transplantation.

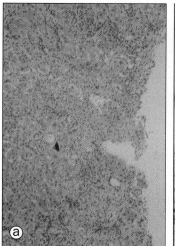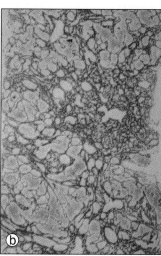

Figure 30.26 Auxiliary transplant. Histologic appearances of the native liver at the time of transplantation.

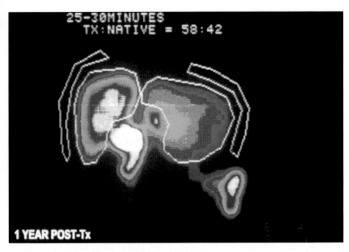

Figure 30.27 Auxiliary transplant. Radionucleotide scan showing 42% of function in the native left lobe 1 year after auxiliary transplantation.

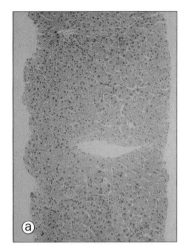
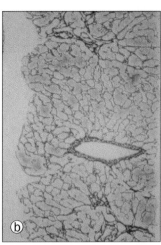

Figure 30.28 Auxiliary transplant. Histologic appearances of the native liver 1 year after auxiliary transplantation showing return to normal morphology.

all results achieved with total hepatectomy followed by standard transplantation. The expectation is that the results of the auxiliary approach should be superior and, at present, it should be considered that the optimal indications for auxiliary transplantation are unclear. The neurologic and hemodynamic benefits derived from the devascularization or removal of the diseased liver are completely or partially lost with this approach, and in unstable patients standard orthotopic transplantation may yield higher survival rates. In the short term, patients who have subacute liver failure may represent better candidates for auxiliary transplantation, but it has been suggested that this group are more likely to develop fibrosis and cirrhosis in the native liver and this has been observed in 30% of medium-term survivors.

The improvement in hemodynamic and neurologic stability that follows hepatectomy was the justification for the development of the two-staged procedure whereby hepatectomy precedes liver transplantation by a variable period of time. The diseased liver is explanted and a portocaval shunt is fashioned pending the availability of a liver graft (Fig. 30.29). It is often used as an act of desperation for very unstable patients in the hope that a liver graft will become available. The longest anhepatic time in an ultimate survivor was 21 hours and 45 minutes in a series of cases predominantly carried out for liver graft failure rather than primary acute liver failure. The risk of sepsis, especially fungal infection, increases as the duration between the two procedures is extended, and was the major cause of death in the largest series described. In that experience, transplantation was achieved in only 59% of cases, and some centers using this technique restrict its application to situations where the availability of an organ appears likely within 24 hours of the hepatectomy.

The profile of sepsis, including fungal infection, seen in acute liver failure extends into the post-transplant period and is further aggravated by the necessary immunosuppressive therapy. Patients transplanted for acute liver failure are routinely included in antimicrobial prophylactic regimens targeted at high-risk patients, together with those undergoing retransplantation and those with prolonged stays in intensive care units. These regimens often include aggressive antifungal prophylaxis with lipid-bound amphoteracin. Renal function may improve dramatically in the immediate postoperative period, but some patients need renal

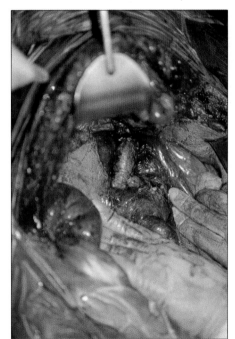

Figure 30.29 Hepatectomy. The liver has been removed in an unstable patient who has acute liver failure to reduce the toxic effects of the vascularized necrotic liver. A portocaval shunt has been fashioned. The patient received a liver transplant 17 hours later and survived.

support for many weeks after successful transplantation. The latter scenario is especially common after transplantation for acetaminophen-induced acute liver failure. The potent immunosuppressive agents and some antimicrobial drugs commonly used are potentially nephrotoxic and the use of these agents should be modified to optimize the return of renal function.

Results

The overall survival rates following transplantation were 63% in the USA and 61% in Europe (Fig. 30.30), and most individual centers that have reported their experience had survival rates falling within the 59–79% range. An exceptional report of a 93% survival rate from one center in the USA suggests that better results are likely to be more routinely attainable. This survival figure was achieved despite transplanting 47% of their overall series and contributing factors may have been the short waiting time (median 1.75 days and 78% within

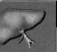

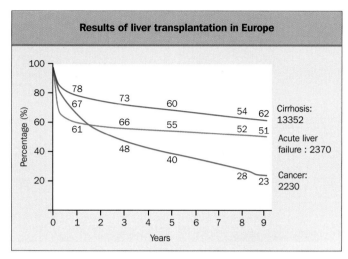

Figure 30.30 Results of transplantation. The results of transplantation for acute liver failure in Europe are inferior to those of elective transplantation, except for patients who have malignant disease at the time of surgery.

3 days, as compared with the USA mean of 5.5 days), deselection of patients who had an unstable neurologic condition (sustained cerebral perfusion pressure <40mmHg), and aggressive support following the use of ABO incompatible grafts (splenectomy, high dose antilymphocyte globulin, plasma exchange).

Patients receiving liver transplants for acute liver failure (median age 28 years) are younger than those undergoing elective transplantation (median age 44 years). The age of the patient influences selection for liver transplantation in acute liver failure more than for elective transplantation. The cumulative effects of age and multisystem disease lead to survival rates that are lower and at a level that questions whether it is justifiable to extend the valuable donor organ rescue to these patients. The European data indicate that the 1-year and 5-year survival rates are 51 and 42%, respectively, for patients aged 60 years or over. These figures compare with survival rates of 61 and 55% at 1 year and 5 years, respectively, for the overall population of patients receiving liver transplants for acute liver failure.

The factors that influence outcome after liver transplantation are multiple. The patient's age has already been addressed. The etiology of the underlying disease correlated with outcome in some centers. The best results were achieved for transplantation for Wilson's disease and the worst for idiosyncratic drug reactions. Patients who survived liver transplantation for acetaminophen-induced liver failure received the graft around the fourth day after drug ingestion, as compared with the sixth day in those who succumbed, and no patient transplanted on or after the seventh day survived. This reflects the role of sepsis in propagating the continued deterioration in these patients and the inability of liver transplantation to ameliorate this complication. Survivors after transplantation also tend to obtain the graft sooner after admission to specialist units, and in one study the average waiting time for survivors was 41 hours compared with 67 hours for those who died after transplantation. The survival rate decreases with progression through the grades of encephalopathy at the time of transplantation; in one series the figures were 90% for grade 1, 77% for grade 2, 79% for grade 3, and 54% for grade 4. As with liver transplantation in general, renal function correlated with outcome and serum creatinine levels above 200μmol/L (1.5mg/dL) were asso-

ciated with a poorer outcome. Acidosis and Apache III score at the time of transplantation were good indicators of the severity of the patients illness and correlated with outcome. However, none of these parameters were sufficiently discriminatory to use as criteria to disqualify individual cases from transplantation.

Management of specific complications
Neurologic complications
The management options for encephalopathy are limited. Patients who have subacute liver failure may benefit from dietary protein restriction, lactulose or bowel decontamination. However, these approaches are ineffective in the treatment of the more rapidly progressive encephalopathy characteristic of the hyperacute and acute syndromes. No convincing data have emerged to support the use of branched chain amino acids. Clinical and electro-encephalograph-assessed responses to flumazenil have been transient and unpredictable, and have not indicated a role for this drug in the management of the encephalopathy of acute liver failure. A transient improvement in encephalopathy has also been noted during many of the studies of the general measures outlined above, for example extracorporeal circuits, but in most of these no ultimate survival benefit was demonstrable.

Mannitol is the mainstay of treatment of surges in intracranial pressure that may compromise brainstem function (Fig. 30.31). The overall beneficial effect of mannitol was established in a controlled trial and the mechanism of action was considered to be its property as an osmotic diuretic. It has also been suggested that the rapidity of action of mannitol is more consistent with its function of increasing cerebral blood flow as being the basis for the therapeutic response. A rapid bolus of 0.3–1.0g/kg is recommended to achieve the maximal diuretic effect, and in anuric patients a diuresis is simulated by ultrafiltrating three times the administered volume over the subsequent 30 minutes. This process is repeated as determined by the pattern of clinical relapses until the serum osmolarity exceeds 320mOsm. More recent studies showed that the administration of mannitol was followed by an increase in cerebral blood flow associated with an increase in cerebral metabolic rate for oxygen and reduced brain lactate formation.

Sodium thiopentone (phenobarbitone) was shown to control cerebral edema that had become unresponsive to mannitol in an uncontrolled study. A priming dose of between 185 and 250mg given over 15 minutes was followed by a 4-hour infusion of between 50 and 250mg/h. Another study documented a 73% response rate to barbiturates, but this was followed by an 80% relapse rate after thiopentone was withdrawn. Thiopentone has neither been subjected to a controlled trial nor shown to improve the survival rate. Its role is limited by loss of efficacy and hemodynamic instability following its administration. There is an additional concern that the use of thiopentone results in an increase in infective complications in those surviving this phase of the illness. Acute, but not chronic, hyperventilation was reported to be of benefit. Nevertheless, hyperventilation to partial pressure of carbon dioxide levels below 25mmHg is routinely incorporated as a first-line treatment in protocols in the USA. Acute hyperventilation using low-tidal volumes (to prevent increases in intrathoracic pressure reducing venous return from the head) combined with 80–100% inspired oxygen may control surges in intracranial pressure that are unresponsive to mannitol and thiopentone. Hypothermia has also been shown in a single study to be effective in the management of severe intracranial hypertension.

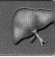

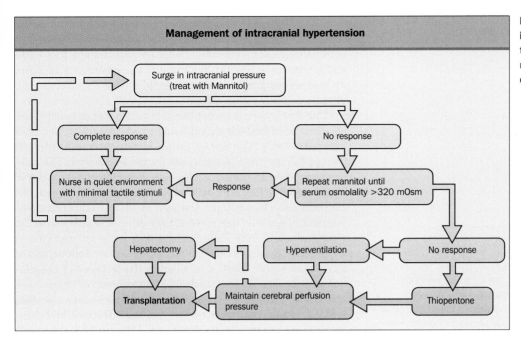

Management of intracranial hypertension

Surge in intracranial pressure
(treat with Mannitol)

Complete response

No response

Nurse in quiet environment with minimal tactile stimuli

Response

Repeat mannitol until serum osmolality >320 mOsm

Hepatectomy

Hyperventilation

No response

Transplantation

Maintain cerebral perfusion pressure

Thiopentone

Figure 30.31 Management of intracranial hypertension. The therapeutic alternatives in the management of this serious complication of acute liver failure.

In the later stages of the neurologic complications, the emphasis of management changes to the preservation of cerebral perfusion pressure, increased oxygen delivery to the brain, and manipulation of the neuronal microcirculation to promote cerebral oxygen extraction. The patient is now nursed with the trunk at 0–10° to the horizontal. The options for increasing the mean arterial pressure and consequently improving cerebral perfusion pressure are outlined in the section dealing with hemodynamics (below). These adjustments are made to maintain a cerebral perfusion pressure greater than 50mmHg where possible. At this stage, spontaneous recovery is unlikely without liver transplantation, and hepatectomy is useful to secure transient improvement.

N-acetylcysteine and prostaglandin I$_2$ infusions have been shown to increase cerebral blood flow and cerebral metabolic rate for oxygen and are considered to improve microcirculatory stability. Occult seizure activity may contribute to neurologic instability in patients who have grade 4 encephalopathy. Phenytoin and diazepam are effective therapies, despite the theoretic consideration that the latter may aggravate the underlying encephalopathy. There is no established role for other diuretics or antihypertensive agents in the management of cerebral edema in acute liver failure.

The use of intracranial pressure monitoring is controversial and has not been subjected to clinical trials. Early detection of cerebral edema and the facility to monitor this complication constantly help to optimize therapeutic interventions. Intracranial pressure monitoring allows earlier and more accurate detection of pressure changes, especially in the ventilated patient in whom most of the clinical signs are masked, and it facilitates careful monitoring of the intracranial pressure during high-risk therapeutic interventions, such as hemodialysis and tracheal suctioning. It is also considered valuable during orthotopic liver transplantation as increases in intracranial pressure often occur during the dissection and reperfusion phases of the transplant operation. The main points of the arguments for and against intracranial pressure monitoring are outlined in Figure 30.32.

The most commonly used system places transducers on or through a small nick in the dura. The risk of intracranial hemorrhage is a deterrent, although the studies that have systematically addressed safety have favored the use of intracranial pressure monitoring, especially using fiberoptic extradural or subdural devices. Proponents argue that it has been shown to be effective and relatively safe, despite the attendant coagulopathy. Epidural transducers were associated with a low complication rate at 3.8%, but subdural and parenchymal devices had higher complication rates at 20 and 22%, respectively.

One study has shown that high intracranial pressures at the time of insertion of the device was the main risk factor for intracranial hemorrhage, rather than the expected coagulopathy (Fig. 30.33). This group recommend the routine use of intracranial pressure monitoring in all patients who have hyperacute and acute liver failure (but not subacute because of the low incidence of cerebral edema) once grade 3–4 encephalopathy develops. Others advocate its use more selectively in patients who have evidence of cerebral edema, or those being considered for transplantation.

Arguments for and against intracranial pressure monitoring in acute liver failure	
For	**Against**
Only way of getting effective insight into condition	Complication rate too high
Allows early diagnosis	Clinical features allow diagnosis
Drives intelligent treatment	Never proven to improve survival
Monitors effect of potentially hazardous interventions	Good management protocols prevent potentially hazardous interventions
Modern devices are easy to place	Requires neurosurgical input
Aggressive correction of coagulopathy not necessary	Aggressive correction of coagulopathy necessary
	False readings may arise and confuse management

Figure 30.32 Intracranial pressure monitoring. The arguments for and against the use of pressure monitoring in acute liver failure are presented.

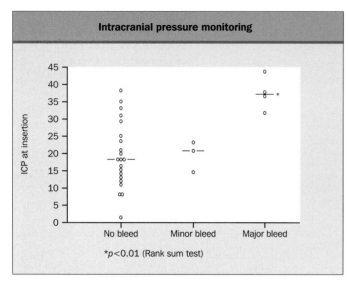

Figure 30.33 Intracranial pressure monitoring (ICP). The initial intracranial pressures are shown for patients developing major and minor intracranial bleeds after insertion of intracranial pressure monitors. High pressures correlated more strongly with risk than prothrombin times. None of the bleeds were fatal and two of the major bleeds were asymptomatic frontal lobe bleeds detected on scanning.

Infection

In the absence of prophylactic antibiotic therapy, bacterial and fungal infection was documented in 82 and 34% of patients with grade 3 and 4 encephalopathy, respectively. Sepsis has been implicated in 50% of deaths. The prophylactic use of the SPEAR regimen [1.5g intravenous cefuroxime every 8 hours, colistin 100mg nasogastric (NG) every 6 hours, tobramycin 80mg NG every 6 hours, amphotericin B 500mg NG every 6 hours, topical antimicrobials to oropharynx and anterior nares] in patients who had at least grade 2 encephalopathy reduced the incidence of culture-positive bacterial infection from 61.3 to 32.1% when the regimen was initiated before there was clinical suspicion of infection. A parallel study in similar patients who had clinical suspicion of infection (temperature >37.5°C, white cell count >15 × 10⁹/L, pulmonary infiltrates on chest radiograph) at the time of entry into the trial showed equivalent reductions in subsequent culture-positive bacterial infections with both the SPEAR regimen and parenteral cefuroxime only (38.1 and 28.6%, respectively). The findings of these studies suggest that any reduction in the incidence of bacterial infection may be due to the parenteral antibiotic alone. However, this study showed no significant impact on major clinical outcomes (mortality, progression to transplantation) or economic considerations [duration of stay in intensive therapy unit (ITU) and hospital stay, overall cost of antimicrobials].

The lack of benefit from the administration of nonabsorbable antibiotics was confirmed in a subsequent study that broadened the parenteral antibiotic regimen (ceftazidime 1g intravenously every 8 hours, flucloxacillin 500mg intravenously every 6 hours) and initiated it earlier in the hospital course. In this study the presence of a coagulopathy, even in the absence of encephalopathy, was adequate for entry to the trial. The incidence of confirmed bacterial infection in the cohort who were or became encephalopathic was 26%, as compared with 42% in the earlier study. The possibility that early antibiotic therapy might inter-fere with diagnosis by positive cultures was recognized, but the combined clinical and confirmed infection rate of 50% was still better than historic controls. However, one drawback of early and aggressive antibiotic therapy was the emergence of three bacteria showing resistance to multiple antibiotics, affecting 9% of the encephalopathic patients.

Topical prophylaxis against fungal infection was included in the regimens described above, and females had cotrimazole pessaries inserted weekly. The use of prophylactic systemic antifungal therapy has not been subjected to formal assessment. This may be appropriate in patients who have risk factors for systemic fungal infection like renal failure, severe cholestasis, previous or concomitant thiopentone therapy or liver transplantation. Systemic fungal infection is notoriously difficult to diagnose in the setting of acute liver failure, and a high index of suspicion is required, especially in the high-risk group outlined above, and in those cases where there is an arrest in the recovery of coagulation activity. The latter is a valuable sentinel marker of infection that often predates clinical manifestations by some days. *Candida* spp. account for the vast majority of fungal infections, and there are no data to show superiority of any of the available therapies.

Hemodynamic instability and oxygen debt

Circulatory failure is considered to be a significant contraindication to transplantation and a common mode of death in acute liver failure, often occurring against the background of sepsis and multiorgan failure. Invasive hemodynamic monitoring is routinely initiated in patients who have grade 3 encephalopathy and filling pressures are normalized with appropriate combinations of colloid, crystalline fluids, and blood products. Hypotension occurring despite adequate intravascular volumes (pulmonary capillary wedge pressure 10–14mmHg) is treated with vasopressor agents, using norepinephrine (noradrenaline) if the cardiac index exceeds 4.5L/min/m² or epinephrine (adrenaline) if the cardiac output needs to be boosted above this threshold. The initial stabilizing dose to achieve a mean arterial pressure above 60mmHg ranged between 0.2 and 1.8mg/kg/min of epinephrine, and 0.2 and 2.0mg/kg/min of norepinephrine. Vasopressor agents may cause or aggravate an oxygen debt and prostacyclin infused at a rate of 5ng/kg/min has been shown to improve parameters of oxygen metabolism (delivery, consumption, and extraction ration) when used in conjunction with both epinephrine and norepinephrine. *N*-acetylcysteine infusion (10mg/kg/min for 15 minutes followed by 0.2mg/kg/min for 4 hours) caused less vasodilatation than prostacyclin, independently increased mean arterial pressure, and was as effective as prostacyclin in improving oxygen metabolism. The combination of prostacyclin and *N*-acetylcysteine was more beneficial to oxygen metabolism than either drug alone (Fig. 30.34).

Renal failure

The prophylactic use of dopamine has been common practice but its benefits have been challenged, especially in the setting of profound vasodilatation that is typical of acute liver failure. The appropriate clinical studies have not been performed in this setting. Extracorporeal renal support was required in 75% of cases of acetaminophen-induced acute liver failure and 30% of other etiologies that progressed to grade 3–4 encephalopathy. The metabolic complexity of combined liver and renal failure suggests

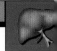

Management of hemodynamic instability

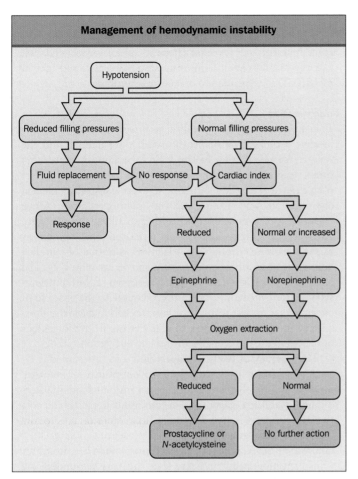

Figure 30.34 Management of hemodynamic instability. A care pathway for the management of hemodynamic instability.

early intervention with hemodialysis, pre-empting standard indications, is prudent. Continuous filtration or dialysis systems are associated with less hemodynamic instability and run a lower risk of aggravating latent or established cerebral edema than intermittent hemodialysis. The coagulopathy of acute liver failure does not negate the need for anticoagulation and, paradoxically, heparin requirements have been shown to be increased during hemodialysis The heparin doses required to prevent platelet depletion showed considerable variation and are best determined by functional assays such as the activated clotting time. Antithrombin III supplementation in a dose of 3000 units before hemodialysis reduced heparin requirements. Prostacyclin infusions in doses between 2 and 5ng/kg/min proved superior to heparin anticoagulation in continuous systems with respect to the functional duration of the filters and the hemorrhagic complications experienced.

Coagulopathy

Prophylactic repletion of coagulation factors with fresh frozen plasma has been practiced and requirements of up to a mean of 40ml/kg/day to maintain the prothrombin time within 5–10s of normal have been reported. The possible potential advantages of reduced bleeding and infection (as a consequence of repletion of opsonins) have not been established by clinical studies. A controlled trial of fresh frozen plasma failed to demonstrate an

improvement in survival, and was thought to be detrimental in a minority of patients who had a consumptive coagulopathy. Fresh frozen plasma administration impedes the use of coagulation studies in the assessment of prognosis and monitoring of disease progression, and other disadvantages associated with aggressive repletion include potential fluid overload and hyperviscosity syndromes. Prophylactic fresh frozen plasma is more commonly used in anticipation of an invasive procedure, for example insertion of cannulae or intracranial pressure monitors, or liver transplantation. However, there is a poor correlation between bleeding tendency and coagulation parameters in acute liver failure, and thrombocytopenia is considered to a more important risk factor for hemorrhage. Maintenance of platelets counts above 50–70 × 10^9/L has been recommended.

Gastric protection is important and hemorrhage was reduced by prophylaxis with cimetidine in a study performed over 20 years ago. Sucralfate, which has the potential advantage of reducing gastric colonization and pulmonary infection by maintaining gastric acidity, has gained favor, even though its efficacy has not been formally assessed. Likewise, the efficacy of ranitidine or proton pump inhibitors, which are also widely used to protect the gastric mucosa, has not been subjected to formal assessment.

Nutrition

Although the standard patient who has acute liver failure is well-nourished at the onset of the illness, it is important to institute nutritional support as soon as possible. The catabolic rate increases in patients who have acute liver failure and this is most apparent in those with complicating sepsis and those undergoing liver transplantation. The theoretic problems that limit nutritional options are legion: gastrointestinal ileus; desire to minimize gastrointestinal protein; difficulty maintaining isoglycemia; fluid restrictions secondary to renal failure; theoretic role of amino acid ratios in mediating encephalopathy; difficulty handling lipids; aggravation of sepsis by intravenous feeding, etc. Despite all of these considerations, adequate nutrition support can be obtained in the majority of patients. An element of enteral nutrition is desirable to help maintain the integrity of the small intestinal mucosa, and this is titrated against the volume of gastric aspirates and the development of diarrhea. Pilot studies showed that parenteral feeding is tolerated considerably better than would be expected from theoretic considerations. Lipid solutions (10%) are cleared from serum and standard amino acid preparations do not appear to have a clinically relevant impact on the encephalopathy profile. Continuous renal support systems give good flexibility with regard to the management of fluid loads and assiduous attention to the maintenance of feeding lines keeps the septic complications within the expected pattern of frequency.

Other complications and management issues

Mechanical ventilation is normally instituted when grade 3 encephalopathy develops, or sooner if airway protection is required. The setting of ventilatory parameters is subsequently determined by both respiratory function and neurologic status. Respiratory function may be compromised by a number of processes, for example infection, fluid overload, and hemorrhage, the treatment of which are considered elsewhere. Nitric oxide inhalation for the treatment of adult respiratory distress syndrome (ARDS) has not been formally assessed in acute liver failure.

PRACTICE POINT

Illustrative case

A 44-year-old woman presented to a gastroenterology clinic in the UK with a 3-week history of jaundice preceded by a 5-day history of nausea and lethargy. There was no significant past medical history. She consumed half a bottle of wine per day at the weekend and worked as a secretary. She used ibuprofen intermittently for headache. Physical examination was normal apart from jaundice and a liver that was palpable 4cm below the costal margin.

The laboratory investigations were as follows: hemoglobin 11.6g/dL, white cell count 6.7×10^9/L, platelet count 178×10^9/L, serum bilirubin 322µmol/L (19g/dL), aspartate aminotransferase (AST) 433IU/L, alkaline phosphatase 122IU/L, and prothrombin time 17s (control 13s). The viral hepatitis screen was negative. Antinuclear factor was positive in a titer of 1:40 and the IgG was raised at 19.6g/L. The ultrasound revealed no significant abnormality. The patient was given a review appointment 1 week later.

At the second consultation the symptoms were unchanged. The liver was no longer palpable and a small amount of dependent edema was present. Laboratory investigations were serum bilirubin 528µmol/L (31g/dL), AST 219IU/L, alkaline phosphatase 136IU/L, and prothrombin time 21s (control 13s). Arrangements were made to review the patient in 1 week, but 2 days later she was brought to the emergency department with confusion. A diagnosis of encephalopathy was made and she was transferred to an institution with a liver transplant program. She was placed on the waiting list within 4 hours of arrival, and was successfully transplanted 5 days later. The post-transplant recovery was uneventful until 2 years later when she became jaundiced again. Investigations revealed a hepatitic process associated with antismooth muscle antibodies in a titer of 1:640 and IgG of 31.6g/L. This responded to oral corticosteroids.

Interpretation

This scenario is very typical of seronegative hepatitis. The modest prolongation of prothrombin time understated the severity of the illness. In the USA, the same prothrombin times would have been more noteworthy because of the narrower range seen. The shrinking liver as assessed by clinical examination was a clue to the poor prognosis. Once encephalopathy developed, the King's College criteria were applicable and these immediately indicated a poor prognosis as she met four criteria (age, diagnosis, duration of jaundice before the onset of encephalopathy, and serum bilirubin). The criteria were satisfied at the initial assessment, but a diagnosis of acute liver failure could not be made in the absence of encephalopathy. However, this is one scenario where the alternative use of a coagulopathy to define acute liver failure does not address the deficiencies of the current definitions.

The etiology of the acute liver failure in this case may be an idiosyncratic drug reaction, autoimmune, or another unidentified mechanism. The original immunologic markers did not establish a diagnosis of autoimmune hepatitis and corticosteroids were not indicated. Corticosteroids are usually ineffective in autoimmune hepatitis presenting as acute liver failure. The development of classic autoimmune hepatitis after transplantation might indicate that this was the underlying pathology, but this can also occur *de-novo* after transplantation.

FURTHER READING

Acharya SK, Dasarathy S, Kumer TL, et al. Fulminant hepatitis in a tropical population: clinical course, cause and early predictors of outcome. Hepatology. 1996;23:1448–55. *Description of acute liver failure in India highlighting distinct differences in this population.*

Bernuau J, Rueff B, Benhamou JP. Fulminant and subfulminant liver failure: definitions and causes. Semin Liver Dis. 1986;6:97–106. *A good overview of acute liver failure highlighting some of the French aspects.*

Davenport A, Will EJ, Davison AM. Continuous vs intermittent forms of haemofiltration and/or dialysis in the management of acute renal failure in patients with defective cerebral autoregulation at risk of cerebral oedema. Contrib Nephrol. 1991;93:225–33. *The basis for recommending continuous renal support systems is outlined in this study.*

Demetriou AA, Rozga J, Podesta E, et al. Early clinical experience with a hybrid bioartificial liver. Scand J Gastroenterol. 1995;30:111–7 (S). *An early clinical experience with a liver support device as a bridge to transplantation.*

Ellis AJ, Wendon J, Hughes R, et al. The extracorporeal liver assist device in acute liver failure: Design and testing of a controlled trial protocol. Hepatology. 1996;24:1446–51. *An early controlled trial with a liver support device using human hepatocytes.*

Harrison PM, Keays R, Bray GP, Alexander GJM, Williams R. Late N-acetylcysteine administration improves outcome for patients developing paracetamol-induced fulminant hepatic failure. Lancet. 1990;335:1572–3. *A study supporting the use of N-acetylcysteine later than its role as an antidote to acetaminophen.*

Hoofnagle JH, Carithers RL, Shapiro C, Ascher N. Fulminant hepatic failure: summary of a workshop. Hepatology. 1995;21:240–52. *Good summary of the key issues with acute liver failure in the USA.*

Lake JR, Sussamn NL. Determining prognosis in patients with fulminant hepatic failure: when you absolutely, positively have to know the answer (Editorial). Hepatology. 1995;21:879–82. *A good assessment of the options for determining prognosis in acute liver failure.*

Makin AJ, Wendon J, Williams R. A 7-year experience of severe acetaminophen-induced hepatotoxicity (1987–93). Gastroenterology. 1995;109:1907–16. *A detailed analysis of acetaminophen-induced liver failure in the UK.*

O'Grady JG, Alexander GJM, Hayllar KM, Williams R. Early indicators of prognosis in fulminant hepatic failure. Gastroenterology. 1989;97:439–45. *The analysis of early prognostic indicators that gave rise to the King's College criteria.*

O'Grady JG, Gimson AES, O'Brien CJ, et al. Controlled trials of charcoal hemoperfusion and prognostic factors in fulminant hepatic failure. Gastroenterology. 1988;94:1186–92. *Large controlled trial of a liver support mechanism that highlights the difficulty in constructing future trials in acute liver failure.*

O'Grady JG, Schalm SW, Williams R. Acute liver failure: Redefining the syndromes. Lancet. 1993;342:273–5. *An updated classification for clinical syndromes of acute liver failure.*

Ringe B, Lubbe N, Kuse E, Frei U, Pichlmayr R. Total hepatectomy and liver transplantation as two-stage procedure. Ann Surg. 1993;218:3–9. *The only major series of patients with liver failure managed by hepatectomy.*

Rolando N, Harvey FAH, Brahm J, et al. Prospective study of bacterial infection in acute liver failure: an analysis of fifty patients. Hepatology. 1990;11:49–53. *Defines the extent of infection in patients with acute liver failure before the use of semi-prophylactic antimicrobial regimens.*

Rolando N, Wade JJ, Stangou A, et al. Prospective study comparing the efficacy of prophylactic parenteral antimicrobials, with or without enteral decontamination, in patients with acute liver failure. Liver Transplant Surg. 1996;2:8–13. *Study highlighting the benefits and disadvantages of prophylactic antimicrobial drugs.*

Wendon JA, Harrison PM, Keays R, Williams R. Cerebral blood flow and metabolism in acute liver failure. Hepatology. 1994;19;1407–13. *An interesting study of cerebral bloodflow abnormalities.*

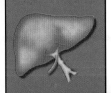

Chapter 31 Hepatobiliary Dysfunction in the Critically Ill

Andrew Rhodes and Julia A Wendon

INTRODUCTION

The finding of deranged liver function in a critically ill patient is a common occurrence in the intensive care unit (ICU). Abnormal liver function tests have been described in over half of the admissions to a general ICU and are associated with an increased mortality. Consequently, a jaundiced patient is a cause of great concern to the intensivist. The investigation and rationalization of the abnormal liver function is one of the more difficult tasks that an hepatologist will face in clinical practice. The etiology underlying the deterioration in liver function is complex, and many factors are potentially involved. The clinical scenarios range from specific pathologic processes that are readily identifiable to situations where many interrelated events are happening, and it is often impossible to elucidate a specific cause for the liver dysfunction.

LIVER BLOODFLOW IN CRITICAL ILLNESS

The vascular supply to, and circulation within, the liver have unique characteristics with important differences from any other organ in the body. Like the lungs, the liver has two inflow systems: the high flow but low pressure portal venous system; and the low flow but high pressure hepatic arterial system. Both drain into the hepatic sinusoidal system and ultimately into a common outflow via the hepatic veins. The liver circulation is the only vascular bed where two separate systems are connected in series, with the portal venous system downstream of the splanchnic vascular compartment (Fig 31.1). The portal vein therefore is important with regard to splanchnic perfusion, hepatic perfusion, and total venous return to the heart.

The regulation of total hepatic bloodflow occurs mainly at the hepatic arterial level. The portal flow is determined mainly by the inflow into the splanchnic beds (mesenteric, splenic, and gastric arteries), and thus the liver can alter the pressure in the portal system but has no control over flow. In health, the liver is able to demonstrate a mild degree of control over its blood supply by means of the hepatic artery buffer response. With decreasing portal inflow, the artery dilates to keep total liver bloodflow constant. The hepatic arteries are also capable of a moderate amount of self autoregulation to compensate for changes in systemic hemodynamics. Normal hepatic flow is maintained until systemic blood pressure drops to a mean arterial pressure below 50mmHg, when autoregulation is no longer sufficient to maintain hepatic perfusion.

The systemic hemodynamic response to sepsis has been well-documented and consists of a diffuse microcirculatory injury associated with arterial vasodilatation and hypotension. There is less known about the hemodynamic response in the venous compartments, but it would appear that in venous beds there is an acute hypertension associated with an increase in vascular resistance. This phenomenon is well characterized in the pulmonary circulation, where sepsis produces pulmonary hypertension, mainly as a consequence of an increase in resistance in the high flow/low pressure pulmonary veins.

The effects of sepsis, or experimental endotoxemia, on the liver are complex. In sepsis, endotoxemia leads to an activation of the Kupffer cells, which swell and partially obstruct the sinusoids. The circulating levels of endothelin, an endothelium-dependent vasoconstricting factor, rise, causing functional postsinusoidal sphincters to contract. The net result is to cause an increase in portal venous pressure as a result of an increase in sinusoidal resistance. The systemic vasculature is affected by massive rises in circulating nitric oxide, which cause a profound arterial vasodilatation. Under control conditions, nitric oxide has very little control over the portal beds, but it seems to have a profound role in endotoxemia by attenuating the responses to endothelin in the portal system. Consequently, nitric oxide appears to play a pivotal role in maintaining the hepatic sinusoidal microcirculation.

Normally, the overall effect of an increase in venous resistance is minimal. However, in sepsis the hepatic arterial inflow

Hepatic vascular supply		
	Pressure/flow characteristics	Vascular control
Hepatic artery	High pressure/low flow	Self autoregulation Hepatic artery buffer response
Portal vein	Low pressure/high flow	Relies on splanchnic inflow

Figure 31.1 Hepatic vascular supply. The concept of the compartmentalization of bloodflow within the liver parenchyma is important in the understanding of the pathogenesis of sepsis and ischemia-related insults.

resistance is dramatically reduced at the same time as the portal venous resistance is increased. This leads to an alteration in the normal control and distribution of regional bloodflow, with venous parameters becoming the dominant factor. This is most dramatically seen in the splanchnic beds where the increases in splanchnic venous pressures result in a pooling of blood, an increase in the formation of edema and third space losses, and are thus a major contributing factor to the hypovolemia of sepsis.

The normal homeostatic response over total liver bloodflow is represented by the hepatic arterial buffer response (HABR). This is where a reduction in portal flow elicits a corresponding increase in the hepatic arterial flow. During endotoxemia, the hepatic arteries are maximally dilated and thus can no longer perform the task of HABR. This appears to be related to a combination of an increase in circulating nitric oxide and an alteration in the normal responses to adenosine. The loss of the active control mechanisms (autoregulation as well as HABR) leads to an inability to compensate for reductions in portal flow and/or systemic arterial hypotension. Thus, in sepsis, even though total hepatic bloodflow is increased, a flow-limiting ischemic state exists as a result of a concomitant increase in liver metabolism, resulting in a state of 'relative ischemia'.

In hemorrhagic shock, there is a lowering of the total cardiac output, with a redistribution of the bloodflow away from the liver. This causes a disproportionately greater reduction in hepatic bloodflow which, when prolonged, can lead to a pronounced ischemic insult to the liver. With prompt and appropriate fluid resuscitation, further hepatic damage and hepatocellular death can be prevented.

The control and regulation of hepatic bloodflow during hemorrhagic shock is complex, and has been the subject of recent research. It appears that, much like the situation in sepsis, there is a precise control over the vascular tone by a combination of endothelium-derived vasoconstrictors and vasodilators. Endothelin levels rise in hemorrhagic hypotension and cause a potent and long-lasting vasoconstriction in multiple vascular beds, including the portal circulation of the liver. It is likely that the endothelins are responsible for the reduced hepatic perfusion seen during hemorrhagic shock. The effects of endothelin can, however, be modulated by nitric oxide. A nitric oxide-mediated vasodilatory process occurs early in resuscitation from hemorrhagic shock and acts to maintain hepatic bloodflow and may help to prevent hepatic ischemia under these conditions. The combination of these two antagonistic pathways contributes towards the fine control of hepatic blood supply during hypovolemia.

Portal venous inflow to the liver can be greatly influenced by the intra-abdominal pressure. Postoperative patients, or patients with intra-abdominal hemorrhage can undergo major changes of pressure within the abdominal cavity. Animal studies have demonstrated that pressures of up to 40cmH$_2$O are associated with reductions in portal flow of 90% and this leads to decreased formation and flow of bile.

Intensive care unit therapy and liver bloodflow

Most drugs that are used in the ICU to influence blood pressure and cardiac output will have some effect on splanchnic and liver bloodflow. The vascular endothelium of the liver is lined with differing vasoactive receptor groups. The hepatic artery is supplied by sympathetic vasoconstrictor nerves and has both α- and β$_2$-

adrenoreceptors as well as dopaminergic receptors, whereas the portal vein has mainly α-adrenoreceptors. The individual effect of differing drugs is thus complex, but to a certain extent may be predicted. Any drug that increases cardiac output should cause a corresponding increase in hepatic arterial bloodflow. However, both norepinephrine (noradrenaline) and epinephrine (adrenaline) in high dose will activate the a vasoconstrictor receptors and thus decrease the proportion of cardiac output that is delivered to the mesenteric and liver vascular beds. Dopamine in low dose (less than 3μg/kg per min) will have a preferentially vasodilating action as will the β$_2$-agonists such as dopexamine or salbutamol, and thus the use of these drugs should result in an increase in liver bloodflow.

Intermittent positive-pressure ventilation (IPPV) with or without positive end-expiratory pressure (PEEP) leads to a reduction in total hepatic bloodflow from a variety of mechanisms. The raised intrathoracic pressure causes a decrease in venous return to the heart and thus a reduction in cardiac output and hepatic arterial flow. This can be compensated for by intravascular volume expansion. The raised intrathoracic pressure also causes an increase in hepatic venous pressure and thus a degree of hepatic congestion. In addition to the pressure effects, alterations in the partial pressure of arterial carbon dioxide (PaCO$_2$) can also lead to states of altered liver perfusion. Hypocapnic hyperventilation leads to a reduction in both portal venous and hepatic arterial bloodflow.

Hepatic ischemia

Although ischemic hepatitis is a discrete syndrome in its own right (see below), ischemia of the liver is almost certainly involved in the hepatic dysfunction that is seen in patients with sepsis, multiple organ dysfunction, acute respiratory distress syndrome, and trauma. Splanchnic hypoperfusion, as measured by gastric tonometry, has been demonstrated in 51% of critically ill patients on admission to ICU, 90% of patients with sepsis, and more than 50% of patients undergoing cardiac surgery. Ischemia is known to be a cause of hepatocellular apoptosis and liver atrophy in experimental animals, and similar mechanisms have recently been demonstrated to be applicable in humans. Animal studies have also demonstrated that reductions in hepatic perfusion are followed by increases in the metabolic markers of hepatic dysfunction and a decrease in the production and flow of bile. Jaundice is a common sequel to major trauma in humans. The severity correlates with the degree of shock that develops, and thus indirectly with the presumed severity of the ischemic insult to the liver.

HEPATIC DYSFUNCTION IN THE SEPSIS SYNDROME

Sepsis, septic shock, and multiple organ failure are commonly encountered in the critically ill patient and have a significant mortality despite modern treatment strategies. Liver dysfunction is usually thought to be a late complication of these syndromes following on from cardiovascular, pulmonary, and renal failure. Hepatic dysfunction is associated with a decrease in hepatic perfusion, hypoxia, lactic acidosis, and an increase in the levels of serum alanine aminotransferase (ALT) and aspartate aminotransferase (AST). The lactic acidosis is due to a combination of impaired hepatic metabolism of lactate as well as increased production of lactic acid in patients with coexisting sepsis. This con-

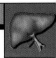

dition may eventually manifest as a progressive cholestatic jaundice, associated with varying degrees and combinations of hypoglycemia, encephalopathy, and impaired synthesis of coagulation factors.

The liver injury seen during sepsis seems to revolve around the function of the fixed hepatic macrophages, which are known as the Kupffer cells. The Kupffer cells are anatomically situated in

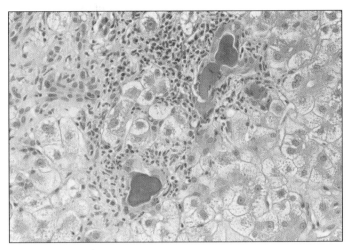

Figure 31.2 Liver in systemic sepsis. Histopathology demonstrating changes in a septic liver including cholestasis, neutrophil infiltration, cell ballooning, and prominent bile plugs.

a strategic position, lining the hepatic sinusoids and thus acting as a filter for the portal circulation. In critically ill or septic patients, bacterial cell overgrowth of the gut is known to occur and it is postulated that bacteria and endotoxin are translocated across the bowel wall into the portal circulation. This exposure to endotoxin and other antigens subsequently leads to the activation of the Kupffer cells, the expression of cytokine messenger RNA, and the release of proinflammatory cytokines including the interleukins, tumor necrosis factor (TNF)-α, leukotriene B$_4$, and the C5 fraction of complement. These agents act as chemoattractants to circulating neutrophils, which upgrade their surface adhesion molecule receptors (CD11β/CD18) and thus adhere to the sinusoidal endothelium. At the same time, the cytokines cause an increase in the density of the endothelial cell adhesion molecules, intercellular adhesion molecule (ICAM)-1 and endothelial leukocyte adhesion molecule (ELAM)-1. The net result of these interactions is to promote the migration of circulating neutrophils into the liver parenchyma (Figs 31.2 & 31.3).

The activated neutrophils are able to cause varying degrees of hepatic damage via the production and release of oxygen-derived free radicals and subsequent lipid peroxidation of cellular membranes. When the liver is subjected to an oxidative stress, xanthine hydrogenase is converted to xanthine oxidase, and when this combines with oxygen it leads to the production of the toxic free radical O_2^{-1}. This reaction can equally well be catalyzed by enzymes from the cyclo-oxygenase and lipo-oxygenase pathways.

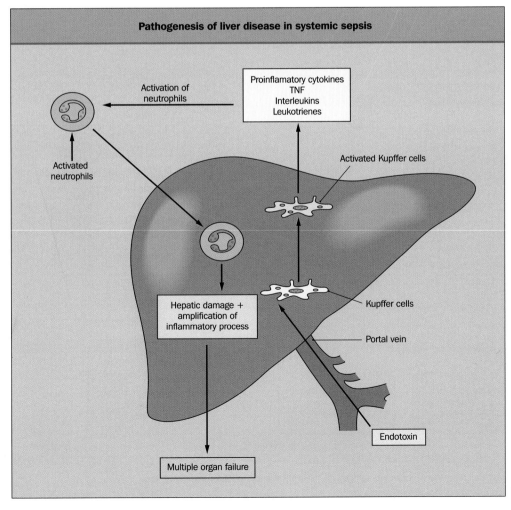

Figure 31.3 Pathogenesis of liver disease in systemic sepsis. The key steps in the pathogenesis of liver disease in sepsis range from the endotoxin mediated trigger through cytokine release to neutrophil activation and cellular damage.

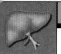

These O_2^{-1} radicals dissolve into water to form hydrogen peroxide, catalyzed by the enzyme superoxide dismutase, and this produces the highly reactive but diffusion-limited hydroxyl radical (OH^1). These radicals cause damage to cellular nucleotides as well as to amino acids and lipids. Lipid peroxidation is the end result of the actions of these radicals on the phospholipid component of the cellular membrane.

Apart from the damage caused by the activated white cells and the release of their toxic intermediaries, it is becoming evident that a variety of drugs may play an important role in the degree of cytotoxicity seen at a cellular level (Fig. 31.4). Drugs that possess adrenoreceptor activity are able to modify the inflammatory process and alter hepatocellular architecture and function. Drugs with β_2-adrenoreceptor activity seem to have anti-inflammatory effects, as opposed to α-adrenoreceptor agonists that have proinflammatory effects. This has been demonstrated in animal models of sepsis where the hepatic architecture can be seen to be profoundly altered following exposure to α-adrenoreceptor agents. These changes are almost completely attenuated by addition of a β_2-adrenoreceptor agonist. The α-agonists act via their cell membrane receptor to cause an activation of phospholipase C (PLC) via a G protein complex. This causes a subsequent

increase in diacylglycerol (DAG) and inositol triphosphate. Diaglycerol can then be further cleaved to form arachidonic acid and the inflammatory mediators such as the lipo-oxygenases and cyclo-oxygenases. Alternatively, DAG may exert an affect via protein kinase C by causing phosphorylation of a variety of important intracellular proteins that produce an increase in the inflammatory capabilities of the cell. Inositol triphosphate acts on intracellular storage organelle membranes to release calcium into the cytosol. The increase in intracellular calcium concentration then activates a variety of calcium-sensitive response mechanisms within the cell, which lead to an activated cytoskeleton and an increase in the permeability across the endothelial membrane. The β_2-adrenoreceptor agonists act via their receptors and G protein complexes to cause an activation of adenyl cyclase and thus an increase in the intracellular concentrations of cyclic AMP. The increases in cyclic AMP concentrations have a variety of effects. They cause an inhibition of phospholipase C and thus downregulate the proinflammatory pathway, but also cause a release of anti-inflammatory mediators such as interleukin-10.

The combination of activated neutrophils together with the fixed and migrating hepatic macrophages, all of which are producing toxic mediators, results in further hepatic damage as a

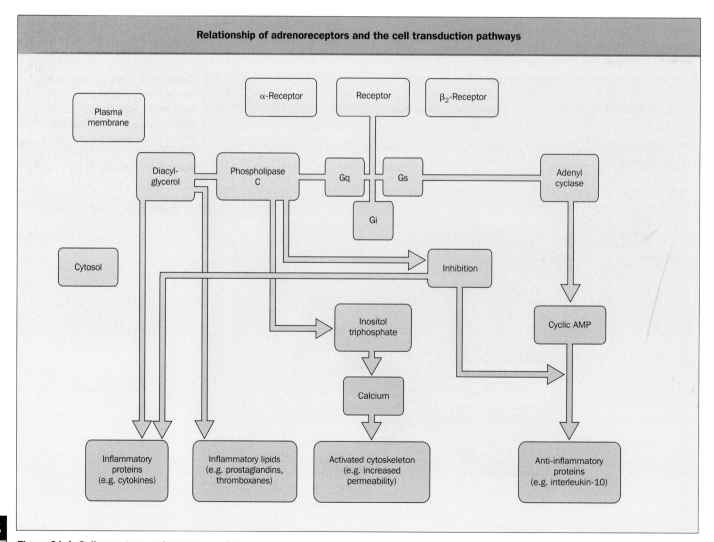

Figure 31.4 Cell receptors and responses. Cell membrane adrenoreceptors with the transduction mechanisms that follow activation of the receptors, highlighting the complexity of the cellular response.

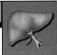

consequence of microcirculatory abnormalities and microthromboses (Fig. 31.5). The plugging of the activated white blood cells and platelets causes microthrombi to block the sinusoids, and as a result induce distal relative hypoxia. This in turn leads to further damage to the hepatocytes. The morphologic changes initially occur in the sinusoids. Kupffer cells become activated and swollen and this is followed by neutrophil and platelet microaggregates becoming adherent to the sinusoid endothelium, with resultant microcirculatory changes. Adjacent and distant hepatocytes rapidly demonstrate dilated organelles and a picture of multifocal hepatocellular necrosis appears, with polymorph infiltration. There are alterations in many of the hepatocyte metabolic pathways, with an inhibition in the adenylate cyclase pathway, alteration in adrenoreceptor distribution and function, decreased gluconeogenesis and cytochrome P450 activity, and increased lipogenesis. There are subsequent alterations in the cellular cytoskeleton with respect to both structure and function, which

are responsible for the decreased bilirubin and fixed anion transport, and the resulting cholestasis that develops in sepsis.

In summary, many of the features of the hepatocellular dysfunction seen with sepsis can be accounted for by the actions of endotoxin and the effects of inflammatory mediators released from activated Kupffer cells. The situation is not quite as simple, however, as Gram-positive infections are able to elicit similar responses to those of Gram-negative infections. Thus, other agents, apart from endotoxin, that are currently unidentified are undoubtedly involved and the nature of these factors will become apparent in due course.

Role of nitric oxide in sepsis-induced hepatic dysfunction

The role of nitric oxide (NO) in the generation of hepatic dysfunction during sepsis remains controversial. Nitric oxide is formed following the conversion of the amino acid L-arginine to L-citrulline through the action of nitric oxide synthase (NOS)

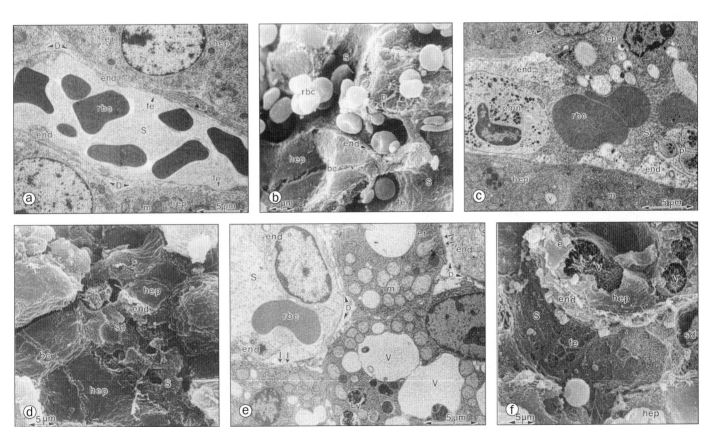

Figure 31.5 Electron micrographs of septic liver. Transmission (a) and scanning (b) electron micrographs of a hepatic biopsy taken from a normal pig. These show patent sinusoids (S) lined by a thin smooth endothelium (end) with fenestrated areas (fe) having free flowing red blood cells (rbc) within the lumen. Normal hepatocytes (hep) with distinct mitochondria (m) and endoplasmic reticulum (er). A narrow perisinusoidal space of Disse (D) can be seen between the apical microvillus hepatocyte surface and endothelium. The scanning image also shows the bile canaliculi (bc) between hepatocytes. Transmission (c) and scanning (d) electron micrographs of a hepatic biopsy taken from a pig with sepsis secondary to fecal peritonitis. These show sinusoids (S) occluded by swollen red cells (rbc), neutrophils (pmn), and platelets (pl). The endothelium (end) is swollen, lucent and bulges into the lumen reducing its area. This swelling has made the perisinusoidal space of Disse indistinct. Hepatocytes (hep) have granular cytoplasm with occasional single membrane-bound vacuoles (v) with both swollen mitochondria (m) and endoplasmic reticulum (er). The scanning image also shows the bile canaliculi (bc) between hepatocytes and sinusoidal debris (sd) forming a luminal plug. Transmission (e) and scanning (f) electron micrographs of an hepatic biopsy taken from a pig with sepsis secondary to fecal peritonitis and treated with α_1-adrenergic receptor agonist methoxamine. These show sinusoids (S) with swollen red blood cells (rbc) and swollen endothelium. The perisinusoidal space of Disse (D) is enlarged and often clearly separates the plasma membraneless apical hepatocyte surfaces (arrowed) from the endothelium (end). Many hepatocytes (hep) show granular cytoplasm full of large lucent vacuoles (V) and swollen mitochondria (m) and lysosomes (Ly). The scanning image also shows the hepatocyte vacuoles (V) with a granular and fibrillar matrix. The sinusoid has occlusive debris (sd) and the endothelium is seen to have an irregular surface with enlarged fenestrations (fe). (Courtesy of Dr R Moss.)

(Fig. 31.6). Once released NO diffuses into adjacent cells where it activates guanylate cyclase, leading to an increase in the intracellular concentration of cyclic cGMP, which is responsible for the majority of its actions. Three distinct isoforms of NOS have been described (Fig. 31.7).

- Brain or neuronal NOS (bNOS or nNOS), a constitutive, calcium-dependent isoform is found in neuronal tissues.
- Endothelial cell NOS (ecNOS or eNOS), a constitutive, calcium-dependent isoform, is found in endothelial tissues. This enzyme plays a major role in the control of systemic blood pressure and the distribution of microcirculatory perfusion. It is also involved in the inhibition of adhesion and aggregation of circulating blood cells. This is activated by a variety of chemical (acetylcholine, bradykinin) and physical stimuli.
- Inducible NOS (iNOS) is a calcium independent isoform. This is not present under normal conditions but is induced in various cell types by stimulation with bacterial cell products (endotoxin and lipoteichoic acid of Gram-positive organisms) and cytokines (TNF, interleukin-1β and interferon). The mechanisms by which this occurs remain unclear, but involve

activation of tyrosine kinase and nuclear factor-κB (NF-κB).

Nitric oxide is released at a low rate under normal conditions by the action of ecNOS, and is important for the control of vascular tone. During sepsis, there is amplification and induction of iNOS in diffuse tissues leading to the release of much higher levels of NO. This enhanced NO synthesis leads to a profound vasodilatation, with a decrease in the systemic vascular resistance and the development of hypotension. At the microcirculatory level, there is a loss of microvascular control, leading to a maldistribution of bloodflow.

High concentrations of NO have been implicated in a variety of tissue injuries by differing mechanisms. The combination of NO with superoxide anions leads to a production of peroxynitrite (OONO⁻), which causes an increase in hydroxyl radical production and thus lipid peroxidation and cell cytotoxicity. Nitric oxide also creates an alteration in the energy handling properties of cells via ADP-ribosylation of glyceraldehyde-3-phosphate dehydrogenase (GAPDH) and modification of the cytoskeletal cell properties via inhibition of actin polymerization. These cytotoxic effects are of paramount importance in the host defense against microorganisms, although are extremely hazardous when targeted against host cells.

The role of NO in preserving hepatic function is not quite so clear-cut. Nitric oxide formation has been detected in Kupffer cells, macrophages, hepatocytes, and sinusoidal endothelial cells following endotoxic stimulation. Nitric oxide is essential in regulating sinusoidal bloodflow and in preventing the aggregation and adherence of white cells and platelets to the sinusoidal walls. With nonselective inhibition of NOS, there is an increase in the number of leukocytes and platelets adherent to the sinusoid wall and a decrease in the number of sinusoids with bloodflow. This disturbance of the hepatic microcirculation then causes several changes in hepatic energy metabolism. Low perfusion causes hepatocyte hypoxia, especially in the pericentral regions, which is associated with a deterioration in hepatic function as assessed by an increase in plasma levels of AST and a decrease in the bileflow rate and hepatic ATP levels. Selective iNOS inhibition has had the opposite effects, however, with a reduction in liver injury following endotoxic shock. The overall effects are thus complex. Nitric oxide at a low dose seems to exert a protective effect on the hepatic microcirculatory function during sepsis, whereas excess production can have a variety of actions depending on both global hemodynamics and local microcirculatory conditions.

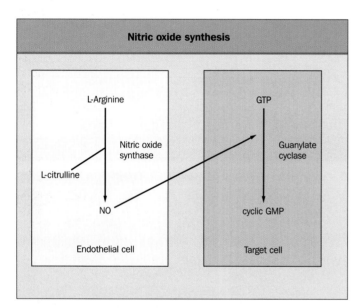

Figure 31.6 Nitric oxide synthesis. An illustration of the synthesis of nitric oxide (NO) within the endothelial cell and its subsequent action on the target cell mediated by the activation of nucleotide GTP (guanine triphosphate) to cGMP (cyclic guanine monophosphate).

Figure 31.7 Nitric oxide synthase isoforms. The nitric oxide synthase isoforms show different patterns of distribution and function.

Nitric oxide synthase isoforms			
Isoform	Enzyme requirements	Normal site	Function
Brain NOS	Calcium dependent	Neuronal tissue	Control of cerebral blood flow, memory, tolerance to opiates, neuronal transmission
Endothelial NOS	Calcium dependent	Endothelial cells	Control of systemic blood pressure, distribution of microfilatory perfusion, inhibits adhesion and aggregation of blood cells
Inducible NOS	Calcium independent	Not present in normal physiologic situations	

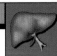

Inhibition of NO production with selective iNOS inhibitors may offer a therapeutic strategy in the future, but much work still needs to be done in this field.

HEPATOCELLULAR DYSFUNCTION AND PARENTERAL NUTRITION

Altered hepatic function is common in patients requiring total parenteral nutrition (TPN), occurring in between 68 and 93% of patients. The precise delineation of the etiologic factors behind TPN-related liver disease is difficult to assess, as other conditions are often present in patients requiring TPN, which may themselves be associated with liver dysfunction. The type of TPN-induced complication that occurs in any given patient appears to be influenced by age. There are three distinct clinical syndromes: cholestasis that occurs mainly in infants; steatosis or steatohepatitis that is seen in adults; and biliary sludge formation and cholelithiasis that occurs in both age groups.

Steatosis is characterized by hepatic fat accumulation without any evidence of inflammation, cholestasis, or hepatocyte necrosis. The fat accumulation is initially periportal in distribution, but as the condition evolves, this extends into either a pan-lobular or centrilobular pattern. Clinically steatosis is usually asymptomatic, although mild abdominal discomfort may occur. Modest elevations in ALT and AST are seen, accompanied less frequently with increases in alkaline phophatase and bilirubin. The increases in these enzymes usually peak following 2 weeks of TPN, are transient, and are associated with spontaneous resolution despite continuation of the infusion. Clinical and animal studies suggest that steatosis is associated with a combination of excess calories in the form of dextrose and glucose and a decreased ability of the liver to secrete triglycerides. There is some evidence to suggest that lipid supplementation of TPN solutions may decrease the incidence of steatosis by decreasing hepatic triglyceride uptake, promoting fatty acid oxidation, and increasing peripheral tissue triglyceride lipolysis. Overall, steatosis seems to be a relatively benign and self-terminating condition that is associated with the delivery of an inappropriate carbohydrate load in TPN. Recent modifications to TPN solutions with balanced glucose, amino acid and lipid solutions, tailoring calorific needs to patient requirements and delivering 10–30% of nonprotein calories in the form of lipid, has led to a significant fall in the incidence of this condition.

Cholestasis induced by TPN occurs mainly in infants, and is characterized by a centrilobular cholestasis with varying degrees of severity. Early in the disease process, the histologic changes demonstrate no evidence of inflammation, necrosis or fat accumulation. At the height of the jaundice, however, portal inflammation, bile duct proliferation, and portal fibrosis can accompany the cholestasis. Individual hepatocytes can be seen to demonstrate mild to moderate swelling with an increase in cytoplasmic glycogen and lipofuscin accumulation. The development of this condition is associated with the amino acid content of the solutions, with the incidence of cholestasis being related to the total volume of amino acids infused. Other associated factors include prematurity, low birth weight, sepsis, a failure to initiate oral nutrition, and the presence of gastrointestinal conditions that necessitate surgery. Immature bile salt secretory mechanisms and immature hepatic mitochondrial function seems to be the reason for the high incidence of this condition in the very young.

Cholestasis can also occur in adult patients on TPN, but this seems to be associated with longer-term feeding regimens. The pathogenesis in adults is poorly understood, but similar etiologic factors as are operative in childhood cholestasis are thought to be implicated. The major concern about TPN-induced cholestasis is the risk of progression of this condition to chronic and irreversible liver disease. Most experts advocate that TPN should be discontinued once cholestasis is apparent, although this is obviously difficult to achieve in patients with short bowel syndromes or chronic intestinal pseudo-obstruction. Small bowel transplantation may become a realistic option for these cases in the future.

Acalular cholecystitis, biliary sludge, gallbladder distension, and gallstones have all been reported in association with TPN in adults and children. Impairment in the flow of bile seems to be a consistent finding in patients with either cholestasis or cholelithiasis. This leads to an increase in the bile acid pool size, although the rate of bile acid synthesis is unchanged. A potential explanation for this would be a stagnation of the bile acids within the enterohepatic circulation during TPN administration. To support this there is some evidence to suggest that severe TPN-induced cholestasis may be partially reversed by the administration of the oral bile acid ursodeoxycholic acid. Along with impaired bileflow, gallbladder stasis seems to be an important contributor to the development of cholelithiasis induced by TPN. Clinical studies have demonstrated that this can be improved by the administration of exogenous cholecystokinin or by stimulating endogenous cholecystokinin through periodic pulsed infusions of large volumes of amino acids, or by the provision of small amounts of enteral nutrition.

ACUTE ACALCULOUS CHOLECYSTITIS

Acute cholecystitis is a recognized complication in the critically ill patient being associated with many clinical entities, including trauma, burns, sepsis, surgery, drug overdose, parenteral nutrition, and the acquired immunodeficiency syndrome. Only 10% of cases of acute cholecystitis seen in the ICU are related to gallstones, with the other 90% being referred to as acute acalculous cholecystitis. Any patient with a prolonged critical illness is at risk of developing this condition, which has a morbidity and mortality rate as high as 66% if left untreated. Diagnosis is difficult and hence presentation is late, often with life-threatening complications such as gangrene, empyema or perforation. With early diagnosis and appropriate management, the mortality rates of this condition can be improved considerably.

Pathogenesis
The pathogenesis of acalculous cholecystitis remains unclear despite the recognition of this syndrome for over 150 years. Many factors have been implicated in the pathogenesis of this condition, which include biliary stasis, gallbladder ischemia, total parenteral nutrition, and substances toxic to the gallbladder wall. It is rare for bacterial infections to be the primary cause of acalculous cholecystitis, but they often develop as a secondary insult invading the already diseased gallbladder. Biliary stasis has been associated with fever, dehydration, fasting, and prolonged infusions of narcotic analgesics. Hypovolemia results in a concentration of bile, which may inspissate in the absence of stimuli for gallbladder emptying. The narcotic analgesics cause an increase in biliary pressure secondary to spasm of the sphincter

of Oddi and thus a functional outlet obstruction. Biliary pressures are also raised by a combination of factors often seen in the critically ill patient, such as increased bile viscosity, positive pressure ventilation, PEEP, edema of the ampulla of Vater, and biliary stasis secondary to TPN and narcotic analgesics. It is proposed that a combination of hypotension with increased gallbladder pressures produce a reduction in the gallbladder perfusion pressure. This results in ischemia with a subsequent ischemia–reperfusion injury leading to necrosis in the gallbladder mucosa. The mucosa is then susceptible to bacterial infection, which if untreated can lead to perforation and pericholecystic abscess formation.

Biliary stasis results in an increase in the concentration of bile, an alteration in its chemical composition, and an increase in substances that may be toxic to the gallbladder. The phospholipid lysophosphatidyl choline is present in bile, and has been implicated in the generation of acalculous cholecystitis by this mechanism. It is known that increased concentrations of lysophosphatidyl choline have potent effects on gallbladder function by disrupting water transport across the gallbladder wall. A variety of other factors or theories have been implicated as being toxic to the gallbladder, including activated factor XII, collagen products, cigarette smoke, reflux of pancreatic juice into the gallbladder lumen, TPN, and a hypersensitivity reaction to broad spectrum antibiotics.

Diagnosis

The diagnosis of acute acalculous cholecystitis is difficult to make in the sick patient. The clinical picture is nonspecific and easily blurs into the background with the myriad of abnormalities seen in this patient population. The classic presentation is of fever, nausea, vomiting, and right upper quadrant abdominal pain, but this is often not apparent in an obtunded patient. Laboratory tests are often unhelpful, but reveal a leukocytosis and mild derangement in serum bilirubin, alkaline phosphatase, and aminotransferases.

For a variety of reasons ultrasonography is frequently the first test performed in this setting (Fig. 31.8). Ultrasound offers a real-time, noninvasive test that can be performed at the bedside and

is of reasonable sensitivity and specificity for the diagnosis, varying from 67% to over 90%. Findings at ultrasound include a diffuse or focal increase in wall thickness, striated intramural gallbladder lucencies, gallbladder dilatation, pericholecystic fluid, pericholecystic sonolucency, and an increased echogenicity within the gallbladder lumen (gallbladder sludge). An increase in the gallbladder wall is a relatively nonspecific finding. A wall thickness of less than 3mm is a normal finding in a fasted patient, but when this increases to greater than 3.5mm cholecystitis is more likely. Increased wall thickness can also be present in other conditions including hepatitis, hypoalbuminemia, right heart failure, renal failure, and myeloma. Striated intramural lucencies are thought to be the most specific abnormality seen on ultrasound for acute cholecystitis. This is where an anechoic area, thought to represent edema and cellular infiltrates, is seen mainly in the perimuscular (subserosal) connective tissues, and is separated from the gallbladder lumen by the mucosa and muscular layers. Other abnormalities seen include pericholecystic fluid which is caused by leakage of inflammatory material out of the gallbladder into adjacent spaces and gallbladder distension. Distension of the gallbladder is one of the initial findings seen when the cystic duct is obstructed. This is neither sensitive nor specific for acute cholecystitis but is found in the majority of cases. Similarly, biliary or gallbladder sludge is seen whenever gallbladder stasis exists and is thus also a fairly nonspecific finding.

Other investigations used for the diagnosis of acute acalculous cholecystitis include hepatobiliary scintigraphy, CT scanning (Fig. 31.9), and percutaneous aspiration of the gallbladder. Cholescintigraphy relies on an obstructed cystic duct preventing radionucleides entering the gallbladder. Delayed or nonvisualization of the gallbladder then implies acute cholecystitis. This technique has an accuracy of between 82 and 97% for gallstone-induced cholecystitis, but the accuracy rates are not as good for the acalculous disease. False-positive scans have been reported in patients with alcoholism, hepatic disease or in patients receiving TPN. The use of intravenous morphine sulfate may increase the accuracy of cholesintigraphy in acalculous cholecystitis.

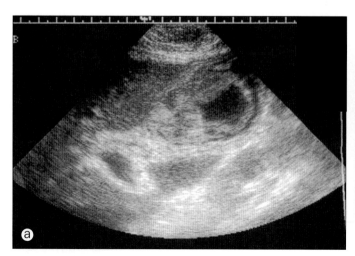

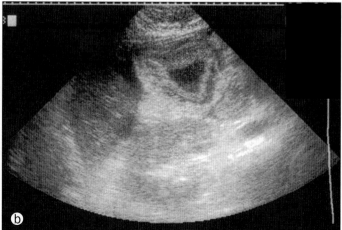

Figure 31.8 Acalculous cholecystitis. Ultrasound scan of the upper abdomen demonstrating findings in acalculous cholecystitis in the longitudinal (a) and transverse (b) sections through the gallbladder fossa. Diffuse thickening of the gallbladder wall with a sonolucent striated appearance due to edema is seen in both sections. Some pericholecystitic fluid is present with sludge in the proximal portion of the gallbladder. (Courtesy Dr Al Rhodes.)

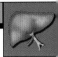

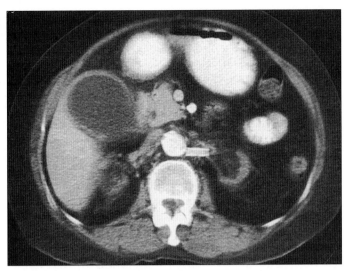

Figure 31.9 Acalculous cholecystitis. CT scan through the upper abdomen taken with intravenous and oral contrast. A distended thick-walled gallbladder is shown with minimal pericholecystitic fluid seen between the gallbladder and the liver. These findings are consistent with acute cholecystitis. (Courtesy of Dr Al Rhodes.)

Scanning by CT is a technique that is often employed in this patient group in search of the source of sepsis. Similar criteria for diagnosis of cholecystitis are used to those described under ultrasound, but the sensitivity and specificity are much higher and figures up to 100% have been quoted for both parameters. Percutaneous aspiration of the gallbladder is a safe technique that can be performed under ultrasound control at the bedside. Positive bacterial cultures may support the diagnosis of acute cholecystitis, but there is a high false-negative rate for this investigation, mainly due to the fact that acalculous cholecystitis is a noninfectious disease with bacterial infection occurring as a secondary event.

Management
Acute acalculous cholecystitis is a serious condition with a mortality as high as 66% if left untreated. Management consists of both medical and interventional therapies and revolves around either drainage or removal of the gallbladder. Even though bacterial infection is a secondary event in this condition, most patients have the systemic features of sepsis and should thus be treated with broad-spectrum antibiotics. Bile cultures when positive usually grow *Escherichia coli*, *Klebsiella*, *Enterobacter*, *Proteus*, and *Streptococcus* spp., enterococci, *Staphylococcus* spp., and anaeobes. The choice of interventional technique required to drain or remove the gallbladder depends primarily on the patient's condition. Often, the general physical state of these patients precludes emergency laparoscopic or open cholecystectomy, and thus drainage procedures are required to temporize and stabilize the patient in preparation for later surgery. Drainage can be performed by a percutaneous ultrasound-guided transhepatic cholecystotomy or from a stent inserted during an endoscopic retrograde cholangiography. Drainage procedures are necessary in order to prevent the potentially fatal complications of perforation, empyema or gangrene of the gallbladder.

DRUG-INDUCED HEPATOBILIARY TOXICITY

Drug-induced hepatotoxicity is a common phenomenon on the ICU, where patients are characteristically on multiple drug therapies. Drug-induced hepatic reactions tend to fall into two main categories: those causing a cholestatic reaction and those causing an hepatitic picture as part of an idiosyncratic drug reaction. Cholestasis presents as a rise in serum alkaline phosphatase along with increases in the transaminases and bilirubin. Drugs responsible for cholestasis include flucloxacillin, chlorpromazine, fusidic acid, warfarin, and erythromycin estolate. An hepatitic picture is characterized by a rise in predominantly the transaminases with lesser increases in the other enzymes. Characteristic drugs commonly used in the ICU setting that cause an acute hepatitis are ketoconazole, isoniazid, rifampin (rifampicin), methyldopa, halothane, phenytoin, sodium valproate, salicylates, nonsteroidal anti-inflammatory agents, allopurinol, furosemide (frusemide), ranitidine, amiodarone, and streptokinase. Occasionally massive hepatic necrosis may occur (Fig. 31.10). This presents with a biochemical picture similar to that of ischemic hepatitis, but the clinical setting should enable a distinction in most cases. Drugs renowned for causing massive necrosis include acetaminophen (paracetamol taken in increased quantities before admission to the ICU), amiodarone, nonsteroidal anti-inflammatory drugs (NSAIDs), antituberculous chemotherapy, and halothane.

ISCHEMIC HEPATITIS

Definition
Ischemic hepatitis, or hypoxic hepatitis, refers to a transient but marked rise in the aminotransferase enzymes in association with circulatory collapse. The syndrome is defined by the following three criteria:
- a clinical setting of circulatory failure;
- a sharp but transient increase in either the ALT or AST enzymes to levels greater than 20 times the upper limits of normal; and
- exclusion of all other causes of acute hepatic necrosis, especially either drug- or viral-induced causes.

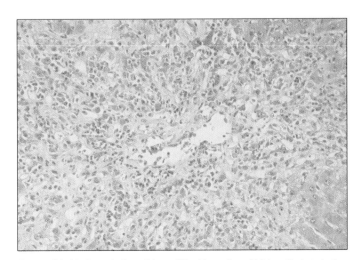

Figure 31.10 Drug-induced hepatitis. The value of histopathology in the assessment of liver dysfunction in the ICU is limited, but the demonstration of drug-induced hepatic necrosis is one of the exceptions. (Courtesy Professor B Portmann.)

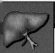

Ischemic hepatitis is thus, in part, a diagnosis of exclusion. Careful scrutiny of the patient's medication is essential to exclude potential drug-related hepatotoxicity. In addition, an extensive screen for viral infections is required, including serology for hepatitis A, B, and C viruses, Epstein–Barr virus (EBV), cytomegalovirus (CMV), and herpes simplex, before the diagnosis can be made with a reasonable degree of certainty.

Incidence

The incidence of ischemic hepatitis was generally considered to be low, although recent prospective studies are consistently indicating that it has been considerably under-reported. A recent study has identified ischemic hepatitis as the single commonest cause of serum transaminases in excess of 500IU/L in hospitalized patients over the age of 50 years. Two influencial retrospective analyses had found only five cases in 12 years in one institution and seven cases over 5 years in another. However, when this condition was studied in a prospective fashion, 29 cases were identified in a 6-month period in one center, while 20 patients were detected over a 1-year period in the specific setting of a coronary care unit, representing 2.6% of all admissions. When the cardiac patients were reanalyzed on the basis of those with low cardiac outputs, the incidence of ischemic hepatititis increased to 21.9%.

Pathophysiology

Ischemic hepatitis occurs in association with cardiovascular compromise and results from a reduction in hepatic bloodflow. The etiology is thought to involve a combination of factors. The hepatic necrosis is ultimately a result of cellular hypoxia, but varying contributions from ischemic hypoxia, passive liver congestion, and arterial hypoxemia have been debated. In cardiac patients, two factors seem to be of importance. Right ventricular failure causes a backflow into the hepatic veins, leading to a limitation of hepatic and portal inflow into the liver whatever the level of systemic pressure or the cardiac output. The combination of this hepatic congestion at the same time as a reduction in hepatic arterial bloodflow, from whatever cause, combines to produce the clinical condition.

The other essential ingredient in producing the biologic and histologic features of ischemic hepatitis is the ischemia–reperfusion injury seen following a period of low flow. Human observations as well as animal experiments demonstrate that the clinical and histopathologic features of this condition are not evident during the ischemic phase, but become apparent later following improvement in the hemodynamic profile. Thus, it seems likely that a number of factors have to combine before the liver injury occurs and the subsequent clinical condition manifests itself.

With decreasing oxygen supply to the cells, the redox state of the mitochondria becomes reduced with an alteration in the ratio between the oxidized and reduced forms of nicotinamide-adenine dinucleotide (NAD^+/NADH). This results in an inhibition of mitochondrial ATPase, a subsequent depletion of cellular ATP, and a resultant cellular acidosis. Further hypoxia leads to a rise in intracellular calcium levels, which in turn activates degradative enzymes for proteins, lipids, and DNA.

Following this period of ischemia, reoxygenation or reperfusion occurs. Early in the reperfusion period neutrophils infiltrate into the hepatic vasculature, but the damage secondary to this does not become apparent for a further 5 hours. During this period there is adherence to the sinusoidal endothelium with extravasation and subsequent parenchymal tissue injury; a series of events that requires expression of adhesion molecules on neutrophils (β-integrins), endothelial cells (ICAM-1), and hepatocytes (ICAM-1). Although there is early upregulation of the β-integrins (CD11β/CD18) on circulating neutrophils, it takes several more hours for full neutrophil activation and subsequent generation of reactive oxygen species and chemotactic factors such as leukotriene B_4. The counter-receptor for the β-integrins, ICAM-1, plays an important role in the transendothelial migration and parenchymal adherence. In the setting of ischemia-reperfusion, increased expression of ICAM-1 is seen on hepatocytes and endothelial cells. In animal studies, monoclonal antibodies against ICAM-1 are beneficial in limiting reperfusion injury. Proteases may also constitute an important injury mechanism, being secreted from both neutrophils and Kupffer cells. Oxygen-derived free radicals can facilitate protease-mediated injury by an inactivation of oxidant-sensitive plasma proteases which results in cell damage. Protease inhibitors may prove to be beneficial in this setting and have also been shown to be effective in reperfusion injury.

Inflammatory mediators largely influence the control and regulation of the cycle of injury during ischemia–reperfusion. Enhanced formation of TNF-α, interleukins (IL-1, IL-6, IL-8), platelet-activating factor (PAF) and complement activation have all been reported in the reperfusion scenario. The effects of individual mediators are difficult to quantify as this syndrome is such a multifactorial entity and all the mediators are produced at the same time in differing concentrations. Complement activation can lead to increased expression of neutrophil β-integrins, resulting in sequestration and subsequent production of oxygen-derived free radicals. Tumor necrosis factor-α and IL-1 can result in transcription of the ICAM-1 gene and hence expression on vascular endothelial cells, as well as production of chemotactic cytokines such as IL-8; PAF is another important mediator in this syndrome of ischemia–reperfusion. It has vasoactive, prothrombotic and proinflammatory effects, leading to activation of white cells and macrophages that trigger release of their cytokines and proteolytic enzymes. It also induces platelet aggregation and promotes adherence of neutrophils to vascular endothelium.

Another significant problem in the reperfusion period is the microvascular dysfunction that may result in further ischemic cell damage or death. Although it was initially thought that capillary plugging might be accounted for by neutrophil accumulation in the sinusoids, it has recently been suggested that sinusoids are not easily obstructed and it is only highly activated neutrophils that contribute to the sequestration process. It is more likely that in areas of endothelial damage there is accumulation of platelets and restriction of bloodflow to adjacent areas. This obstruction takes place on top of an imbalance between vasodilating (NO) and vasoconstricting (endothelins) mediators, which have the capacity to result in stasis in some areas, while in other areas the flow is so rapid that substrates have little time to equilibrate between tissues.

Clinical features and diagnosis

The clinical picture of ischemic hepatitis closely resembles that of either viral or drug-induced hepatitis. The condition manifests itself superimposed on a picture of decompensated circu-

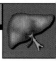

latory collapse. The patients will be shocked, often requiring vasopressor support, demonstrate an alteration in mental status and renal function, and will rapidly develop a metabolic acidosis. Hepatomegaly occurs in 50% of patients. Plasma AST and ALT are commonly greater than 1000 IU/L (greater than 20 times and sometimes up to 200 times the upper limit of normal), and lactate dehydrogenase peaks at 16–28 times the upper limit of normal. Peak concentrations occur within 24 hours of the insult and then decline to normal over the next 7–10 days. Plasma levels of alkaline phosphatase and bilirubin are commonly normal or only mildly elevated in the early stages, but the bilirubin may rise later as a secondary event. Hypoglycemia and prolongation of the prothrombin time commonly occur. Ischemic hepatitis progresses to acute liver failure in rare instances.

The dominant histopathologic feature of this condition is centrilobular necrosis. There is also marked congestion of the central veins and a distortion of the sinusoids in the central areas, with neutrophil infiltration, and nuclear abnormalities (Fig. 31.11). A liver biopsy is not usually necessary in this condition however, as the features are readily recognized on clinical grounds and the morbidity and mortality from the procedure in this patient group is high.

Treatment

There is no specific treatment for the condition apart from general supportive intensive care. Correction of the underlying circulatory collapse is necessary as well as prevention of further complications. Specific measures to monitor hepatic and splanchnic perfusion can be employed with either gastric tonometry or continuous hepatic vein oximetry to demonstrate the balance between hepatic oxygen delivery and consumption. The liver compensates for reduced oxygen delivery by increasing extraction, and this can be seen by decreasing levels of oxygen saturation in the hepatic veins. An intravenous infusion of dobutamine hydrochloride has been reported to be useful by increasing the cardiac output as well as improving hepatic perfusion. Right ventricular failure can be improved by decreasing the hypervolemia and more specifically by the administration of a pulmonary vasodilator such as inhaled NO.

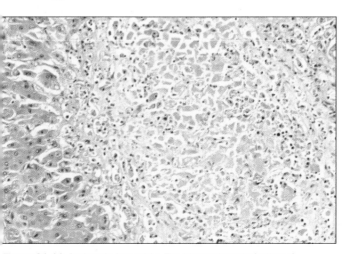

Figure 31.11 Ischemic hepatitis. The histopathologic finding of centrilobular necrosis is very suggestive of ischemic hepatitis. (Courtesy Professor B Portmann.)

Nitric oxide will preferentially vasodilate the pulmonary arteries, thereby reducing the right ventricular afterload and improving the performance.

This condition has a high mortality with reported rates varying between 50 and 60%. The overall prognosis is not primarily due to the hepatic failure, but relates to the cause, and response to treatment, of the underlying circulatory derangement. The consequences of ischemic hepatitis are often reported as minimal providing the patient survives. However, it is often involved in the later development of jaundice and contributes to the complexity of abnormal liver function in the ICU patient.

BLUNT HEPATIC TRAUMA

Abdominal trauma is a relatively common reason for admission to the ICU and a considerable proportion of these patients have a degree of liver injury (Fig. 31.12). Patients with sharp penetrating injuries obviously require immediate operative intervention, but the more common scenario is a blunt injury to the abdomen. Although the liver is the abdominal organ most commonly injured after blunt trauma, the majority of injuries are relatively minor. The more severe injuries, however, are associated with a significant mortality. Traditionally these patients have undergone a laparotomy to explore the severity of the injury, but recent studies are beginning to modify practice to a nonoperative management strategy. This change in surgical philosophy has come about as a result of the increasing sophistication of radiologic assessment for these patients. It is now also appreciated that up to 67% of all operations for blunt hepatic trauma had been nontherapeutic and that 86% of these hepatic injuries had stopped bleeding by the time of laparotomy. Modern high-speed CT scanners can accurately delineate the severity of hepatic injury and degree of hemoperitoneum, and provide a reliable evaluation of the integrity of gastrointestinal and retroperitoneal structures (Fig. 31.13).

The first priority in the management of these patients is resuscitation, and with appropriate fluid replacement many potential complications can be avoided. The best predictor of the need to operate in these patients is the degree of hemodynamic stability. For any patient with cardiovascular compromise, urgent surgical exploration is necessary. If the patient is hemodynamically stable, a nonoperative strategy should be employed. The patient should be admitted to an appropriate ICU for observation. This unit must have an immediate access to specialist hepatobiliary surgery services, should the need arise. Repeated CT scan evaluation is indicated when transfusion requirements do not abate, especially when the trauma impacted on multiple sites. When the hepatic lesion is unchanged and the cause of the falling hematocrit is not deemed to be the liver, other sources of blood loss should be sought. When the hepatic lesion has extended, additional treatment is necessary and angiography should be performed with the objective of embolizing the bleeding vessel (Fig. 31.14).

The advantages of nonoperative intervention strategies for these patients are that the overall mortality is unchanged (5–8%) while there is a decrease in the incidence of complications. The incidence of bleeding in patients with blunt hepatic injuries is low, between 2.8 and 3.5%, and can usually be controlled by angioembolization. Laparotomy at this stage is rarely therapeutic and can often precipitate further hemorrhage.

Hepatic Injury Scale		
Grade*		**Injury description****
I	Hematoma	Subcapsular, nonexpanding, <10% surface area
	Laceration	Capsular tear, nonbleeding, <1cm parenchymal depth
II	Hematoma	Subcapsular, nonexpanding, 10–50% surface area; or intraparenchymal, <2cm in diameter
	Laceration	Capsular tear, active bleeding, 1–3cm parenchymal depth, <10cm in length
III	Hematoma	Subcapsular, <50% surface area or expanding ruptured subcapsular haematoma with active bleeding; intraparenchymal hematoma <2cm or expanding
	Laceration	<3cm parenchymal depth
IV	Hematoma	Ruptured intraparenchymal haematoma with active bleeding
	Laceration	Parenchymal disruption involving 25–50% of hepatic lobe
V	Laceration	Parenchymal disruption involving >50% of hepatic lobe
	Vascular	Juxtahepatic venous injuries (ie. retrohepatic vena cava, hepatic veins)
VI	Vascular	Hepatic avulsion

Figure 31.12 Liver trauma: The Hepatic Injury Scale. The Hepatic Injury Scale was devised by the American Association for Trauma Surgery and is used to stratify the severity of liver injury. *Advance one grade for multiple injuries to the same organ. **Based on the most accurate assessment at autopsy, laparotomy, or radiologic study. (With permission, Pachter HL, Knudson MM, Esrig B, et al.)

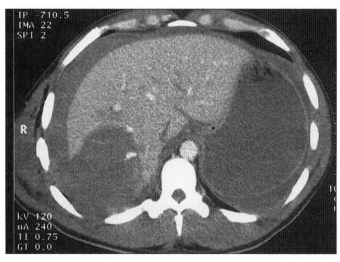

Figure 31.13 Liver trauma. CT scan showing an hepatic hematoma with extracapsular hemorrhage following trauma to the upper abdomen.

Other complications encountered in these patients include a collection of bile (biloma), biliary leak or fistula and abdominal abscess or infections. Control of biliary leaks can usually be maintained via stent placement at endoscopic retrograde cholangiopancreatography (Fig. 31.15). With severe injuries (grade IV, V), a prolonged period of observation and treatment in the ICU is necessary. These patients are prone to other interrelated complications, and the cholestasis is involved with sepsis and critical illness.

PRACTICAL APPROACH TO LIVER DYSFUNCTION IN THE ICU

The development of abnormal liver function in the patient has two management implications, prognostic and therapeutic. The required skill is to investigate the patient as extensively as nec-

essary to identify remediable causes while not subjecting unstable patients to investigations that may precipitate further deterioration without offering any benefit. The transport of critical patients to radiology departments is not always well-tolerated and intravenous contrast material may be another insult to precarious renal function, even though newer contrast agents and optimal intravascular repletion have reduced this risk.

Liver biochemistry and ultrasound examination form the basis of the preliminary assessment of liver dysfunction. An isolated hyperbilirubinemia usually reflects the functional cholestasis secondary to sepsis or a component of multiorgan dysfunction, and does not require extensive investigation if the ultrasound examination shows no biliary dilatation. The coexistence of hyperbilirubinemia and anemia should trigger a screen for hemolysis, especially if the hyperbilirubinemia is predominantly unconjugated. A serum transaminase level in excess of 300IU/L suggests a hepatitic process that may be ischemic, viral or drug-related. The most likely diagnosis will be suggested by the clinical situation with particular regard to circulatory dysfunction, comprehensive viral serology, and a review of the medication administered. Additional diagnostic information is rarely forthcoming from a liver biopsy in this situation. The coexistence of a coagulopathy points to a severe insult to the liver and is of greater prognostic value than the other components of the liver function profile.

Cholestatic profiles are the most difficult of the patterns of liver dysfunction to categorize. An early ultrasound is essential to screen for biliary dilatation and aseptic cholecystitis. More extensive radiologic investigation is indicated when there is a coexisting fever and this may include CT scanning or cholangiography to exclude biliary leak, biliary obstruction, hemobilia or previously undiagnosed aseptic cholecystitis in different clinical settings. In the absence of a fever and diagnostic radiology, a liver biopsy may be useful. This will frequently show a pattern of cholestasis with or without bile plugs that is typical of 'ICU' cholestasis and possible hepatic response to systemic sepsis. More precise diagnoses made on liver biopsy include steatosis (which may be

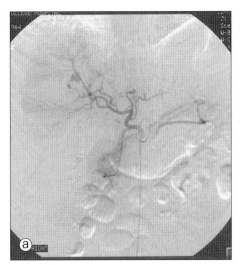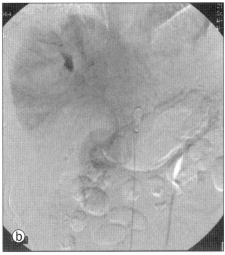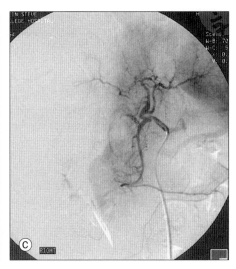

Figure 31.14 Liver trauma. The case illustrated in Fig. 31.13 underwent hepatic angiography which demonstrated the bleeding point in the arterial phase (a) and venous (b) phases. The hemorrhage was arrested after selective embolization without further ischemic insult to the liver (c).

related to parenteral nutrition), drug-induced ductopenia, and biliary obstruction or cholangitis (that may not have been detected by preliminary radiologic investigation). The liver biopsy may also be very useful in specific clinical settings (e.g. in bone-marrow transplant recipients) to differentiate veno-occlusive disease from graft-versus-host disease.

The combination of liver dysfunction and ascites suggests either coexisting and often previously undiagnosed chronic liver disease or venous outflow obstruction. Cirrhosis is much more frequent in the ICU patient population than in hospitalized patients in general because of the propensity for these patients to develop organ failure and the higher incidence of trauma in alcohol consumers. The clinical features or ultrasound assessment may provide clues to the presence of cirrhosis, especially the presence of splenomegaly and a small or nodular liver. The presence of a low albumin or prolonged prothrombin time at the time of admission to the ICU also suggests chronic liver disease, but these parameters become abnormal during the ICU stay for many reasons and therefore lose their diagnostic value with time. The nature of the ascites should be examined for diagnostic clues particularly relating to the protein content, culture, white cell count and cytology. Severe ascites should concentrate the investigations on establishing the patency of the hepatic veins and excluding venous outflow obstruction. This assessment will include an echocardiogram to screen for right ventricular dilatation, tricuspid regurgitation, pericardial effusion, and constrictive pericarditis.

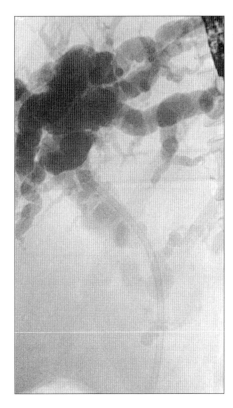

Figure 31.15 Biliary obstruction. The finding of biliary obstruction that is remediable by stent insertion is one of the most effective interventions in the management of hepatobiliary dysfunction in the ICU.

PRACTICE POINT

Illustrative Case

A 34-year-old man was admitted to the ICU following a road traffic accident in which he sustained a head injury, a fractured xiphisternum, rib fractures, and blunt trauma to the upper abdomen. The CT scan of the head revealed a right-sided subdural hematoma; the chest radiograph was normal apart from a pneumothorax; and the CT scan of the abdomen showed a subcapsular hematoma with a linear tear extending through the liver tissue towards the right hepatic vein. The subdural hematoma was evacuated, a chest drain was inserted, and he was commenced on flucloxacillin and gentamycin as antibacterial prophylaxis. Two days later he was commenced on parenteral nutrition.

On the fourth day the AST increased to 156IU/L and the serum bilirubin increased to 41μmol/L (2.4mg/dL). An ultrasound of the liver showed no significant change from the original findings on CT scan and there was no evidence of free fluid within the abdomen. On day 5, he developed a high fever and the antibiotics were changed empirically to ceftazidime and vancomycin. Blood cultures performed during the fever grew *Escherichia coli*. On day 6 the hemoglobin fell by 1.1g/dL to 10.6g/dL, the platelet count fell from the normal range to 90×10⁹/L and the prothrombin time became prolonged by 3 seconds.

By day 10, most of the liver and hematology parameters had become grossly abnormal: hemoglobin 7.9g/dL, white cell count 23.8×10^9/L, platelet count 34×10^9/L, prothrombin time 8 seconds prolonged, serum bilirubin 298μmol/L (17.5mg/dL), AST 324IU/L, alkaline phosphatase 940IU/L, and γ-glutamyltransferase 566IU/L. The ultrasound of the liver showed no major change. A CT scan of the abdomen indicated that the capsule of the liver remained intact, the liver parenchyma adjacent to the tear had an altered perfusion pattern, and a mild degree of bile duct dilatation had developed.

Interpretation

The initial abnormality in the liver function profile was subtle and could have been explained solely on the basis of resorption of the large subcapsular hematoma. The ultrasound was the appropriate investigation at that time and in the absence of a new finding, further intervention was not required. Day 6 saw some changes in the hematology profile that were not singularly impressive but in combination raised the possibility of hemorrhage in association with a low-grade syndrome of disseminated intravascular coagulation.

The multiplicity of change by the tenth day created a difficult clinical problem. There was some evidence to support a wide range of possible diagnoses including sepsis (culture proven), drug reaction (flucloxacillin), parenteral nutrition, regional or generalized hepatic ischemia, biliary obstruction, and cholangitis.

FURTHER READING

Barie PS, Fischer E. Acute acalculous cholecystitis. J Am Coll Surg. 1995;180:232–44. *Good clinical review of this condition.*

Boland G, Lee MJ, Mueller PR. Acute cholecystitis in the intensive care unit. New Horizons. 1993;2:246–60. *Review of a difficult clinical diagnosis to make in the ICU.*

Brienza N, Ayuse T, Robotham JL. Pressure-flow relationships in liver vascular beds during sepsis. In: Vincent JL, ed. Yearbook of intensive care and emergency medicine. Berlin: Springer;1996:321–32. *Broad review of complex topic that is central to the understanding of liver pathophysiology.*

Gibson PR, Dudley FJ. Ischemic hepatitis: clinical features, diagnosis and prognosis. Aust NZ J Med. 1984;14:822–25. *Good clinical description of this condition.*

Hawker F. Liver dysfunction in critical illness. Anaesth Intens Care. 1991;19:165–81. *Excellent review of the subject.*

Herrera JL. Hepatobiliary abnormalities in the critically ill. Curr Opin Crit Care. 1995;1:147–51. *Authoritative review.*

Losser MR, Payen D. Mechanisms of liver damage. Semin Liv Dis. 1996;4:357–67. *Excellent summary of the scope of the problem and the underlying mechanisms.*

Liaudet L, Schaller MD, Feihl F. Selective pharmacological inhibition of inducible nitric oxide synthetase in experimental septic shock. In: Vincent JL, ed. Yearbook of intensive care and emergency medicine. Berlin: Springer; 1998;161–77. *Simply, a very good review.*

Pachter HL, Knudson MM, Esrig B, et al. Status of nonoperative management of blunt hepatic injuries in 1995: a multicenter experience with 404 patients. J Trauma. 1996;40:31–8. *Very extensive clinical experience.*

Pannen BHJ, Bauer M, Noldge-Schomberg GFE, et al. Regulation of hepatic blood flow during resuscitation from haemorrhagic shock: role of nitric oxide and endothelins. Am J Physiol. 1997;272:H2736–45. *Good clinical study that gives important insights into liver bloodflow.*

Quigley EMM, Marsh MN, Shaffer JL, Markin RS. Hepatobiliary complications of total parenteral nutrition. Gastroenterology. 1993;104:286–301. *A very broad study of parenteral nutrition and related problems.*

Tighe D, Moss R, Bennett ED. Cell surface adrenergic receptor stimulation modifies the endothelial response to SIRS. New Horizons. 1996;4:426–42. *Excellent paper incorporating interesting hypotheses.*

Wang P, Chaudry IH. Mechanism of hepatocellular dysfunction during hyperdynamic sepsis. Am J Physiol. 1996;270:R927–38. *Excellent review of topic.*

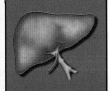

Section 3 Specific Diseases of the Liver

Chapter 32 The Liver in Systemic Disease

Rolland C Dickson

INTRODUCTION

The liver is arguably the most diverse and interactive organ in the body. It receives one quarter of the resting cardiac output, provides major metabolic functions, and is important in detoxification and in the immunologic response. Thus, the liver is potentially vulnerable to a vast array of systemic diseases. In this chapter those systemic diseases that are commonly found to involve the liver will be discussed. The wide variety of diseases affecting the liver attests to the diversity and importance of this remarkable organ. Figure 32.1 lists the systemic disorders that produce significant liver disease.

CIRCULATORY FAILURE

The vascular connections of the liver make it particularly vulnerable to circulatory failure as a result of various causes. In Fig. 32.2 these mechanisms are schematically represented.

Decreased hepatic bloodflow, increased hepatic venous pressure, and arterial hypoxia are the principal factors. Thus, in cases of severe shock, the acute fall in blood pressure can lead to a situation of acute hepatic injury or 'ischemic hepatitis'. Alternatively, constrictive pericarditis causes hepatic venous congestion and a clinical picture similar to the Budd–Chiari syndrome. Most frequently, however, a number of these mechanisms come into play concur-

rently. Thus, in a patient who has chronic heart failure there will be a reduced cardiac output, arterial hypotension, and right and left ventricular failure leading to hepatic venous congestion and hypoxia.

Congestive heart failure
Clinical features
Congestive hepatopathy can occur as a complication of any form of heart disease that produces right ventricular failure. It can either be acquired or congenital, and can occur in the severe acute or chronic setting. Symptoms of congestive heart failure (CHF) such as dyspnea, orthopnea, or paroxysmal nocturnal dyspnea may give clues to a cardiac etiology, but may be absent. Signs of right-sided heart failure, including a cardiac gallop, distended jugular veins, and the hepatojugular reflex, should generally be present. Peripheral edema is common, and ascites when present is usually secondary to the heart failure rather than liver dysfunction. It should be noted that, particularly in an obese patient, findings such as a gallop and jugular venous distension may be subtle; thus, even more vigilance is required when these patients are admitted for evaluation of ascites or hepatic failure. A jaundiced patient who has ascites and hepatomegaly but no stigmata of chronic liver disease such as telangiectasia, palmar erythema, and dilatated superficial abdominal veins should evoke consideration of congestive hepatopathy. Patients almost universally have a large tender liver, although with time and the development of 'cardiac cirrhosis' the liver may decrease to near normal size. Splenomegaly is present in about 20%, but may be seen in up to 80% of those who have cardiac cirrhosis.

Investigations
The laboratory tests that will usually precipitate hepatologic investigation are a moderate elevation of the serum bilirubin and eleva-

Systemic disorders affecting the liver	
Systemic disorder	**Specific disease process**
Circulatory failure	Congestive heart failure Ischemic hepatitis Constrictive pericarditis
Amyloidosis	Hepatic amyloid
Connective tissue disorders	Systemic lupus erythematosis Scleroderma
Granulomatous disease	Sarcoidosis Hepatic granulomas
Endocrine disorders	Hyperthryoidism Hypothyroidism
Lymphoma	Hodgkin's disease Non-Hodgkin's lymphoma
Gastrointestinal disorders	Inflammatory bowel disease Malabsorption syndromes

Figure 32.1 Systemic disorders that affect the liver.

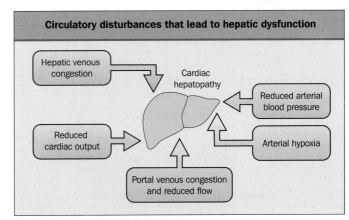

Figure 32.2 Circulatory disturbances that lead to hepatic dysfunction.

tion of the prothrombin time that does not respond to vitamin K. Alkaline phosphatase tends to be normal or minimally elevated, although pronounced elevations have been correlated with very large distended livers. In a patient who has right-sided failure and elevated bilirubin or prothrombin time, a normal alkaline phosphatase would be suggestive of congestive hepatopathy. Transaminases are more unreliable, although they tend to be elevated more often and more dramatically with acute rather than chronic worsening of right-sided failure. No clinical parameter of severity of CHF has been correlated with the degree of transaminase elevation. The aspartate aminotransferase (AST) will usually be greater than the alanine aminotransferase (ALT), but again this is not absolute. A mild elevation of bilirubin can be present with normal transaminases, although with more marked elevations the transaminases are also raised. The ascitic fluid should have a serum ascites–albumin gradient (serum albumin minus ascites albumin) of >1.1, as seen in cirrhotic portal hypertension; however, a high ascites protein (>2.5g/100mL) strongly suggests cardiac rather than cirrhotic portal hypertension. Chest radiograph should reveal cardiomegaly, although pulmonary edema may be absent. Liver biopsy may provide the clue that leads to diagnosis in a previously unsuspected case, but percutaneous biopsy carries the risk of increased bleeding secondary to elevated venous pressure. A summary of the clinical and biochemical findings is shown in Figs 32.3 & 32.4.

Pathologic findings

The histology of congestive hepatopathy is as would be expected from a physiologic standpoint. The elevated right-sided pressure is first transmitted to the central veins leading to dilatation

and engorgement, with dilatation of adjacent sinusoids. The centrilobular (zone 3) hepatocytes become compressed, distorted, and atrophied, with dropout of hepatocytes, granular cytoplasmic changes, and pyknotic fragmented nuclei. This zone 3 damage is exacerbated by the relative hypoxia resulting from a poor cardiac output. With more severe congestion the changes move in the direction of the portal tracts, with the most severe changes closest to the central veins. Necrosis may be accompanied by a brownish pigment in cells, which appears to be related to bile. While the architecture is usually maintained, in cases of prolonged severe congestion bands of fibrous tissue and collapsed reticulin may begin to extend from central vein to central vein. This 'reverse lobulation' constitutes cardiac cirrhosis (Fig. 32.5).

The possible mechanisms for the hepatic pathology in heart failure are shown in Fig. 32.6.

Prognosis

The prognosis of congestive hepatopathy is generally dependent on the underlying cardiac disease. With clinical improvement of right-sided failure the transaminases rapidly return to normal, although the prothrombin time may require 2–3 weeks. Even the rare event of the development of cardiac cirrhosis (present in 4–10% of patients dying of right heart failure) does not appear to worsen the prognosis. Cardiac cirrhosis is not associated with ascites if the right-sided failure is controlled, and varices are rarely present. Encephalopathy may be present but is usually related to decreasing cardiac output, or in the acute setting to hypoglycemia, rather than to hepatic insufficiency.

Ischemic hepatitis

Ischemic hepatitis or shock liver results from anoxic damage to the hepatocytes secondary to acute hepatic circulatory failure. The most commonly described clinical scenario is an 8- to 100-fold AST elevation within 1–3 days of an episode of acute systemic hypotension or clinical signs of left ventricular failure. Sepsis, hemorrhage, trauma, dehydration, heat stroke or burns have also been reported as precipitating events. The serum bilirubin is often increased, but rarely more than four-fold. Alkaline phosphatase is usually less than two-fold. Acute viral hepatitis and drug toxicity are the most common other causes of an acute significant transaminase elevation in this setting. However, a concomitant marked rise in serum lactate dehydrogenase (LDH) and glucose, along with a rapid normalization of these parameters (within 8 days) would strongly suggest ischemic hepatitis. Acute renal insufficiency and altered mental state have also been associated with this condition. The diagnosis should be made on clinical grounds without the need

Clinical features of congestive hepatopathy and hepatic failure		
Clinical features common to both conditions	Features suggestive of congestive hepatopathy	Features suggestive of hepatic failure
Fatigue	Dyspnea	–
Altered Mental Status	Orthopnea	–
Hepatomegaly	Neck venous distension	Spider angiomata
Ascites	Hepatojugular reflex	Palmar erythema
Edema	Cardiac gallop	Caput medusae
Jaundice	Cardiomegaly on radiograph	–
Transaminasemia	–	–

Figure 32.3 A comparison of the clinical features showing the similarities and differences between congestive hepatopathy and hepatic failure due to chronic liver disease.

Liver function test abnormalities in congestive hepatopathy					
Liver test	Abnormal	Right-sided CHF: acute versus chronic	Correlation with clinical or pathologic findings	Improvement with CHF resolution	Normalization with CHF resolution
AST	Common	acute > chronic	Centrilobular necrosis	1 – 3 days	3 – 7 days
ALT	Less common	acute > chronic	Centrilobular necrosis	1 – 3 days	3 – 7 days
Alk phos	Uncommon	acute = chronic	Hepatomegaly	No	No
Bilirubin	Common	acute > chronic	Centrilobular necrosis	1 – 3 days	3 – 7 days
PT	Common	acute = chronic	No	Yes	2 – 3 weeks
Alb	Less common	acute = chronic	No	1 – 2 months	Less common

Figure 32.4 Liver function test abnormalities in congestive hepatopathy. CHF, congestive heart failure; AST, aspartate aminotransferase; ALT, alanine aminotransferase; PT, prothrombin time; Alb, albumin.

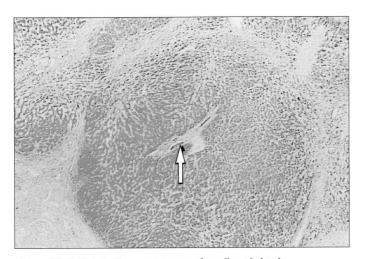

Figure 32.5 Histologic appearances of cardiac cirrhosis.
Regenerative nodules form within the liver, due to fibrous linking of
perivenular areas that come to surround the unaffected portal tract
(arrow). This is associated with atrophy of the zone 3 hepatocytes, and
sinusoidal dilatation, in contrast to regenerative activity in periportal
hepatocytes. (By kind permission of Dr. J. Wyatt.)

of a liver biopsy, which may carry an increased risk of bleeding. The
overall prognosis is almost always dependent on the precipitating
event, but overall the mortality is high, being more than 50%. The
typical bland centrilobular necrosis seen histologically will resolve
without long-term histologic sequelae if there is reversal of the
underlying problem. Treatment is confined to management of the
precipitating event and care should be taken not to cause too aggressive a diuresis, which could exacerbate the hepatic injury. Fulminant
liver failure has been described, but is exceedingly rare.

Constrictive pericarditis

In this condition there is a diffuse thickening of the pericardium
with a consequent restriction in ventricular filling and a rise in
right atrial and vena caval pressures. The clinical features and
hepatic changes are similar to those in the Budd–Chiari syndrome
and there is also confusion with hepatic cirrhosis. All three conditions produce hepatomegaly, and frequently splenomegaly, ascites,
and jaundice in the latter stages. The diagnosis of hepatopathy
due to constrictive pericarditis is made clinically, based on the
presence of a small volume, paradoxic pulse, an increased jugular
venous pressure with a paradoxic rise and characteristic wave form
(prominent 'x' and 'y' descents), and a loud third heart sound. A
chest radiograph may show pericardial calcification, but computed tomography scanning or magnetic resonance imaging, together
with cardiac catheterization, are usually required. Cardiac Doppler
studies may demonstrate abnormalities of ventricular filling.

Treatment is the same as that of the pericarditis. A list of
causes is shown in Fig. 32.7.

If pericardectomy is possible, the prognosis of the liver disease
is good, although recovery is slow. Even the fibrosis of cardiac cirrhosis can partially resolve.

SYSTEMIC AMYLOIDOSIS

Etiology and pathology

Amyloidosis is a disease syndrome that involves the systemic extracellular deposition of an eosinophilic, glassy, hyaline, amorphous

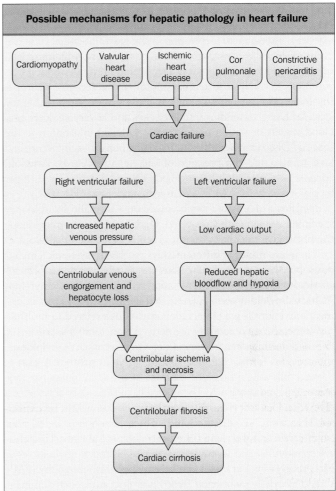

**Figure 32.6 Possible mechanisms for hepatic pathology in heart
failure.** Cardiac failure leads to hepatic congestion and relative ischemia.
The centrilobular areas (zone 3) are affected most, but cardiac cirrhosis
rarely develops.

Causes of constrictive pericarditis	
Infections	Viral Bacterial (including tuberculosis) Toxoplasma Amebic *Histoplasma* Actinomycosis
Other inflammatory	Post cardiotomy Dressler's syndrome
Neoplastic	Primary mesothelioma Secondary – lung, breast, lymphoma
Connective tissue disease	Rheumatoid arthritis, SLE
Chronic renal failure (uremia)	
Physical agents	Trauma, radiotherapy
Idiopathic	

Figure 32.7 Causes of constrictive pericarditis.

material. With sufficient deposition of amyloid, organs such as the liver, kidney, heart and spleen can become enlarged and take on a 'rubbery' appearance. Deposition in the gastrointestinal tract can occur in the submucosa, muscularis, or subserosa, which can lead to malabsorption or ulceration. Deposition in the peripheral nervous system can lead to sensory, motor, and autonomic neuropathy. In hepatic amyloidosis, amyloid fibrils are deposited within the space of Disse, extending into liver cells and in varying degrees in blood vessels or within portal tracts. Amyloid infiltration in the space of Disse may be sufficient to distort hepatic architecture and lead to atrophic compression of the hepatic chords. Amyloid appears as a pale pink homogenous amorphous protein on liver biopsy when stained with hematoxylin and eosin (Fig. 32.8).

Diagnosis of amyloid can be made on a formalin-fixed biopsy specimen stained with Congo red. Under a polarizing microscope the fibrils give the characteristic green refringence of amyloid.

There are multiple different ways to classify systemic amyloidosis, but three major subdivisions are usually described: primary amyloidosis, or light-chain amyloidosis (AL), secondary amyloidosis from amyloid protein A (AA), and familial amyloidosis. In primary amyloidosis, which includes amyloidosis related to multiple myeloma, the amyloid fibrils are derived from a variable portion of the immunoglobulin light chain (κ or λ). In secondary amyloidosis, the amyloid fibrils contain a unique amyloid protein A that is formed following proteolytic cleavage of the acute phase reactant serum amyloid protein A. The etiologies of secondary amyloid are diverse and include rheumatoid arthritis, osteomyelitis, tuberculosis, Hodgkin's disease and other lymphomas, familial Mediterranean fever, long-term heroin abuse, subclinical ankylosing spondylitis, and lepromatous leprosy. Familial amyloidosis is exceedingly rare, but type I familial amyloid polyneuropathy (FAP) should be briefly mentioned. Type I FAP is an autosomal dominant disorder caused by a mutation on chromosome 18 that leads to hepatic production of a variant prealbumen (TTR variant). The disease state is manifested by a progressive mixed chronic polyneuropathy (sensory, motor, and autonomic) that presents after the age of 20 years and is universally fatal. Early recognition is important as liver transplantation has been demonstrated to halt progression and even improve neurologic symptoms.

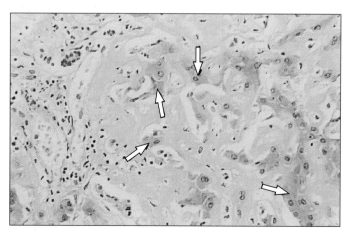

Figure 32.8 Histologic appearances of hepatic amyloidosis. Autopsy specimen of patient with diffuse amyloid infiltration of the liver. Homogeneous pale eosinophilic material fills the sinusoidal space of the liver, resulting in atrophy of the surviving hepatocytes (arrows). An affected tract is to the left side. (By kind permission of Dr. J. Wyatt.)

In AL and AA amyloidosis the fibrils can be differentiated by specific antibody staining, and by the ability of AL fibrils but not of AA fibrils to stain with Congo red despite pretreatment with potassium permanganate. Differences in hepatic deposition patterns are not sufficiently sensitive to be of value. In autopsy series the liver was the third most affected organ (56%) after the spleen (87%) and kidney (81%). However, in series where diagnosis of liver involvement was based on autopsy histology, there was a low incidence of reported clinically significant liver involvement and there were no pathognomonic signs of liver involvement. Hepatomegaly was the most common sign, although it did not reliably differentiate amyloid patients with hepatic involvement from those without.

Clinical features

The best clinical description of hepatic amyloidosis was from a large series of patients who had the premortem diagnosis of primary amyloidosis by liver biopsy. The majority presented between ages 40–80 years old with an approximately equal ratio of men to women. The most common presenting symptoms were bloating, early satiety, or weight loss. The primary physical finding was a palpable liver (90%) from 1–20cm below the costal margin, with approximately 75% having livers 5–14cm below the margin. Splenomegaly (9/80) and a macroglossia (6/80) were the next most common signs. However, hepatomegaly does not always imply hepatic involvement with amyloid. The autopsy series mentioned above have shown that 20% of amyloid patients who have hepatomegaly do not have amyloid deposits, suggesting other etiologies such as congestive hepatopathy. Clinical syndromes in patients diagnosed with hepatic amyloid are listed in Fig. 32.9.

Clinical stigmata of chronic liver disease such as spider angiomata, esophageal varices, or ascites are unusual.

Laboratory findings

The most common laboratory finding in primary amyloid was proteinuria (88%) with nephrotic range proteinuria (median 7.1g/24 hours) in approximately 50%. Liver biochemistry was surprisingly minimally disturbed, even in the presence of hepatomegaly. Alkaline phosphatase was the most commonly elevated test, but was normal in 32% and less than two-fold elevated in 55%. The AST was less than two-fold elevated in 79%, and the serum bilirubin was almost always normal. However, patients with an alkaline phosphatase more than four-fold elevated, an AST level more than two-fold elevated, or a total bilirubin greater than 26μmol/L (1.5mg/dL) all had median survivals of less than 5 months. Thus, in patients who have hepatomegaly and low level liver biochemistry abnormalities, systemic amyloidosis should be considered. Those who have suspected amyloid and a significant disturbance of liver biochemistry may have a poor prognosis. Serum protein studies reveal a globulin spike in up to 50% by immunoelectrophoresis, but this is often missed by protein electrophoresis alone. A monoclonal spike is found in either the serum or urine in up to 70%. Interestingly, 30% have hypogammaglobulinemia, which is rare in chronic liver disease. This may be secondary to urinary globulin loss from the nephrotic syndrome or suppression of normal immunoglobulin synthesis by an abnormal clone of plasma cells. Evidence of hyposplenism, rather than hypersplenism, secondary to massive amyloid deposits in the spleen may be present. This results in thrombocytosis (>500,000/μL) in 30% and Howell–Jolly bodies on the peripheral smear in 62% (secondary to the spleen's inability to 'cull and pit' erythroblast nuclear remnants).

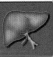

Syndromes in patients diagnosed with primary hepatic amyloid					
	At/before diagnosis of amyloid		After diagnosis of amyloid		Total
Syndrome	Patients % (no.)	Median duration	Patients % (no.)	Median duration	Patients % (no.)
Nephrotic syndrome	28 (22/80)	2 months	9 (7/80)	2 months	36 (29/80)
Congestive heart failure	13 (10/80)	3 months	8 (6/80)	4.5 months	20 (16/80)
Orthostatic hypotension	6 (5/80)	0 months	6 (5/80)	6 months	13 (10/80)
Carpal tunnel syndrome	5 (4/80)	25 months	1 (1/80)	2 months	5 (4/80)
Peripheral neuropathy	5 (4/80)	8.5 months	3 (2/80)	5, 52 months	8 (6/80)

Figure 32.9 Syndromes in patients diagnosed with primary hepatic amyloid. (Adapted from Gertz and Kyle. Am J Med. 1988;85:73–80.)

Diagnosis

Premortem diagnosis of hepatic amyloidosis requires an astute clinician. Listed below are clues to a potential diagnosis in a patient who has hepatomegaly:

- Presence of proteinuria, rare in chronic liver disease;
- monoclonal gammopathy or hypogammaglobulinemia, versus hypergammaglobulinemia in chronic liver disease;
- hyposplenism with elevated platelets or Howell–Jolly bodies versus hypersplenism in end-stage liver disease;
- low-level liver biochemistry abnormalities except in patients who have less than 1-year survival; and
- multisystemic involvement.

Once amyloid is suspected it is usually best diagnosed with biopsy. Rectal, small bowel, skin, and gingival biopsies all have yields of more than 75%. Liver biopsy also has a high yield, but may have an increased risk of hemorrhage due to hepatic fracture. Since documentation of hepatic involvement generally does not affect management, and there is usually other more easily accessible tissue, liver biopsy generally is not required. However, recent series have suggested liver biopsy to be relatively safe in the absence of coagulopathy. Thus, if liver biopsy is to be performed it should be done with careful attempts to correct any underlying coagulopathy (see Fig. 32.8).

Prognosis

The overall survival of patients diagnosed with primary hepatic amyloid is poor. The median survival is less than 1 year, 5-year survival is 13%, and 10-year survival is 1%. Mortality is most commonly secondary to CHF, sudden death (probable arrhythmia), progressive renal insufficiency, or progression of malignancy, rather than portal hypertension or hepatic failure. Thus, clinical evidence of hepatic involvement may be considered evidence of advanced systemic disease.

Treatment

The approach to treatment of systemic amyloid should be as follows:

- supportive care for those organs or tissues with failure secondary to amyloid deposition; and
- recognition and treatment of the underlying conditions in secondary amyloid or myeloma in primary amyloid.

Thus far, management has been primarily limited to supportive care or treatment of underlying conditions as successful approaches for treatment of amyloid itself remain limited. Liver transplantation may be of benefit in the rare patient who has familial amyloid related to the liver.

CONNECTIVE TISSUE DISORDERS

Systemic lupus erythematosus

Transient abnormal liver tests in systemic lupus erythematosus (SLE) are relatively common, but may relate to systemic disease activity rather than to significant hepatic involvement. However, up to 20% of patients who have SLE are found to have significant liver biochemistry abnormalities. The majority have elevations of transaminases and/or alkaline phosphatase in the mild-to-moderate range. These patients are found to have hepatomegaly (39%), splenomegaly (6%), and jaundice (24%) at time of diagnosis of liver disease. In fact the diagnosis of liver disease preceded the diagnosis of SLE by up to 5 years in 27% of patients in one series. In 45% the diagnosis of liver disease occurred within 1 year of diagnosis of SLE and in 28% it was made 1 or more years after the diagnosis of SLE. Patients who had SLE and liver disease differed from those without liver disease by having a higher number of mucosal ulcers (73 versus 18%), more thyroid gland involvement (24 versus 4%), and less arthritis (30 versus 95%). The most common hepatic histologic finding in SLE is steatosis, often not accounted for by steroid use or other risk factors for steatosis. Additional histologic findings without known etiology other than SLE are granulomatous hepatitis, centrolobular necrosis, chronic active and persistent hepatitis (CAH and CPH), and cirrhosis. In one series the cirrhosis described was peculiar, with 3/4 having a cholestasis typified by a canalicular cast (bile cast in bile duct). Secondary histologic findings that have been described have included microabscesses from bacterial infection, hemosiderosis from blood transfusion, primary biliary cirrhosis (PBC), and drug toxicity. Patients who have SLE are especially prone to salicylate toxicity from prolonged high-dose treatment. Salicylate toxicity in this setting has been typified by diffuse hepatocyte injury, with poor definition of the limiting plate, early stellate fibrosis, a plasma cell predominant chronic portal infiltrate, and occasional lymphoid follicles. A more acute injury pattern can also be present with centrilobular ballooning without lobular disarray, scattered acidophilic bodies, and moderate portal inflammation.

It has been clearly shown that SLE is not related to the classic type 1 autoimmune hepatitis (AIH), previously given the misnomer of 'lupoid hepatitis'. Currently, both SLE and AIH have criteria that allow a presumptive diagnosis. Authors have emphasized the importance of differentiating patients who have SLE and liver abnormalities from patients who have AIH. This is because patients who have AIH are thought to have more severe liver disease than patients who have SLE. However, significant liver disease including cirrhosis has been described in SLE. While criteria for treatment and treatment options are currently not well defined for those patients found to have SLE-related liver disease, the majority of patients treated with steroids in one series had an improvement in liver biochemistry. In patients who have persistent liver test abnormalities, however, the diagnosis of SLE should not prevent thorough evaluation, including liver biopsy. Attention should be paid to the medication history, particularly salicylate therapy. Overall, therefore, up to 25% of patients who have SLE will have an abnormality of liver function tests and a relatively minor lesion on liver biopsy. Rarely, however, SLE *per se* does cause serious hepatic disease.

Scleroderma (systemic sclerosis)

Scleroderma is a multisystemic disease characterized by fibrosis of skin, blood vessels, and visceral organs including the heart, lungs, kidneys, and gastrointestinal tract. The two major subsets of scleroderma are diffuse cutaneous scleroderma and limited cutaneous scleroderma. Diffuse cutaneous scleroderma is associated with a rapid development of symmetric skin thickening of the face, trunk, and distal and proximal extremities. This subset is associated with early development of renal and other visceral disease. Limited cutaneous scleroderma is associated with symmetric skin thickening limited to the face and fingers or distal extremities. This subset is frequently accompanied by features of the CREST syndrome (calcinosis cutis, Raynaud's phenomenon, esophageal dysmotility, sclerodactyly, and telangiectasia).

Limited cutaneous scleroderma with the CREST syndrome has been described in association with PBC in 3–17% of cases, with most series in the 3–4% range. Importantly, the age of onset of scleroderma preceded the diagnosis of PBC in the majority of patients by a mean of 12 years (36 years versus 48 years). Raynaud's phenomenon was the most common presenting symptom. The anticentromere antibody is relatively specific for the CREST syndrome. It has been found in the serum of 10–29% of PBC patients but in up to 100% of PBC patients who have CREST. Thus, in patients who have PBC and evolving features of CREST, this may be of benefit in the diagnosis. Up to 90% of patients who have scleroderma and PBC also have evidence of keratoconjunctivitis sicca (Sjogren's syndrome) leading to the proposal of the acronym 'PACK' (PBC, Anticentromere antibody, CREST, and keratoconjunctivitis sicca). Differentiation between diffuse and limited cutaneous scleroderma is important in determining potential adverse outcomes. In diffuse cutaneous scleroderma the major causes of morbidity and mortality are from cardiac, renal, or pulmonary involvement, while in limited cutaneous scleroderma malabsorption and complications of liver disease are the major causes.

GRANULOMATOUS DISEASE

Sarcoidosis

Sarcoidosis is a chronic multisystemic disorder that is characterized by an accumulation of T lymphocytes and macrophages leading to granuloma formation in affected organs. The etiology is unknown, but the disease process is driven by an exaggerated T-helper lymphocyte immune process. Organ dysfunction occurs from distortion of the normal architecture by the inflammatory infiltrate or by development of fibrosis associated with chronic inflammation (Fig. 32.10).

Hepatic involvement with sarcoid

Hepatic involvement is seen in up 60–90% of patients with sarcoidwhen liver biopsy is performed. Biochemically, serum immunoglobulin G is usually raised, bilirubin is normal, and alkaline phosphatase is mildly elevated. The serum angiotensin-converting enzyme is increased. While the vast majority of these patients have asymptomatic hepatic granulomas in the parenchyma and portal tracts, significant liver disease can rarely develop. Hepatomegaly, cholestasis, and the development of portal hypertension have been described. It is important to note that in sarcoid patients the presence of splenomegaly does not always imply portal hypertension, nor does ascites always imply primary hepatic disease. Splenomegaly is most commonly secondary to granulomatous infiltration rather than portal hypertension. Ascites formation can be secondary to right heart failure secondary to pulmonary hypertension, hypoalbuminemia secondary to hepatic dysfunction, or rarely from peritoneal sarcoid granulomas.

Clinical features of portal hypertension

In a literature review, patients who had portal hypertension more commonly had mild extrahepatic disease, had less frequent pulmonary involvement, and had marked constitutional symptoms. Extrahepatic disease in these patients rarely required corticosteroid treatment and was an infrequent cause of morbidity or mortality. Patients who had portal hypertension presented in several different ways. Rarely one group presented first with pruritus and/or jaundice, hepatosplenomegaly, and markedly elevated alkaline phosphatase. Evidence of portal hypertension and hepatic insufficiency occurred later in the course of the disease and was generally associated with cirrhosis or severe portal fibrosis. Antimitochondrial antibodies were positive in over 50% of patients tested, raising the question of a possible overlap with PBC. The second group presented with

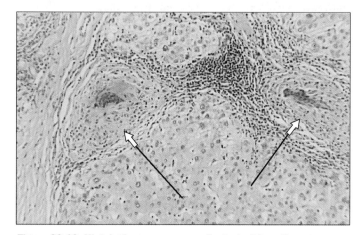

Figure 32.10 Histologic appearances of a typical hepatic granuloma. Granulomas composed of epithelioid macrophages, including some multinucleated giant cells, are seen adjacent to fibrous septa (granulomas indicated by arrows). This is in a patient who has sarcoidosis who has developed cirrhosis. (By kind permission of Dr. J. Wyatt.)

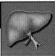

hepatomegaly, gastrointestinal bleeding, or rarely ascites in the absence of clinical manifestations of cholestasis such as jaundice and pruritus. Serum alkaline phosphatase was increased but less marked than in the first group, and transaminases were moderately elevated. In almost all of these patients portal hypertension was the only complication of hepatic sarcoid. A smaller group of patients has been described with a course more typical of a chronic hepatitis with active hepatic inflammation. All developed evidence of liver failure (jaundice, ascites, encephalopathy, or bacterial infection) a few months to several years after onset, with six out of the eight patients reported to have died from complications of liver disease. In these patients another etiology of liver disease such as hepatitis C may need to be entertained, as the series reviewed were all prior to the availability of serologic testing.

Etiology, pathology, and management of portal hypertension

The etiology of the portal hypertension in sarcoidosis has been found to be due to cirrhosis, diffuse nodular hyperplasia, or from presinusoidal portal hypertension. Increasing paucity of bile ducts in association with increasing fibrosis has been described in some patients. The pathogenesis is unclear. Granulomatous phlebitis involving the portal and hepatic venules causing ischemic injury has been described. Progressive fibrosis caused by conversion of granulomas to avascular hyaline fibrosis is a known mechanism of injury in chronic sarcoid and could occur in portal and periportal areas. Both mechanisms could cause a paucity of bile ducts and increase in fibrosis along with distortion and rearrangement of the hepatic architecture. Thrombosis of the main portal vein has also been described but could be secondary to underlying cirrhosis and decreased portal flow. Either way, primary therapeutic options are limited. In a review of the literature, none of 31 patients who had hepatic sarcoid responded to corticosteroid treatment, with severe complications of steroid treatment developing in 50%. Treatment in the past has been relegated to management of the portal hypertension by medical means or surgical shunting. However, in patients who have primary liver disease and no significant extrahepatic disease, liver transplantation should be considered.

Hepatic granulomas
Etiology
Although sarcoidosis is a disease entity typified by widespread granulomatous lesions, granuloma formation in the liver represents a nonspecific reaction to a wide spectrum of noxious stimuli of diverse etiologies. The liver is a prime target for granuloma formation. It has a vast number of reticuloendothial cells, clears a variety of substances from the circulation including microorganisms, and detoxifies and degrades endogenous and exogenous chemical substances. Thus, it is not surprising that hepatic granulomas are common and have been described in 2–15% of liver biopsy specimens. A granuloma has at its core a small collection of modified macrophages or histiocytes called epithelioid cells (see Fig. 32.10). The epithelioid cells are surrounded by a rim of mononuclear cells, which are primarily lymphocytes. Langerhans cells or foreign body type giant cells are often present within the granuloma and are derived from the fusion of epithelioid cells. The key process is the transformation of the macrophage into epithelioid cell. This can be secondary to persistence of a phagocytized substance within the macrophage or a hypersensitivity reaction. Lipogranulomas are to be distinguished from the above. They are generally associated with marked hepatic steatosis that is secondary to diabetes melli-

tus, obesity, malnutrition, and alcohol abuse. They are typified by small fat vacuoles surrounded by granulomas.

The evaluation of hepatic granulomas should proceed in a logical and orderly manner, given the vast array of potential diagnosis. A number of potential causes is listed in Fig. 32.11, although given the nonspecific nature of hepatic granulomas, the list is not complete.

A careful history and physical examination together with review of the liver biopsy are particularly important and can help direct the evaluation. A haphazard approach could amount to an exponential number of unnecessary tests, and a more methodic approach is outlined in Fig. 32.12.

The history may provide pertinent clues to the diagnosis. A careful review of all medications is important and all potential contributing medications should be discontinued. The most commonly associated medications are listed in Fig. 32.11; however, all medications could be considered as potential causes. Significant weight loss may be suggestive of tuberculosis, neoplasm, or inflam-

Etiology of hepatic granulomas	
Primary liver diseases	**Hypersensitivity diseases**
PBC	Erythema nodosum
PSC	Berylliosis
Biliary obstruction	Foreign body (Talc, suture)
Autoimmune hepatitis?	Drug reaction
Granulomatous hepatitis?	Sulfonamide
Hepatitis C virus	Phenylbutazone
Nonspecific reactive hepatitis	Allopurinol
	Quinidine
Infectious	Chlorpropamide
	Halothane
Fungal	Hydralazine
Histoplasmosis	Penicillin
Coccidiomycosis	Chlorpromazine
Others	Oral contraceptives
Aspergillosis	
Actinomycosis	**Hematologic/oncologic**
Candidiasis	
Blastomycosis	Lymphoma
Nocardiosis	Hodgkin's disease
	Idiopathic hypogammaglobulinemia
Viral	
HIV	**Obscure etiology**
Epstein–Barr virus	
Cytomegalovirus	Sarcoidosis
Chicken pox (herpes zoster)	Allergic granulomatosis
	Polymyalgia rheumatica
Parasitic	Psoriasis
Schistosomiasis	Vasculitis
Visceral larva migrans (*Toxocara*	Giant-cell arteritis
canis and cati)	Polyarteritis nodosa
Others	Wegner's granulomatosis
Ascariasis	
Clonorchiasis	**Gastroenterology**
Strongyloidiasis	
	Jejunoileal bypass operation
Protozoan	Inflammatory bowel disease
Amoebiasis	Whipple's disease
Bacterial	
Brucellosis	
Lepromatous leprosy	
Tularemia	
Listeriosis (granulomatosis	
infantisepticum)	
Mycobacteria (typical and atypical)	
Ricettsial	
Coxiella burnetti (Q-fever)	
Spirochetal	
syphilis	

Figure 32.11 Etiology of hepatic granulomas.

matory bowel disease. Headaches and myalgia may suggest arteritis. Occupational history may lead to a consideration of brucellosis (farmers and vets) or chronic beryllium poisoning (electrical and atomic energy industries). Many of the infectious causes of disease can either be considered or excluded depending on geographic location or history of travel. Figure 32.13 offers clues in the diagnosis of the most commonly described infectious causes of hepatic granulomas. The clinical examination may be of value in the assessment for systemic disease, and may provide clues to the primary diagnosis. Often the primary disease process is diagnosed by its other systemic involvement. On other occasions, the hepatic granulomas may be the only clue to a disease process with a variety of nonspecific systemic signs and symptoms.

Granulomatous pathology

The granuloma itself is rarely of diagnostic value with a few exceptions. The presence of acid-fast bacilli in association with extensive caseous necrosis or a positive tuberculous culture are relatively specific, but rarely occur (≤10%). Fungal cultures may reveal *Histoplasma capsulatum* in up to 50% of such cases. *Toxocara* larvae or schistosomiasis ova may be identified within the granuloma. The presence of florid duct lesions can help diagnose PBC. *Coxiella burnetti* (Q-fever) can cause a typical eosinophilic fibrinoid ring with a clear central space that is most likely a fat vac-

uole. While suggestive, this lacks specificity as it has been described in the liver and bone marrow of patients who have Epstein–Barr virus (EBV) or cytomegalovirus (CMV) infection, acute typhoid fever, visceral leishmaniasis, toxoplasmosis, and Hodgkin's disease. Large numbers of eosinophils can suggest drug reactions, parasites, Hodgkin's disease or, in rare instances, sarcoidosis. Granulomas in association with extrahepatic biliary obstruction should be readily identified. These granulomas are associated with bile pigment and necrotic hepatocytes. The bile duct proliferation, cholestasis, and polymorphonucleocyte (PMN) infiltrate should be further factors that suggest the diagnosis.

Diagnosis

The most common causes of hepatic granulomas are sarcoidosis, mycobacteria, medications, or idiopathic, depending on the geographic and referral bias of the series. Sarcoidosis and mycobacterial infections generally account for the majority of patients who have generalized granulomatous disease. Sarcoidosis should be accompanied by other clinical features such as pulmonary infiltrates, uveitis, lymph adenopathy, rash, polyarteritis, elevated erythrocyte sedimentation rate, mild eosinophilia, hypercalciuria ± hypercalcemia (rare), and granulomas in other organs (most commonly lungs, spleen, or lymph nodes). Serum angiotensin-converting enzyme should only be performed if

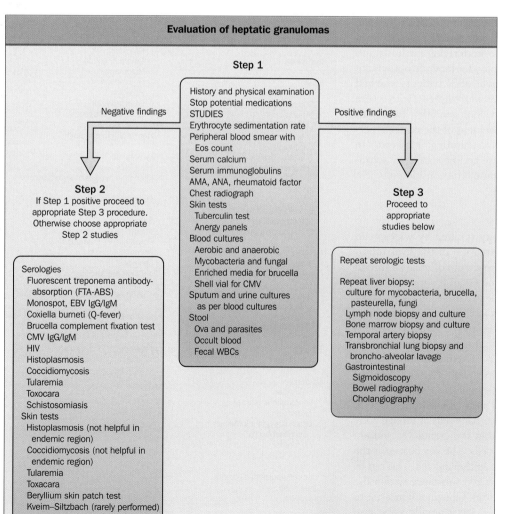

Evaluation of heptatic granulomas

Step 1

History and physical examination
Stop potential medications
STUDIES
Erythrocyte sedimentation rate
Peripheral blood smear with
  Eos count
Serum calcium
Serum immunoglobulins
AMA, ANA, rheumatoid factor
Chest radiograph
Skin tests
  Tuberculin test
  Anergy panels
Blood cultures
  Aerobic and anaerobic
  Mycobacteria and fungal
  Enriched media for brucella
  Shell vial for CMV
Sputum and urine cultures
  as per blood cultures
Stool
  Ova and parasites
  Occult blood
  Fecal WBCs

Negative findings

Positive findings

Step 2
If Step 1 positive proceed to appropriate Step 3 procedure. Otherwise choose appropriate Step 2 studies

Step 3
Proceed to appropriate studies below

Serologies
  Fluorescent treponema antibody-absorption (FTA-ABS)
  Monospot, EBV IgG/IgM
  Coxiella burneti (Q-fever)
  Brucella complement fixation test
  CMV IgG/IgM
  HIV
  Histoplasmosis
  Coccidiomycosis
  Tularemia
  Toxocara
  Schistosomiasis
Skin tests
  Histoplasmosis (not helpful in endemic region)
  Coccidiomycosis (not helpful in endemic region)
  Tularemia
  Toxacara
  Beryllium skin patch test
  Kveim–Siltzbach (rarely performed)

Repeat serologic tests

Repeat liver biopsy:
  culture for mycobacteria, brucella, pasteurella, fungi
Lymph node biopsy and culture
Bone marrow biopsy and culture
Temporal artery biopsy
Transbronchial lung biopsy and broncho-alveolar lavage
Gastrointestinal
  Sigmoidoscopy
  Bowel radiography
  Cholangiography

Figure 32.12 Evaluation of hepatic granulomas. If all studies are negative and patient nontoxic, consider 'test of time'.

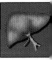

another feature is present as it lacks sufficient positive or negative predictive value to make or exclude the diagnosis. If pulmonary findings are present, bronchoscopy with bronchoalveolar lavage (increased T lymphocytes, primarily helper-inducer), and biopsy would be of benefit. The Kveim–Siltzbach skin test, although having a 70–80% sensitivity and less than 5% false positive rate, is rarely done and is mostly of historic interest.

The diagnosis of idiopathic granulomatous hepatitis as a primary disease should be made with caution. It is typified by hepatic granulomas in association with liver test abnormalities, often

Infection	Location	Risks	Signs	Diagnosis/clues
Fungal				
Histoplasmosis	Central USA to Virginia/Maryland	Exposure to fowl excreta (clean chicken houses, bird roosts) Demolition/construction	Systematic symptoms, nodes, pulmonary	Chest radiograph, serology, cu
Coccidiomycosis	California, Texas, Mexico, Central/South America	Dry weather, dust	Primary pulmonary history of 'valley fever'	Chest radiograph, serology, cu
Aspergillosis	Worldwide	Unfiltered air	Pulmonary, may disseminate	Chest radiograph, peripheral serology, serum immunoglobu tissue invasion
Blastomycosis	North America and rarely Africa, Mexico, Central/South America	Inhalation from decomposed vegetation, rotting wood, soil	Pulmonary/skin, may disseminate	Chest radiograph, culture sm of skin, pus, urine, sputum
Bacterial				
Brucellosis	Worldwide	Farmers, abattoir workers, veterinarians, exposure to infected animal tissue/products	Fever, constitutional symptoms	Culture blood, bone marrow serology
Tularemia	Arkansas, Illinois, Missouri, Texas, Virginia, Tennessee	Hunters, trappers, game wardens, veterinarians, lab workers. Contact with animal/arthropod	History of skin ulcer, fever, adenopathy	White blood cell count, serol
Mycobacteria (M. tuberculosis)	Worldwide	Elderly, urban poor, HIV immunosuppressed	Fever, pulmonary	Culture/smear, chest radiogra skin test
Viral				
HIV	Worldwide	Blood transfusion, high-risk sexual behavior	Opportunistic infection, lymphoma, sarcoma	Serology
Epstein–Barr virus	Worldwide	Salivary contact (kissing)	Mononucleosis	'Monospot', atypical virus, lymphocytosis, serology
Cytomegalovirus	Worldwide	Prolonged intimate exposure, poor hygiene	Heterophil-antibody (–) mononucleosis	Serology, shell vial culture
Chicken pox (varicella-zoster)	Worldwide	Exposure to infected individual	Systemic + rash	Tissue culture, Tzanck smear serology
Ricettsial				
Coxiella burnetti (Q-fever)	North America, elsewhere	Slaughterhouse workers, reservoirs, cattle, sheep, goats, ticks	Fever, hepatitis, hepatomegaly	Serology, biopsy
Parasitic				
Schistosomiasis		Exposure to infested water	Abdominal pain, diarrhea	Stools, rectal biopsy, eosinophilia, serology
S. mansoni	South America, Caribbean, Africa, Middle East			
S. japonicum	Far East (China, Phillipines)			
Visceral larva migrans (Toxocara)	Worldwide	Intimate association with dogs and cats	Fever, tender hepatomegaly	Leukocytosis, eosinophilia, serology (ELISA)
Ascaris lumbricoides	Worldwide	Contaminated soil	Abdominal colic, fever, tender hepatomegaly	Stools, eosinophilia
Strongyloidiasis stercoralis	Tropics, rural southern USA	Contaminated soil, food or drink	Pulmonary or gastrointestinal symptoms	Stools, eosinophilia, serology (ELISA)
Protozoan				
Amebiasis	Worldwide	Poor sanitation	Intermittent diarrhea, cramping, flatulence	Stools, serology

Figure 32.13 Clues to infectious causes of hepatic granulomas. ELISA, enzyme-linked immunosorbent assay.

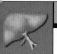

with nonspecific generalized signs (fever, hepatomegaly) and symptoms (malaise, anorexia, weight loss, abdominal pain) after exclusion of all other disease etiologies. The diagnosis often requires a test of time. Series reporting follow-up of these patients have revealed that they fall into several groups.

- Resolution of hepatitis and symptoms without treatment.
- Diagnosis of an uncommon manifestation of sarcoid or infectious etiology often mycobacteria or Q-fever depending on series.
- True idiopathic granulomatous hepatitis. True idiopathic granulomatous hepatitis often has a benign, short-term course and treatment should be undertaken only if persistent or more toxic symptoms are present.

Management

In those who have persistent symptoms with unrevealing repeat biopsies and cultures, there are two basic approaches. Some have advocated a trial of antituberculous therapy because of the difficulty in diagnosing mycobacterial infection. The few patients that still have persistent illness and remain without a diagnosis may have true idiopathic granulomatous hepatitis, and could benefit from immunosuppressive therapy. Others have advocated a trial of indomethacin and if this fails a trial of steroids. Prednisone could be started at 0.75–1.0mg/kg/day and tapered after 3–4 weeks until the fever returns or steroids have been discontinued. If the fever returns the prednisone can be increased if there is no evidence of infection. Generally steroids can then be tapered after several months, although in some cases long-term treatment is required. In a recent series, seven patients who had granulomatous hepatitis were treated with methotrexate (15–20mg per week). All had evidence of symptomatic granulomatous hepatitis for at least 1.5 years (mean 9.4) and had failed steroid therapy due to complications (three patients), no response (three patients), or refusal to undergo treatment (one patient). All patients had a successful response to methotrexate therapy within 3–6 months. The minimal effective dose was 0.2mg/kg per week, and all those on steroids were successfully tapered. Six of six febrile patients defervesced, and four of four patients with follow-up biopsies demonstrated loss of granulomas. Three patients demonstrated stable or decreased inflammation, and one patient demonstrated chronic hepatitis and bridging fibrosis 3 years after discontinuation of methotrexate therapy. Mean duration of methotrexate treatment was 1.3 years with three patients successfully tapered and four patients remaining on maintenance therapy.

Thus, in summary, patients who have granulomatous hepatitis at high risk for mycobacterial infection or with a positive skin test for tuberculosis or unexplained anergy should undergo antituberculous therapy prior to considering immunosuppressive therapy. If symptoms persist or there is nothing to suggest a potential infectious etiology, a trial of corticosteroid therapy should be considered. Methotrexate can be considered in patients who have steroid failure or in patients that are steroid dependent. A trial of methotrexate requires close follow-up, repeat liver biopsies, and an understanding that the data are preliminary and there is potential significant toxicity from methotrexate therapy.

ENDOCRINE DISORDERS

Thyroid disease

Screening for thyroid disease should be an essential component in the evaluation of patients who have abnormal liver tests or who have known liver disease. Abnormal thyroid function has been well-described in association with autoimmune liver diseases such as autoimmune hepatitis and PBC. More recently thyroid disease has been associated with hepatitis C and as a complication of interferon therapy, most commonly in those with antithyroid antibodies prior to treatment. In addition, abnormal thyroid function itself can affect the liver and will be addressed in the following section. Thyroid-stimulating hormone (TSH) and free tetraiodothyronine are thought to be the most reliable thyroid tests in liver disease, given the possible decrease in conversion of tetraiodothyronine to triiodothyronine due to hepatic insufficiency.

Hyperthyroidism

Disturbances of liver biochemistry are seen in 15–76% of hyperthyroid patients. The most common hepatic abnormality is a cholestatic picture with elevation of the alkaline phosphatase and serum bilirubin. Cases of clinical jaundice have been reported to occur in 5.3–50% of published series. Clinically, ascites should not occur in uncomplicated hyperthyroidism and should raise concerns of a concomitant underlying liver disease or CHF. Hepatomegaly, jaundice, and a more markedly elevated prothrombin time are more common in patients who have concomitant CHF. Markedly elevated serum transaminases (>500IU/L) would suggest a search for autoimmune or viral hepatitis. However, even with an unrevealing evaluation, an underlying liver condition cannot be excluded until hyperthyroidism has been successfully treated.

There have been a wide variety of findings reported on liver biopsy in hyperthyroid patients. The most common findings described are fatty change and centrilobular necrosis. Other findings include vacuolization of hepatocytes, balloon degeneration, nuclear glycogen, mild infiltration by mononuclear cells, centrilobular intrahepatocytic cholestasis, and Kupffer cell hyperplasia. The etiology of the cholestasis is unknown. The hypermetabolic state could lead to an increase in oxygen consumption without a concomitant increase in hepatic blood supply. Tissue hypoxia could result in damage to the centrilobular zones leading to dysfunction and cholestasis. A direct toxic effect of thyroxine is also a possibility, as are contributions from other coexisting conditions. Successful treatment and return to the euthyroid state should result in the normalization of the transaminases, bilirubin, and albumin. The alkaline phosphatase may rise during the first 3–5 months of therapy due to a rise in the bone isoenzyme associated with increased osteoblastic activity. Normalization of alkaline phosphatase may take up to 20 months.

Antithyroid therapy itself can also cause liver test abnormalities. Treatment with methimazole or carbimazole can be a rare cause of reversible cholestasis, primarily in women over 50 years of age. Propylthiouracil most commonly causes a mild transient asymptomatic hepatitis. However, severe hepatitis leading to jaundice and even liver failure has been reported. This most commonly occurs in the first few months of therapy in women under 30 years of age. The etiology is thought to be an allergic host reaction. Thus, while propylthiouracil can generally be continued in patients who have low level transaminase abnormalities, they must be followed closely with frequent laboratory testing.

Hypothyroidism

Hypothyroidism affects nearly every organ in the body including the liver. There is decreased hepatic oxygen consumption, and a decrease in bile acid production, bile flow, and bile salt excre-

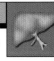

tion. These changes may lead to an increased proportion of conjugated bilirubin, although jaundice in adults is less common than in hyperthyroidism. An increase in serum cholesterol and low-density lipoprotein (LDL) cholesterol may also result. Hypercholesterolemia could contribute to hepatic steatosis or, in a prolonged setting, atherosclerotic disease. There may be an increased risk for gallstone formation due to the decrease in biliary excretion and hypercholesterolemia. An increased peritoneal membrane permeability to protein and mucopolysaccharides and a decreased rate of peritoneal lymph flow may lead to accumulation of a protein rich 'myxedematous' ascites. Pleural and pericardial effusions may also accompany myxedematous ascites. Elevations of AST and lactate dehydrogenase (LDH) from myopathy may occur, which could lead to a misdiagnosis of primary liver disease. Creatine phosphokinase (CPK) should also be elevated with myopathy and may help to make this diagnosis. Alanine aminotransferase may be elevated in hypothyroidism, and so will not help to differentiate between primary thyroid and liver disease. The protein rich ascitic fluid on diagnostic paracentesis should help differentiate myxedematous ascites from that due to portal hypertension. Accurate diagnosis and treatment with thyroid replacement should lead to a reversal of all of the above.

LYMPHOMA

Hodgkin's disease

The liver, as part of the reticuloendothelial system, may be affected by lymphomas. Hepatic histologic abnormalities in Hodgkin's disease are common and have been described in up to 60% of patients. Early in the course of disease the majority of findings are benign and can be transient. In a series of 308 patients with 459 biopsies the following findings were described. Fifty-six per cent of patients had lymphocytic infiltrate in the portobiliary space without histiocytes present. Severe inflammation was rare and findings persisted on repeat biopsies in only 50%. Twenty-four per cent of patients had focal necrosis that was present on repeat biopsy in only 35%. Additional findings included Kupffer cell hyperplasia in 52%, slight increased iron deposition in 23%, moderate-to-severe steatosis in 20%, pleomorphic cell infiltrates in 4%, and epithelioid granulomas in 2%. Thirty per cent of patients had a normal biopsy. Reed–Sternberg cells, which are diagnostic of Hodgkin's disease, were found in only 2.4% of liver biopsies, often associated with abnormal histiocytic cells in a background of lymphocytes, neutrophils, and eosinophils. A similar infiltrate without Reed–Sternberg cells was also found. However, hepatic involvement in Hodgkin's disease has been reported to increase with progression of the disease: 2–5% at diagnosis, 30% during the course of disease, and up to 50% at the time of autopsy. The method of biopsy does not appear to increase the frequency of diagnosis as sequential liver biopsy and peritoneoscopy detected liver involvement with the same frequency as laparotomy. Hepatomegaly occurred in 9% of patients who had stage I–II disease and in approximately 45% who had stage III–IV disease. The majority of patients who had hepatomegaly had an increase in ALT and alkaline phosphatase (23/34), but the elevation was nonspecific for hepatomegaly. In addition, neither increased ALT, alkaline phosphatase, hepatomegaly, splenomegaly, or lymphadenopathy were able to predict Hodgkin's infiltrate in the liver. However, patients with hepatic involvement leading to jaundice had hepatomegaly in 86% of cases.

Non-Hodgkin's lymphoma

In non-Hodgkin's lymphoma (NHL) lymphomatous infiltration of the liver is more common. It has been described in 16–43% of cases, although it is generally not clinically significant. Hepatic involvement is more common with small cell varieties and less frequent with large cell types. It can be associated with abnormal liver tests, primarily an increase in alkaline phosphatase and clinical evidence of hepatomegaly. Rarely NHL can present as a primary hepatic lymphoma. Apart from human immunodeficiency virus-associated lymphomas, primary hepatic lymphomas have a better prognosis due to the ability to obtain a cure with a successful resection. Unlike Hodgkin's disease, laparotomy significantly increases the yield for hepatic involvement over laparoscopy and percutaneous needle biopsy.

Features of hepatic involvement by lymphoma
Jaundice
Jaundice is a relatively rare event in patients who have lymphoma and in the past was considered part of the terminal event. The potential causes of jaundice are listed in Fig. 32.14.

Extrahepatic obstruction is more commonly seen in NHL (1.2%) than in Hodgkin's disease (0.3%), although it is still rare. Biliary obstruction most commonly occurs at the porta hepatitis or intrapancreatic duct given the presence of lymph nodes and decreased mobility of the bile ducts at these sites. Primary lymphomatous involvement of bile ducts has been reported, but is very rare. These causes may be difficult to differentiate from gallstones or pancreatic adenocarcinoma, and may require surgical biopsy. Jaundice in Hodgkin's disease patients is secondary to intrahepatic disease in approximately 40–50% and extrahepatic disease in 3–10%.

Acute liver failure
Rarely malignant infiltration from lymphoma can cause acute liver failure (ALF). Malignant infiltration accounted for 0.44% of all ALF seen at King's College Hospital from 1978 to 1995. Non-Hodgkin's lymphoma accounted for 9/18 and Hodgkin's for 3/18 malignancies in this series. Malignant histiocytosis, acute and chronic leukemias, adenocarcinoma, melanoma, and anaplastic tumors from various primary sites have also been reported as causes. The majority in the King's series presented with hyperacute liver failure (encephalopathy within 7 days of jaundice in the absence of previous liver disease) while the remainder progressed within 28 days.

Etiology of jaundice in lymphoma patients	
Cause	Possible mechanism
Extrahepatic biliary obstruction	Hilar nodes Pancreatic obstruction
Intrahepatic causes	Tumour masses/infiltration including acute liver failure Idiopathic cholestasis
Hemolysis	Autoimmune hemolytic anemia
Treatment-related	High-dose chemotherapy High-dose radiotherapy
Infection	Reactivation of viral hepatitis (B, C etc.) Opportunistic infections, especially in immunocompromised individuals

Figure 32.14 Etiology of jaundice in lymphoma patients.

Prodromal symptoms usually occurred 2–4 weeks (range 5 days to 2 months) prior to onset of liver failure and were nonspecific. The patients had a mean age of 40.7 years (16–73 years) with an equal distribution of males and females. The most common symptoms were malaise (50%), weight loss (39%), right upper quadrant pain (39%), and fever (33%). Significant physical signs included fever in 50%, palpable nodes in 5/9 NHL patients, and all patients had firm palpable livers 2–5 finger breadths below the costal margin, a rare finding with other causes of ALF. Laboratory tests could not separate these patients from other patients who had ALF, although transaminases tended to be less elevated. Patients had a rapid clinical deterioration with death from multiorgan failure in 94% at a median 6 days from admission (range 1–54 days). The one survivor was a patient with NHL who received aggressive chemotherapy despite presenting with palpable hepatosplenomegaly, international normalized ratio 3.9, alkaline phosphatase >1000IU/L, and grade 3 encephalopathy.

Histologic evaluation by needle biopsy or autopsy demonstrated that the malignant infiltration was diffusely spread through the liver parenchyma with large areas of necrosis that was present in both infiltrated and noninfiltrated areas alike. Potential etiologies for ALF include massive hepatic replacement by nonfunctioning malignant cells, malignant cell release of cytokines, hepatotoxicity from Kupffer cell activation, and ischemia from leukocyte and platelet recruitment to hepatic sinusoids. Prompt diagnosis and treatment is the key to a successful outcome. All patients had a prodromal syndrome of at least 2 weeks. The diagnosis can be made from bone marrow or lymph node biopsies. However, the absence of peripheral adenopathy in some patients and the predilection for the liver emphasizes the importance of the liver biopsy in making the diagnosis. It is essential to differentiate these patients from other patients who have nonmalignant causes of ALF. Transplantation in the latter may be life saving, but is contraindicated in the former.

'Idiopathic' intrahepatic cholestasis

Cholestasis has been described in the absence of extrahepatic obstruction or significant tumor infiltration. The majority of the cases had Hodgkin's disease and jaundice was the most common presenting feature. The etiology is unclear, but may represent a paraneoplastic phenomenon or defect in hepatic microsomal function. A recent review of three cases of idiopathic cholestasis in Hodgkin's disease patients discovered a loss of small intrahepatic bile ducts that was not noted on initial assessment. Cholestasis was most pronounced in zone 3 and was not associated with hepatitis. The authors proposed a vanishing bile duct syndrome as the cause in these cases and also in other cases of idiopathic cholestasis. Toxic cytokine release from lymphoma cells was proposed as a mechanism. Jaundice has been shown to resolve with successful treatment of underlying lymphoma in some patients, but persistence in the absence of primary disease in other patients may imply permanent injury from bile duct loss.

Hepatic radiation injury

Radiation-induced hepatitis occurs 1–3 months after radiation therapy. Patients present with ascites, hepatomegaly, and jaundice. Laboratory tests are significant for transaminase, alkaline phosphatase and bilirubin elevation with hypoalbuminemia. Hepatic histology in the first 60 days reveals sinusoidal congestion, hyperemia, hemorrhage, and hepatocyte atrophy. Biopsies after 180 days demonstrate resolution except for atrophy of the central

lobular chords and thickening of the central vein wall. Autopsies of patients who had died demonstrated massive hemorrhage and loss of architecture. Risk of hepatic injury appeared to be dose-related. Whole liver radiation tolerance is thought to be 2400 rad (in 300 rad doses) and up to 3000 if smaller daily doses are used (200 rad). Radiation exposure greater than 3500 rad led to a significant risk for hepatitis, and at 4000 rad there was a 50% risk of death from hepatitis.

GASTROINTESTINAL DISEASES

Hepatobiliary complications of inflammatory bowel disease

The association between inflammatory bowel disease (IBD) and liver disease has been known for over 100 years and the close relationship is well established. Those hepatobiliary disorders associated with IBD include:

- primary sclerosing cholangitis (PSC),
- pericholangitis,
- chronic active hepatitis,
- cirrhosis,
- cholangiocarcinoma,
- hepatocellular carcinoma,
- fatty liver,
- granulomas,
- amyloid,
- gallstones,
- hepatic abscess,
- drug reactions, and
- PBC.

Some of these are rare complications of IBD, but the major hepatobiliary disorders (i.e. pericholangitis, primary sclerosing cholangitis, cholangiocarcinoma) and chronic active hepatitis probably represent a spectrum of one disease process. The prevalence of significant hepatobiliary disease in IBD is approximately 5%.

Primary sclerosing cholangitis

Primary sclerosing cholangitis (PSC) is a chronic cholestatic disease due to obliterative inflammatory fibrosis involving the intra- and extrahepatic biliary system. Approximately 70% of patients who have PSC have ulcerative colitis. The colitis is usually total but relatively asymptomatic. There is a male preponderance (2:1). The progression of the PSC is independent of the course of the colitis. There is an increased risk of cholangiocarcinoma. Primary sclerosing cholangitis is less common in Crohn's disease than in ulcerative colitis.

Pericholangitis

This is traditionally a histologic diagnosis of periductular inflammation and fibrosis in the portal zones of the liver. Large duct sclerosing cholangitis may be present in the majority of cases, but a significant minority only have disease of the small bile ducts as typified by fibrosis of zone 1 ducts on liver biopsy. Both types of lesion may develop cholangiocarcinoma and the distinction between the conditions is somewhat artificial, one merging into the other.

Cholangiocarcinoma

The prevalence of cholangiocarcinoma in IBD is reported at 0.5%, giving a relative risk in patients who have ulcerative colitis of approximately 20 times that of the normal population. The major-

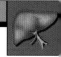

ity of patients have evidence of either PSC or pericholangitis. The development of the carcinoma is somewhat independent of the activity of the colitis, even occurring after colectomy. Clinically the patients present with a progressive cholestatic jaundice. The prognosis is very poor.

Chronic active hepatitis

This may be a difficult diagnosis to make in patients who have IBD, and most patients probably have underlying sclerosing cholangitis. Patients may develop cirrhosis with typical complications. Although probably a result of end-stage PSC, the cirrhosis may result from other viral or nutritional factors.

Hepatobiliary disorders due to malabsorption syndromes

A number of primary bowel disorders cause hepatic dysfunction:
- celiac disease,
- Crohn's disease,
- tropical sprue,
- Whipple's disease,
- cystic fibrosis,
- jejuno-ileal bypass, and
- anorexia nervosa.

There have been few comprehensive studies of hepatobiliary disorders in these diseases but celiac disease and cystic fibrosis are common disorders worthy of comment.

Celiac disease

Abnormalities of liver function are found in up to 40% of patients who have celiac disease. These are elevations of liver enzymes and they almost always resolve on adequate treatment of the celiac disease with a gluten-free diet. The incidence of PBC and PSC in celiac disease is probably greater than expected, although very rare. Gallbladder function is reduced in untreated celiac disease but there is no evidence of an increased incidence of gallstones.

Cystic fibrosis

Up to 20% of patients who have cystic fibrosis develop fatty change and portal fibrosis in the liver, going on to develop biliary cirrhosis. Patients usually have respiratory disease and pancreatic insufficiency before cirrhosis becomes apparent. Its usual presentation is with variceal hemorrhage due to portal hypertension. Liver transplantation, together with lung transplantation, has been successful in such patients.

PRACTICE POINT

Illustrative case

A 45-year-old woman was admitted with a productive cough, pleuritic chest pain and a fever. She had a long history of recurrent chest infections between the ages of 15 and 25 years when she had been diagnosed as having common varied immunodeficiency (CVID). Since that time she had been relatively well with regular intravenous immunoglobulin G every 4 weeks.

On examination she was febrile, and she had signs of consolidation in the left base and coarse crepitations on the right. There was hepatosplenomegaly but no signs of chronic liver disease or peripheral lymphadenopathy. Her initial investigations revealed a mild normochromic anemia, a moderate neutrophil leukocytosis, and mild thrombocytopenia. Albumin was 30g/L (3g/dL), bilirubin 40μmol/L (2.4mg/dL), ALT 60U/L, and alkaline phosphatase 600U/L. Chest radiograph showed a left basal pneumonia and chronic changes of bronchiectasis in the right base.

She was treated with broad-spectrum antibiotics, additional intravenous immunoglobulin G, and her chest symptoms resolved. However, she failed to improve clinically with generalized weakness and a continuing fever. Her liver function tests remained abnormal with a rising level of alkaline phosphatase. Her condition was static for 3–4 weeks and causes for her continuing fever were sought. The acute findings on her chest radiograph resolved. There was no hilar lymphadenopathy. Multiple cultures were negative, as was serology for HBV and hepatitis C virus (HCV). An abdominal ultrasound showed an enlarged liver with coarse echotexture, but no focal lesion and a normal biliary system. There was splenomegaly and normal vascular flow in the hepatic and portal systems. Computed tomography scans did not reveal any other abnormalities nor any thoracic or abdominal

lymphadenopathy. Serum angiotensin-converting enzyme (ACE) level was elevated at 120U/L (normal 5–35) and the alkaline phosphatase continued to rise, but otherwise the liver function tests were relatively unchanged.

A liver biopsy showed mild chronic hepatitis with scattered noncaseating granulomas. Culture was negative, particularly for tubercle bacilli. She was eventually treated with oral steroids, and within 2 days her fever began to resolve. Over the ensuing 2–3 weeks the serum ACE level returned to normal levels and the alkaline phosphatase returned to almost normal.

Interpretation

This patient who has CVID presented with pneumonia (which was adequately treated) on a background of chronic lung damage. She had several reasons for hepatic granulomas and a prolonged fever. Patients who have CVID can develop chronic hepatitis associated with HBV or HCV. Such patients are also prime candidates to develop chronic bacterial infections (e.g. tuberculosis). The findings of a raised ACE and alkaline phosphatase raise the possibility of sarcoidosis, although such enzymes can be raised in other causes of hepatic granulomas. Patients who have CVID can also develop a chronic granulomatous hepatitis of no etiology.

In this patient no evidence was found for tuberculosis or sarcoidosis. The patient did not have chronic HBV or HCV liver disease and other infective causes of granulomatous hepatitis were excluded. There was no evidence of complications of CVID such as abdominal carcinoma or lymphoma, or of other causes of chronic liver disease. It was concluded that this patient had granulomatous hepatitis in the context of CVID, which was responsive to steroids.

FURTHER READING

Bayraktar M, Van Thiel DH. Abnormalities in measures of liver function and injury in thyroid disorders. Hepatogastroenterology. 1997;44:1614–18. *Best overall review on the effect of thyroid function alteration on the liver.*

Birrer MJ, Young RC. Differential diagnosis of jaundice in lymphoma patients. Semin Liver Dis. 1987;7:269–7. *A well organized systematic review of the different etiologies of jaundice in lymphoma patients.*

Brinckmeyter LM, Skovsgaard T, Thiede T, Vestergager L, Nissen NI. The liver in Hodgkin's disease – I. Clinicopathologic relations. Eur J Cancer Clin Oncol. 1982;18:421–6. *A retrospective review of the clinical and pathologic findings on 308 patients presenting with unstaged Hodgkin's disease.*

Dunn GD, Hayes P, Breen KJ, Schenker S. The liver in congestive heart failure: a review. Am J Med Sci. 1973;265:174–89. *The best overall review on the liver in congestive heart failure.*

Gertz MA, Kyle RA. Hepatic amyloidosis (AL), immunoglobulin light chain: The natural history in 80 patients. Am J Med. 1988;85:73–80. *Review of the clinical and laboratory features of 80 patients with a premortem diagnosis of hepatic amyloid along with a complete discussion on the topic. Most comprehensive article available on the subject.*

Gibson PR, Dudley FJ. Ischemic hepatitis?: clinical features, diagnosis and prognosis. Aust NZ J Med. 1984;14:822–5. *Reviews the clinical and laboratory features of ischemic hepatitis in 19 patients.*

Gitlin N, Seriio KM. Ischemic hepatitis: widening horizons. Am J Gastroenterol. 1992;87:831–836. *Retrospective analysis of nine patients with ischemic hepatitis and includes an excellent review of the topic.*

Hubscher SG, Lumley MA, Elias E. Vanishing bile duct syndrome: A possible mechanism for intrahepatic cholestasis in Hodgkin's lymphoma. Hepatology. 1993;17:70–77. *This paper proposes vanishing bile duct syndrome as a new potential mechanism of cholestasis in Hodgkin's disease, and adds Hodgkin's disease as a potentially new cause of vanishing bile duct syndrome. Three cases are presented and the potential mechanisms of vanishing bile duct syndrome development are discussed.*

Irani SK, Dobbins WO. Hepatic granulomas: A review of 73 patients from one hospital and a review of the literature. J Clin Gastroenterol. 1979;1:131–43. *Retrospective review of 73 cases of hepatic granulomas with a review of the literature.*

Jaffe ES. Malignant lymphomas: pathology of hepatic involvement. Semin Liver Dis. 1987;7:257–68. *Clinical and pathologic review of the different malignant lymphomas involving the liver.*

Knox TA, Kaplan MM, Gelfand JA, Wolff SM. Methotrexate treatment of idiopathic granulomatous hepatitis. Ann Intern Med. 1995;122:592–5. *Reports the successful use of methotrexate for patients who have idiopathic granulomatous hepatitis and suggests a treatment algorithm for these patients.*

Kushimoto K, Nagawawa K, Ueda A, et al. Liver abnormalities and liver membrane autoantibodies in systemic lupus erythematosus. Ann Rheum Dis. 1989;48:946–52. *Presents data suggesting liver test abnormalities in lupus patients are related to overall disease activity rather than significant underlying liver disease.*

Levine RA. Amyloid disease of the liver. Correlation of clinical, functional and morphologic features in forty-seven patients. Am J Med 1962;33:349–57. *Autopsy series of 47 patients with a review of the clinical and pathologic features of patients with hepatic amyloid.*

Mills PR, Russell RI. Diagnosis of hepatic granulomatous: a review. J Roy Soc Med 1983;76:393–7. *Provides a table with an extensive differential for hepatic granulomas and a table for useful investigations. In addition there is a short review on idiopathic hepatic granulomas.*

Moreno-Merlo F, Wanless IR, Shimamatsu K, Sherman M, Greig P, Chaisson D. The role of granulomatous phlebitis and thrombosis in the pathogenesis of cirrhosis and portal hypertension in sarcoidosis. Hepatology. 1997;26:554–60. *Proposes a novel mechanism for development of portal hypertension in sarcoidosis patients.*

Parrilla P, Ramirez P, Bueno RS, et al. Clinical improvement after liver transplantation for type I familial amyloid polyneuropathy. Br J Surg. 1995;82:825–8. *Long-term results of 13 patients transplanted for type I amyloid polyneuropathy.*

Perrett AD, Higgins G. Johnson HH, Massarella GR, Truelove SC, Wright R. The liver in Crohn's disease: the liver in ulcerative colitis. Quart J Med. 1971;40:187–238. *Two early studies describing the hepatic abnormalities in IBD. Hepatic histologic abnormalities were found in up to 20% of cases of IBD.*

Powell FC, Schroeter AL, Dickson ER. Primary biliary cirrhosis and the CREST syndrome: A report of 22 cases. Quart J Med. 1987;237:75–82. *Provides strong evidence for an association of PBC and CREST syndrome, and includes a thorough discussion of the syndrome.*

Richman SM, Delman AJ, Grob D. Alterations in indices of liver function in congestive heart failure with particular reference to serum enzymes. Am J Med. 1961;Febuary:211–25. *Best data available regarding liver test abnormalities in congestive heart failure.*

Rowbotham D, Wendon J, Williams R. Acute liver failure secondary to hepatic infiltration: a single center experience of 18 cases. Gut. 1998;42:576–80. *A complete description and discussion of the clinical patterns and diagnostic factors of acute liver failure secondary to malignant infiltration.*

Runyan BA, LeBrecque DR, Anuras S. The spectrum of liver disease in systemic lupus erythematosis. Report of 33 histologically-proved cases and review of the literature. Am J Med. 1980;69:187–94. *A thorough review of liver disease in patients who have SLE.*

Seaman WE, Ishak KG, Plotz PH. Aspirin-induced hepatoxicity in patients with systemic lupus erythematosus. Ann Intern Med. 1974;80:1. *Most widely referenced paper on aspirin-induced hepatotoxicity in lupus patients.*

Skovsgaard T, Brinckmeyter LM, Vestergager L, Thiede T, Nissen NI. The liver in Hodgkin's disease-II. Histopathologic relations. Eur J Cancer Clin Oncol. 1982;18:429–35. Companion article to that by Brinckmeyter et al. (1982). *This article reviews the histopathologic findings in 459 liver biopsies performed on the 308 patients with Hodgkin's disease described in the first paper.*

Valla D, Pessegueiro-Miranda H, Degott C, Lebrec D, Rueff B, Benhamou JP. Hepatic sarcoid with portal hypertension. A report of seven cases and a review of the literature. Quart J Med. 1987;242:531–7. *Describes clinical syndromes associated with portal hypertension in patients who have hepatic sarcoidosis and speculates on the mechanisms.*

Volta U, Franceschi LD, Lari F, Molinaro N, Zoli M, Bianchi FB. Coeliac disease hidden by cryptogenic hypertransaminase Lancet. 1998;352:26–9. *A useful summary of hepatic transaminase levels in celiac disease.*

Zoutman DE, Ralph ED, Frei JV. Granulomatous hepatitis and fever of unknown origin. An 11-year experience of 23 cases with three years' follow-up. J Clin Gastroenterol. 1991;13:69–75. *A comprehensive paper describing the clinical course of patients who have idiopathic granulomatous hepatitis.*

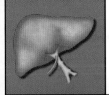

Chapter 33 Non-transplant Surgery and the Liver

J Michael Henderson and David Vogt

INTRODUCTION

As early as 2000–3000 BC, the Assyrian and Babylonian cultures used the livers of sacrificed animals to divine the future. Over the ensuing centuries, battle surgeons debrided small bits of liver protruding from abdominal wall stab and gunshot wounds. However, formal entry into the peritoneal cavity to control hemorrhage due to trauma or to remove tumors and drain cysts had to await the development of general anesthesia and antisepsis.

A burst of early activity occurred between 1880 and 1910. The first successful liver resection was performed in Berlin by Dr Carl von Langenbuch in 1887. He removed a pediceled tumor from the left lobe of a 30-year-old woman. Later that evening, however, the patient required re-exploration to control hemorrhage. Dr William Keen is credited with the first liver resection performed in the USA when in 1892 he removed a pediceled cystadenoma from the right lobe of a young woman. After this flurry of pioneering activity, little progress was made until after the Second World War.

Liver surgery entered the modern era in the 1950s, and remarkable progress has occurred over the past 40 years. The factors responsible for the progress include an understanding of the segmental anatomy of the liver as described by Couinoud in 1954, advances in the techniques of liver resection, a better understanding of liver diseases, the dramatic improvements in techniques to image the liver, and the ability to support patients metabolically both intraoperatively and postoperatively.

LIVER TRAUMA

Many advances have been made in the past century in the management of liver trauma, particularly severe injuries. The role of radiographic modalities such as CT scanning and ultrasonography have become much more prominent both in the assessment and in the treatment of liver injuries. Angiographic embolization is the therapy of choice in selected patients with hemobilia as a result of trauma. The current trends in the evaluation and management of liver trauma include CT staging of the injury, nonoperative management (NOM) in stable patients, temporary packing to control bleeding, and the technique of mesh hepatorrhaphy. Hemorrhage and infection continue to be the major lethal consequences associated with liver trauma.

Nature of the injury
The liver is partially protected from injury by the overlying ribs of the lower chest. Yet, as the largest solid organ in the abdomen, the liver is particularly vulnerable to the ability of compressive

blows to rupture the relatively thin capsule. It is, therefore, not surprising that 45% of patients who suffer blunt abdominal trauma and 40% of those injured by penetrating trauma sustain a liver injury. The current grading of liver injuries as defined by the American Association for the Surgery of Trauma has been outlined in Chapter 31. Injuries of grade III and higher are considered severe.

Diagnostic issues
The appropriate evaluation and management of liver injury results from an organized approach to abdominal trauma. The patient's physiologic status determines the most effective treatment; that is, hemodynamically unstable patients require immediate operative intervention. Stable patients can be evaluated more thoroughly using imaging techniques, and perhaps observed and managed nonoperatively.

For several years, diagnostic peritoneal lavage (DPL) has been the 'gold standard' in assessing patients with blunt abdominal trauma, particularly in conjunction with a head injury. This method is also very sensitive in the detection of liver trauma, with a false-negative and false-positive incidences of 1.2 and 0.2%, respectively. More recently, CT scanning has become the preferred method in many centers to evaluate a patient who has sustained blunt abdominal trauma. The CT scan is useful in delineating the nature and severity of the liver injury. However, the accuracy of CT scanning in assessing the grade of liver injury has been challenged. A recent study observed only a 16% correlation when the CT staging was compared with the operative findings. The scans both overestimated and underestimated the degree of injury. An associated injury, particularly a gastrointestinal perforation, may not be apparent on a CT scan.

Management
The current trend in liver trauma is NOM, even in selected patients with severe (grade III or higher) injuries. The evolution of NOM for isolated liver trauma began in pediatric patients. The lessons learned and the guidelines that developed in the NOM of splenic injuries in the pediatric population were applied to liver trauma. The successful experience in the pediatric patients was then cautiously extended to adult patients. Currently, approximately 24–55% of adults with blunt liver injuries are managed nonoperatively. Figures 33.1 & 33.2 show the marked decrease in size of a subcapsular hematoma over the course of several weeks in a teenage boy who sustained an injury while playing soccer. The two major reasons for this transition to NOM include the shift to CT scanning rather than DPL in evaluating trauma patients, and the comfort that

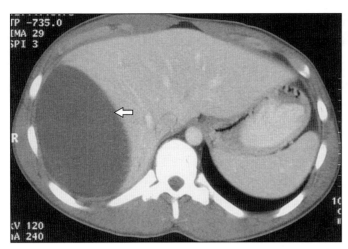

Figure 33.1 Liver trauma. A CT scan demonstrating a subcapsular hematoma (arrow) of the liver caused by a soccer injury in a teenage boy. The injury was treated nonoperatively because of clinical stability.

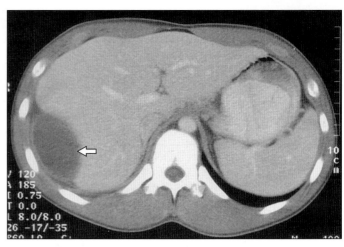

Figure 33.2 Liver trauma after nonoperative management (NOM). A repeat CT scan performed several weeks later in the same patient as shown in Fig. 33.1; the hematoma (arrow) is significantly smaller.

has accumulated with the nonoperative approach. The criteria for NOM of liver trauma include hemodynamic stability, absence of associated injuries, availability of intensive care unit monitoring, 24-hour operating room availability, and a normal neurologic examination.

Hemodynamically unstable patients or those with associated injuries require immediate operative intervention. The two major goals of surgery are to control hemorrhage and prevent infection. The hemorrhage associated with liver injuries can be massive, and is the most frequent cause of death. Injuries that are no longer bleeding at the time of laparotomy require no treatment. External drainage may be indicated if there is evidence of a bile leak.

The initial efforts to control bleeding usually begin with a 'Pringle' maneuver, which consists of temporarily occluding the hepatic artery and portal vein in the hepatoduodenal ligament. The maneuver can be performed by either digital compression, or, by means of a noncrushing vascular clamp. This temporary occlusion can be applied safely for up to an hour in a stable patient with normal liver parenchyma. However, since the most troublesome bleeding associated with liver injuries is venous, the 'Pringle' maneuver is often relatively ineffective. Therefore, the liver wound must be explored, debrided, and individual vessels ligated while the inflow has been controlled (Fig. 33.3). The area is then drained externally.

Bleeding that persists can be managed by a major resection, temporary packing, or mesh hepatorrhaphy. A major liver resection is performed in less than 5% of patients, and is reserved as the last option because of a mortality rate of approximately 50% and the complications of hemobilia, secondary hemorrhage, and intrahepatic cavitation. Temporary packing fell into disfavor when it was first introduced during the Second World War because of the resultant sepsis and secondary bleeding. Currently, however, temporary packing is enjoying a re-emergence because of better results. The packing is performed in a perihepatic, rather than an intrahepatic fashion (Fig. 33.4). The rationale is to provide adequate compression to control hemorrhage in an expedient manner, particularly in a hypothermic and acidotic patient. The packs are then removed 48 hours

later after further resuscitation, with some risk of recurrent bleeding. A liver injury that is severe enough to require packing to control hemorrhage carries a 30% mortality.

The results with mesh hepatorrhaphy were first reported in the early 1990s. This technique uses absorbable mesh to sufficiently compress the parenchyma to control hemorrhage without causing ischemic injury. The 'Pita Pocket' technique is best suited to injuries that involve the major portion of an anatomic lobe, such as a large stellate lesion (Fig. 33.5). Unlike packing, mesh hepatorrhaphy does not require a second laparotomy to remove the mesh, and there is less pulmonary compromise because of less intra-abdominal pressure. However, the technique cannot be performed quickly and therefore may not be the best approach in a cold, coagulopathic patient. The associated mortality is similar to packing, about 30–40%.

Retrohepatic vena cava and hepatic vein injuries can still thwart surgical efforts to control hemorrhage. Even the results of using shunts introduced into the right atrium, as described by Schrock, are disappointing. Total vascular exclusion (TVE) in conjunction with a venovenous bypass, as is used in liver transplantation, is another technique that may have some promise; it is a technique of occluding the vena cava both above and below the liver in addition to controlling the hepatic artery and portal vein. However, there is currently little experience with this option in the trauma setting. Recently, good results have been reported with perihepatic packing even with this particularly severe injury. The mortality rate reported with these challenging injuries approaches 80%.

PYOGENIC ABSCESS

Liver abscesses remain a significant problem and are responsible for 13–20 per 100,000 hospital admissions annually with an associated mortality of up to 30%. Over the past 20 years, several trends have emerged. The major source of liver abscesses is now the biliary tree rather than pyelophlebitis. Approximately 50% of patients have a malignancy, 80% of which are hepatobiliary. More patients, particularly those who are immunosuppressed either because of transplantation or

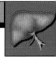

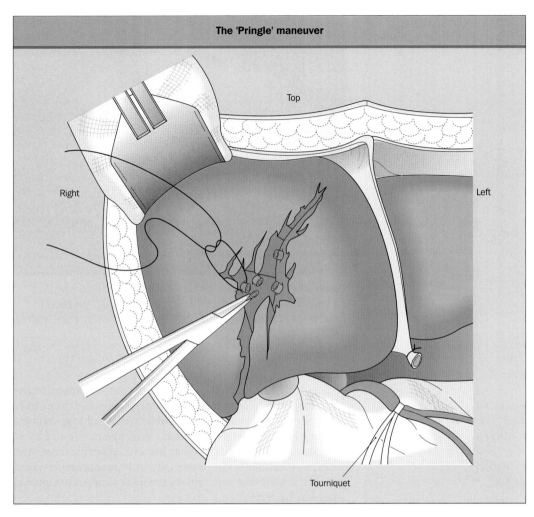

Figure 33.3 The 'Pringle' maneuver. A large, deep laceration in the right lobe of the liver which requires control of individual vessels to arrest bleeding. The tourniquet is occluding the vascular inflow (hepatic artery and portal vein); the 'Pringle' maneuver.

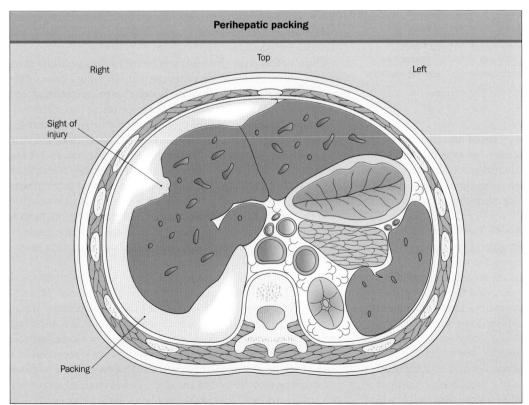

Figure 33.4 Perihepatic packing. An axial view of perihepatic packing to control hemorrhage.

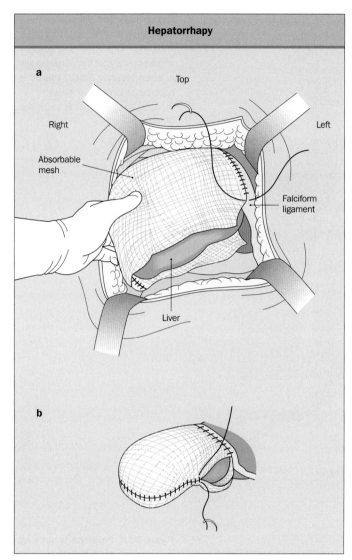

Hepatorrhapy

a

Top

Right

Left

Absorbable
mesh

Falciform
ligament

Liver

b

Figure 33.5 Hepatorrhapy. Performing a hepatorrhapy to control
bleeding from a major injury to the right lobe. (a) Demonstration of how
the absorbable mesh is anchored to the retroperitoneum and the falciform
ligament. (b) Almost complete wrapping is shown.

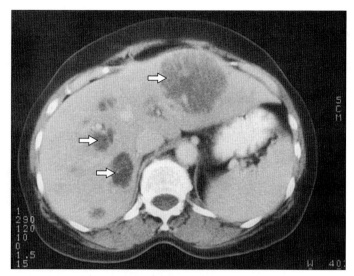

Figure 33.6 Liver abscess. An axial image from a CT scan that
demonstrates multiple septated liver abscesses (arrows). This patient
required operative drainage because of the loculated nature of the lesions.

intense therapy for malignancy, have mixed bacterial and fungal
abscesses. Up to 50% of liver abscesses can now be successfully drained nonoperatively with catheters placed by CT or ultrasound. The mortality associated with liver abscesses has
decreased from 65 to 30%. The biggest decline has occurred in
patients with multiple lesions.

The clinical features associated with liver abscesses have not
changed appreciably over the past several years. Fever (90%),
pain (50%), and weight loss (50%) are the major symptoms; an
enlarged, tender liver and jaundice are present in approximately 50% of patients. Leukocytosis is found in 80% of patients;
hyperbilirubinemia and hypoalbuminemia are also frequently
seen. At least half of the patients with a liver abscess have a positive blood culture.

Since the symptoms, physical findings, and laboratory studies
are nonspecific, a high index of suspicion and imaging studies
are the key to making the diagnosis of a liver abscess. Computed
tomography is 93% accurate in confirming the presence of a liver

abscess (Fig. 33.6). Although *Escherichia coli* and *Streptococcus*
spp. remain the most frequent bacteria cultured from liver
abscesses, *Pseudomonas* spp., probably because of long-term indwelling biliary stents, are increasing in incidence. Up to 25% of
abscesses contain fungi as well as bacteria, generally associated
with prior antibiotic use, especially in immunocompromised
patients. *Bacteroides* spp. remain the most frequently cultured
anaerobic bacteria.

Obstruction of the biliary tree, particularly in patients with
malignancy, is currently the most frequent cause of a liver abscess.
Other etiologies include hepatic metastases, diverticulitis, hepatic necrosis and infection as a result of chemoembolization, and
bacterial endocarditis.

Over 50% of liver abscesses can be treated successfully nonoperatively by drainage via a catheter placed under either ultrasound or CT guidance. Drainage is superior to aspiration alone,
which is associated with a 37% recurrence rate.

Surgery and percutaneous drainage should be viewed as complementary, and not competitive means to treat liver abscesses. Surgical drainage is reserved for those cases where
percutaneous drainage fails, or may not be possible because of
the location of the abscess (dome of the liver) and the possibility of pleural cavity contamination. Other indications for
surgery include the presence of infarcted hepatic tissue which
requires debridement, or the source of the abscess requires
concomitant surgical treatment, such as a sigmoid colon resection for diverticulitis.

Surgical drainage is best accomplished by a transabdominal
approach. The procedure tends to be bloody because of the associated inflammatory condition of the liver. Intraoperative ultrasound may be necessary to locate the abscess, which is unroofed
and gently debrided. A drain, either a penrose or closed-suction
type, is left in place for several days. A CT scan is repeated in a
week to 10 days to assess the size of the abscess cavity. The drain
can safely be removed when the drainage has stopped and either
an ultrasound or CT scan has confirmed that the cavity has

resolved. If the drainage persists or becomes bilious, a contrast study through the drain is necessary in an effort to document a communication with the biliary tree. If a biliary fistula is present, an endoscopic sphincterotomy, with or without the placement of a stent, often results in more rapid healing by lowering the pressure in the biliary tree.

Although the mortality associated with liver abscesses has declined significantly over the past 20 years, it remains at about 30%. Factors predictive of a poor outcome include multiple abscesses, malignancy, malnutrition, abnormal liver function, leukocytosis, sepsis, fungus, advanced age, and polymicrobial infections.

CYSTIC DISEASE

Simple, benign cysts of the liver occur in about 5% of the general population; however, only 5% of these patients become symptomatic. Although most patients have a solitary cyst, some patients may have several simple cysts. The pathogenesis of these presumed congenital, slow growing cysts is not clearly defined, but congenital lymphatic obstruction and faulty bile duct development are the two leading proposed mechanisms. The right lobe is most frequent site of these lesions, which are lined by cuboidal epithelium and most often contain clear liquid. Occasionally, they may contain bloody, milky, or bile-stained fluid.

While most simple cysts are asymptomatic, when symptoms occur, they do so because of the very large the size of the cyst, or hemorrhage into it, which occurs in 2% of patients with simple cysts. Physical examination may reveal a soft upper abdominal mass; a tender mass may be appreciated if hemorrhage has occurred. Liver function tests are generally normal. Ultrasound and CT reveal a homogenous cystic lesion(s) (see Chapter 24).

Treatment is required only if the cyst is symptomatic or if the diagnosis is uncertain. Percutaneous aspiration alone results in prompt recurrence of the cyst. Placement of a percutaneous catheter may also result in infection of the cavity. Removing as much of the cyst wall as possible is the surgical procedure of choice. More recently, excellent results have been obtained by excising the cyst wall laparoscopically (Fig. 33.7).

Complete excision or a liver resection is not necessary and may be hazardous because of bleeding. Any fluid that is produced by the remaining cyst wall is reabsorbed by the peritoneum. If the cyst is infected, external drainage is necessary. A cyst that contains bile must communicate with the biliary tree. Formerly, the recommendation was to sew a Roux limb to the cyst. However, the sterile cyst was then converted to an abscess. The current approach is to identify the communication with the bile duct by performing an intraoperative cholangiogram and then closing the fistula by suturing. The morbidity and mortality associated with procedures to treat simple liver cysts is extremely low and the long-term prognosis is excellent.

Polycystic liver disease

Adult polycystic liver disease (APLD) is inherited as an autosomal dominant and occurs in 0.6% of the population. Of patients with APLD, 50% have polycystic kidney disease as well. The pancreas is infrequently cystic. The disease has been classified into three types, depending on the extent of cystic involvement.

The clinical manifestations of APLD are related to the massive size of the cystic liver. Abdominal distention, discomfort, early satiety, supine dyspnea, leg edema from compression of the vena cava, and hepatomegaly are the major symptoms and findings. Less frequent complications include portal hypertension and biliary obstruction. In spite of the massive cystic changes, the

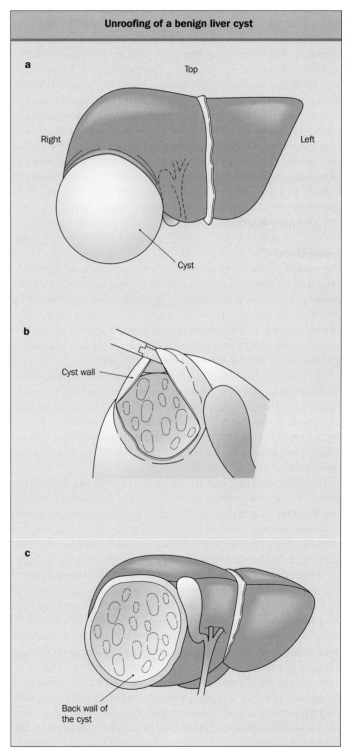

Figure 33.7 Unroofing of a benign liver cyst. (a) A cyst in the right lobe. (b) The lesion is being partially excised laparoscopically; the same procedure could be performed open. (c) Final appearance after much of the cyst wall has been excised.

liver maintains its functional capability; these patients do not progress to liver failure. Computed tomography is the most helpful imaging study.

Therapy for APLD is reserved for patients who have severe symptoms that are significantly affecting their quality of life. The goal of surgical therapy is to reduce the bulk of the cystic liver. Two surgical approaches that have resulted in some success include resection of the most involved portion of the liver, and extensive fenestration or unroofing of as many cysts as possible. A recent review of 46 patients from eight series reported that combining resection and fenestration resulted in 82% of the patients becoming symptom free. The associated morbidity and mortality were 33 and 4.3%, respectively. Some authors have reported progression of the cysts in the unresected portion of parenchyma over the next several years. Liver transplantation has been successfully performed in a small number of patients. However, the technical difficulty of performing the transplant is much greater in a patient who has previously had a resection and/or fenestration. A combined kidney and liver transplant has been advocated for patients with both APLD and polycystic kidney disease in whom renal failure seems eminent.

Hydatid cysts

Although hydatid cysts of the liver are uncommon in the USA, they are endemic in South America, New Zealand, and the Mediterranean. Approximately 95% of infections are caused by *Echinococcus granulosa*; the remaining 5% are from *E. multilocularis*, which is more virulent and difficult to control because of its diffuse nature and invasive characteristics. Three-quarters of the infections involve the right lobe of the liver.

Although hydatid cysts can be asymptomatic for several years, hepatomegaly, jaundice, bloating, and indigestion may eventually develop. The complications associated with hydatid cysts usually result from either the cyst becoming secondarily infected with bacteria, or it ruptures into the peritoneal cavity, pleural space, pericardium, or biliary tree. Cholangitis can result from infestation of the bile ducts.

The diagnosis of hydatid disease of the liver requires a high index of suspicion, especially if the patient is either a native or has recently traveled to an endemic area. The current serum immunoelectrophoresis is 85–90% accurate. The most helpful study is a CT scan which demonstrates a cystic lesion in the liver that either has a calcified wall, contains daughter cysts, or both.

Surgery remains the mainstay of therapy for hydatid cysts of the liver. Medical therapy includes the antihelmintics such as albendazole and mebendazole. However, these agents have limited success. They are used preoperatively in an effort to sterilize the cyst and reserved as definitive treatment for patients with inoperable, diffuse, or recurrent disease. The principles of surgical therapy include complete evacuation of the cyst, destruction of the germinal lining, and avoiding spillage of daughter cysts. The surgical options consist of a liver resection, pericystectomy, and nonresectional procedures. A liver resection is considered radical and reserved for peripheral lesions or diffuse involvement of a lobe. A pericystectomy involves removing the entire cyst; the procedure is difficult to perform and carries significant morbidity. The current preferred procedure involves complete evacuation of the cyst, instillation of 30% hypertonic saline to sterilize any remaining scolices, removing

the endocyst (contains the germinal layer), and either leaving the cavity open or packing it with omentum. With the nonresectional approach, the mortality in uncomplicated cases is 5% and the recurrence rate is 5–10%.

Neoplastic cysts

Cystadenoma and cystadenocarcinoma are rare cystic tumors of the liver. Of these tumors, 75% occur in women. Upper abdominal fullness and/or discomfort and a palpable mass are the presenting clinical manifestations. An ultrasound and/or CT scan are the most helpful imaging studies. A cystadenoma appears as a cystic mass with smooth walls and internal septa (Fig 33.8); a cystadenocarcinoma has a similar appearance but with a solid component (Fig. 33.9). A cystadenoma requires complete excision because of its malignant potential. However, enucleation without liver resection of these lesions is sufficient. A cystade-

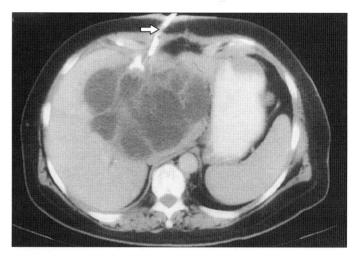

Figure 33.8 Hepatic cystadenoma. A CT scan image that shows a large, multiseptated cystic mass in the central portion of the liver. Attempts to drain (arrow) the lesion were unsuccessful. The benign lesion was excised using total vascular exclusion because of its central location.

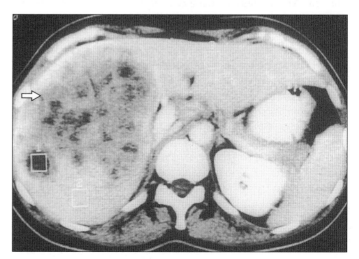

Figure 33.9 Hepatic cystadenocarcinoma. A large lesion (arrow) that involves the right lobe and the medial portion of the left lobe. The patient was a Jehovah's witness. The lesion was resected without blood products using total vascular exclusion.

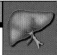

nocarcinoma, on the other hand, does require a formal resection with a margin of normal liver. The prognosis following surgical removal of either type of tumor is very good.

BENIGN TUMORS

Cavernous hemangioma

Cavernous hemangioma is the most frequently encountered benign tumor of the liver, occurring in 2–7% of the population. This tumor is of mesenchymal origin and is seen more often in women, suggesting that estrogen may play a role in its pathogenesis. The majority of cavernous hemangiomas are small, incidental, and require no intervention. However, very large lesions may be associated with upper abdominal fullness or discomfort and early satiety. Bleeding, either into the hemangioma or the peritoneal cavity, is rare. A palpable mass may be present in the upper abdomen. The Kasabach–Merritt syndrome, which is a low-grade local consumptive coagulopathy usually associated with hemangiomas of the extremities, has also been reported with cavernous hemangiomas of the liver.

Several imaging studies are available to differentiate hemangioma from other liver tumors. Although often suggestive, an ultrasound may not be diagnostic. A dynamic CT scan typically shows incomplete early filling of the lesion with intravenous contrast, and subsequent filling from the periphery toward the center. Scanning by MRI is 90% sensitive and 92% accurate (Fig. 33.10). A technetium-labeled red blood cell scan is also reported to be highly accurate. Because of the accuracy of other modalities, angiography is rarely necessary as a diagnostic study.

Only symptomatic hemangiomas need to be excised, regardless of their size. The majority of patients are referred because of nonspecific upper abdominal symptoms and an imaging study which reveals a 5–6cm hemangioma. These patients require no treatment. However, patients who return on more than one occasion because of upper abdominal pain for which no other cause is uncovered may be candidates for excision. Massive lesions that are clearly responsible for pain should also be excised. Older literature suggested that hemangiomas greater than 5–6cm in size had a 4–21% incidence of spontaneous rupture. However, a series from the Mayo Clinic which included 36 patients with heman-

giomas with an average size of 8cm followed for a mean of 12 years reported no spontaneous bleeding. Therefore, asymptomatic hemangiomas, regardless of size, can be followed safely by yearly imaging studies. In our series, only one patient presented with bleeding into a large hemangioma in the left lobe; another patient had pain and the Kasabach–Merritt syndrome. Both of these hemangiomas were excised.

Enucleation is the procedure of choice for removing a cavernous hemangioma. A 'friendly plane' can be developed between the hemangioma and the normal liver parenchyma. Blood loss can be minimized if the enucleation procedure is combined with control of vascular inflow (Pringle maneuver), or, if the hemangioma is massive, total vascular exclusion (TVE). Enucleation is associated with a 50% reduction of blood loss when compared with a formal resection. Resection is indicated only if the diagnosis is in doubt and there is concern that the lesion is a hemangiosarcoma. Long-term survival after removal of a cavernous hemangioma is excellent.

Hepatic cell adenoma

In 1973, the first article that described the association between oral contraceptives and hepatic cell adenomas was reported by Baum. He found that women who took oral contraceptives had a 25% higher risk of developing an adenoma than the general population. The mean age at the time of diagnosis is 32 years with a range of 21–57 years.

Up to 50% of patients have upper abdominal pain and as many as 30% may present acutely with bleeding, either into the tumor, or freely into the peritoneal cavity. Malignant degeneration has also been reported with hepatic adenomas. Laboratory studies are usually normal, although the serum alkaline phosphatase and gamma-glutamyl phosphatase (γGT) activities may occasionally be elevated. Ultrasound, CT, and MRI are no more than 50–60% specific. Angiography reveals a vascular mass that is not necessarily diagnostic of an adenoma. Up to 25% of adenomas may show uptake on a sulfur colloid scan, which is supposed to differentiate focal nodular hyperplasia from adenoma. No imaging study is completely specific for an adenoma. The histologic appearance of these tumors is sheets of hepatocytes, devoid of bile ducts and reticuloendothelial cells.

All symptomatic hepatic cell adenomas and those greater

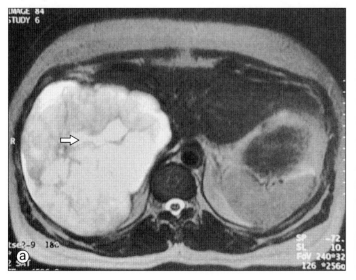

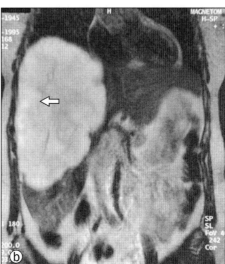

Figure 33.10. Cavernous hemangioma. (a) An axial MRI image showing a large, symptomatic hemangioma (white area; arrow). (b) A coronal view of the same lesion. The hemangioma was enucleated.

than 5cm require resection because of the risk of hemorrhage and malignant degeneration. Asymptomatic lesions that are less than 5cm may be observed by serial scans if the patient discontinues the oral contraceptives. However, a low threshold to resect the adenoma must be maintained if the lesion does not significantly reduce in size within a few months. Because of the possibility of malignancy, a liver resection with a 1–2cm margin of normal parenchyma is required for adequate treatment. The overall mortality associated with hepatic cell adenomas is 2–3%, which is virtually limited to those women who present with intraperitoneal rupture and hemorrhage; 20% of these women die.

Focal nodular hyperplasia

In contrast to hepatic cell adenomas, focal nodular hyperplasia (FNH) is not associated with oral contraceptives. It is usually found incidentally, and no cases of spontaneous hemorrhage have been reported. Laboratory studies are normal. Computed tomography, MRI, and a technicium sulfur colloid scan are the most helpful imaging studies. Scanning by CT and MRI may reveal the typical 'central scar' (Fig. 33.11). Virtually all cases of FNH should have a positive sulfur colloid scan because of the presence of nonparenchymal cells as well as hepatocytes in these lesions

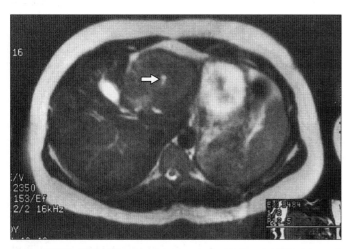

Figure 33.11 MRI of focal nodular hyperplasia. An axial MRI picture of the characteristic central scar (arrow) of FNH.

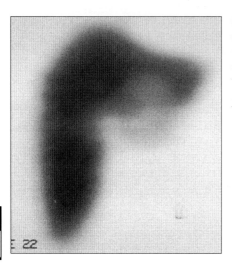

Figure 33.12 Sulfur colloid scan of focal nodular hyperplasia. A sulfur colloid scan on the same lesion as depicted in Fig. 33.11. The FNH takes up the isotope because of the presence of Kupffer cells in the tumor.

(Fig. 33.12). A biopsy reveals all the elements of normal liver tissue, not just hepatocytes.

Unlike adenomas, FNH rarely requires resection because there is little risk of either hemorrhage or malignant degeneration. Asymptomatic lesions, even very large ones, can be followed safely. Indications for resection include pain or increasing size as demonstrated by repeated imaging.

MALIGNANT NEOPLASMS

Primary hepatocellular carcinoma

Hepatocellular carcinoma (HCC), once relatively uncommon in the USA, is increasing in incidence; the reported incidence is approximately 2/100,000, or 9000 new cases per year. By contrast in parts of Asia and sub-Sahara Africa, HCC is the most frequently encountered intra-abdominal malignancy, with an incidence of 30 cases per 100,000 population. Risk factors associated with the development of HCC include cirrhosis, hepatitis B virus (HBV) or hepatitis C virus (HCV) infection, male sex, thorotrast, aflatoxin B1, parasites, and certain metabolic liver diseases (e.g. hemochromatosis).

The clinical presentation of HCC varies considerably. The spectrum includes asymptomatic patients with an abdominal mass discovered by screening as well as those who present with fever, malaise, pain, weight loss, jaundice, and even liver failure. The laboratory studies most likely to be abnormal include alkaline phosphatase, γGT, and bilirubin. Alpha-fetoprotein can be a valuable serum marker, although it is elevated in only 75–80% of patients in the USA. Both CT and MRI are excellent imaging studies. However, of the two, MRI is more sensitive in that it is more likely to reveal multicentric disease or a more extensive tumor than demonstrated by CT (Fig. 33.13). A needle biopsy, either a core, or an aspiration for cytology are often diagnostic. If a needle biopsy of the tumor is performed, a biopsy of the nontumor bearing portion of the liver should also be carried out to rule out the presence of cirrhosis, particularly if splenomegaly is demonstrated on the imaging studies. Splenomegaly suggests the diagnosis of portal hypertension and cirrhosis. The key issues in the surgical man-

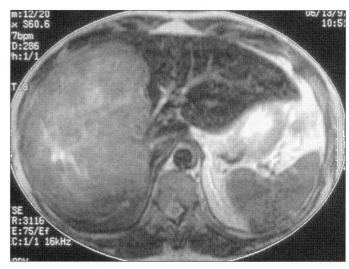

Figure 33.13 Hepatoma. An MRI image of a large hepatoma that required an extended right lobectomy.

agement of HCC is to confirm the diagnosis quickly with the least invasive techniques; and to assess whether the patient is a candidate for liver transplantation, and if not to determine whether a resection can be performed safely and with a good chance of success.

Once the diagnosis of HCC has been made, further studies are necessary to rule out metastatic disease. A CT scan of the chest, or, at least, a chest X-ray is required to eliminate the possibility of pulmonary spread. A bone scan may also be indicated. The indications for and appropriate selection of candidates for liver transplantation are presented in Chapter 34. If no metastatic disease is detected, and the patient is not a transplant candidate, the patient should be further worked up for a possible resection, assuming the patient does not have any other comorbid conditions, such as heart or lung disease, that would preclude a major surgical procedure.

The resectability rate for HCC is approximately 30%. The operative mortality for a major liver resection for HCC ranges from 2 to 15%. Factors that increase operative morbidity and mortality include cirrhosis, significant fatty change, prolonged (greater than 1 hour) vascular occlusion (warm ischemia), major blood loss, a major resection, coronary artery disease, and an elevated preoperative bilirubin. The incidence of cirrhosis in patients with resectable HCC in the USA ranges from 4 to 24%; the associated mortality ranges from 14 to 23% in Child's class A patients. Death is usually from liver failure or severe dysfunction and multiorgan failure. A major liver resection carries a morbidity rate of 25–40%. Complications are discussed in more detail later in this Chapter.

The ranges of 1- and 5-year survival for patients resected for potential cure are 42–71 and 20–45%, respectively. Blumgart reported 5- and 10-year survivals of 41 and 32%, respectively. The favorable determinants of survival by univariate analysis include no vascular invasion, asymptomatic status, a solitary tumor, histologically negative margin, an encapsulated tumor, and a tumor less than 5cm. Lack of vascular invasion is the most reliable favorable factor by multivariate analysis.

There is a role for a repeat liver resection for recurrent HCC in a very select group of patients. Approximately 10% of patients who have a liver resection will develop a solitary recurrence that is amenable to a second resection. The same preoperative evaluation that was performed before the first resection is repeated. Although the operative procedure may be more demanding technically and associated with more blood loss than the first resection, the short- and long-term survival are the same. The morbidity is also similar to the initial resection.

The role of preoperative hepatic artery chemoembolization (HAC) in the treatment of HCC is not clear. A recent series reported 140 patients who had liver resections; 105 had HAC preoperatively. Approximately 50% of patients had significant reduction in the size of the tumor, particularly tumors greater than 5cm. However, 53% of patients had complications related to the HAC including bile duct necrosis, necrotizing cholecystitis, pancreatitis, liver injury as reflected by a worsening Child–Pugh score, and hilar adhesions. Overall, there was no significant difference in postoperative morbidity, mortality, or survival. Patients with tumors that border on not being resectable before HAC may benefit from the procedure. However, more studies are necessary.

The role of cryosurgery for treating HCC is also not well defined. A series of 27 patients with HCC and cirrhosis treated by cryosurgery reported 1-, 3-, and 5-year survival rates of 33, 13, and 4%, respectively. Another small report of 12 patients with HCC and cirrhosis treated with cryosurgery revealed almost 100% recurrence at a mean of 9 months. Survival was not prolonged. The authors concluded that cryosurgery may benefit patients with one or two lesions that are less than 5cm in diameter.

Fibrolamellar HCC (FLHCC) is a rare variant of hepatoma that was first described in 1956. In contrast to the more common type of HCC, FLHCC is found in young patients (mean age 23 years), is not associated with either hepatitis or cirrhosis, and α-fetoprotein is not a serum marker. The variant FLHCC is thought to be biologically relatively more indolent than HCC because it usually becomes quite large before it is detected. Neurotensin may be a serum marker.

Two series reporting FLHCC have been published recently. In one series there were 10 patients with a mean tumor size of 8cm. The 5- and 10-year survival rates were 70%. Half of the patients recurred and three had a repeat liver resection. Of the 20 patients in the other report, 14 were resected and six underwent liver transplantation. The 5-year survival was 36%. A review of the literature reveals a 5-year survival of 56%. When matched stage for stage, the survival in patients with FLHCC is no better than non-FLHCC. No patient with stage III disease survived for 5 years. However, all agree that recurrences should be treated aggressively.

METASTATIC TUMORS

The most frequently encountered liver tumor is one that is metastatic. The metastatic lesions currently most often treated by liver resection include colorectal and neuroendocrine tumors. Other tumors that have been treated by liver resection include breast, melanoma, genitourinary, and sarcoma. However, the results have been poor and patients with these primary tumors should be highly selected for a liver resection.

The majority of liver resections in the USA are performed for metastatic colorectal carcinoma. Approximately 150,000 new cases of colorectal carcinoma occur in the USA annually. Of these, about one-third will develop liver metastases, 20% of whom will have their metastatic disease confined to the liver. Approximately a quarter of this 20% (about 2000 patients) may be candidates for liver resection.

Potential candidates for a liver resection for metastatic colorectal carcinoma must have no evidence of extrahepatic spread, lesion(s) confined to one lobe, and have no comorbid conditions to preclude a major operative procedure. The preoperative evaluation consists of a thorough history and physical examination, routine blood studies, chorio-embryonic antigen (CEA), a colonoscopy if one has not been performed within the past year, chest CT, and either a abdominal CT or MRI that demonstrates no more than three lesions, all contained in one lobe (Fig. 33.14). The operative mortality ranges from 3 to 8%. The overall, average 5-year survival following a liver resection for metastatic colorectal carcinoma ranges from 25 to 30%; the disease-free survival ranges from 15 to 20%. The 10-year overall and disease-free survivals are 26 and 18%, respectively. The factors that do not appear to affect survival include the size of the lesion, synchronous versus metachronous lesions, and DNA aneuploidy.

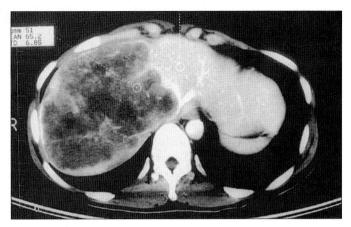

Figure 33.14 Metastatic colorectal carcinoma. Axial CT image of a large metastatic lesion that was resected by an extended right lobectomy.

The variables that do affect survival include a 1cm negative resection margin, the number of lesions, and bilobar disease. Although there is conflicting data regarding the number of lesions and survival, recent reports reveal a significantly improved outlook if the patient has a solitary lesion. The 5-year survival drops from 47 to 16% if more than one lesion is present. None of the patients in our series with bilobar disease survived for 3 years.

Approximately 10–15% of patients are candidates for a second liver resection for recurrent disease. Almost 65–85% of patients who have a liver resection for metastatic colorectal carcinoma will develop a recurrence. About 20–30% of these patients will recur in the liver alone and 10% may be a candidate for another resection. The preoperative evaluation is the same as before the first resection; the operative morbidity and mortality are also the same. The operative blood loss is higher because of the adhesions from the prior surgery. The prognostic factors are also the same: obtaining a 1cm tumor free margin and a solitary lesion. The survival is also equal to that obtained from the first resection (Fig. 33.15). Patients with a metastatic neuroendocrine tumor, such as carcinoid or an islet cell tumor of the pancreas, may also be candidates for a liver resection. The patients most likely to benefit from a resection are those who have symptoms from a functioning tumor that is overproducing a biologically active hormone, such as is associated with the carcinoid syndrome or a gastrinoma. The severity of symptoms is proportional to the volume of tumor. A series from the Mayo Clinic included 74 patients, 50 with carcinoid and 23 with islet cell tumors. The operative morbidity and mortality were 24 and 2.7%, respectively. About 90%

Survival after repeat liver resection for colorectal metastases				
Resection	1 Year (%)	3 Years (%)	5 Years (%)	10 Years (%)
First	78	30	16	16
Second	85	39	25	11

Figure 33.15 Metastatic tumors. A repeat liver resection for colorectal metastases has a survival comparable with that of the initial resection.

of patients had improvement in their symptoms related to hormone overproduction for a mean of 19 months. The 4-year survival was 73%. The authors concluded that in select patients liver resection was safe and effective palliation for patients with metastatic neuroendocrine tumors. A small percentage of patients may also gain a survival advantage from a liver resection.

PREOPERATIVE PREPARATION

The preoperative preparation for a potential liver resection depends on the diagnosis, the overall health of the patient, and the magnitude of the planned resection. Coagulation parameters must be checked and normalized. Patients with significant pulmonary or cardiac problems require the appropriate consultations to optimize the intraoperative and postoperative course. Bowel preparation is used routinely in patients with metastatic colorectal carcinoma. Prior surgery and the associated adhesions increase the risk of an enterotomy; a bowel resection may be necessary if a local recurrence is found at the time of exploration. All patients receive broad spectrum prophylactic antibiotics. If a major resection is planned, four units of packed red cells and two units of fresh frozen plasma are set aside.

ANATOMY AND DEFINITION OF RESECTIONS

The liver is divided into a left and right half based on the incoming vascular structures. Externally, a plane between the gallbladder and the inferior vena cava (IVC) divide the right and left lobes; the falciform ligament further divides the left lobe into a medial and lateral segment. The liver has segmental anatomy as defined by Couinoud (Fig. 33.16). A right lobectomy or hepatectomy removes segments V–VIII; a left lobectomy excises segments II–IV. Removal of segments IV–VIII comprise an extended right lobectomy; the medial segment of the left lobe is resected in addition to the entire right lobe. Segments II–VI are excised in an extended left lobectomy; the anterior portion of the right lobe in addition to the entire left lobe. A wedge resection removes the tumor along with a 1–2cm margin of normal parenchyma in a nonanatomic manner.

INTRAOPERATIVE MONITORING AND RESUSCITATION

Precise intraoperative monitoring and resuscitation are crucial for the success of a liver resection. A mean arterial pressure (MAP) line and central venous pressure line (CVP) are added to the routine monitoring of the heart rate, blood pressure, electrocardiogram, and oxygen saturation. A Swan–Ganz catheter is reserved for patients with cardiac problems who require even more precise monitoring. The Foley catheter and nasogastric tube are placed after the induction of general anesthesia. Initial volume replacement consists of crystalloid fluids; blood components are administered as necessary.

SURGICAL TECHNIQUES

Laparoscopy is performed initially in patients with primary HCC who have not had previous upper abdominal surgery. If laparoscopy reveals metastatic disease, bilobar disease, cirrhosis

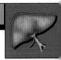

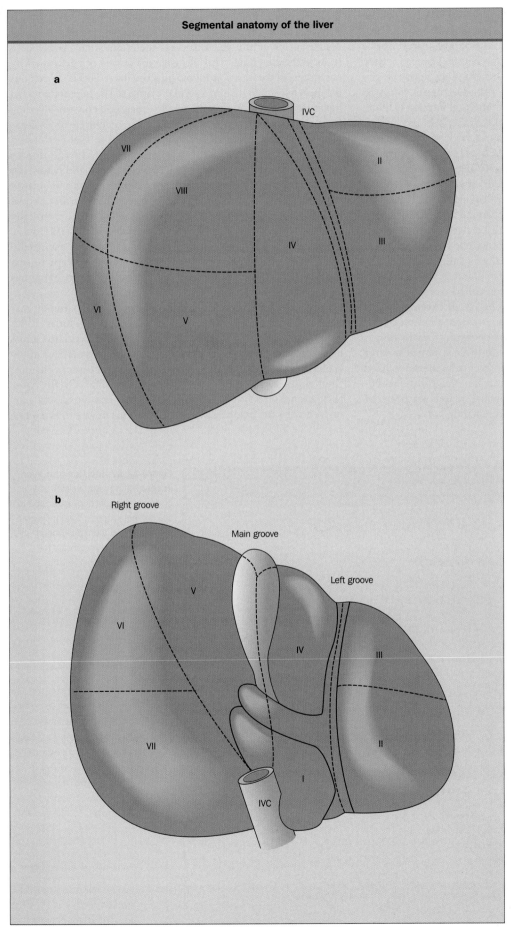

Figure 33.16 Segmental anatomy of the liver. (a) Anterior view of the segments II–VIII. (b) Inferior aspect of the segmental anatomy.

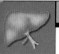

or significant fatty change in the nontumor-bearing portion of the liver, the procedure is terminated. The patient is spared a laparotomy and can be discharged within 24 hours. Laparoscopy is less useful in patients who have metastatic disease since they have adhesions from prior surgery. The adhesions limit the visibility of laparoscopy and increase the risk of iatrogenic injury to the bowel. Therefore, a limited right subcostal incision is made in patients with metastatic disease. If extrahepatic and bilobar disease are not found, the incision is extended into a chevron with a midline extension (Fig 33.17).Once the laparotomy has been performed, the abdomen is again inspected for any extrahepatic disease. The liver is mobilized by dividing the right and left triangular ligaments, and the falciform ligament. The mobilization facilitates intraoperative ultrasound and parenchymal transection later. If a lobectomy is to be performed, the gallbladder is removed and the artery to the lobe being resected is ligated and divided; dividing the portal vein and bile duct to the lobe may also be carried out at this time, but is not absolutely necessary. These structures can be controlled from within the parenchyma at the time of transection. If an extended right lobectomy is the planned procedure, however, division of the portal vein and bile duct prior to parenchymal transection is necessary to reduce the risk of injury to these structures. After completion of the hilar dissection, the liver is further mobilized by taking down the retroperitoneal attachments. If total vascular exclusion is planned during parenchymal transection, both the suprahepatic and infrahepatic IVC are encircled.

Controlling the bleeding from the parenchyma at the time of its transection remains the most challenging portion of a liver resection. Over the years, several techniques have evolved to reduce the bleeding. The 'Pringle' maneuver is performed by occluding all the vascular inflow into the liver. This is carried out by applying a noncrushing vascular clamp to the hepatoduodenal ligament. However, this maneuver does not control bleeding from the hepatic veins. More recently, the technique of TVE has gained popularity. The dissection is identical to that performed for a total hepatectomy for a liver transplant. In addition to occluding the portal inflow, the IVC both above and below the liver are controlled. Therefore, all the vascular inflow and outflow are occluded. The technique of TVE does reduce cardiac output by 25–30%, but the majority of patients remain hemodynamically stable with additional volume (approximately 500–1000cm³). The technique allows parenchymal transection in a virtually bloodless field. However, clamp times should be kept to less than 60 minutes, particularly if the remaining parenchyma has either fibrosis or fatty change.

Several methods are used to transect the parenchyma, including 'finger fracture', suction knife, a hemostat or Kelly clamp, or the cavitron ultrasonic aspirator (CUSA). The CUSA uses ultrasound waves to dissolve the parenchyma and allow skeletonization of the vessels and biliary structures which are then clipped or tied prior to being divided (Fig. 33.18). After the parenchyma has been transected, the raw surface is cauterized with the argon beam coagulator; this device uses a jet of

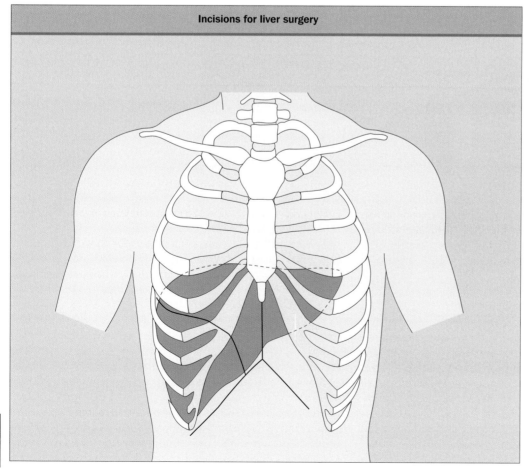

Incisions for liver surgery

Figure 33.17 Incisions for liver surgery. The major incision is a chevron with a midline extension to the xiphoid process. Seldomly, an extension into the right chest or the sternum may be necessary for adequate exposure.

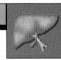

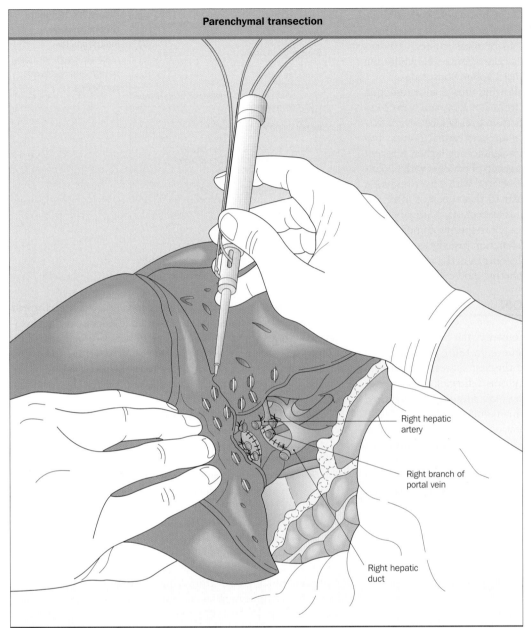

Parenchymal transection

Right hepatic artery

Right branch of portal vein

Right hepatic duct

Figure 33.18 Parenchymal transection. A right hepatic lobectomy is depicted. The right branches of the hepatic artery, portal vein, and bile duct have been ligated and divided. The liver parenchyma is being transected with the CUSA, which is an instrument that uses ultrasound to melt away the parenchyma and expose the vessels and bile ducts which are then clipped or ligated, depending on their size, and divided.

argon gas to conduct an electric current. The result is tissue desiccation. When there is no further bleeding from the raw surface, an attempt is made to approximate the capsule with sutures and drains are left in the subphrenic and subhepatic areas. The abdomen is then closed.

POSTOPERATIVE CARE

The majority of patients who undergo a liver resection enjoy a relatively uncomplicated postoperative course. That is particularly true if the intraoperative effort was problem free. Relatively few patients require more than an overnight stay in a monitored unit. Intravenous fluids and blood products are given as needed; antibiotics are continued for the first 24 hours. The nasogastric tube is removed on the first postoperative day and the diet is advanced as tolerated. The majority of patients have an epidural catheter inserted for pain control; this is removed on the fourth or fifth postoperative day, if the coagulation profile is normal. The Foley catheter is removed on the same day.

Laboratory studies, which include a complete blood count, liver and renal tests, and a prothrombin time, are obtained daily for at least the first 3 days. Initially, the transaminases are elevated, ranging from a few hundred to more than a thousand; however, they should normalize rapidly over the next 5–7 days. The prothrombin time and serum bilirubin level may also become elevated; the former may require the administration of vitamin K or fresh frozen plasma. The severity of the derangement of the postoperative liver studies depends on the magnitude of the resection, the duration of the clamp time (warm ischemia), the integrity of the remaining parenchyma, and the intraoperative course. A bloody resection associated with hypotension and the administration of large volumes of fluid and blood products results in more postoperative liver dysfunction. The cholestatic enzymes, alkaline phosphatase, and γGT are initially normal and then tend to rise toward the end of the first week. Both of these tests are markers of regeneration and may stay elevated for a few weeks. The most worrisome biochemical profile 7–10 days following a major liver resection includes a rising serum bilirubin and prothrombin time, and a normal alkaline phosphatase.

The mortality and morbidity following a major liver resection in patients without cirrhosis range from 2 to 15%, and from 24 to 40%, respectively. Mortality results from liver failure/severe dysfunction, infection, multisystem failure, and cardiac events. The mortality in patients with cirrhosis is significantly higher. A recent series reported a 14% mortality in a group of patients with Child's class A cirrhosis. The morbidity associated with a liver resection can be procedure specific, or similar to that reported after any major abdominal operation, such as atelectasis, a urinary tract infection, or a wound infection. Procedure specific complications include liver dysfunction, renal dysfunction (usually as a result of the liver dysfunction), bile leaks, bleeding from the operative site, pleural effusions, ascites, and subphrenic fluid collection.

BILIARY RECONSTRUCTION

The early efforts to bypass or reconstruct the biliary tree were most often to deal with bile duct stones. In 1880, Alexander von Winiwarter of Belgium performed the first successful cholecystoenterostomy for persistent symptoms following aspiration of the gallbladder. The first choledochoduodenostomy was achieved in 1891 by Oskar Sprengel in Germany following a cholecystectomy and common bile duct exploration that was unsuccessful in clearing the duct of stones. Halsted reconstructed the biliary tree with a choledochoduodenostomy in 1898 after locally excising an ampullary tumor. By 1913, choledochoduodenostomy had become established as an operation with acceptable mortality and morbidity. Its proponents claimed that cholangitis and stone formation were prevented. An important innovation was introduced by Robert Dahl of Sweden in 1909: the Roux-en-Y hepaticojejunostomy. Since those early years, choledochoduodenostomy and Roux-en-Y drainage have become the most frequently used procedures for biliary reconstruction or bypass.

Indications for biliary reconstruction

Figure 33.19 lists the indications for biliary reconstruction or bypass. An iatrogenic injury resulting from a cholecystectomy is the leading cause of benign strictures. Other benign problems include recurrent or retained bile duct stones and chronic pancreatitis. However, the highly successful endoscopic and radiographic approaches to bile duct stones has virtually eliminated the need for surgical intervention. Biliary obstruction as a result of either a cholangiocarcinoma or a periampullary malignancy is the other major indication for biliary reconstruction. Unresectable periampullary lesions may be amenable to a biliary-enteric bypass, thus eliminating the need for indwelling stents that require changing on a regular basis to prevent cholangitis.

Operative techniques

Choledochoduodenostomy and Roux-en-Y biliary reconstruction are the methods used most frequently to reconstruct or bypass

Figure 33.19 Biliary reconstruction.
Indications for reconstruction, including benign and malignant conditions.

Indications for biliary reconstruction
Benign conditions
Strictures/injuries:
Iatrogenic
Ampullary stenosis secondary to stone disease
Chronic pancreatitis
Stone disease
Recurrent or persistent stone disease not amenable to endoscopic or radiographic intervention
Malignant disease
Unresectable periampullary carcinomas
Cholangiocarcinoma
Proximal lesions
Mid-duct lesions

the biliary tree. Primary duct-to-duct repairs, even if performed at the time of the cholecystectomy and bile duct injury, are associated with a high rate of subsequent stricture and therefore should be avoided. The high incidence of stricture formation results from bile duct ischemia due to the tenuous nature of the arterial blood supply to the extrahepatic biliary tree, and the tension on the anastomosis.

Choledochoduodenostomy is an excellent bypass procedure for unresectable periampullary malignancies. The procedure is relatively easy to perform and requires only one anastomosis. The anastomsis is within easy reach of the endoscope therefore allowing both diagnostic and therapeutic endoscopic intervention. Benign, iatrogenic strictures are not usually amenable to a choledochoduodenostomy because of the high location of the obstruction and the associated scarring in the area of the duodenum. Ascending cholangitis was cited as a complication of choledochoduodenostomy. However, an anastomosis 2.5cm in length will prevent this problem. Other disadvantages include the sump syndrome which results from inadequate drainage of the distal duct. This complication can also be prevented by performing a large anastomosis. An endoscopic sphincterotomy usually eliminated the sump syndrome.

Construction of a Roux limb provides an excellent conduit for biliary reconstruction. The limb may be sewn to any accessible portion of the biliary tree, particularly the common bile duct (choledochojejunostomy) or the hepatic duct (hepaticojejunostomy). A Roux limb is the best option for either an immediately recognized bile duct injury or a subsequent benign stricture because it will easily reach the hepatic bifurcation and the anastomosis is tension free (Fig. 33.20). An anastomotic stricture results in cholangitis and occurs in 15–20% of patients. Many of these recurrent strictures can be successfully treated by radiographic dilatation and stenting. If stenting is not successful, the biliary-enteric anastomosis can be revised with a good long-term result in 90% of patients. Roux limb reconstruction is also the procedure of choice to restore biliary drainage following the resection of a proximal cholangiocarcinoma.

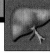

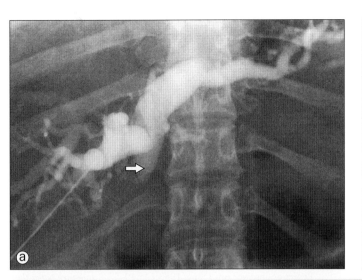

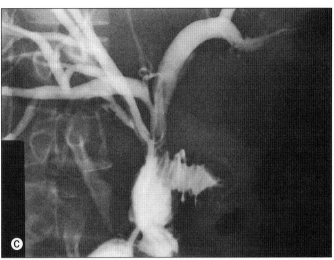

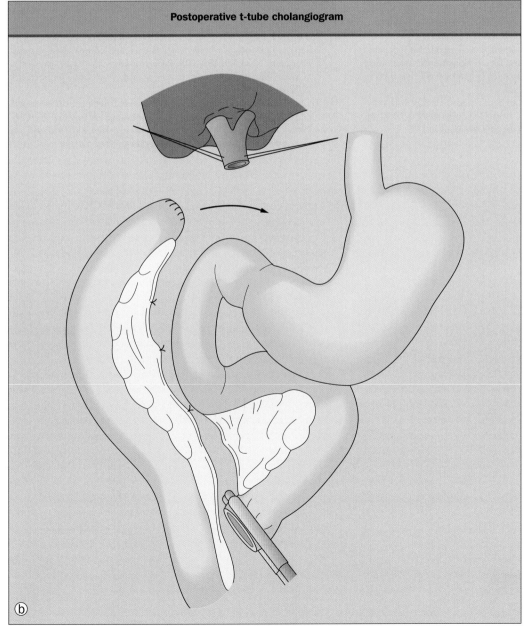

Postoperative t-tube cholangiogram

Figure 33.20
Choledochojejunostomy. (a) A percutaneous transhepatic cholangiogram demonstrating a benign stricture (arrow) which developed several months following a cholecystectomy. (b) A Roux limb has been created and will be sewn to the common hepatic duct. (c) A t-tube cholangiogram obtained one week postoperatively after reconstruction of the bile duct depicted in (a).

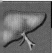

FURTHER READING

DeCarlis L, Pirotta V, Rondinara G, et al.. Hepatic adenoma and focal nodular hyperplasia: diagnosis and criteria for treatment. Liver Transpl Surg. 1997;3:160–5. *Good review of the diagnostic dilemmas associated with these two benign liver tumors.*

Foster JH. History of liver surgery. Arch Surg. 1991;126:381–7. *Excellent review of the history of liver surgery by one of the experts.*

Gigot J, Jadoul P, Que F, et al. Adult polycystic liver disease. Is fenestration the most adequate operation for long-term management ? Ann Surg. 1997;225:286–94. *Good review and current experience in the treatment of a rare but difficult clinical problem.*

Hemming A, Langer B, Sheiner P, et al. Aggressive surgical management of fibrolamellar hepatocellular carcinoma. J Gastrointest Surg. 1997;1:342–46. *A large experience with a rare variant of HCC.*

Huang C, Pitt H, Lipsett P, et al. Pyogenic hepatic abscess. Changing trends over 42 years. Ann Surg. 1996;223:600–9. *A large experience with liver abscesses over a long time period. The trends are clear.*

Hughes K, Simon R, Adson M, et al. Resection of the liver for colorectal carcinoma metastases: A multi-institutional study of indications for resection. Surgery. 1988;103:278–88. *The first and largest multicenter report of the results of liver resection for colorectal metastases.*

Jamison R, Donohue J, Nagorney D, et al. Hepatic resection for metastatic colorectal cancer results in cure for some patients. Arch Surg. 1997;132:505–11. *This paper provides long-term follow-up from an institution with extensive experience.*

Kelly D, Emre S, Guy S, et al. Resection of benign hepatic lesions with selective use of total vascular isolation. J Am Coll Surg. 1996;183:113–16. *Reviews both benign liver tumors and the technique of TVE.*

Kern K, Foster J. Surgical approach to hydatid cysts of the liver. Surg Rounds. 1993;March:181–92. *Discusses the various surgical approaches to hydatid disease of the liver along with the authors' experience.*

McEntee G, Nagorney D, Kvols K, et al. Cytoreductive hepatic surgery for neuroendocrine tumors. Surgery. 1990;108:1091–6. *The results demonstrate the value of an aggressive surgical approach to patients with symptomatic functioning islet cell tumors.*

Reed R, Merrell R, Meyers W, et al. Continuing evolution in the approach to severe liver trauma. Ann Surg. 1992;216:524–38. *Excellent review article on the management of liver trauma.*

Taylor M, Forster J, Langer B, et al. A study of prognostic factors for hepatic resection for colorectal metastases. Am J Surg. 1997;173:467–71. *Recent experience of a large number of patients in an established liver unit. Supports other recent studies which show that patients with solitary lesions benefit the most from liver resection.*

Trastek V, van Heerden J, Sheedy P, et al. Cavernous hemangiomas of the liver: Resect or observe? Am J Surg. 1983;145:49–52. *Landmark paper that reported the safety of observing asymptomatic cavernous hemangiomas, regardless of size.*

Tsao J, Loftus J, Nagorney D, et al. Trends in morbidity and mortality of hepatic resection for malignancy. A matched comparative analysis. Ann Surg. 1994;220:199–205. *Reports a large experience over several years. Major liver resections can be performed safely in units with sufficient experience.*

Wanebo H, Chu Q, Avradopoulos K, et al. Current perspectives on repeat hepatic resection for colorectal carcinoma: A review. Surgery. 1996;119:361–71. *This report reviews the experience of 29 papers; the data supports a second resection in highly selected patients.*

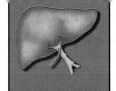

Chapter 34

Indications and Patient Selection

Didier Samuel, José Figueiro and Henri Bismuth

INTRODUCTION

Liver transplantation is the ultimate therapy for various liver diseases, and it has greatly changed the field of hepatology and the clinical care of patients suffering from liver disease. This procedure is now widely accepted as an effective therapeutic modality for a large number of irreversible acute and chronic liver diseases for which there were formerly no other treatment options (Fig. 34.1).

As the goals of liver transplantation are to prolong life and to improve the quality of life, it is essential to define optimal patient selection and the ideal timing of transplantation during the course of advanced liver disease. In recent years there has been an enormous increase in the number of liver transplant operations performed (Figs 34.2 & 34.3).

In the USA, 4167 liver transplant operations were carried out in 1997, while the equivalent figure for Europe was 3601. However, there are clear signs that the rate of expansion is slowing on both sides of the Atlantic.

The results of liver transplantation have improved due to advances in perioperative technique, a better understanding of the course and prognosis of several liver diseases, and more effective postoperative care. In recent years there has also been

Indications for liver transplantation in adults	
Chronic liver disease	Cholestatic diseases Primary biliary cirrhosis Primary sclerosing cholangitis Secondary biliary cirrhosis Viral-related cirrhosis Viral B cirrhosis Viral B-δ cirrhosis Viral C cirrhosis Alcoholic cirrhosis Autoimmune cirrhosis Budd–Chiari syndrome
Parasitic diseases	Echinococosis
Metabolic diseases	With liver disease Wilson's disease Congenital hemochromatosis α_1-antitrypsin deficiency Protoporphyria Gaucher's disease Glycogenosis type 1 Without liver disease, but secondary to a liver metabolic defect Primary hyperoxaluria Essential hypercholesterolemia Familial amyloid polyneuropathy secondary to a variant transthyretin
Primary malignant tumor of the liver	Hepatocellular carcinoma Fibrolamellar hepatocellular carcinoma Epitheloid hemangioendothelioma Cholangiocellular carcinoma
Various	Adenomatosis of the liver Polycystic liver diseases Caroli's disease

Acute liver failure	Fulminant and subfulminant hepatitis
	Wilson's disease (fulminant)
	Budd–Chiari syndrome (fulminant)
	Other causes of acute liver failure:
	  post-trauma, postsurgery,
	  postarterial embolization
	Acute alcoholic hepatitis (?)

Figure 34.1 Indications for liver transplantation in adults.

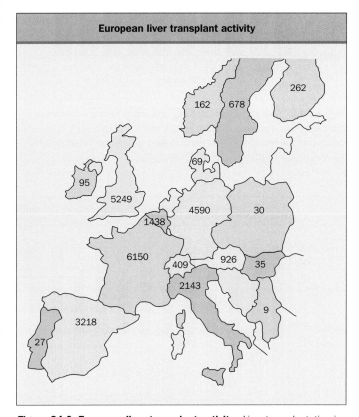

Figure 34.2 European liver transplant activity. Liver transplantation is performed in 19 European countries with 103 transplant centers, 26,538 transplants in 23,476 patients. (From The European Liver Registry Report, 5/1968–6/1997.)

a significant change in the indications for liver transplantation, so that nowadays the procedure is being offered in a wider range of more complicated conditions as well as to younger and older patients.

The most common indication is end-stage chronic liver disease in adults, which accounts for 69 and 70% of liver transplant activity in the USA and Europe, respectively (Fig. 34.4).

The main differences between the USA and Europe relate to the higher proportion of patients who have acute liver failure in Europe and the lower proportion of patients who have malignant disease receiving transplants in the USA (see Fig. 34.4). However,

the proportion of patients receiving liver transplants for malignant disease in Europe is now decreasing (Fig. 34.5).

Among patients who have cirrhosis, chronic viral hepatitis and alcoholic liver disease are more frequent indications than they were a decade ago, while in Europe, primary biliary cirrhosis is a contracting indication for transplantation (Fig. 34.6).

This expansion in indications contrasts with a shortage in liver donors and the constriction in health care budgets. This precipitates the need for continuous refinement of the selection for, and timing of, transplantation to obtain the most suitable and cost-effective outcome.

TIMING OF LIVER TRANSPLANTATION

The success and increase in the number of liver transplants as a treatment option for end-stage liver disease has led to a marked shortage in donor organs and has greatly lengthened the waiting time for this procedure. As the waiting list grows, there has been an increase in the number of patients dying while awaiting the procedure. In the USA there was an almost five-fold increase in the number of patients dying while listed for liver transplantation between 1988 and 1996, with the number rising from 195 to 954. This trend is forcing transplant physicians to list patients earlier in the course of the disease than was the case several years ago. Ideally, liver transplantation should be performed at a sufficiently late phase of the disease to give the patient maximal opportunity for spontaneous stabilization or recovery, but also in a condition that does not prejudice the outcome after transplantation. In other words, the patient's referral should occur when the anticipated survival is no more than 1–2 years, but before the onset the complications of end-stage disease that increase the risks and/or costs of liver transplantation. Patients who have more advanced liver disease are the ones most likely to develop operative complications and have longer postoperative hospitalization. On the other hand, although patients who have less advanced liver disease have excellent survival rates after the procedure, they could also be expected to survive with a reasonable quality of life for extended periods without liver transplantation.

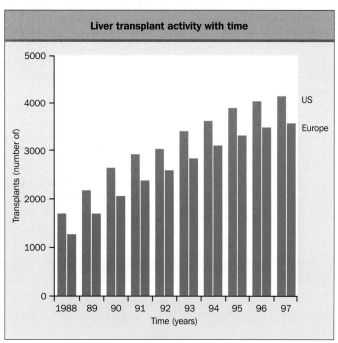

Figure 34.3 Liver transplant activity with time. Annual increases of the number of liver transplantations in Europe and the US are decreasing as a function of the limited supply of donor organs. (Data from UNOS and The European Liver Registry Report, 5/1968–6/1997.)

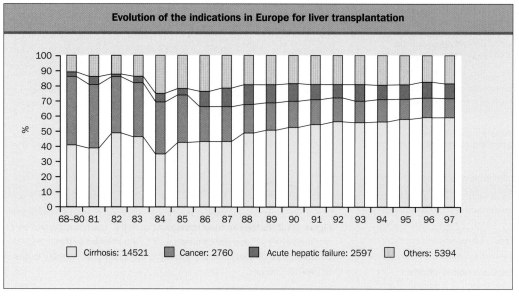

Figure 34.4 Evolution of the indications in Europe for liver transplantation. The main changes have been the progressive decrease of the patients transplanted for malignancy, the emergence of acute liver failure in the indications in 1986, and the increase of the number of patients transplanted for cirrhosis. (From The European Liver Registry Report, 5/1968–6/1997.)

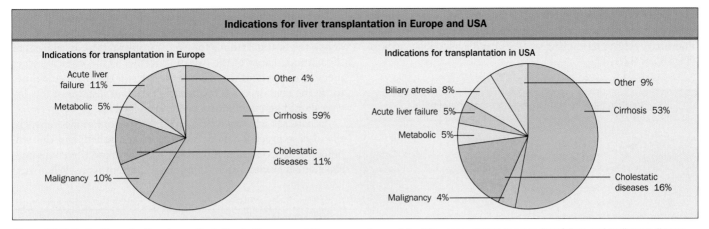

Figure 34.5 Indications for liver transplantation in Europe and the USA. The main indications for liver transplantation in Europe and the USA show subtle differences relating to acute liver failure and malignant disease. (Data from UNOS and The European Liver Registry Report, 5/1968–6/1997.)

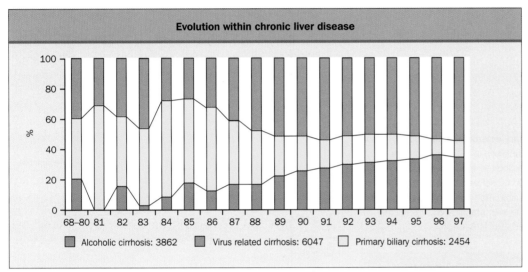

Figure 34.6 Evolution within chronic liver disease. Changes in the indications among patients transplanted for primary biliary cirrhosis, alcoholic cirrhosis and viral cirrhosis. Note the progressive decline of PBC as an indication and the increase of alcoholic and viral cirrhosis, which are now the two main indications for transplantation. (From The European Liver Registry Report, 5/1968–6/1997.)

Guidelines for referral or performance of the transplant in patients who have chronic liver disease are not yet adequately defined. The aim is to optimize the timing of liver transplantation in order to increase survival and decrease the postoperative morbidity and the total cost of the procedure. Survival models have been applied to liver transplantation for a number of diseases such as primary biliary cirrhosis and alcoholic cirrhosis, and these have shown that a survival benefit may not be apparent for up to 5 years after transplantation when the operation was performed relatively early in the disease. One model was developed at the Mayo Clinic for primary biliary cirrhosis (PBC), the liver disease with the most predictable natural history, and this identified five independent prognostic variables predictive of survival: serum levels of both bilirubin and albumin; age; prothrombin time; and the presence or absence of peripheral edema (including response to diuretic therapy). These five variables are used to determine a risk score that can be translated into a survival function to estimate survival for the individual PBC patient (Fig. 34.7).

The application of this model has demonstrated that liver transplantation improves survival when compared with supportive therapy in patients who have PBC. The survival benefit with liver transplantation is greater in the highest risk group, even though the survival rate is poorer in this high risk group due to the higher postoperative mortality (see Fig. 34.7).

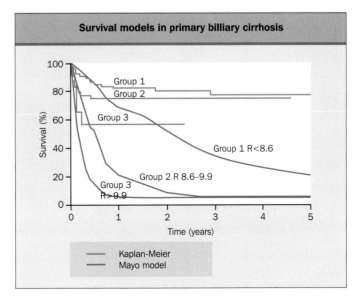

Figure 34.7 Survival models in primary biliary cirrhosis. Estimated Kaplan–Meier survival after liver transplantation in three groups of patients who had primary biliary cirrhosis versus estimated survival without liver transplantation as predicted by the Mayo model. Group 1, low risk; group 2, medium risk; group 3, high risk. (From Markus et al. N Engl J Med. 1989;320:1709–1713.)

Effective prognostic models are not yet well-developed for other chronic liver diseases, although attempts have been made in primary sclerosing cholangitis (PSC) and in alcoholic cirrhosis (Figs 34.8–34.10).

No model will be perfect, and they apply to a group of patients rather than an individual who has that particular disease. To define the optimal timing for liver transplantation, an analysis of the natural history of the disease, together with a clinical judgement of the patient's quality of life are still the main guidelines to aid the final decision. In addition, the clinical status of the disease should be taken into account (Fig. 34.11).

In patients who have PBC, PSC, and autoimmune hepatitis, the disease process may or may not be controlled, and this will influence the decision. Likewise, in viral-related liver disease, the control of viral replication is an important issue. When viral

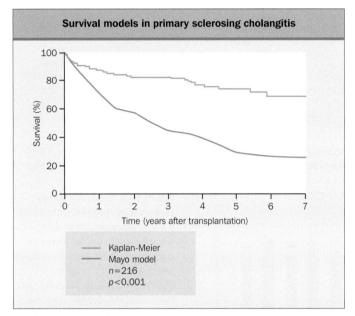

Figure 34.8 Survival models in primary sclerosing cholangitis. Actual Kaplan–Meier survival after liver transplantation in patients who have primary sclerosing cholangitis and the estimated survival without transplantation as predicted by the Mayo model simulated control. (From Wiesner et al. Prognostic models to assist in the timing of liver transplantation. In: Transplantation of the liver. Maddrey WC, Sorrell MF, eds. Newark (NY), Appleton and Lange; 1995:123–44.)

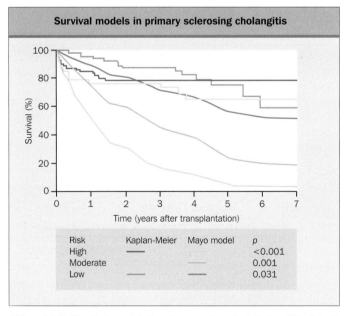

Figure 34.9 Survival models in primary sclerosing cholangitis. Actual Kaplan–Meier survival after liver transplantation in three risk groups of patients with PSC and their estimated survival without transplantation as predicted by the Mayo model. (From Wiesner et al. Prognostic models to assist in the timing of liver transplantation. In: Transplantation of the liver. Maddrey WC, Sorrell MF, eds. Newark (NY), Appleton and Lange; 1995:123–44.)

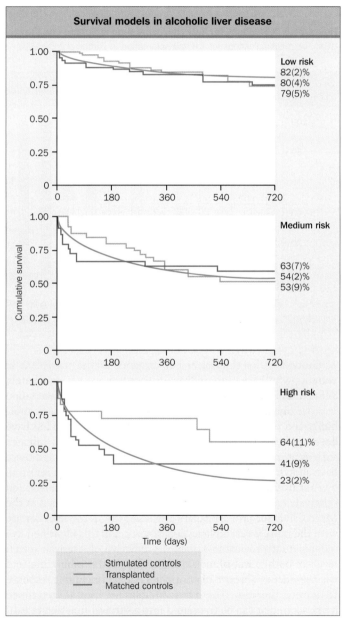

Figure 34.10 Survival models in alcoholic liver disease. Survival observed in patients transplanted for alcoholic cirrhosis, in matched and simulated controls, in a French multicenter trial. A higher survival after liver transplantation versus matched and simulated control was observed only in the high risk group. Figures in brackets represent percent of survival. (From Poynard et al. Lancet. 1994;344:502–7.)

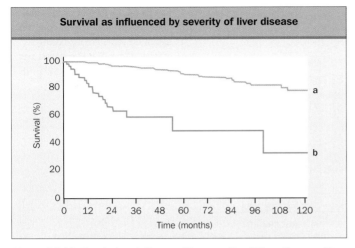

Figure 34.11 Survival as influenced by severity of liver disease. The probability of survival in patients who have compensated viral C cirrhosis (a) is greater at 91% at 5 years than after the appearance of the first major complication in patients who have decompensated viral C cirrhosis (b), which is 50% at 5 years. (From Fattovich et al. Gastroenterology. 1997;112;463–72.)

replication is controlled, the severity of the liver disease is usually mild and the clinical course is either stable or evolving slowly. In contrast, if viral replication persists and is associated with severe liver disease, liver function can be expected to deteriorate further. Sometimes, independent of any therapeutic intervention, either spontaneous arrest of the viral replication or spontaneous viral reactivation may occur. In both cases, particularly for chronic hepatitis B virus (HBV) carriers, the liver disease may deteriorate and the prognosis is difficult to assess. In some cases, liver function will return to baseline values after a transient period, but in others liver function will continue to deteriorate. In patients who have alcoholic cirrhosis, the discontinuation of alcohol may dramatically improve the prognosis. This improvement may take several months, and this is one of the reasons to recommend a 6-month period of abstinence from alcohol before performing transplantation in alcoholic patients. The timing of transplantation is necessarily influenced by access to donor organs. The most sophisticated system has been developed by the United Network for Organ Sharing (UNOS) in the USA. The organs are allocated primarily on the clinical status of the patient:

- status 1 – patients who have acute liver failure (fulminant hepatic failure) with a life expectancy of no more than 7 days without transplantation; acute decompensated Wilson's disease; or primary nonfunction or hepatic artery thrombosis within 7 days of implantation of the graft;
- status 2a – patients who have chronic liver disease who have a life expectancy of no more than 7 days with a Childs–Pugh score greater than nine, complicated by unresponsive active variceal hemorrhage; hepatorenal syndrome; spontaneous bacterial peritonitis; refractory ascites or hydrothorax; or grade 3–4 encephalopathy;
- status 2b – patients who have a Childs–Pugh score greater than nine or a score greater than six, but complicated by active variceal hemorrhage; hepatorenal syndrome; spontaneous bacterial peritonitis; refractory ascites; or hydrothorax; and
- status 3 – patients who have a Childs–Pugh score greater than six.

CONTRAINDICATIONS TO LIVER TRANSPLANTATION

As more experience has been gained with liver transplantation, the number of contraindications has decreased over the years. Nowadays, there is general consensus about a number of contraindications to liver transplantation, although these are not universally agreed by all transplant centers:

- extrahepatic organ failure (heart, lungs), unless multiorgan transplantation is envisaged;
- uncontrolled extrahepatic infection;
- extrahepatic malignant disease – the only potential exception to metastatic disease is for neuroendocrine tumors;
- diffuse thrombosis of the portal venous system (including the three main veins of the portal system – portal vein, superior mesenteric vein, and splenic vein);
- uncontrolled congenital immune deficiency;
- acquired immune deficiency – infected patients with the human immunodeficiency virus should be selectively regarded, although more recently the dramatic improvement observed in patients treated with combined antiretroviral therapy may modify this approach; and
- inability to withstand the surgical procedure.

Previous contraindications no longer applicable include: an upper age limit of 55 years; previous multiple upper abdominal operations or previous portocaval surgical anastomosis; isolated thrombosis of the portal venous vein; and the presence of hepatitis B surface antigen (HBsAg) in patient's serum. Other clinical conditions, such as active chronic alcoholism, noncompliance with medical treatment, critical clinical status, and active viral replication are selectively considered. The ultimate decision depends mainly on protocol within each transplant center. There is no absolute upper limit for age and, as defined by the Conference Consensus held in Paris 1993, the physiologic age is more important than the chronologic age. The proportion of recipients over the age of 60 years has been increasing steadily, but in candidates over the age of 65 years the indication should still be considered very carefully (Fig. 34.12).

An older patient receives a transplant, but his or her ability to overcome postoperative complications is lower than a 20-year-old patient, despite the apparent absence of specific risk factors such as coronary artery disease.

CHOLESTATIC DISEASES

Primary biliary cirrhosis

Primary biliary cirrhosis is a cholestatic liver disease, characterized by the destruction of small interlobular bile ducts due to an inflammatory process, probably autoimmune, that mainly affects women between 40 and 60 years of age. The course of the disease comprises three periods: an asymptomatic phase, lasting from 1 to 20 years and detected by an anicteric cholestasis or extrahepatic signs; a symptomatic phase with mild jaundice, itching, and lethargy, also lasting from 1 to 20 years; and a third and final stage, lasting a few months to 2 years, with marked jaundice, relentless increase in serum bilirubin levels, and clinical complications of portal hypertension. The course of the disease is smoothly progressive, with clinical manifestations such as disabling lethargy, itching, variceal bleeding, ascites, spontaneous

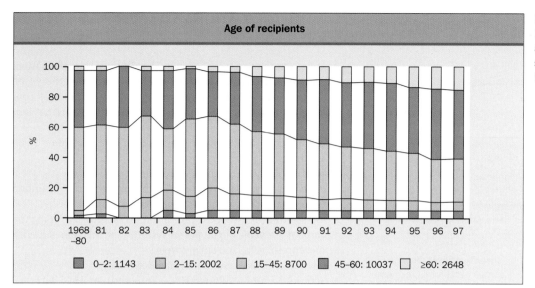

Figure 34.12 Age of recipients. Liver transplant recipients over the age of 60 years are increasing steadily. (From The European Liver Registry Report, 5/1968–12/1998.)

bacterial peritonitis, and osteodystrophy. It is clear that liver transplantation dramatically improves the prognosis of PBC, with better survival rates and quality of life.

In contrast with most of the liver diseases that require liver transplantation, the natural history of PBC is relatively well-known, and some centers have attempted to develop prognosis indices for these patients. The most widely used prognosis index was developed at the Mayo Clinic, but an alternative model that utilizes histologic and clinical data was developed in Europe. The prognostic models have also been used to evaluate objectively the efficacy of the procedure. Estimated survival of PBC patients who had undergone liver transplantation was better than the simulated survival of these same patients if they had been treated conservatively without transplantation (see Fig. 34.7). The overall benefit has been clearly demonstrated for these patients. The benefit was greater in patients who had the highest risk score, but in this high risk group the post-transplant mortality rate was higher. Furthermore, it was shown that patients who have lower risk scores using the Mayo model had a better early post-transplant survival rate. A reasonable option is to consider the patient for transplantation when the expected survival is between 1 and 2 years, taking into account the period of time on the waiting list and the risk of deterioration of the liver disease.

Primary biliary cirrhosis was the first disease to be universally accepted as an indication for liver transplantation, and presently it is considered that the timing of intervention should be set at the onset of the third clinical stage, when there is no prospect of spontaneous stabilization or recovery of the disease, but sufficiently early so as not to prejudice the outcome of transplantation. The major indication for liver transplantation is a serum bilirubin level over 100μmol/L (6mg/dL). At this level, the risk of death awaiting transplantation is under 15% and the median survival when serum bilirubin level is over 100μmol/L (6mg/dL) and 150μmol/L (9mg/dL) is of 24 and 17 months, respectively. Other indications include variceal bleeding not controlled by sclerotherapy or drug treatment, intractable ascites, and intolerable pruritus or lethargy, even if the latter symptoms are present in patients who have relatively early disease by other criteria.

The most common indications are related to jaundice and/or the complications of portal hypertension, and these account for approximately 50% of cases referred for transplantation. With the more widespread use of ursodesoxycholic acid as a medical treatment, the indication for liver transplantation has become less frequently determined by the serum bilirubin level and more frequently by the complications of portal hypertension and by liver failure. A few patients are transplanted because their quality of life is so poor despite all medical therapies that liver transplantation is considered to be indicated, mainly relating to severe lethargy and/or intolerable pruritus. In these cases, a cautious psychologic appraisal of the quality of life, and of the lethargy should be performed before referral for liver transplantation. Another small group of patients are transplanted primarily because of accelerated severe osteopenia.

The 10-year survival rate in these patients after transplantation is 80–90% and the risk of recurrence seems to be less than 10% at 5 years, even though the immunologic manifestations of the disease persists after transplantation. Whether or not the risk of recurrence is real, its impact on liver graft function is low, and in our own series of more than 100 patients transplanted for PBC since 1984, none have been retransplanted for PBC recurrence. Interestingly, there is a disappearance of pruritus immediately after transplantation in 100% of cases and of lethargy in 90% of cases. Clearly, liver transplantation not only increased survival, but also dramatically improved the quality of life.

Primary sclerosing cholangitis

Primary sclerosing cholangitis is a rare idiopathic cholestatic disease of unknown cause, characterized by a chronic fibrosing inflammation of the bile ducts. It is commonest in men under the age of 50 years, and is often associated with inflammatory bowel disease. It appears insidiously with pruritus, lethargy, and jaundice initially, but later leads to cholangitis, biliary cirrhosis, and portal hypertension. There is also an increased risk of cholangiocarcinoma, which is difficult to diagnose, with a prevalence over 30% after a 10-year disease course. Biliary drainage or biliary surgical reconstruction have been attempted with limited success only in those patients who have dominant extrahepatic strictures. The improvement is transient, and does not prevent evolution towards cirrhosis. Treatment with steroids or urso desoxycholic acid does not seem to modify the course of the disease. Primary sclerosing cholangitis has become a common indication for liver transplantation and accounts for nearly 10% of

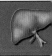

transplant activity in the USA, and it is the fourth most common indication in Europe in adults. Currently the main indications are:

- patients who have long-standing severe jaundice [bilirubin level over 100μmol/L (6mg/dL)], cholestasis, and pruritus not related to an acute episode of cholangitis;
- repeated episodes of cholangitis not controlled by antibiotics;
- established cirrhosis resulting in portal hypertension (ascites/esophageal varices) and/or liver failure (prothrombin less than 50% of normal value); and
- significant deterioration in the patient's quality of life.

There are still some remaining questions and limitations regarding liver transplantation for PSC. The natural course of the disease and the optimal timing of liver transplantation are not totally clear. Five independent clinical variables predictive of survival in PSC were identified: age; histologic stage on liver biopsy; serum bilirubin level; hemoglobin concentration; and presence or absence of inflammatory bowel disease. A recent report showed a 73% 5-year post-transplant survival rate, whereas the expected survival rate without transplantation was 28% (see Fig. 34.8). On the other hand, liver transplantation in PSC is still associated with higher morbidity and mortality due to prior surgical interventions (reported by most transplant centers), uncontrolled infection, undiagnosed cholangiocarcinoma, and, possibly, a higher risk of graft loss from chronic rejection.

Latent cholangiocarcinoma remains a problem. Cholangiocarcinoma can be a difficult differential diagnosis of PSC, while the latter can be complicated by the development of cholangiocarcinoma. Progression of the tumor is usually silent despite routine ultrasound examination and computed tomography (CT) scan, and patients who are otherwise good candidates for transplantation may have extrahepatic spread that precludes transplantation. In surgical specimens, the incidence of cholangiocarcinoma varied from 8 to 18%, and most of these tumors were not diagnosed before transplantation. Currently, accurate tools are lacking for the recognition of cholangiocarcinoma developing in PSC-affected livers and there is no particular clinical, morphologic or epidemiologic pattern associated with this increased risk. Rapid development of persistent jaundice and pruritus, a recent clinical deterioration with weight loss, increased CEA or CA 19–9 levels, and a long course of the disease (over 10 years) could suggest the development of malignancy, but better methods are still needed to diagnose malignancy at an early stage (Fig. 34.13 and 34.14). Patients who have coexisting inflammatory bowel disease should also have a colonoscopy at the time of assessment for transplantation to exclude colonic malignancy.

Primary sclerosing cholangitis associated with persistent jaundice, repeated episodes of cholangitis, established biliary cirrhosis (and its complications), and a long clinical course of the disease are the main guidelines to indicate transplantation. In addition, since the results of liver transplantation are good and the procedure radically changes the prognosis of the disease, patients should be referred early after the onset of liver symptoms in order to reduce the operative risk and to prevent the development of hepatobiliary malignancy. Cases of recurrence of PSC have been described, but this does not seem to affect the outcome of the graft. In contrast, PSC-like symptoms have also been observed after liver transplantation in patients transplanted for diseases unrelated to PSC, and the real significance of recurrent disease will only become apparent with long-term follow-up.

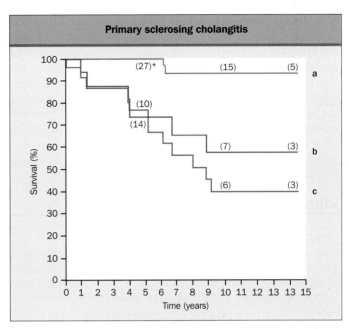

Figure 34.13 Primary sclerosing cholangitis. Survival from the time of onset of primary sclerosing cholangitis in patients not undergoing transplantation (c); in patients not undergoing transplantation after exclusion of those who had bile duct carcinoma at time of examination (b); and in patients treated by liver transplantation (a) at the Paul Brousse Center. (* actual patient numbers at that time point). (From Farges et al. Surgery. 1995;117:146–55.)

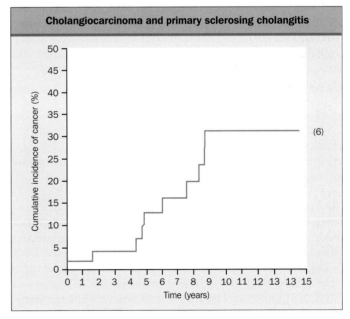

Figure 34.14 Cholangiocarcinoma and primary sclerosing cholangitis. Cumulative actuarial incidence of cholangiocarcinoma from time of onset of primary sclerosing cholangitis, emphasizing the increasing risk of developing cholangiocarcinoma. 6: number of patients at 15 years. (From Farges et al. Surgery. 1995;117:146–55.)

Secondary biliary cirrhosis

The main causes of secondary biliary cirrhosis are anatomic abnormalities of the bile ducts, intrahepatic gallstones or perioperative trauma of the extrahepatic bile ducts. Liver transplantation is indicated if surgical repair is not possible or after the development of secondary biliary cirrhosis when there is uncontrolled clinical cholestasis, jaundice, repeated episodes of cholangitis, and/or portal hypertension. The timing of liver transplantation can be particularly difficult, as relief of the underlying obstruction can lead to a dramatic stabilization of the liver disease. On the other hand, the timing of liver transplantation ideally should be before the occurrence of severe portal hypertension or severe liver failure with ascites. The highest operative risk is now seen in patients who have coexisting extensive intra-abdominal adhesions and portal hypertension, and these patients are prime candidates for this unfavorable combination.

VIRAL HEPATITIS

Chronic viral hepatitis is one of the most common causes of end-stage liver disease worldwide, and it is a frequent diagnosis in patients referred for liver transplantation. However, viral recurrence after liver transplantation is a major issue and viral reinfection may lead to graft failure, retransplantation or death.

Hepatitis B

Patients with cirrhosis due to HBV constitute a large group of candidates for liver transplantation (5–10% of all indications), although this is still controversial because of the risk of HBV persistence and infection of the graft after transplantation. The spontaneous prognosis of HBV cirrhosis may be difficult to determine. Although it is a progressive disease in the majority of cases, some patients present with an acute clinical deterioration at the time of viral reactivation or during the process of hepatitis B e antigen (HBeAg)/anti-HBe seroconversion. This can result in either irreversible liver failure and death, or a transient deterioration that is followed by an dramatic improvement of the liver disease. The main indications are similar to those for other liver diseases:

- recurrent ascites;
- spontaneous bacterial peritonitis;
- recurrent episodes of gastrointestinal bleeding not successfully controlled by medical treatment or ablative therapy;
- recurrent encephalopathy; and
- liver failure with a low level of albumin, elevated serum bilirubin, and low prothrombin level.

Recurrent HBV infection is one of the most severe complications after liver transplantation, and strategies to prevent reinfection have been developed. The spontaneous risk of HBV reinfection after transplantation is around 80%. The pretransplant HBV DNA status detected using conventional hybridization technique rather than HBeAg positivity is the best predictor of HBV recurrence after transplantation. Hepatitis B virus reinfection is the consequence of either an immediate reinfection of the graft due to circulating HBV particles, or of a reinfection of the graft from HBV particles coming from extrahepatic sites. Reinfection of the graft in patients receiving anti-HBs immunoglobulin (Ig) is probably related to HBV in extrahepatic sites. It may be the consequence of HBV overproduction at these extrahepatic sites, a low protective titer of anti-HBs Ig, or of emergence of escape mutants. This latter mechanism is probably important since mutations in the pre-S/S genome of HBV and in the 'a' determinant have been described.

Hepatitis B virus reinfection is characterized by the appearance of HBsAg and HBV DNA in the serum. After HBsAg reappearance, HBV replication levels are usually high, and large amounts of HBV particles are present in the graft. This HBV reinfection has a major deleterious impact on graft and patient survival. Almost all patients reinfected with HBV will develop graft disease, mostly an acute lobular hepatitis with evolution to chronic active hepatitis. Some cases follow a particularly severe clinical course leading to acute liver failure, probably related to the high amount of HBsAg, HBeAg, and hepatitis B core antigen (HBcAg) in the nuclei and cytoplasm of the hepatocytes. This is called fibrosing cholestatic hepatitis and is a unique clinical and histologic disease that is only seen in immunosuppressed patients.

HBV recurrence rate in relation to initial liver disease and HBV Ig administration			
Liver disease	No Ig (%)	Short-term Ig (%)	Long-term Ig (%)
HBV cirrhosis*	78	90	56
HBV DNA, HBeAg+	75	71	70
HBV DNA, HBeAg–	66	92	37
HDV cirrhosis*	70	56	17
FHF B	56	ND	0

Figure 34.15 Hepatitis B virus recurrence rate in relation to initial liver disease and HBV Ig administration. *$p<0.001$. FHF, fulminant hepatic failure B. (From Samuel et al. N Engl J Med. 1993;329:1842–7.)

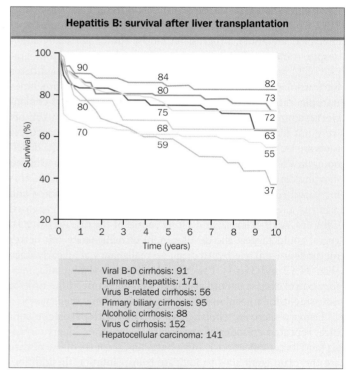

Figure 34.16 Hepatitis B: survival after liver transplantation. Actuarial 10-year survival after liver transplantation at Paul Brousse Hospital in 1106 patients transplanted from June 1984 to June 1997 in relation to the initial liver disease. Observe that using a policy of giving long-term administration of anti-HBs Ig, patients with B–D cirrhosis have the highest survival and those with B and C cirrhosis have the same survival. Patients who have hepatocellular carcinoma have the lowest survival and those with fulminant hepatitis have the lowest short-term survival due to higher postoperative mortality, but a relative stable survival curve in the long term. Numbers in key refer to number of patients in each group.

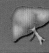

Since the natural history of recurrent HBV infection can be so devastating, particularly in patients who have active post-transplant viral replication, the administration of anti-HBs Ig as a prophylactic measure was proposed. Early studies of the use of anti-HBs Ig during the anhepatic phase and short-term post-transplant period yielded disappointing results as most of the patients developed HBV reinfection (Fig. 34.15).

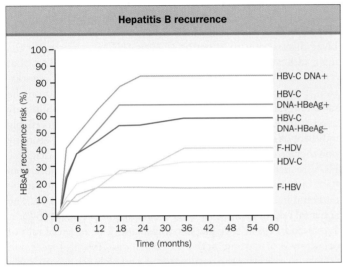

Figure 34.17 Hepatitis B recurrence. Hepatitis B virus recurrence risk in relation with the initial liver disease in a multicenter European trial on 372 patients. Note that patients with fulminant hepatitis B (F-HBV) have a 17% risk, those with B–D cirrhosis (HDV-C) a 32% risk, those with fulminant B–D hepatitis (F-HDV) a 40% risk, and those with B cirrhosis (HBV-C) a 67% risk (*p*<0.01). Among the group of patients with HBV-C, the risk of recurrence was significantly higher in those who were HBV DNA-positive (80%), than in those who were HBV DNA and HBeAg-negative. (From Samuel et al. N Engl J Med. 1993;329:1842–7.)

In contrast, the long-term administration of high doses of anti-HBs Ig dramatically reduced the rate of HBV recurrence. In a European multicenter study, the effect of long-term administration of anti-HBs Ig was clearly demonstrated by showing a dramatic decrease of the rate of HBV recurrence from 75% in patients receiving no or short-term administration of anti-HBs Ig, to 33% in those receiving long-term administration of anti-HBs Ig. In the most aggressive protocols, up to 10,000IU of anti-HBs Ig are given during the anhepatic phase, and repeated daily during the first six postoperative days. Then the level of anti-HBs is assessed weekly and doses of anti-HBs Ig readministered when anti-HBs is less than 100IU/L. This approach reduced the overall actuarial rates of reappearance of HBsAg in patients who had HBV cirrhosis to 17 and 29% at 1 and 2 years, respectively (Figs 34.16–34.19).

It is important to inhibit viral replication with antiviral therapy before transplantation, in order to clear HBV DNA from serum. An ideal treatment should have a rapid and potent antiviral action without provoking a deterioration of liver function. Alpha recombinant interferon is difficult to manage in many transplant candidates, and does not reduce HBV recurrence after liver transplantation. In a few cases, intravenous ganciclovir cleared HBV DNA from serum, but further evaluation in a controlled clinical trial is necessary to determine the safety and efficacy of this therapy. Lamivudine, a nucleoside analog, is the most effective currently available drug to clear HBV DNA from the serum in patients who have cirrhosis awaiting liver transplantation. The drug has also been given for 1 year after transplantation with promising short-term results and a low rate of HBV reinfection. The level of anti-HBs antibody that needs to be maintained in serum is a subject of debate. There was a general agreement that it should be at least 100IU/L, but this level may be insufficient in patients at high risk of recurrence such as HBV DNA-positive cirrhotic patients.

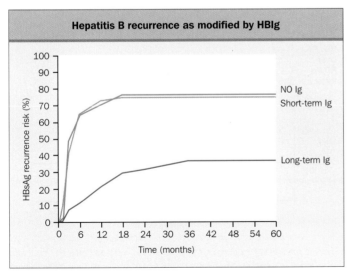

Figure 34.18 Hepatitis B recurrence as modified by HBIg. HBV recurrence risk in relation to the administration of anti-HBs immunoglobulin (HBIg) in a multicenter European trial. Note that patients receiving at least 6 months of HBIg have a significantly lower risk of HBV recurrence (32%) in contrast to those who receive either no or short-term prophylaxis (80% rate of HBV recurrence). (From Samuel et al. N Engl J Med. 1993;329:1842–7.)

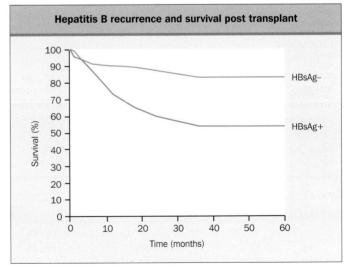

Figure 34.19 Hepatitis B recurrence and survival post transplant. Actuarial survival in patients in relation to HBV recurrence in a multicenter European trial. Those with HBV recurrence (HBsAg+) have a significantly lower survival rate, mostly due to HBV recurrence, than those without recurrence. This underlines the importance of prophylaxis against HBV. (From Samuel et al. N Engl J Med. 1993;329:1842–7.)

In this setting, the maintenance of anti-HBs antibody over 500IU/L may be able to prevent HBV recurrence, but this approach is both unproven and expensive. The consensus on the indications for liver transplantation for patients who have HBV-related liver disease is that those without HBV replication could be candidates if they receive a passive immunoprophylaxis against HBV for a minimum of 1 year and that patients who have active viral B replication should be included in protocols including antiviral treatment before transplantation followed by a combination of anti-HBs passive immunoprophylaxis and antiviral treatment after transplantation.

Hepatitis B and D

Patients chronically infected with HBV and hepatitis D virus (HDV) are at lower risk of HBsAg reappearance than patients chronically infected with HBV alone, and if reinfection does occur, the disease is less devastating than in patients who have solitary HBV infection. The rate of HBsAg reappearance in patients who have hepatitis B and D-associated cirrhosis was around 50–60% in patients who did not receive long-term administration of anti-HBs Ig, and was 13–17% in those receiving long-term anti-HBs Ig. The overall lower HBV recurrence rate in these patients compared with HBV cirrhotic patients is probably due to the fact that almost all patients who have HDV cirrhosis are HBV DNA-negative at the time of liver transplantation and that HDV has an inhibitory effect on HBV replication.

In this group of patients, there is a risk of reinfection with either HBV or HDV or with both viruses. The course of HDV reinfection and its consequences on the graft are different depending on whether HBsAg reappears or not. In the first post-transplant months, HDV reinfection assessed by the presence of HDV RNA in the serum or in the liver was observed in 80% of cases. With HBV recurrence, there is viral reactivation of both viruses(Fig. 34.20), but HBV–HDV recurrence is in general less severe than HBV recurrence alone. In patients who remained HBsAg negative after transplantation, HDV RNA was found transiently in serum and HDV antigen was detected in the liver. However, the amount of HDV antigen in the graft was low, the graft was histologically normal, and ultimately HDV markers progressively disappeared from the liver and serum (Fig. 34.21).

Hepatitis C

Liver disease due to hepatitis C virus (HCV) is currently the main indication for liver transplantation due to the fact that chronic HCV infection is a frequent cause of end-stage liver disease. Patient selection for liver transplantation is based on the same criteria as other causes of viral cirrhosis. Anti-HCV antibody persists in 90% of cases after transplantation and is not a reliable indicator of recurrence. The detection of HCV RNA in serum by polymerase chain reaction (PCR) is the best method to diagnose HCV recurrence. Hepatitis C virus RNA is found in more than 95% of patients transplanted for HCV cirrhosis, and it can be detected in serum as soon as the first post-transplant week. The actuarial rate of occurrence of acute lobular hepatitis was 57% at 1 year and 72% at 5 years post-transplant. The actuarial rate of occurrence of chronic active hepatitis was 25% at 1 year and 60% at 4 years after the occurrence of acute lobular hepatitis; 8% of the patients developed liver cirrhosis within 5 years of follow-up (Fig. 34.22).

In some series, the rate of HCV cirrhosis on the graft was as high as 20% at 5 years, and 26% at 8 years. It should be emphasized that the majority of the reinfected patients have a benign course and 20–40% of the patients have minimal or no lesions on

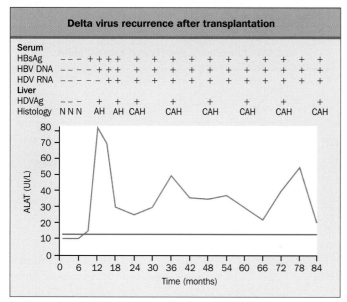

Figure 34.20 Delta virus recurrence after transplantation. Classic course of a patient transplanted for B–D liver cirrhosis with HBV recurrence. Note the concomitant reactivation of B and D infection and the development of chronic B–D hepatitis on the graft. This outcome is present in 10–15% of cases when HBIg is administered after transplantation. (From Samuel personal communication.)

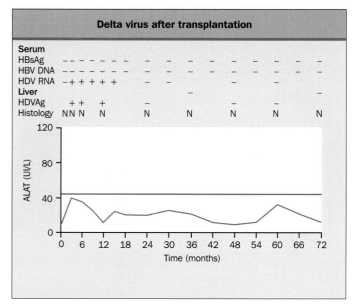

Figure 34.21 Delta virus after transplantation. Classical course of a patient transplanted for B-D liver cirrhosis without HBV recurrence. Note the presence of D antigen in the liver and HDV RNA in serum in the first months, despite the absence of HBsAg in serum; however there are no graft lesions and HDV markers disappeared after 2 years. This outcome is present in 90–85% of cases when HBIg is administered after transplantation. (From Samuel personal communication.)

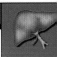

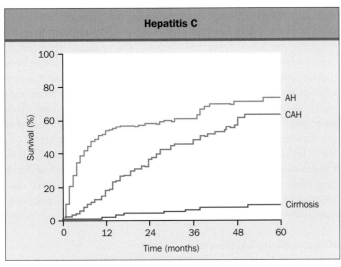

Figure 34.22 Hepatitis C. Actuarial rate of acute hepatitis (AH), chronic hepatitis (CAH), and cirrhosis in 140 patients transplanted at Paul Brousse hospital for HCV cirrhosis. Despite a 75% survival rate at 5 years, this emphasizes the need for a prevention of HCV recurrence after transplantation. (From Feray et al.. Hepatology. 1994;20:1137–43.)

histologic assessment of the graft. The actuarial 5-year patient survival rate is in the order of 75–80%.

After transplantation, HCV RNA levels may be increased by 10- to 100-fold, as a consequence of immunosuppressive therapy. The severity of HCV recurrence appears to be related to the level of HCV viremia after transplantation. An association between the genotype 1b and the occurrence of severe hepatitis was also observed. The rate of acute and chronic hepatitis was higher in patients infected with genotype 1b than with the other genotypes in several European centers, but the deleterious effect of the genotype 1b was not confirmed in the USA experience. Methods to prevent HCV infection after transplantation have yet to be identified and the long-term outcome remains unclear. Treatment of HCV reinfection in the graft using interferon or ribavirin or both are under evaluation, as are prophylactic regimens with these drugs.

ALCOHOLIC LIVER DISEASE

Alcoholic cirrhosis is the most frequently occurring liver disease and, although it accounted for a small proportion of liver transplant activity in the past, an increasing number of patients who have alcoholic liver disease are undergoing transplantation. It is believed that end-stage alcoholic liver disease will become the most common indication for transplantation in the USA in the near future. Alcohol is already the second most common indication for liver transplantation in USA and Europe after HCV related liver disease, and is now the leading indication in France. Nevertheless, current data indicate that with 11,000 deaths from alcoholic cirrhosis in the USA per year, only 6% of cases are receiving liver transplants. Given the limited supply of donor organs and some reluctance to transplant patients who have a 'self-inflicted' illness, several centers have developed an evaluation process (based on medical and psychiatric criteria) to identify patients who would most benefit from transplantation. The number of patients from the population who have

alcohol-related cirrhosis who are candidates for liver transplantation is still limited. There are several reasons for this.

- Although alcoholic disease itself is not a contraindication, many physicians do not select these patients for liver transplantation, and some centers are reluctant to transplant these patients, due to a concern about the ethics and legitimacy of the procedure and the risk of recidivism.
- In many patients, cirrhosis develops at a later age when transplantation is contraindicated.
- Alcohol is also the cause of extrahepatic diseases that will not be treated by transplantation.
- Most centers demand a 6-month alcohol abstinence before intervention.
- Some patients may show behavior patterns that suggest the compliance with long-term immunosuppressive therapy may be erratic.
- It is still difficult to determine the spontaneous prognosis of patients who have alcoholic liver disease and a dramatic clinical improvement can occur after 6 or more months of abstinence from alcohol.

In this context, guidelines for patient selection are currently directed at cirrhotic patients whose liver disease remains life-threatening despite a minimal period of 6 months of abstinence. This permits the re-evaluation of the need for, and timing of, liver transplantation and gives some insight into the patient's ability to control alcoholism when it coexists with alcoholic liver disease. This interval is neither a consensus nor an absolute requirement. Some period of sobriety is important, but it should not be used as the sole criterion and should be considered along with other psychosocial predictors of abstinence. In some cases the required duration of abstinence may allow some patients to escape transplantation because of a marked improvement of liver function. Patients participating in an alcohol counseling program with a stable and favorable psychosocial supportive environment are most often capable of avoiding recidivism and noncompliance with immunosuppressive therapy.

Acute alcoholic hepatitis is currently regarded as a contraindication in most centers because the majority of the patients with this condition are actively drinking at the time of presentation and have a higher risk of recidivism. Consequently, scarce donor organs would be allocated to patients who have a predictably inferior medical and psychiatric outcome. In selected cases, in whom the 6-month period of abstinence will be impossible to achieve because of the severity of the liver disease, candidacy for liver transplantation should be discussed on an individual basis. A positive selection decision needs to be supported by a self-recognition of alcoholism with a real desire for long-term cessation of alcohol consumption, in addition to a strong psychosocial and family support network and a positive appraisal by a psychiatrist.

Several reports suggest that the short-term outcome of liver transplantation in alcoholic cirrhosis is equivalent to that in non-alcoholics, although it remains unclear in patients who have acute alcoholic hepatitis. The risk of recidivism of alcoholism is estimated between 15 and 40%, and it seems to be related to the duration of abstinence before transplantation and the duration of follow-up after transplantation. Most patients with recidivism have a moderate drinking pattern after transplantation without consequences for the graft, but 5–10% of patients have severe recidivism with loss of compliance with medication, steatosis, and ultimately loss of the graft. The recidivism rates indicate the importance of stringent selection criteria in this context. Psychosocial support after transplantation is clearly needed. Additional studies of large numbers of patients are needed to determine the medical outcome of alcoholic liver disease and liver transplantation, as well as the long-term relapse rate with regard to alcohol consumption. An increased rate of de-novo cancer has been observed in patients transplanted for alcoholic cirrhosis, but the significance of this is unclear.

AUTOIMMUNE HEPATITIS AND CIRRHOSIS

Autoimmune hepatitis is more common in young women and is classified in three main groups:
- type 1 autoimmune hepatitis with positive antismooth muscle antibody;
- type 2 autoimmune hepatitis with positive antiliver, kidney, microsome-1 (anti-LKM-1) antibody; and
- type 3 autoimmune hepatitis with positive anti-soluble liver antigens (SLA) antibody.

The clinical presentation of the disease is variable, classically presenting as chronic hepatitis, but may also present as established cirrhosis and in a few cases as acute liver failure. The main characteristic of this disease is a good response to immunosuppressive treatment with steroids and azathioprine, particularly in type 1 patients.

Liver transplantation is indicated when there is clinical deterioration including the development of cirrhosis, esophageal varices, and impaired coagulation despite long-term adequate immunosuppressive treatment. More urgent clinical conditions include resistant ascites, spontaneous bacterial peritonitis, and encephalopathy. In this condition, it is essential to evaluate the severity as well as the activity of the disease. The level of liver enzymes and the histologic evaluation of the inflammatory infiltrate, together with intensity of hepatocyte necrosis and fibrosis, help to decide whether additional immunosuppressive treatment might improve the clinical condition and as a result postpone the need for transplantation. A short course of immunosuppressive treatment could be introduced under cautious supervision by transplant physicians, and in the absence of an improvement liver transplantation is indicated. Acute liver failure, in which immunosuppressive treatment is usually ineffective and potentially deleterious, is an indication for emergency liver transplantation.

The results of liver transplantation for autoimmune hepatitis are usually excellent with a 5-year survival rate over 80%. A higher risk of rejection has been reported and the role of corticosteroid treatment before transplantation in the occurrence of rejection has been debated. Some well-documented cases of recurrence have been described, but they usually respond to an increase in the corticosteroid component of the immunosuppressive regimen and rarely lead to graft failure and retransplantation of the liver.

HEPATOBILIARY MALIGNANCY

From the earlier days of liver transplantation, hepatobiliary malignancy was a favored indication for liver transplantation (Fig. 34.23). However, it is now a matter of some controversy because of the uncertain long-term benefit and results that are statistically inferior to those of liver transplantation for other diseases. The key concepts in the evaluation of the role of transplantation are the different tumor types and volumes, risk of tumor recurrence, donor organ shortage, and the role of immunosuppression in promoting tumor growth. In addition, there is debate about the use of liver transplantation as a curative treatment for liver malignancy, as opposed to its use as a palliative treatment which gives some patients additional years of good quality life. In the context of organ shortage, and an analysis of the results of transplantation, the latter view is not currently widely accepted. Contraindications to liver transplantation are advanced primary liver tumors with any extrahepatic spread, cholangiocellular carcinoma, hemangiosarcoma, and liver metastases from non-neuroendocrine primary tumors.

Hepatocellular carcinoma

Hepatocellular carcinoma (HCC), when left untreated, has an extremely poor prognosis with only 1–24 months survival from the time of diagnosis. Early enthusiasm for this indication for transplantation was frustrated by the high incidence of tumor recurrence, in excess of 50%, over 1–2 years of follow-up. Although there is a degree of variation, most centers currently practise a restrictive policy for transplantation for HCC (Fig. 34.24).

Improved criteria for patient selection have led to better results. The procedure is offered to patients who have fewer than three nodules that are smaller than 3–5cm in diameter, in the absence of lymph node metastases or vascular invasion (Fig. 34.25). Tumor size is a characteristic that has been reported by some centers, but not others, to influence prognosis. A series of 20 patients who have HCC and cirrhosis who underwent liver transplantation for tumors less than 6cm in diameter revealed that only two had died as a result of recurrent HCC over a median follow-up of 30 months, and that 60% of the patients had survived for at least 1 year. Others were able to demonstrate a significant effect of tumor size on survival after liver transplantation. The tumor diameter predicting survival without recurrence ranged from 3 to 5cm. Tumor invasion of the portal vein leading to intrahepatic metastasis is the most common means of HCC spread. A relationship between the risk of tumor recurrence and the presence of portal vein involvement has been established. The risk of recurrence was 100% when the tumor involved

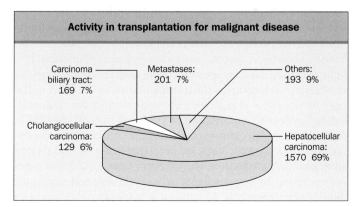

Figure 34.23 Activity in transplantation for malignant disease. The breakdown of indications shows a predominance of patients with hepatocellular carcinoma. (From The European Liver Registry Report, 1/1968–12/1997.)

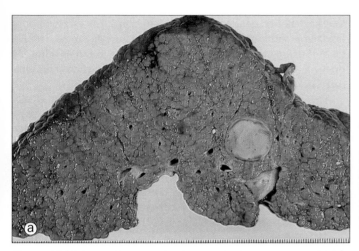

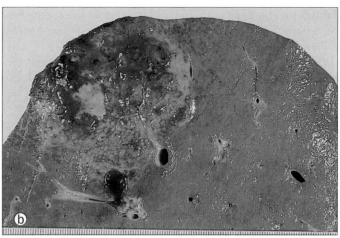

Figure 34.24 Transplantation for hepatocellular carcinoma. (a) The small, singular, circumscribed tumor in a patient with cirrhosis is an ideal candidate for transplantation, but the large tumor arising in a noncirrhotic liver (b) is no longer considered a good risk patient. (Courtesy of Professor B. Portmann.)

Overall 3-year survival rate and survival without recurrence in patients with hepatocellular carcinoma				
Liver disease	Resection (n=60)		Transplantation (n=60)	
	Survival (%)	Recurrence free survival (%)	Survival (%)	Recurrence free survival (%)
All patients	52	27	49	46
Size				
<3cm	39	18	60	56*
>3cm	56	32	43	39*
No. nodules				
1	53	28	46	20
>1	46	20	51	49
Combination				
< 3cm and 1–2 nodules	41	18	83	83
>3cm and >2 nodules			46	44

Figure 34.25 Overall 3-year survival rate and survival without recurrence in patients with hepatocellular carcinoma treated by resection or transplantation in relation to the size and the number of nodules. Note the excellent survival in those transplanted with less than three nodules of <3cm. *$p<0.05$. (From Bismuth et al. Ann Surg. 1993;218:145–51.)

the main portal vein or the two main intrahepatic portal branches. Although the recurrence rate was lower in cases of involvement of a smaller portal branch, the risk remained significant and this should be considered as a negative prognostic factor. For this reason, the possible involvement of the portal vein or its branches with a tumor needs to be carefully evaluated in potential transplant candidates.

Preoperative evaluation must include at least a CT scan of the abdomen and chest, and a bone isotope study. In the USA, patients are restaged at 3-month intervals after registering on the UNOS waiting list. Some centers perform an exploratory laparotomy before transplantation, in order to confirm the absence of extrahepatic spread. As soon as the transplant procedure begins,

it is essential to look for any sign of extrahepatic disease and to carefully inspect the hepatic pedicle for the presence of pathologic lymph nodes. A perioperative histologic analysis of suspicious tissue is mandatory, and the procedure should be stopped before the hepatectomy in cases of confirmed extrahepatic spread. Despite the uncertain long-term benefit in some cases, and the need to compare carefully the results obtained with liver transplantation with those of other methods (e.g. early resection, alcohol injection, chemoembolization), it is clear that liver transplantation is the only possible curative option in many cases of HCC associated with cirrhosis. The procedure in patients who have early disease is associated with a recurrence rate of 10% and a 5-year survival rate of 75%, which is similar to that achieved for other indications for liver transplantation. The size, the number of lesions, and the presence of portal involvement are the most important factors related to long-term survival.

Fibrolamellar carcinoma

This is a particular histologic variant of HCC that is more common in young women who have normal liver function. When a partial hepatectomy is not possible, liver transplantation is a good option, although there is a significant risk of recurrence since these tumors tend to be large at presentation and at transplantation. However, the slower tumor growth rates result in significant periods of survival, even when the tumor eventually recurs.

Cholangiocarcinoma

Cholangiocarcinoma is the second most common cancer among the primary hepatic neoplasms, accounting for 5–20% of liver malignancies. The ones that arise from the epithelium of the intrahepatic bile ducts are called 'true' cholangiocarcinoma as opposed to those that arise from the extrahepatic biliary tree. A clear association between cholangiocarcinoma and PSC has been established, and the occurrence of cholangiocarcinoma seems to correlate with the duration of the latter disease. Nowadays there is considerable debate about the indications for, and results of, transplantation for this kind of tumor. Liver transplantation does not offer either a cure or a significant duration of palliation in the majority of patients, except when the tumor is small and intrahepatic. This may be due to the fact that many of these tumors are diagnosed at an advanced stage, when the disease has metastasized to the lymph nodes. In the absence of lymph node disease, 1-year, 2-year, and 3-year survival rates of 77, 64, and 51% were observed, respectively. On the other hand, with lymph node disease the 1-year survival rate dropped to 14%, and the 2-year survival rate was 0%. Due to its high probability of recurrence, most centers no longer consider transplantation appropriate for cholangiocarcinoma.

Epithelioid hemangioendothelioma

Epithelioid hemangioendothelioma is a rare tumor of the liver that is generally multifocal and has an endothelial origin. It is more common in younger adults and is usually thought to be indolent in nature. In the absence of extrahepatic dissemination, liver transplantation should be considered. In an experience of 10 patients, the 3-month survival rate was 89%, with 3-year survival rates of 76%. The recurrence rate was 30%, although little is known about the factors affecting survival and recurrence following liver transplantation. It should be noted that metastatic spread at the time of surgery does not appear to be a contraindication to transplantation, and this is distinctly different from the situation in patients who have HCC or cholangiocarcinoma.

Metastatic liver disease

Classically, metastatic tumors of the liver have been considered a poor indication for liver transplantation, although some centers have performed this procedure in conjunction with other therapies, such as chemotherapy and radiotherapy. Several series demonstrated an unacceptably high recurrence rate with nonendocrine metastases that did not justify the cost of the procedure and utilization of scarce donors organs. On the other hand, in metastases from neuroendocrine tumors, liver transplantation could be indicated for patients who have symptoms related to massive hepatomegaly and syndromes related to hormone production. Effective therapeutic alternatives are usually not available and the typical candidate for transplantation has diffuse metastases of the liver, slow-growing tumors, and no extrahepatic disease. The main advantages of transplantation are a significant improvement of the quality of life in many patients and a possible cure in some of them. However, an inadequate knowledge of specific biologic and pathologic prognosis factors, the possibility of tumor growth as a consequence of immunosuppression, and the shortage of donor organs are key issues that counterbalance the argument in favor of transplantation. It is believed that long-term follow-up will confirm or refute the promising preliminary results obtained in liver transplantation for neuroendocrine liver metastases.

BUDD–CHIARI SYNDROME

The Budd–Chiari syndrome is a clinical disorder with a broad clinical spectrum resulting from the occlusion of the main hepatic veins at their junction with the inferior vena cava. The diagnosis is suggested by the absence of flow in the hepatic veins on ultrasonography and confirmed by the demonstration of thrombus on retrograde hepatic venography, together with changes in liver morphology.

Surgical portasystemic shunt, principally mesocaval, is the most commonly used treatment in all acute and subacute forms

that have not responded to other treatments. The effect of portasystemic shunting is to reduce portal pressure and induce reversal of the flow in the portal vein. The liver congestion is relieved, preserving hepatocytes and allowing liver regeneration. This ultimately leads to a reduction in the ascites.

The first liver transplantat for Budd–Chiari syndrome was performed in 1974, and the European Liver Transplant Registry records 224 liver transplantat for this disease from January 1988 to June 1997. In this context the indications for liver transplantation are the fulminant form of the disease associated with liver failure, which usually does not respond to mesocaval shunt surgery, and the chronic stage with established cirrhosis and its complications despite shunt procedures including transhepatic intrahepatic portal systemic shunt (TIPSS).

Although the choice of transplantation is appropriate for end-stage cirrhotic disease, it is difficult to ignore the efficacy of the long-term results of portasystemic shunting. Conclusions on the benefits of one treatment over another might be difficult due to the rarity of the disease, the wide variety of precipitating diseases, and the diversity of the clinical conditions. The final decision should be made taking into account the causative disease, a careful assessment of the degree of hepatic venous occlusion, and a precise grading of the clinical form of the disease and the hepatic dysfunction. If liver transplantation is performed, it is essential to identify and treat associated prothrombotic disease and adhere to a rigid protocol for long-term anticoagulant therapy.

ALVEOLAR ECHINOCOCCOSIS

Alveolar echinococcosis of the liver is an uncommon parasitic disease, endemic in Eastern France, Southern Germany, Western Austria, and large parts of Western Asia, Japan, Alaska, and Canada. Because of the very slow growth of the parasite, death occurs 10–15 years after the diagnosis has been established. The indications for liver transplantation are not clearly defined, but it should be considered in patients who have parasitic Budd–Chiari syndrome, patients who have complicated secondary biliary cirrhosis and in some cases where a radical hepatectomy cannot be performed due to extensive hepatic involvement. The optimal time for transplantation is difficult to define. However, uncontrolled biliary infections, previous abdominal surgery, lung metastases, portal vein and hepatic artery thrombosis are the main factors that increase the operative risks and may constitute contraindications to the procedure. Recurrence may occur related to the use of immunosuppressive therapy.

CYSTIC FIBROSIS

Cystic fibrosis is a multisystemic genetic disease with a gene carrier rate of 5% in the population. In spite of new medical therapies, life expectancy is approximately 50% at 30 years. Cirrhosis occurs in 5–15% of patients who have cystic fibrosis, with an onset in the first decade of life and later progression to portal hypertension, hypersplenism, and variceal bleeding. For these patients, liver transplantation, isolated or in combination with lung or heart–lung transplantation, is the only effective treatment option to prolong survival and the quality of life. Questions have been raised regarding the suitability of such candidates for liver transplantation, because these patients are often in a poor nutritional condition as a result of severe intestinal malabsorption

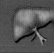

and chronic infection with highly resistant bacteria. However, postoperative management does not differ significantly from that of other patients undergoing liver transplantation, except for special attention to pulmonary care and the risk of malabsorption of immunosuppressive drugs.

CAROLI'S DISEASE

Caroli's disease is an uncommon congenital disorder of the intrahepatic biliary tree. It is characterized by multiple and segmental dilatations of the bile ducts. The clinical course is often complicated by recurrent episodes of cholangitis that seriously impair the patient's quality of life. Treatment is difficult and depends on the location and extent of the disease. Medical treatment is worthless because bile duct dilatation and gallstone formation favor bacterial persistence after the initial colonization of the biliary tree. Antimicrobial agents provide temporary improvement, but recurrence is the rule after cessation of this therapy. Bacterial cholangitis is the most frequent and life-threatening complication of the disease. Consequently, due to poor results of both medical and surgical therapies, liver transplantation has been proposed in complicated Caroli's disease that is diffuse within the liver, but to date only a small number of cases have been reported.

LIVER METABOLIC DISEASES

Wilson's disease

In this disease, there is copper deposition in the liver, the central nervous system, and the kidneys. This autosomal recessive hereditary disease is secondary to a gene mutation on chromosome 13 and results in hepatocyte inability to excrete copper in bile and consequently copper accumulates in the liver. There are four main clinical presentations of liver disease:

- active chronic hepatitis with a moderate increase in transaminases;
- decompensated liver cirrhosis with ascites and liver failure;
- acute liver failure with impaired coagulation, hemolytic anemia, and encephalopathy; and
- asymptomatic, when the diagnosis is made during the investigation of neurologic or other manifestations or following the diagnosis of Wilson's disease in a sibling.

Most frequently, this disease is medically treatable and the drug of choice is D-penicillamine, which acts as a chelant of copper and as a detoxificant of copper overload in hepatocytes. This therapy may arrest further progression of the disease and promote possible reversal of the clinical manifestations. However, liver transplantation may be indicated in the following situations:

- a fulminant course that almost invariably requires urgent transplantation;
- patients who have cirrhosis who fail to respond to 2–3 months of D-penicillamine therapy and supportive therapy for associated complications;
- progression of the disease despite D-penicillamine therapy; and
- severe hepatic failure and hemolysis after discontinuation of D-penicillamine therapy.

Generally, after liver transplantation, the copper balance is restored and there might be a reversal in both the neurologic and renal complications of the disease. The prognosis is good with no evidence of reaccumulation of hepatic copper.

α₁-Antitrypsin deficiency

The diagnosis is made by the finding of a significant reduction of serum α_1-antitrypsin levels, a positive Pi ZZ phenotype, and a diagnostic liver biopsy with periodic acid–Schiff-positive diastase-resistant cytoplasmic globules. One quarter of children who have Pi ZZ phenotype will develop neonatal cholestasis and among this group, 50% will develop progressive liver failure at some time during childhood or adolescence. More than 50% of adults have coexistent pulmonary disease associated with α_1-antitrypsin deficiency, but the lung disease is usually mild. Clinical signs of neonatal cholestasis appear during the first days of life and are usually evident before 10 weeks of age. As there is no effective replacement therapy, liver transplantation is indicated in patients who have cirrhosis and progressive hepatic decompensation. After liver transplantation, α_1-antitrypsin level returns to normal and the 5-year actuarial survival rate after transplantation is higher than 80%.

Hereditary tyrosinemia

This disease is characterized by progressive hepatocellular damage, renal tubular dysfunction, hypophosphatemia, and urinary excretion at concentrations of more than 100 times the normal rate of the tyrosine metabolite succinylacetone. Hepatic fibrosis develops with prominent regeneration nodules, leading to cirrhosis. Survival beyond the age of 10 years is rare. Up to 37% of children over the age of 2 years will develop HCC.

Medical treatment has not proved to be effective. Consequently, liver transplantation was suggested in order to correct the biochemical abnormalities and allow patients to have a normal protein intake. In patients presenting with the disease in early infancy, transplantation should be postponed for as long as possible to allow the baby to grow. In those who have a later onset of symptoms, the timing of grafting is difficult as delay may increase the risk of developing HCC. The UNOS criteria recommend pre-emptive transplantation before the second birthday. Prospective screening with ultrasound examination of the liver and serum α-fetoprotein estimates may be useful to detect tumors early enough to allow liver transplantation.

Crigler–Najjar syndrome

This is an inherited disorder that occurs in two forms (type I and II), characterized by severe, life-long, nonhemolytic, unconjugated hyperbilirubinemia. Liver transplantation is not indicated in the type II syndrome, which can be treated with continuous phenobarbital (phenobarbitone) therapy. In type I syndrome, the serum bilirubin concentration does not decrease when phenobarbital is administered. The majority of infants will develop kernicterus and die in the first 18 months of life, but the onset of kernicterus and progressive brain damage may be delayed until puberty or the early twenties. Liver transplantation may be indicated when there is failure to control the kernicterus despite extensive phototherapy, or in cases of poor quality of life due the need for prolonged phototherapy. Auxiliary partial orthotopic liver transplantation has also been performed successfully. As irreversible brain damage has been described, the optimal timing for liver transplantation is important, in order to reduce neurologic sequelae and improve survival after transplantation.

Hereditary hemochromatosis

Hereditary hemochromatosis is a recessive autosomal disorder leading to iron overload with a disease frequency of 5 per 1000 population. The disease is secondary in 95% of cases to a point mutation (Cys 282Y) in the H gene located on chromosome 6. It is characterized by increased intestinal iron absorption with deposition of parenchymal iron in the liver, heart, pancreas, pituitary and joints, and a potential risk for developing cirrhosis and HCC. Liver transplantation is indicated for hemochromatosis complicated by liver failure or the presence of HCC not treatable by resection. However, the survival of patients undergoing liver transplantation for hemochromatosis is less favorable, due to cardiac problems and the frequent coexistence of HCC. Pretransplant phlebotomy to reduce cardiac complications needs to be carefully evaluated, to determine whether it can improve survival after liver transplantation. The risk of reappearance of iron deposits in the liver is debatable.

Protoporphyria

This is an autosomal dominant disorder characterized by photosensitivity and elevated levels of protoporphyrin in erythrocytes, plasma and feces. It is secondary to a deficiency in an enzyme responsible for heme synthesis called heme synthase or ferrochelatase. The pathogenesis of liver disease is still unclear, but is probably the consequence of accumulation of protoporphyrin pigments in the liver. Liver transplantation should be considered when jaundice, recurrent cholangitis or liver failure occur. After transplantation a dramatic, but partial, decrease in plasma and erythrocyte levels of protoporphyrins is obtained, and this leads to a partial or complete resolution of photosensitivity. Some patients may develop recurrent disease in the graft, but long-term survival without recurrence has also been described.

Gaucher's disease

This is the most common inherited glycolipid storage disease and is due to lysosomal B-glucocerebrosidase deficiency. This autosomal recessive disorder is characterized by excessive accumulation of glucocerebrosidase in mononuclear phagocytic lysosomes throughout the body. The adult chronic form has no central nervous system involvement and can be compatible with a normal life span in the absence of cirrhosis. Although liver transplantation is not a definite treatment for Gaucher's disease, it seems to be useful in the management of the complications of cirrhosis, resulting in a marked clinical and biochemical improvement. Post-transplantation morphologic studies did not demonstrate evidence of recurrent deposits in a short-term follow-up.

Primary hyperoxaluria

Primary hyperoxaluria is a rare autosomal recessive disorder characterized by hyperoxaluria, calcium oxalate urinary lithiasis, nephrocalcinosis and early death from renal failure. There are at least two types, and type 1 is much more common and well-studied. Type 1 primary hyperoxaluria is secondary to a hepatic deficit in alanine-glyoxylate aminotransferase deficiency. Renal transplantation in isolation results in almost universal recurrence of oxalosis in the kidney graft and a return to hemodialysis. Combined liver and kidney transplantation treats both the renal failure and cures the cause of the disease, and this approach may avoid recurrence of oxalosis in the kidney graft. However, this presumes the kidney graft functions sufficiently well to clear the excess pool of calcium oxalate, but this does not necessarily occur before further damage to the graft occurs. Combined liver and kidney transplantation should be performed before the occurrence of severe complications, and the ideal timing is just before or immediately after the patients are initiated on hemodialysis. Long periods of hemodialysis will significantly increase the pool of calcium oxalate in the body. Some authors have advocated an isolated liver transplantation early in the course of the disease before the occurrence of renal failure, but this pre-emptive therapeutic approach remains controversial.

Familial amyloid polyneuropathy

This is a hereditary systemic condition with an autosomal dominant pattern, usually involving the peripheral nervous system. The genetic defect is a single mutation located on chromosome 18, leading to the synthesis of a variant transthyretin (also called prealbumin) that is found in plasma. It takes an amyloid form and is deposited in neural and visceral tissues. The disease usually starts between 30 and 40 years of age. There is no medical treatment and patients usually die at a median of 10 years after the onset of symptoms. The principle of liver transplantation to treat familial amyloid polyneuropathy is to suppress the production of the transthyretin variant which is mainly of hepatic origin, thus stopping the evolution of the disease leading to clinical improvement. The main indication is when the disease is at an early stage clinically. Liver transplantation is not indicated in asymptomatic patients or advanced cases.

PEDIATRIC LIVER TRANSPLANTATION

Liver transplantation is a well-accepted treatment for children with end-stage liver disease (Fig. 34.26). Evaluation and appropriate patient selection for transplantation are becoming

Indications for liver transplantation in children	
Chronic liver disease	Cholestatic diseases Extrahepatic biliary atresia Byler's disease Ductopenia (nonsyndromic) Alagille syndrome Primary sclerosing cholangitis Autoimmune chronic active hepatitis Viral B cirrhosis Budd–Chiari syndrome
Metabolic liver disease	α_1 antitrypsin 1 defect Hereditary tyrosinemia Criggler–Najjar type 1 Protoporphyria Type 1 and 4 glycogenosis Galactosemia
Primary malignant tumor of the liver	Hepatocellular carcinoma Hepatoblastoma Cholangiocellular carcinoma
Acute liver failure	Fulminant and subfulminant hepatitis Wilson's disease (fulminant) Budd–Chiari syndrome (fulminant)

Figure 34.26 Indications for liver transplantation in children.

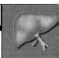

increasingly important issues as more and more children are submitted to the procedure (Fig. 34.27). The main selection criteria for liver transplantation are:

- severe jaundice;
- intractable variceal hemorrhage;
- liver failure manifested as vitamin K-resistant coagulopathy, malnutrition, and hypoalbuminemia;
- hepatic encephalopathy; and
- severe malaise, weakness, and failure to grow.

The results of transplantation in children are better than those in adults, with a 1-year survival rate of over 90% and with little further change in up to 5-years of follow-up. In addition, liver transplantation results in a dramatic improvement in quality of life, resumption of daily activities including education, psychologic transformation, and a complete reintegration into society. In some critical clinical situations, such as age under 1 year, congenital anatomic abnormalities, multiple organ injuries, and malnutrition, the outcome is not as good.

The small number of pediatric donors available has necessitated the use of partial or reduced adult grafts or grafts from living related donors. There is a higher incidence of hepatic artery thrombosis after liver transplantation, and this is the main difference between pediatric and adult transplantation The exact timing of the procedure may be difficult, but if possible it should be performed in children at least 1-year-old and over 10kg in weight. On the other hand, delayed intervention can be associated with progressive complications and clinical deterioration of the patient.

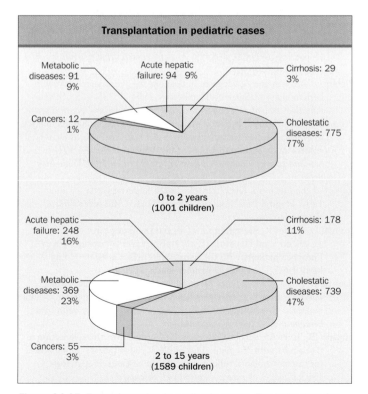

Figure 34.27 Transplantation in pediatric cases. The indications for liver transplantation up to the age of 2 years and in older children. (From The European Liver Registry Report, 5/1968–6/1997.)

Extrahepatic biliary atresia

Biliary atresia is the most frequent cause of chronic cholestasis in infants, affecting 1:8,000 to 1:12,000 live births. It is a panbiliary disease of both the intrahepatic and extrahepatic biliary tree, probably the end result of a destructive inflammatory process leading to fibrosis and obliteration of the biliary tract. When left untreated, this condition leads to death from liver failure in early childhood, with an average survival of 12–19 months. Fewer than 10% of patients not undergoing surgery survive beyond 3 years.

The best primary treatment of biliary atresia remains controversial because of the limited efficacy of Kasai portoenterostomy, the success of liver transplantation, and the greater technical difficulty of transplantation in patients who have multiple previous surgical procedures. Currently, liver transplantation for biliary atresia represents 35–67% of the reported series of pediatric liver transplantation and between 5–10% of the total indications for the procedure. The first-line treatment should be a Kasai portoenterostomy before the age of 8–10 weeks by an experienced pediatric surgical team. Generally speaking, 25–30% of children who underwent a Kasai procedure had a restoration of bile flow, with resolution of cholestasis and no progression to cirrhosis. The remaining 70–75% are potential candidates for liver transplantation because restoration of bile flow was not obtained.

The current criteria for liver transplantation are an immediate failure of the Kasai procedure (30–40% of the total), leading to transplantation before 3 years of age or secondary failure (30–35% of the total) with recurrence of jaundice, leading to transplantation at a variable age. These patients develop portal hypertension and uncontrolled bleeding, uncontrolled cholangitis, intolerable pruritus, and liver failure.

The timing of liver transplantation is based on the patient's clinical condition. The procedure must be performed before the onset of liver failure, irreversible complications, and deteriorating nutritional status. If possible, it is preferable to postpone the procedure until the infant reaches 1 year of age or weighs 10kg, because the survival rates increase from 50–60% to 80% if the transplant is performed after 1 year of age. Recurrence of the disease after liver transplantation has not been observed. It has become clear that the Kasai procedure and liver transplantation are complementary treatments for biliary atresia and that transplantation should be considered for cases of early or late failure of portoenterostomy. The ultimate aims of liver transplantation in these patients are the return to full quality of life and normal development.

Interlobular bile duct paucity

Two types of paucity of interlobular bile ducts are described: a syndromic type, the most common being called Alagille's syndrome, with the presence of at least two major extrahepatic associated features; and a nonsyndromic type that is secondary to multiple viral or metabolic insults to the liver. As liver failure is rarely responsible for death in the syndromic type, liver transplantation is rarely indicated. On the other hand, there is a progressive biliary cirrhosis and liver failure in the nonsyndromic type, and liver transplantation is the only available therapy, being indicated at any age in which liver failure becomes clinically manifest.

Byler's disease

This is a poorly understood disease for which the biochemical basis is still unknown. Clinically, it is characterized by hepatocyte failure to excrete bile, without any anatomic or histologic biliary abnormalities. Recently the use of ursodesoxycholic acid has been shown to improve cholestasis and liver function in some patients. When secondary biliary cirrhosis and liver failure develop, liver transplantation should be considered.

RETRANSPLANTATION

Due to the shortage of organ donors, the indications for retransplantation are controversial. Survival after retransplantation is lower than that after primary transplantation at around 50% at 1 year. Emergency retransplantation during the first week should be differentiated from later retransplantation. The indications for the former are in general primary graft nonfunction, thrombosis of the hepatic artery and, more rarely, acute rejection. The causes of later retransplantation are chronic rejection, long-term biliary consequences of arterial thrombosis, and hepatitis C or B recurrence in the graft. In these cases, survival is more dependent on the condition of the patient at the time of retransplantation, rather than on the indication for retransplantation. In general the transplant should not be done too late, in order to offer the patient a reasonable chance of success. Retransplantation for HBV recurrence is generally considered to be contraindicated, due to a very high risk of HBV recurrence and of an accelerated and fatal course of reinfection in the second graft. However, an aggressive antiviral approach may improve the prognosis.

FURTHER READING

Alagille D. Liver transplantation in children . Indications in cholestatic states. Transplant Proc. 1987;vol XIX:3242–8. *Pioneering description of role of liver transplantation in pediatric cholestatic liver disease.*

Belle SH, Beringer KC, Detre KM. Liver transplantation for alcoholic liver disease in the United States: 1988 to 1995. Liver Transplant Surg. 1997;3:212–9. *Detailed analysis of issues related to transplantation for alcohol related liver disease in the US.*

Benhamou JP. Indications for liver transplantation in primary biliary cirrhosis. Hepatology. 1994;20:11S–3S. *Thoughtful assessment of the role of liver transplantation in primary biliary cirrhosis.*

Bismuth H, Chiche L, Adam R, Castaing D, Diamond T, Dennisson A. Liver resection versus transplantation for hepatocellular carcinoma in cirrhotic patients. Ann Surg. 1993;218:145–51. *Useful experience in what is still a controversial area.*

Farges O, Malassagne B, Sebagh M, Bismuth H. Primary sclerosing cholangitis: liver transplantation or biliary surgery. Surgery. 1995;117:146–55. *Another controversial topic.*

Feray C, Gigou M, Samuel D, et al. The course of hepatitis C virus infection after liver transplantation. Hepatology. 1994;20:1137–43. *Early study of the impact of hepatitis C after transplantation.*

Feray C, Gigou M, Samuel D, et al. Influence of the genotypes of hepatitis C virus on the severity of recurrent liver disease after liver transplantation. Gastroenterology. 1995;108:1088–96. *Valuable data on the effect of genotype on outcome after transplantation for hepatitis C.*

Hadni SB, Franza A, Miguet JP, et al. Orthotopic liver transplantation for incurable alveolar echinococcosis of the liver: report of 17 cases. Hepatology. 1991;13:1061–9. *A good discussion of a rare indication for liver transplantation.*

Harrison J, McMaster P. The role of liver transplantation in the management of sclerosing cholangitis. Hepatology. 1994; 20:14S–9S. *A good insight into a difficult topic.*

Holmgren G, Ericzon BG, Groth CG, et al. Clinical improvement and amyloid regression after liver transplantation in hereditary transthyretin amyloidosis. Lancet. 1993;341:1113–16. *Early description of an interesting indication for liver transplantation.*

Jury of The Conference of Consensus on the Indications of Liver Transplantation. Consensus statement on indications for liver transplantation: Paris, June 22–3 1993. Hepatology. 1994;20:63S–8S. *A summary of attempts to reach consensus in a number of controversial areas in liver transplantation.*

Markus BH, Dickson ER, Grambsch PM, et al. Efficacy of liver transplantation in primary biliary cirrhosis. N Engl J Med. 1989;320:1709–13. *An early example of a critical analysis of the results of liver transplantation in a particular indication.*

O'Grady JG, Polson RJ, Rolles K, Calne RY, Williams R. Liver transplantation for malignant disease. Results in 93 consecutive patients. Ann Surg. 1988;207:373–9. *An early clinical experience that outlined many of the principles that still apply in malignancy.*

Otte JB, De Ville de Goyet J, et al. Sequential treatment of biliary atresia with Kasai portoenterostomy and liver transplantation: a review. Hepatology. 1994;20:41S–8S. *A useful contribution to what is still a controversial debate.*

Pichlmayr R, Weimann A, Ringe B. Indications for liver transplantation in hepatobiliary malignancy. Hepatology. 1994;20:33S–40S. *Another valuable clinical experience in transplantation for malignant disease.*

Poynard T, Barthelemy P, Fratte S, et al. for a multicentre group. Evaluation of efficacy of liver transplantation in alcoholic cirrhosis by a case-control study and simulated controls. Lancet. 1994;344:502–7. *Seminal paper on the role of liver transplantation in alcoholic liver disease.*

Report of the European Liver Transplantation Registry; Updating June 1997. Hopital Paul Brousse, Villejuif, France. *Valuable source of data in Europe.*

Samuel D, Muller R, Alexander G, et al. and the European Concerted Action on Viral Hepatitis (EUROHEP). Liver transplantation in European patients with the hepatitis B surface antigen. N Engl J Med. 1993;329:1842–7. *Another seminal paper.*

Samuel D, Zignego AL, Reynes M, et al. Long-term clinical and virologic outcome after liver transplantation for cirrhosis due to chronic delta hepatitis. Hepatology. 1995;21:333–9. *A good study on delta virus behaviour after liver transplantation.*

Smanik EJ, Tavill AS, Jacobs GH, et al. Orthotopic liver transplantation in two adults with Niemann–Pick and Gaucher's disease: implications for the treatment of inherited metabolic diseases. Hepatology. 1993;17:42–9. *A rare indication well discussed.*

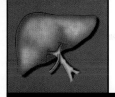

Chapter 35

The Transplant Operation

Milan Kinkhabwala and Jean Crawford Emond

INTRODUCTION

The evolution of the liver transplant operation over the past 30 years has required the resolution of a spectrum of physiologic and technical problems. The first description of experimental liver transplantation is attributed to CS Welch, who performed transplantation of the whole canine liver. These initial experimental efforts were based on the assumption that total removal of the native liver would be a prohibitive undertaking and therefore the graft was placed next to the native liver in an *auxiliary* position. The general procedure of *orthotopic* liver replacement in humans was defined within a decade of the initial attempt by Starzl in 1963, but the transition to gradual acceptance was associated with continued technical modifications, leading to more dependable outcomes.

Because the early attempts at liver transplantation in humans were uniformly unsuccessful, clinical liver transplantation was halted in a self-imposed moratorium until 1967, when improvements in surgical technique, organ preservation, and intraoperative management led to renewed attempts. Although success was achieved, consistent long-term survival remained elusive and liver replacement remained an impractical therapy for the majority of patients with liver disease, until cyclosporine became available for clinical use. Cyclosporine, introduced in 1979, improved 1-year graft survival from less than 50% to over 70%, spurring a proliferation of liver transplant programs worldwide. In 1983 liver transplantation was reviewed at a US National Instituties of Health Consensus Conference and designated as the optimal therapy for end-stage liver disease.

Modifications in liver transplantation technique continue to this day. Among the most important developments was the introduction of venous bypass in 1983, in response to the significant hemodynamic instability that was common during the anhepatic phase of the transplant procedure. While some centers no longer use routine venous bypass, its widespread acceptance in the 1980s contributed to a reduction in operative mortality and allowed liver transplantation to achieve greater acceptance as a therapeutic modality. In addition to venous bypass, other key developments in liver transplantation included simplification of the multiorgan retrieval operation in the donor, and the introduction of the University of Wisconsin preservation solution. These advances collectively mitigated the logistic constraints of the transplant procedure and facilitated training of new transplant surgeons.

Living-related and split liver transplantation were developed in the 1980s as a result of a stepwise progression of surgical innovations driven by a scarcity of donors for small children. Both of these modalities are now accepted worldwide; in many centers they account for the majority of liver transplants performed in children. More recently these techniques in partial liver transplantation have been further extended to adults, a trend that has also been driven by a scarcity of donor organs. Auxiliary liver transplantation, in which part or all of the native liver is preserved, has been rediscovered in recent years with several potential applications. In this chapter these diverse procedures are reviewed, thus displaying the range of possibilities available to the transplant surgeon. In addition, a flexible approach is described, in which the array of procedures can be adapted to address specific indications in liver disease, although the detail of a technical atlas is beyond the scope of this text.

ORGANIZATION OF THE OPERATING ROOM FOR LIVER TRANSPLANTATION

Because of the unpredictable and often urgent nature of liver transplantation, most transplant centers utilize dedicated liver transplant operating rooms with surgical teams available around the clock. The complexity of the procedure demands a complete understanding of the operation and its potential complications by specialized nursing and anesthetic teams. While costly in terms of personnel, the expense is well justified, because even small errors in functional efficiency can lead to disastrous outcomes. The consistently high survival rates in current practice have been achieved by widespread adherence to these standards. Nowhere is this high standard in the operating room more dramatic than in the role of the liver transplant anesthetist, whose interventions must address profound alterations in homeostasis caused by the failing liver, support the circulation during periods of massive blood loss, and overcome the occasional bouts of cardiac dysfunction and arrhythmias associated with reperfusion.

Immediate access to support services for the liver transplant operating room is essential. These services include clinical laboratory, blood bank, telephone links for in-hospital and out-of-hospital calls, refrigeration for preservation solutions and stored vascular conduits, and access to advanced monitoring devices such as transesophageal echocardiography. The operating room itself should be large enough to accommodate all of the equipment, instrumentation, and personnel that are present during the transplant operation; 900 square feet is a desirable operating room size. The patient table must be electrically controlled rather than manual in order to facilitate rotation of the patient during the operation. Two modern electrosurgical units and an argon beam coagulator should be available and functional at all times. A rapid infusion system permits rapid correction of volume losses,

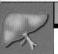

and when bypass is used the bypass pump can also serve as a reservoir for rapid infusion of blood products. We also utilize a cell saver system to reduce blood product requirements. A sterile slush machine is required, particularly if extensive *ex vivo* surgery is required to prepare the allograft. A spectrum of cannulas and other supplies for cardiovascular procedures is required when venous bypass is used

The instrument trays should include both vascular and general surgical instruments: these trays should be open on the field for every case. Vascular trays should include instruments for fine anastomoses such as the portal vein and artery, as well as larger instruments for the vena cava. We have added a microvascular instrument set to our instrument list, which has been particularly useful for small hepatic arterial and biliary anastamoses. Several sets of mechanical retractors should be available in the inventory so that there are no delays for sterilization when multiple cases are performed. For pediatric cases, an operating microscope should be available, as it has become standard for arterial anastamoses in many centers, particularly for living donor transplants

CADAVERIC DONOR HEPATECTOMY

Most organs for transplantation are now procured from multiple-organ donors. Consequently, abdominal transplant surgeons must be skilled in the safe procurement of the liver, kidneys, and pancreas. The donor operation has evolved greatly from the classical method, in which most of the dissection was performed *in situ* ('warm') before cooling and removal of the organs. Today most donor surgeons utilize variations of the rapid flush/en-bloc retrieval technique, in which cold perfusion of the organs with preservation solution is performed first, followed by dissection and removal of the organs under asanguinous conditions. Additionally, organs are retrieved 'en bloc', in groups of grape-like clusters that are based on common vascular pedicles. The individual organs can then be separated on the back table under controlled conditions. These modifications have greatly simplified the abdominal donor operation, which has facilitated utilization of cadaver organs.

In performing donor hepatectomy, the surgeon is faced with two general tasks: first, direct assessment of the donor liver for suitability; second, removal of the liver and its hilar structures without injury. Hypoxic injury due to donor hemodynamic instability, macrovesicular steatosis, cirrhosis, and carcinoma are potential conditions for which the surgeon may choose to discard the liver during direct assessment. When additional information is required, an intraoperative frozen section biopsy may be obtained to investigate suspected liver pathology.

Donor hepatectomy is performed through a long midline abdominal incision and median sternotomy (Fig. 35.1). The pericardium and right pleural spaces are opened for later exsanguination through the vena cava. The abdomen is explored to exclude incidental malignancy. The suprahepatic vena cava is exposed by division of the falciform and triangular ligaments. The left lateral segment is mobilized, exposing the gastrohepatic ligament. An accessory left hepatic artery, if present, is carefully protected. Limited dissection of the porta hepatis is then performed in order to expose the common bile duct, which is divided distally. The extrahepatic biliary tree is flushed with saline through an incision in the gallbladder, in order to

prevent bile-induced autolysis of the biliary epithelium during storage (Fig. 35.2).

The terminal ileum, right colon and duodenum are mobilized medially by sharp dissection along the peritoneal reflection. This maneuver affords complete exposure of the retroperitoneum. The origins of the renal veins are identified on the vena cava, and the distal aorta is encircled with a tape for later cannulation. In conventional retrieval, precooling of the liver with cold crystalloid solution is accomplished by introduction of a small catheter in the portal circulation, usually the inferior mesenteric vein (IMV) (Fig. 35.3). This same catheter is then used later in the procurement as a conduit to flush the portal vein with preservation solution. Some centers, including our own, perform neither 'precool' nor *in situ* portal flush during en-bloc liver/pancreas procurement, avoiding the need for an IMV catheter. In this modification the *in situ* flush is performed only through the arterial circulation, with the portal flush performed on the back table immediately after retrieval.

In the final step before *in situ* flush, the supraceliac aorta is encircled with a tape at the level of diaphragmatic crus. The donor is then fully heparinized and a large-bore cannula inserted into the distal aorta (see Fig. 35.3). The donor is exsanguinated through a large venting incision in the vena cava, while the supraceliac aorta is simultaneously clamped and cold preservation solution flushed through the aortic and portal cannulae, allowing rapid core cooling of the abdominal organs. Concomitantly, topical cooling is accomplished by instilling ice slush into the peritoneum. Once the caval effluent has cleared, the organs have been adequately flushed. The organs can now be removed sequentially: thoracic organs first, liver/pancreas second, and kidneys last.

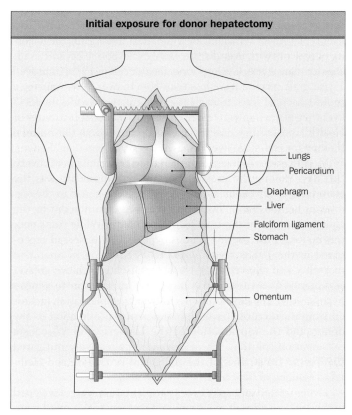

Initial exposure for donor hepatectomy

Lungs
Pericardium
Diaphragm
Liver
Falciform ligament
Stomach
Omentum

Figure 35.1 Initial exposure for donor hepatectomy.

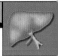

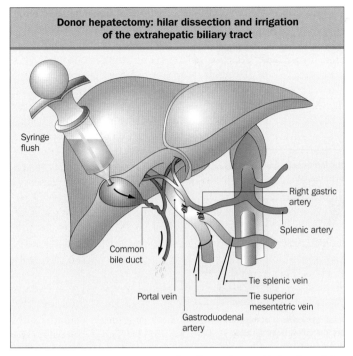

Donor hepatectomy: hilar dissection and irrigation of the extrahepatic biliary tract

Syringe flush

Right gastric artery

Splenic artery

Common bile duct

Portal vein

Tie splenic vein

Tie superior mesentetic vein

Gastroduodenal artery

Figure 35.2 Donor hepatectomy: hilar dissection and irrigation of the extrahepatic biliary tract.

The liver is removed by first dividing the diaphragm circumferentially, encompassing the suprahepatic vena cava and the dome of the liver. The circular cuff of diaphragm is removed from the liver and cava during back-table preparation of the liver. The common hepatic artery is identified along the superior border of the pancreas and dissected proximally to the celiac trunk, sequentially ligating the principal branches: gastroduodenal, left gastric, and splenic arteries. The origin of the celiac trunk on the aorta is identified and a circular patch of aorta is fashioned around the origin ('Carrell patch'). Knowledge of variations in hepatic arterial anatomy is crucial to safe hepatectomy (Fig. 35.4).

The portal vein is divided at its origin behind the pancreas, ensuring adequate length for the recipient operation. The remainder of the porta hepatis is then divided, with careful attention to identification and preservation of an accessory right hepatic artery. In our technique, the existence of an accessory right hepatic artery is investigated by mobilizing the superior mesenteric artery (SMA) at the root of the mesentery; the SMA can be dissected along its right border in order to identify any vessels that emerge from within the first few centimeters of the aorta. If an accessory right hepatic artery is identified, the entire length of the vessel together with a trunk of SMA can be procured in order to facilitate back-table reconstruction.

In the final step, the infrahepatic vena cava is divided above the renal veins. The liver is then removed and placed in storage containers for transport. Before closing the abdomen, lengths of iliac artery and vein are procured for potential use as vascular conduits in the recipient.

ORTHOTOPIC LIVER TRANSPLANTATION

As described above, orthotopic liver transplantation (OLT) has largely evolved from Starzl's pioneering efforts in the 1960s. Like most difficult operative endeavors, technical success requires

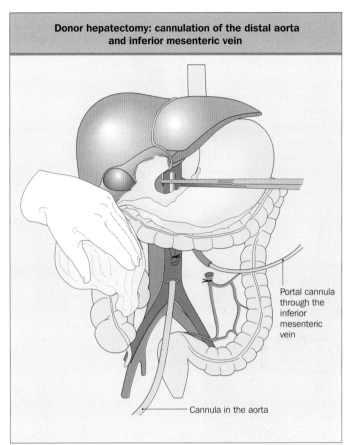

Donor hepatectomy: cannulation of the distal aorta and inferior mesenteric vein

Portal cannula through the inferior mesenteric vein

Cannula in the aorta

Figure 35.3 Donor hepatectomy: cannulation of the distal aorta and inferior mesenteric vein in preparation for in situ flush with preservation solution.

complete mastery of anatomy, efficient surgical technique that minimizes unnecessary movement, and seamless communication between team members. Refinements in technique continue to this day, although events can be identified that have had broad impact in shaping the liver transplant operation. For example, the technique of dissection has evolved with the introduction of improved electrocautery units and the argon beam coagulator, devices that have reduced operative time and facilitated hemostasis. Second, it has become standard practice to utilize mechanical retractors for exposure during liver transplantation, facilitating anatomic exposure during the liver transplant operation.

General approaches to the operation

Three general operative strategies are available during OLT: the traditional dissection without bypass, the traditional dissection with bypass, and 'piggyback' placement of the liver. Each offers advantages and risks. Traditional dissection without bypass is the most challenging, requiring both an experienced surgeon and an anesthetic team. The principal advantages are simplicity and short anhepatic times, as little as 30 minutes. In addition, complications associated with bypass, such as morbidity related to the cannulation sites, are avoided. Hemodynamic instability can be more severe, however, increasing demands on the anesthetic team during the anhepatic phase. Addition of bypass prolongs the operation and the anhepatic time, but mitigates the volume-associated hemodynamic changes associated with portal and caval clamping.

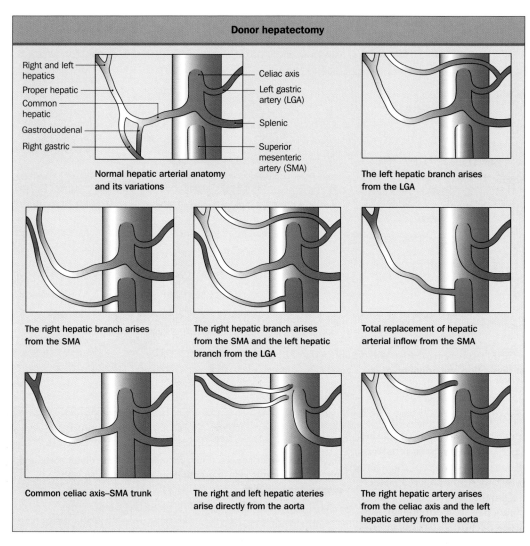

Donor hepatectomy

Figure 35.4 Donor hepatectomy: variations in hepatic arterial anatomy.

Right and left hepatics
Proper hepatic
Common hepatic
Gastroduodenal
Right gastric

Celiac axis
Left gastric artery (LGA)
Splenic
Superior mesenteric artery (SMA)

Normal hepatic arterial anatomy and its variations

The left hepatic branch arises from the LGA

The right hepatic branch arises from the SMA

The right hepatic branch arises from the SMA and the left hepatic branch from the LGA

Total replacement of hepatic arterial inflow from the SMA

Common celiac axis–SMA trunk

The right and left hepatic ateries arise directly from the aorta

The right hepatic artery arises from the celiac axis and the left hepatic artery from the aorta

The piggyback technique is designed to circumvent the hemodynamic risks of traditional dissection without bypass by removing the native liver with preservation of the vena cava, avoiding the need to cross-clamp the vena cava during the anhepatic phase, and thereby preserving venous return to the heart (Fig. 35.5). This technique adds additional time and complexity during the hepatectomy and introduces an increased risk of hepatic outflow complications related to the single hepatic venous anastomosis. However, advocates of the piggyback technique have been pleased with a decrease in volume-related instability during the anhepatic time. The piggyback technique may be most appropriate in patients with compromised cardiovascular reserve as an alternative to bypass.

Three phases of orthotopic liver transplantation

The liver transplant operation is described in three phases: hepatectomy, anhepatic phase, and reperfusion phase. The patient is prepared for operation by positioning in the supine position with the right arm tucked to facilitate placement of an assistant. Upon induction of anesthesia, vascular access lines are placed by the anesthetist. At least one large sheath introducer is placed in the central venous circulation, which serves as a large volume access and as a portal for a pulmonary artery catheter. An additional large volume access, usually a sheath introducer, is placed either centrally or peripherally. When venovenous bypass is used, the bypass cannulae are placed surgically after preparing and draping the entire chest, abdomen, and groins. A femoral cannula is placed by cut-down on the saphenous vein. The axillary cannula, through which blood is returned to the central circulation, can be placed either percutaneously or by open cut-down on the axillary vein (Fig. 35.6).

Hepatectomy

The hepatectomy is performed through a bilateral subcostal incision with extension in the midline to the xiphoid process, which is often excised. The incision should be carried as far laterally to the right as possible in order to allow complete and unobstructed view of the liver, especially the retrohepatic and suprahepatic vena cava. Mechanical retraction under both costal margins elevates and spreads the aperture of the rib cage in order to create a horizontal rather than convex costal margin, thereby maximizing access to the suprahepatic vena cava (Fig. 35.7). It should be remembered that the cirrhotic liver is often extremely small and difficult to access in its location high above the costal margin. The exposure is completed by inferior traction on the viscera, thereby clearly exposing the porta hepatis for dissection.

The falciform ligament is divided with electrocautery along the anterior margin of the liver until the leaves of the triangular ligaments, which form the anterior fascial covering of the suprahepatic vena cava, are reached. The left lobe is then mobilized

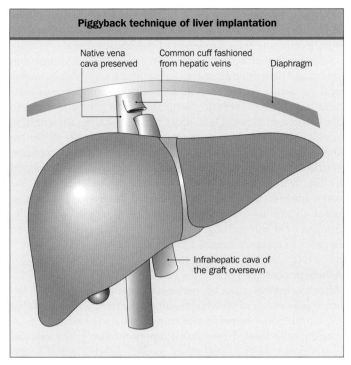

Figure 35.5 Piggyback technique of liver implantation. The native vena cava is preserved.

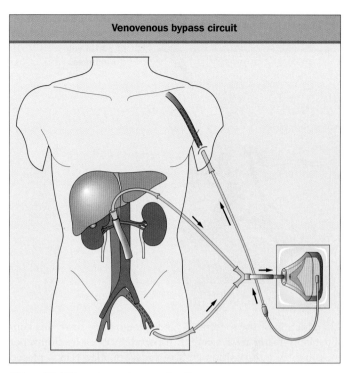

Figure 35.6 Venovenous bypass circuit.

by division of the left triangular ligament and reflected anteriorly in order to expose the gastrohepatic ligament. The gastrohepatic ligament can be divided with cautery, although when large venous collaterals are present this tissue must be ligated. An accessory left hepatic artery, when present, is ligated in this plane of tissue.

The hilar dissection is performed after the porta hepatis is exposed by an assistant, who maintains anterior and superior reflection of the liver edge. The goal of the hilar dissection is identification and ligation of the structures in the porta hepatis (hepatic artery, bile duct, and portal vein). The general principle is that portal structures must be ligated as high in the hilum as possible in order to preserve length, which may be important during implantation of the liver allograft.

The hilar dissection is adapted to the particular anatomic situation since previous surgery, hepatic atrophy and rotation of the liver, and vascular anomalies require changes in strategy. In patients who have had previous hepatobiliary surgery (most commonly cholecystectomy), densely vascularized adhesions of the colon, stomach, duodenum, and omentum present an obstacle to exposure of the porta. In such cases, the adhesions and adherent structures must be 'shaved' off the liver surface using cautery. It may be easiest to remove the gallbladder as the initial step of the hilar dissection, facilitating the exposure and division of the bile duct. Identification, exposure, and ligation of the hepatic arteries above the bifurcation of the proper hepatic artery is usually performed after duct transection. Some surgeons delay ligation of the hepatic artery until mobilization is complete, since it is thought that the end-stage liver is predominantly dependent upon the arterial supply and the patient becomes functionally anhepatic after arterial ligation.

The portal vein is skeletonized in its entirety from the border of the pancreas to the bifurcation, taking care to ligate the dorsal

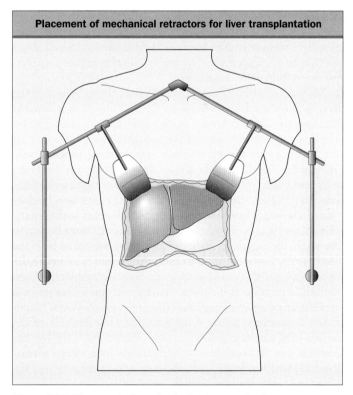

Figure 35.7 Placement of mechanical retractors for liver transplantation.

pancreatic branch of the portal vein. If the portal vein is thrombosed, it is usually possible to re-establish flow by transecting it and removing the inner layers of organized thrombus and scar, in a procedure that is analagous to endarterectomy for atherosclerosis (Fig. 35.8). This dissection can be carried proximally to

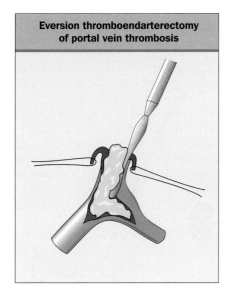

Eversion thromboendarterectomy of portal vein thrombosis

Figure 35.8 Eversion thromboendarterectomy of portal vein thrombosis.

the junction of the mesenteric and splenic veins since this confluence is nearly always patent. If portal revascularization is not possible, an interposition graft of cadaveric iliac vein is placed from the mesenteric vein to the portal vein of the graft. Preoperative imaging of the portal vein is essential in planning the strategy in response to portal anomalies. This is crucial in patients with previous portosystemic shunts, who pose an array of problems that can be overcome with good planning. If the piggyback technique is to be used, an end-to-side portocaval shunt is made to decompress the visceral circulation before completing the retrohepatic dissection.

After completion of the hilar dissection, the right lobe of the liver is mobilized by division of the peritoneal attachments between the inferior border of the liver and the right kidney. The diaphragmatic attachments on the right lobe are elevated off the bare area of the liver with electrocautery, progressively 'rolling' the right lobe to the left until the retrohepatic vena cava is exposed. The retrohepatic cava is fully dissected on the right side from the infrahepatic cava to the right hepatic vein by division of the flimsy lateral and posterior attachments with cautery. The adrenal vein is encountered in this plane and must be suture ligated. In the piggyback technique the liver is separated from the vena cava by ligation of all the small hepatic vein branches to the right lobe and the caudate until the liver is completely freed with the exception of the three main hepatic veins. This permits application of a partial occlusion clamp to preserve caval blood-flow during implantation of the new liver. The left side of the retrohepatic cava is exposed by anterior reflection of the left lateral segment and retraction of the caudate lobe with a narrow hand-held malleable retractor, allowing cautery dissection of the left side of the retrohepatic cava.

If bypass is to be used, the portal bypass cannula can be placed as the final step in the hepatectomy, after high ligation of the portal vein close to or above its bifurcation in the hilum (see Fig. 35.6). When the portal vein cannot safely be dissected because of dense scar tissue, or when portal vein thrombosis is present, it may be preferable to gain access for portal bypass using the IMV. When no bypass is used, the portal vein is simply clamped proximally, near the pancreatic border. Before clamping, however, we perform a test clamp of the infrahepatic vena cava to

determine whether the patient will tolerate the anhepatic phase. If the blood pressure falls, additional volume loading is required before clamping and completion of the hepatectomy.

Finally, the infra- and suprahepatic vena cava are clamped in traditional dissection techniques (Fig. 35.9). Correct placement of these clamps is important in facilitating subsequent caval anastamoses; the suprahepatic clamp should be placed as close to the diaphragm as possible in order to gain as much cuff length as possible for use in the suprahepatic caval anastomosis. We secure the suprahepatic clamp with a vascular tape in order to minimize accidental release. The infrahepatic caval clamp should be placed as distally as possible, without occlusion of the renal veins. We often transect the hepatic veins within the liver substance, in order to gain as much suprahepatic caval length as possible. Similarly, the infrahepatic cava is transected high into the liver, in order to preserve length, and the liver is removed.

Anhepatic phase

After the liver is removed, hemostasis is achieved by suture ligature and cautery of bleeding tissues in the retroperitoneum (see Fig. 35.9). Some surgeons also reapproximate the edges of peritoneum to facilitate hemostasis ('reperitonealize'). The vascular anastamoses are then performed in the following order: suprahepatic cava, infrahepatic cava, and portal vein. The hepatic arterial anastomosis is usually performed after portal reperfusion. The duration of the anhepatic phase, ending in portal venous reperfusion, is approximately 30–45 minutes. The physiologic consequences of the anhepatic phase include progressive coagulopathy, fibrinolysis, and acidosis. Before reperfusion, preservation solution in the liver graft must be flushed out to prevent hyperkalemia-induced arrythmias. We accomplish this task by flushing the portal vein of the graft on the back table with cold colloid solution (hetastarch), although this can also be performed during implantation.

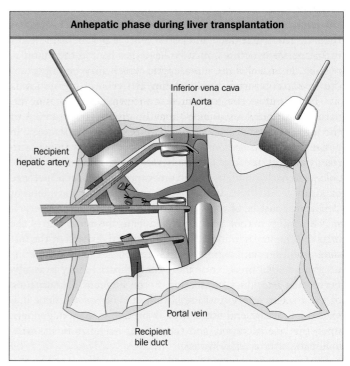

Anhepatic phase during liver transplantation

Inferior vena cava
Aorta
Recipient hepatic artery
Portal vein
Recipient bile duct

Figure 35.9 Anhepatic phase during liver transplantation.

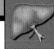
The recipient suprahepatic vena cava is prepared for anastomosis by division of the right and left hepatic veins, in order to fashion a single large cuff. The liver graft is then brought to the operative field and placed in an iced laparotomy pad. An iced sponge is also placed in the hepatic fossa. The liver is supported by the assistant, allowing the surgeon to place corner stitches on the horizontal corners of the suprahepatic cava. The liver graft is parachuted into the hepatic fossa and the corners tied. The posterior (back wall) aspect of the anastomosis is performed first, through the inside of the cava. The anastomosis is performed in an everting fashion to optimize intimal approximation. Care is taken to prevent constriction at the anastomosis upon reperfusion. The infrahepatic vena cava anastomosis is performed in a similar fashion. Assessment of the proper length of the infrahepatic cava and maintenance of the alignment of the cava on its axis are important considerations in performing the infracaval anastomosis. In the piggyback technique, the suprahepatic cava of the graft is directly anastomosed to the confluence of the recipient hepatic veins or to a long anterior incision on the recipient vena cava, utilizing partial occlusion of the recipient vena cava to preserve venous return. The infrahepatic vena cava of the graft is then simply oversewn.

The portal vein anastomosis is performed after removal of the portal vein bypass cannula, if bypass has been used. A crucial aspect of the portal anastomosis is estimation of the proper donor portal vein length that allows a straight anastomosis. Care is taken to avoid constriction, by tying the sutures loosely ('growth factor') to allow the vein to distend after reperfusion.

Reperfusion phase

Metabolic products accumulate in both the graft liver and the gut during implantation of the liver, especially when the portal vein has been clamped without bypass. Reperfusion is sometimes associated with significant hemodynamic instability ('reperfusion syndrome') due to the hypothermic, hyperkalemic, and acidotic effluent that is flushed into the right heart upon revascularization. The anesthetist must be prepared to administer hemodynamic support, including catecholamines, bicarbonate, and calcium on reperfusion. The technique of reperfusion varies between centers, but most surgeons reperfuse the liver by sequential removal of the suprahepatic clamp, infrahepatic clamp, and finally the portal venous clamp. Between clamp removals any obvious suture line leaks can be oversewn. Upon releasing the portal vein clamp, some blood may be discarded ('vented') to eliminate some of the detrimental substances which accumulate in the mesenteric circulation during the cross-clamp. It is not clear that venting reduces the reperfusion syndrome and probably has no advantage, except in the circumstance where the patient is known to be hyperkalemic before reperfusion.

The appearance of the liver upon reperfusion may often give an early indication of graft function. Severe reperfusion injury may be manifest by a bright red color and a firm, swollen appearance. The liver with good initial function and minimal reperfusion injury will rapidly and homogeneously fill with blood upon portal reperfusion and appear a dark salmon color. To palpation, the liver will remain soft and retain the sharpness of its edges. Bile may be seen at the common duct. Finally, the functioning liver will readily clear lactic acid and plasminogen activators, resulting in a correction of acid–base abnormalities and resolution of the complex coagulopathy that is due to a combination of fibrinolysis and dilution of platelets and coagulation factors.

Arterial anastomoses

After portal reperfusion the vascular suture lines are rapidly inspected for preliminary hemostasis before beginning the hepatic arterial anastomosis. If an accessory right hepatic artery is present in the liver graft, reconstruction of this vessel is performed *ex vivo* on the back table before implantation. The most common technique for hepatic arterial anastamosis is an end-to-end anastamosis of the donor aortic Carrel patch to the recipient hepatic artery (Fig. 35.10). The hepatic arterial anastamosis can be facilitated by preparation of the recipient hepatic artery as a 'branch patch', in which a common cuff is fashioned from a bifurcation, usually the hepatic–gastroduodenal bifurcation (Fig. 35.11). The recipient hepatic artery tends to be fragile and is prone to intimal dissection with even small trauma. If the recipient hepatic artery is unsatisfactory the splenic artery can be used as an alternative, or an interposition graft can be taken directly off the aorta. Before the introduction of microvascular techniques, direct aortic implantation was in fact the most common approach in pediatric recipients.

While there has been some debate about the etiology of hepatic artery thrombosis in the past, it is now clear that precision in fashioning the arterial anastomosis is the most important factor in decreasing the risk of this complication. Fine atraumatic clamps and fine monofilament sutures are used in the anastomosis, and growth factors are occasionally used to prevent constriction. High-power magnification has clearly been shown to decrease the thrombosis rate in pediatric liver transplantation, in which reconstruction of 2 or 3mm arteries may be required. After releasing the arterial clamp, adequacy of flow is assessed by palpation, Doppler examination, and, in some cases, direct measurement with a flow probe. Causes of inadequate arterial flow include technical flaws in the anastomosis, clamp injury to the

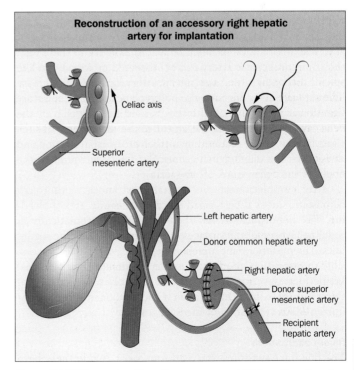

Figure 35.10 Reconstruction of an accessory right hepatic artery for implantation.

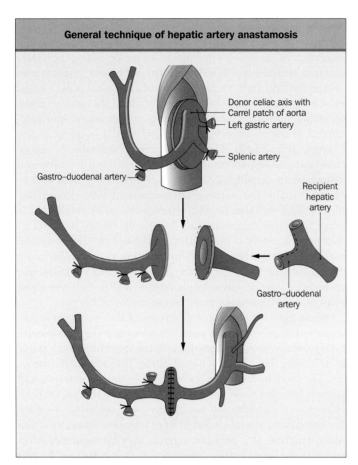

General technique of hepatic artery anastamosis

Donor celiac axis with
Carrel patch of aorta
Left gastric artery

Splenic artery

Gastro–duodenal artery

Recipient
hepatic
artery

Gastro–duodenal
artery

Figure 35.11 General technique of hepatic arterial anastomosis utilizing a donor aortic Carrel patch to the recipient hepatic artery branch patch.

intima of the artery proximal to the anastomosis, or inadequate inflow due to alterations in the recipient, such as celiac arterial disease. When arterial flow seems inadequate in the absence of any clear anastamotic problem or anatomic injury to the artery, the common hepatic artery can be dissected proximally to the splenic artery. In some cases splenic artery ligation will increase inflow to the liver. We have also observed occasional respiratory variation in hepatic arterial inflow caused by occlusion of the celiac artery by the arcuate ligament of the diaphragm. In such cases, inflow can be restored by further proximal dissection and division of the diaphragmatic muscular fibers surrounding the origin of the celiac trunk off the aorta.

After completion of the arterial anastomosis, a thorough hemostatic survey is performed in order to identify sites of bleeding. The hemostatic survey should be done systematically in order to inspect all the surfaces of the liver and all of the suture lines. The posterior right suprahepatic vena cava is the least accessible to inspection, requiring anterior rotation of the right lobe. We perform this maneuver as often as necessary to achieve hemostasis, but try to limit the duration of the rotation in order to minimize venous congestion of the liver graft.

Biliary anastomosis

The bile duct anastomosis is performed last. While there have been many variations in bile duct reconstruction that have been described, the two most commonly performed reconstructions

are simple end-to-end choledochocholedochostomy and biliary–enteric drainage into a Roux-en-Y (defunctionalized) limb of intestine. Choledochocholedochostomy is preferable because it avoids the need for an enteric anastomosis and is less likely to cause ascending cholangitis. In either case, cholecystectomy is performed first and the donor bile duct is prepared for anastomosis above the cystic duct junction, in most cases. Choledochocholedochostomy is performed using fine monofilament absorbable suture. Size mismatches may be corrected by ductoplasty with a running suture, or by spatulation of the smaller duct. In the past, a choledochal drainage tube (T-tube) was always left in the bile duct, with one limb of the tube stenting the anastomosis. The tube allowed collection of bile during the postoperative period, which facilitated clinical management of dysfunctional livers and allowed cholangiography. However, T-tubes are associated with complications in up to one-third of patients. The most common complications are leaks and bile peritonitis associated with tube removal several months after transplantation. Bile peritonitis almost always requires hospitalization, endoscopic placement of biliary stents, and in some cases operation. As part of a general trend toward greater operative simplicity, therefore, many centers have abandoned the routine use of T-tubes.

Hepatojejunostomy is preferred when primary choledochocholedochostomy is not possible, as in sclerosing cholangitis or when the recipient bile duct is too small to allow effective biliary drainage (Fig. 35.12). Hepatojejunostomy is also performed in almost all pediatric patients, who may already have an existing Roux-en-Y limb from a Kasai procedure for biliary atresia. The original Roux limb can be revised for use in the hepato–enteric anastomosis. When a new Roux-en-Y must be constructed, the proximal jejunum is divided 20–30cm distal to the ligament of Treitz with a stapler. The distal intestine is then used to construct a 40cm defunctionalized limb. Bowel continuity is restored with a jejunojejunostomy. The distal end of the Roux limb, containing the staple line, is oversewn. The Roux can be brought up to the donor liver through either an antecolic or retrocolic approach. The biliary–enteric anastomosis is performed with a single interrupted layer of absorbable suture to reapproximate mucosa to mucosa. If desired, a small stent can be left across the anastomosis, usually an infant feeding tube. The stent can be cut at either end or the distal end can be brought out through a second enterotomy, allowing access for postoperative imaging.

Before closure a final hemostatic survey is performed (Fig. 35.13). When the liver graft is functioning well, hemostasis is generally accomplished without much difficulty, but in cases of poor initial graft function the surgical surfaces and suture lines can bleed profusely from fibrinolysis, coagulopathy, and hypothermia. This situation can markedly prolong the operation because the surgeon cannot close in the presence of gross hemorrhage. Coagulopathy is treated with fresh frozen plasma, cryoprecipitate, and platelets. Epsilon aminocaproic acid can be used to treat fibrinolysis. In some cases aprotinin has also been used to treat fibrinolysis, but in general this drug is most efficacious when it is started at the beginning of the case. While aprotinin has been lauded for its beneficial effects on hemostasis, concerns regarding an increased risk of vascular thrombosis have limited widespread acceptance. When hemostasis has been accomplished, closed suction drains are left in the peritoneum (Fig. 35.14). We generally use one or two drains, which are useful in

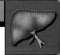

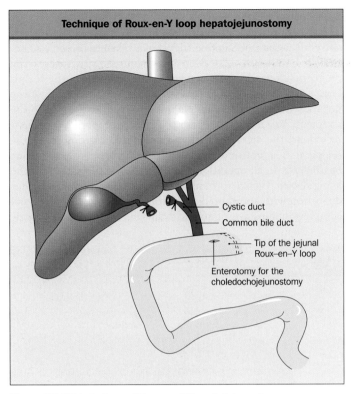

Technique of Roux-en-Y loop hepatojejunostomy

Cystic duct

Common bile duct

Tip of the jejunal Roux–en–Y loop

Enterotomy for the choledochojejunostomy

Figure 35.12 Technique of Roux-en-Y hepatojejunostomy.

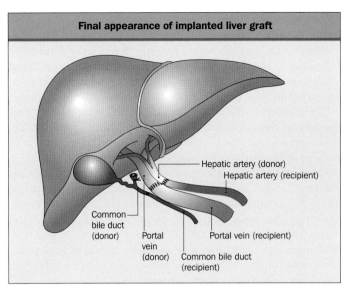

Final appearance of implanted liver graft

Hepatic artery (donor)
Hepatic artery (recipient)

Common bile duct (donor)

Portal vein (donor)

Portal vein (recipient)

Common bile duct (recipient)

Figure 35.13 Final appearance of implanted liver graft.

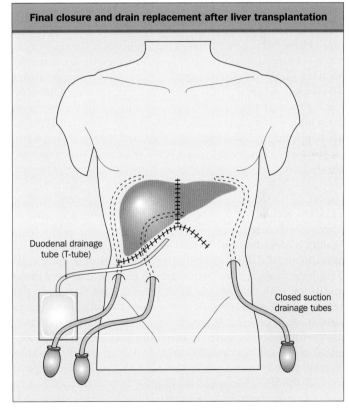

Final closure and drain replacement after liver transplantation

Duodenal drainage tube (T-tube)

Closed suction drainage tubes

Figure 35.14 Final closure and drain placement after liver transplantation.

evacuating postoperative serosanguinous fluid and facilitating early diagnosis of a bile leak, but they are not reliable indicators of intraperitoneal hemorrhage as their small size usually results in early occlusion by clot.

SPECIAL OPERATIVE CONSIDERATIONS: PEDIATRIC AND REDUCED-SIZE LIVER TRANSPLANTATION

Standard cadaveric transplantation in children is quite similar to the adult transplant, utilizing smaller instruments and sutures. Bypass is not used in children, and hepatojejunostomy is the preferred method of biliary reconstruction in all except larger teenage children. Experienced anesthesiology is of paramount importance in successful pediatric transplantation. Because of the difficulty of establishing large volume access in infants, central venous and arterial lines may sometimes require open surgical placement before beginning the transplant operation. In this decade, techniques of reduced-size liver transplantation have become routine in the transplantation of children. The incentive for development of these techniques was the shortage of small donors, which lead to a waiting list mortality for children approaching 50%. Initially, when the adult waiting list was small in the 1980s, livers from adult donors could be readily diverted to children. A small liver was fashioned *ex vivo* on the back table, usually from the left lateral segment, while the remainder was discarded. Shortly thereafter, the technique was extended to create two grafts from a single liver, the 'split liver' procedure. The appeal of splitting livers was the possibility of doubling the organ supply, but initial experiences with split livers were fraught with technical complications, thereby limiting application of this technique. More recently, there has been a renewed interest in split livers with the introduction of several innovations that have improved the results, most importantly the development of techniques to perform the dissection *in vivo* (*in situ*), borrowing directly from the experience with living donor liver transplantation.

We introduced living donors in children in the 1980s, with rapidly improving results throughout the 1990s. Living donation has now become routine in pediatrics, although with improvements in split liver transplantation there are additional options available to pediatric transplant surgeons than in the past.

Widespread application of split liver transplantation as a replacement for living donor transplantation has been limited, however, by intercenter sharing issues. Currently, in regions with multiple liver centers there is little incentive on the part of nonpediatric centers to share their full size organs for splits. Equitable resolution of this issue must be achieved before splitting can achieve its full potential, which would largely eliminate the need to perform living donor transplants in children. For the present time, however, we continue to rely on living donor transplantation to achieve optimal results for our pediatric patients.

More recently, increasing concern over liver transplant waiting time-related morbidity has fostered interest in developing living donation for adults, which requires a greater hepatic resection from the donor than living donation in pediatrics. Ethical issues over indications for adult living donation, patient selection, techniques, and outcomes now dominate debate in liver transplantation forums, although the overall role of this modality in improving outcomes remains controversial.

Technique of graft size reduction

Standard donor hepatectomy is performed in the cadaveric donor. The graft reduction (or splitting) is performed *ex vivo* with the liver kept cold on the back table (Fig. 35.15). The size of liver required will determine the plane of the dissection. For a very small infant (with a donor to recipient size disparity of 10 to 1), the left lateral segment (Couinaud segments II and III) is used; whereas, if the disparity is less, the entire left lobe can be used. If the right lobe is to be discarded, the common structures of the porta hepatis are kept with the graft. The dissection is best initiated from a dorsal direction with exposure of the confluence of the portal vein. Several caudate veins are divided and the right portal vein is divided at its origin. The caudate lobe may be removed to enhance access to the posterior aspect of the portal vein. The right hepatic artery is then exposed and divided at its origin. Finally, the bile duct is approached. After division of the cystic duct, the right hepatic duct is identified and divided in the hepatic parenchyma. At this point, the hilar plate is separated from segment IV (quadrate lobe), and the parenchyma is entered. The liver tissue is divided with clips or fine sutures being used to control the small vascular structures. As noted above the hilar dissection is similar whether a left lateral or full left lobe graft is required. If the full left lobe is to be used, the liver is divided in the plane of the gallbladder fossa (Fig. 35.15a – plane B), and the parenchyma is transected to the right of the middle hepatic vein. If the lateral segment is used, the liver is divided just to the right of the round ligament (Fig. 35.15a – plane A). Superiorly, the dissection of the hepatic veins varies depending on whether the vena cava of the recipient is to be replaced by the donor vena cava. For lateral segment grafts, it is best to remove the vena cava and the caudate lobe and position the graft directly on the recipient vena cava. If the whole left lobe is used, it is more convenient to preserve the entire vena cava and replace it in the recipient as in whole organ transplantation. At the completion of parenchymal transection, it is necessary to treat the section with a hemostatic surface. Despite meticulous preparation, the cut section will generally pose a hemostatic problem. Several strategies have been utilized, including fibrin glue, or reinforcement of the surface with a mesh, which permits direct control of the bleeding sites.

Split liver graft preparation

The split liver is prepared in much the same way as the reduced size graft with the exception that care is taken to preserve structures of both lobes. Allocation of the common structures to the recipients depends upon anatomic considerations in the recipients. The side which does not receive the common trunk of the hepatic artery will generally be more difficult to implant in the recipient. Vascular grafts from the cadaver donor may be used to extend the arterial length to facilitate anastomosis in the recipient. The entire dissection can be performed in the heart beating donor, an operation analogous to the dissection for the living donor: the *in situ* split. The advantages include a safer dissection with accurate identification of ducts and vessels, and complete hemostasis. The disadvantages are primarily logistic

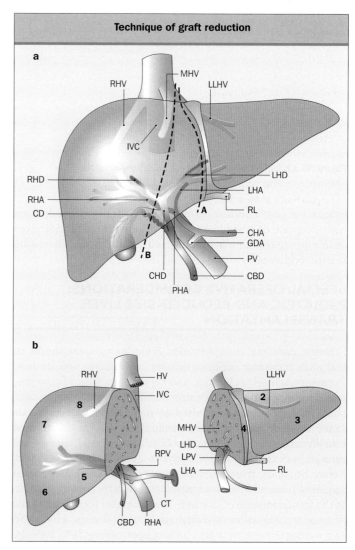

Figure 35.15 Technique of graft reduction. (a) There are two planes of potential parenchymal transection, for either a segment II/III graft (plane A) or for a full lobar split (plane B). (b) Dissected lobes. HV, hepatic vein; RHV, right hepatic vein; MHV, middle hepatic vein; LLHV, left lobe hepatic vein; IVC, inferior vena cava; CBD, common bile duct; CHD, common hepatic duct; CD, cystic duct; RHD, right hepatic duct; LHD, left hepatic duct; CHA, common hepatic artery; GDA, gastroduodenal artery; PHA, proper hepatic artery; LHA, left hepatic artery; RHA, right hepatic artery; GDA, gastroduodenal artery; CT, celiac trunk; PV, portal vein; RPV, right portal vein; LPV, left portal vein; RL, round ligament.

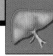

since it prolongs the donor operation and may complicate recovery of the other organs.

Reduced-size liver transplantation: the recipient operation

The recipient hepatectomy for the reduced size liver is a conventional dissection. The principal deviation from the standard technique is the need to preserve the recipient vena cava for implantation. This requires meticulous suture ligation of each hepatic vein branch to the caudate lobe, eventually mobilizing the entire retrohepatic vena cava with the liver attached only by the three main hepatic veins. The portal vein and cava are then clamped and the liver removed. The orifices of the hepatic veins are combined into a cuff that receives the hepatic vein of the graft for anastomosis. If the vena cava has been preserved with the graft, it is interposed end-to-end as in a standard transplant. The portal vein is anastomosed end-to-end but requires careful positioning since the course of the vessel is altered by the shape of the partial graft. The artery is then reconstructed according to the local situation. If the recipient hepatic artery is of adequate caliber, it is used for the anastomosis, using the microscope if needed. Otherwise, an interposition graft can be taken to the aorta. Reconstruction of the bile duct requires a Roux-en-Y anastomosis since the orientation of the partial graft is generally distorted to the right.

Implantation of the left lobe of a split liver graft is comparable to the technique described above. The right lobe graft usually contains the vena cava and is implanted in a fashion that is nearly identical to a standard adult liver transplant. If common structures were allocated to the left lobe, reconstruction of the artery or bile duct may be more complex and require either an interposition graft or a microvascular anastomosis. Reconstruction of the bile duct may require creation of one or more anastomoses to segmental bile ducts. Although some authors favor use of small stents for these anastomoses, we perform a direct mucosa-to-mucosa anastomosis under high magnification without intubation. Two or, occasionally, three small ducts may be anastomosed. Whenever possible, small ducts are incorporated into a single anastomosis, but if they are too far apart separate anastomoses are constructed.

Abdominal closure

The use of reduced grafts often creates a scenario in which the graft is either too large, or too small for the recipient. Both these situations can create lethal complications that must be detected and prevented at the time of abdominal closure. If the graft is too small, it can rotate on the axis of its vessels and acutely obstruct the circulation. Hepatic venous outflow is particularly prone to this complication. The graft's position must be assured by appropriate planning of the vascular anastomoses, and by positioning the intestines to occupy any empty space in the right upper quadrant into which the liver can rotate. Mechanical fixation of the liver is usually not helpful. If the liver is too large, closure under tension can result in a compression syndrome, leading to liver ischemia, and renal and pulmonary compromise. This is managed by temporary prosthetic closure of the abdomen.

Living related donor transplantation
Living donor hepatectomy

Living donor hepatectomy has become common in pediatrics, since the initial description of the procedure in 1989. The graft is usually segments II and III of Couinaud, comprising 15–20% of the donor's hepatic volume, generally between 200 and 250g of liver tissue. This is ideal for infants, but as the recipient becomes larger, outcomes are compromised by the small size of the graft. For this reason, several authors have proposed right lobe donor hepatectomy for use in adult recipients.

Segmentectomy of segments II and III for a pediatric recipient can be readily performed through a midline incision (Fig. 35.16a). The porta hepatis is dissected to expose the origin of the left hepatic artery. The left portal vein is then encircled, and the posterior branches to the caudate lobe are divided. The left bile duct is approached anteriorly and encircled. The left duct should be divided with a minimum of dissection to preserve the blood supply of the duct wall. Superiorly, the confluence of the left and middle hepatic veins is exposed; this is the terminal point of the dissection. The parenchyma is then divided just to the right of the falciform ligament with meticulous division of the biliary and vascular branches to segment IV. If a larger graft is to be obtained, the parenchyma can be divided in the principal fissure just to the right of the middle hepatic vein. The full left lobe graft weighs between 350 and 500g in adults and is sufficient for a small adult or an older child. After the parenchyma is divided the graft is attached only by its vessels, which are then divided, and the liver is rapidly flushed with heparinized preservation solution.

Right lobe donor hepatectomy

A graft of sufficient volume for an adult recipient can be obtained by right hepatectomy. This requires a more extensive incision similar to that used for the transplant recipient. The portal dissection requires cholecystectomy with identification of the right hepatic artery near its origin. The right border of the common hepatic duct is exposed until the right bile duct is encountered. A common trunk of the right bile duct is absent in the majority of cases with the duct of segments V and VIII encountered first and then, more superiorly, the duct to segments VI and VII. After the ducts are transected, the right portal vein is encircled at its origin. The liver is completely mobilized, then the small hepatic vein branches to the caudate lobe are encircled and divided to free completely the right lobe from its attachments to the vena cava. The right hepatic vein is freed and encircled. After completion of the dissection the parenchyma is divided in the plane just to the right of the middle hepatic vein. Operative sonography is used to localize the vessels and guide the dissection. After completion of the parenchymal transection, the vessels are clamped and divided, and the graft flushed with heparinized preservation fluid.

Implantation of the lobe grafts

The left lobe graft is implanted as described above for reduced size liver transplantation. The hepatic veins are anastomosed directly onto the vena cava at the confluence of the right and middle hepatic veins. The portal vein is anastomosed end-to-end; if greater length is need, the internal jugular vein provides an excellent conduit. The artery is anastomosed directly using microvascular technique and the operating microscope. The bile duct anastomosis is performed using microvascular technique to the Roux-en-Y jejunal limb. The closure should be uneventful, although careful positioning of the graft is essential to avoid postoperative complications (Fig. 35.16b & c).

Technique of living donor hepatectomy and implantation of a segment II/III graft

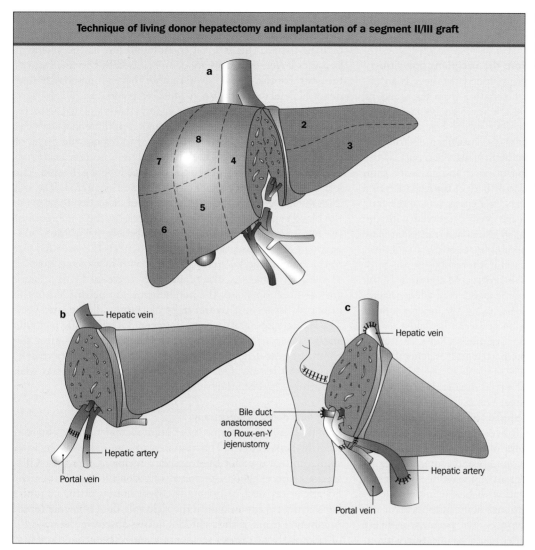

Figure 35.16 Technique of living donor hepatectomy and implantation of a segment II/III graft.

The right lobe graft is used if the donor is the same size, or smaller than the recipient. The right hepatic vein of the graft is anastomosed end-to-side to the recipient hepatic vein orifice with partial occlusion of the vena cava. The portal vein is anastomosed end-to-end with reperfusion of the liver. Microvascular technique is used to anastomose the artery, but if needed the recipient's saphenous vein can be used to create an arterial conduit for a more convenient anastomosis to a larger vessel. The biliary anastomosis is most difficult in the adult recipient, particularly if the recipient had large volume losses and resuscitation leading to bowel edema. It is extremely difficult to create a fine anastomosis between the tiny segmental ducts and massively edematous jejunum. Fortunately, these cases can be done electively, with careful volume replacement to minimize these technical difficulties. The right lobe graft is much easier to position than the left, creating fewer difficulties with closure (Fig. 35.17).

AUXILIARY LIVER TRANSPLANTATION

Replacement of part of the liver has been used in cases of fulminant hepatic failure or metabolic liver diseases. It has also been proposed for living related liver transplantation in which a small left lobe graft is implanted next to the residual function-

Implantation of a right lobe graft

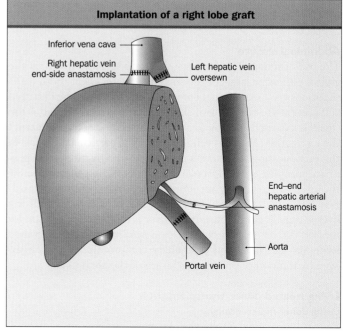

Figure 35.17 Implantation of a right lobe graft.

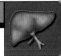

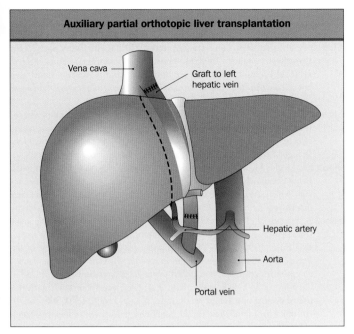

Figure 35.18 Auxiliary partial orthotopic liver transplantation. A left lobe graft has been implanted in the bed (orthotopically) of the resected native left lobe.

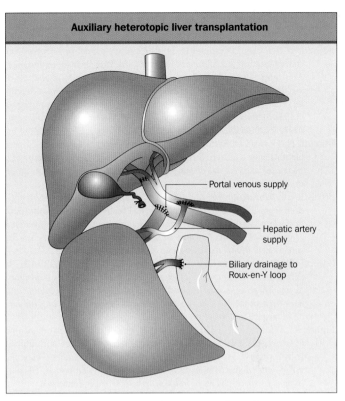

Figure 35.19 Auxiliary heterotopic liver transplantation.

ing native liver. Auxiliary liver transplantation involves a group of diverse techniques that are too complex to be covered in this section. Early experiences established the need for portal blood and adequate hepatic venous outflow for successful grafting. This is most readily accomplished by placing the liver graft in an *orthotopic* position, in which a specific lobe is replaced by an anatomically similar graft (Fig. 35.18).

Most commonly used is replacement of the left lobe of the diseased liver with a left lobe graft from a cadaveric or living donor, requiring partial hepatectomy in the recipient as the first step. The hepatic vein is reconstructed in an end-to-end fashion, as are the portal vein and hepatic artery. The bile duct generally requires hepatojejunostomy. An older technique involves place-

ment of the graft in the hepatic fossa inferior to the native liver with attachment of the portal and hepatic veins onto the side of the recipient vessels (Fig. 35.19). The principal technical challenge involves managing the competition for portal blood between the two livers. The recipient liver tends to be favored for portal perfusion and successful grafting depends upon modifying portal perfusion to favor the graft, leading to relative hypertropy of the graft. Optimal techniques for auxiliary liver transplantation remain under development as the eventual role of this technique remains uncertain.

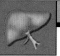
FURTHER READING

Bismuth H, Azoulay D, Samuel D, et al. Auxiliary partial orthotopic liver transplantation for fulminant hepatitis: the Paul Brousse experience. Ann Surg. 1996;224:712–24. *An excellent description of the use of auxiliary partial orthotopic liver transplantation in fulminant hepatitis. Five cases underwent the procedure. The results were encouraging but the authors express great caution before the procedure is to be routinely recommended.*

Bismuth H, Houssin D. Reduced size orthotopic liver graft in hepatic transplantation in children. Surgery. 1984;95:367–70. *The first report of a successful reduced-size orthotopic liver graft for hepatic transplantation in children.*

Broelsch CE, Whitington PF, Emond JC, et al. Liver transplantation in children from living related donors. Surgical techniques and results. Ann Surg. 1991;214:428–37. *A detailed description of hepatic segmented graft transplants in 20 young children. The early results show a 75% success rate in this difficult group of patients.*

Busuttil RW, Goss JA. Split liver transplantation. Ann Surg. 1999;229:13–21. *A review of the experience of ex vivo and in situ split liver transplantation. These techniques expand the pool of donor organs available and have been successful. The in situ splitting technique results in graft survival as good as that of whole organs.*

Emond JC, Whitington PF, Thistlethwaite JR, et al. Reduced size orthotopic liver transplantation: use in the management of children with chronic liver disease. Hepatology. 1989;10:867–72. *The authors review the use of reduced-size liver grafts in children over a 2-year period. The outcome is as successful as in full-size orthotopic transplantation.*

Kalayoglu M, Sollinger HW, Stratta RJ, et al. Extended preservation of the liver for clinical transplantation. Lancet. 1988;1:617–9. *The original description of the use of University of Wisconsin preservation solution in human liver transplantation.*

Millis JM, Melinek J, Csete M, et al. Randomized controlled trial to evaluate flush and reperfusion techniques in liver transplantation. Transplantation. 1997;63:397–403. *An interesting trial describing different flushing techniques to enhance graft survival in liver transplantation.*

Raia S, Nery JR, Meis S. Liver transplantation from live donors. Lancet. 1989;ii:497. *An important letter from Brazil describing two liver transplants in young children from living donors. There was a successful outcome. Due to the shortage of donors, the waiting list mortality at the time was 73%.*

Randall HB, Wachs ME, Somberg KA, et al. The use of the T tube after orthotopic liver transplantation. Transplantation. 1996;61:258–61. *A paper showing that biliary anastomoses had as successful an outcome whether or not they were constructed over a T-tube.*

Shaked A, Busuttil RW. Liver transplantation in patients with portal vein thrombosis and central portacaval shunts. Ann Surg. 1991;214:696–702. *Portal vein thrombosis and portacaval shunts are not a contraindication to successful liver transplantation, although careful patient selection is needed.*

Shaw BW Jr, Martin DJ, Marquez JM, et al. Venous bypass in clinical liver transplantation. Ann Surg. 1984;200:524–34. *A trial demonstrating the effectiveness of venous bypass in maintaining the transplant recipient in a good cardiovascular and metabolic state during surgery.*

Singer PA, Siegler M, Whitington PF, et al. Ethics of liver transplantation with living donors. N Engl J Med. 1989;321:620–2. *An interesting discussion paper stressing the need for 'open display, public evaluation and discussion' as regards the ethical conduct of therapeutic innovation.*

Soin AS, Friend PJ, Rasmussen A, et al. Donor arterial variations in liver transplantation: management and outcome of 527 consecutive grafts. Br J Surg. 1996;83:637–41. *This paper showed that anomalies of the hepatic arterial anatomy occur in one-third of all livers but do not compromise graft function unless difficult anastomoses are required.*

Starzl TE, Klintmalm GBG, Porter KA, et al. Liver transplantation with the use of cyclosporin A and prednisone. N Engl J Med. 1981;305:266–9. *An important trial showing the benefit of cyclosporin in hepatic transplantation over the previously used immunosuppressive regimens.*

Starzl TE, Marchioro TL, Von Kaulla KN, et al. Homotransplantation of the liver in humans. Surg Gynecol Obstet. 1963;117:659–76. *An important historical record of the first three patients undergoing hepatic transplantation by Starzl.*

Starzl TE, Miller C, Broznick B, et al. An improved technique for multiple organ harvesting. Surg Gynecol Obstet. 1987;165:343–8. *A description of the technique for rapid organ removal from the donor with improved results for hepatic graft function.*

Todo S, Nery J, Yanaga K, Podestra L, Gordon RD, Starzl T. Extended preservation of human liver grafts with UW solution. JAMA. 1989;261:711–4. *This paper describes the major impact of the University of Wisconsin solution on graft preservation and subsequent successful grafting. This development was a major advance.*

van Hoek B, de Boer J, Boudjema K, et al. Auxiliary versus orthotopic liver transplantation for acute liver failure, EURALT Study Group, European Auxiliary Liver Transplant Registry. J Hepatol. 1999;30:699–705. *Auxiliary partial OLT is a potentially advantageous technique in acute liver failure. Further work is necessary to reduce the early complications.*

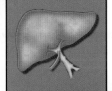

Section 4 Liver Transplantation

Chapter 36

Immunology and Immunosuppression

Geoffrey W McCaughan

INTRODUCTION

This chapter includes a detailed account of the immune response, particularly in relation to organ transplantation. An understanding of these basic mechanisms will allow the reader to appreciate the use of immunosuppressive drugs and specific aspects of graft rejection.

GENERAL OVERVIEW OF THE IMMUNE RESPONSE

Cellular aspects

Traditionally the immune response has been divided into antigen-specific and nonspecific responses. Antigen-specific responses are also known as the adaptive immune system, while nonspecific responses are known as the innate immune system.

The antigen-specific immune response is dictated by specific receptors for antigen which are restricted to T- and B- lymphocyte populations. These antigen receptors are part of a large family of molecules known as the immunoglobulin (Ig) superfamily. The T-cell receptors consist of heterodimers and are of two types ($\alpha\beta$ and $\gamma\delta$). These heterodimers join to form a single antigen binding site. The B-cell antigen receptor consists of two identical antigen-binding sites that are formed by the interaction of heterodimers of so-called heavy and light Ig chains. These T-cell and B-cell antigen receptors are highly polymorphic in their antigen-binding regions, as each receptor is derived from a variable set of exons in the genome. The specific immune system at the T-cell level is triggered by the presentation of antigen via cells from the innate or nonspecific immune system (Fig 36.1). These are usually dendritic cells or macrophages. Once T cells are triggered, they perform various functions. Cells of the CD4+ phenotype provide help to B cells and produce various mediators that activate cells of the nonspecific immune system such as macrophages, neutrophils and eosinophils. They also stimulate and provide help to other T cells, particularly CD8+ T cells. CD8+ cells are usually effector cells, particularly involved in cellular lysis and apoptosis [cytotoxic T lymphocytes (CTLs)]. Activation of these pathways results in protective immunity against specific antigens, but also may result in tissue damage via delayed-type hypersensitivity (DTH) reactions and direct cellular cytotoxicity (see below).

The nonspecific immune system is characterized by immune effector cells that do not have antigen-specific receptors. These cells include macrophages, natural killer (NK) cells, polymorphonuclear leukocytes and the complement system. It is beyond this chapter to discuss the activation and regulation of these cells.

However, it is increasingly recognized that the interaction between the antigen-specific and nonspecific immune systems is blurred. Triggering of antigen-specific T cells may activate cells within the innate immune system. Also, it has recently become clear that activation of NK cells and macrophages, when exposed particularly to infectious organisms, may be crucial in triggering antigen-specific cells themselves, particularly T cells. Furthermore, it has been recognized that the binding of complement components to receptors on B cells is important in regulating antibody production.

Cytokines

Key components in the regulation of the antigen-specific and nonspecific systems are soluble mediators known as cytokines (Fig. 36.2).

Cytokines are relatively low molecular weight polypeptides that are secreted from cells and act upon other cells in the immune system via specific cell surface receptors. They may also act in an autocrine fashion on the cytokine-producing cell itself, in an enhancing or inhibitory way. Cytokines are pleiotropic in their action and often display redundancy for some functions. Cytokines can be grouped into various sub-

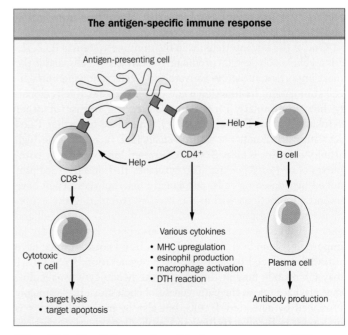

Figure 36.1 Simplistic overview of the immune response. DTH, delayed type hypersensitivity; MHC, major histocompatibility complex.

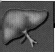

Key cytokines in antiallograft responses		
Cytokine	Main source	Main actions
IL-1	Many cells (macrophages)	Lymphocyte co-stimulation, acute phase protein response, fever, neutrophil/endothelial cell activation, decreased bile flow
IL-2	Activated T cells (Th1)	T-cell proliferation
IL-4	Activated T cells (Th2) Mast cells	B-cell activation and antibody production (particularly IgE)
IL-5	Activated T cells (Th2)	Eosinophil differentiation and proliferation, B-cell antibody production (IgA)
IL-6	Many cells (T-cells, macrophages)	Acute phase protein production, B-cell antibody production (IgA), liver regeneration
IL-8	Multiple	Neutrophil chemotaxis and activation
IL-10	Multiple T cells (Th2) Macrophages	B-cell activation, inhibition of DTH (Th1) responses
IL-12	Macrophages NK cells	Stimulation (T1-type cells), DTH responses and IFN-γ production, NK stimulation
IL-13	Activated T cells	B-cell activation, inhibition of Th1 pathway, stimulation of NK cells
IFN-γ	Activated T cells NK cells	Upregulation of MHC class I and MHC class II expression, macrophage activation, stimulation of NK cells, B-cell activation, class switching, inhibits IL-4 activation, chemokine induction

Figure 36.2 Summary of major cytokines that play a role in inflammatory responses seen in allograft rejection. Ig, immunoglobulin; NK, natural killer.

families, namely the interleukins (ILs), interferons (IFNs), tumor necrosis factor (TNF) family, chemokines and growth factors. The important cytokines that play a role in rejection and tolerance are discussed below.

One of the key interleukins in the immune system is IL-2. IL-2 is a 15kDa polypeptide produced by activated T cells, and is the most important autocrine activator of T cells following initial T-cell stimulation. Its function is not only to expand T cells clonally, but to stimulate T cells to produce the release of other cytokines such as TNF-α and IFN-γ, which lead to further T-cell activation. IL-2 acts via a three-chain IL-2 receptor. The high affinity receptor is an α/β/γ heterotrimer, but low affinity complexes of α/γ or β/γ exist. The cytokines IL-1 and IL-6 are produced by numerous cells, particularly macrophages. They have important functions within the liver by stimulating the acute-phase protein response, but also play a role in T- and B-cell and endothelial cell activation. IL-6 has also been shown to play an important role in liver regeneration, as IL-6 knockout mice have markedly reduced capacity for liver regeneration. Excess IL-1 may inhibit bile flow at the level of the hepatocyte canaliculus, thus playing a role in the pathogenesis of cholestasis. IL-4 is mainly produced by activated T cells, but also by mast cells and it is important in B-cell activation and antibody production, particularly of the IgE subclass. It also activates antigen-presenting cells by increasing expression of major histocompatibility complex

(MHC) class II and CD40, which are important co-stimulatory molecules. IL-5 is produced by a large range of cells, particularly by activated T cells. IL-5 plays a role in B-cell antibody production, particularly of the IgA isotype, and is crucial to eosinophil differentiation and growth. IL-10 has immunosuppressive properties and inhibits IFN-γ and IL-2 production from activated T cells. It also inhibits monocytes and the expression of adhesion molecules on antigen-presenting cells. It is largely produced by macrophages and by T cells of the so-called Th2 type. More recently identified interleukins such as IL-13, IL-15 and IL-18 have also been shown to play important regulatory roles in the immune response. IL-12 is produced by NK and by T cells, and is important in stimulating IL-2 and IFN-γ production during the early phases of T-cell activation. It is crucial in the induction of the Th1-type cytokine response. IL-13 shares similar properties with IL-10, in that it inhibits T-cell activation, production of IL-2 and IFN-γ. IL-15 has similar properties to those of IL-2 and triggers through the same receptor. IL-18 has been recently shown to have profound IFN-γ-inducing properties, particularly in macrophages.

A key group of cytokines is the chemokine family. They have been broadly divided into α (CXC) and β (CC) cytokine families. The prototype member of the CXC chemokine family is IL-8, which is crucial in neutrophil activation and migration. Eotaxin is a CXC chemokine, important for eosinophil chemotaxis. The β subfamily (the CC cytokines) includes macrophage inflammatory protein (MIP)-1α, MIP-1β, inteferon-inducible protein (IP)-10 and RANTES. These molecules are thought to play major roles in monocyte activation and migration, and they also have a chemotactic role for T cells. Chemokines act via a family of receptors known as the chemokine receptors that have been recently linked to HIV co-entry into macrophages and CD4+ T cells. There are now over 30 different chemokines, although functional data on some is limited.

The interferon families consist of the α and β subclasses, which are homologous to each other and are produced by numerous cell types following stimulation by infectious organisms or other inflammatory responses. These molecules increase the cellular expression of major histocompatibility molecules, and stimulate macrophage and NK cell activation. They are known to have antiviral properties. Interferon-γ shares no homology with α or β interferon, and is produced by T cells of the Th1 phenotype following antigen presentation via macrophages or dendritic cells. Interferon-γ is a powerful activator of macrophages and also inhibits IL-10 and IL-4 production from other cell types. Interferon-γ results in upregulation of MHC, particularly class II molecules.

Tumor necrosis factor-α is produced mainly by macrophages but also by other cell types, including activated T cells. The molecule exists as a homotrimer and not only exists in soluble but also in cell surface forms. It binds to two receptors, TNF receptor type 1 (p75) and TNF receptor type 2 (p55). Tumor necrosis factor-α has many pleomorphic reactions, including the triggering of nitric oxide release from endothelium resulting in systemic vasodilatation, and it plays a role in septic shock. At the hepatocyte level it is crucial in priming for hepatocyte proliferation in liver regeneration, but also may trigger cell death and apoptosis via the apoptotic cell death cascade.

Important growth factors in the inflammatory response include transforming growth factor (TGF)-β. This is an important anti-inflammatory cytokine that also has the potential to inhibit hepatocyte proliferation. Furthermore, it is the key player in hepatic stellate cell stimulation, and in the production of extracellular matrix which is important in tissue remodeling within the liver and the hepatic fibrosis response which occurs in chronic allograft rejection. It is produced by many cells including macrophages, hepatic stellate cells and fibroblasts.

MAJOR HISTOCOMPATIBILITY COMPLEX

The MHC was recognized initially in mice, when it was realized that the time to rejection of experimentally transplanted organs and tumors in animals depended on the degree of genetic relationship between the donor and recipient. The closer the animals were related, the longer the graft survival. These initial experiments took place in the 1930s and 1940s, but were soon followed in the late 1940s and early 1950s through to the mid-1970s by skin transplantation in humans. In parallel with these studies it had been recognized that polymorphic antigens on leukocytes were recognized by serum from patients who had received multiple blood transfusions, or patients who had a history of multiple pregnancies. These leukocyte antigens were then used to define human subjects that underwent experimental skin transplantation, and they were linked to the survival of allograft tissue. This work led to the molecular definition of the MHC complex, particularly in humans and mice, that has now been characterized by molecular techniques.

The MHC gene complex is located on the short arm of human chromosome 6 (Fig. 36.3). The complex consists of over 50 genes spanning an area of 3500kb. Genes in the area have been classified as class I, class II, class III, and class IV loci. The MHC class I locus consists of MHC A, B, and C regions. MHC class I molecules are heterodimers. The α-chain possesses three domains α1, α2 and α3, and the β-chain is a single domain consisting of β₂ microglobulin. The β₂ microglobulin and the α3 domain show very strong homology to single Ig-related domains of the immunoglobulin superfamily. The α1 and α2 domains each interact, forming two parallel α-helical loops (one derived from each domain). These two helices form the sides of a cleft that binds peptide antigens. The protein structures of each molecule are highly polymorphic, varying from individual to individual, with the main heterogeneity occurring in amino acid residues around the antigen-binding cleft.

The MHC class II region consists of four sets of molecules: DR, DQ, DP, and DM. These are heterodimers of α- and β-chains which consist of two immunoglobulin-like domains each. Similar to MHC class I molecules, two parallel α-helices (one derived from each α1 and β1 Ig domain) form an antigen-binding cleft.

Major histocompatibility complex class II molecules are highly polymorphic, with the major amino acid heterogeneity in the vicinity of the antigen-binding cleft. The DP, DQ, and DM genes are encoded by single α- and single β-chain genes, while there are two β-chain genes in the DR region. The MHC class II region between the DQ and DM genes also consists of the transporters associated with antigen processing (TAP) genes and large multicatalytic protease (LMP) genes. The LMP genes encode the proteosome complex, while TAP genes encode peptide transporters. Both of these gene complexes are associated with the function of peptide ligand binding to MHC molecules. Class III genes consist of TNF family, complement molecules and steroid hydroxylase. This region may be eventually split into class III and IV genes, with the latter including the TNF family and other inflammatory mediators.

Understanding the MHC complex is important in transplantation. These molecules are crucial in regulation of antigen presentation to the immune system, and the polymorphisms are crucial in the recognition of foreign antigen during the effector phase of the immune response. Matching of polymorphisms within the MHC complex plays a role in clinical transplantation, particularly in renal and bone marrow transplantation.

T-CELL RECOGNITION OF ANTIGEN

The recognition of antigen, including alloantigen, by the T-cell system occurs via the specific T-cell receptor (TCR) molecules on both CD4⁺ and CD8⁺ T cells. Recognition mostly occurs via the αβ rather than the γδ set of T-cell receptors, and is fundamentally different between CD4⁺ cells and CD8⁺ cells. CD8⁺ cells recognize antigen in association with MHC class I molecules, while CD4⁺ cells recognize antigen in association with class II molecules. In both situations small peptides, generated from whole antigens, bind to these molecular complexes, then make their way to the cell surface and are recognized by the TCR as an MHC/peptide complex.

Peptides associated with class I molecules are usually derived from antigens that are processed intracellularly in the cytoplasmic compartment (Fig. 36.4). Such antigens are degraded by a large 26S multicatylitic, 700kDa, protease known as the proteasome. This is a complex, cylindrical-shaped structure consisting of outer rings of α and β subunits. Following this interaction, peptides, usually 8–11 amino acids in length (predominantly nine amino acids), are generated and then transported from the cytoplasmic proteasome complex to the endoplasmic reticulum, usually in association with various chaperones of the heat shock protein (HSP) family (HSP70 and HSP90). These peptides are transported into

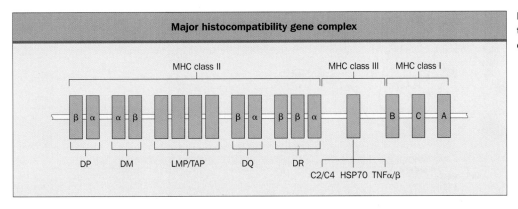

Figure 36.3 Schematic diagram of the major histocompatibility gene complex on human chromosome 6.

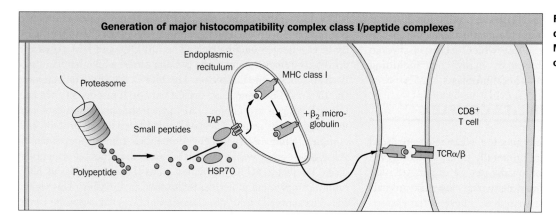

Generation of major histocompatibility complex class I/peptide complexes

Figure 36.4 Schematic diagram of the generation of MHC class I/peptide complexes.

the endoplasmic reticulum by the TAP-1/TAP-2 molecules. Transporters associated with antigen processing are a superfamily of adenosine triphosphate (ATP) multimembrane cassette transporters, and transport of peptides into the endoplasmic reticulum is ATP-dependent. These peptides then bind to the MHC class I complex via an MHC peptide-binding groove. The peptides are anchored at the carboxyl terminus, usually by an hydrophobic amino acid (although this may vary depending on the MHC class I allele). This complex is then sorted through the Golgi complex, and appears on the cell surface where the antigenic peptide in association with its MHC groove is recognized by the $\alpha\beta$ T-cell receptor on CD8$^+$ cells. The β_2 microglobulin and peptide binding to the MHC groove are essential for the transport of the class I/peptide complex to the cell surface.

MHC class II peptide generation and binding to MHC class II molecules is more complex than described for the peptide/MHC class I pathway (Fig. 36.5). As mentioned earlier, MHC class II molecules are $\alpha\beta$ heterodimers. These are synthesized and form a nonameric complex with another molecule known as the invariant chain. This complex is targeted to the endocytic pathway within the transgolgi network via sorting signals that are present within the cytoplasmic tail of the invariant chain. It is here that the interaction with antigenic peptide takes

place. Antigenic peptides that become associated with MHC class II molecules are usually generated by the endocytic pathway following the ingestion of extracellular antigen. The endocytic pathway where this interaction takes place has been defined as having multivesicular structures. Antigen is degraded by lysosomal type proteases into small peptides of varying lengths. At the same time, the MHC class II invariant chain complex is degraded by other proteases (including cathepsin) into single $\alpha\beta$ structures with a small individual peptide of the invariant chain (clip) remaining associated in the MHC class II peptide binding groove. This clip peptide is then exchanged for antigenic peptides by a process catalyzed by human leukocyte antigen-DM (HLA-DM) molecules. The peptide requirements for binding to the MHC class II groove are not as stringent as that for class I ligands. The peptides are usually longer, ranging between 14 and 18 amino acids in length (even up to 28 amino acids). These peptides extrude from the binding groove at both the amino- and carboxyl-terminal ends. The peptides are anchored in the MHC class II groove by various anchor residues, the most important one being at the beginning of the groove where the amino acid at this position is often hydrophobic in nature (but may be charged, once again depending on the MHC class II allele with which it is actually associating). Once the $\alpha\beta$ heterodimer and peptide

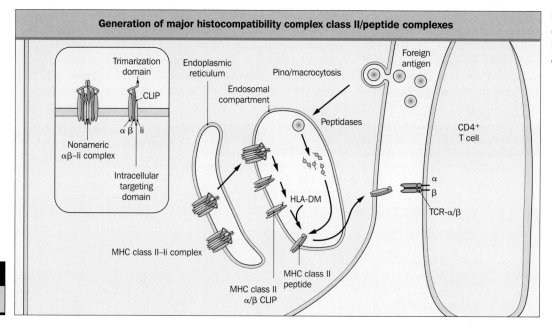

Generation of major histocompatibility complex class II/peptide complexes

Figure 36.5 Schematic diagram of the generation of MHC class II/peptide complexes.

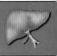
complex is stabilized, this is then transported and appears on the cell surface where the antigenic determinants in the groove are recognized by the $\alpha\beta$ T-cell receptor on CD4$^+$ cells.

EARLY EVENTS IN ACTIVATION OF T CELLS BY ANTIGEN (G0–G1 TRANSITION)

Activation via the T-cell receptor
Following the recognition of antigen by the TCR, there are complex signaling pathways that lead to the induction of lymphocyte activation, division, and clonal proliferation. The T-cell receptor is associated at the cell surface with a group of molecules known as the CD3 complex (Fig. 36.6).

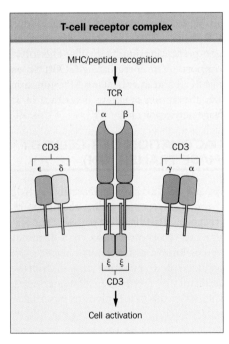

Figure 36.6 Schematic diagram of T-cell receptor complex that recognizes MHC/peptide complexes resulting in T-cell activation and proliferation.

This complex consists of $\epsilon\gamma\delta$ heterodimers and an important $\zeta\zeta$ homodimer. In particular, the $\zeta\zeta$ homodimer has a long cytoplasmic tail, part of which is a repetitive 16 amino acid motif known as the immunoreceptor tyrosine-base activation motif (ITAM). Following antigen binding to the receptor and oligomerization of the receptor and the CD3 complex, phosphorylation of the ITAM takes place by tyrosine kinase molecules associated with CD4 (lck) or the T-cell receptor itself (fym) (Fig. 36.7).

Phosphorylation of the ITAM leads to the generation of a specific binding site for other protein tyrosine kinase (PTK) molecules, in particular ZAP-70 and Syk. These molecules become activated, generating further multiple tyrosine phosphorylation sites that serve as binding sites for other proteins that regulate two major pathways of cellular activation, finally leading to transcription of IL-2 and other cytokine genes. One of the key mediators in one of the pathways is phospholipase Cγ (PLCγ). Following triggering of the T-cell receptor complex PLCγ is recruited to the cell membrane, is phosphorylated and results in the hydrolysis of inositol phospholipids, generating inositol polyphosphates (IP-3) and diglycerols (DG) from the cell membrane. Inositol polyphosphate-3 stimulates the mobilization of calcium from intracellular stores. The increase in intracellular cytoplasmic calcium leads to the activation of the calmodulin-dependent serine phosphatase calcineurin. This is a crucial molecule in T-cell activation, and is a target for immunosuppressive drugs such as cyclosporine and tacrolimus. Activation of calcineurin has two main effects. It leads to the activation of the cytoplasmic form of nuclear factor for activated T cells (NFAT$_c$), resulting in its transfer to the nucleus where it combines with NFAT$_n$ to form an active nuclear transcription activator which binds to various gene promoters, including the promoter for the IL-2 gene. This transcription factor acts together with other transcription factors of the AP-1 family such as FOS and JUN. Calcineurin also plays a major role in the phosphorylation status of other pathways, in particular the mitogen-activated protein kinase (MAPK) cascade at the site of the JNK (JUN N-terminal

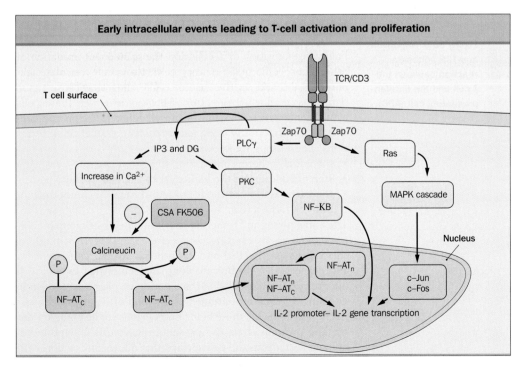

Figure 36.7 Schematic diagram of the main early intracellular events leading to T-cell activation and proliferation. Sites of drug interactions outlined in the text are labeled. PKC, protein kinase C.

kinase) molecule. The other product of phospholipid breakdown, DG, is important in the activation of another transcription factor nuclear factor-κB (NF-κB).

The second main pathway following the initial events at the TCR is activation of the MAPK cascade. This cascade is characterized by the successive phosphorylation of various cytoplasmic kinases which may act on themselves and finally lead to cytokine gene transcription. Mitogen-activated protein kinases phosphorylate at proline χ-threonine/serine-proline sequences where x is often a leucine residue. They require dual phosphorylation at both serine/threonine and a tyrosine residue for activation. Activation through this cascade results in activation of c-JUN, c-FOS and NF-κB transcription factors, as well as optimally activating the NFAT transcription factor. Early activation of the MAPK cascade occurs via the RAS pathway and RAS-mediated recruitment of Raf-1 to plasma membrane. Raf-1 is one of the MAPKK (MAPK kinase) molecules that form part of the MAPK cascade itself. It is important to note that activation via both of these cascades (i.e. the PLCγ/calcineurin pathway and the MAPK pathway) is needed for optimal T-cell activation.

Co-stimulatory pathways

Apart from activation via the T-cell receptor, there are various cell surface molecules that are also crucial in optimal T-cell activation. These include the CD8 and CD4 molecules themselves which interact with MHC class I and class II proteins respectively on the cell surface of the antigen-presenting cell, the CD58/CD2 interaction, and the CD54/intercellular adhesion molecule (ICAM) interaction (Fig. 36.8).

However, the most important adhesion molecule is CD28, which interacts with the CD80/CD86 molecules on the antigen-presenting cell. These molecules are both members of the immunoglobulin superfamily. CD28 is a two-domain structure, while CD80/CD86 has a single immunoglobulin domain. Following T-cell receptor interaction, CD28 is rapidly expressed at increased levels on the cell surface, and ligation of CD28 with CD80/CD86 results in activation of the protein tyrosine kinase

complex, including the MAPK cascade. It is at this point that the calcineurin pathway via the T-cell receptor and the activation pathway via CD28 meet. This process leads to the optimal activation of various gene transcription factors, which rapidly upregulate IL-2 itself, the IL-2 receptor, and the CD40 ligand. The pathway of CD28 signaling also leads to the upregulation of a molecule known as cytotoxic T-lymphocyte antigen (CTLA)4. This molecule has approximately a 10- to 100-fold higher avidity for CD28 than for CD80/CD86. It has been recently recognized that CTLA4 may have an important negative influence on T-cell activation.

Another recently identified adhesion co-stimulatory pathway for T-cell activation is the CD40/CD40 ligand (CD40L) interaction. CD40 ligand is a member of the TNF cytokine family, while CD40 is a member of the tumour necrosin factor receptor (TNFR) family. CD40 ligand is expressed on T cells following activation via the TCR, while CD40 is widely expressed on cell types including antigen-presenting dendritic cells. This interaction is thought to be important in upregulating CD80/86 on antigen-presenting cells (APCs) and in enhancing APC function itself. The CD40/CD40L interaction seems to be critical in T-cell-dependent macrophage activation.

LATER EVENTS IN ACTIVATION OF T CELLS BY ANTIGEN (G1–S PHASE TRANSITION)

The early activation steps and production and secretion of IL-2 lead to the induction of the IL-2 receptor and subsequent signaling through the IL-2 receptor. This signaling pathway and signaling through other cytokine receptors occurs via a different set of cytoplasmic molecules known as the Janus kinase (JAK) proteins and signal transducers and activation of transcription (STAT) molecules. This results in progression of lymphocyte activation in the cell cycle from the G1–S phase. These latter events are important as the STAT/targets of rapamycin (TOR) molecules are important targets of the rapamycin group of immunosuppressant drugs.

HOW DO ACTIVATED CELLS ENTER TISSUES?

Following activation of T cells and the subsequent induction of other nonspecific inflammatory cells, these cells circulate and enter tissues and, in the case of organ allografts, cause tissue damage and allograft rejection. The way in which these cells actually enter tissues has now been well defined. The process consists of three steps involving leukocyte–endothelial cell interactions. These steps are known as:

- the initial tethering and rolling step;
- step of adhesion of the leukocyte to the endothelium; and
- the extravasation of the leukocyte through the endothelium into the tissues (Fig. 36.9).

The initial rolling and tethering step is initiated by a group of molecules known as selectins. These are expressed on leukocytes themselves (L-selectin) and endothelial structures (E-selectin and P-selectin). Selectins are 'long' molecules that extend well out from the endothelial surface and have plant C-type lectin domains, which are positioned on the end of repetitive consensus repeat domains, these being homologous to the complement binding proteins. It is the presentation of this C-type lectin domain away from the cell surface that allows interaction with

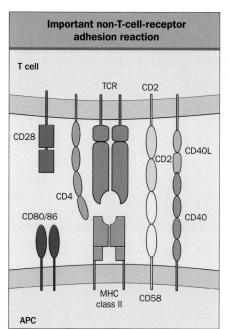

Figure 36.8 Important non-TCR adhesion reaction between the T cell and the antigen-presenting cell (APC).

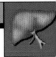

Important molecules involved in lymphocyte and neutrophil endothelial interaction

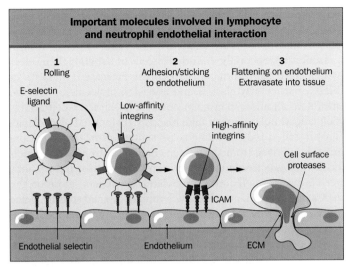

Figure 36.9 Important molecules involved in lymphocyte and neutrophil endothelial interaction resulting in cellular chemotaxis into inflamed tissues. ECM, extracellular matrix; ICAM, intercellular adhesion molecule; PCAM, platelet-cell adhesion molecule.

selectin ligands. The selectin ligands are a class of complex oligosaccharides known as lactosaminoglycans, and these contain the core tetrasaccharide structure sialyl Lewis-X (SLEX). Binding of selectins to their ligands is calcium dependent, and the initial tethering and rolling steps are relatively loose and reversible. Selectins are upregulated quite rapidly by various cytokines which also lead to the induction of a high affinity group of molecules known as integrins, in particular lymphocyte function-associated antigen (LFA)-1, very late antigen (VLA)-4 and α4β7 on the leukocyte cell surface. Integrins mediate the second step of leukocyte–endothelial interaction. The integrins bind to endothelial adhesion molecules such as the ICAMs (ICAM-1/ICAM-20), vascular adhesion molecule (VCAM-1) and mucosal addressin cell adhesion molecule (MAD CAM)-1. The interactions between integrins and the integrin receptors mediate firm adhesion of leukocytes to the vascular endothelium. Another recently described molecule, vascular adhesion protein (VAP)-1, may play an important role in leukocyte–endothelial interactions within the liver. The second step of firm adhesion to the endothelium leads to leukocyte flattening, and the development of cell surface pseudopodia which insinuate themselves between endothelial junctions, and result in leukocyte extravasation into tissues. This last step involves the platelet endothelial cell adhesion molecule (PECAM)-1 and leukocyte cell surface proteinases, which are involved in the breakdown of endothelial cell junctions and extracellular matrix degradation. The above processes of extravasation and chemotaxis are driven by various cytokines, particularly the α and β chemokines.

MECHANISMS OF TISSUE INJURY

Once the activated cell enters tissues further activation of antigen-specific and nonspecific effector mechanisms may take place resulting in tissue damage. One of the important cell interactions involved in tissue damage involves the cytotoxic T cell. Cytotoxic T-lymphocytes (CTLs) are predominantly of the CD8+ phenotype, which interact with antigen in association with class I MHC expressed on tissue cells. Cell surface MHC class I is rapidly upregulated by any inflammatory response, particularly by mediators such as TNF and IFN-γ <19>. This increased expression is important in clearance of viral antigen from tissues but also potentiates tissue damage in allograft rejection. Cytotoxic T cells express important cell surface molecules such as Fas ligand, CD40, and cell-surface TNF. These molecules interact through their respective ligands such as Fas and the TNF receptor and may induce cells to undergo programmed cell death or apoptosis. Activation of these pathways may also result in intracellular oxidative stress and cell necrosis. The pathways of apoptosis are similar in many cells, and have been described in great detail over the past 1–2 years. They are not discussed in detail here. Cellular apoptosis is triggered via a 'death domain' amino acid motif on the cytoplasmic tail of TNF receptors (e.g. FAS), which are members of a larger family sharing these motifs. Cytotoxic T cells also produce various enzymes such as granzymes and perforin, which attack target cells and cause cell injury and death through apoptotic and necrotic pathways. Cells triggered in nonspecific effector responses include NK cells, which were initially described *in vitro* and whose role *in vivo* has been difficult to define. They recognize and kill targets that do not express MHC class I molecules, and therefore their role in allograft rejection is probably minimal. They in fact carry receptors for MHC class I molecules, so that their activation is inhibited, once the interaction between that receptor and MHC class I takes place.

Activated T cells, particularly of the CD4+ phenotype, produce significant amounts of IFN-γ, and other molecules which turn on and activate macrophages. These are cells which are primarily involved in the DTH reaction, and they produce numerous cytokines such as TNF-α, IL-1, IL-6, IL-10, and TGF-β. All these molecules are important in cell injury via various mechanisms. The specific molecular pathways that are important in allograft rejection itself are discussed on page 36.6.

Antibody production within nonlymphoid organs is probably minimal, but serum-derived antibody produced in lymph nodes and spleen may enter organs, activate complement, and cause cellular injury. Such events are important in hyperacute allograft rejection and xenoallograft-associated rejection. The cellular target of serum antibody is likely to be the endothelial cell.

Th1 VERSUS Th2 CYTOKINE RESPONSE

One of the paradigms that is important in tissue injury, inflammation, and regulation of the immune response, including outcomes from allograft rejection, has been the Th1/Th2 paradigm. This refers to the existence in some experimental systems of polarized cytokine responses following T-cell activation. The Th1 cytokine response involves the production of predominantly INF-γ, IL-2, and TNF-β (lymphotoxin), and results in macrophage activation and DTH reactions. In contrast, the Th2 response involves the production of IL-4, IL-5, IL-10, and IL-13, is associated with strong antibody responses including IgE production, and results in cross-inhibition of the Th1 response, predominantly via IL-4 and IL-10. Although the paradigm was initially worked out on isolated CD4+ T-cell clones *in vitro* , it has been observed *in vivo* following various immunization schedules and during experimental and clinical infectious states. For example, human tuberculoid leprosy is associated with a strong Th1 response at the site of the lesion, while lepromatous leprosy is associated with Th2-type responses. In experimental leishmaniasis, the BALB/c mouse is associated with systemic infection and progressive disease and a Th2-type response, while in the CH3B6 mouse leishmania is controlled and associated with a DTH Th1-type response. It is unclear how these responses are diverted at the early stages of T-cell activation. It is thought that IL-12 production and IFN-α production from perhaps macrophages and NK cells are important in the induction of the Th1 response. In contrast, IL-4, either produced from macrophages, T cells themselves, or mast cells, is crucial in directing the response towards a Th2 phenotype. In some experimental situations, the Th1 response has been associated with allograft rejection, while the Th2 response has been associated with allograft tolerance.

ALLOANTIGEN RECOGNITION

The description of the immune response is formulated on the recognition of foreign antigen, consisting of foreign protein or infectious organisms, by the immune system. However, the response against an organ allograft is complicated by the presence of allo-MHC as well as self-MHC cell surface molecules. This has led to the concept that T-cell stimulation following allograft transplantation can occur by direct and indirect pathways (Fig. 36.10).

The direct T-cell response is defined as the stimulation of T cells by the allogeneic MHC antigen on allogeneic APCs. This response does not require intracellular processing and presentation of peptides in order to stimulate the T-cell response. Quite extraordinarily, when this response is measured *in vitro*, the frequency of precursor T cells for a direct alloimmune response is about 100-fold greater than that for a response to individual peptides derived from environmental antigens. The

direct pathway is likely to involve two kinds of APCs. First, initially in tissues such as the liver, true APCs such as dendritic cells or macrophages are likely to be the main source of antigen presentation. Secondly, endothelial cells of the graft themselves which have been induced to express increased amounts of MHC, particularly class II and adhesion molecules, may also stimulate an alloresponse. In contrast to direct T-cell activation, allostimulation may take place by the normal physiologic. This is called indirect antigen presentation. In this situation, peptides derived from alloantigen combine with self-MHC molecules and are presented to the immune system as foreign antigen. Indirect T-cell activation is likely to depend more on the APCs in the recipient's draining lymph nodes and spleens, being primed either by soluble antigen or cellular antigen itself, following degradation into allopeptides.

Although it is thought that the direct pathway is crucial in allograft recognition, there is evidence that indirect antigen presentation actually does occur, as it is possible to immunize with allo-MHC peptides and induce recognition responses and even accelerate experimental rejection. The process may not be as efficient as the direct pathway.

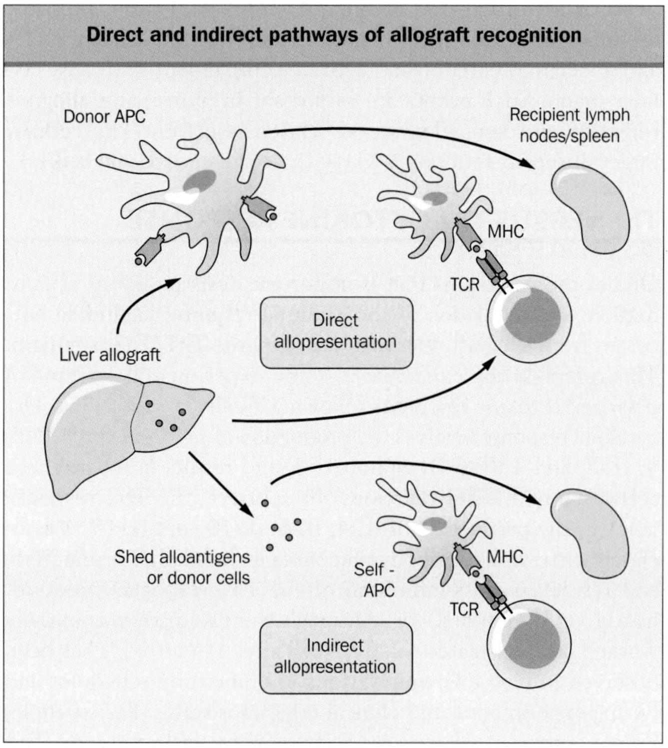

CELLULAR AND MOLECULAR BASIS OF ACUTE AND CHRONIC ALLOGRAFT REJECTION

Acute allograft rejection

The initial target of the acute allograft rejection response in vascularized allografts is the microvasculature. The microvasculature has high constitutive expression of MHC molecules and other adhesion molecules. Furthermore, the microvasculature has a very narrow lumen. This combination predisposes to leukocyte–endothelial cell interactions. The predominant cells that mediate acute rejection are T cells, particularly the T-helper CD4+ subset. The molecular mechanisms particularly involve a DTH reaction, with macrophage activation and production of cytokines such as IL-2, INF-γ, TNF-α and lymphotoxin. The T-helper subset also triggers alloreactive CTL production. Alloreactive CTLs have been isolated from allografts during rejection, and there is evidence of increased messenger RNA and protein for granzyme and perforin, major components of the CTL effector pathway. These CTLs are predominantly CD8+ and have been shown to be important, not so much in determining whether rejection occurs, but in the speed of the rejection process. As well as the recruitment of macrophages, there is evidence for the recruitment of other components of the nonspecific immune system. In particular the presence of eosinophils and eosinophil protein products (eosinophilic cationic protein) and IL-5 have been correlated with acute rejection. Recently much interest has been shown in studying 'final common pathways' in tissue damage during acute rejection, particularly the role of nitric oxide and oxidative stress.

Chronic allograft rejection

Chronic allograft rejection usually results from uncontrolled acute rejection episodes, but it does have some distinct pathogenic mechanisms not seen in acute rejection. The microvasculature, an initial target during acute rejection, is totally obliterated in the chronic rejection process. In conjunction with obliteration of the microvasculature, there is the development of a process known as 'transplant vasculopathy' which affects

Direct and indirect pathways of allograft recognition

Donor APC

Recipient lymph nodes/spleen

MHC

TCR

Direct allopresentation

Liver allograft

Shed alloantigens or donor cells

Self - APC

MHC

TCR

Indirect allopresentation

Figure 36.10 Direct and indirect pathways of allograft recognition.

medium-sized arteries. This vasculopathy is a result of antigen-specific and antigen nonspecific damage to arterial endothelium. The initiating stimulus is a cell-mediated immune response directed against allo-MHC molecules. This results in the accumulation of CD4$^+$- and CD8$^+$-activated T cells within the vessel wall and the consequent activation of macrophages. The release of chemotactic factors such as membrane cofactor protein (MCP)-1, MIP-1α, and MIP-1β seems to be crucial in the resulting macrophage activation and proliferation. The release of platelet-derived growth factor from macrophages, adherent platelets, and damaged endothelium is a major stimulator for smooth muscle proliferation. Transforming growth factor-β production by macrophages leads to the transition of smooth muscle cells to the myofibroblasts which secrete significant extracellular matrix protein resulting in vessel (subintimal) fibrosis. Similar processes also take place in the interstitium of various organs resulting in organ fibrosis.

DRUGS THAT INHIBIT THE IMMUNE SYSTEM: PHARMACOLOGY AND MECHANISMS OF ACTION

Corticosteroids

Corticosteroids are chemically modified derivatives of natural adrenal hormones and are used in various forms, such as prednisolone, hydrocortisone, and methylprednisolone. They have similar efficacy apart from hydrocortisone, which acts at 1:5 strength compared with prednisolone and methylprednisolone. Corticosteroids have numerous mechanisms of action in inhibiting the immune system. At very high doses they cause lympholysis/apoptosis and margination of lymphocytes resulting in significant lymphopenia. They also inhibit macrophage/dendritic cell antigen presenting function via inhibition of transcription of cytokines such as IL-1 and TNF-α, and by inhibiting arachidonic acid metabolism. Corticosteroids inhibit the first enzyme of the arachidonic acid metabolic pathway: phospholipase A2. This leads to blockage of the cyclo-oxygenase and 5-lipo-oxygenase pathways with the resulting inhibition of thromboxane and prostacyclin production. Corticosteroids also inhibit interferon-dependent adhesion molecule expression including MHC class II. Furthermore, there is some evidence that corticosteroids stimulate TGF-β production, a known inhibitory cytokine resulting in a more Th2-type cytokine profile (anti-inflammatory) rather than Th1 cytokine production.

Azathioprine

Azathioprine is an imidazole derivative of 6-mercaptopurine, and is well-absorbed and converted to 6-mercaptopurine and to 6-thio-ionosine monophosphate in the liver. Xanthine oxidase is required for azathioprine metabolism with conversion to 6-thiouric acid, followed by excretion in the urine. These chemicals are alkaloid DNA precursors and azathioprine leads to reduced bioavailability of purine molecules by inhibition of inosine monophosphate and the de-novo purine pathway. Azathioprine also blocks phosphoribozyl pyrophosphate (PRPP), thus blocking purine synthesis via the salvage pathway. The overall affect of azathioprine is to inhibit lymphocyte proliferation at the G1–S phase transition, (i.e. following signaling via the T-cell receptor/adhesion molecule cascade).

Cyclosporine

Cyclosporine (CSA) was isolated from the fungus *Trichoderma polysporum*. It is a cyclic endecapeptide. It is currently available as a microemulsion (Neoral). Before this microemulsion form was available, absorption of CSA (Sandimmune) showed large individual variation with an average oral bioavailability of only 30%, but varying between 5 and 90%. Cyclosporine (Sandimmune) is highly lipid-soluble, and dependent on bile salt availability in the gastrointestinal lumen. The microemulsion form (Neoral) has an improved overall bioavailability, with less individual variation and less dependence on bile salts for absorption. The area under the curve following absorption of Neoral compared with Sandimmune is increased by 1.5 to three-fold. Cyclosporine is highly metabolized in the gastrointestinal tract and the liver by the cytochrome P450 complex, mainly cytochrome P450 3A4. This results in numerous metabolites which are excreted in the bile. Less than 1% of CSA is excreted unchanged. There is evidence for enterohepatic circulation.

Cyclosporine exerts its immunosuppressive actions by binding to a cytoplasmic protein called cyclophilin, the prototype member of the immunophilin family. Cyclophilin is a highly basic, abundant protein present in many tissues. It is an 18kDa CIS transpeptidyl-propyl isomerase ('rotamase') which plays a role in protein folding. However, this action is not related to the drug's immunosuppressive property. Cyclosporine forms a complex with cyclophilin and this complex binds with high affinity to calcineurin (a cytoplasmic calcium-dependent phosphatase) resulting in inhibition of its phosphatase function. The phosphatase function of calcineurin is crucial in the activation of the NFAT$_C$ transcription factor resulting in its translocation into the nucleus to act as a transcription factor for the IL-2 molecule. This step is effectively blocked by the CSA cyclophilin/calcineurin complex. Cyclosporine has two domains: one involved in the drug interaction with cyclophilin itself; and the effector domain which is a composite of the CSA and the cyclophilin itself, which interacts with calcineurin. The interaction between cyclophilin and CSA is highly dependent on the hydrophobic side chain of the 6-methyl leucine in CSA. Also, it has been shown that tryptophan at position 121 in cyclophilin itself is required for calcineurin inhibition. The overall effect of CSA is to block the early cytokine transcription gene and G0–G1 transition following T-cell activation.

Tacrolimus (FK506)

Tacrolimus is a cyclic macrolide antibiotic similar to erythromycin. It was derived from the soil micro-organism *Streptomyces tsukubaensis*. It is well-absorbed from the gastrointestinal tract, not influenced greatly by the presence or absence of bile in the gastrointestinal lumen, and like CSA is extensively metabolized by the cytochrome P450 system and excreted in bile. The mechanism of immunosuppressive function is very similar to that of CSA. It also binds to a cytoplasmic immunophilin. This immunophilin, known as FK-binding protein (FKBP), is a 12kDa protein consisting of many isoforms, the most important of which is FKBP-12. In mice a recent isoform FKBP-51 has been shown to be mainly restricted to T cells. Its importance is currently under study. Like CSA, the FK/FKBP complex then binds to calcineurin resulting in inhibition of its phosphatase activity, inhibition of translocation of NFAT$_C$ to the nucleus, and inhibition of early transcription of genes such as IL-2. FK/FKBP and CSA/cyclophilin bind at two overlapping but distinct sites within a region on calcineurin.

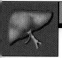

Therefore, they do compete with each other for immunosuppressive function and thus are unable to be used simultaneously. There are three-dimensional crystal structures of the tacrolimus/immunophilin complex available, indicating a similar formation of an immunophilin-binding domain and an effector domain, as in the CSA/immunophilin complex.

Rapamycin

Rapamycin is also a cyclic macrolide. It is derived from the soil micro-organism *Streptomyces hygroscopicus*. It is well-absorbed and metabolized by the cytochrome P450 system. Rapamycin, like CSA and tacrolimus, mediates its action by binding to an immunophilin. In fact it binds to the FKBP immunophilin, particularly FKBP-12. However, it has no effect on the phosphatase activity of calcineurin. In contrast to tacrolimus, rapamycin, when it binds to FKBP-12, does not undergo a dramatic conformational change. Instead of binding to calcineurin, the complex of rapamycin/FKBP targets two cytoplasmic proteins associated with G1–S phase cell cycle progression. These molecules are known as targets of rapamycin (TOR)-1 and TOR-2. These 200kDa proteins are highly expressed in human tissues, particularly in the testis and skeletal muscle. The two proteins have 67% identity. The exact function of these proteins has not been totally defined, but they seem to be cytoplasmic kinases involved in activation cascades that eventually turn on cytokine genes. The rapamycin/FKBP complex has been shown to bind to a 90 amino acid region adjacent to a lipid kinase domain within TOR-1/TOR-2. A crucial serine motif in this complex seems important in blocking TOR-1/TOR-2 function. Apart from the affect on TOR-1/TOR-2, there is evidence that rapamycin may also inhibit the promoter activity of proliferating cell nuclear antigen which is important in cell cycle progression within many cells. Apart from its affect on lymphocytes in blocking immune function, rapamycin also inhibits the proliferation of other cell types and, in terms of allograft rejection, inhibition of smooth muscle proliferation may be important in its effects on chronic rejection. Thus, rapamycin blocks the second set of phosphorylation events following the binding of IL-2 to the IL-2 receptor and the release of other cytokines, thereby acting later in the phase of lymphocyte activation than CSA and tacrolimus.

Mycophenolate mofetil

Mycophenolic acid (MPA) was originally isolated from the fungal genus *Penicillium* and has been modified by a synthetic morpholinoethyl side chain ester resulting in the production of mycophenolate mofetil (MMF). This modification significantly improved oral bioavailability of MPA. Mycophenolate is converted back to MPA and undergoes conjugation in the liver. The drug is well-absorbed and primarily (87%) eliminated in the urine. Its half-life is approximately 12 hours. Mycophenolic acid is a noncompetitive inhibitor of inosine monophosphate dehydrogenase (IMPDH), the key enzyme that converts inosine monophosphate (IMP) to adenosine monophosphate (AMP), thus effectively blocking the rate-limiting enzyme step in the de-novo purine synthetic pathway. The drug seems more selective for lymphocytes because the IMPDH isoform-2 is 5–6 times more sensitive to MPA than the IMPDH isoform-1 enzyme. The IMPDH isoform-2 is predominantly expressed in lymphocytes and monocytes and this, in conjunction with the fact that lymphocytes tend not to use the salvage pathway for purine metabolism, results in the relative selective action of MMF on lymphocyte activation. The depletion of guanosine purine-type precursors also results in the inhibition of transfer of fructose and manose to the cell surface of various glycoproteins. This seems particularly to affect adhesion molecules. Thus a further action of mycophenolate may be to inhibit lymphocyte binding to endothelium and extravasation into inflamed tissues. Mycophenolate mofetil not only has an affect on T- and B-cell proliferation, but also inhibits smooth muscle cell proliferation and thus has potential in the treatment of chronic rejection.

Antibodies (ALG, OKT3, IL-2 receptor)

Antibodies directed against antigens on human leukocytes are used as immunosuppressive therapy. Antithymocyte globulins (ATGs) or antilymphocyte globulins (ALGs) are raised in horses, goats or dogs and have been extensively used in human renal transplantation. Currently they have largely been replaced by the mouse monoclonal antibody OKT3 directed against the ε-chain of the human CD3 complex and is thus specific for human T cells. OKT3 is given as a bolus intravenous injection and leads to the disappearance of all T cells in the peripheral blood within 30–60 minutes (Fig. 36.11).

This effect is due to a combination of cell apoptosis/lysis, cell marginalization, opsonization, and antigenic modulation of CD3/TCR from the cell surface. After 2–3 days of therapy, a small number of antigenically modulated cells appear in the peripheral blood, but these cells are nonfunctional. Other monoclonal antibodies (mAbs) against other T-cell antigens have been used experimentally, but have not met with significant clinical use. Mouse mAbs against the IL-2 receptor have been studied in human transplantation. Their effects have been disappointing. However, the recent synthesis of 'humanized' mAb directed against the IL-2 receptor α-chain has resulted in high affinity reagents with powerful immunosuppressive properties. These are currently under study and preliminary evidence suggests that they result in a significant decrease in acute rejection episodes in renal transplant recipients. These agents have a half-life of approximately 20 days, and may be administered monthly.

Future clinical therapies

These include the pyrimidine pathway inhibitor brequinar, a new agent called deoxyspergillin (DSG), and another drug called leflunomide. There is also considerable interest in the development of

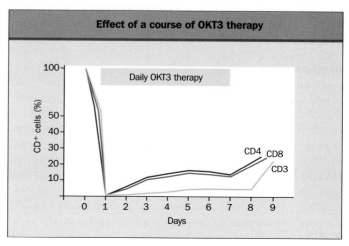

Figure 36.11 Effect of a course of OKT3 therapy on peripheral blood T-cell markers.

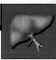

new mAbs against other adhesion molecules such as the CD28/CD80 pathway and against molecules involved in lymphocyte endothelium interactions such as selectins. Brequinar has been shown experimentally to inhibit T and B cells *in vitro* and graft rejection *in vivo*. Deoxyspergillin seems to block the immune response at the level of antigen presentation and has been shown experimentally to reverse corticosteroid-resistant rejection and chronic rejection. Leflunomide inhibits IL-2 receptor transcription and inhibits experimental allograft rejection. It may have effects on chronic rejection.

USE OF IMMUNOSUPPRESSIVE DRUGS TO PREVENT ACUTE REJECTION

The prototype prophylactic therapeutic combination that has been used in the majority of liver transplant units is based around triple immunosuppressive therapy with corticosteroids, azathioprine, and CSA. High dose induction corticosteroid regimens usually consist of 500mg at the time of transplant, reducing to 20–30mg within 7–10 days. Lower dose regimens consist of just 1mg/kg in tapering fashion. Some units withdraw corticosteroids at 3 months without any significant increase in acute rejection. Azathioprine is usually given at 1–1.5mg/kg and CSA initially given orally at 10mg/kg day. Recent studies have shown that liver allograft rejection is reduced with Neoral therapy compared with the original Sandimmune preparation of CSA. Absorption of Neoral in the first 24–48 hours is variable, but this does not seem to decrease the effectiveness of this agent. Cyclosporine is usually given as a q12h dose, and doses are adjusted according to drug levels. Cyclosporine is usually measured in whole blood by monoclonal immunoassays which detect only parent compound or by high performance liquid chromatography (HPLC). Drug levels are usually maintained in the 100–300ng/mL) range in the early postoperative period. Improvement on CSA-based triple immunosuppressive regimens has been examined in several studies. The addition of prophylactic OKT3 or ALG therapy, so-called 'quadruple therapy' has not led to a significant decrease in eventual rejection rates or alterations in outcomes. Controlled clinical trials that have compared the Sandimmune preparation of CSA with tacrolimus in a triple therapy regimen have shown a significant decrease in the acute rejection rate, significant decrease in the use of OKT3 for rescue therapy, and a decrease in the need for long-term corticosteroids and the maintenance corticosteroid dose with tacrolimus. Thus, improvements in 'baseline' or prophylactic immunosuppression can be achieved with the substitution of tacrolimus for Sandimmune, and many units prefer tacrolimus instead of CSA as baseline immunosuppression. Side effects of tacrolimus were slightly worse in these two studies, although tacrolimus was used at doses that are slightly higher than would currently be recommended. The recommended dosage for tacrolimus for prophylaxis is 0.1–0.15mg/kg daily. Similar to CSA, tacrolimus doses are adjusted according to drug levels. Tacrolimus levels should be 5–15pg/ml, although the lower limit of the therapeutic range is unclear. Direct comparisons of Neoral versus tacrolimus are not yet available, but multicenter trials in Europe and in the USA and Canada are currently underway.

The next major alternative in immunosuppressive therapy is the substitution of azathioprine by mycophenolate on a background of corticosteroid and CSA therapy. Mycophenolate has been shown, in renal transplantation in three multicenter control trials, to decrease the acute rejection rate and decrease the incidence of use of OKT3 rescue therapy for acute rejection. The dose recommended in liver transplantation is 2–3g/day. There is currently a multicenter international trial directly comparing mycophenolate and azathioprine in liver transplantation. Rapamycin has now entered clinical trials in renal transplantation. Rapamycin cannot be used with tacrolimus. Results are keenly awaited from these studies.

DRUGS WHICH INHIBIT THE IMMUNE SYSTEM: SIDE EFFECTS AND DRUG INTERACTIONS

General side effects of immunosuppressive agents
All immunosuppressive drugs predispose the organism to infection and the development of neoplastic disease.

It should be always realized that there is a close correlation between suppression of the immune system and these two side effects. The infections that are generally predisposed to by immunosuppressive drugs include the activation of the herpes viruses [cytomeglovirus (CMV), herpes simplex virus (HSV) and herpes zoster]. There is also the predisposition to fungal infections and bacterial infections. General immunosuppression leads to the development of lymphoproliferative diseases and the development of epithelial tumors. Lymphoproliferative disease occurring relatively early post-transplant in the setting of immunosuppression is often associated with reactivation or primary infection with Epstein–Barr virus (EBV). Apart from these general side effects, each individual immunosuppressive drug has particular side effects that are exacerbated or decreased by certain drug interactions (Fig. 36.12).

Summary of major side effects and drug interactions of immunosuppressive therapies		
Drug	**Side effects**	**Drug interaction**
Corticosteroids	Glucose intolerance, delirium, hypertension, osteoporosis, cataracts	N/A
Azathioprine	Thrombocytopenia, neutropenia 'allergic' reaction, pancreatitis	Allopurinol
Cyclosporine	Hypertension, renal dysfunction, headaches, hair growth, central nervous system problems, hyperkalemia	Increased levels: diltiazem doxycyline erythromycin itraconazole omeprazole Decreased levels: rifampin phenytoin carbamazapine
Mycophenolate mofetil	Diarrhea, dyspepsia, neutropenia, thrombocytopenia, headache, skin rash	Not known
Rapamycin	Hyperlipidemia	Not known
OKT3/ALG	'Cytokine release' syndrome: aseptic meningitis bronchospasm fever, chills, rigors myalgias hypotension	Nil significance

Figure 36.12 Summary of major side effects and drug interaction of main immunosuppressive therapies.

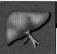
Corticosteroids

The side effects of corticosteroids are numerous and well known. The most common effects involve the musculoskeletal problems of osteoporosis, osteonecrosis, and myopathy. Associated with these are the endocrine effects of glucose intolerance with the development of overt diabetes, hypokalemia, and fluid retention often associated with hypertension. There are effects on the neuropsychiatric system, such as psychosis, insomnia, and depression, which are usually associated with high doses. Cataracts commonly occur with prolonged use. Apart from these side effects, the common gastrointestinal effects of dyspepsia, the predisposition to peptic ulcer and the skin effects of easy bruising, atrophy, stria, and acne occur in many patients. All of the above effects are almost routine with the prolonged use of these agents in doses above 10mg/day. Corticosteroids are not contraindicated in pregnancy.

Azathioprine

The main side effect of azathioprine is associated bone marrow depression, particularly leukopenia and thrombocytopenia. Other side effects include mild alopecia, gastrointestinal upset, and retinopathy. It should be also recognized that azathioprine may cause pancreatitis, cholestatic hepatitis, and vascular abnormalities within the liver with the development of nodular regenerative hyperplasia and veno-occlusive disease. Its major toxicity is increased by interaction with allopurinol, a xanthine oxidase inhibitor. Xanthine oxidase is important in the metabolism of azathioprine. These drugs should not be used together in clinical practice. Azathioprine may also cause an allergic reaction in <1% of individuals resulting in high fevers, arthralgias, and myalgias. Reintroduction of the azathioprine in these circumstances reproduces the syndrome. Azathioprine is not contraindicated in pregnancy.

Cyclosporine

Cyclosporine has quite a narrow therapeutic window. Its most common side effects include hypertension (over 30% of cases) and nephrotoxicity which is associated with almost a universal decrease of 30% in the glomerular filtration rate. The nephrotoxicity is associated with structural changes within the kidney, particularly the development of interstitial fibrosis. Cyclosporine also has a tendency to cause hyperkalemia. Its other toxicities include effects on the central and peripheral nervous systems. It commonly causes tremor and headache, predisposes patients to convulsions, and may also cause peripheral neuropathy. It has been associated with leukoencephalopathy, which mainly involves the occipital cortical pathways and may result in coma and the development of cortical blindness. Its effect on the skin may result in features of hirsutism and hair growth. The latter is associated with extension of the length of the individual hair fibers, making them less brittle and therefore less prone to breakage. It may also cause gingival hyperplasia, and breast adenofibromatosis, and commonly causes respiratory side effects that resemble sinusitis and sinus congestion. Patients often complain of nasal stuffiness.

The above side effects of CSA are directly dose related, and drug levels may be altered by significant drug interactions. Calcium channel blockers, particularly diltiazem and verapamil; antibiotics such doxycycline and erythromycin; and the antifungal agents itraconazale and ketoconazole all increase levels and predispose to toxicity. Apart from these direct drug interactions on levels, neurotoxicity seems to be increased with the interaction with the antibiotic imipenem, and nephrotoxicity is increased with the use of aminoglycosides, nonsteroidal anti-inflammatory drugs, amphotericin, and intravenous bactrim. Angiotensin-converting enzyme inhibitors, used for the treatment of CSA-associated hypertension, increase the hyperkalemic effect of CSA.

Although increased CSA levels predispose to toxicity, decreased levels may predispose to allograft rejection. Decreased levels may be brought about by cytochrome P450 enzyme inducers such as the anticonvulsants (phenytoin, barbiturates), the antituberculous drugs [isoniazid (INAH) and rifampin (rifampicin)], and octreotide and bactrim. Cyclosporine is not contraindicated in pregnancy.

Tacrolimus

The side effects of tacrolimus are very similar to those of CSA, apart from a few significant differences. The renal nephrotoxicity is almost identical, although the neurotoxicity seems to be worse. There seems to be less hypertension, but there is increased glucose intolerance with tacrolimus. There is certainly less effect on gingival hyperplasia, hirsutism or hair growth compared with CSA. Tacrolimus is thought to be associated with a 'less cardiovascular risk' lipid profile than CSA. The drug interactions with tacrolimus are very similar to those of CSA. Tacrolimus is contraindicated in pregnancy.

Mycophenolate mofetil

The main side effect is on the gastrointestinal tract, resulting particularly in diarrhea. There may be associated nausea and vomiting. Headache seems to be a common problem. Bone marrow suppression with leukopenia and thrombocytopenia is less common than with azathioprine, but does occur. Mycophenolate mofetil is contraindicated in pregnancy.

Rapamycin

The main side effect of rapamycin is the development of hypertriglyceridemia, which may be quite profound. It also has effects on the gastrointestinal tract with nausea, vomiting, and diarrhea. It is contraindicated in pregnancy.

OKT3

The main effect of this drug is the development of the cytokine release syndrome, resulting in high fevers, arthralgia, and myalgia. This syndrome can be quite severe and may be associated with aseptic meningitis, coma, adult respiratory distress syndrome, and systemic hypotension. Cardiac arrest has been described with the use of OKT3. It is particularly important that the patient is not fluid overloaded at the time of the injection. Side effects are modified by the initial use of 1g of methyl prednisolone during the first injection and the regular use of antihistamines and acetaminophen (paracetamol) with each subsequent injection. The cytokine release syndrome is most severe during the first 1–2 injections. OKT3 causes profound immunosuppression. There is clinical reactivation of herpes viruses (HSV, CMV) in over 70% of cases. Total doses of >75mg predispose to lymphoproliferative diseases.

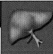

LIVER ALLOGRAFT REJECTION

Hyperacute liver allograft rejection

This is an uncommon event in liver transplantation with only a small number of cases reported in the literature. It may come on within the first 1–2 days after transplantation, but usually does not appear until the second week (Fig. 36.13).

It is characterized by a rapid deterioration of graft function, often with the clinical picture of acute liver failure. There is usually a high fever, right upper quadrant pain, rapidly deteriorating liver function tests with asparate aminotransferase (AST) and alanine aminotransferase (ALT) at levels of >1000U/L. The international normalized ratio (INR) becomes rapidly prolonged and there is profound thrombocytopenia and acid/base disturbances.

Hyperacute rejection is mediated by an antibody and complement mediated attack on the vascular endothelium. The antibodies that result in the hyperacute rejection syndrome are either preformed HLA antibodies against the donor MHC antigens, or against blood group antigens. The characteristic pathologic finding is that of massive hemorrhagic necrosis associated with complement, fibrin, and immunoglobulin deposition in arteries, veins, and sinusoids (Fig. 36.14).

There may be segmental infarction of the graft, together with necrosis of the biliary tract. The management is very difficult. Plasmapheresis, cyclophosphamide and OKT3 therapies have been attempted with little success. The only really effective management is that of urgent retransplantation.

Acute liver allograft rejection

Acute liver allograft rejection occurs at varying frequencies (30–70%). It occurs at a mean of 7–9 days after transplant, and is often clinically silent. Occasionally there may be right upper quadrant discomfort and fever. Biochemically there is derangement of the serum bilirubin, alkaline phosphatase (AP), γ-glutamyltranspeptidase (γ-GT), AST, and ALT levels. However, these do not form a characteristic pattern, and cannot be used to distinguish acute rejection from other causes of liver graft dysfunction. The coagulation status is usually not disturbed and there is usually not a fall in the platelet count.

The diagnosis of acute liver allograft rejection is made on liver biopsy and has been recently defined by an international panel as 'inflammation of the allograft, elicited by a genetic disparity between the donor and recipient, primarily affecting interlobular bile ducts and vascular endothelia, including portal veins and hepatic venules and occasionally the hepatic artery and its branches'. Hence, there are three predominant features:
- portal inflammation;
- bile duct damage; and
- endothelitis.

At least two of these three features are required for a histopathologic diagnosis of acute rejection (AR).

First, a 'mixed' portal tract infiltrate consisting of lymphocytes, neutrophils, monocytes, and eosinophils is present (Fig. 36.15). The percentage of eosinophils is usually determined by the prophylactic corticosteroid dose at the time of the acute rejection. If the corticosteroid dose has been high and acute rejection occurs, then the eosinophils are not often seen.

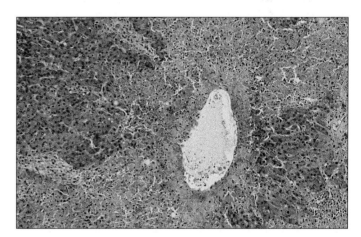

Figure 36.14 Liver biopsy features of hyperacute liver allograft rejection showing widespread hemorrhegic necrosis. (Hematoxylin and eosin.)

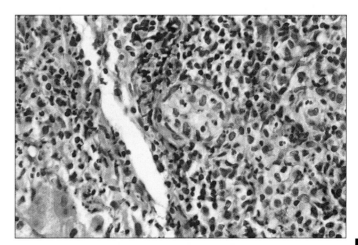

Figure 36.15 Liver biopsy features of acute liver allograft rejection with portal tract infiltrate and bile duct damage with invading inflammatory cells.

Patterns of liver allograft rejection

Type of rejection	Clinical	Biochemical changes	Biopsy features	Molecular/cellular pathways
Hyperacute	Within 10 days of transplant, acute liver failure	AST >1000μ/L AST >1000μ/L INR prolonged hypoglycemia	Hemorrhagic necrosis	Antibody and complement
Acute	Any time, average day 9 post-transplant, nonspecific symptoms (if any)	Any pattern	Mixed portal infiltrate, endothelitis, bile duct damage	DTH, T cells, cytokines
Chronic	Any time after the first month post-transplant, jaundice and cholestasis	AP, γ-GT markedly elevated, hyper-bilirubinemia	Loss of inter-lobular bile ducts, portal tract fibrosis, a decrease in cellular filtrate	T cells, macrophages, growth factors, stellate cells

Figure 36.13 Patterns of liver allograft rejection.

The second feature is that of vascular endothelitis, particularly of the portal tract venules, but sometimes including central veins (Fig. 36.16). This is characterized by activated lymphocytes and monocytes adhering to the vascular endothelium, invading underneath and sometimes lifting off the endothelial structures.

The third feature is inflammation of the interlobular bile ducts with infiltration of the epithelium with lymphocytes and monocytes (see Fig. 36.15). In more advanced cases, there is flattening of the epithelium and an increasing eosinophilic component to the cytoplasm and loss of nuclei from individual cells. Immunohistochemical studies have shown that the lymphocytic infiltrate within portal tracts is of both the CD4$^+$ and CD8$^+$ subsets, while infiltration of the biliary epithelium is predominantly by CD8$^+$ cells. The molecular pathogenesis of acute liver allograft rejection is associated with increased intrahepatic expression of IL-2, INF-γ, and IL-5 (particularly if eosinophils are present). Studies have also indicated that there is loss of portal tract microvascular structures during acute rejection (Fig. 36.17).

Although the three key pathologic changes described above are the basis of diagnosis, other changes may occur. In lobular areas there may be cell necrosis/apoptosis and a lobular portal tract infiltrate consisting mainly of CD8$^+$ cells. The presence of centrizonal ballooning and particularly fallout of hepatocytes in zone three of the hepatic lobule suggests that the rejection is severe and may have a vascular component (Fig. 36.18).

Very rarely there may be an arteritis of small arterioles in portal tracts.

Actual grading systems of acute liver allograft rejection have been provided by many groups. More recently a grading system has been developed by an international panel to classify and grade liver allograft rejection (Fig. 36.19).

This system essentially grades the level of acute rejection as indeterminate, mild, moderate or severe dependent on the degree of portal tract infiltrate. As part of this, a rejection activity index (RAI) can be derived by scoring each of the three main features (i.e. portal tract infiltrate, bile duct damage, and endothelitis) on a score of 0–3 (Fig. 36.20).

It is generally thought that all episodes of AR with RAI $\geq$ 6 should be treated, although many units treat milder forms of AR.

The management of acute rejection consists of a pulse of corticosteroid therapy, 1g daily on three successive days with a rapid taper back to maintenance corticosteroid doses. Such therapy is usually successful in 60–70% of cases. In cases that are slow to respond or do not respond to such a pulse of corticosteroids, different plans of management exist that depend on the baseline immunosuppressive regimen. For example, in a

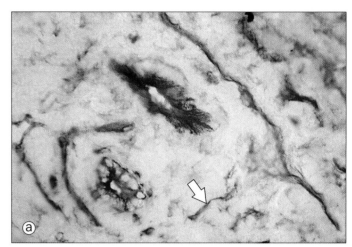

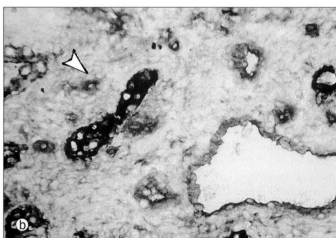

Figure 36.17 Identification of microvascular portal tract structures (brown staining). (a) In normal liver and (b) their reduction during acute liver allograft rejection.

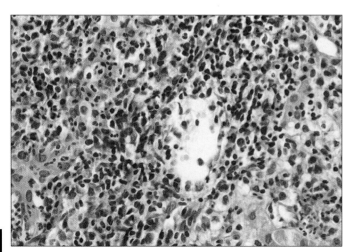

Figure 36.16 Liver biopsy features of acute liver allograft rejection showing endothelitis.

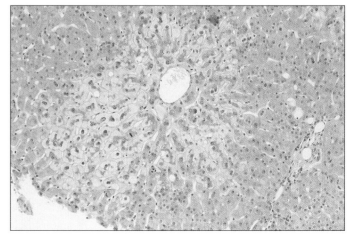

Figure 36.18 Centrizonal ballooning during acute liver allograft rejection suggesting vascular involvement and severe rejection.

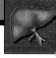

Grading of acute liver allograft rejection

Global assessment	Criteria
No rejection	No infiltrate present or the inflammation is related to other causes of dysfunction (viral hepatitis, biliary obstruction, etc).
Indeterminate for rejection	Rejection-type portal inflammatory infiltrate that fails to meet the criteria for the diagnosis of rejection because of lack of direct bile duct damage, or involvement of an insufficient percentage of portal triads.
Mild rejection	Evidence of a mixed portal infiltrate (usually lymphocytic with blasts and often with eosinophils and neutrophils) in at least one-third of the triads, that is generally mild and confined within the portal spaces. Clearly defined bile duct damage is present and subendothelial inflammation of portal or central vein branches is often seen.
Moderate rejection	As above for mild, with the rejection infiltrate expanding most or all of the triads.
Severe rejection	As above for moderate, with spillover of the infiltrate into the periportal areas and moderate to severe perivenular inflammation that extends into the hepatic parenchyma and is associated with hepatocyte necrosis.

Figure 36.19 Diagnosis of acute graft rejection – Banff International Consensus Schema. This table shows the grading of acute liver allograft rejection.

The acute liver allograft rejection activity index

Category	Criteria	Score
Portal inflammation	Mostly lymphocytic inflammation involving, but not noticeably expanding, a minority of the triads.	1
	Expansion of most or all of the triads, by a mixed infiltrate containing lymphocytes with occasional blasts, neutrophils and eosinophils.	2
	Marked expansion of most or all of the triads by a mixed infiltrate containing numerous blasts and eosinophils with inflammatory spillover into the periportal parenchyma.	3
Bile duct inflammation damage	A minority of the ducts are cuffed and infiltrated by inflammatory cells and show only mild reactive changes such as increased nuclear cytoplasmic ratio of the epithelial cells.	1
	Most or all of the ducts infiltrated by inflammatory cells. More than an occasional duct shows degenerative changes such as nuclear pleomorphism, disordered polarity and cytoplasmic vacuolization of the epithelium.	2
	As above for 2, with most or all of the ducts showing degenerative changes or focal lumenal disruption.	3
Venous endothelial inflammation	Subendothelial lymphocytic infiltration involving some, but not a majority of the portal and/or hepatic venules.	1
	Subendothelial infiltration involving most or all of the portal and/or hepatic venules.	2
	As above for 2, with moderate or severe perivenular inflammation that extends into the perivenular parenchyma and is associated with perivenular hepatocyte necrosis.	3
Total score	(Sum of components) =	9 (max)

Figure 36.20 Diagnosis of acute graft rejection – Banff International Consensus Schema. This table shows the rejection activity index (RAI). Criteria that can be used to score liver allograft biopsies with acute rejection, as defined by the Banff International Consensus scheme.

CSA-based regimen, nonresponsiveness at this stage may lead to the introduction of tacrolimus, replacing CSA. Alternatively, if the corticosteroid-resistant rejection is mild, then a further pulse of corticosteroids may occur. In severe corticosteroid-resistant rejection, OKT3 is effective in reversing ongoing rejection in over 90% of cases. The decision whether to use OKT3 in corticosteroid-resistant rejection or convert to tacrolimus will often be dependent on the severity of the cellular infiltrate. These two approaches have not been directly compared, but both seem effective in reversing corticosteroid-resistant rejection. Tacrolimus is probably less effective than OKT3 if the serum bilirubin is >200μmol/L (Fig. 36.21).

Chronic liver allograft rejection

Chronic liver allograft rejection (CR) occurs at a low frequency in human liver transplantation. Currently, experience in most centers indicates a frequency of less than 10%. Several factors

have been shown to predispose to chronic liver allograft rejection (Fig. 36.22).

These include low cyclosporine (CSA) levels, multiple episodes of acute rejection, late episodes of acute rejection, CMV infection, positive lymphotoxic antibody cross-matching, HCV infection and gender mismatching between donor and recipient.

Clinically, CR is associated with progressive cholestasis, a rise in the serum bilirubin with clinical jaundice, an enlarged liver, increasing alkaline phosphatase and γ-GT with only moderate elevations in AST and ALT levels. The INR and the platelet count are usually normal. The diagnosis is based on liver histology and is characterized by two predominant lesions. First, is the loss of interlobular bile ducts, the so-called 'vanishing bile duct syndrome'. This is associated with loss of microvasculature and arteriolar structures within the portal tract and a decreasing rather than increasing inflammatory infiltrate. The portal tracts often become small and fibrotic (Fig. 36.23).

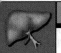
The second major change occurs in the hepatic lobule with progressive ballooning in zone three of the hepatic lobule and cellular fallout with hepatocyte necrosis (Fig. 36.24).

There is marked upregulation of MHC and adhesion molecules on hepatocytes and remaining bile ducts. CD8+ T cells can still be found attacking bile duct remnants and in lobular zone three areas (Fig. 36.25).

Although often not seen on needle biopsy specimens there is a marked transplant vasculopathy in medium-sized arteries in liver explants or at autopsy (Fig. 36.26). This consists of thickening of the arterial intimae, destruction of the internal elastic lamina, and the presence of macrophages (arterial foam cells), smooth muscle cells (myofibroblasts), and thickening and fibrosis of the intimae. There is also continuing infiltrate in these lesions of CD4+, and CD8+ cells, as well as macrophages (Figs 36.27 & 36.28).

These lesions show increased expression of adhesion molecules on the endothelium. The process is not dissimilar to classic atherosclerosis, although the lesions tend to be concentric, effect medium-sized vessels, and have intact endothelium (Figs 36.29 & 36.30).

Risk factors for chronic rejection
Persistently low CSA levels
Gender (M/F) allograft mismatch
CMV mismatch
Multiple episodes of acute rejection
Severity of acute rejection
Late acute rejection
HCV infection
Positive lymphocytotoxic crossmatch with donor

Figure 36.22 Risk factors for chronic rejection.

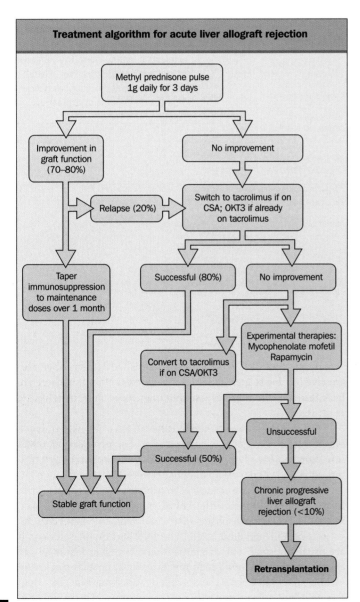

Figure 36.21 Treatment algorithm for acute liver allograft rejection.

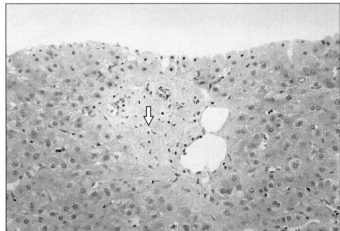

Figure 36.23 Liver biopsy features of chronic allograft rejection. Hematoxylin and eosin stained section of portal tract (arrow) showing lack of inflammatory infiltrate and portal tract fibrosis, severe bile duct damage, and loss of portal tract arterioles.

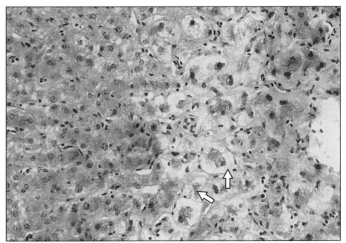

Figure 36.24 Liver biopsy features of chronic allograft rejection. Hematoxylin and eosin stained section of liver lobule showing ballooning of hepatocytes in zone III of hepatic lobule (arrows).

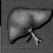

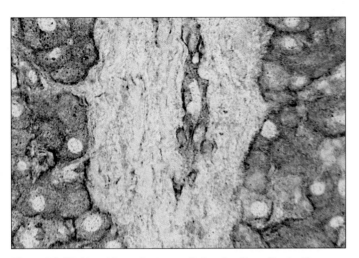

Figure 36.25 Liver biopsy features of chronic allograft rejection.
Remnant of damaged bile duct (blue) being attacked by CD8+ T cells
(pink). (With permission of WB Saunders, Hepatology. 1990;12:1305.)

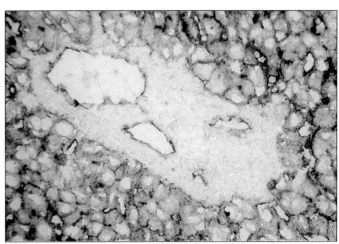

Figure 36.26 Liver biopsy features of chronic allograft rejection.
Total loss of microvascular structures in chronic rejection.

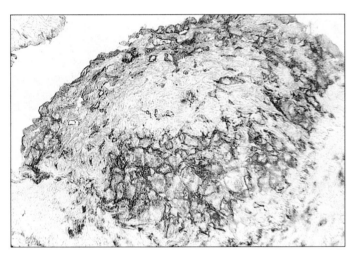

Figure 36.27 Liver biopsy features of chronic allograft rejection.
Macrophage infiltrate in allograft atherosclerosis. (With permission of WB
Saunders, Hepatology. 1990;12:1305.)

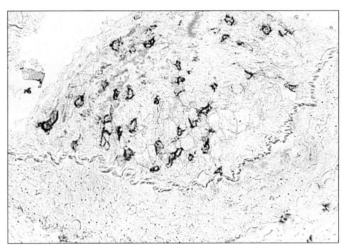

Figure 36.28 CD3+ T cells in allograft atherosclerosis. (With
permission of WB Saunders, Hepatology. 1990;12:1305.)

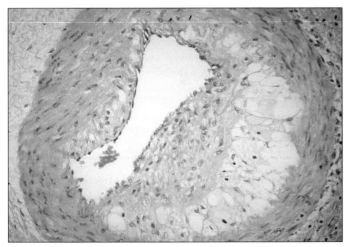

Figure 36.29 Liver biopsy features of chronic allograft rejection.
Evidence of 'allograft atherosclerosis'.

The process of CR once fully established is invariably progressive leading to graft failure. However it is clear that there are
intermediate cases and reversibility may occur. It is thought that
tacrolimus therapy may be effective at early stages of CR, particularly when the serum bilirubin is <200μmol/L. Also
mycophenolate mofetil may be useful in this situation, although
this has not been proven or recognized clinically at the moment.
Both these drugs inhibit smooth muscle proliferation as well as
T- and B-cell proliferation. Smooth muscle proliferation is an
important feature of the chronic liver allograft response particularly at the level of the medium-sized transplant vasculopathy.
Eventually rapamycin may also prove useful in CR.

XENOTRANSPLANTATION

The possibility of xenotransplantation, (i.e. the transplantation of
organs from one species to another) (Fig. 36.31) has been an
ongoing area of research for several decades. The major problem

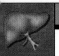

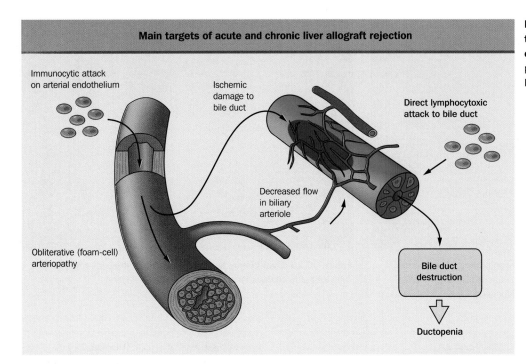

Main targets of acute and chronic liver allograft rejection

Immunocytic attack
on arterial endothelium

Ischemic
damage to
bile duct

Direct lymphocytoxic
attack to bile duct

Obliterative (foam-cell)
arteriopathy

Decreased flow
in biliary
arteriole

Bile duct
destruction

Ductopenia

Figure 36.30 Schematic summary of the main targets of acute and chronic liver allograft rejection. (With permission of WB Saunders, Hepatology. 1991;14:721.)

Current approaches to xenotransplantation

Modification type	Example
Recipient	Depletion of anti-Galα1–3Gal antibodies
Donor	Knockout of α1,3-galactosyltransferase gene Creation of human CD55 (decay accelerating factor) transgenics Creation of human CD59 (membrane inhibitor of reactive lysis) transgenics Creation of combined human CD55/CD59 double transgenics

Figure 36.31 Current approach to xenotransplantation.

with organ xenotransplantation has been hyperacute rejection characterized by interstitial hemorrhage and widespread vascular thrombosis leading to necrosis and destruction of the organ within minutes or hours after revascularization. This process is mainly mediated by the binding of xenoreactive antibodies to recipient endothelium, leading to the activation of the complement system. Natural inhibitors of the complement system are species specific and are unable to dampen down this process.

Recent studies have identified that 85% of xenoreactive antibodies (>90% of the IgM subclass) in human serum recognize a single structure: Galα1–3Gal. The synthesis of this sugar on various glycoproteins is catalyzed by α1,3-galactosyl transferase. Approaches to overcome hyperacute xenograft rejection have involved the depletion from recipient serum of these antibodies by various columns, and this has been shown to prevent hyperacute rejection of some xenografts. The other approach has been to produce 'knock-out' organ donors. In mice, xenografted organs in which the α1,3-galactosyl transferase gene has been ablated survive significantly longer than do 'normal' xenografts. A third approach has been the generation of transgenic xenograft donors which express a galactosyl transferase that catalyzes the addition

of an extra sugar other than α-galactose onto the terminus of various oligosaccharide chains. Currently all of these processes remain at the experimental level, and have not been applied to the human situation.

A further critical event during hyperacute xenograft rejection is that of complement activation. This is regulated by complementary regulatory proteins such as decay-accelerating factor (CD55) and membrane inhibitor of reactive lysis (CD59). These control proteins are species specific. For example, pig CD55 and CD59 are unable to break down human complement. Thus, when human complement is activated on pig endothelium, the process is ongoing. Approaches to overcome this have included the production of transgenic animals that express human CD55 and CD59. Such experiments have recently shown that significant delays in hyperacute rejection after xenotransplantation can be obtained.

Apart from the problem of hyperacute rejection there are other layers of acute vascular rejection that are mediated by a significant cellular component, as well as an antibody/complement component. There is increasing interest in the possible role of NK cells in acute vascular xenograft rejection. Other hurdles to be overcome include further cellular responses resulting in T-cell-mediated xenograft rejection. Finally, concerns about infectious agents and the transfer of endogenous retroviral infections from other species into the human need to be overcome before xenotransplantation becomes a clinical reality.

LIVER ALLOGRAFT TOLERANCE

There are four main general mechanisms of tolerance:
- First, there is anergy where the antigen is ignored by the immune system.
- Second, there is regulation away from an active immune response towards a nonactive immune response. The Th1/Th2 paradigm has been implicated in such regulation with a predominant Th1 response occurring in rejection, and a Th2 response occurring in tolerance to the liver allograft.

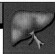
- Third, there is deletion of antigen-specific cells.
- Fourth, there is activation-associated tolerance which may or may not be related to the deletional processes.

It has been recognized in human clinical studies that a select group of patients can be weaned off immunosuppression without loss of their liver allograft, thus implying that a subset of humans in fact have become tolerant. The mechanisms of liver transplant tolerance have, however, been best studied in models of spontaneous tolerance, which have been identified between inbred rat strains, inbred mouse strains, and some outbred pig strains. One of the important observations in clarifying the mechanisms of spontaneous liver allograft tolerance was the recognition that there was a migration of a significant number of donor leukocytes from the transplanted liver to the recipient lymph nodes and spleen. This led to the concept of the establishment of microchimerism and 'minigraft-versus-host disease' as a suppressor mechanism of the recipient immune response. While this process may definitely occur, it seems to evolve over a long period of time, while acceptance of livers in the experimental spontaneous tolerance systems occurs very rapidly within the first few days.

Recently, the mechanism of this early tolerance process has been defined to a significant extent. It seems that the early rapid migration of donor leukocytes from the liver allograft to recipient lymphoid tissues results in 'hyperactivation of recipient lymphocytes' (Fig. 36.32).

This has been shown by the demonstration of increased messenger RNA production for IL-2 and IFN-γ by these cells. In subsequent events, it has been shown that within the liver

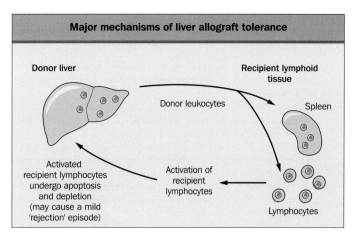

Figure 36.32 Major mechanism of liver allograft tolerance.

allograft itself there is increased apoptosis of infiltrating lymphocytes in tolerant animals compared with animals undergoing rejection. These two observations imply that spontaneous liver allograft tolerance is an activation-associated event, resulting in apoptosis and probable deletion of alloreactive cells. The above concept has important implications for approaches designed to increase the chances of liver allograft tolerance in the clinical setting. It would imply that donor leukocytes are crucial in establishing the process and that early heavy immunosuppression at the time of transplantation or in the 24–48 hours afterwards may inhibit the tolerance process, not enhance it. Such concepts need to be tested in the clinical setting.

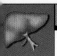

FURTHER READING

Abraham RT, Wiedernecht GJ. Immunopharmacology of rapamycin. Ann Rev Immunol. 1996;14:483–510. *Up-to-date, detailed overview of actions of rapamycin and experimental evidence for inhibition of the immune response.*

Auchincloss H, Sultan H. Antigen processing and presentation in transplantation. Curr Opin Immunol. 1996;8:681–7. *Summary of the main arguments for indirect alloantigen presentation.*

Azuma H, Tilney NL. Chronic graft rejection. Curr Opin Immunol. 1994;6:770–6. *Summary of pathogenic mechanisms in chronic allograft rejection.*

Baggioline M, Dewald B, Moser B. Human chemokines: an update. Ann Rev Immunol. 1997;15:675–706. *Overview of the chemokine family and their receptors.*

Bishop GA, Sun JH, Sheil AGR, McCaughan GW. High dose/activation associated tolerance: a mechanism for allograft tolerance. Transplantation. 1997;64:1377–83. *Evidence for the mechanisms of activation associated tolerance as the mechanism in spontaneous liver allograft tolerance.*

Brady LM, Watson SR. Lymphocyte migration into tissue: the paradigm derived from CD4 subsets. Curr Opin Immunol. 1996;8:312–20. *Discussion of mechanisms of lymphocyte entrance into tissues.*

Brazelton T, Morris RE. Molecular mechanisms of action of new xenobiotic immunosuppressive drugs: tacrolimus (FK506), sirolimus (rapamycin), mycophenolate mofetil and leflunomide. Curr Opin Immunol. 1996;8:710–20. *Summary of current knowledge of molecular action of the new immunosuppressive drugs.*

Cantrell D. The T cell antigen receptor signal transduction pathways. Ann Rev Immunol. 1996;14:259–74. *Detailed description of intracellular pathways following TCR recognition responses leading to T-cell activation.*

Chambers CA, Allix JP. Co-stimulation in T cell responses. Curr Opin Immunol. 1997;9:396–404. *Current description of T-cell co-stimulatory pathways important in T-cell activation.*

Chan AC, Shaw AS. Regulation of antigen receptor signal transduction by protein tyrosine kinases. Curr Opin Immunol. 1997;9:394–401. *Review of current knowledge on the intracellular kinase pathways that are important in T-cell activation.*

European FK 506 Multicentre Liver Study Group. Randomised trial comparing tacrolimus (FK 506) and cyclosporine in prevention of liver allograft rejection. Lancet. 1994;344:423–8. *The European study of a direct comparison of tacrolimus with CSA (Sandimmune) for prophylaxis of acute and chronic liver allograft rejection.*

Fulton B, Markham A. Mycophenolate mofetil. A review of its pharmacodynamic and pharmacokinetic properties and clinical efficacy in renal transplantation. Drugs. 1996;51:278–98. *Detailed description of the new immunosuppressive drug MMF.*

Hendrick JA, Zlotnick A. Chemokines and lymphocyte biology. Curr Opin Immunol. 1996;8:343–54. *Summary of chemokine structure and function.*

Holt DW, Johnstone A. Cyclosporin microemulsion. A guide to usage and monitoring. Biodrugs. 1997;7:175–97. *Detailed description of the new microemulsion form of CSA.*

Kahan BD. Cyclosporine. N Engl J Med. 1989;321:1725–38. *Detailed description of clinical efficacy and side effects of CSA.*

Karnitz LM, Abraham RT. Cytokine receptor signalling mechanism. Curr Opin Immunol. 1995;7:320–6. *Summary of T-cell activation events at the level of various cytokines.*

Koopman J-O, Hämmerling GJ, Momburg F. Generation, intracellular transport and loading of peptides associated with MHC Class I molecules. Curr Opin Immunol. 1997;9:80–88. *Summary of the current state of knowledge of MHC class I peptide processing.*

Lechler R, Bluestone J. Transplant tolerance – putting the pieces together. Curr Opin Immunol. 1997;9:631–3. *General overview of allograft tolerance.*

Liu J. FK506 and cyclosporine molecular probes for studying intracellular signal transduction. Immunol Today. 1993;14:290–5. *Summary of molecular analysis of CSA and tacrolimus immunosuppressive properties.*

McCaughan GW, Bishop GA. Atherosclerosis of the liver allograft. J Hepatol. 1997;27:592–8. *Comparison of pathogenesis of allograft atherosclerosis versus conventional atherosclerosis.*

Orosz C, Pelletier R. Chronic remodelling pathology in grafts. Curr Opin Immunol. 1997;9:676–80. *Summary of pathogenic mechanisms in chronic allograft rejection.*

Pieters J. MHC Class II restricted antigen presentation. Curr Opin Immunol. 1997;9:89–95. *Summary of MHC Class II peptide processing.*

Platt JL. Xenotransplantation: recent progress and current perspectives. Curr Opin Immunol. 1996;8:721–8. *Summary of current status of xenotransplantation.*

Rossiter H, Alan R, Kupper TS. Selectins, T-cell rolling and inflammation. Mol Med Today. 1997;3:214–22. *Review of mechanisms involved in T cell/endothelial adherence.*

Rumagnani S. The TH1/TH2 paradigm. Immunol Today. 1997;18:263–6. *Review of polarized cytokine responses.*

Strom TB, Roy-Chaudhury P, et al. The TH1/TH2 paradigm and the allograft response. Curr Opin Immunol. 1996;8:688–93. *Summary of the relationship of polarized cytokine responses in allograft rejection.*

Su B, Karin M. Mitogen activated protein kinase cascades and regulation of gene expression. Curr Opin Immunol. 1996;8:402–411. *Summary of intracellular kinase responses involved in T-cell activation.*

US Multicentre FK 506 Liver Study Group. A comparison of tacrolimus (FK506) and cyclosporine for immunosuppression in liver transplantation. N Engl J Med. 1994;331:1110–15. *USA study comparing cyclosporines (Sandimmune) and tacrolimus in prevention of acute and chronic liver allograft rejection.*

Wiesner RH, Ludwig J, vanHaek B, Krom RAF. Current concepts in cell-mediated hepatic allograft rejection leading to ductopenia and liver failure. Hepatology. 1991;14:721–9. *Definitive summary of the cellular pathogenesis of acute and chronic liver allograft rejection.*

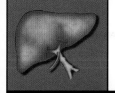

Chapter 37 Infective Complications

Carlos V Paya and Irene G Sia

INTRODUCTION

Despite remarkable progress in liver transplantation, infection is still a constant threat for all liver transplant recipients. The incidence of infections after liver transplantation is generally higher than that after kidney or heart transplantation. In addition to the T- and B-cell immunodeficiencies that are common to any patient receiving high doses of immunosuppressive agents, the complex surgical procedure in a potentially contaminated environment within the abdominal cavity, confounded by the extremely poor medical condition of many recipients, contributes to a high incidence of liver transplantation-specific infectious complications.

Infection affects up to 70% of liver allograft recipients. It is the one of the most serious and common complications of transplant surgery, followed by rejection and allograft dysfunction. The decline in infection-related mortality from more than 50% before 1980 to less than 10% in the 1990s largely reflects refinement of surgical techniques, improved immunosuppressive regimens, and a greater appreciation of the common infectious complications, with the implementation of effective strategies to prevent and treat these infections.

PRETRANSPLANTATION INFECTIOUS DISEASE EVALUATION

Before transplantation, candidates should be evaluated for the presence of factors that may require therapy or preclude transplantation and/or enhance the patient's risk for infection after surgery. Moreover, latent infections might reactivate post-transplantation. Evaluation includes a complete infectious disease history with emphasis on previous infections, vaccinations and endemic exposures; serologic tests, tuberculin skin test with control skin antigens; and chest radiography (Fig. 37.1). Further investigations are pursued depending on elicited risks. When possible, necessary dental evaluation and treatment should be completed before transplantation. If the patient has been exposed to an area endemic for dimorphic fungi, fungal serologies are performed. Vaccinations for tetanus, diphtheria, influenza, pneumococci, hepatitis A and B viruses, and *Haemophilus influenzae* type B infection in pediatric patients, are given if the candidate has not been previously vaccinated. Live vaccines including measles and varicella vaccines may be considered in those candidates with a significant likelihood of exposure, and should be administered prior to transplantation.

TIMING AND EPIDEMIOLOGY OF INFECTIONS AFTER TRANSPLANTATION

The risk of infection after liver transplantation is largely determined by the interaction of host factors, surgical complications, environmental exposures, and the host's net state of immunosuppression. To arrive at a meaningful differential diagnosis for a potential infectious disease syndrome after transplantation, several factors need to be considered. These include the presence of any pre-existing or latent infection in the allograft recipient; possible transmission of infection from the donor organ; knowledge of the anatomic complexities in each individual; actual dosages and duration of immunosuppressive agents; occurrence of acute or chronic rejections; and knowledge of donor and recipient sero-status for various pathogens, particularly for the herpesviruses. These factors also influence the timing of infections after trans-

---

Infectious diseases evaluation before orthotopic liver transplantation

Pretransplant evaluation

History
Immunosuppressive therapy: type and duration
Antibiotic allergies
Past medical history of infectious diseases

Exposure history
Travel history: endemic regions for dimorphic fungi, parasitic diseases; foreign travel
Tuberculosis exposure or prior disease, previous tuberculin skin testing, chest radiography, treatment information
Animal and pet exposures
Occupational exposures
Risk factors for transfusion transmissible viruses (e.g. hepatitis B and C viruses, HIV)
Dietary habits, source of drinking water

Tests
Tuberculin skin test and anergy panel
Chest radiography
Stool examination for ova and parasites
Serologic tests: CMV, HSV, VZV, EBV, HBV, HCV, anti-HIV, anti-HTLV1; rapid plasma reagin; dimorphic fungi (if exposure history is positive); toxoplasmosis

Vaccinations

Tetanus-diphtheria
Pneumococcus
Hepatitis B
Influenza
Haemophilus influenzae type B (in pediatric candidates)

Figure 37.1 Infectious disease evaluation before orthotopic liver transplantation.

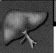

plantation. Post-transplant infections can be best conceptualized by considering three time frames: the first month; the second through the sixth month; and beyond the sixth month. The occurrence of specific infectious syndromes and other diagnostic possibilities vary during each of these time periods, although overlap may occur (Fig. 37.2). Moreover, the routine administration of prophylactic antimicrobial agents such as trimethoprim–sulfamethoxazole (TMP-SMX) to prevent *Pneumocystis carinii* pneumonia has remarkably decreased the occurrence and may have altered the natural history of some of the opportunistic infections that afflict the liver transplant population.

First month (early period)
Major infectious disease problems occurring in the first month after transplantation are related to surgical complications and nosocomial infections. The majority of these infections are due to bacterial followed by fungal pathogens, and, rarely, herpes simplex virus infection. Fever due to wound infections, nosocomial pneumonia, urinary tract infections, line sepsis, and infections of biliary and other drainage catheters often presents during this period. Specific risk factors for early infections include prolonged duration of surgery, graft failure requiring retransplantation, additional abdominal surgeries for treatment of surgical complications, and stays in the intensive care unit, specifically if artificial ventilation and renal dialysis are required. Furthermore, biliary anastomosis with the Roux-en-Y choledochojejunostomy predisposes to reflux into the biliary system, resulting in a higher risk of infection (Figs 37.3 & 37.4). In addition, infections such as chronic cholangitis with small peritoneal abscesses that are present in the allograft recipient before surgery may continue after transplantation if they are not recognized and treated at the

time of surgery. Reactivation of infections due to *Mycobacterium tuberculosis*, the endemic mycoses, *Strongyloides stercoralis*, the viral hepatitides and herpes simplex virus may occur early, but also can present during the middle postsurgical period. Fever in the first month after transplantation may also be from noninfectious causes. Potential etiologies include acute allograft rejection and antilymphocyte therapy; pulmonary embolism and drug fevers also need to be considered.

Months two through six (middle period)
The period from the second to the sixth month after transplantation represents the time of greatest risk for the development of life-threatening opportunistic infections. It is the time during which infections with the immunomodulating viruses exert maximal effects, and when infections with opportunistic pathogens manifest. The type and degree of immunosuppressive therapy used to prevent and/or treat graft rejection and, to a lesser degree, surgical re-exploration due to retransplantation or complications of biliary anastomosis are the major risk factors. The kind of immunosuppressive medication(s) used may also influence the incidence of infectious complications after transplantation. Corticosteroid boluses, OKT3 monoclonal antibody, and antilymphocyte globulin use significantly increase the risk of infection. Marked depression of cell-mediated immune response places patients at an especially high risk for cytomegalovirus (CMV), *Pneumocystis carinii*, *Aspergillus* spp., *Nocardia* spp., *Toxoplasma gondii* and *Listeria monocytogenes* infections. The middle period also witnesses occasional reactivation disease syndromes. Clinical illness may result from the recrudescence of *M. tuberculosis*, an occult focus of bacterial infection, viral hepatitis or one of the dimorphic fungi. Post-transplant lymphoprolif-

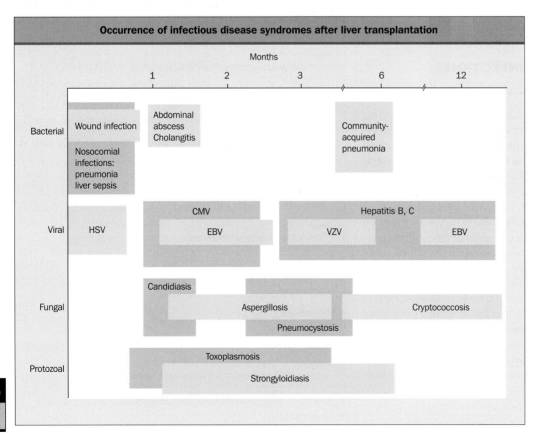

Figure 37.2 Occurrence of infectious disease syndromes after liver transplantation. Note that the occurrence of the specific syndromes follows relatively well-defined periods after transplantation.

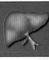
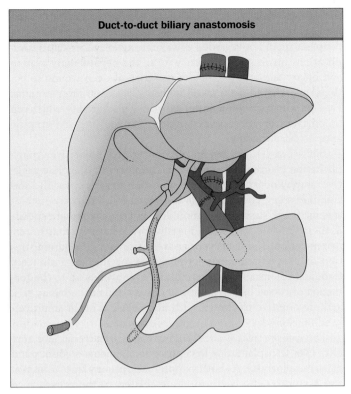

Figure 37.3 Duct-to-duct biliary anastomosis (choledochocholedocostomy).

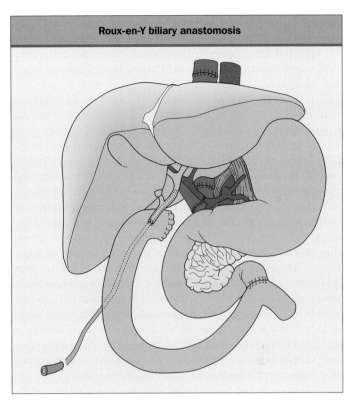

Figure 37.4 Roux-en-Y biliary anastomosis (choledochojejunostomy).

erative disease associated with Epstein–Barr virus is also occasionally seen during this period.

Beyond six months (late period)

The late post-transplant period is associated with relatively few infections among patients with good allograft function because of the lower level of immunosuppression. However, transplant recipients remain more susceptible to the common community-acquired infections seen in the general population. These include influenza virus infection, urinary tract infection, and pneumococcal pneumonia. In contrast, patients with poor allograft function who are maintained on higher doses of immunosuppressive drugs, and patients with biliary strictures or hepatic vascular complications remain at risk for bacterial, fungal, and viral infections. Those with chronic infections such as viral hepatitis suffer increased morbidity associated with these agents.

BACTERIAL INFECTIONS

Bacteria are the most common causes of infections in liver transplant recipients, affecting 35–70% of patients, most of which occur within the first 2 months of transplantation (Fig. 37.5). Many of these infections are related to technical problems with the liver graft, such as bile leaks or biliary obstruction. Significant risk factors associated with bacterial infections are prolonged surgical time, transfusion of large amounts of blood and blood products, repeat abdominal surgeries, CMV infection, rejection, renal dysfunction, and prolonged hospitalization. Liver abscesses are associated with biliary strictures and allograft ischemia from hepatic artery thrombosis. The presence of a choledochojejunostomy rather than a choledochocholedochostomy increas-

es an individual's risk for sepsis, infectious complications related to liver biopsies, and enterococcal and *Pseudomonas* bacteremia.

Commonly encountered bacterial pathogens include aerobic Gram-positive organisms (*Staphylococcus aureus*, coagulase-negative *Staphylococcus* spp., *Streptococcus* spp.) and aerobic Gram-negative bacilli (Enterobacteriaceae, *Pseudomonas aeruginosa*). Whereas antimicrobial agents used for prophylaxis, especially oral agents given to decontaminate the gastrointestinal tract, eliminate most aerobic Gram-negative bacilli and *Candida* organisms while sparing the anaerobic gut flora, selective bowel decontamination has little effect on eliminating Gram-positive bacterial flora. A preponderance of Gram-posi-

Incidence of infectious disease complications after liver transplantation	
Etiology	Frequency (%)
Bacterial	24–68
Viral	5–53
CMV	24–40
HSV	13–30
VZV	5
Fungal	2.8–25
Candida spp.	4–25
Aspergillus spp.	1.5–5
Pneumocystis carinii	4–11
Mycobacterium tuberculosis	0.3–1.2
Protozoal	12

Figure 37.5 Incidence of infectious disease complications after liver transplantation.

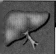

tive infections has been noted after liver transplantation when selective bowel decontamination is used; anaerobic pathogens are reported less frequently. An obvious advantage is the relatively lower incidence of serious Gram-negative bacterial sepsis and its associated mortality.

The abdomen is the most common site of bacterial infections in the liver transplant patients. Infectious complications include wound infections, intrahepatic and extrahepatic abscesses, peritonitis, and cholangitis. The major determinant of wound infections is the complexity of the technical aspect of the operative procedure. Intra-abdominal bleeding and contamination with upper gastrointestinal microbial flora are not uncommon events. Re-exploration for bleeding, retransplantation, and/or biliary leak further increases the risk of acquiring postoperative wound infections. Ischemia of the liver allograft following hepatic artery thrombosis is often complicated by the development of intrahepatic abscesses. Peritonitis and extrahepatic abscesses may arise from biliary anastomotic leaks. Cholangitis usually results from a stricture in the biliary tract. Ultrasound and CT scan are useful aids in identifying the presence of intra-abdominal abscesses (Fig. 37.6). Radiographically guided percutaneous aspiration and culture of a fluid collection is warranted to confirm the presence of infection since sterile fluid loculations are common early after liver transplantation. The anatomy of the biliary tract and the integrity of the hepatic vasculature can be evaluated by Doppler ultrasound, cholangiography, and hepatic angiography.

Nosocomial bacterial pneumonia after liver transplantation is commonly caused by aerobic Gram-negative bacilli including *Pseudomonas aeruginosa* and *Enterobacter* spp. most frequently. Chest radiography is useful for the evaluation of pneumonia; however, right-sided pleural effusion and right lower lobe atelectasis are almost always present in liver transplant patients immediately after surgery, making differentiation of an infected pleural space from reactive pleuritis difficult.

Bacteremia may arise from either a known or unknown source. Most commonly, an intra-abdominal focus and intravascular catheters are the main sources, followed by wounds, lungs, and the urinary tract as additional foci. The appearance of unexplained fever or Gram-negative bacteremia in a liver transplant recipient should be regarded as a manifestation of technical complications involving the vascular tree, the hepatobiliary system and biliary anastomosis, or the presence of deep wound infections, and should prompt immediate diagnostic interventions. Patients with bacteremia suffer a high overall mortality, which can be obviated by appropriate surgical interventions and empiric antimicrobial therapy.

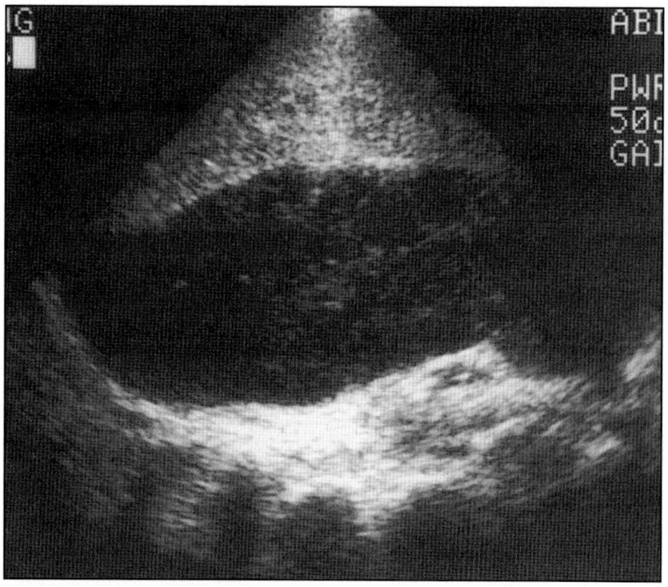

Bile from T-tubes left in place after orthotopic liver transplantation is often colonized with streptococci, coagulase-negative staphylococci, a variety of Gram-negative bacilli, and *Candida* spp. that originate in the bowel. With the exception of specific fungi, such colonization does not usually require specific therapy. However, when invasive procedures such as biliary manipulations and liver biopsies are anticipated, the administration of prophylatic antimicrobial therapy may be indicated. Candidal colonization in the bile can eventually lead to the formation of fungal balls resulting in obstruction of the biliary tree and pre-emptive treatment with fluconazole is often empirically administered.

The urinary tract is a less frequent site of bacterial infection after liver transplantation in contrast to recipients of kidney and pancreas allografts. As both symptomatic urinary tract infection and asymptomatic bacteriuria are related to the presence of indwelling catheters, the prolonged and unnecessary use of bladder catheters is discouraged. Infections of the urinary tract in the absence of Foley catheters, especially if recurrent, should prompt an aggressive and invasive diagnostic work-up to exclude the presence of upper tract infection and/or anatomic abnormalities that may require other therapeutic interventions in addition to antimicrobial therapy.

In patients with suspected bacterial infection, an empiric antimicrobial regimen may be started to cover the most likely pathogens. Before culture results are available, the initial choice of agents should be guided by the most likely site(s) of infection, the antimicrobial susceptibility patterns of the microorganisms in the transplant center, the patient's renal function, and the possibility of existing resistant bacterial species. However, due to the many etiologies of fever in the recipient of an hepatic allograft, especially during the first two months after transplantation, the initiation of empiric treatment in the absence of an overt source of infection is discouraged, unless the patient is clinically and hemodynamically unstable. Aminoglycosides are generally avoided because most liver transplant patients have underlying renal dysfunction, and because the potential cumulative nephrotoxicity with cyclosporine or tacrolimus. Most centers use a third generation cephalosporin as imitial treatment of a suspected pneumonia or abdominal infection. The β-lactam/β-lactamase inhibitor combinations are also often utilized. Some liver transplant groups avoid the use of agents with anaerobic activity when selective bowel decontamination is used to prevent disruption of the Gram-negative anaerobic flora. In a transplant center where the incidence of Gram-negative infection is low and the frequency of Gram-positive bacteremia is high, the appropriate treatment of the latter becomes difficult due to the rapid emergence of resistant microorganisms, notably vancomycin-resistant enterococci (VRE). Because of the relatively low morbidity of infections caused by these organisms, awaiting the results of culture and susceptibility studies before initiating treatment may be

Figure 37.6 Liver abscess. Ultrasound of the abdomen demonstrates the presence of an intrahepatic abscess in the liver allograft.

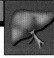

appropriate. Other currently available broad-spectrum antimicrobial agents are the carbapenems, quinolones, and the new fourth-generation cephalosporins. Once the source of infection is identified and the diagnosis established, the antimicrobial coverage should be tailored to an agent that is safe and with the narrowest spectrum of microbial coverage. Surgical or radiologic evacuation of infected fluid collections and debridement of necrotic tissues should not be inadvertently delayed once these are identified.

At the time of transplant surgery, general principles of surgical antimicrobial prophylaxis are observed. Prophylaxis should be adjusted to reflect the vast spectrum of infectious etiologies and the antimicrobial susceptibility patterns of microorganisms typically encountered in a particular transplant center. Most centers use a third-generation cephalosporin either alone or in combination with an aminoglycoside. Regimens that include ampicillin and metronidazole are also used in some centers. Perioperative antibiotic prophylaxis is routinely initiated just before the surgery, and for no longer than 24–48 hours thereafter, although durations of up to 5 days may be acceptable. The major concern about the administration of antibiotics for prophylaxis is the selection of antibiotic-resistant bacteria and the replacement of Gram-negative with Gram-positive bacteria as the major pathogens.

Considerable interest and debate have been focused on the use of selective bowel decontamination (SBD) to prevent postoperative infections. The concept of selective bowel decontamination evolved from the belief that preservation of anaerobic bacteria in the gut would limit colonization or overgrowth by the Gram-negative bacilli, the major nosocomial pathogens. While no large randomized prospective studies have been performed in the liver transplant recipients, several reports have noted a low level of serious Gram-negative infections when SBD regimens are used. The combination of oral nonabsorbable antibiotics (e.g. polymixin E, gentamicin, and nystatin in a solution), is administered four times daily from the time of activation for transplantation until 3–4 weeks after transplantation. To achieve oropharyngeal decontamination more effectively, the same antibiotics have been added to a sticky paste that is then applied topically on the buccal mucosa. Further studies are needed to determine whether SBD decreases mortality in the liver allograft recipients.

Other bacterial infections

Infections with *Legionella* spp. can be community-acquired or nosocomial. While *Legionella pneumophila* is the most common pathogen implicated, infections with *L. micdadei*, *L. bozemanii* and *L. dumoffii* have been reported. Typically presenting with a pneumonia, patients often complain of fever, chills, headache, diarrhea, chest pain, malaise, dyspnea, and cough. The chest radiograph usually reveals pulmonary infiltrates, but lung abscess and cavitation may be seen. Involvement of the hepatic allograft has also been reported to occur.

Direct fluorescent-antibody testing, culture of sputum or bronchoalveolar lavage fluid, and urinary antigen testing often confirm the diagnosis. Mortality due to this infection in transplant patients is high; the institution of empiric treatment with erythromycin when *Legionella* infection is suspected improves the patient's chances of survival. Nosocomial transmission should prompt a search for sources of *Legionella* spp. in the environment, especially in the ventilation systems and hot-water supply.

Infections with *Nocardia asteroides*, *N. nova*, *N. trans-valensis*, *N. brasiliensis*, *N. otitidis cavarium*, and *N. farcinica* are usually localized in the lung, presenting as febrile episodes with cough, pulmonary infiltrates, pleural effusion, and cavitary lesions or nodules. Brain abscesses need to be ruled out in transplant patients with a nocardial infection elsewhere. Cutaneous lesions, meningitis, and ventriculitis may also occur. Examination of the sputum or bronchoalveolar lavage specimen by direct microscopy following Gram and modified acid-fast staining, and microbial cultures are useful for diagnosis. Sulfonamides alone or in combination with TMP is the agent of choice in the treatment of nocardial infections; therapy should be prolonged to prevent disease relapse. Alternative agents include minocycline, chloramphenicol, amikacin, ceftriaxone, cefuroxime, cefotaxime, erythromycin, ampicillin, amoxicillin/clavulanate, and ciprofloxacin.

The first 2 months after liver transplantation is a high risk period for infection with *Listeria monocytogenes*. The portal of entry of the organism is the gastrointestinal tract via ingestion of contaminated food. The majority of infected patients have central nervous system (CNS) involvement. Meningitis, meningoencephalitis, and encephalitis can manifest as headache, fever, meningeal irritation, altered state of consciousness, seizures, and/or focal neurologic deficits. *Listeria monocytogenes* may also cause a primary bacteremia, peritonitis, pneumonia, and endophthalmitis. It is imperative to consider *L. monocytogenes* as a potential cause of meningitis in the liver transplant recipient. Lumbar puncture should be performed in a timely fashion, to prevent a fatal outcome. Direct cerebrospinal fluid (CSF) examination will often fail to show the organism; CSF pleocytosis with polymorphonuclear predominance and a low glucose content are seen in CNS listerial infection. Intravenous penicillin or ampicillin and gentamicin are effective agents for the treatment of this Gram-positive bacillary infection; TMP-SMX is an alternative drug for patients who are intolerant to the penicillins. Prevention is best achieved by meticulous attention to food preparation and the avoidance of drinking unpasteurized milk. Moreover, TMP-SMX, routinely used for *Pneumocystis carinii* pneumonia prophylaxis, is very effective is preventing listerial and other bacterial infections.

VIRAL INFECTIONS

Cytomegalovirus

Cytomegalovirus is the single most important pathogen in liver transplant recipients, contributing directly to morbidity and mortality. Infection usually develops within the first 3 months after transplantation. Without antiviral prophylaxis, the overall incidence of CMV infection is 50–60%, and of CMV disease is 20–30% (Fig. 37.5). The clinical effects of CMV in transplant recipients include the direct causation of infectious disease syndromes, production of an added immunosuppressed state resulting in superinfection with opportunistic pathogens, and a possible role in chronic allograft rejection.

The sources of CMV infection following organ transplantation include allografts from CMV-seropositive donors, leukocyte-containing blood products, reactivation of endogenous virus in seropositive transplant recipients, and, infrequently, acquisition from the general community. Three patterns of viral transmission are therefore observed. Primary infection develops in a CMV-seronegative individual who receives blood products and/or an

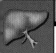

organ from a seropositive donor. Secondary infection or reactivation disease occurs when latent CMV reactivates after transplantation in a CMV-seropositive recipient. Superinfection or reinfection with CMV occurs in a CMV-seropositive recipient who receives cells and/or organ from a seropositive donor, with reactivation of latent virus of donor origin.

Immunosuppressive treatments administered following transplantation may lead to uncontrolled viral replication and symptomatic CMV infection. The type and intensity of immunosuppression is an important factor influencing the course of CMV infection after transplantation. The use of antilymphocyte antibody therapy in addition to conventional immunosuppression increases the incidence of CMV disease in the transplant population. As new and more potent immunosuppressive agents are developed and used in the clinical management of transplant patients, the incidence, severity, and relapse rates of CMV infection will be modified. The risk factors for CMV disease include the following: CMV-seronegative recipient of an organ from a CMV-seropositive donor, use of antilymphocyte antibody preparations, and fulminant hepatic failure at the time of transplant. A positive CMV donor serology is the single most important risk factor for the subsequent development of CMV infection.

Cytomegalovirus infection exhibits a wide range of clinical manifestations (Fig. 37.7). In over half of infected patients, CMV is isolated from bodily samples without evidence of disease. In one quarter of patients the isolation of the virus is accompanied by mild and self-limited febrile syndromes that include anorexia, malaise, fever, myalgias, arthralgias, and sometimes arthritis. Organ involvement with CMV develops in 20–25% of patients with CMV infection and most commonly occurs in the transplanted organ (i.e. CMV hepatitis in liver transplant recipients), especially in the CMV donor seropositive–recipient seronegative situation. Cytomegalovirus hepatitis typically manifests with greater elevations of γ-glutamyltransferase and alkaline phosphatase activities as compared with aminotransferase activities, and minimally elevated bilirubin levels. Other sites of CMV organ involvement are the gastrointestinal tract, gallbladder, pancreas, epididymis, biliary tract, retina, skin, endometrium, and CNS. Any segment of the gastrointestinal tract may be affected with a variety of clinical manifestations including hemorrhage, discrete ulcerations, perforation, hemorrhoiditis, and possibly pneumatosis intestinalis. Symptoms include dysphagia, odynophagia, nausea, vomiting, sense of abdominal fullness, delayed gastric emptying, abdominal pain, bleeding, and diarrhea. Findings on endoscopy are not specific and biopsy is essential for diagnostic confirmation.

Cytomegalovirus pneumonitis results in fever, dypsnea, cough, hypoxemia, and pulmonary infiltrates. The radiographic manifestations vary: bilateral, symmetric, interstitial, and alveolar processes predominantly affecting the lower lobes is the most common form; unilateral lobar and nodular infiltrates are also known to occur. In the liver transplant patient, lung involvement is relatively uncommon. On occasion, it can present as a subacute process that evolves over several days – a presentation similar to that of *Pneumocystis carinii* infection.

During the course of CMV infection, hematologic abnormalities are common. Atypical lymphocytes may be detected on peripheral blood smears. Leukopenia with or without thrombocytopenia occurs in up to a third of patients with CMV infection. The presence of leukopenia and fever during CMV infection is often an indication of serious clinical disease. Chorioretinitis occurs distinctly later in the post-transplant period (beyond 6 months), and is extremely rare. Patients may be asymptomatic or, more commonly, may experience blurring of vision, scotoma, and/or decreased visual acuity. The initial retinal lesion may be restricted to one eye that later progresses to involve the contralateral eye. Funduscopic examination reveals gradually expanding white dots or granular patches with irregular sheathing of the retinal vessels.

An important effect of CMV infection in the transplant patient is its potentiation of the individual's immunosuppression, which can result in bacterial and fungal superinfections. The clinical markers that identify the patient with the greatest risk are viremia and CMV-induced leukopenia. Pulmonary superinfection occurs with *Pneumocystis carinii*, *Aspergillus fumigatus*, and various Gram-negative pathogens. Sepsis with Gram-negative microorganisms, *L. monocytogenes* and *Candida* spp. may also occur. Without specific antiviral therapy, mortality is high. Cytomegalovirus infection has also been reported to play a role in chronic ductopenic rejection. The indirect association of CMV in the pathogenesis of malignancies in transplant patients have been difficult to establish and remains controversial.

The diagnosis of CMV infection can be established by serologic and virologic techniques. Serology is most useful in assessing the past exposure to CMV in both the donor and recipient. Moreover, serial testing with documentation of either seroconversion or rising IgG titers is an indirect measure of active viral infection, although these are not routinely tested after transplantation. The cornerstone for CMV diagnosis remains the demonstration of the virus in the blood, respiratory specimens, urine, or tissue (Fig. 37.8). The traditional method of isolating the virus is by tube cell culture. This has the disadvantage of a prolonged incubation period (7–14 days) for a cytopathic effect to be visible. The rapid shell vial culture

Incidence of cytomegalovirus infection in liver transplant patients				
	Huddinge Hospital	University of Pittsburgh	Pittsburgh VAMC	Mayo Clinic
Number of patients	48	101	79	53
Asymptomatic infection	8 (17%)		14 (18%)	12 (23%)
Symptomatic viremia	5 (5%)	15 (15%)	5 (6%)	7 (13%)
Hepatitis	2 (4%)	1 (<1%)	2 (3%)	9 (17%)
Pneumonitis	–	–	–	1 (<1%)
Disseminated	–	6 (6%)	2 (3%)	1 (<1%)
Enteritis	–	–	2 (3%)	–
Retinitis	–	–	1 (<1%)	–

Figure 37.7 Incidence of cytomegalovirus infection in liver transplant patients.

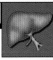

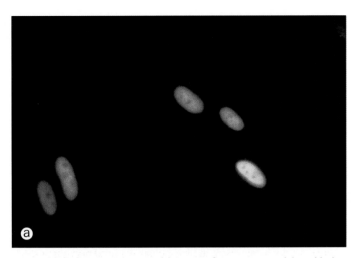

Figure 37.8 Cytomegalovirus. (a) Immunofluorescence staining with the CMV immediate-early monoclonal antibody following 16 hours of inoculation by shell vial culture. (b) Cytopathic effects caused by CMV on human fibroblast cells on conventional tube cell culture.

technique, by contrast, allows the detection of the major immediate early protein by monoclonal antibody staining after only 16 hours of incubation. Another rapid technique that facilitates early diagnosis of CMV infection is the CMV antigenemia assay in blood polymorphonuclear leukocytes from transplant patients. The technique is more sensitive than rapid shell vial culture, and has the advantage of not requiring cell culture methodologies. The use of polymerase chain reaction (PCR) technology is the most sensitive technique in establishing the presence of viral particles, but has a low specificity, particularly in identifying patients with CMV disease. Quantitation of CMV-DNA by PCR-based techniques is being studied and may help improve the specificity of this test in the diagnosis of CMV disease.

Typical histologic features from tissue biopsies including the presence of 'cytomegalic' cells with intranuclear inclusions and the associated acute, focal inflammation aid in confirming CMV involvement of the target organ. Additionally, the demonstration of the presence of CMV antigens by monoclonal antibody staining or by DNA *in situ* hybridization further supports the diagnosis of CMV organ involvement (Fig. 37.9).

Currently available antiviral agents, that are effective for the treatment of CMV infection, include ganciclovir, foscarnet, and cidofovir, all of which have excellent activity against all herpesviruses. Common side effects of ganciclovir include bone marrow suppression, which is infrequently observed in liver transplant recipients. While there is much less experience with the use of foscarnet and cidofovir in this solid organ transplant population, the major adverse effect of both agents is nephrotoxicity. Thus, their use is restricted to liver transplant patients who fail to respond to ganciclovir therapy due to acquired viral resistance. A far more complex question is the appropriate duration of therapy for both asymptomatic infection and CMV disease. Despite the usual practice of treating CMV infections with 2–3 weeks of intravenous ganciclovir, much debate remains on the optimum treatment duration. Another vague area in CMV therapeutics is the issue of longer term maintenance therapy. This topic is being carefully scrutinized by various transplant groups, particularly since the introduction of the well-tolerated oral ganciclovir formulation.

The prevention of CMV infection has generated intense interest in transplantation medicine. Numerous studies using a variety of treatments have been published in the literature; these include the use of acyclovir, ganciclovir, intravenous immunoglobulin, and CMV hyperimmune globulin. These agents can be administered in a universal prophylaxis approach, or alternatively, pre-emptively to patients at risk of CMV disease, identified by markers of early viral replication or epidemiologic tools. Using the former approach, at least three randomized studies have demonstrated that it is possible to reduce CMV disease in CMV recipients of donor positive organs. Universal prophylaxis is achieved through the prolonged administration of intravenous globulin or oral ganciclovir, or sequential use of ganciclovir followed by oral acyclovir. Pre-emptive prophylaxis with ganciclovir based on CMV detection by surveillance cultures or at the time of OKT3 use are also effective. The results of trials using pre-emptive oral ganciclovir therapy based on earlier markers of viral replication in liver transplant patients are expected soon.

Epstein–Barr virus

Primary Epstein–Barr virus (EBV) infection in transplant patients may be acquired from the allograft, leukocyte-containing blood

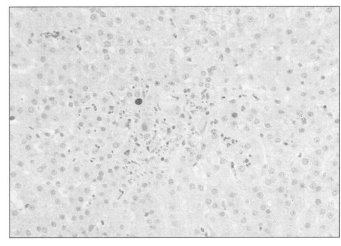

Figure 37.9 Cytomegalovirus hepatitis. *In situ* hybridization shows the presence of CMV inclusion bodies in a liver biopsy tissue.

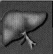

products, or from the community. However, the great majority of EBV-related illnesses in adults represents reactivation infection in individuals who are EBV-seropositive, most likely reflecting the high prevalence of EBV-seropositivity in this age population. Clinical presentations of EBV infection after liver transplantation include asymptomatic infection, mononucleosis syndromes, hepatitis and post-transplant lymphoproliferative disease (PTLD). The reported incidence of PTLD following liver transplantation varies from 2–4%. The main risk factors for the development of PTLD are EBV seronegativity before transplantation, use of OKT3 therapy for rejection treatment, CMV donor positive-recipient negative serostatus, and the development of CMV disease following hepatic transplantation.

The clinical presentation of EBV-associated PTLD is also variable. Unexplained fevers with adenopathy, tonsillitis and pharyngitis are common symptoms of the mononucleosis-like syndrome. In addition, more severe forms of presentations with abdominal pain, bleeding, bowel perforation or obstruction; hepatocellular dysfunction; impairment of renal function; weight loss; pulmonary infiltrates; and CNS involvement with seizure, change in the state of consciousness, or focal neurologic disease are encountered clinically. Histologically, the spectrum of PTLD represents a continuum: from a polyclonal nonspecific reactive hyperplasia that generally follows a benign course, to a malignant monoclonal polymorphic B-cell lymphoma.

The diagnosis of PTLD relies on the demonstration of abnormal lymphoid proliferation in biopsy material or on the identification of cellular clonal abnormality by cytologic analysis. Serologic evidence of EBV infection or reactivation may be supportive. The best therapy remains to be defined. Drastic reduction or cessation of immunosuppression appears to be the most effective measure. The addition of high-dose acyclovir or ganciclovir inhibits viral replication in the oropharynx but has not been shown to improve disease prognosis, especially in those cases in which cell transformation by EBV has occurred. Patients with extranodal, multifocal and brain involvement may require further therapy; including surgical extirpation of tumor masses, cytotoxic chemotherapy and/or radiation therapy. Other therapeutic possibilities that have been explored include the use of anti-B-cell monoclonal antibody and interferon-α, with also equivocal beneficial effects.

Clearly, prevention is much to be preferred. Decreased immunosuppression, especially avoiding the use of antilymphocyte therapy, should be used in patients at risk, if possible. Moreover, given the association of CMV disease with PTLD, strategies to prevent CMV disease may be useful. Anecdotally, in nonrandomized trials, the incidence of PTLD was reported to be reduced with the use of prophylactic antiviral therapy in high-risk patients. Unfortunately, a single effective strategy to prevent the evolution of this process needs to be established. The goal would be to detect early viral replication using PCR-based techniques and intervening when increases in EBV-DNA levels are first demonstrated.

Herpes simplex virus
Virtually all of the infections caused by herpes simplex virus (HSV) result from reactivation of latent virus. In the absence of prophylaxis, about half of HSV-seropositive recipients experience active infection during the first 3 weeks during surgery. Primary infection can be transmitted by person to person contact or via the allograft. Oral mucocutaneous lesions commonly occur during the first month after transplantation, and are aggravated by anti-rejection therapy. Most orolabial lesions are mild, but can be considerably severe with large, painful, crusted ulcerations that bleed and interfere with nutrition. Furthermore, these can be complicated by bacterial superinfection and esophageal involvement. Anogenital infection may occur; this usually presents as large, coalescing, and ulcerating lesions.

In liver transplant patients, HSV pneumonia is an uncommon event, occurring as a secondary infection in intubated patients with other forms of primary lung injury or severe pneumonia caused by other pathogens. More severe forms of HSV infections are less frequent. Disseminated cutaneous disease occurring at sites of previous skin injury (eczema herpeticum) may develop. Herpes simplex virus also causes hepatitis in the liver allograft recipient, which can result in liver failure. Central nervous system involvement with meningoencephalitis is rare.

During the evaluation of lesions caused by HSV, routine bacteriologic cultures and Tzanck preparations may not give the appropriate diagnosis. Rapid diagnosis can be made by direct immunofluorescence study performed on swabs taken from the lesion. Visible cytopathic effects may be seen 24–48 hours after viral culture of tissue and/or body fluids. A positive IgM titer or a fourfold or greater rise in IgG titers observed between acute- and convalescent-phase sera by serologic techniques are suggestive of the diagnosis.

Acyclovir, ganciclovir, and famciclovir are all effective anti-HSV drugs. Mucocutaneous infections may be treated by oral medications, while disseminated or deep HSV disease require the use of the intravenous formulations of these drugs. The recent availability of oral valacyclovir, an ester formulation of acyclovir that produces high serum drug levels, may be a valid alternative to the intravenous medications. While usually treatment-responsive, the advent of antiviral prophylaxis has had a remarkable effect on the occurrence of HSV infections in the liver transplant recipient. The use of acyclovir for the first month post-transplant is quite successful in preventing disease.

Varicella-zoster virus
Clinical disease with varicella-zoster virus (VZV) is uncommon earlier than 2 months after transplantation. Primary infection occurs in a minority of liver transplant recipients; the vast majority of disease represents reactivation infection in VZV-seropositive individuals. Primary infection occurs after exposure to the virus of a susceptible VZV-seronegative transplant recipient, and can be encountered at any time after transplantation0. The disease may be characterized by life-threatening hemorrhagic pneumonia, skin lesions, encephalitis, hepatitis, pancreatitis, and disseminated intravascular coagulation. Localized dermatomal reactivation results in herpes zoster. Typically, two or three adjoining dermatomes are involved with a few distant sites of cutaneous dissemination. A syndrome of unilateral pain without cutaneous lesions has also been described to occur in the transplant patient.

The diagnosis is made by the characteristic vesicular lesions distributed in a dermatomal pattern. Microbiologic confirmation of the diagnosis is made by direct immunofluorescence of a swab taken from a lesion, culture, or demonstration of multinucleated giant cells on Tzanck smear. High-dose intravenous acyclovir is usually effective, especially if the disease is recognized early and treatment is initiated within 24 hours of the

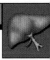

eruption of skin rash. Both valacyclovir and famciclovir may be valid alternative therapeutic agents. Because of the high mortality associated with severe primary VZV infection in organ transplant recipients, varicella-zoster immune globulin (VZIG) and antiviral agents should be administered promptly after a documented or suspected exposure. It is hoped that pretransplant VZV vaccination will eliminate the problems associated with severe infections.

Hepatitis viruses

Hepatitis B virus (HBV)-induced fulminant hepatitis and cirrhosis are important indications for liver transplantation. Unfortunately, reinfection with HBV is almost inevitable, with a frequency of up to 90%, resulting in significant morbidity and indirectly contributing to mortality. Recurrent disease typically begins with the appearance of hepatitis B surface antigen (HBsAg) and HBV-DNA 2–6 months after transplantation, followed thereafter by evidence of hepatocellular injury. The liver injury can be mild and self-limited; however, aggressive chronic hepatitis and fulminant liver failure are not uncommon complications. Clinical manifestations include a rapidly progressive liver disease with graft dysfunction leading to graft loss in a few months. Recurrent infection of the liver allograft portends a poor post-transplant life expectancy. Evidence of active viral replication at the time of transplantation increases the risk of HBV reinfection post-transplant, whereas patients with fulminant hepatitis B or coexistent chronic hepatitis D infection have a lower risk. The primary acquisition of HBV occurs via transmission from an infected donor organ or transfusion of infected blood products. The currently employed techniques for HBsAg detection are extremely sensitive and specific, leading to only isolated cases of post-transfusion HBV infection.

The optimal treatment for hepatitis B recurrence is evolving. Interferon therapy, in an effort to reduce HBV viral DNA load before transplantation, has been studied without much success. The administration of high doses of anti-HBs hyperimmune globulin to patients undergoing liver transplantation for HBV-related end-stage liver disease confers long-term protection and improved survival rates. Newer and more potent antiviral agents such as lamivudine, lobucavir, and famciclovir exhibit antihepatitis B activity and are being studied in transplant patients with very promising results.

Hepatitis C virus (HCV)-induced liver disease is the most common indication for liver transplantation in the USA. Moreover, it is the cause of more than 80% of progressive liver disease that occurs after transplantation. Hepatitis C virus is spread via parenteral contact with infected blood and via the liver allograft with a high degree of efficiency. Organs from donors with a positive HCV antibody are highly likely to transmit the virus. Reinfection of the hepatic allograft with HCV after liver transplantation occurs almost universally. Indeed, it is a major cause of post-transplant hepatitis; while the majority of those reinfected experience relatively benign disease, a small number of patients will have an accelerated deterioration of graft function. Nonetheless, compared with untreated HBV-infected patients, liver transplantation in those with HCV infection has a much better prognosis, as shown by the fact that recipients with recurrent infection have a 5-year survival not different from that of noninfected recipients.

Hepatitis C virus infection is diagnosed by detecting HCV-RNA in serum using reverse transcriptase PCR. Liver biopsy is essential in delineating disease severity. The use of interferon-α and ribavirin in transplant recipients has shown preliminary encouraging results, although more studies are needed to confirm their potential therapeutic efficacy and to support their use.

Hepatitis A virus can cause fulminant hepatic failure that requires transplantation. Chronic disease does not occur, and transmission by blood transfusion or the organ is extremely rare. Similarly, hepatitis E virus, a frequent cause of epidemic hepatitis in developing countries, has failed to have an impact on liver transplant recipients. The defective hepatitis D virus requires the presence of HBV to cause liver disease. Coinfection can result in either acute liver failure or chronic hepatitis leading to liver transplantation; after transplantation, an acute hepatitis D virus has been described, but the post-transplant course is largely dictated by whether HBV infection recurs.

Hepatitis G virus is a newly described virus that is parenterally transmitted. It has been found frequently in patients with chronic HCV infection, although it does not appear to influence the clinical outcome after liver transplantation.

Other viruses

Human immunodeficiency virus (HIV) is effectively transmitted by organ transplantation. However, with currently utilized tools for donor screening, transmission is virtually interrupted, except when the donor is in the 'window period' of HIV infection when replicating viruses are present but an immunologic response has not yet appeared. The natural history of HIV infection in transplant patients who either experience a primary infection at the time of transplantation or who acquire HIV infection after transplantation demonstrate that while some may do well and survive for prolonged periods, others have an accelerated course towards the acquired immune deficiency syndrome. Whereas HIV positivity has long been considered a strong contraindication to organ transplantation, the advent of potent antiretroviral regimens resulting in improved patient survival raises the issue of whether asymptomatic HIV infected individuals with end-stage liver disease should be offered transplantation. At the present time, no guidelines have been set for determining which HIV-infected patients might be candidates for organ transplantation.

The human polyoma JC virus is the cause of progressive multifocal leukoencephalopathy, a subacute, progressive demyelinating disease of the CNS in immunocompromised hosts. Unfortunately, there is no effective treatment and the only measure that may confer some advantage is to drastically decrease immunosuppression.

Papillomavirus infection in liver transplant recipients results in the production of extensive warty growths, some of which undergo malignant transformation especially in sun-exposed areas. Similarly, cervical papillomavirus infection is more extensive in this population and has been linked to squamous cell cancer of the cervix. Most of the effects of papillomavirus infections in transplant patients are modulated by the intensity of immunosuppressive therapy. The introduction and the use of systemic and topical interferon are accepted treatment modalities. Newer antivirals such as cidofovir are being evaluated for topical administration as well.

Respiratory virus infections in the community have a serious impact on the transplant population. During the influenza season, the transplant recipient can be at an increased risk for serious disease with respiratory failure or complicating bacterial pneumonia with *Streptococcus pneumoniae*, *Haemophilus influenzae*, and *Staphylococcus aureus*. The virus can be isolated readily from nasal swabs or other respiratory specimens. Paired serum specimens tested serologically are also commonly collected for diagnostic purposes. Postexposure administration of amantadine or rimantadine in unvaccinated patients is effective in preventing infection transmission in most instances. Respiratory syncytial virus (RSV) infections are uncommon but are associated with a higher rate of pneumonia and mortality in this vulnerable population. Common symptoms are fever, tachypnea, cough, and respiratory congestion with interstitial or lobar lung infiltrates. Diagnosis is made by viral isolation or by one of the plethora of rapid diagnostic techniques, such as the direct and indirect immunofluorescence and enzyme immunosorbent assays. Severe RSV infection is treated with aerosolized ribavirin.

While adenovirus infection predominantly causes a benign illness in the general population, it has a propensity for causing life-threatening lung and gastrointestinal tract disease in pediatric liver recipients. An aggressive hepatitis leading to graft loss requiring retransplantation has been reported following infection with adenovirus. There is no effective treatment.

The pathogenic potential of human herpesvirus (HHV)-6 in liver transplant recipients is just now being better understood. Most infections are caused by reactivation of the latent virus in the recipient, although donor transmission also occurs. Febrile illness with profound thrombocytopenia after liver transplantation has been associated with HHV-6 infection; skin rash may accompany the febrile illness. A notable feature of HHV-6 is its propensity for neural invasion, presenting clinically as encephalitis/encephalopathy. Laboratory tools that are essential in the diagnosis of this potentially serious infection include viral isolation by culturing peripheral blood mononuclear cells, immunohistochemical staining of tissue specimens, PCR assays, and serologic studies. The virus is susceptible to ganciclovir and foscarnet, although the role of antiviral therapy and prophylaxis in this setting remains to be determined. The clinical relevance of additional viruses including the HHV-7 and HHV-8 are currently being studied.

FUNGAL INFECTIONS

Fungal infections occur in 2–25% of liver transplant patients (see Fig. 37.5). Pathogenic fungi cause different patterns of illness: pulmonary and/or disseminated infection with one of the endemic mycoses, or opportunistic infections with organisms that rarely cause invasive disease in the normal hosts. The latter includes *Candida* spp., *Pneumocystis carinii*, *Aspergillus* spp. and *Cryptococcus neoformans*. Cases of mucormycosis and infection with *Pseudoallescheria boydii* may occur, but are less common. A large number of risk factors have been identified that predispose the liver transplant recipient to develop invasive fungal diseases. These include increased age; urgent transplantation, duration of surgery, high intraoperative transfusion requirement, type of biliary reconstruction; reintubation, retransplantation, abdominal or intra-thoracic reoperation; vascular complications, postoperative hemorrhage with re-exploration; preoperative steroid and antibiotic use, large doses of steroid after transplantation; high creatinine level, requirement for dialysis; bacterial and CMV infections; rejection episodes, the vanishing bile duct syndrome, and the use

of OKT3 monoclonal antibody. Using multivariate time-dependent analysis in a large cohort of patients, it has been possible to discern between the risk factors that predispose an individual to candidal versus noncandidal infections. Prolonged surgical time at transplantation, reoperation, bacterial infection, and/or increased antibiotic use are the main risk factors for candidal infections. For the other fungal infections such as cryptococcal and aspergillal infections, the degree of immunosuppression indicated by the use of OKT3, a pretransplant diagnosis of fulminant hepatic failure, and the development of symptomatic CMV infection are the most significant risk factors.

More than half of fungal infections occurring in these individuals originate from the abdominal cavity. Compared with bacterial and viral infections, mortality associated with fungal infections in the liver transplant population is significantly higher, and approaches 100% in patients with invasive aspergillosis. The presentations of fungal infections in the immunosuppressed liver transplant recipients are quite nonspecific and may be obscured by other infectious and noninfectious processes. Thus, the clinician must maintain a high index of suspicion for this type of infection and pursue an aggressive diagnostic approach.

Candida spp.

Most candidal infections occur in the first 2 months after organ transplantation. *Candida albicans* is the most frequently implicated pathogen. Moreover, C. *krusei*, C. *glabrata*, and C. *tropicalis* can all cause disease. Portals of entry include the gastrointestinal tract, urinary and intravenous catheters, and diseased skin. Fungal overgrowth and colonization of the mucocutaneous surfaces that occurs with antibiotic use and the elimination of normal bacterial flora, gut mucosal disruption by the surgical procedure, presence of indwelling urinary and intravascular catheters, and metabolic factors such as diabetes and corticosteroid use that affect phagocytic function are all of pathogenic importance.

The most common presentation of candidal infection in the organ transplant recipient is mucocutaneous disease manifesting as oropharyngeal thrush, esophageal candidiasis, vaginitis, intertrigo, and paronychia or onychomycosis. Technical complications during surgery can lead to the spillage of candidal organisms from the gastrointestinal tract into devitalized tissues, hematoma or ascites, giving rise to bloodstream invasion with subsequent dissemination and visceral seeding in at least half of the transplant patients. Disseminated candidal infection can present in diverse ways, ranging from the subtle manifestations of end-organ involvement such as skin lesions, osteomyelitis, and endophthalmitis, to sepsis. Other clinical entities caused by infections with *Candida* spp. include intra-abdominal abscesses, pulmonary infection, urinary tract infection with ureteral obstruction from fungus balls, arthritis, endocarditis, aortitis, brain abscess, meningitis, and invasive cutaneous/subcutaneous infections. Catheter-related candidal sepsis is a common presentation in the transplant setting.

Although a number of liver transplant recipients are colonized with candidal organisms, most patients do not develop clinically significant infections. The utility of routine surveillance cultures in this patient population is of little clinical relevance due to its poor positive predictive value and low specificity. The performance of fungal staining and culture from appropriate specimens usually yields the diagnosis. Topical therapy with

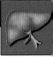

nonabsorbable fungal agents such as nystatin and clotrimazole are usually effective in treating mild mucocutaneous candidiasis. If therapeutic response is not achieved, fluconazole is the subsequent agent of choice.

The therapeutic approach to invasive candidal infection is to initiate therapy with amphotericin B, and then switch to fluconazole for completion of treatment. Although effective in many instances, the use of amphotericin B is wrought with numerous difficulties. Bone marrow and renal toxicities are common. Moreover, the immunosuppressive regimen of these patients commonly includes agents such as cyclosporine or tacrolimus, which can potentiate the nephrotoxicity caused by amphotericin. Despite the toxicities associated with the administration of amphotericin, the development of renal dysfunction should not necessitate the discontinuation of therapy in a patient with a life-threatening fungal infection. Furthermore, a step-wise increase in drug dosage is not recommended. The introduction of the liposomal formulations of amphotericin allows for the administration of larger amounts of the drug with fewer adverse effects. Although its efficacy in the treatment of severe fungal infections appears to be as effective as the nonliposomal formulation, it is not routinely used as a first-line agent unless significant renal toxicity is present or is developing. It should be remembered that while most C. albicans and C. tropicalis are azole-sensitive, C. krusei and C. glabrata should be considered fluconazole-resistant and treatment with amphotericin is imperative in these instances.

The use of the azole antifungal agent fluconazole for treating fungal infections has been increasing. It is well-absorbed, is available in both oral and parenteral formulations, and has good CSF penetration. Furthermore, its use is associated with a low incidence of adverse reactions but it has an important effect, inhibiting the metabolism of both cyclosporine and tacrolimus, leading to higher drug levels. It is effective against most Candida spp., and is used in the treatment of oropharyngeal and esophageal candidiasis, deep-seated candidal infections, cryptococcal meningitis, and in some cases of candidal bloodstream infection. Oral fluconazole has an important niche in the continuing treatment of immunocompromised patients who require chronic maintenance therapy with an antifungal agent. Prophylaxis of candidal infection with low-dose fluconazole or a short course of liposomal trypcoterinium following liver transplantation should be restricted to those transplant centers with a high incidence of this infectious complication.

Cryptococcus neoformans

Infection with C. neoformans in organ transplant recipients occurs almost exclusively in the late post-transplant period (beyond 6 months). Its classic presentation is of subacute to chronic meningitis in this population. A primary pulmonary infection often follows inhalation of the organisms, presenting as pneumonia, pleural effusion, or as an asymptomatic pulmonary nodule discovered on chest radiography. Post-primary fungal dissemination follows, with organisms seeding the CNS, skin, the urinary tract and bone. Symptoms suggestive of CNS involvement can be indolent with headache, memory loss, disorientation, confusion, dysphasia, muscle weakness, unsteadiness, tremors, urinary incontinence, behavioral disturbances, and seizures or focal neurologic deficits. Skin lesions can be the initial indication of a systemic infection and may take one of different forms: ulcers, papules or pustules, subcutaneous swelling, vesicles, necrotizing vasculitis, and cellulitis (Fig. 37.10). Alternatively, in men, cryptococcal infection can present as sterile pyuria; the prostate gland may be a source of hematogenous infection.

Fungal stains such as calcofluor white, India ink, and methenamine silver stains are valuable in supporting a presumptive diagnosis, but the detection of the organism by culture is necessary for diagnosis of cryptococcal infection (Fig. 37.11). Cryptococcosis may also be diagnosed from histologic sections. Detection of the cryptococcal polysaccharide capsular antigen by latex agglutination is also widely used to guide further diagnostic effort and therapy. The test is positive in the blood of individuals with systemic infection and in the CSF of patients with cryptococcal meningitis. It is also useful in the evaluation of patients with undiagnosed skin lesions, and in monitoring response to therapy. Examination of the CSF shows lymphocytic pleocytosis, hypoglycorrhachia and an elevated protein level. The presence of unexplained papules, nodules or areas of atypical cellulitis in a transplant patient should prompt a tissue biopsy.

As in all cases of life-threatening fungal infections, intravenous amphotericin B remains the standard of care for treatment of cryptococcosis in the liver transplant patients. If tolerated, 5-flucytosine should be used in combination with amphotericin B for initiating therapy of serious cryptococcal infections. The organism is also sensitive to fluconazole, although this may not be the first agent of choice in immunocompromised patients. The oral imidazole, however, makes the long-term treatment of this infection easier to maintain with much less concern for adverse drug effects. The best way to deal with cryptococcal CNS infection is by preventing pulmonary infection; this may be possible by eliminating exposure to soil contaminated with pigeon droppings.

Aspergillus spp.

Aspergillus fumigatus is the second most common fungal agent causing CNS infection in the transplant recipient. Infections caused by Aspergillus spp. occur most frequently in the first 3 months after transplantation. Invasive aspergillosis occurs in up

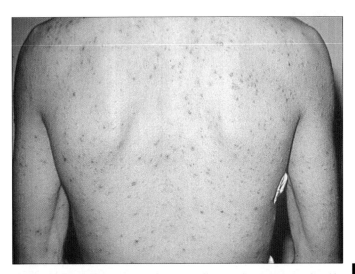

Figure 37.10 Cryptococcal infection. Diffuse erythematous papular skin eruptions may be the initial manifestation of disseminated cryptococcal infection.

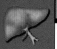

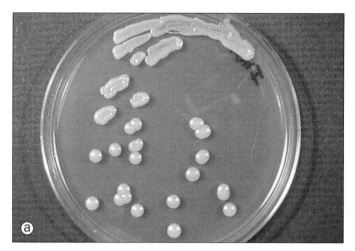

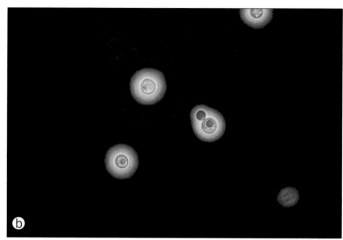

Figure 37.11 *Cryptococcus neoformans.* (a) Fungal colonies grow as smooth, convex, yellow or tan areas on solid culture media.

(b) Calcofluor white stain shows cryptococci with distinct cell walls and polysaccharide capsules.

to 20% of liver transplant recipients and is invariably fatal. In addition, other disease-causing mycelial fungi include *A. flavus*, *A. niger*, *A. terreus*, *Pseudoallescheria boydii*, *Sporothrix schenkii*, as well as a number of other fungi.

Inhalation of aerosolized fungal organisms is the usual route of transmission, resulting in a primary infection of the lungs and/or paranasal sinuses. Pulmonary symptoms with nonproductive cough, pleuritic chest pain, dyspnea, and low-grade fever predominate. The chest radiograph may appear normal, or may show nodular opacities, interstitial infiltrates or cavitary disease. Persistent fever despite conventional antimicrobial therapy, and a progressive pulmonary infiltrate should raise the suspicion of aspergillal pneumonia, particularly in a liver transplant patient with a poorly functioning allograft.

Metastatic infection to the brain occurs via hematogenous spread (Fig. 37.12). Dissemination may involve almost any organ including the liver, spleen, kidneys, heart, pericardium, blood vessels, gastrointestinal tract, bones, and joints. Central nervous system involvement can present as alteration in the mental status,

seizures, cerebrovascular accidents, and headache. Blood vessel invasion invariably follows tissue infection. Pathologically, this results in tissue infarction, hemorrhage, and metastatic seeding.

The recovery of *Aspergillus* spp. from respiratory and wound specimens may represent fungal colonization without invasive disease. However, repeated isolation of the organism should alert the clinician to the possibility of organ involvement. An aggressive diagnostic approach should be pursued; this may include a bronchoalveolar lavage or, ideally, a transbronchial or open lung biopsy. Histologic examination of tissues from extrapulmonary sources will often reveal the presence of branching septate hyphal elements and angioinvasion (Fig. 37.13).

Management of invasive aspergillosis is similar to the therapy of other serious fungal infections (i.e. amphotericin B). *In vitro* studies have shown poor susceptibility of *Aspergillus* spp. to fluconazole. Another oral imidazole drug that is effective against this filamentous fungus is itraconazole. In addition to its demonstrated efficacy in the treatment of aspergillal infections, the antifungal spectrum of itraconazole covers most *Candida*

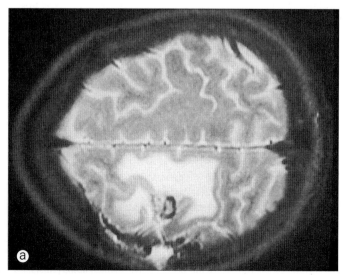

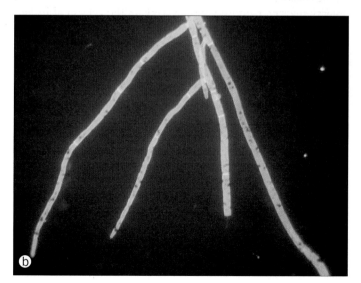

Figure 37.12 Aspergillosis. (a) Cranial MRI of a transplant patient with CNS aspergilloma demonstrates a focal lesion with surrounding edema.

(b) Broad-based branching hyphal elements characteristic of *Aspergillus fumigatus*.

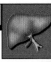

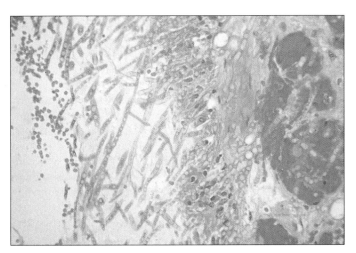

Figure 37.13 Angioinvasion. Tissue biopsy shows fungal elements invading blood vessels and contiguous areas.

spp. The major drawback to the use of oral itraconazole is its erratic absorption and unpredictable plasma levels. Additionally, CNS penetration of the drug is poor. A new and improved oral solution of itraconazole has recently become available. Pharmacokinetic data indicate that it has improved bioavailability when compared with itraconazole capsule. The efficacy of intravenous itraconazole in the treatment of severe fungal infections is currently being studied in clinical trials. Although the use of high-efficiency particulate air filter has been suggested, there is no practical and easy method for preventing invasive aspergillosis.

Dimorphic fungi

The geographically restricted endemic mycoses can cause disease in the transplant patient at any period after transplantation. Such agents include *Histoplasma capsulatum*, *Coccidioides immitis*, *Blastomyces dermatitidis*, and, less frequently, *Paracoccidioides brasiliensis*. Two different patterns of disease occur in the immunosuppressed patient–primary infection with progressive disease and reactivation infection – both of which can cause systemic disease.

Histoplasma capsulatum is endemic in the central USA and certain other river valleys of the world. Infection is acquired by inhalation of infectious microconidial spores. Typically, patients present with nonspecific signs and symptoms such as fever, night sweats, chills, cough, headache, arthritis, myalgias, and a variety of cutaneous and mucosal lesions may be seen on physical examination. Hepatosplenomegaly can occur, or CNS signs may predominate. Chest radiography may show hilar adenopathy, focal or diffuse infiltrates and pleural effusion; however, a normal radiograph can not exclude pulmonary histoplasmosis. Urine antigen testing and cultures of respiratory secretions and other specimens can all provide the diagnosis. Serology is rarely of value due to the high likelihood of a negative result, despite active infection in an immunocompromised individual; alternatively, a positive test may be a poor indicator of active disease because of its high prevalence in endemic areas. In some instances, histopathologic examination of the bone marrow, skin, respiratory specimen, and other tissues is necessary to establish a rapid and confirmatory diagnosis.

Infection with *Coccidioides immitis* occurs in residents of the desert areas of the southwestern USA and northern Mexico; individuals who have traveled to these areas are also susceptible. Most cases of coccidioidomycosis are seen within the first post-transplant year. Isolated pulmonary involvement can present with fever, nonproductive cough, and chest radiographic abnormalities that range from a nodular infiltrate, interstitial disease, lobar involvement, and hilar adenopathy to, rarely, cavitation. Dissemination is common; frequent sites of extrapulmonary disease are the spleen, liver, joints, brain, urinary tract, thyroid gland, blood, muscle, myocardium, and skin. Coccidioidomycosis can further depress the cell-mediated immunity of the transplant patient who is already on an immunosuppressive regimen after liver transplantation. Serologic testing does not always give a positive result despite active infection. Cultures and histopathologic examination of respiratory secretions, blood, bone marrow, and other tissues aid in confirming the diagnosis.

Endemic in the southern USA along the Mississippi and Ohio River Valleys, the upper Midwestern states, and the Canadian provinces adjacent to the Great Lakes and the Saint Lawrence River, *Blastomyces dermatitidis* is an uncommon infectious disease problem encountered by the liver transplant patient. The most common sites of disease are the lungs and skin. The diagnosis is made by fungal staining and cultures of appropriate clinical specimens, including the skin.

With the exception of *Pseudoallescheria boydii*, which is inherently resistant to the drug, amphotericin B is still regarded as the first-line agent for serious fungal infections, including the endemic mycoses. Oral antifungal preparations with activity against the dimorphic fungi are limited to itraconazole and ketoconazole. A novel antifungal agent that shows promise is voriconazole; *in vitro* susceptibility studies indicate that voriconazole is a potent agent with activity against a number of opportunistic fungal pathogens, as well as dimorphic fungi.

The amount of immunosuppression should be reduced as tolerated for those with serious and deep fungal infections. In some instances, surgical extirpation and debridement are an integral part of the management. While surgical extirpation and debridement is beneficial for the prevention of *Candida* infection, it has no demonstrable efficacy in reducing the incidence of other fungal infections in liver recipients. Prophylactic low-dose amphotericin, given to patients at high risk for developing fungal infections, may reduce the incidence and severity of these infections. The potential beneficial role of liposomal formulations of amphotericin B needs to be clearly established due to its extreme cost. The use of interferon-γ, colony-stimulating factors, and immunoglobulin preparations need to be thoroughly investigated before their use can be recommended.

Pneumocystis carinii

Among patients who are not receiving prophylactic therapy, pneumonia related to *P. carinii* occurs in approximately 5–10% of liver transplant recipients. The incidence of this infection is highest from the second to the sixth post-transplant month; it occurs most commonly in those who suffer from chronic allograft rejection who have received an inordinately high amount of immunosuppressive therapy.

Pneumonia caused by *P. carinii* usually has a subacute presentation with fever, dyspnea, nonproductive cough, hypoxemia, and radiographic findings consistent with an interstitial process. In addition, asymptomatic infection has been observed in transplant recipients, and an increased association with the development of pneumothorax has been reported. Pneumocystosis is often linked to the occurrence of CMV infection; invasive diagnostic studies are needed to rule out coinfection.

Examination of bronchoalveolar lavage fluid or a lung biopsy specimen often confirms the diagnosis of *P. carinii* infection. Monoclonal antibody staining has a high yield for rapid diagnosis, as does staining with calcofluor white, methenamine silver, and Wright–Giemsa stains (Fig. 37.14). Treatment is with high-dose TMP-SMX or intravenous pentamidine. At therapeutic doses however, these medications are associated with a high incidence of adverse effects. High-dose TMP-SMX causes anorexia, nausea, vomiting, hyponatremia, and elevated creatinine levels; furthermore, drug interactions with cyclosporine may result in renal failure. Side effects of intravenous pentamidine are bone marrow depression, hypoglycemia, hypocalcemia, seizure, and impairments in kidney and liver functions that can confound pre-existing renal and hepatic dysfunctions common in recipients of liver allografts. Because of the potential morbidity associated with pneumocystosis and the availability of an effective drug, it is clear that preventive strategies should take precedence. Doses of TMP-SMX given daily during the first 6 months after liver transplantation has been very successful in preventing *P. carinii* infections.

MYCOBACTERIAL INFECTIONS

Mycobacterium tuberculosis

Liver transplant recipients are at an increased risk for the acquisition of both primary and reactivation tuberculous infections. Although the incidence of mycobacterial infection in liver transplant recipients is less than 1%, the associated mortality is high. Disease onset does not conform to any specific timetable. Residence outside the USA and extensive travel in foreign countries are identified risk factors.

Tuberculosis can present at any time and a variety of forms can be observed in the immunocompromised patients. Primary infection is acquired by the aerosol route. Symptomatic disease may present as an atypical pneumonia, tuberculous pleurisy, fever and cough, or as disseminated tuberculosis. Reactivation of an old tuberculous lesion occurs in the transplant patient whose host defenses cannot contain a previously dormant focus. Symptoms of reactivation disease are cough, malaise, fever, weight loss, night sweats, pleuritic chest pain, and blood-streaked sputum production. Pulmonary tuberculosis can be associated with concurrent disease in almost any organ system, or with disseminated infection. The liver, spleen and bone marrow are commonly involved; other extrapulmonary sites of disease include the intestine, musculoskeletal system, CNS, pericardium, serosal surfaces, and skin.

Both primary and reactivation pulmonary disease in the transplant patient may have protean radiographic presentations. Radiologically, the disease may be seen as a classic apical fibronodular infiltrate or cavity, a lower lobe infiltrate, miliary pattern, pleural effusion, or mediastinal masses. Smears for acid-fast bacilli and mycobacterial cultures of appropriate specimens are the standard methods for diagnosing mycobacterial infection. A high index of suspicion should be maintained and early invasive procedures pursued in any transplant recipient with undefined pulmonary infiltrates. This could include bronchoscopy with bronchoalveolar lavage, transbronchial and open lung biopsies, and biopsies of such organs as the liver, lymph node, and bone marrow. Histopathologic evidence of granuloma formation is highly indicative of *M. tuberculosis* infection, although the identification of acid-fast bacilli remains the hallmark of tuberculous disease. A positive tuberculin skin test is helpful; however, less than half of infected transplant patients react to skin testing.

Treatment of active infection should consist of at least two bactericidal agents such as isoniazid, rifampin (rifampicin), and

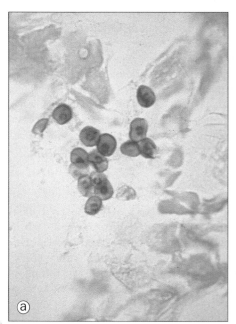
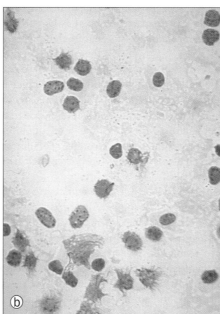
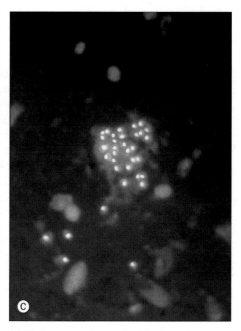

Figure 37.14 *Pneumocystis carinii*. A variety of stains can be used to identify *P. carinii* in respiratory tract secretions, all of which are highly efficient in detecting the organism. (a) Methenamine silver stain. (b) Wright–Giemsa stain. (c) Calcofluor white stain.

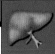

pyrazinamide to which the organism is susceptible for a minimum duration of 12 months. Antimycobacterial therapy has important drug interactions and toxicities that may be more pronounced in the transplant patient. Renal impairment dictates dosage adjustments for isoniazid, streptomycin, and ethambutol. The induction of hepatic enzymes by rifampin, and possibly isoniazid, increases the catabolism of tacrolimus and cyclosporine, necessitating increased dosing and careful monitoring of cyclosporine and tacrolimus levels. Isoniazid and, to a lesser degree, rifampin and pyrazinamide are potentially hepatotoxic; the evaluation of abnormalities in liver function tests may require a liver biopsy to differentiate drug toxicity from allograft rejection and other etiologies of impaired hepatic function.

Controversy exists among transplant physicians on the issue of chemoprophylaxis for tuberculosis. Whereas the administration of isoniazid to tuberculin-positive patients on immunosuppression is generally recommended, the potential hepatotoxic effects of the drug raise concerns. However, chemoprophylaxis is justified in all high-risk patients; these include patients from developing countries or with a history of inadequately treated tuberculosis, conversion of tuberculin skin test, exposure to patients with active tuberculosis, or a suggestive chest radiograph.

Nontuberculous mycobacteria

In addition to tuberculous mycobacterial infection, diseases caused by atypical mycobacteria have been observed in liver transplant recipients. Nontuberculous mycobacteria include *M. kansasii*, *M. avium-intracellulare*, *M. fortuitum*, *M. xenopi*, *M. haemophilum*, *M. marinum*, *M. chelonae*, *M. abscessus*, *M. gastri*, *M. scrofulaceum*, and *M. thermoresistibile*. These organisms are ubiquitous in the environment and infection classically occurs late in the post-transplant period. Chronic infections with these mycobacterial organisms frequently manifest as cutaneous lesions of the extremities, tenosynovitis, and joint infections. A painful erythematous or violaceous subcutaneous nodule may be the initial presentation of an abscess caused by nontuberculous mycobacteria; cutaneous ulcers develop with the exudation of seropurulent fluid. Bacterial superinfection may occur following skin breakdown. Joint involvement is most commonly seen on the digits, wrists, elbows, ankles, and knees.

Suspicion for the presence of this type of infection should be heightened when lesions fail to respond to standard antimicrobial therapy. Performance of mycobacterial staining and culture, and histopathologic examination of appropriate specimen or tissue are essential for diagnosis. Granulomas may be seen on tissue slides; a predominance of polymorphonuclear cells, however, does not exclude mycobacteriosis. The optimal therapeutic regimen for these infections is not well-defined. Surgical debridement is often necessary and immunosuppression may need to be reduced. Empiric antimycobacterial treatment is initiated in most instances, pending the results of *in vitro* susceptibility testing. Mainstays of treatment include rifampin, ethambutol, streptomycin, and isoniazid. The extended-spectrum macrolides such as clarithromycin and azithromycin, and the fluoroquinolones have proven efficacy against mycobacterial organisms as well.

PARASITIC INFECTIONS

Toxoplasma gondii

Toxoplasmosis is uncommon in liver allograft recipients. It most frequently presents within the first 2 months of transplantation; however, infection has been reported as long as several years after transplantation. The use of OKT3 monoclonal antibody has been associated with the development of disseminated toxoplasmosis. Clinically presenting as meningoencephalitis, brain abscess, pneumonia, myocarditis, pericarditis, hepatitis or chorioretinitis, the diagnosis of toxoplasmosis rests on the histologic demonstration of toxoplasma trophozoites in tissues. Biopsy specimen may be examined following staining with Wright, Giemsa, periodic acid–Schiff stains, or with specific antibody (Fig. 37.15). Serologic testing with a positive IgM or a fourfold rise in IgG titers supports the diagnosis. Antigen detection and PCR techniques may become useful diagnostic tools for toxoplasmosis. Treatment of *Toxoplasma* infection requires a combination of pyrimethamine with folinic acid and sulfadiazine, or clindamycin and pyrimethanime with folinic acid.

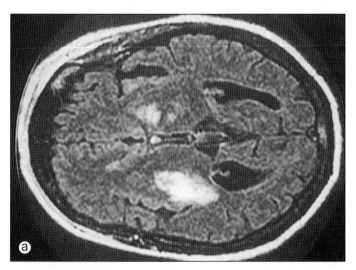

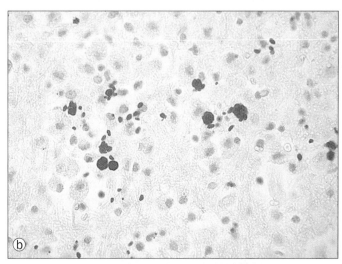

Figure 37.15 *Toxoplasma gondii*. (a) Toxoplasmosis in immunocompromised patients often present with CNS lesions that are best evaluated by MRI. (b) Immunoperoxidase stain of brain biopsy tissue shows toxoplasma cysts and tachyzoites.

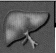
Strongyloides stercoralis

An individual harboring the helminth *S. stercoralis* in the intestinal tract may be asymptomatic for decades, only to present with severe disseminated disease with immunosuppression after liver transplantation. Symptomatic infection develops within 6 months of transplantation in most cases. The isolation of the larval form of parasite in the stool or duodenal secretions indicates intestinal parasitism. Symptoms can include nausea, vomiting, abdominal pain, diarrhea, and abdominal distention; adynamic ileus, small bowel obstruction, and gastrointestinal bleeding may also be seen. The autoinfection cycle of the organism allows the filariform larvae to invade the intestinal mucosa or perianal skin. This phenomenon may result in the hyperinfection syndrome, characterized by an increased worm burden. Predominant complaints are referable to the gastrointestinal and pulmonary systems; these include tachypnea, dyspnea, cough, and hemoptysis, with radiographic changes consistent with alveolar or interstitial infiltration in the lungs. Enterocolitis and widespread migration of the larvae to extraintestinal sites typifies disseminated strongyloidiasis. Consequent Gram-negative bacteremia and meningitis have an exceedingly high mortality rate.

Several stool samples should be examined for the larval form of the parasite in high-risk individuals. Examination of duodenal aspirates, urine, ascitic fluid, wound specimen, sputum, and jejunal biopsy samples may reveal the presence of the larval organism. Thiabendazole and ivermectin are both efficacious in eradicating intestinal parasitism. Infected patients who live in areas of endemicity may require monthly suppressive courses of thiabendazole. Of note, cyclosporine possesses some activity against *S. stercoralis*, and may diminish the threat of disseminated infection in transplant recipients receiving the drug.

CONCLUSION

Despite considerable progress in organ procurement and preservation, marked improvements in the complex liver transplant procedure, and remarkable advances in the immunosuppressive and antimicrobial armamentarium, infection continues to be a major source of transplant morbidity and mortality. As the clinician achieves mastery in the knowledge of the timing and patterns of infectious disease syndromes that occur after liver transplantation, the emphasis in the field of transplantation-associated infectious diseases has shifted from the diagnosis and management of established infections to disease prevention.

The prevention of infectious diseases begins with a detailed and comprehensive pretransplant medical evaluation. The importance of a detailed medical history can not be overemphasized. Meticulous attention to achieving technical perfection during transplant surgery is of paramount importance. While routine antibiotic administration beyond the perioperative period is discouraged, a number of universally accepted prophylactic antimicrobial prophylactic protocols have well-established efficacy in the prevention of serious bacterial, viral, and, to a lesser extent, fungal infections (Fig. 37.16). Careful surveillance should be maintained for the early identification of the presence of an infectious process. While surveillance cultures are routinely undertaken by some transplantation programs, their predictive value remains unknown. Results of these cultures may, however, guide therapy in transplant patients presenting with fever.

Once discharged from the hospital, the liver transplant recipient can lead a normal life. However, because of their increased risk for acquiring infections, patients should be well-advised on strategies for infectious disease prevention. Avoidance of close contact with individuals with respiratory tract infection can diminish the likelihood of disease transmission. In order to prevent food-borne illnesses from a number of microbial pathogens, avoidance of consumption of raw meat, meat products and eggs, as well as unpasteurized milk and water from wells, rivers or lakes, should be emphasized. Precautionary measures are advised when the handling of pets cannot be avoided.

In conclusion, advances in immunosuppressive therapy, surgical techniques and in the treatment of established infections have remarkably improved the survival and quality of life after liver transplantation. However, infection remains a serious problem for the transplant recipient. The management of these infectious complications and more importantly, disease prevention certainly remain evolving challenges in transplantation medicine.

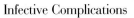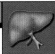
Infectious diseases prophylaxis for liver transplant recipients

Infection	Regimen	Comments
Bacterial	Cephalosporin + aminoglycoside, i.v.; Cephalosporin + ampicillin, i.v.	Antibiotics are given for 2–3 days perioperatively Expert surgery required; discontinuation of catheters
	Polymixin E + gentamicin + nystatin, p.o.; erythromycin + neomycin + nystatin, p.o.	SBD: decreases Gram-negative infections early posttransplant
Pneumococcal infections	Vaccination; penicillin; TMP-SMX	Immunization every 5–6 years
Listeriosis	TMP-SMX	Meticulous food preparation
Legionellosis		Decontamination of water supply
Nocardiosis	TMP-SMX	
Viral		
Herpes simplex	Acyclovir, p.o. or i.v.	During the first post-transplant month
Cytomegalovirus	Use of blood products from seronegative donors or leukocyte-filtered blood	Some use high dose acyclovir, i.v. ganciclovir, CMVIg during anti-lymphocyte antibody therapy; studies with oral ganciclovir, CMV vaccines are pending
Varicella-zoster	Vaccination; varicella-zoster immune globulin	Prior to transplantation Given when exposure has occurred
Hepatitis B, recurrence	Anti-HBs hyperimmune globulin	Long-term treatment necessary to achieve sustained benefit
Hepatitis C, recurrence	? interferon	
Influenza	Vaccination; amantadine or rimantadine	Annual vaccination For postexposure prophylaxis in unvaccinated patients
Fungal		
Candidiasis	Oral nystatin; clotrimazole troches	For the first 4weeks post-transplant, during rejection and additional broad-spectrum antimicrobial therapy
Aspergillosis	HEPA filter	?Low-dose amphotericin in high-risk patients
Pneumocystosis	TMP-SMX; aerosolized pentamidine	Given for 6 months post-transplant. Prevention of CMV infection
Mycobacterial		
Tuberculosis	Isoniazid	Prophylaxis controversial; if given, careful monitoring of liver function tests necessary
Protozoal		
Strongyloidiasis		Pretransplant screening.

Figure 37.16 Infectious diseases prophylaxis for liver transplant recipients. TMP-SMX is also effective in preventing listerial, nocardial, toxoplasma, and other bacterial infections. SBD, selective bowel decontamination; TMP-SMX, trimethoprim-sulfamethoxazole.

FURTHER READING

Arnow PM. Prevention of bacterial infection in the transplant recipient. The role of selective bowel decontamination. Infect Dis Clin N Am. 1995;9:849–62.

Badley AD, Seaberg EC, Porayko MK, et al. Prophylaxis of cytomegalovirus infection in liver transplantation. Transplantation. 1997;64:66–73.

Barkholt L, Ericzon BG, Tollemar J, et al. Infections in human liver recipients: different patterns early and late after transplantation. Transpl Int. 1993;6:77–84.

Basgoz N, Preiksaitis JK. Post-transplant lymphoproliferative disorder. Infect Dis Clin N Am. 1995;9:901–21.

Castaldo P, Stratta RJ, Wood RP, et al. Clinical spectrum of fungal infections after orthotopic liver transplantation. Arch Surg. 1991;126:149–56.

Collins La, Samore MH, Roberts MS, et al. Risk factors for invasive fungal infections complicating orthotopic liver transplantation. J Infect Dis. 1994;170:644–52.

Darenkov IA, Marcarelli MA, Basadonna GP, et al. Reduced incidence of Epstein–Barr virus-associated posttransplant lymphoproliferative disorder using preemptive antiviral therapy. Transplantation. 1997;64:848–52.

Gane E, Saliba F, Valdecasas GJC, et al. Randomized trial of efficacy and safety of oral ganciclovir in the prevention of cytomegalovirus disease in liver-transplant recipients. Lancet. 1997;350:1729–33.

George DL, Arnow PM, Fox AS, et al. Bacterial infections as a complication of liver transplantation: Epidemiology and risk factors. Rev Infect Dis. 1991;13:387–96.

Gorensek MJ, Carey WD, Washington II JA, et al. Selective bowel decontamination with quinolones and nystatin reduces gram-negative and fungal infections in orthotopic liver transplant recipients. Cleve Clin J Med. 1993;60:139–44.

Grauhan O, Lohmann R, Lemmens, et al. Mycobacterial infection after liver transplantation. Langenbecks Arch Chir. 1995;380:171–5.

Hibberd PL, Tolkoff-Rubin NE, Conti D, et al. Preemptive ganciclovir therapy to prevent cytomegalovirus disease in cytomegalovirus antibody-positive renal transplant recipients. A randomized controlled trial. Ann Intern Med. 1995;123:18.

Karchmer AW, Samore MH, Hadley S, et al. Fungal infections complicating orthotopic liver transplantation. Trans Am Clin Climatol Assoc. 1994;106:38–47.

Kusne S, Dummer JS, Singh N, et al. Infections after liver transplantation. An analysis of 101 consecutive cases. Medicine. 1988;67:132–43.

Patel R, Snydman DR, Rubin RH, et al. Cytomegalovirus prophylaxis in solid organ transplant recipients. Transplantation. 1996;61:1279–89.

Paya CV, Hermans PE, Washington II JA, et al. Incidence, distribution, and outcome of episodes of infection in 100 orthotopic liver transplantations. Mayo Clin Proc. 1989;64:555–64.

Singh N, Gayowski T, Wagener M, Yu VL. Infectious complications in liver transplant recipients on tacrolimus. Prospective analysis of 88 consecutive liver transplants. Transplantation. 1994;58:774–8.

Singh N, Yu VL, Mieles L, et al. High-dose acyclovir compared with short-course preemptive ganciclovir therapy to prevent cytomegalovirus disease in liver transplant recipients. A randomized trial. Ann Intern Med. 1994;120:375–81.

Wiesner RH, Hermans P, Rakela J, et al. Selective bowel decontamination to prevent gram-negative bacterial and fungal infection following orthotopic liver transplantation. Transplant Proc. 1987;19:2420–23.

Winston DJ, Winn D, Shaked A, et al. Randomized comparison of ganciclovir and high-dose acyclovir for long-term cytomegalovirus prophylaxis in liver transplant recipients. Lancet. 1995;346:43.

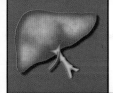

Chapter 38

Technical Complications

Peter Neuhaus, Andrea R Mueller and Klaus-Peter Platz

INTRODUCTION

Liver transplantation has evolved as a successful treatment for patients with end-stage chronic liver disease and acute liver failure. Improvements in immunosuppression, perioperative management, and surgical techniques have led to 1-year patient survival figures of greater than 90% for elective transplants in many programs. Although the surgical technique is highly standardized, technical complications are reported to occur in 5–10% of liver transplant patients (Fig. 38.1).

Factors that influence the pattern of complications include the preoperative condition of the patient, the presence of a severe coagulopathy and a history of previous upper abdominal surgery. The spectrum of possible technical complications is broad, ranging from simple reoperation for postoperative hemorrhage to the requirement for urgent retransplantation. Most of the technical complications are related to the transplant procedure itself, but the donor operation can also have a significant influence on the surgical outcome, especially when arterial reconstruction is necessary.

The most frequent technical complications affect the biliary tract, including biliary leaks which may develop in the presence or absence of a T tube, and strictures at the common bile duct anastomosis. The second group of complications affects the vasculature. Stenosis and thrombosis of the hepatic artery and portal vein are observed more frequently than stenoses of the infra- and suprahepatic vena cava. Postoperative hemorrhage is also commonly

observed after liver transplantation and may be due to technical factors in a number of patients (see Fig. 38.1). According to the heterogeneity of these complications, the time-frame of occurrence can vary from immediately post-transplant to months or even years after transplantation. Furthermore, the severity of technical complications can range from minor to severe, with the latter compromising the patient's condition and outcome.

POSTOPERATIVE HEMORRHAGE

Incidence and predisposing factors for postoperative hemorrhage

Approximately 10–15% of liver transplant patients require reoperation for control of postoperative hemorrhage. Paradoxically, the severe disorder in coagulation associated with acute liver failure usually does not result in severe bleeding, either during or after surgery. Nevertheless, one of the most important risk factors for the development of early postoperative hemorrhage is the presence of a severe clinical coagulopathy, especially when associated with thrombocytopenia or disseminated intravascular coagulation. These patients may develop diffuse bleeding after reperfusion, and further surgery to control the bleeding after stabilization of the patient's clinical condition may be necessary. This is especially the case in patients with poor early graft function, when synthesis of coagulation factors is deficient and any tendency to disseminated intravascular coagulation is accentuated.

Surgical reasons for recurrent postoperative bleeding most frequently result from the donor procedure or the recipient hepatectomy. During the donor procedure, lacerations of the right hepatic lobe may occur and predispose to postoperative hemorrhage, especially when early graft function is not optimal. The gallbladder bed, cystic artery, and undetected small veins draining into the vena cava are other sources of postoperative hemorrhage. During the recipient hepatectomy, caution should be paid to the adrenal gland, as failure to do so may lead to repeated postoperative hemorrhage. Furthermore, postoperative hemorrhage can originate from any of the vascular anastomoses. Late intra-abdominal hemorrhage is mostly associated with surgical interventions including percutaneous liver biopsy. A few patients are very sensitive to heparin treatment, and may develop severe bleeding despite normal coagulation factors shortly after initiation of heparin treatment, (e.g. following liver transplantation for the Budd–Chiari syndrome). Some cases of acute bleeding as a consequence of rupture of a mycotic aneurysm of the hepatic artery have been observed. These aneurysms have a predilection for the site of the arterial anastomosis and these require urgent reoperation with resection of the mycotic aneurysm and reconstruction of the arterial anastomosis.

Technical complications after liver transplantation	
Type of complication	**Examples (onset)**
Abdominal bleeding	Anastomoses (immediate) Size of implantation (immediate)
Vascular complication	Hepatic artery thrombosis (early) Hepatic artery stenosis (late) Portal vein thrombosis (early) Portal vein stenosis (early/late) Suprahepatic/infrahepatic vena cava obstruction
Biliary complications	Biliary leakage (early) Biliary strictures (late) Stenosis of papilla of vater (early)
Nonspecific surgical complications	Infections (early/late) Small bowel obstruction (early/late) Injury to intra-abdominal organs (immediate)

Figure 38.1 Technical complications after liver transplantation.

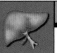

Diagnosis and management of postoperative hemorrhage

The diagnosis of postoperative bleeding is predominantly on clinical grounds. Percutaneous abdominal drains are usually inserted at the end of the transplant procedure unless excellent hemostasis has been secured. Intra-abdominal hemorrhage may become evident on the basis of drainage of frank blood from these drains or when the effluent has a hemoglobin concentration in excess of 3mmol/L (5mg/dL) in patients with severe ascites preoperatively. However, it needs to be considered that these percutaneous drains may fail to function when the hemorrhage occurs more than 2 days after transplantation, even when the drains are properly positioned within the abdominal cavity. Increasing distension of the abdomen may be the main clinical feature in such cases. The patient can present with classic signs of shock, including hypotension and tachycardia, a reduction in filling pressures detected by monitoring or a deterioration in renal function. Liver function is usually unaffected, especially during the early phase of postoperative hemorrhage, even in the presence of intense bleeding.

The presence of intra-abdominal hemorrhage may be detected by ultrasound examination of the abdomen showing sub- or perihepatic hematoma and intraperitoneal fluid. However, such observations are common after transplantation and when suspicion of active bleeding exists, angio-computed tomography (CT) scanning should be performed. Using the angio-CT-scan, intrahepatic hematoma can be sensitively differentiated from the less dangerous extrahepatic hematoma as well as from other intrahepatic pathologies like liver abscess or areas of poor perfusion.

Guidelines for reoperation include the use of more than 4–6 units of packed red blood cells within 24 hours, and hemodynamic instability in the patient. In the latter situation, severe hemorrhage in combination with severely impaired coagulation may require a two-step procedure, with packing of the abdomen to control the bleeding in the first instance. Following stabilization of the patient, the packs are normally removed after approximately 48 hours. However, in most instances, removal of the hematoma and control of the bleeding can be achieved during one laparotomy. In patients with poor early graft function and severe hemorrhage without signs of hemodynamic instability, delaying surgery for 1 or 2 days can be advantageous if liver function and coagulation improve over that period of time. In all patients with postoperative hemorrhage, coagulation studies should be closely monitored and the appropriate combinations of fresh frozen plasma, cryoprecipitate, specific coagulation factors (including antithrombin III and factor XIII), and platelets given to correct the coagulopathy. Functional studies like thromboelastography (TEG) may be useful in monitoring and correcting complex coagulation disorders.

HEPATIC ARTERY STENOSIS AND THROMBOSIS

Although the native liver may function very well without an arterial blood supply, this does not apply to the transplanted liver. Failure to detect and reconstruct an aberrant right hepatic artery during the donor procedure and later during transplantation will invariably lead to necrosis of the right hepatic lobe and the need for urgent retransplantation (Fig. 38.2).

In general, hepatic artery stenosis and thrombosis are more dangerous in terms of graft and patient survival the earlier the complication arises postoperatively.

Incidence and predisposing factors of hepatic artery thrombosis

Age

The incidence of hepatic artery thrombosis ranges between 2.5 and 10% in adults and up to 15–20% in children (Fig. 38.3).

Children are more susceptible to the development of hepatic artery thrombosis simply because of the small diameter of arterial vessels. The majority of hepatic artery thromboses occur during the early postoperative period, but they may also occur several months after transplantation. The type of arterial reconstruction significantly affects the incidence of arterial thrombosis. The need for vascular extension grafts increased the risk of the development of arterial thrombosis up to 70% in children. This was especially the case when the extension graft was attached to the infrarenal aorta. The use of the supraceliac aorta as an anastomotic site reduced the incidence of hepatic artery thrombosis to 12.5% in children, and this was not significantly higher than the incidence of arterial thrombosis after primary anastomosis in adults.

Recipient anatomy

The recipient anatomy also influences the incidence of arterial thrombosis. When the recipient has multiple aberrant arteries, seen in approximately 28% of patients, the arterial inflow into the graft may be seriously compromised. The arterial graft should then be placed to the celiac trunk of the recipient or to the supraceliac aorta (Fig. 38.4a).

The latter approach requires an arterial extension graft using the common and external iliac artery. This procedure has the added advantage that the use of a Carrel patch has significantly reduced the incidence of hepatic artery thrombosis, while using the right and left hepatic artery separately has been associated with a higher incidence of hepatic artery thrombosis. The placement of the celiac trunk with a small Carrel patch to the confluence of the recipient's common hepatic and gastroduodenal artery will further reduce the incidence of hepatic artery stenosis and thrombosis, as blood flow will be supplied by two main arteries, the recipient celiac trunk and the mesenteric artery (Fig. 38.4b).

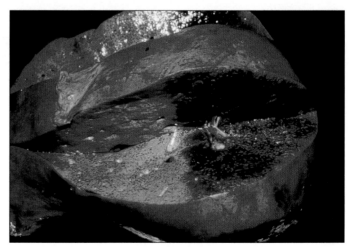

Figure 38.2 Explanted liver allograft following primary transplantation for hepatitis C, 3 days previously. Complete necrosis of the right hepatic lobe due to undetected right hepatic artery which was not reconstructed at transplantation. Normal perfusion of the left hepatic lobe.

Anatomy of donor

The anatomy of the donor also has an influence on the incidence of hepatic artery thrombosis. Aberrant left and right hepatic arteries have to be carefully reconstructed. In some cases, these are small in diameter (2–3mm) and have a fragile intima requiring atraumatic surgical handling and care (Fig. 38.5).

The anastomoses of these reconstructions predispose to the development of hepatic artery stenosis and thrombosis during the early postoperative period. In these cases, anticoagulation with heparin and hemodilution maintaining a hemoglobin below 9mmol/L (12g/dL) during the early postoperative period may reduce the risk of thrombosis. In the presence of impaired early graft function, anticoagulation increases the risk of postoperative hemorrhage.

Other factors

Other factors predisposing to the development of arterial thromboses are arteriosclerosis with plaques involving the celiac trunk

Treatment of vascular complications				Figure 38.3 Treatment of vascular complications.
	Time of occurrence	Leading features	Treatment	
Hepatic artery Thrombosis	Early	Rapid deterioration in graft function Acute liver failure Hemodynamic instability	Urgent thrombectomy or urgent retransplantation	
	Late	Biliary complications Strictures, intrahepatic abscesses Cholangitis and sepsis	Management of biliary complications using ERC, PTCD Rt-PA lysis therapy Elective retransplantation	
Stenosis	–	Slight increase in LFT Mild or late biliary complications	Ballon angioplasty Reoperation with resection of the anastomosis and end-to-end reconstruction	
Portal vein Thrombosis	Early	Rapid deterioration in graft function Acute liver failure Hemodynamic instability Ascites Variceal bleeding	Urgent thrombectomy Urgent retransplantation	
	Late	Slight increase in LFT Portal hypertension Ascites Variceal bleeding Splenomegaly	Endoscopic treatment Rt-PA lysis therapy Elective retransplantation*	
Stenosis	–	Slight incease in LFT Portal hypertension Ascites Variceal bleeding Splenomegaly	Balloon dilation Resection and end-to-end reconstruction	

Figure 38.3 Treatment of vascular complications. ERC, endoscopic retrograde cholangiography; Rt-PA, recombinant tissue-type plasminogen activator; PTCD, percutaneous transhepatic cholangio-drainage; LFTs, liver function tests. *If technically possible.

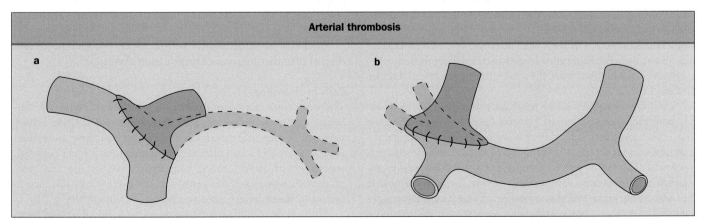

Arterial thrombosis

a   b

Figure 38.4 Arterial thrombosis. (a) Arterial reconstruction using the celiac trunk of the recipient for anastomosis with the donor celiac trunk including a Carrel patch. Hypoplastic common hepatic artery of the recipient. (b) Standard reconstruction of the hepatic artery. Anastomosis of the donor celiac trunk including a Carrel patch to the recipient's common hepatic artery at the confluence of the hepatic artery and the gastroduodenal artery. By this technique, arterial blood supply for the graft originates from two main arteries: the recipient's celiac trunk and the mesenteric artery.

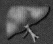

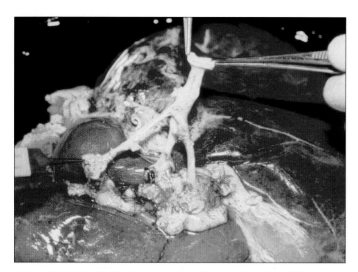

Figure 38.5 'Backtable' (extracorporeal) reconstruction of the donor liver. Two aberrant arteries, a left and a right aberrant artery, were reconstructed with 7/0 proline running sutures. Skilful microsurgical techniques will diminish the risk of postoperative hepatic artery stenosis and thrombosis at the side of these anastomoses.

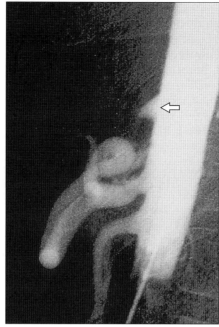

Figure 38.6 Angiography of the aorta, the celiac trunk, and the supraceliac extension graft. Complete thrombosis of the supraceliac extension graft, barely seen above the celiac trunk. Arterial perfusion stops abruptly after the insertion of the extension graft into the aorta.

of either the donor or recipient, stenosis of the hepatic artery anastomosis, aneurysms of the donor hepatic artery, splenic steal syndromes, and reduced diameters or size disparity involving the anastomosed vessels. Depending on the severity of the anatomic variations, an arterial extension graft may be necessary. In patients with steal syndromes with preferential arterial flow to the spleen, ligation of the splenic artery or reduction of the blood flow by subtotal ligation of the splenic artery may be a safe and effective intervention. This approach avoids the need for an extension graft while providing sufficient arterial inflow to the common hepatic artery.

Mechanical factors including internal flaps, prolonged clamping of the hepatic artery during the fashioning of the anastomosis, redundancy or kinking of a long artery, and intra-arterial hematoma also predispose to the development of hepatic artery thrombosis. However, in many cases no anatomic or technical cause can be identified. Although impaired coagulation and thrombocytopenia reduce the risk of thrombosis in many liver graft recipients, some patients have a prothrombotic state either related to the primary indication for transplantation, (e.g. Budd–Chiari syndrome), or to overly aggressive correction of the coagulation defects. These clinical situations may predispose to hepatic artery thrombosis, especially in combination with the anatomic or technical factors detailed above.

A number of complications involving the graft may contribute to thrombosis of the hepatic artery. Graft edema associated with poor early graft function may increase vascular resistance and consequently reduce arterial blood flow. A similar effect is seen with the use of potent vasopressor agents, especially epinephrine (adrenaline) and norepinephrine (noradrenaline). It has also been suggested that episodes of rejection may trigger hepatic artery thrombosis. Although the existence of hyperacute rejection is not universally acknowledged, some of the cases described highlighted complete thrombosis of intrahepatic arteries and the intrahepatic portal venous system without signs of extrahepatic thrombosis or other recognized predisposing fac-

tors. Hyperacute rejection remains difficult to diagnose, since this type of rejection is predominantly humoral in nature and less strongly associated with the typical morphologic features of acute cellular rejection. The latter may also compromise the hepatic artery by reducing blood flow and thus predisposing to thrombosis. In chronic rejection, the hepatic artery becomes occluded by a process characterized by infiltration of the arterial wall with foamy macrophages and this can lead to almost complete de-arterialization of the graft.

Diagnosis and management of hepatic artery stenosis and thrombosis

Doppler ultrasound is reasonably effective for the monitoring of early postoperative stenosis and patency, with a reported inaccuracy rate of less than 10%. This noninvasive investigation is easy to perform and can be repeated frequently in any intensive care unit at a low cost. However, the potential for false-positive and false-negative results is well-recognized, and when hepatic artery thrombosis is suspected on clinical grounds angiography should be performed to confirm or refute the diagnosis (Fig. 38.6).

Furthermore, angiography will facilitate the technical planning of retransplantation or urgent thrombectomy.

Early presentation

There are three dominant presentations of hepatic artery thrombosis – liver necrosis, hepatic abscesses, and diffuse biliary stenoses. A dramatic increase in transaminases [aspartate aminotransferase (AST) and alanine aminotransferase (ALT) levels], together with deteriorating coagulation studies are the most prominent features of early postoperative hepatic artery thrombosis and these reflect massive necrosis of the graft (Fig. 38.7).

This can be accompanied by a decrease in bile flow and lightening of bile color, fever, and a clinical scenario similar to septic shock. During this early postoperative period, the diagnosis of hepatic artery thrombosis usually requires urgent retransplantation caused by the rapid deterioration in liver function and the

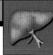

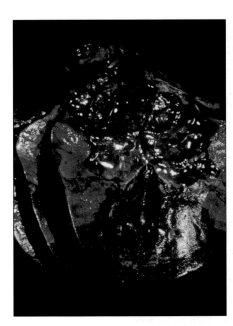

Figure 38.7 Explanted liver of a patient with fulminant liver failure following primary transplantation due to early postoperative hepatic artery thrombosis. Complete necrosis of the liver allograft.

patient's condition (see Fig. 38.3). Within the first 10 days after transplantation, acute thrombectomy is an alternative therapeutic option to retransplantation and a number of programs have reported success rates of 50–88% in adults. However, these results were achieved in the setting of very early detection of the thrombosis, probably within 6 hours of the event. Although the short-term results of acute thrombectomy are reported to be excellent, the long-term patient survival rate was decreased when compared with patients who did not develop arterial thrombosis.

Early postoperative hepatic artery stenosis, often occurring at the site of the anastomosis, presents with a slower and less severe clinical progression. Anastomotic stenosis may be suggested by the detection of high velocity flow across the anastomosis during Doppler ultrasound examination. Angioplasty has been described with inconsistent results and surgical reconstruction of the arterial anastomosis may be the preferred intervention.

Second and third month presentation

The second presentation of hepatic artery thrombosis is with intrahepatic abscesses, most typically during the second and third months after transplantation. These patients present with fever and upper abdominal pain or discomfort. The diagnosis is usually suggested by ultrasound or CT scan appearances. This type of presentation tends to occur in the absence of a significant deterioration in liver graft function and frequently the liver function tests are entirely normal at the time of diagnosis. This should not lead to a false sense of security as these cases cannot be successfully managed using antibiotics and drainage techniques. These patients invariably require urgent retransplantation.

Late presentation

The third clinical scenario is seen when the hepatic artery thrombosis presents several months after transplantation and biliary complications are the most prominent feature (see Fig. 38.3). Nonanastomotic strictures, especially those occurring at the hilum, are most likely to have an underlying ischemic etiology. The biliary assessment is usually performed using endoscopic retrograde cholangiography and pancreatography (ERCP) or percutaneous cholangiography, but magnetic resonance (MR) cholangiography may emerge as the diagnostic test of choice in this situation. About 80% of patients with late hepatic artery thrombosis will develop biliary complications and only a minority of patients will escape clinical complications in the long term. Thrombosis of the hepatic artery should be excluded in all patients presenting with severe cholestasis of unknown origin and repeated cholangitis or biliary sepsis. In addition to Doppler ultrasound and angiography, CT-scan of the liver and abdomen is recommended to exclude other causes of graft dysfunction, biliary and infectious complications (Figs 38.8 & 38.9).

The arterial perfusion of the liver can be sensitively detected using angio-CT-scans. The pathogenesis of these biliary complications is related to the loss of arterial blood supply to extrahepatic and/or intrahepatic bile ducts. Effective arterial collateralization is occasionally observed, more commonly in children than in adults.

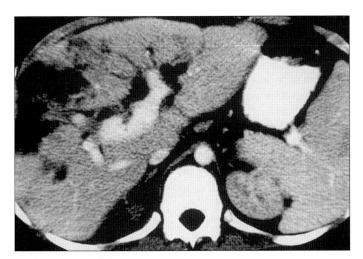

Figure 38.8 Angio-CT-scan of a transplanted liver in a patient with multiple bile duct strictures, dilatation of intrahepatic bile ducts, and biliary abscesses, predominantly within the right lobe of the liver. These changes to the biliary tract resulted from hepatic artery thrombosis.

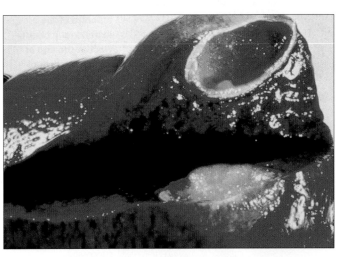

Figure 38.9 Explanted liver allograft from a patient with ischemic-type biliary lesion, who developed multiple liver abscesses. Encapsulated abscess in the explanted liver.

The clinical picture of late hepatic artery thrombosis ranges from asymptomatic cholestasis detected on blood tests to biliary sepsis with intrahepatic abscesses, bile duct dilatation or stenoses. These changes can occur separately or in combination. Depending on the different manifestations, patients may present with increased bilirubin and cholestatic enzymes (alkaline phosphatase, γ-GT). However, severe graft dysfunction with an increase in AST and ALT, severe infection and sepsis, fever, elevated C-reactive protein levels, and secondary organ dysfunction (including acute renal failure, pulmonary, and circulatory insufficiency) are also possible.

Multiple ischemic strictures, which can be so severe as to present with complete destruction of the intrahepatic biliary tract, require retransplantation after resolution of the septic complications. Temporary bile duct drainage and decompression of the biliary tract can be achieved by ERCP with dilatation of the stenoses with or without stent implantation. External drainage via percutaneous trans-hepatic catheter insertion may be necessary in patients with biliary sepsis, when ERCP is not successful, and in patients with Roux-en-Y biliary anastomoses. This approach carries the risk of secondary cutaneous infection and seriously compromises the patient's quality of life. In a few cases, when the extrahepatic bile duct is predominantly affected, ERCP and dilatation of the common bile duct in combination with stent implantation can prove successful in the medium to long term (Fig. 38.10).

In others with destruction largely confined to the extrahepatic and second order intrahepatic bile ducts, a Roux-en-Y surgical reconstruction may be effective.

Long-term management

Following the establishment of effective biliary drainage, a long-term management strategy is required. This may involve early elective retransplantation or it may be possible to defer this for several months or years when the clinical response is excellent. While children with late hepatic artery thrombosis often develop sufficient collateralization to obviate the need for retransplanta-tion, this is less likely to occur in adults. The administration of fibrinolytic agents like recombinant tissue-type plasminogen acti-vator (rt-PA) has been used on occasion for lysis of late hepatic artery thrombosis. However, in most instances this therapy was not successful because of the delay between the occurrence of the thrombosis and the diagnosis as a result of the slow progres-sion of the related symptoms.

PORTAL VEIN STENOSIS AND THROMBOSIS

As with the arterial blood supply, effective perfusion of the portal vein is very important during the early postoperative period. Thrombosis of the portal vein is most detrimental during this time period and potentially leads to severe allograft dysfunction, variceal hemorrhage, oliguria, and hemodynamic instability. The mortality in these patients is high. During the later follow-up period, the sequelae to portal vein thrombosis are less severe and are frequently associated with good liver function for variable periods of time.

Incidence and predisposing factors of portal vein thrombosis

The incidence of portal vein thrombosis is low at 0.3–2.2%. However, the incidence of portal vein thrombosis increased to approximately 15% in patients with pre-existing portocaval shunts. Risk factors for the development of portal vein throm-bosis include pre-existing portal vein thrombosis, hypoplastic portal vein, mismatch in size of the donor and recipient portal veins, and large portosystemic collaterals. The latter may cause a steal phenomenon and thereby decrease portal venous blood flow. Previous splenectomy may also decrease portal venous blood flow and predispose to portal vein thrombosis. Thrombectomy of pre-existing portal vein thrombosis at the time of transplantation is commonly practised, but this may lead to denudation of the epithelium and increase the susceptibility to recurrent throm-bosis. Technical factors that predispose to portal vein thrombo-sis include redundancy of portal vein, kinking, torsion, and stenosis of the portal vein at the site of anastomosis. Severe allo-graft edema and prothrombotic states are less common causes of portal vein thrombosis but may contribute in association with other predisposing factors.

Diagnosis and management of portal vein stenosis and thrombosis

Doppler ultrasound of the portal vein is the most effective screening technique to detect portal vein stenosis and thrombo-sis (Fig. 38.11).

During the early postoperative period, Doppler ultrasound should be performed daily and subsequently whenever graft dys-function occurs. If portal vein thrombosis is suggested by Doppler ultrasound, angiography and an angio-CT-scan should be per-formed to confirm the diagnosis. This not only defines the anatomic extent of the stenosis or thrombosis but also assesses any abnormality in the perfusion pattern of the liver.

Early clinical scenarios

The most frequent clinical scenarios following thrombosis of the portal vein include signs of portal hypertension, variceal bleeding, ascites, and graft failure (see Fig. 38.3). The latter occurs when the portal vein thrombosis develops during the early postopera-

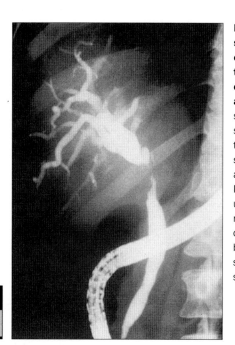

Figure 38.10 Isolated stricture of the extrahepatic biliary tract at the site of common bile duct anastomosis. This stricture occurred several months after transplantation (late stricture) due to hepatic artery thrombosis. Interventional endoscopy using endoscopic retrograde cholangiography with balloon dilatation and stent implantation was successful.

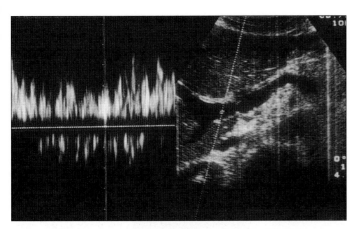

Figure 38.11 Doppler ultrasound of the portal vein. This shows a significant portal vein stenosis in a patient with stable graft function.

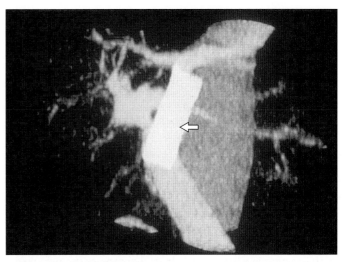

Figure 38.12 Angiography of a patient with transjugular intrahepatic portosystemic shunt (TIPS) implantation following liver transplantation. TIPS was performed because of a clinically significant portal vein thrombosis. The patient has previously developed recurrent variceal bleeding and ascites. Liver function was good. Direct perfusion of the portal venous blood into the right hepatic vein (arrow).

tive period. A deterioration in the liver function tests will invariably be observed in addition to the development of a coagulopathy and other features of acute liver failure to varying degrees of severity. Early postoperative portal vein thrombosis in patients with good liver function may be treated with immediate thrombectomy. This procedure is most effective after early and rapid diagnosis of the compromise to portal venous flow. However, this approach is not suitable for patients with early postoperative graft failure, and in this situation urgent retransplantation is usually required (see Fig. 38.3).

Later clinical scenarios

During the later post-transplant period, portal vein thrombosis may be cured by rt-PA lysis therapy. This approach will be most effective if the time interval between the diagnosis of portal vein thrombosis and the commencement of treatment is short. Late portal vein thrombosis can be treated symptomatically, (e.g. by controlling variceal bleeding using endoscopic techniques). Splenectomy and distal renal shunt (Warren shunt) may be required if variceal hemorrhage is refractory to other treatment modalities. In some cases with predominantly intrahepatic portal vein thrombosis, transjugular intrahepatic portosystemic shunt (TIPS) can be an effective treatment, but it may also lead to a deterioration in graft function as a consequence of reduced parenchymal perfusion (Fig. 38.12).

Surgical procedures with thrombectomy and direct repair are difficult and therefore in general not recommended. When the portal vein thrombosis involves the superior mesenteric vein, neither direct surgical repair, nor retransplantation may be feasible for technical reasons. Extensive collaterals will prohibit the effective drainage of mesenteric blood into the donor portal vein, despite the use of extension grafts.

Stenosis of the portal vein at the site of the anastomosis may cause clinical problems similar to those complicating portal vein thrombosis, but the most frequent are manifestations of portal hypertension, including esophageal varices and splenomegaly. Doppler ultrasound detects increased velocity of blood flow across the anastomosis and turbulent blood flow distal to the anastomosis. In many instances these ultrasound findings are of no significance in the early postoperative period and no intervention is required. However, when the stenosis is symptomatic or severe, it should be treated to reduce the risk of secondary

portal vein thrombosis. Most cases are amenable to angioplasty and dilatation of the stenosis using a trans-hepatic approach. Occasional cases require surgical reconstruction and revision of the end-to-end portal vein anastomosis (see Fig. 38.3).

VENOCAVAL STENOSIS AND OBSTRUCTION

Two patterns of complications involving the vena cava are seen. The removal of the intrahepatic vena cava with the explant is followed by the construction of two end-to-end caval anastomoses between the native and donor cavas. Of these, the superior anastomosis is more susceptible to stenosis. The sparing of the native cava that is a feature of the 'piggy-back' technique is more likely to be associated with outflow problems involving kinking or stenoses of the main hepatic veins. Stenosis or obstruction of the infrahepatic or suprahepatic vena cava are generally unusual complications that occur with different degrees of severity. However, this complication is important as it can be associated with mortality rates as high as 50–75%. This is especially the case when serious stenosis or complete obstruction of the vena cava develops early in the postoperative period. Stenosis and obstruction of the suprahepatic vena cava are more dangerous than stenosis and obstruction of the infrahepatic vena cava, since suprahepatic venocaval stenosis and obstruction can seriously affect the venous outflow and function of the liver graft as well as cardiac function, leading to severe hemodynamic instability.

Incidence and predisposing factors for venocaval stenosis and obstruction

Stenosis or obstruction of the infrahepatic or suprahepatic vena cava were observed in 1–2% of liver transplant patients. The causes of venocaval stenosis and obstruction are predominantly technical in nature or result from recurrence of the Budd–Chiari syndrome. Technical reasons include narrowing and stenosis of the supra- or infrahepatic venocaval anastomosis, excessive

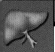

length and kinking of the supra- or infrahepatic vena cava, and mechanical obstruction due to the use of a large graft in a small recipient. In rare cases, poor graft function can result in swelling of the liver allograft with subsequent obstruction and thrombosis of the vena cava. Anatomic variations with severe narrowing of the infrahepatic vena cava are occasionally observed. These may present either in the donor or the recipient, although they usually have developed adequate collaterals and are therefore asymptomatic. In these cases (anatomic variation of the donor or recipient), the 'piggy-back' technique should be used for the transplantat procedure and the reconstruction of the venocaval anastomosis.

Diagnosis and management of venocaval stenosis and obstruction

Stenosis and obstruction of the suprahepatic vena cava presents with massive swelling of the liver, hepatomegaly, peripheral edema, deterioration in renal function and the development or persistence of ascites. Arterial and portal venous perfusion of the graft are impaired and this usually results in a modest increase in serum bilirubin and other liver function tests. If there is a significant suprahepatic venocaval stenosis or if the obstruction of the vena cava is complete, liver failure may ensue. This is usually accompanied by acute renal failure and severe hemodynamic instability of the patient. Urgent reoperation with resection and reconstruction of the venocaval anastomosis or urgent retransplantation will be required. The latter is preferred, since a direct surgical approach may be difficult to perform, as a result of the seriously compromised clinical condition of the patient. Stenosis and obstruction of the infrahepatic vena cava are usually less dangerous. Patients present with edema of the lower extremities and impaired renal function without signs of hepatomegaly and ascites. The venous outflow of the kidney may also be seriously compromised, especially after complete obstruction of the infrahepatic vena cava with an increased risk of thrombosis of the renal vein.

Scanning

As with other vascular complications, Doppler ultrasound has been valuable in diagnosing decreased blood flow as a result of venocaval stenosis or obstruction. Angio-CT-scan may show an edematous liver graft with compromised arterial and portal venous blood flow and may indicate suprahepatic venocaval stenosis and obstruction. Liver biopsy typically reveals nonspecific cholestasis and centrilobular necrosis. The definitive diagnosis, however, can be only made by contrast venography. The inferior venacavogram allows diagnosis and visualization of vena cava stenosis, kinking, or obstruction (Fig. 38.13). Although there is a concern regarding anastomotic rupture, especially during the early postoperative period, balloon dilatation has been successfully performed for both supra- and infrahepatic venocaval stenosis. Some patients have been managed to good effect with the insertion of expansile metal stents. If these approaches are not successful, direct surgical intervention or occasionally retransplantation may be required, especially in those patients with suprahepatic venocaval obstruction. In patients with infrahepatic stenosis or obstruction, retransplantation is usually not necessary and if interventional therapy fails, surgical treatment is usually feasible with correction and resection of the stenosis following thrombectomy.

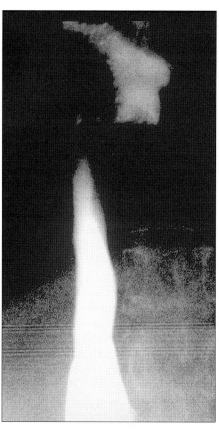

Figure 38.13 Venacavogram of a liver transplant patient with suspected venocaval obstruction. The patient presented with severe deterioration of liver function, severely swollen liver, hemodynamic instability, acute renal failure, ascites, and severe edema of the distal extremities. Kinking of the vena cava with near complete obstruction of the vena cava at the site of the suprahepatic venocaval anastomosis was observed. The outflow of the hepatic veins was seriously compromised. Urgent reoperation with resection and end-to-end reconstruction of the vena cava was performed.

Budd–Chiari syndrome

Immediate postoperative anticoagulation with heparin is mandatory to prevent the recurrence of Budd–Chiari syndrome leading to obstruction and thrombosis of the hepatic veins and the vena cava. Once the patient is stable and the need for liver biopsy and other invasive procedures is reduced the patients are converted to warfarin or other coumarins. The autoanticoagulation that is commonly seen immediately after liver transplantation does not give adequate protection against devastating thrombosis and heparin should be commenced even when the prothrombin time, international normalized ratio (INR), or other coagulation tests are prolonged. Recurrence of the Budd–Chiari syndrome usually means that retransplantation has to be considered. Urgent retransplantation is only required in the rare cases in whom the thrombosis leads to complete or almost complete obstruction of the vena cava. Otherwise elective retransplantation is usually feasible. The potential to manage recurrent Budd–Chiari syndrome with percutaneously placed shunts (TIPS) has not yet been defined in the transplant population.

The 'piggy-back' technique

The 'piggy-back' technique of caval preservation appears to be associated with an increase in problems with venous outflow from the graft. The clinical manifestations include hepatomegaly, ascites, and persistence of abnormal liver function tests. Alternatively the problem may be suggested by histologic changes that include congestion and perivenular cell drop-out. Caval venography permits an anatomic definition of the anastomoses between the cava and the hepatic veins as well as the measurement of the pressure gradients across these anastomoses. In some cases this procedure can be extended to dilatation and correction of significant stenoses.

BILIARY TRACT COMPLICATIONS

Biliary complications are the most frequent of the technical problems encountered after liver transplantation. Calne and Starzl have called the biliary tract the 'Achilles' heel' of liver transplantation, because of the high risk of complications at the anastomotic site and/or biliary obstruction or leaks which are frequently accompanied by serious infection. Despite attempts to repair the biliary tract, morbidity and mortality remained high in this group of patients. Historically, patients tended to die between 1 and 6 months after diagnosis of these complications, mostly as a consequence of the sequelae to infection. Modern techniques and a lower reliance on corticosteroids were probably important in greatly improving this problem, but it is still true that great attention should be paid to the quality of biliary tract reconstruction during the transplant procedure.

Incidence and predisposing factors for biliary tract complications

Incidence

Although the overall incidence is around 15%, biliary tract complications were observed in 2.3–50% of liver transplant recipients, depending on the type of biliary anastomosis and reconstruction. Biliary tract complications can be innocuous and may resolve with conservative management. However, they may also cause significant morbidity and mortality. The incidence of bile leaks ranges between 1.3 and 10%. Bile leaks frequently occur at the site of anastomosis and are often T tube related, (i.e. leakage with a T tube in place, displaced T tube or leak after removal of the T tube) (Fig. 38.14).

Leaks are also observed at the site of the anastomosis in the absence of a T tube, or may originate from the cystic duct (Fig. 38.15) or aberrant bile ducts within the bed of the gallbladder. Surgical factors that predispose to the development of bile leaks are surgical dissection of the common bile duct, too many sutures placed at the common bile duct anastomosis, or a long donor common bile duct. All these technical factors will compromise arterial blood supply and may eventually lead to necrosis of the biliary anastomosis and a bile leak.

The incidence of stenosis of the biliary tract is reported at between 2.6% and more than 20%. Stenoses of the biliary tract are also predominantly found at the site of anastomosis but nonanastomotic strictures occur at the papilla of Vater, hilum, and diffusely within the extra- and/or intrahepatic bile ducts. The development of a stenosis of the choledochocholedochostomy largely depends on the type of biliary reconstruction. The introduction of the side-to-side technique significantly reduced the incidence of stenoses at the anastomosis to less than 3% (Fig. 38.16).

This technique provides an uninterrupted bile flow, despite contraction of the bile duct anastomosis, which is a regular phenomenon of the healing process. Using this technique, early stenoses of the anastomosis are virtually absent. Despite these findings end-to-end biliary anastomoses are more routinely performed. Late stenoses at the site of anastomosis are more closely related to other factors, including hepatic artery thrombosis (as mentioned earlier in this chapter) and ischemic-type biliary lesion (ITBL).

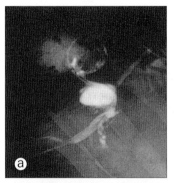
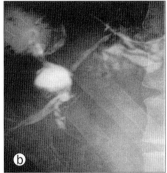
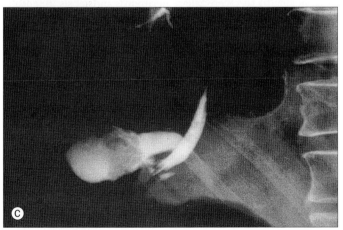

Figure 38.14 T-drain cholangiogram. (a) Bile leak at the site of the T-tube insertion observed during the early postoperative period. Reopening of the T tube resolved this complication. (b) Endoscopic retrograde cholangiography and pancreatography (ERCP)-guided cholangiography after T-tube removal showing a leak from the biliary tract at the side of T-drain insertion. The patient presented with upper abdominal pain and fever. (c) ERCP-guided stent implantation in combination with percutaneous drainage of the bilioma resolved this complication.

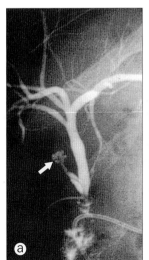
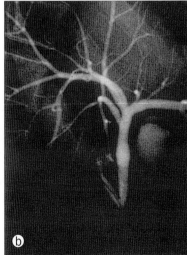

Figure 38.15 T-drain cholangiography performed during the early postoperative period. (a) Leakage from the cystic duct was observed (arrow). (b) Reopening of the T tube was effective in resolving this complication.

Techniques for the common bile duct anastomosis

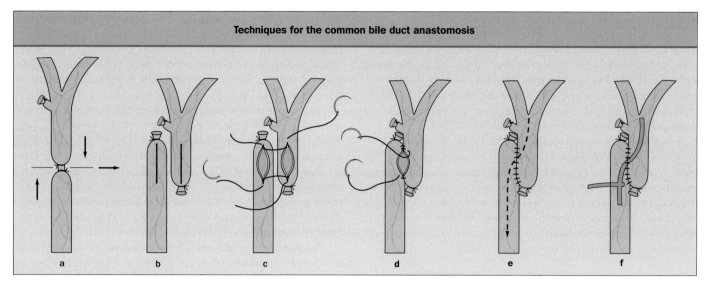

a   b   c   d   e   f

Figure 38.16 Techniques for bile duct anastomosis. (a) Typical stricture of the common bile duct anastomosis after end-to-end choledochocholedochostomy. Technique for side-to-side choledochocholedochostomy (b–e) with insertion of a T tube drained via the recipient's common bile duct (f). Running sutures with 5/0 poly-dioxanone sutures (PDS) were used.

Influencing factors

Donor and recipient factors, as well as the type and quality of liver preservation will have an influence on the incidence of biliary tract complications. During the donor procedure, it is important to preserve the tissue surrounding the bile duct to optimize the arterial blood supply to the bile ducts. Cholecystectomy prior to perfusion and preservation of the liver will reduce bile contamination and thereby reduce the toxicity of bile within the biliary tract during preservation. Furthermore, an effective arterial perfusion optimizes preservation of the biliary tract. These approaches, together with maintaining the duration of cold preservation below 10–12 hours, may reduce the incidence of postoperative bile duct complications, especially the incidence of ITBL.

The indication for liver transplantation also has an influence on the development of biliary tract complications. Patients with primary or secondary sclerosing cholangitis often have abnormal intra- and extrahepatic biliary tracts and a choledochojejunostomy or choledochoduodenostomy is usually recommended. The incidence of biliary tract complications following these surgical procedures ranged from between 4 and 30%. In general, leaks are more frequently observed after choledochojejunostomy and choledochoduodenostomy, while stenosis and strictures occur more frequently after choledochostomy. Furthermore, reduced-size and split-liver techniques are associated with a higher incidence of biliary tract complications. Secondary hemorrhage is also more common following Roux-en-Y anastomoses.

Diagnosis and management of biliary tract complications
Bile leaks

The clinical picture of biliary tract complications can present with a broad spectrum ranging from asymptomatic cholestasis and cholangitis to severe biliary peritonitis and sepsis. Bile leaks can be asymptomatic or may cause biliary peritonitis (Fig. 38.17).

Figure 38.17 Biliary tract complications. ANV, acute renal failure; ARI, acute respiratory insufficiency; CI, cardiocirculatory insufficiency; ERCP, endoscopic retrograde cholangiography and pancreatography; PTCD, percutaneous transhepatic cholangio-drainage.

	Biliary tract complications		
	Type and onset	Leading features	Treatment
Leak	T-tube insertion (early)	Cholestasis, fever, biliary peritonitis	Reopen T tube Drainage of biloma
	T-tube removal (late)	Cholestasis, fever, biliary peritonitis	ERCP and stent implantation Percuntous drainage
	Anastomasis (early)	Cholestasis, fever, biliary peritonitis	ERCP and stent implantation Reoperation: Roux-en-Y loop
Stricture	Anastomosis, extrahepatic (late)	Severe cholestasis, cholangitis, sepsis	ERCP: dilatation and stent implantation Reconstructive surgery
	Multiple strictures, intrahepatic, abscesses (late)	Severe cholestasis, cholangitis, sepsis Secondary organ dysfunction ANV, ARI, CI	ERCP: dilatation and stent implantation PTCD of liver abscesses Elective retransplantation

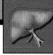

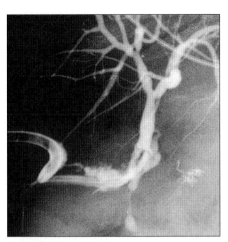

Figure 38.18 T-drain cholangiography showing a bile leak from the common bile duct anastomosis. CT-guided percutaneous drain was placed into the subhepatic area, which effectively drained the collection of bile. The T tube was reopened and the leak closed after several weeks of conservative treatment.

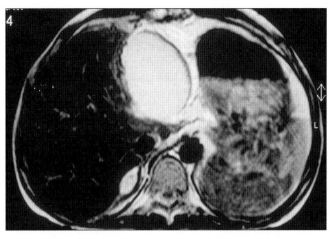

Figure 38.19 CT-scan of a large subhepatic bilioma prior to percutaneous drainage.

T-tube cholangiography is a useful diagnostic tool in those patients in whom a T tube has been placed. A leak from the T-tube insertion site usually does not require surgical intervention. Unclamping of the T tube, together with percutaneous drainage of the subhepatic biloma – if the perioperative percutaneous drain(s) have already been removed – are sufficient in most cases that present after the T tube has been clamped or spigoted (Figs 38.18 & 38.19).

Alternatively, or when the aforementioned approaches have failed, ERCP and placement of a stent may be required. This approach is also taken when leaks complicate removal of the T tube. If the leak develops at the site of the bile duct anastomosis, the aforementioned procedures may not be effective and surgical intervention will be required. Secondary choledochocholedochostomy may be feasible, but more usually conversion to a Roux-en-Y loop anastomosis will be necessary. This is especially true when the arterial blood supply to the bile duct anastomosis is compromised.

In the absence of a T tube, ERCP is required for the diagnosis of a bile leak and in this setting it is usually found at the site of the anastomosis. Magnetic resonance cholangiography and radionucleotide scans may be useful in some patients, but these approaches lack the therapeutic potential of ERCP. In patients with choledochojejunostomy or choleduodenostomy, ERCP is difficult unless an access loop has been fashioned and percutaneous transhepatic cholangiography (PTC) may be necessary. When the leak develops during the early postoperative period and a percutaneous drain is still in place, the presence of a bile leak may be indicated by bile staining of the effluent. Occasionally contrast placed via the drain may provide reasonable definition of the site and extent of the leak.

Biliary stenosis and strictures

Biliary stenosis and strictures may present in a similar manner to bile leaks, but jaundice and ascending cholangitis are more prominent features. Impairment of liver function, severe cholangitis with sepsis and/or intrahepatic abscesses may occur (see Fig. 38.17). These patients may also develop secondary organ dysfunction, including acute renal failure, pulmonary complications and/or circulatory insufficiency. Decompression of the biliary tract is the major therapeutic goal in these patients. This will be

accompanied by antibiotic medication and specific intensive care treatment to cope with secondary organ dysfunction. The extent of the stricturing is visualized using T-tube cholangiography or ECRP. The latter is also used to achieve dilatation of the stenoses and the implantation of stents to maintain bile flow. Intraluminal material including sludge, stones, and casts of necrotic epithelium may have to be removed from the bile ducts before the stents can be placed (Fig. 38.20).

The hilar stricture characteristic of ischemia is amenable to dilatation, but retransplantation may be needed because of the underlying pathology. In patients with cholestatic complica-

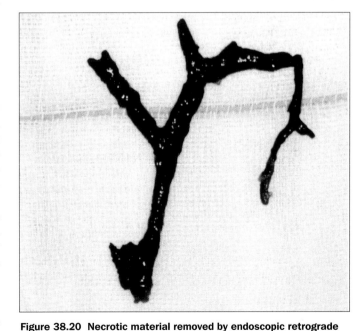

Figure 38.20 Necrotic material removed by endoscopic retrograde cholangiography (ERC) from the extrahepatic biliary tract. Late hepatic artery thrombosis was the cause for necrosis of the epithelium of the biliary tract, resulting in multiple biliary strictures and poststenotic dilatations. These changes led to severe recurrent cholangitis and biliary sepsis. Repeated interventional ERC procedures with removal of necroses, dilatation of bile duct strictures, and stent implantations controlled the sepsis. Elective retransplantation was performed.

tions presenting with stenosis of the papilla of Vater, papillotomy should be performed in addition to any other procedures that are required. Patients with intrahepatic abscesses will require radiologically guided percutaneous aspiration. Using this aggressive interventional management, septic complications usually resolve within days or weeks. However, in general endoscopic approaches are most effective when the time interval between the development of stenoses and ERCP-directed therapy is short. Success also depends on the severity of disease and extensive or recurrent stricturing may be best managed by surgical revision and conversion to a Roux-en-Y anastomosis. Recourse to retransplantation is needed when the hepatic artery is compromised, chronic rejection coexists, and in cases of very extensive disease associated with severe preservation injury (see Fig. 38.17).

Multiple stenosis and strictures

The most serious and complex biliary tract complications occur in conjunction with ITBL, which presents with multiple stenoses and strictures of the extra- and intrahepatic biliary tract system, intrahepatic bile duct dilatation or abscesses (Fig. 38.21).

It is supposedly associated with preservation injury to the bile duct epithelium, stasis of bile due to papilla of Vater stenosis, stricturing of the bile duct anastomosis, and damage secondary to acidic bile composition, compromised arterial blood supply (hepatic artery stenosis or thrombosis), and possibly immunologic factors (including acute and chronic rejection). Clinical features of ITBL develop over several months and will be aggravated by recurrent cholestasis and cholangitis. The management is similar to biliary tract stenosis and strictures of other causes (Figs 38.22 & 38.23).

However, this type of biliary complication frequently involves the intrahepatic bile duct system and retransplantation is eventually necessary in the majority of patients. Effective interventional endoscopy, aggressive treatment of infection and

ursodeoxycholic acid (UDCA) may delay the requirement of retransplantation for months or years with a good quality of life for the transplanted patient. A similar pattern of diffuse stricturing develops more commonly in patients transplanted for primary sclerosing cholangitis than for any other etiology. Whether this represents true recurrence of the disease is difficult to determine. These patients are managed in a similar fashion to diffuse stricturing occurring after transplantation for other etiologies.

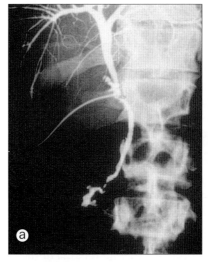
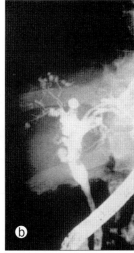

Figure 38.22 T-drain cholangiography performed 5 days after transplantation. (a) Normal anatomy of the intra- and extrahepatic biliary tract. (b) After 1 year, ischemic-type biliary lesion (ITBL) with stenosis of the distal common bile duct and poststenotic dilatation. Intrahepatic bile ducts are not well-visualized.

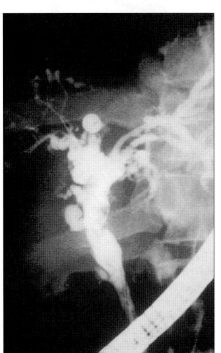

Figure 38.21 Endoscopic retrograde cholangiography in a patient with severe ischemic-type biliary lesion predominantly affecting the extrahepatic biliary tract. Stenosis of the distal common bile duct and dilatation of the proximal common and right and left bile duct. Visualization of the intrahepatic bile ducts in the left lobe is also reduced. Dilatation and stent implantation was performed. Elective retransplantation was indicated 1 year later.

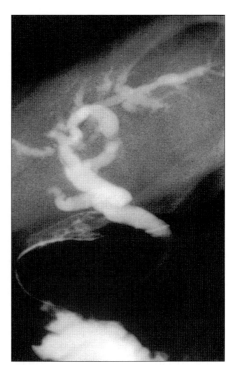

Figure 38.23 Percutaneous transhepatic cholangiography in a patient with ischemic type biliary lesion. Near complete stenosis of the distal common biliary tract, poststenotic dilatation, strictures, and dilatations of the intrahepatic biliary tract. Elective retransplantation was performed after decompression of the biliary tract and treatment of the infectious complications.

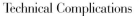
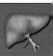
MISCELLANEOUS TECHNICAL PROBLEMS

In addition to the complications specific for liver transplantation, various other complications observed after major abdominal surgery may also occur (see Fig. 38.1). These complications include perforation of intestinal organs due to mobilization of adhesions, especially in patients with previous abdominal surgery.

Leaks from intestinal anastomoses performed in patients receiving Roux-en-Y loops, and postoperative small bowel obstruction are also seen. The diagnosis of these complications may be delayed because of masking of symptoms due to the immuno-compromised status of the patient. However, the diagnosis and management follow standard surgical guidelines with the proviso that early surgical intervention is usually the preferred option.

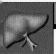

FURTHER READING

The following articles describe in detail the diagnosis and management of many of the complications discussed in this chapter. The article titles are self-explanatory.

Dodd GD, Memel DS, Zajko AB, Baron RL, Santaguida LA. Hepatic artery stenosis and thrombosis in transplant recipients: Doppler diagnosis with resistive index and systolic acceleration time. Radiology. 1994;192:657–62.

Gordon RD, van Thiel DH, Starzl TE. Liver transplantation. In: Schiff L, Schiff E, eds. Diseases of the liver, vol 2. Philadelphia: JP Lippincott; 1993;1210–35.

Greif F, Bronsther OL, Van-Thiel DH, et al. The incidence, timing, and management of biliary tract complications after orthotopic liver transplantation. Ann Surg. 1994;219:40–5.

Lebeau G, Yanago K, Marsh JW, et al. Analysis of surgical complications after 397 hepatic transplantations. Surg Gynaecol Obstet. 1990; 170:317–21.

Lerut J, Tzakis AG, Bron K, et al. Complications of venous reconstruction in human orthotopic liver transplantation. Ann Surg. 1987; 205:404–414.

McDonald M, Perkins JD, Ralph D Carithers RL. Postoperative care: immediate. In: Maddrey WC, Sorrell MF (eds). Transplantation of the liver. Conneticut: Appleton and Lange; 1995:171–206.

Neuhaus P, Blumhardt G, Bechstein WO, et al. Technique and results of biliary reconstruction using side-to-side choledochocholedochostomy in 300 orthotopic liver transplants. Ann Surg. 1994;219:426–34.

Nghiem HV, Tran K, Winter TC 3rd, et al. Imaging of complications in liver transplantation. Radiographics. 1996;16:825–40.

Northover JMA, Terblanche J. The importance of the blood supply to the bile duct in human liver transplantation. Transplantation. 1978;26:67.

Orons PD, Sheng R, Zajko AB. Hepatic artery stenosis in liver transplant recipients: prevalence and cholangiographic appearence of associated biliary complications. Am J Roentgenol. 1995;165:1145–9.

Osorio RW, Freise CE, Stock PG, et al. Nonoperative management of biliary leaks after orthotopic liver transplantation. Transplantation. 1993; 5:1074–7.

Pinna AD, Smith CV, Furukawa H, Starzl TE, Fung JJ. Urgent revascularization of liver allografts after early hepatic artery thrombosis. Transplantation. 1996;62:1584–7.

Randall HB, Wachs ME, Somberg KA, et al. The use of the T-tube after orthotopic liver transplantation. Transplantation. 1996;61:258–61.

Rolles K, Dawson K, Novell R, et al. Biliary anastomosis after liver transplantation does not benefit from T-tube splintage. Transplantation. 1994;57:402–4.

Sanchez-Bueno F, Robles R, Ramirez P, et al. Hepatic artery complications after liver transplantation. Clin Transplant. 1994;8:399–404.

Shackleton CR, Goss JA, Swenson K, et al. The impact of microsurgical hepatic arterial reconstruction on the outcome of liver transplantation for congenital biliary atresia. Am J Surg. 1997;173:431–5.

Sherman S, Shaked A, Cryer HM, Goldstein LI, Busuttil RW. Endoscopic management of biliary fistulas complicating liver transplantation and other hepatobiliary operations. Ann Surg. 1993;218:167–75.

Stratta RJ, Wood RP, Langnas AN, et al. Diagnosis and treatment of biliary tract complications after orthotopic liver transplantation. Surgery. 1989;106:675–84.

Tzakis AG, Gordon RD, Shaw BW, Iwatsuki S, Starzl TE. Clinical presentation of hepatic artery thrombosis after liver transplantation in the cyclosporine era. Transplantation. 1985;40:667–71.

Valente JF, Alonso MH, Weber FL, Hanto DW. Late hepatic artery thrombosis in liver allograft recipients is associated with intrahepatic biliary necrosis. Transplantation. 1996;61:61–5.

Zajko AB, Claus D, Clapuyt P, et al. Obstruction to hepatic venous drainage after liver transplantation: treatment with balloon angioplasty. Radiology. 1989;170:763–5.

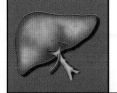

Section 4 Liver Transplantation

Chapter 39 Graft Dysfunction

Federico G Villamil and Fernanda G Zingale

INTRODUCTION

Orthotopic liver transplantation (OLT) is the most effective therapy for adults and children with severe acute or chronic hepatic failure. Following this formidable operation the majority of patients are able to return to a productive life and resume pretransplant activities. However, the price of the new life offered by transplantation is the morbidity and mortality associated with graft dysfunction or unwanted side effects of immunosuppression. The spectrum of graft dysfunction after OLT is quite varied. Technical complications, preservation injury, rejection, infectious complications, drug-induced hepatotoxicity or recurrence of the native disease are the most common causes of allograft dysfunction (Fig. 39.1). Virtually all liver allografts are injured after OLT and most patients develop at least one significant postoperative complication. Fortunately, accurate diagnosis and prompt institution of therapy, coupled with the ability of the liver to recover from injury, results in long-term survival for both allografts and patients in most instances. The purpose of this chapter is to provide an overview of the assessment and differential diagnosis of early and late causes of graft dysfunction after OLT. The reader is referred to other chapters of this book for a more detailed analysis of specific postoperative complications in transplant recipients (see Chapters 36–38).

GENERAL CONSIDERATIONS

Assessment of early graft function

Fortunately, most liver allografts function well from the beginning. The earliest parameters of successful engraftment are appreciated by the transplant surgeon during the operation. Intraoperative evidence of adequate graft function includes the production of bile after the liver is reperfused, improvement in coagulopathy allowing satisfactory hemostasis and completion of the operation and adequate rewarming with increase in body temperature after closure of the wound. Following a successful OLT, the patient should be fully awake shortly after arrival in the intensive care unit (ICU) due to the rapid clearance of the anesthetic agents by the newly implanted liver. The quality and quantity of bile output in patients with a T-tube or transjejunal biliary catheter is a good barometer of the excretory function of the allograft. Drainage of more than 100mL/day of a viscous, dark golden-brown bile is an encouraging sign. Serum lactate and prothrombin time (PT) are the most valuable biochemical parameters of early graft function; PT is measured two or three times/day during the first few days following OLT. Peak PT should ideally be less than 20 seconds, but it is the progressive improvement in coagulopathy rather than the absolute value that indicates adequate early function of the new liver. Serum

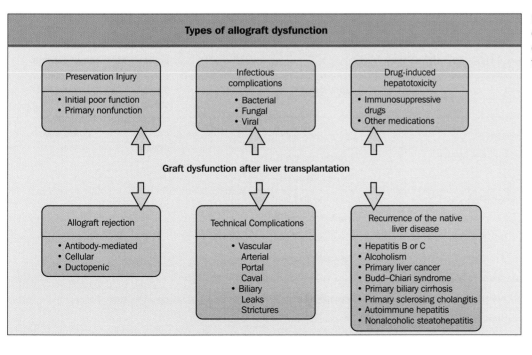

Figure 39.1 Types of allograft dysfunction. Spectrum of graft dysfunction following liver transplantation.

lactate levels usually normalize within 12 hours of OLT in patients with good allograft function. Serum aminotransferases, asparate aminotransferase (AST) and alanine aminotransferase (ALT), are considered indirect markers of the severity of preservation injury. In transplant recipients with good early function, AST peaks at less than 2000IU/L and decreases rapidly over the subsequent hours or days in parallel with the improvement in coagulopathy. Hyperbilirubinemia during the first postoperative days is usually not indicative of graft dysfunction. This early increase in serum bilirubin is mostly due to resorption of hematomas or blood accumulated in the abdomen and hemolysis of transfused erythrocytes. Canalicular enzymes, alkaline phosphatase and γ-glutamyl transferase (γ–GT), remain in the normal range during the first postoperative days and are of no value for the differential diagnosis of early graft dysfunction. Adequate function of the newly implanted liver is usually evident within 24–72 hours after OLT, at which time most patients are discharged from the ICU.

Monitoring and diagnostic work-up of graft dysfunction

Following early successful engraftment, a variety of insults can damage the allograft. Host–graft interactions are quite variable from patient to patient and are mostly unpredictable. While some patients are never hospitalized following discharge from the initial transplant admission, others develop almost the whole spectrum of graft dysfunction, require multiple hospitalizations, and are at higher risk of long-term liver damage. The differential diagnosis of graft dysfunction after OLT is a major medical challenge, even for physicians with experience in the postoperative management of transplant recipients. The key for success is a high index of suspicion, prompt investigation of any abnormality, and early institution of effective therapy. Ideally, transplant physicians should anticipate the occurrence of certain complications to minimize morbidity and mortality after OLT. A higher risk for complications such as poor initial function, sepsis, cytomegalovirus (CMV) or Epstein–Barr (EBV) infection, technical problems, and recurrent or acquired viral

hepatitis can be predicted based on the analysis of donor and recipient variables (Fig. 39.2).

As an example, patients transplanted for hepatitis C virus (HCV) infection usually develop recurrent infection and hepatitis following OLT. When elevated aminotransferases are found after the first postoperative month in such patients, recurrent HCV infection should be placed high in the list of the differential diagnoses, and unless liver biopsy shows typical features of rejection, intensified immunosuppression should be avoided. Similarly, increased post-OLT radiologic surveillance is required in small children who are at increased risk of developing hepatic artery thrombosis (HAT) or bile leaks from the cut edge of reduced-size grafts. These technical complications should be diagnosed ideally in the early postoperative period when they are most easily corrected. In addition, anticipating certain complications allows effective therapeutic interventions. Examples of this are ganciclovir prophylaxis for CMV-seronegative recipients transplanted with CMV-seropositive donor organs or administration of hepatitis B hyperimmune globulin (HBIg) and/or lamivudine when hepatitis B core antibody (anti-HBc)-positive donors are utilized.

The differential diagnosis of graft dysfunction mostly relies on the combination of clinical parameters, serum biochemical tests, noninvasive and invasive radiologic procedures, and liver biopsy.

Clinical parameters

Patients may manifest a variety of clinical symptoms following OLT. It should be noted that clinical parameters lack sensitivity and specificity and are thus more important in providing a signal to alert the physician, rather than being a valuable tool for the diagnosis of a specific type of allograft dysfunction. Fever, malaise, increasing jaundice, and failure to thrive are frequent findings in patients with rejection, infection with opportunistic organisms, or biliary obstruction–processes that differ markedly in their pathophysiology and therapy. Similarly, increased ascites and a large and tender liver can be found both in rejection and poor initial graft function. A large proportion of OLT

Expected postoperative complications		
Donor	**Recipient**	**Expected complication**
CMV seropositive	CMV seronegative	CMV infection and disease
EBV seropositive	EBV seronegative	EBV infection and PTLD
Anti-HBc (+)	HBsAg (–) and Anti-HBc (–)	Acquired hepatitis B
Anti-HCV (+)	Anti-HCV (–)	Acquired hepatitis C
Steatosis or old age	High medical status	Initial poor graft function
Blood type A	Blood type B (incompatible)	Accelerated rejection
Living-related	–	Biliary complications
	Small child (<10kg)	Vascular thrombosis
	Intubated and comatose cirrhotic	Bacterial and fungal sepsis
	HBsAg or anti-HCV (+)	Recurrent infection and hepatitis
	Primary sclerosing cholangitis	Intrahepatic biliary strictures, ductopenic rejection

Figure 39.2 Expected postoperative complications. Donor and recipient variables that may predict the occurrence of specific postoperative complications. PTLD: post-transplant lymphoproliferative disease

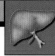

recipients with graft dysfunction, particularly beyond 3 months of transplantation, remain completely asymptomatic. Thus, clinical parameters are neither sensitive nor specific.

Serum biochemical tests

Liver tests including total and conjugated bilirubin, alkaline phosphatase, γ–GT, AST, and ALT are obtained daily until hospital discharge, usually from 2 to 4 weeks after OLT. Once normalized, it is unnecessary to repeat PT at frequent intervals except during episodes of allograft injury that may compromise liver synthetic function. Following discharge, clinic visits and laboratory tests are scheduled biweekly or weekly for 3 months, monthly for 6 months, and at 3–6 month intervals thereafter in most transplant centers. As mentioned earlier, host–graft interactions and the incidence and severity of postoperative complications are quite variable among transplant recipients. Consequently, outpatient consultations and biochemical monitoring of graft function can be spaced further apart in stable OLT recipients with no significant clinical problems and rapid normalization of liver tests. After a successful transplant operation, serum bilirubin and liver enzymes decrease progressively over the following days and often reach the normal range within 3 weeks. Rise in serum bilirubin, aminotransferases, or alkaline phosphatase after the initial postoperative decline is usually indicative of some type of allograft injury (Fig. 39.3).

Liver tests are sensitive markers of graft dysfunction but have a relative inability to discriminate effectively between the different types of injury. However, any unexplained elevation in liver function tests in transplant recipients deserves attention. Neither the degree of biochemical abnormalities nor the pattern of enzyme elevation are specific for any given cause of graft dysfunction. During the first postoperative weeks, common causes of graft dysfunction such as rejection, infection, or biliary com-

plications should be suspected in patients with isolated increase in bilirubin, ALT, or alkaline phosphatase, or more commonly when a mixed hepatocellular/cholestatic pattern of enzyme elevation is present, with or without hyperbilirubinemia. Liver tests are relatively more specific in the long-term follow-up of transplant recipients. In this scenario, a predominantly cholestatic pattern of enzyme elevation is suggestive of biliary complications or ductopenic rejection, whereas an isolated increase in aminotransferases is more frequently encountered among patients with hepatocellular causes of graft dysfunction such as recurrent or acquired viral hepatitis. Poor correlation exists between the degree of biochemical abnormalities and the severity of histologic findings. Significantly elevated liver tests are often found in patients with mild histologic disease and vice versa. In addition, persistently normal bilirubin and liver enzymes are found in many asymptomatic patients with biopsy-proven graft dysfunction. Clinical and biochemical parameters are important to alert the physician that something is going wrong and to establish the need for additional studies to identify the specific cause of graft dysfunction (see Fig. 39.3). Therapeutic decisions based on clinical suspicions alone are not to be recommended. Wrong decisions such as administering supplemental immunosuppression to patients with infection, or withholding immunosuppression in patients with significant rejection, may jeopardize the graft.

Noninvasive radiologic procedures

Ultrasonography (US) with Doppler examination is the most utilized noninvasive imaging study following OLT due to its accuracy, low cost, and availability at the bedside if necessary. Doppler-US is routinely performed at different intervals following OLT to assess the hepatic parenchyma, abdominal cavity, biliary tree, and status of vascular anastomoses. In our transplant center, the site of entry for percutaneous liver biopsy is selected by US and the procedure is subsequently performed at the bedside. Bilomas, liver abscesses or infarcted tissue appear on US as areas of heterogeneous liver parenchyma. The presence of periportal fluid or edema, better assessed by CT than by US, is considered an indirect radiologic sign of allograft rejection. Ultrasonography has good sensitivity for the detection of abdominal fluid collections, which are commonly present during the first weeks post-OLT. However, it is not always helpful in differentiating loculated ascites from other types of fluids such as blood, bile, or pus. The demonstration of bile duct dilatation on US is almost diagnostic of biliary obstruction and should be further characterized by cholangiography in most cases. Unfortunately, US is an insensitive method to diagnose biliary complications in many transplant recipients, particularly in the early postoperative period. Normal studies are found in as many as 50% of patients with partial or complete biliary obstruction on cholangiography.

Doppler-US is an effective method to evaluate the patency of the arterial, portal, and caval vascular anastomoses. In most centers, a bedside study is performed in the ICU within the first postoperative day to detect technical problems that may require surgical revision. Subsequently, Doppler-US is used whenever graft dysfunction is suspected. In a normal study, nonturbulent flow should be detected below and above the vascular anastomoses and in both the right and left intrahepatic branches of the hepatic artery and portal vein.

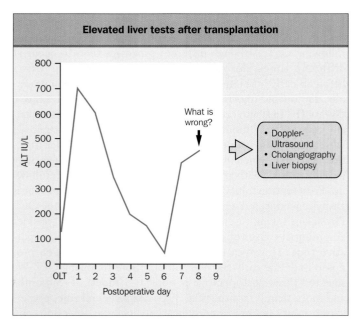

Figure 39.3 Elevated liver tests after transplantation. Requirement of specific studies following the biochemical diagnosis of graft dysfunction.

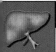
Accuracy of Doppler-US to detect vascular thrombosis or stenosis after OLT is around 90%. A confirmatory angiogram is necessary when arterial or portal bloodflow is not demonstrated by Doppler-US and whenever hepatic artery thrombosis (HAT) or portal vein thrombosis (PVT) are suspected but not confirmed by Doppler examination. Normal Doppler-US following OLT is clinically relevant because it indicates in most cases a nonvascular cause of graft dysfunction. Technetium-99m hepatoiminodiacetic acid (HIDA) scan is utilized in some centers as a screening test for bile leaks or biliary obstruction in patients without indwelling biliary catheters or after removal of the T-tube.

Direct cholangiography is the gold standard for the diagnosis of biliary complications following OLT. Indwelling biliary catheters, a T-tube in patients with duct-to-duct anastomosis, or a transjejunal catheter in those with a Roux-en-Y choledocojejunostomy provide easy access for visualization of the biliary system. In addition, a normal cholangiogram by the end of the first postoperative week allows clamping of the T-tube. Cholangiography is repeated during episodes of graft dysfunction and around 3 months after OLT before removal of the T-tube.

Invasive radiologic procedures

Percutaneous transhepatic cholangiography or endoscopic retrograde cholangiography are indicated whenever biliary complications are suspected in transplant recipients without indwelling biliary catheters. The most appropriate cholangiographic technique is selected according to the type of biliary anastomosis performed and the location of the presumed complication. The percutaneous route is preferred in patients with a Roux-en-Y choledocojejunostomy, or biliary lesions located at or above the confluence of the right and left ducts. Conversely, the endoscopic route is indicated for more distal lesions located at the anastomosis or below.

Liver biopsy

Liver biopsy is the single most useful test for the differential diagnosis of graft dysfunction. Results of liver biopsy are available on the day following the procedure for patients with mild clinical injury or those studied during long-term follow-up. However, when significant graft dysfunction is suspected and histologic results are needed with special urgency, biopsies are processed by a rapid technique with a turnaround time of 4–6 hours. Most liver biopsies are performed percutaneously. The transjugular technique is reserved for patients with contraindications for percutaneous biopsy such as severe coagulopathy or massive ascites. Another safe approach in these cases is to open a small window in the abdominal wound that provides good exposure of the graft surface and the possibility of performing direct hemostasis after the biopsy. Most causes of graft dysfunction are identifiable by routine light microscopy with hematoxylin and eosin stained specimens. Trichrome, iron, and diastase-periodic acid–Schiff stains are helpful in some cases. Immunohistochemistry studies of liver tissue are of great value to confirm some specific causes of allograft injury such as hyperacute rejection or viral infections. Liver biopsy is routinely performed whenever graft dysfunction is suspected. In addition, protocol biopsies are obtained in some transplant centers at fixed intervals following OLT. The usefulness of protocol biopsies during the first postoperative weeks is controversial.

Histologic features of cellular rejection are often found in protocol biopsies obtained from patients with normal or improving liver tests. It is unclear whether these findings are clinically relevant and whether supplemental immunosuppression should be used. On the one hand, treatment of rejection with isolated histologic expression may potentially prevent more serious injury that will become manifest on subsequent days as clinical or biochemical abnormalities. On the other hand, it has been demonstrated that most rejection episodes found on protocol biopsies resolve spontaneously. Moreover, experimental OLT in certain strains of rats that develop tolerance without immunosuppression has shown that most animals suffer a self-limited and reversible episode of rejection. This suggests that some degree of host–graft immune interaction appears necessary for achievement of successful engraftment. Protocol biopsies performed at yearly intervals in the long-term follow-up are much less controversial. As an example, most cases of recurrence of primary biliary cirrhosis (PBC) following OLT have been diagnosed on protocol biopsies obtained in asymptomatic patients with normal liver tests. Liver biopsy interpretation in OLT recipients is much more difficult than in nontransplant patients because more than one process may affect the allograft simultaneously. Examples of this are the frequent coexistence of rejection with preservation injury, biliary complications, CMV infection, or viral hepatitis. The major challenges for the pathologist and transplant physician are not only to identify the causes of graft dysfunction, but also to place them in order of clinical relevance to select the best treatment strategy. Follow-up biopsies are recommended after a specific therapeutic intervention to see 'what is left'. Not infrequently, histologic abnormalities found in transplant recipients do not fulfill diagnostic criteria for any specific cause of graft dysfunction. As a general rule, when doubts exist, it is preferable to do nothing. A simplified algorithm for the differential diagnosis of graft dysfunction after OLT is shown in Fig. 39.4.

Classification of graft dysfunction

From a teaching perspective, the best approach to classify graft dysfunction is according to the time of onset of complications following OLT. Although different processes tend to occur at different times during follow-up, marked overlap exists between early and late causes of graft dysfunction. For example, ductopenic rejection, post-transplant lymphoproliferative disease (PTLD) and recurrent hepatitis C, conditions that usually occur several months following OLT, have been diagnosed within the first postoperative weeks. Conversely, cellular rejection and HAT, which in most cases are early complications, may initially present with graft dysfunction during long-term follow-up. Preservation injury is perhaps the only complication that is always encountered within the same time frame following OLT. Physicians taking care of transplant recipients should consider all potential causes of graft dysfunction at any given postoperative time. However, different time intervals have been proposed to define early and late complications following OLT. We selected three postoperative periods: 0–1 month, 1–3 months and more than 3 months (Fig. 39.5). As a general rule, preservation injury, technical complications, cellular rejection, and viral infections are encountered mainly within the first 3 postoperative months, whereas the prevalence of ductopenic rejection, biliary strictures, and recurrent disease increase in the

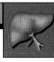

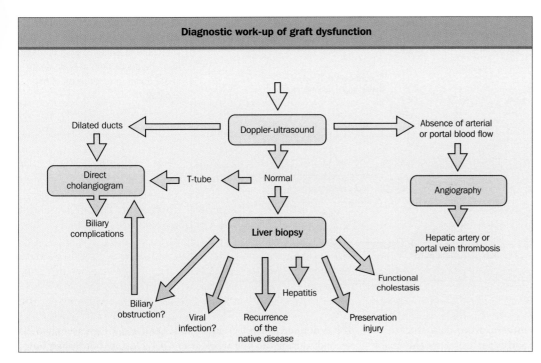

Diagnostic work-up of graft dysfunction

Figure 39.4 Diagnostic work-up of graft dysfunction. Simplified algorithm for the differential diagnosis of graft dysfunction in transplant recipients.

long term. Good clinical judgment and knowledge of the most frequent time of onset of each postoperative complication are essential to select the most appropriate diagnostic strategy for the individual case.

SPECIFIC TYPES OF GRAFT DYSFUNCTION

Preservation injury and primary graft dysfunction

Some degree of ischemic damage occurs in all liver allografts as reflected by the postoperative increase in aminotransferases and PT. The term preservation injury or harvesting injury is commonly used to describe the additive effects of several sequential steps in which the donor organ is damaged after being exposed to periods of cold and warm ischemia followed by reperfusion (Fig. 39.6). The spectrum of preservation injury is quite varied and ranges from mild and rapidly reversible clinical and histologic abnormalities to primary nonfunction (PNF), a life-threatening complication leading to death or emergency retransplantation. Ischemic damage resulting from donor events *in situ* and during the harvesting operation is called prepreservation injury. Pre-existing donor diseases such as alcoholic or nonalcoholic steatosis or drug-induced hepatotoxicity can render the liver more susceptible to the deleterious effects of cold and warm ischemia. In addition, endocrine abnormalities described in brain-dead donors, such as the euthyroid sick syndrome, and altered mitochondrial function and contribute to liver damage. Episodes of hypotension or hypoxia occurring after the declaration of brain death or during surgical removal of the donor organ may also result in graft injury due to the unwanted effects of warm ischemia. Following organ retrieval, cold preservation of the

Early and late causes of graft dysfunction		
First postoperative month	1–3 postoperative months	Late follow-up
Primary nonfunction	Cellular rejection	Ductopenic rejection
Preservation injury	Biliary complications	Biliary complications
Antibody-mediated rejection	CMV infection	Recurrent hepatitis B or C
Hepatic artery thrombosis	EBV infection	Acquired hepatitis B or C
Bacterial or fungal infection	Recurrent hepatitis B or C	EBV infection
Functional cholestasis	Adenovirus hepatitis	Lymphoproliferative disease
Biliary complications		Drug-induced hepatotoxicity
Cellular rejection		Recurrence of the native disease
HSV or VZV hepatitis		

Figure 39.5 Early and late causes of graft dysfunction. Expected types of graft dysfunction at different time periods after liver transplantation.

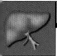

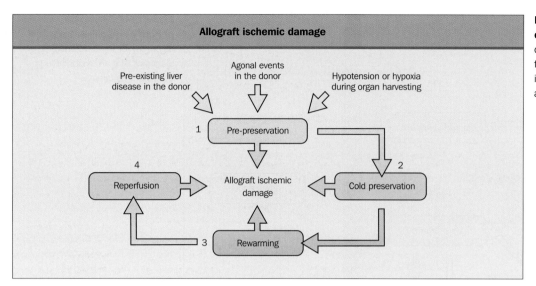

Figure 39.6 Allograft ischemic damage. Sequential steps that may contribute to ischemic graft damage from the declaration of brain death in the donor to reperfusion of the allograft.

graft, and rewarming during the interval from cold storage to resumption of hepatic circulation and reperfusion are the major events leading to ischemic allograft injury.

Pathogenesis of preservation injury

The pathogenesis of preservation injury is multifactorial. The mechanisms of liver damage during cold preservation and following reperfusion have been extensively studied. Stored ATP is rapidly consumed during cold anoxia. Cellular energy needs in this setting are obtained through anaerobic glycolysis and glycogenolysis. The main consequences of these metabolic changes are intracellular acidosis, which can produce cell damage, and accumulation of xanthine oxidase, a precursor of reactive oxygen intermediates, triggering rapid oxidative stress following reperfusion. Cooling the organ results also in inhibition of the enzyme sodium/potassium-ATPase with increased intracellular sodium concentration and cell swelling. The earliest morphologic abnormality during cold ischemia is damage to endothelial cells. Increased body temperature during the rewarming phase is associated with a parallel increase in the metabolic rate with activation of proteases that contribute to graft injury. The major mechanisms of reperfusion-induced ischemic damage are loss of viability of sinusoidal endothelial cells and Kupffer cell activation. Denudation of the sinusoidal cell lining triggers leukocyte and platelet adhesion resulting in a profound disruption of the liver microcirculation with intravascular coagulation and ischemic hepatocyte necrosis. Activated Kupffer cells generate a variety of proinflammatory mediators such as cytokines, eicosanoids, and reactive oxygen intermediates, which aggravate hepatic damage and mediate multiorgan failure. The extent of reperfusion injury is directly related to the duration of cold storage. Thus, to minimize the risk of severe preservation injury, cold and warm ischemic times should be kept as short as possible. In children undergoing living-related OLT, where cold ischemia time is minimal, PNF is extremely rare.

Primary graft dysfunction

Severe preservation injury leading to graft failure is called primary graft dysfunction, a syndrome with two similar but distinct variants: initial poor function (IPF) and PNF. In most reported series,

IPF is defined as AST greater than 2000, and PT greater than 20 seconds during the first week after OLT. Despite borderline function, grafts with IPF are able to support life, although some patients will require retransplantation at a later time. PNF is defined as death or need for emergency retransplantation within 2 weeks of OLT in patients with IPF. In addition to coagulopathy and marked increase in aminotransferases, patients with PNF usually display other clinical features of severe liver failure such as persistence of encephalopathy or slowed awakening, absence of bile flow or production of watery bile, hypoglycemia, lactic acidosis, hyperkalemia, and renal impairment. PNF is evident on the first postoperative day in the majority of patients, but can occur several days after a period of adequate initial function. The incidences of IPF and PNF is approximately 15 and 5–10%, respectively. The major challenge for the transplant physician is to differentiate, as early as possible, reversible from irreversible primary graft dysfunction. An optimal decision has to be made rapidly because delay in emergency retransplantation may result in the death of the patient. PNF is the principal indication for retransplantation during the first 2 weeks after OLT.

Histologic findings

Perivenular hepatocyte ballooning or hemorrhagic necrosis are the main histologic features of preservation injury (Fig. 39.7). Submassive or massive coagulative necrosis is often found in the explanted livers of patients with PNF undergoing retransplantation. Portal tracts are usually unremarkable. Ductular proliferation and cholangiolitis, simulating biliary obstruction, are frequently observed in cases with severe ischemic necrosis. Complete histologic recovery is the usual outcome of preservation injury. However, follow-up biopsies may show portal or perivenular fibrosis in patients who recovered from severe ischemic damage.

Risk factors for poor graft function

The profound alteration of the liver microcirculation after cold storage and reperfusion may render the allograft more vulnerable to vascular thrombosis and biliary complications. Several relative risk factors for IPF and PNF have been identified. Donor-related factors are age greater than 50 years, moderate or

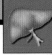

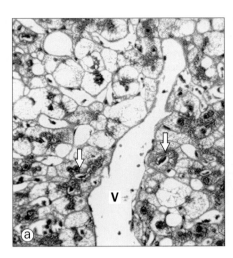

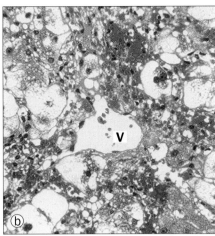

Figure 39.7 Preservation injury. Perivenular (V) area with (a) ballooning of hepatocytes and canalicular cholestasis (arrows) and (b) congestion and hemorrhagic necrosis.

severe steatosis, and cold preservation times greater than 12 hours. Warm ischemia time greater than 1 hour is the major perioperative risk factor. Among the recipient's factors, pre-OLT medical status and retransplantation are the ones with a proven relationship to outcome. A combination of risk factors should be avoided. As an example, transplantation of old or steatotic donor livers into medically unstable recipients significantly increases the risk of IPF and PNF. Protocol donor biopsies obtained after cold storage and 1 or 2 hours following reperfusion have been utilized to predict the severity of preservation injury following OLT. Most 'back table' biopsies are normal or show minimal histologic abnormalities such as liver cell swelling. However, zonal coagulative necrosis encountered in biopsy specimens obtained after reperfusion is a good predictor of significant preservation injury following OLT. Despite the availability of better preservation solutions and the continuous search for more accurate risk factors, PNF is still unpredictable in most cases. Other causes of early graft failure such as HAT, PVT, antibody-mediated rejection, and accelerated cellular rejection are the main differential diagnoses of PNF.

Functional cholestasis

The term 'functional cholestasis' is used to describe the occurrence of progressive jaundice in the early post-OLT period in the absence of biliary obstruction, rejection, and viral hepatitis. Patients with this complication develop a gradual increase in serum bilirubin with normal or mildly elevated hepatocellular and canalicular enzymes. Histologic examination reveals prominent cellular and canalicular cholestasis with feathery degeneration and absence of significant portal or lobular inflammation. Functional cholestasis is a benign and reversible condition of unknown cause for which there is no specific therapy.

Vascular thrombosis

Thrombosis or stenosis of the hepatic artery, portal vein, or inferior vena cava may occur at any time after OLT, but are more commonly encountered during the early postoperative period.

Hepatic artery thrombosis

The incidence of HAT is approximately 5% in adults and 10% in children. Small pediatric recipients are at higher risk of developing technical complications of the arterial reconstruction due to the small diameter, frequently less than 3mm, of the donor and recip-

ient vessels. The impact of HAT on the allograft depends on the ability of the parenchyma and biliary system to survive on portal flow alone. Liver cells have a dual blood supply from the hepatic artery and portal vein. Some transplant recipients who have sufficient portal bloodflow or rearterialization from collaterals can tolerate HAT without significant parenchymal changes. Bile ducts are devoid of portal blood supply and are thus entirely dependent on arterial flow from branches of the gastroduodenal and retroportal arteries that are divided in the transplant operation. Thrombosis of the hepatic artery often results in bile duct necrosis. Ischemic injury occurs mostly in donor bile ducts that are largely dependent on bloodflow supplied by the arterial anastomosis. Reduced hepatic bloodflow in preservation injury or rejection arteriopathy may compromise the arterial supply of the peribiliary arteriolar plexus and result in ischemic bile duct injury. The clinical presentation of HAT is variable. Early thrombosis in grafts that are unable to survive on portal bloodflow alone results in infarction of the liver parenchyma and acute liver failure requiring prompt retransplantation. In less dramatic cases, HAT produces bile duct necrosis of the extrahepatic or intrahepatic biliary tree expressed as anastomotic leaks or parenchymal bilomas, respectively. Emergency surgical revascularization procedures may save the graft, but in most cases retransplantation is required. Patients who tolerate early HAT with no major sequelae usually have a more insidious clinical presentation with late development of multiple intrahepatic biliary strictures. It should be noted that HAT is discovered incidentally in some children and a few adults who are completely asymptomatic with normal graft function and no biliary complications.

Hepatic artery stenosis

Hepatic artery stenosis is less frequent than thrombosis and usually occurs at the anastomotic site or within arterial grafts utilized for vascular reconstruction (Fig. 39.8). Doppler-US is the screening test of choice for HAT or stenosis. Angiography is necessary when no arterial flow signal or persistent turbulent flow is found on Doppler examination and in patients with clinical suspicion of HAT or stenosis not confirmed by noninvasive techniques.

Portal vein thrombosis

Portal vein thrombosis (PVT) occurs in 1–2% of OLT recipients. Prior splenectomy or portosystemic shunts, preoperative PVT, hypercoagulable states, and OLT in small children with reduced or living-related grafts and marked size differences between the

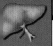

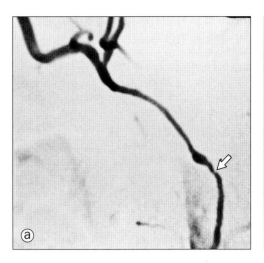

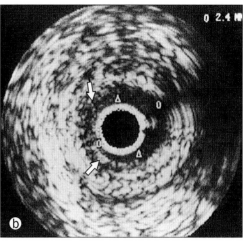

Figure 39.8 Hepatic artery stenosis.
(a) Angiogram showing stenosis (arrow) and beading of an iliac homograft utilized for arterial reconstruction. (b) Intravascular ultrasound with abnormal soft tissue within the lumen of the arterial graft (arrows).

donor and recipient portal veins are considered risk factors for this vascular complication. Early and complete PVT can be a catastrophic event with rapid onset of acute liver failure, shock, and massive ascites. Emergency portal vein thrombectomy with successful restoration of portal bloodflow may salvage the graft, but many patients will still require retransplantation. Patients with late PVT or stenosis, occurring months or years following OLT, usually present with variceal hemorrhage or ascites due to reappearance of portal hypertension. Absence of portal bloodflow on Doppler-US requires angiographic confirmation of PVT. When turbulent flow is demonstrated on Doppler examination, portal vein stenosis should be suspected. Balloon dilatation may restore normal portal circulation in some cases. Gradual development of portal hypertension triggers the formation of hepatopetal venous collaterals appearing as a cavernous transformation of the portal vein on Doppler-US.

Vena caval thrombosis

Thrombosis of the caval anastomosis following OLT is a rare but severe vascular complication. Complete outflow obstruction results in marked liver congestion with graft enlargement, ascites, and hepatic failure requiring prompt retransplantation. Balloon dilatation is effective in some patients with partial or less severe thrombosis or stenosis of the inferior vena cava.

Biliary complications

Some type of biliary complication occurs in as many as a third of transplant recipients at variable times following surgery. Bile duct obstruction or leaks are due to a technically imperfect anastomosis or bile duct ischemia resulting from HAT, ductopenic rejection, donor cold ischemia times greater than 12 hours, or utilization of ABO incompatible donors.

Bile leaks

The majority of bile leaks occur in the early postoperative period from ischemic dehiscence of the anastomosis. Patients usually present with variable degrees of abdominal pain, jaundice, fever, and leukocytosis according to the severity of bile peritonitis. The presence of bile in the suction drains, particularly when bilirubin levels are higher in the drains than in the serum, is almost diagnostic of a bile leak. Detection of abdominal fluid collections on US in association with clinical features that are suggestive of bil-

iary complications establish the need to obtain a prompt direct cholangiogram in order to define the severity and location of the bile leak. A HIDA scan is useful as a screening test for leaks in patients without indwelling biliary catheters and to select the most appropriate cholangiographic procedure. Most early leaks require surgery for either revision of the anastomosis or conversion of an end-to-end to a Roux-en-Y anastomosis. Conversely, the majority of bile leaks that occur after removal of the T-tube are treated nonoperatively.

Biliary obstruction

Strictures are the most common cause of biliary obstruction following OLT and may be located anywhere in the biliary tree from intrahepatic ducts to the sphincter of Oddi. Anastomotic strictures usually occur within the first 2 postoperative months, result from technical failure or ischemia, and are more frequent in patients with a duct-to-duct biliary reconstruction. Nonanastomotic strictures are strongly associated with the duration of cold ischemia, affect the hilar or intrahepatic ducts, and in the majority of cases are diagnosed >2 months following OLT, when late HAT or ductopenic rejection are likely to occur. Sludge or stone formation increase further the degree of obstruction in patients with bile duct strictures. In severe cases, large intrabiliary casts are removed at the time of reoperation (Fig. 39.9). OLT recipients with biliary obstruction can present in a variety of ways. Increasing jaundice, abdominal pain, and fever from bacterial cholangitis are frequently found in patients with severe obstruction. When obstruction is incomplete, an asymptomatic rise in liver enzymes with a predominant cholestatic pattern is the most common presentation. Histologic abnormalities suggestive of biliary complications are the first clue to the diagnosis in some cases. Ultrasonography may show ductal dilatation, particularly in patients with long-standing biliary obstruction. However, US is not sufficiently reliable in OLT recipients, and a normal study does not exclude biliary obstruction. Although HIDA scan can help in ruling out obstruction, most patients require direct cholangiography to assess the type, severity, number, and location of biliary strictures. Liver biopsy is often unremarkable in early bile duct obstruction. As time elapses, variable degrees of portal edema, ductular proliferation, and centrilobular cholestasis may appear, allowing the pathologist to suggest the diagnosis of biliary obstruction and assist the transplant physician in the selection of

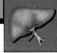

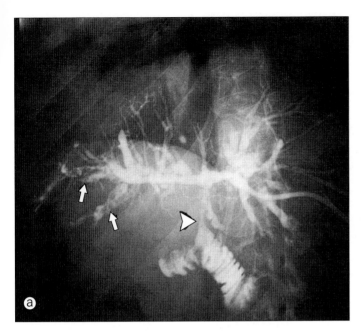

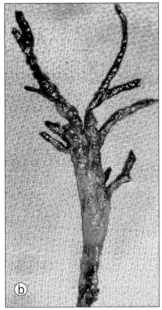

Figure 39.9 Biliary obstruction.
(a) Percutaneous cholangiogram with narrowing of the common hepatic duct above the anastomosis (arrowhead) and diffuse intrahepatic strictures with luminal filling defects (arrows). (b) Large biliary cast extracted from the biliary tree at the time of reoperation.

other diagnostic procedures. Most bile duct strictures are initially treated with transhepatic or endoscopic balloon dilatation or stenting. Surgical procedures are reserved for endoscopic or interventional radiologic treatment failures.

Allograft rejection

Classically, allograft rejection has been classified in hyperacute, acute, and chronic forms according to the time of onset following OLT. However, hyperacute rejection may manifest in the second postoperative week, acute (cellular) rejection may occur at any time during follow-up, and chronic rejection has been recognized after a few weeks following OLT. The terms antibody-mediated, cellular, and ductopenic rejection have been proposed to replace hyperacute, acute, and chronic rejection, respectively.

Antibody-mediated rejection

Antibody-mediated or humoral rejection is extremely uncommon in OLT recipients. Binding of preformed antibodies to donor antigens expressed on the vascular endothelium results in diffuse small vessel thrombosis, widespread hemorrhagic necrosis, and rapid graft failure requiring emergency retransplantation. The majority of cases are found when OLT is performed across the ABO blood group barrier. Deposition of immunoglobulins and complement along the sinusoids, veins, and arteries, as assessed by immunohistochemistry, helps to differentiate antibody-mediated rejection from PNF or other causes of severe ischemic graft injury.

Cellular rejection

Cellular rejection is the most common early complication after OLT and occurs in around 50–80% of patients. The vast majority of rejection episodes are diagnosed between 6 days and 8 weeks after surgery. The incidence of early cellular rejection is lower when polyclonal or monoclonal antilymphocyte preparations are used as initial immunosuppression, but these patients are at risk of developing delayed rebound rejection. Late cellular rejection is associated in most cases with a state of underimmunosuppression due to either noncompliance, intercurrent illnesses, or administration of drugs that decrease blood levels of cyclosporine. Patients

with cellular rejection may be asymptomatic or present with a variety of symptoms and signs such as unexplained fever, malaise, increasing ascites, graft tenderness, or changes in the quantity and quality of the bile output. Increased serum bilirubin or liver enzymes are found in the majority of patients with rejection. However, neither the absolute level nor the pattern of enzyme elevation is specific for this condition. Imaging studies are more helpful to exclude other causes of graft dysfunction than to suggest or confirm the occurrence of rejection.

Liver biopsy is the gold standard for the diagnosis of rejection and provides an objective assessment of the interaction of the host immune response with donor antigens predominantly displayed on the bile duct epithelial cells and vascular endothelium. The histologic hallmarks of cellular rejection are portal inflammation, bile duct damage, and endotheliitis or phlebitis (Fig. 39.10). Portal inflammation is characteristically polymorphous with large activated or blastic lymphocytes, small lymphocytes, macrophages, neutrophils, plasma cells, and eosinophils (see Fig. 39.10a). The limiting plate is usually preserved, although in severe cases periportal inflammation is frequently observed. The mixed nature of the portal infiltrates is helpful to distinguish rejection from recurrent or acquired viral hepatitis. Portal edema and ductular proliferation are histologic features of rejection that mimic biliary obstruction. Nonsuppurative cholangitis, also called rejection cholangitis or lymphocytic cholangitis, is the most frequent and reliable histologic feature of cellular rejection. The epithelium of small interlobular bile ducts is infiltrated by lymphocytes or other inflammatory cells, producing degenerative changes such as cytoplasmic eosinophilia and vacuolization or nuclear pyknosis (see Fig. 39.10b). In severe cases, necrosis of epithelial cells results in bile duct loss. Endotheliitis is defined as the attachment of inflammatory cells to the endothelial surface of portal or terminal hepatic veins. The term phlebitis is used by some pathologists to describe the infiltration of the vein wall by inflammatory cells with lifting of the endothelium (see Figs. 39.10c & d). The histologic abnormalities described as phlebitis are included under the definition of endotheliitis in most series.

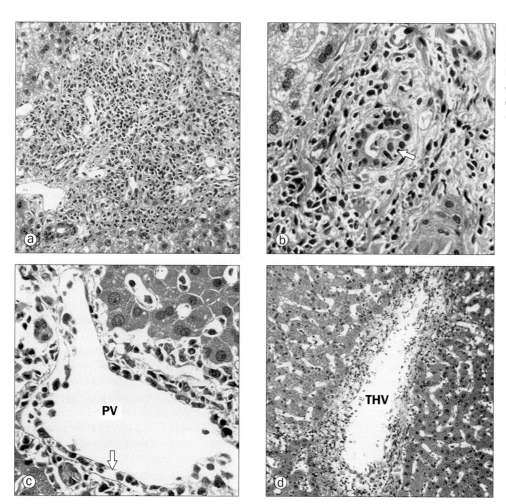

Figure 39.10 Cellular rejection. (a)
Mixed portal inflammation. (b)
Nonsuppurative cholangitis (arrows). (c)
Portal vein (PV) phlebitis with lifting of the
endothelium (arrow). (d) Severe
endotheliitis of terminal hepatic venule
(THV) with perivenular necrosis.

Both phlebitis and endotheliitis are not specific for rejection and may be observed particularly in some viral infections, both in OLT recipients and in patients who are not immunosuppressed. Cellular rejection is reversible in most circumstances. No correlation exists between the exuberance of the portal inflammatory infiltration and response to therapy or outcome. However, duct loss and centrilobular ischemic necrosis may announce the occurrence of irreversible rejection requiring retransplantation.

Ductopenic rejection
Ductopenic rejection is a major cause of late graft failure. Early ductopenic rejection, occurring weeks after OLT, usually follows episodes of cellular rejection that are unresponsive to immunosuppression. In this setting, duct loss is found in portal tracts with prominent inflammation. Ductopenic rejection diagnosed several months after OLT, also called vanishing bile duct syndrome, has a more indolent presentation with asymptomatic increase in canalicular enzymes, followed by progressive elevation of serum bilirubin and clinical jaundice. Duct loss in these cases is found in the absence of significant portal inflammation.

The histologic hallmarks of ductopenic rejection are occlusive or rejection arteriopathy and paucity or disappearance of interlobular bile ducts. Rejection arteriopathy is characterized by the subendothelial deposition of lipid-laden macrophages with narrowing of the arterial lumen. As this process affects mostly the hilar vessels, rejection arteriopathy is infrequently found in routine subcapsular liver biopsies. Ductopenia is defined as absence of interlobular bile ducts in at least 50% of portal tracts in an adequate biopsy specimen. Both direct immunologic damage and ischemia contribute to the loss of bile ducts. Severe centrilobular cholestasis, resulting from the complete loss of bile ducts and ischemic parenchymal necrosis due to arteriopathy, are late histologic features of ductopenic rejection associated with a poor prognosis. Conversion of cyclosporine-based immunosuppression to tacrolimus may rescue the graft, but many patients will still require retransplantation. To be effective, medical or surgical therapy should be considered early in the course of ductopenic rejection. Recurrence of vanishing bile duct syndrome following retransplantation is frequent, particularly in patients undergoing OLT for primary sclerosing cholangitis (PSC).

Infectious complications
Infectious complications are among the leading causes of death following OLT. The majority of patients experience at least one episode of infection, particularly during the early postoperative period when immunosuppression is maximal. Infection may be present in the patient before OLT, result from the major surgical procedure itself, or be acquired from the donor.

A case of donor-transmitted tuberculosis is shown in Fig. 39.11. The patient presented 1 month after OLT with elevated liver tests and was found to have large granulomas with caseation on liver biopsy. As a general rule, bacterial infections occur early after OLT and affect mostly extrahepatic organs, whereas viral infections are found later in the follow-up and frequently involve the allograft. Pediatric recipients without exposure to childhood illnesses at the time of OLT have a high risk of primary infection with opportunistic viruses. Reactivation of endogenous latent viral infections by immunosuppression is more prevalent among adult recipients. Primary infection is usually more severe than reactivated infection. The risk of developing infectious complications significantly decreases 6 months after OLT, except for patients who require supplemental immunosuppression to treat repeated bouts of late allograft rejection. Graft dysfunction is infrequent in bacterial and fungal infections. Jaundice or subclinical increase in bilirubin levels are usually found in patients with bacterial infections and systemic signs of sepsis.

Histologic features of sepsis are cholangiolar proliferation, acute cholangiolitis, large bile plugs in dilated ductules, and variable degrees of centrilobular cholestasis. Ascending cholangitis in patients with biliary complications is the most frequent bacterial infection affecting the allograft. Necrotic liver tissue or infarction following HAT may become seeded with bacteria or fungi leading to hepatic gangrene or abscess formation.

Opportunistic viruses such as CMV, EBV, herpes simplex virus (HSV), varicella-zoster virus (VZV), and adenovirus may produce graft dysfunction at variable times following OLT (Fig. 39.12). The diagnosis of viral infections in transplant recipients mostly relies on assays to detect viremia or antigenemia and histologic examination of liver specimens with routine stains,

immunohistochemistry, or *in situ* hybridization techniques. Serologic tests are unreliable because they lack sensitivity in this patient population.

Cytomegalovirus infection

Cytomegalovirus is the most common microbial pathogen encountered in OLT recipients and causes significant morbidity. Most infections occur 4–12 weeks postoperatively. Risk factors for CMV infection and disease are transplantation of a seropositive-donor into a seronegative-recipient, intense immunosuppression, use of OKT3, and retransplantation. Antilymphocyte globulins produce reactivation of latent CMV infection, whereas cyclosporin and tacrolimus increase viral replication of previously activated virus. Clinical presentation of patients with CMV infection is variable and ranges from asymptomatic viral shedding to lethal systemic disease with multiorgan involvement. Low-grade fever, malaise, arthralgias, myalgias, leukopenia, thrombocytopenia, and elevated liver tests are frequent clinical findings. Sensitive and rapid diagnostic assays are available to detect the presence of replicating CMV in serum samples or other body fluids. The shell vial leukocyte culture technique utilizes a labeled monoclonal antibody that binds to an early viral antigen and has a turnaround time of 24–48 hours. Cytomegalovirus antigenemia is as sensitive as the shell vial culture and has the advantages of being more rapid, with results available in around 5 hours, and semiquantitative. The antigenemia assay is based on the reaction of a monoclonal antibody with a structural CMV antigen (pp65) located in the nuclei of polymorphonuclear leukocytes. The level of antigenemia correlates with the severity of infection and decreases following effective therapy. Polymerase chain reaction (PCR) for CMV DNA allows the detection of even minimal concentrations of the virus in serum or other clinical specimens. The demonstration of CMV viremia or antigenemia should strongly suggest active infection and the need for antiviral treatment. In addition, these techniques may detect replicating virus several days before the onset of clinical disease, allowing pre-emptive ther-

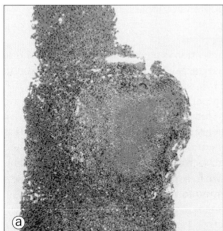

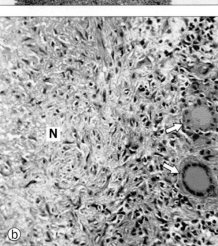

Figure 39.11 Donor transmitted tuberculosis. (a) Large hepatic granuloma with caseation. (b) Langhans giant cells (arrows) surrounding the area of central necrosis (N).

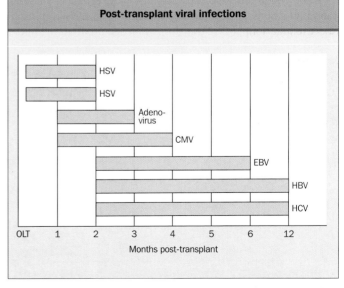

Figure 39.12 Post-transplant viral infections. Most frequent time of onset of viral infections after liver transplantation.

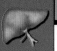
apy. The histologic diagnosis of CMV hepatitis mostly relies on the presence of characteristic inclusion bodies in hepatocytes or mesenchymal cells, surrounded by clusters of neutrophils (microabscesses) or microgranulomas (Fig. 39.13a).

Immunostaining of biopsy specimens with monoclonal antibodies to early CMV antigens or *in situ* hybridization with specific DNA probes are useful to confirm the diagnosis, especially when cytomegalic inclusion bodies are not found. Allograft rejection and CMV hepatitis often coexist (Fig. 39.13b). It should be noted that the virus itself is immunosuppressive. Reduction of the level of immunosuppression is safe, and when combined with ganciclovir therapy, results in resolution of both rejection and CMV hepatitis in most cases. Cytomegalovirus infection has been proposed as a risk factor for ductopenic rejection, but this association remains controversial.

Epstein–Barr virus infection

Epstein–Barr virus produces a spectrum of abnormalities in OLT recipients ranging from asymptomatic infection to diffuse lymphomatous infiltration of multiple organs. Small children are at particular risk of developing primary EBV infection because around 50% are seronegative at the time of OLT. Reactivated infection occurs in approximately 30% of EBV-seropositive allograft recipients. The majority of episodes of EBV infection are diagnosed from 2 to 6 months following OLT, but the risk of developing EBV-related post-transplant lymphoproliferative disease (PTLD) continues thereafter. Productive EBV infection with active release of viral particles often results in a mononucleosis-like syndrome with fever, malaise, circulating atypical lymphocytes, and mild and reversible hepatitis. Seroconversion or detection of IgM antibodies to EBV are helpful to confirm the diagnosis. Liver biopsy usually shows polymorphous portal inflammation with portal and sinusoidal atypical lymphocytes, but with minimal hepatocellular necrosis. Endotheliitis of portal and central veins may be present in EBV infection, mimicking rejection. The disproportion between the intensity of the portal infiltrate and the mild or absent bile duct damage favors the diagnosis of EBV hepatitis over rejection. Uncomplicated EBV infection is self-limited and reversible unless supplemental immunosuppression is administered. Epstein–Barr virus produces life-long latent infections, has unique tropism for B cells, and has the ability to induce lymphocyte transformation and proliferation under the effects of immunosuppressive therapy. Around 2% of patients experience PTLD between 2 months and 2 years following OLT. The intensity of immunosuppression, particularly if OKT3 is used, and EBV infection are the major risk factors for PTLD. As many as 25% of pediatric recipients develop PTLD after the administration of OKT3 for intractable rejection, associated in many cases with primary EBV infection.

Localized tumors or systemic disease resulting from lymphomatous infiltration of multiple organs are typical presentations of PTLD. As the graft itself is involved in 20–30% of cases, some patients initially present with allograft dysfunction. Serologic tests are of little help for diagnosis of this nonproductive type of EBV infection. Computed tomography of head, chest, abdomen, and pelvis is indicated to search for discrete masses both in the allograft and extrahepatic sites. Histologically, PTLD appears as intense monomorphic or polymorphic portal inflammation. Polymorphous lymphoid infiltration may mimic rejection. Distinction between these two entities is crucial because administration of additional immunosuppression to patients with PTLD may result in rapidly progressive and fatal lymphoma. Monomorphic appearance on light microscopy is often associated with clonality. Tumor cells are generally of B-cell origin and express several EBV antigens. Staining for immunoglobulins in biopsy specimens and southern blot hybridization techniques to detect rearrangement of immunoglobulin genes are utilized to establish clonality. Around 50% of PTLD are monoclonal, 25% are polyclonal, and 25% are mixed. The majority of lymphomas occurring after OLT are of non-Hodgkin type. If detected early enough, PTLD is potentially reversible following temporary withdrawal or reduction of immunosuppression.

Herpes simplex virus infections

Herpes simplex virus infection is unusual in OLT recipients due to the prophylactic use of aciclovir in most centers. Around 75% of adults are HSV-seropositive at the time of OLT. Reactivation of virulent strains of HSV may produce a severe, rapidly progressive and fatal hepatitis in the early postoperative period. Cutaneous lesions may or may not be present. Hepatitis caused by HSV is characterized histologically by circumscribed areas of coagulative necrosis with nonzonal distribution. Ground glass nuclei or Cowdry type A inclusions are often found in viable hepatocytes in the periphery of the necrotic

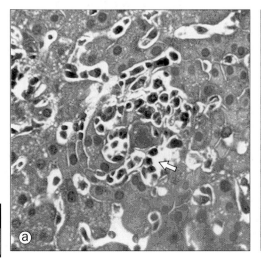

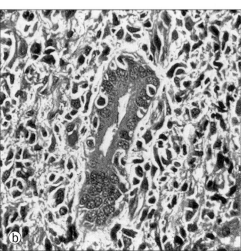

Figure 39.13 Coexistence of CMV hepatitis and allograft rejection. (a) Microabscess surrounding a necrotic hepatocyte with a CMV inclusion body (arrow). (b) Portal inflammation and rejection cholangitis.

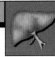

areas. Immunohistochemistry is utilized to confirm the presence of HSV antigens in infected hepatocytes. Intravenous aciclovir therapy followed by retransplantation is the only hope for the few patients destined to survive this devastating infectious complication.

Other viral infections

The large majority of adult patients have antibodies to VZV before OLT. However, primary infection or varicella in pediatric recipients may cause severe illness early after OLT with hemorrhagic rash, hepatitis, and multiorgan failure. Adenovirus infection is mostly restricted to pediatric recipients who usually present with fever and elevated liver tests approximately 1 month following OLT. The severity of hepatitis ranges from mild and self-limited disease to fulminant hepatic failure. Liver biopsy shows areas of parenchymal necrosis with no particular zonal distribution, collections of inflammatory cells with a granulomatoid appearance, and characteristic nuclear inclusions in the periphery of necrotic areas. Immunostaining of specific viral antigens in liver specimens is required to confirm the diagnosis.

Drug-induced hepatotoxicity

The diagnosis of drug-induced hepatotoxicity in nontransplant patients is mostly based on the exclusion of other causes of liver injury that may explain the clinical or histologic abnormalities that are attributed to the specific medication. This is almost impossible in transplant recipients who receive several potentially hepatotoxic drugs simultaneously, and usually have alternative causes to explain graft dysfunction.

Cyclosporine hepatotoxicity has been reported in renal, cardiac, and bone marrow transplant recipients. A dose-dependent increase in liver enzymes and histologic cholestasis without inflammation have been the most frequent abnormalities attributed to cyclosporine. However, the potential hepatotoxicity of cyclosporine in OLT recipients has not been defined. It is unclear whether this drug may contribute to the increase in serum bilirubin during some episodes of graft dysfunction such as the functional cholestasis observed in the early postoperative period. Similarly, tacrolimus hepatotoxicity has been suggested but not proven.

More information is available regarding azathioprine hepatotoxicity in renal and OLT recipients. Patients presented with elevated liver tests and were found to have pericentral hepatocyte degeneration or congestion on liver biopsy. Most abnormalities reversed upon discontinuation of the drug. In addition a few patients developed benign liver tumors or tumor-like lesions such as focal nodular hyperplasia or nodular regenerative hyperplasia causing portal hypertension.

Despite our inability to decipher the role of most drugs in producing liver damage following OLT, a careful review of all potential hepatotoxic medications should be considered in the differential diagnosis of graft dysfunction. Several antimicrobial agents and many medications commonly utilized in OLT recipients to treat hypertension, hyperlipidemia, or other complications have proven hepatotoxicity. When a toxic reaction is suspected, the medication should be discontinued unless it is essential for the treatment of life-threatening complications.

Recurrence of the native disease

With the increased success of OLT, recurrence of the native liver disease has become an important source of morbidity and mortality. The routine performance of protocol liver biopsies following OLT has allowed the diagnosis of recurrent disease at a preclinical stage.

Primary biliary cirrhosis

The diagnosis of PBC in nontransplant patients relies on the combination of symptoms, elevated cholestatic enzymes, positive mitochondrial antibodies, and chronic nonsuppurative and destructive cholangitis on liver biopsy. These features lose their diagnostic value following OLT because they can be found alone or in combination in a number of conditions other than disease recurrence. Elevated alkaline phosphatase and γ-GT are seen in most causes of graft dysfunction; mitochondrial antibodies may be present after OLT in patients with or without PBC recurrence; and nonsuppurative cholangitis is one of the typical histologic features of allograft rejection. However, granulomatous cholangitis or a florid duct lesion, the most characteristic morphologic finding of PBC, has not been found in patients with cellular or ductopenic rejection and is thus the only reliable finding to diagnose recurrent disease. The majority of patients with recurrent PBC are asymptomatic and have normal liver tests. In a few cases, progression to the fibrotic stage has been described. Despite that, the diagnosis depends almost exclusively on biopsy findings. It appears that PBC does recur following OLT in around 10% of patients. Long-term histologic follow-up of patients with PBC recurrence in necessary to establish the rate of progression and the need for retransplantation.

Primary sclerosing cholangitis

The diagnosis of PSC before OLT is based on the demonstration of multiple areas of stenosis and dilatation of the extrahepatic and intrahepatic biliary system on cholangiography. The first limitation to diagnose disease recurrence is that the common bile duct of the recipient is resected in the majority of patients grafted for PSC, mostly to prevent cholangiocarcinoma. Second, diffuse PSC-like intrahepatic biliary strictures often result from bile duct ischemia in recipients with extended cold preservation times, ductopenic rejection, or HAT. It appears then that cholangiographic abnormalities are not enough to confirm recurrent PSC. However, fibro-obliterative cholangiopathy, a near-diagnostic histologic feature of PSC, has only been found in transplant recipients with putative disease recurrence. Unfortunately, this lesion is not frequently present in needle biopsy specimens, even in nontransplant patients with well-documented PSC. It has recently been shown that patients transplanted for PSC have a significantly increased prevalence of biliary strictures diagnosed more than 90 days after OLT and/or fibro-obliterative cholangiopathy in the absence of ductopenic rejection. At present it appears likely that PSC may recur following OLT.

Autoimmune hepatitis

Recurrence of autoimmune hepatitis has been described in the late follow-up of female OLT recipients who developed clinical and histologic hepatitis, hypergammaglobulinemia and positive autoantibodies following withdrawal of corticosteroids. More importantly, reinstitution of appropriate doses of corticosteroids resulted in rapid resolution of the disease. Histologically, florid interphase hepatitis with minor bile duct damage favors the diagnosis of recurrent autoimmune hepatitis over cellular rejection. Other causes of hepatocellular graft dysfunction such as viral

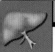
hepatitis or drug-induced hepatotoxicity should be excluded as well. HLA DR3-positive recipients transplanted with HLA DR3-negative donors have the highest risk of developing recurrent autoimmune hepatitis.

Alcoholic liver disease

Approximately 20–30% of patients undergoing OLT for alcoholic liver disease return to drinking, usually defined as any postoperative use of alcohol. The rate of recidivism increases with the duration of follow-up and is greater in patients with pre-OLT sobriety less than 6 months and those found to have alcoholic hepatitis on histologic examination of the explanted liver. Return to continuous abusive drinking may result in several medical problems related to alcoholism itself or to lack of compliance with immunosuppressive medications, jeopardizing the graft from uncontrolled rejection.

Although rapid progression to severe liver disease has been described in some cases, mild and nonspecific inflammatory changes are the most common histologic finding in patients with moderate drinking after OLT. It is unclear whether alcoholic liver disease progresses faster in transplant recipients compared with in patients who are not immunosuppressed. The incidence of rejection does not differ in abstinent and nonabstinent alcoholic patients, except for those who are noncompliant with immunosuppression. Long-term follow up appears necessary to define the natural history of alcoholic liver disease following OLT. For the time being, complete abstinence should be strongly recommended to all patients transplanted for alcoholic cirrhosis.

Budd–Chiari syndrome

The majority of patients with Budd–Chiari syndrome treated with OLT have an underlying myeloproliferative disease or hypercoagulable state. As these extrahepatic disorders persist after OLT, patients are at risk of developing recurrent hepatic vein thrombosis mostly during the early postoperative period. Lifetime anticoagulation or administration of hydroxyurea and aspirin to treat platelet disorders are essential to prevent recurrent disease. Exceptions to this general rule are patients with Budd–Chiari secondary to liver-based disorders corrected by OLT such as protein C or antithrombin III deficiencies. Retransplantation is required for most patients with recurrent hepatic vein thrombosis.

Primary hepatic malignancies

Hepatocellular carcinoma, cholangiocarcinoma, and epithelioid hemangioendothelioma are the primary malignant liver tumors most frequently treated with OLT in adults. Hepatoblastoma is the leading indication of OLT for liver neoplasms in the pediatric population.

Hepatocellular carcinoma

In the early days of OLT, HCC was a frequent indication for liver replacement. Experience over the past two decades has shown that OLT for 'all comers' with HCC is associated with tumor recurrence in 60–80% of cases and poor long-term survival, not exceeding 20% at 5 years in most centers. Several factors may explain these disappointing results. First, patients may have extrahepatic metastases before surgery not detected by US, CT, or bone scan performed during the pre-OLT evaluation or at vari-

able intervals after inclusion on the waiting list. Second, manipulation of the liver during the operation may cause dissemination of viable malignant cells resulting in multiple micrometastases. Finally, occult malignant disease becomes clinically evident following OLT due to the dramatic effects of immunosuppression on tumor growth and spread. It should be stressed that OLT is the only option for cure or extended palliation for patients with unresectable HCC. A major challenge for transplant physicians is to identify accurate preoperative predictors of tumor recurrence, allowing selection of candidates who will benefit most from OLT.

In patients with a small HCC discovered incidentally in the resected liver, results of OLT are excellent and similar to that of patients transplanted for cirrhosis without malignancy. Patients with either large or multiple tumors, vascular invasion or lymph node metastases, representing the opposite end of the clinical spectrum of HCC, are destined to have early postoperative recurrence and dismal survival in the majority of instances. Results of OLT for patients with the more benign fibrolamellar variant of HCC have been slightly better than those in patients with the 'usual' histologic tumor types. As fibrolamellar HCC occurs in noncirrhotic livers, major resections are well tolerated in most cases. However, patients with unresectable fibrolamellar HCC referred for OLT often have multilobar and advanced disease resulting in frequent postoperative tumor recurrence. Which patients with HCC diagnosed before surgery should be transplanted? There is no conclusive answer for this key question. However, those with solitary tumors less than 5cm or fewer than 3 nodules of less than 3cm in size, without microscopic vascular invasion and absence of lymph node or extrahepatic metastases, are accepted as OLT candidates in the majority of centers. Post-OLT recurrence of HCC occurs mostly within the first year after surgery. The graft itself and lungs are the most common sites of recurrence. Preoperative and/or postoperative adjuvant chemotherapy protocols have been utilized in an attempt to decrease recurrence and improve survival. The potential benefit of these therapeutic strategies is still controversial and should be investigated in randomized trials.

Other malignant tumors

In children with unresectable hepatoblastoma, OLT appears justified. Tumor recurrence occurs in one-third of patients and 5-year disease-free survival averages 50%. The vast majority of patients transplanted for cholangiocarcinoma develop early tumor recurrence and die within 1 year of surgery from florid carcinomatosis. Unlike HCC, many incidental cholangiocarcinomas discovered in the explanted liver are already at advanced stages and have a similar and dismal prognosis as the tumors diagnosed before OLT. Cholangiocarcinoma is regarded as a contraindication for OLT in many centers.

Epithelioid hemangioendothelioma is a slow but aggressive malignant tumor more commonly found in young adults. Results of OLT in unresectable epithelioid hemangioendothelioma are quite good, even in cases with metastatic spread. Tumor recurrence is found in around one-third of cases, usually beyond 1 year of OLT, and 5-year survival is approximately 50%.

Angiosarcoma should be considered a contraindication for OLT. Postoperative early recurrence and rapidly progressive tumor spread and death are almost inevitable.

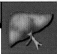

Viral hepatitis B and C

Patients with hepatitis B or hepatitis C have a high risk of recurrent infection and hepatitis usually between 2 and 12 months following surgery (see Fig. 39.12). However, the morbidity associated with disease recurrence and the availability of strategies to prevent or treat graft reinfection markedly differs in patients with hepatitis B virus (HBV) or hepatitis C virus (HCV) infection (Fig. 39.14).

Hepatitis B virus

Recurrence of HBV infection is almost universal in hepatitis B surface antigen (HBsAg)-positive patients transplanted without immunoprophylaxis. The vast majority of patients with recurrent infection develop a rapidly progressive form of chronic hepatitis evolving to cirrhosis within 3 years of OLT and jeopardizing long-term patient and allograft survival. Until recently, hepatitis B was considered a relative or even absolute contraindication for OLT in many centers. Continuous clinical research over the past decade has resulted in the development of effective adjuvant treatment protocols to decrease HBV recurrence and increase survival. Currently, long-term administration of HBIg is the most established strategy to prevent graft reinfection.

Prophylaxis with HBIg prevents HBV recurrence in 80–90% of patients with fulminant hepatitis B, concurrent HBV and hepatitis delta infection, or HBV-cirrhosis without pre-OLT viral replication. Results of immunoprophylaxis in HBV-cirrhosis with active viral replication, as indicated by a positive hepatitis B e antigen (HBeAg) or HBV DNA in serum, are not as good with around 50–70% of patients developing recurrence despite HBIg administration. Lamivudine, a second-generation nucleoside analog, produces intense and rapid suppression of HBV replication in the vast majority of patients with hepatitis B and is well-tolerated in advanced cirrhosis. On a practical basis, HBsAg-positive patients before OLT are now divided into those with spontaneous or lamivudine-induced absence of viral replication. It can be speculated that pre-OLT lamivudine therapy may improve further the results of HBIg prophylaxis in patients with active viral replication. The HBIg is administered intravenously during the anhepatic phase of OLT and the first postoperative days when large doses are required.

The most utilized protocol consists of fixed doses of 10,000IU of HBIg given during surgery and daily for the first postoperative week, independently of the serum concentrations of hepatitis B surface antibody (anti-HBs) obtained. Our approach is to measure daily post-OLT titers of anti-HBs and administer enough HBIg intravenously to achieve the putative protective concentration of greater than 500IU/L (Fig. 39.15). After clearance of HBsAg and stable anti-HBs titers are obtained, indefinite HBIg prophylaxis is required, either with fixed intravenous doses given at monthly intervals or small repetitive doses by the intramuscular route. In our center, 1000IU of HBIg are administered intramuscularly, initially at weekly intervals and subsequently every 2 or 3 weeks, to maintain serum anti-HBs concentrations above 200IU/L (see Fig. 39.15). Treatment with HBIg is expensive and in many countries intravenous preparations are not commercially available. The efficacy of long-term HBIg prophylaxis appears similar for intravenous or intramuscular preparations, but the cost is significantly less utilizing the intramuscular route. Lamivudine monotherapy has also been utilized for prophylaxis of HBV recurrence. The disadvantage of this strategy is that many patients develop escape HBV mutants after 6 months of therapy with reappearance of HBsAg in serum. Theoretically, combined lamivudine and HBIg therapy should be the most effective regimen to prevent HBV recurrence. However, well-designed randomized trials are needed to confirm this observation.

Nucleoside analogs such as lamivudine or famciclovir, alone or in combination with interferon, are currently the best treatment options for patients destined to develop HBV recurrence despite HBIg prophylaxis. Survival of patients with hepatitis B undergoing OLT with long-term immunoprophylaxis is similar to that of patients transplanted for HBsAg-negative liver diseases.

Hepatitis C virus

The vast majority of patients transplanted for HCV infection develop recurrent infection following OLT, as indicated by a positive HCV RNA in serum. However, the morbidity and mortality associated with recurrence is substantially less in patients

Recurrent viral hepatitis B and C		
	Hepatitis B	**Hepatitis C**
Recurrence of infection without prophylactic therapy	90–100%	90–100%
Histologic hepatitis in patients with recurrent infection	90–100%	50–70%
Characteristics of recurrent hepatitis	Severe Rapidly progressive	Mild Slowly progressive
Pre-OLT therapy	Lamivudine Famciclovir	None
Prophylaxis of recurrence	HBIg Lamivudine HBIg + lamivudine	Interferon? Interferon + ribavirin?
Treatment of recurrent hepatitis	Lamivudine Famciclovir Interferon	Interferon Interferon + ribavirin?

Figure 39.14 Recurrent viral hepatitis B and C. Prevalence, clinical course, prophylaxis, and therapy of recurrent HBV or HCV infection after liver transplantation.

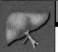

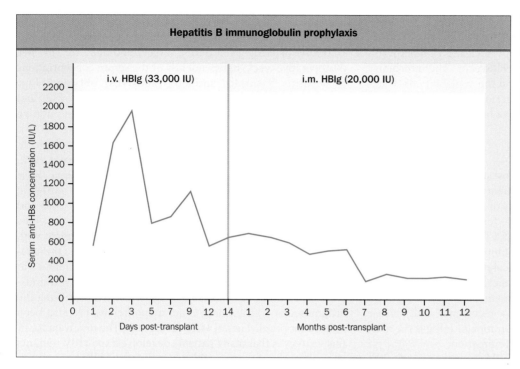

Figure 39.15 Hepatitis B immunoglobulin prophylaxis. Serum anti-HBs concentrations during intravenous and intramuscular HBIg therapy in a patient who remained HBsAg-negative following liver transplantation for hepatitis B.

undergoing OLT for hepatitis C compared with that of patients transplanted for hepatitis B. The prevalence of histologic hepatitis in patients with recurrent HCV infection is around 50–70%, but graft injury is mild and slowly progressive in most cases. Long-term survival is the rule rather than the exception. Severe cholestatic hepatitis or rapid progression to cirrhosis leading to death or retransplantation occur in only 10% of patients with recurrent disease.

The mechanisms of graft damage in HCV infection after OLT are poorly understood. In some studies, but not in others, the prevalence and severity of recurrent hepatitis C was associated with viral factors such as infection with the HCV genotype 1b and/or the concentration of HCV RNA in serum or liver, suggesting a direct cytopathic effect of HCV. It should be noted, however, that many patients with extremely high levels of HCV RNA in serum, or infection with genotype 1b, have normal histology. Host factors have been much less studied. A polyclonal immune response to HCV has been described in nontransplant patients with acute or chronic hepatitis C. However, the effects of immunosuppression and mismatch of HLA on the immune response to HCV antigens in transplant recipients has not been investigated.

Understanding the pathogenesis of hepatobiliary damage in post-OLT HCV infection appears essential to select the timing for antiviral therapy and the need to modify the immunosuppressive regimen. Before OLT, interferon therapy of patients with advanced HCV-cirrhosis is mostly ineffective and potentially dangerous. In this patient population interferon is poorly tolerated, induces profound cytopenias, and may trigger life-threatening infectious complications. Pre-OLT therapy with low doses of interferon and ribavirin should be investigated in future trials. At present there is no effective immunoprophylaxis for recurrence of HCV infection. Administration of standard immune globulin to experimentally infected primates failed to prevent HCV infection and hepatitis. Development of specific hepatitis C immunoglobulin preparations appears unlikely, mostly because

protective antibodies have not been identified in animals or humans with resolved HCV infection. Recent preliminary data suggest that therapy with interferon alone or combined with ribavirin, initiated a few days after OLT, may be effective to prevent HCV recurrence. These observations require further confirmation. Experience with interferon-α therapy in OLT recipients with recurrent hepatitis C is limited. Normalization of aminotransferases and decrease in serum HCV RNA levels occur in around one-third of patients. However, these beneficial effects of interferon are transient in the vast majority of treated patients. It has recently been shown that combination therapy with interferon and ribavirin was associated with biochemical and virologic response in approximately 50% of patients with recurrent hepatitis C. One of the major limitations of interferon therapy in immunosuppressed OLT recipients is the potential risk of precipitating ductopenic rejection, which occurred in up to 30% of treated patients in some reported series but was nonexistent in others. Five-year survival is similar in HCV-positive or HCV-negative cirrhotics treated with OLT in most series. However, long-term histologic follow-up is required to determine the rate of progression of recurrent hepatitis C leading to retransplantation or death.

Acquired viral hepatitis

Acquisition of HBV infection after OLT is mostly related to the use of liver grafts from anti-HBc-positive cadaveric or living-related donors. Post-OLT lamivudine therapy and/or HBIg immunoprophylaxis may prevent HBV graft infection in this setting. Some HBsAg-negative patients before OLT who become HBsAg-positive recipients postoperatively may not have acquired infection, but have developed recurrence of an occult infection, defined by the presence of HBV DNA in serum or liver without serologic markers of hepatitis B.

Infection with HCV following OLT may be acquired from infected donors or transfused blood products. Almost all HCV RNA-negative recipients transplanted with HCV RNA-positive

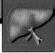

donors develop HCV infection after OLT. The incidence of acquired HCV infection was as high as 40% before the advent of serologic assays to detect anti-HCV in serum. Routine screening of blood and organ donors for anti-HCV resulted in a substantial decrease in the rate of acquisition of HCV infection following OLT. However, liver transplant recipients are still at risk of acquiring infection from anti-HCV-negative donors with detectable HCV RNA in serum or liver.

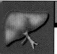
FURTHER READING

Clavien P-A, Harvey PRC, Strasberg SM. Preservation and reperfusion injuries in liver allografts. An overview and synthesis of current studies. Transplantation. 1992;53:957–78. *Excellent review of the mechanisms underlying liver injury during cold storage and reperfusion.*

Demetris AJ, Batts KP, Dhillon AP and International Panel. Banff schema for grading liver allograft rejection: an international consensus document. Hepatology. 1997;25:658–63. *A panel of experts reviewed the histopathologic features of acute allograft rejection and proposed a simple and reproducible classification and grading system that will facilitate comparison between different series.*

Gane EJ, Naoumov NV, Qian K-P, et al. A longitudinal analysis of hepatitis C virus replication following liver transplantation. Gastroenterology. 1996;110:167–77. *Infection with genotype 1b and high levels of viremia were associated with more severe allograft damage in European patients with recurrent hepatitis C.*

Hubscher SG, Elias E, Buckels JAC, Mayer AD, McMaster P, Neuberger JM. Primary biliary cirrhosis. Histological evidence of disease recurrence after liver transplantation. J Hepatol. 1993;18:173–84. *Histopathologic analysis of a large number of liver biopsies obtained more than 1 year after OLT showed recurrence of PBC in 16% of cases.*

Lake JR. Long-term management of biliary tract complications. Liver Transplant Surg. 1995;1(Suppl 1):45–54. *This review focuses on the diagnosis and management of biliary complications presenting beyond the index hospitalization.*

Ludwig J. Histopathology of the liver following transplantation. In: Maddrey WC, Sorrell MF, eds. Transplantation of the liver, second edition, Chapter 13. East Norwalk, Connecticut: Appleton & Lange; 1995:267–95. *The histopathologic features of early and late causes of graft dysfunction following OLT are described in this chapter.*

Rubin RH. Infection in the organ transplant recipient. In: Rubin RH, Young LS, eds. Clinical approach to infection in the compromised host, third edition, Chapter 24. New York: Plenum Publishing Corporation; 1994:629–705. *This chapter provides a detailed analysis about the prevalence, clinical course, diagnosis, prophylaxis and therapy of infectious complications following OLT.*

Samuel D, Bismuth A, Mathieu D, et al. Passive immunoprophylaxis after liver transplantation in HBsAg-positive patients. Lancet. 1991;337:813–15. *This study confirmed that long-term HBIg prophylaxis prevents HBV recurrence following OLT and established the association between preoperative status of viral replication and risk of graft reinfection.*

Sanchez-Urdazpal L, Gores JG, Ward EM, et al. Ischemic-type biliary complications after orthotopic liver transplantation. Hepatology. 1992;16:49–53. *Nonanastomotic biliary strictures appear to be the result of bile duct ischemic injury associated with the duration of cold storage.*

Strasberg SM, Howard TK, Molmenti EP, Hertl M. Selecting the donor liver: factors for poor function after orthotopic liver transplantation. Hepatology. 1994;20:829–38. *The authors provide clear definitions of IPF and PNF and analyse the predictive value of donor, perioperative, and recipient risk factors for primary graft dysfunction.*

Wright H, Bou-Abboud CF, Hassanein T, et al. Disease recurrence and rejection following liver transplantation for autoimmune chronic active liver disease. Transplantation. 1992;53:136–9. *This study showed post-OLT recurrence of autoimmune hepatitis in 25% of cases, particularly when donor and recipient were mismatched for HLA-DR3.*

Zhou S, Terrault NA, Ferrell L, et al. Severity of liver disease in liver transplantation recipients with hepatitis C virus infection: relationship to genotype and level of viremia. Hepatology. 1996; 24:1041–6. *In this large series of patients with recurrent hepatitis C from the USA, infection with HCV genotype 1 or 1b and serum levels of HCV RNA had no impact on disease severity or survival.*

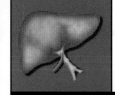

Chapter 40

Retransplantation

Peter J Friend

INTRODUCTION

During the early days of clinical liver transplantation, retransplantation was infrequently and not often successfully performed. For a number of reasons retransplantation subsequently became a practical possibility and now accounts for a substantial amount of liver transplant activity. The major reasons for this change are, first, the development of the surgical and anesthesic techniques and intensive care support to enable this often more complex surgery to be carried out in patients who are frequently in very poor condition. Second, it became possible to obtain a second graft for a patient within the time constraints because of the improved organization of donor organ retrieval and allocation.

Patients who require retransplantation of the liver fall broadly into two categories: urgent and semielective. In a patient whose primary liver transplant has failed acutely, very little time is available to carry out a retransplant before the patient either dies or deteriorates to such an extent that transplantation would be unsuccessful. Urgent retransplantation requires access to an appropriate donor organ within a few days of making the decision to retransplant, and success depends therefore upon an effective system of organ sharing that enables priority to be given to urgent cases. The results of transplantation for highly urgent cases, either for primary liver transplants or retransplants, are poorer than transplantation for patients with nonacute disease. As the availability of liver donors has increasingly become the limiting factor in the provision of liver transplant services in most countries, a system whereby priority is given to patients who are less likely to benefit does raise important ethical and logistic issues.

INCIDENCE OF RETRANSPLANTATION

The incidence of retransplantation varies considerably between centers. This reflects a number of factors including differences not only in patient selection, but also in early postoperative complication rates and immunosuppressive strategies. An important additional variable is the willingness of a clinician to submit a patient to a further transplant when the results of retransplantation may be poor and to do so may deprive a primary transplant recipient of the opportunity of a transplant with a much higher probability of success. This latter factor has become more prominent with lengthening transplant waiting lists and the resulting increased risk of dying before a donor organ becomes available. The incidence of retransplantation is probably falling, due mainly to improved immunosuppression and patient management and partly to the need to optimize the benefit from an increasingly limited resource.

In the 1980s, retransplant rates of 20–25% were standard, but these have now fallen considerably. There has been a marked reduction in the need for retransplantation for primary graft nonfunction and for chronic rejection. On the other hand the increasing pediatric activity may increase the need for retransplantation because the rates decrease as the recipient population gets older (Fig. 40.1).

In the UK in 1996, 12% of recipients had previously received a liver transplant, compared with 14% in 1995. A total of 9% of patients on the waiting list (in 1996) were awaiting retransplantation, the discrepancy presumably being related to the higher proportion of urgent patients in the retransplant group.

INDICATIONS FOR RETRANSPLANTATION

The overall indications for retransplantation are shown in Fig. 40.2, and include primary nonfunction, rejection, vascular and other technical complications, and disease recurrence.

Primary nonfunction and poor early function of the graft

Immediate function of a transplanted liver is necessary for the survival of the patient, and the assessment of this involves a range of clinical and laboratory parameters (Fig. 40.3).

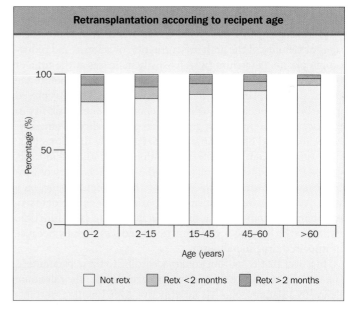

Figure 40.1 Incidence of liver retransplantation with age. The highest retransplant (retx) rates, especially in the first 2 months, are seen in pediatric cases. (Data from European Liver Transplant Registry.)

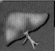

Indications for retransplantation			
Europe (%)		**USA (%)**	
Technical complications	31.3	Primary nonfunction	30.0
Rejection	28.8	Vascular complications	26.6
Primary nonfunction	28.6	Chronic rejection	11.3
Disease recurrence	4.2	Acute rejection	10.7
Sepsis	1.1	Nonthrombotic ischemia	9.6
Others	6.0	Disease recurrence	5.0

Figure 40.2 Indications for retransplantation. There are some differences between the frequencies of the indications for retransplantation in Europe and the USA.

Early indicators of graft function	
Indicator	**Interpretation**
Bile quality	Good bile indicates good function; poor bile at the end of the transplant should increase the suspicion of PNF
Arterial pH	Persistent acidemia is an early indicator of poor function, but is not specific
Serum potassium	Good graft function reverses hyperkalemia
Blood sugar	Insulin resistant hyperglycemia indicates poor graft function
Prothrombin time	Initial values are nonspecific, but a failure to improve indicates poor function. Non-discriminatory with respect to determining need for retransplantation
Transaminanses	Values in first 12 hours are of no value - thereafter trends are important, but absolute results are not discriminatory
Drug metabolism	Best assessed by ability to metabolise drugs given for sedation – failure to reverse sedation is a good indicator of poor function
Clinical complications	Hypoptension, increasing inotrope requirements, cerebral edema, *de novo* renal failure suggest poor graft function if sepsis has been excluded

Figure 40.3 Early indicators of graft function. Factors that are helpful in assessing possible early graft dysfunction that may require emergency retransplantation (PNF, primary non-function).

Following reperfusion of the transplanted liver, the earliest signs of viability of the graft are correction of acidosis and reduction in plasma potassium (which usually increases at the time of reperfusion). The quality of bile may also be assessable before the end of the transplant operation or afterwards if a T-tube is placed in the biliary tree. Good quality bile eliminates the possibility of primary nonfunction of the graft, while poor quality bile increases the likelihood of this complication. Poor early function of the graft is subsequently manifest by prolonged prothrombin time, persistent hyperglycemia, oliguria, and impaired recovery of consciousness following the operation. If the patient remains on a ventilator following transplantation, the drug requirements to maintain sedation can be a further indication of liver function. Patients who have poor graft function need less therapy because of impaired drug metabolism.

In a liver that is not functioning according to these parameters, the decision to replace the graft must be made with the minimum delay. In a patient who has no effective liver function, retransplantation must be carried out within 1–2 days if the patient is to have a realistic chance of survival. Primary nonfunction of a liver transplant is an accepted criterion for a patient being listed for urgent transplantation in most organ allocation systems. In the UK such a patient would be given a very high level of priority, alongside patients who have acute liver failure and ahead of patients awaiting transplantation for chronic liver failure. United Network for Organ Sharing (UNOS) status 1 is also accorded to patients developing primary nonfunction of the implanted graft or hepatic artery thrombosis within 7 days of implantation.

More commonly, however, there is evidence that the transplanted liver is providing some function, but that this is suboptimal. Poor initial function cannot be predicted with any certainty, although in many such cases the appearance of the reperfused liver will give cause for concern. Significant fatty infiltration is an important cause of poor initial function of a transplanted liver, this being diagnosed by the appearances of the liver at surgery or by the extent of fatty deposition on histologic examination. However, even livers with histologic evidence of moderately severe steatosis are used for transplantation. Although in these cases there is a significant incidence of poor early graft function, this has not always been shown to affect outcome, and resolution of fatty change is well documented. Thus, although fatty infiltration is generally regarded as an adverse prognostic indicator, the degree to which this is acceptable in a donor liver remains an issue of individual opinion among liver transplant surgeons.

In a patient who has a poorly functioning liver, there is a very slow recovery of measurable liver function, manifest by a prolonged prothrombin time and very high levels of transaminase enzymes for several days, indicating extensive hepatocyte injury. In such a case the decision as to whether to await recovery or to plan urgent retransplantation may be difficult. Although such livers are potentially recoverable, there is a significant risk to the patient of developing a life-threatening complication such as sepsis or renal failure On balance, listing for emergency retransplantation may be in the best interests of the patient, and the final decision to proceed is made when a liver becomes available.

A major problem in liver transplant surgery is the lack of a reliable means to determine whether a donor liver is likely to function well after transplantation. Although many techniques for assessing liver function have been studied in an attempt to identify a means by which primary poor function may be predicted, the most widely used reliable indicator is that of the appearance of the liver at the time of donor hepatectomy. If the liver appears to be poorly perfused or fatty, the risk of post-transplant dysfunction is significant. Other techniques have been used and shown to be of variable usefulness. The measurement of the ability of a donor liver to metabolize lidocaine (lignocaine), the monoethylglycinexylidide assay, was believed to provide valuable information about the metabolic function of the liver, but this technique has not been found consistently to be clinically useful. The other donor parameters that have been associated with poor outcome include hypernatremia, death from cerebral trauma, and

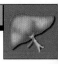

total ischemia time. Prolonged ventilation of the donor and the use of powerful inotropic agents [particularly epinephrine (adrenaline)] are also negative prognostic factors. The issue of donor age remains controversial, some studies demonstrating this to be an adverse risk factor and others showing no effect on outcome.

The liver is relatively resistant to humoral injury and, in contrast to renal transplantation, it is normal practice to undertake liver transplantation without ensuring a negative lymphocyte cross-match. The phenomenon of hyperacute rejection is exceedingly rare in liver transplantation, but if it is encountered the need for immediate retransplantation is obvious. However, because of the degree of sensitization these patients should receive organs from donors for whom there is a negative cross-match and this may be logistically difficult in the short period of time available. Alternatively, antibody depletion by means of plasmapheresis may be beneficial.

Vascular complications

Although in a nontransplant environment occlusion of the hepatic artery is frequently well tolerated, in the transplanted liver early thrombosis of the hepatic artery usually leads to acute ischemia associated with a massive rise in transaminase levels and loss of liver function. Such patients therefore rapidly progress to acute liver failure, behaving in a similar manner to those patients who have acute hepatic failure. Under such circumstances emergency retransplantation is invariably indicated and the decision to proceed is easy.

Less frequently early occlusion of the hepatic artery does not lead to massive hepatocyte necrosis and may present with a more modest elevation of transaminase levels. The diagnosis of hepatic artery occlusion is usually made by Doppler ultrasound and confirmed by arteriography. There is some experience of emergency exploration and vascular reconstruction under such circumstances, although this procedure is often unsuccessful in avoiding the need for retransplantation. These patients should probably be registered for retransplantation as it is almost inevitable that further complications of de-arterialization of the graft will develop.

Hepatic artery occlusion some months after transplantation presents in a less acute manner. Some degree of liver dysfunction may be noted at the time of vascular occlusion, but the patient is likely to present with the more chronic manifestations of arterial ischemia, particularly biliary complications – the biliary tree is particularly dependent on the arterial supply. The development of nonanastomotic biliary strictures or liver abscesses following liver transplantation should raise the question of arterial stenosis or occlusion. Although some patients who have hepatic arterial strictures may be managed successfully by angioplasty or arterial reconstruction, the majority of such patients require retransplantation. The patients presenting with liver abscesses often have liver function profiles that are entirely normal, giving rise to the temptation to try and manage these cases conservatively. This approach usually fails because of failure to eradicate the infection or later development of biliary complications.

Complications much less frequently involve the portal vein than the hepatic artery. Portal vein thrombosis may present with acute graft dysfunction, in a manner similar to that of hepatic arterial thrombosis; this complication most commonly requires retransplantation. However, in a patient in whom liver function is well-maintained, reconstruction of the portal vein may be undertaken. Alternatively however there may be no acute symptoms and

the presentation is that of portal hypertension with gastroesophageal variceal bleeding. The need for retransplantation is much less clear-cut in this situation.

Biliary complications

Intractable biliary complications, particularly intrahepatic biliary strictures, are an important indication for retransplantation. Biliary stenoses may be a manifestation of infection or ischemia of the biliary tree, immunologic complications, or the delayed effects of injury at the time of transplantation. The biliary complications that occur early after transplantation, particularly biliary leakage, are usually managed by surgical biliary reconstruction or endoscopic stenting and rarely necessitate retransplantation. However, perioperative ischemia or infection may lead to longer term problems with biliary stenosis.

Intrahepatic strictures are less likely to be of direct surgical etiology, although hepatic arterial thrombosis or stenosis should be excluded at an early stage. There is concern, supported by some studies, but not others, that cold ischemia times in excess of 15 hours are associated with a substantial increase in the risk of this complication. Similarly, it is believed in some centers that during the period between reperfusion through the portal vein and reperfusion through the hepatic artery the biliary epithelium is relatively ischemic and that the practice of reperfusing the liver through the portal vein before constructing the arterial anastomosis is, therefore, an avoidable cause of biliary injury. A more widely held view, however, is that intrahepatic biliary strictures for which no other specific cause is found may represent an immunologic injury; indeed biliary tract disease is frequently associated with other manifestations of chronic rejection of the liver. The need for retransplantation is clearest when the biliary stricturing coexists with another complication, especially chronic rejection, hepatic artery thrombosis, and intractable recurrent cholangitis. In cases where the degree of damage may not progress (e.g. preservation injury), the decision is more difficult and should be made on an individual basis.

Chronic rejection

The syndrome of chronic rejection is manifest by a progressive deterioration in biochemical liver function in association with characteristic histologic features, particularly of loss of bile ducts in the portal tract and intimal hyperplasia of the small arteries (Fig. 40.4).

Although the diagnosis can be made on needle biopsy, this is not always the case and it may be necessary to undertake retransplantation of the liver for presumed chronic rejection, the diagnosis being confirmed only when the explanted liver is examined histologically. Chronic rejection can occur as early as 6 weeks after the initial transplant but typically occurs between 3 and 12 months. It is assumed to be of immunologic origin, although its precise mechanism remains unclear. The incidence of chronic rejection has fallen dramatically from around 15 to 5%, or even as low as 2% in some series.

The decision to undertake retransplantation in a patient who has proven or presumed chronic rejection depends upon the level of liver function and its rate of deterioration in association with an assessment of risk factors in the individual case. In the 1980s, the decision to retransplant was relatively easy as chronic rejection with more than 50% ductopenia almost invariably progressed to loss of the graft. Subsequently, however, spontaneous recovery was documented and the introduction of tacrolimus and other

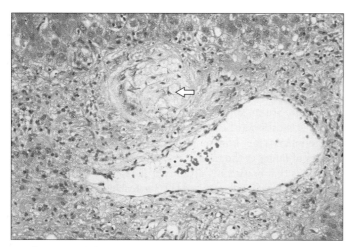

Figure 40.4 Chronic rejection. The relatively acellular portal tract that is devoid of bile ducts is typical of advanced chronic rejection. The obliteration of the artery with foam cells is highly suggestive that the process is irreversible and retransplantation is indicated (arrow).

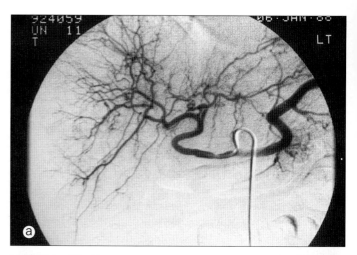

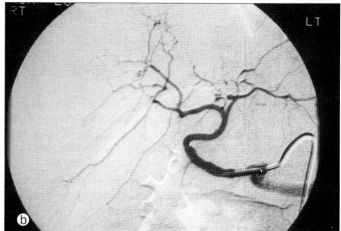

Figure 40.5 Chronic rejection. The obliterative arteriopathy of chronic rejection may be more sensitively detected by angiography. The normal arteriogram a week after transplantation (a) has changed to severe pruning of the arterial tree (b) 3 months later after the development of chronic rejection.

potent immunosuppressive drugs increased considerably the percentage of patients who had apparent chronic rejection in whom the graft could be salvaged. While a serum bilirubin greater than 200μmol/L or 12g/dL was usually indicative of eventual graft loss, the discriminatory value of these levels no longer applies. The development of an obliterative arteriopathy is the most specific indicator of irreversible chronic rejection (Fig. 40.5).

Other cases should be considered on the basis of the liver function tests as observed over a period of time. It should be remembered that a response to tacrolimus or other changes in immunosuppression may not become apparent until 3–4 weeks after the change was instituted.

Recurrent disease

With the increasing experience and long-term success of liver transplantation, it has become clear that a number of conditions which necessitate transplantation may recur in the transplanted liver. These include primary biliary cirrhosis, sclerosing cholangitis, hepatitis B, and hepatitis C. In addition, patients transplanted for alcoholic liver disease are at risk of recurrence of alcohol abuse and further liver damage.

Autoimmune liver disease

It has been recognized for some years that a minority of patients who undergo liver transplantation for primary biliary cirrhosis will develop recurrence of their disease. It is difficult to distinguish histologically between recurrence of primary biliary cirrhosis and the development of chronic rejection before retransplantation. In patients who undergo liver transplantation for primary sclerosing cholangitis recurrent disease has been reported. However, patients who undergo liver transplantation for other conditions may develop post-transplant (secondary) sclerosing cholangitis as a consequence of biliary stasis and/or recurrent episodes of ascending cholangitis, particularly in patients in whom biliary drainage has been established with a hepaticojejunostomy (Roux loop). Nevertheless, patients who have primary sclerosing cholangitis are much more likely to develop 'onion ring' fibrosis of the portal tract, which comes close to being pathognomonic for primary sclerosing cholangitis (Fig. 40.6).

Whatever the academic considerations, recurrent primary biliary cirrhosis and primary sclerosing cholangitis are rarely cited as causes for retransplantation. However, the natural history of these diseases is such that the real extent of this potential problem will not be apparent until a large number of patients have survived for 10–20 years or more after liver transplantation.

Viral hepatitis

Patients originally transplanted for hepatitis B-related liver disease may need to be considered for retransplantation in three clinical scenarios, two of which involve recurrent hepatitis B virus (HBV) infection. The first, and previously the commonest, is aggressive graft disease secondary to HBV reinfection, including fibrosing cholestatic hepatitis. These patients have very high levels of viral replication, and retransplantation is almost invariably followed by even more rapid destruction of the graft. Consequently, these patients are generally not considered for retransplantation. However, anecdotal cases of successful transplantation have been described using new antiviral drugs including lamivudine.

The second scenario is where the reinfection of the graft leads to cirrhosis over a longer period of time than that seen with fibrosing cholestatic hepatitis. These patients are likely to have

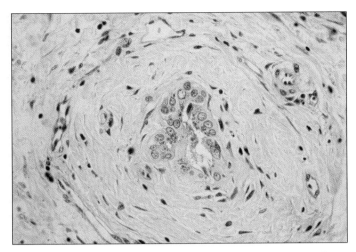

Figure 40.6 Recurrent primary sclerosing cholangitis. The clinical, radiologic, and histologic features of primary sclerosing cholangitis may be mimicked by other conditions after transplantation. However, the concentric fibrosis known as 'onion ring' fibrosis, which is almost pathognomonic of primary sclerosing cholangitis, occurs in up to 10% of patients after transplantation.

developed reinfection despite treatment with hepatitis B immunoglobulin or lamivudine, or both agents. Where this occurs because of the development of mutations, these agents are no longer available for prevention of reinfection after retransplantation. However, if the breakthrough is the consequence of poor compliance, these may be of value after retransplantation. Suppression of viral replication, to render the patient HBV DNA negative in serum, is essential before the second transplant is performed. This may be achievable with drugs not normally used for maintenance antiviral therapy (e.g. ganciclovir). The decision to retransplant these patients depends on whether a strategy that has a reasonable degree of success can be constructed to prevent or control reinfection of the graft.

Patients may need transplantation for any of the standard indications that apply to other etiologies. These cases should be assessed for transplantation in the standard way. This comment also applies to the occasional patient who is infected with HBV,

but whose primary transplant was for an unrelated condition. These patients might have had HBV infection at the time of transplantation or acquired it afterwards. There is some evidence that the implication of HBV reinfection is not as grave in these cases.

Recurrence of hepatitis C virus infection of the liver following transplantation is almost universal. However, the consequence of reinfection of the graft is less severe than is the case with HBV. Acute graft loss is uncommon, but occasional cases have been reported that are similar to the clinical syndrome of fibrosing cholestatic hepatitis that is associated with recurrent hepatitis B. Although the medium-term results of liver transplantation for hepatitis C are satisfactory, up to 20% of patients do develop cirrhosis by 5 years after transplantation. Although this has not yet translated to a large experience of retransplantation for recurrent hepatitis C, it should be anticipated that this may occur in the future. There are no clear guidelines at present regarding if and when these patients should be retransplanted. The preliminary studies suggest that retransplantation is justifiable, but it is not known whether the 5–10 year cycle of disease leading to graft failure will be repeated or accelerated following retransplantation. Although the currently available antiviral drugs for treating hepatitis C are suboptimal, it is likely that more effective remedies will become available in the future. These considerations would suggest that, until data to the contrary are available, these patients should be considered for retransplantation.

TIMING OF RETRANSPLANTATION

The peak period for retransplantation ranges from the first week up to 6 months after transplantation (Fig. 40.7).

In those patients who require retransplantation shortly following the primary transplant, the need for a second graft is usually extremely urgent. The most common indications for this are primary nonfunction or poor initial function of the graft or acute arterial thrombosis. In those patients in whom there is no evidence of liver function following revascularization of the liver, replacement of the graft is required within 24–48 hours. Similarly a patient in whom hepatic arterial thrombosis has occurred is likely to survive for only a few days in the absence of a retransplant. These patients therefore are of similar urgency to patients awaiting transplantation for acute hepatic failure and are accorded the

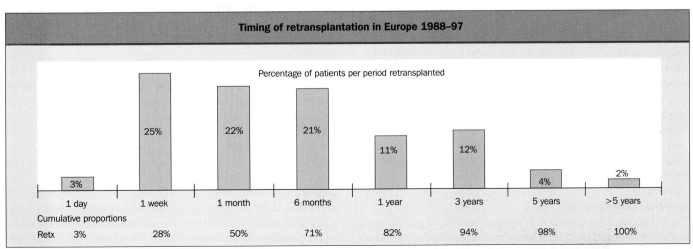

Figure 40.7 Timing of retransplantation. The distribution of retransplants (retx) by time after the primary transplant indicates that most occur within 6 months. (Data from European Liver Transplant Registry.)

same level of priority for organ allocation. In the UK a separate category exists for such 'super urgent' patients who take priority over all other liver transplant recipients. Other countries have comparable systems for patients whose likely survival without a transplant is no more than a few days.

Other patients awaiting retransplantation (for chronic rejection, recurrent disease, late arterial complications, etc.) are given the same level of priority as all other patients awaiting non-emergency transplantation. Thus, the priority accorded to such a patient depends upon the relative urgency of the individual case in the context of the other patients awaiting liver transplantation at a particular transplant center. In many cases this decision over relative priorities depends not only upon the relative urgency of the patients, but also upon the likely outcome following transplantation. In the context of a shortage of donor organs, there is an increasing view that the available organs should be directed to those patients who are most likely to benefit. In effect the decision, which is made locally, usually reflects a compromise of these factors.

TECHNICAL ASPECTS

Postoperative adhesions

One of the factors that complicates the surgery of liver transplantation is the presence of adhesions following previous upper abdominal surgery. These may be very dense and very vascular, particularly in the context of a patient who has extensive high pressure venous collateral vessels secondary to portal hypertension. This, combined with a coagulopathy secondary to poor synthetic liver function, may lead to severe intraoperative hemmorhage.

Patients who undergo retransplantation months or years following surgery nearly always have dense adhesions around the liver. The liver is firmly adherent to the diaphragm, the omentum, stomach, duodenum, and, often, transverse colon. However, the majority of these patients have not developed the stigmata of advanced portal hypertension. Thus, although the surgery is time consuming and technically demanding, the surgical outcome is usually satisfactory. A number of postoperative complications, however, may reflect the more extensive nature of the dissection required in such cases. In particular mobilization of the liver from the diaphragm may be difficult, leading to a substantial risk of diaphragmatic perforation. In some cases it is preferable that the liver should be mobilized inside its capsule to reduce the risk of damage to the diaphragm. Dissection of adherent loops of intestine from the liver may lead to the risk of subsequent intestinal perforation due to local devitalization of tissue. Surgical technique is important in reducing this risk, which appears to be substantially greater in children.

In patients undergoing retransplantation within days or a few weeks of the first transplant, postoperative adhesions have not developed and mobilization of the liver is rapid and usually uncomplicated. From a technical perspective, early retransplantation is uncomplicated and rapid because very little dissection is required to mobilize the liver before hepatectomy.

Arterial reconstruction

In patients who require retransplantation because of hepatic arterial occlusion, the arterial reconstruction of the second graft may be complex. It is important that an adequate vessel is used to revascularize the new graft. This may entail dissection of the recipient's common hepatic artery proximally towards the celiac artery. If no adequate vessel is found for revascularization, it is necessary to carry out arterial reconstruction directly from the aorta. This can be approached above the celiac artery (particularly in children), but more commonly (particularly in adults) requires an arterial conduit interposed between the infrarenal aorta and the donor celiac artery. The conduit may be of donor iliac artery, recipient saphenous vein or prosthetic material (polytetrafluoroethylene). It is recognized that multiple arterial anastomoses do constitute a risk factor for hepatic arterial complications, but the use of an arterial conduit is, nonetheless, associated with satisfactory outcomes.

Dissection of the portal vein in a patient who has undergone a previous liver transplant may prove difficult. The portal vein is sometimes friable and is often encased in dense adhesions. It is preferable, if possible, to dissect the portal vein proximally towards the confluence of the superior mesenteric and splenic veins, avoiding the area of the previous anastomosis. However, this may not be practical. In a difficult situation, it is possible to institute venovenous bypass at an early stage by cannulation of the inferior mesenteric vein, allowing decompression of the portal venous system and reduction in blood loss. This is helpful in enabling earlier division of the portal vein. If the portal vein is occluded it may be possible for thrombectomy to be carried out at the time of retransplantation. If this is not possible or if the portal vein is not deemed to be suitable for reconstruction for any other reason, it may be necessary to use a conduit of donor iliac vein from the recipient superior mesenteric vein to the donor portal vein. This conduit is usually placed anterior to the neck of the pancreas.

In a few patients who have undergone previous transplantation, access to the suprahepatic inferior vena cava (IVC) is inadequate below the diaphragm. If the previous suprahepatic caval anastomosis is of good caliber, this is commonly retained during retransplantation such that a short cuff of IVC from the first graft remains; it is difficult to mobilize an adequate length of suprahepatic IVC to excise the previous anastomosis. However, stenosis at the site of the previous anastomosis might lead to complications if not resected at the time of retransplantation. In such cases, it is occasionally advantageous to open the diaphragm into the pericardium in order to control the IVC above the diaphragm. This enables resection of the previous anastomosis.

Biliary problems

In the majority of primary liver transplants, biliary reconstruction is carried out by direct anastomosis of the common bile ducts of the donor and recipient. In early retransplantation, it may be possible to reconstruct the bile duct once more using a duct to duct technique. It is important, however, that the previous donor bile duct is resected completely; to leave a short length of the previous donor bile duct would, inevitably, leave a length of ischemic duct and lead to either early biliary leakage or later stenosis. In the majority of retransplanted livers, therefore, a Roux loop of jejunum is constructed to enable a choledochojejunostomy to be performed. A 50cm Roux loop of jejunum is used in order to minimize the risk of enteric reflux into the biliary system. Usually the end of the Roux loop is closed and the donor common bile duct anastomosed to the side of the jejunum, close to its end. Increasingly this anastomosis is carried out without the use of a stent, although many surgeons still prefer an external stent (brought out through a seromuscular tunnel in the wall of the Roux loop), to enable cholangiography to be carried out subsequently. There is little evidence to support the use of a biliary stent for reasons other than access for cholangiography.

In those patients in whom a choledochojejunostomy was used for the first transplant, it is usually possible for the existing Roux loop to be reused for the second graft. It is important, however, to ensure that the Roux loop is still of adequate length. If this is not the case, it is preferable to reconstruct the Roux loop appropriately.

Venovenous bypass

Liver transplantation requires the cross-clamping of the IVC, which causes a large reduction in the venous return to the heart. This is well tolerated in many patients, but in some it leads to hemodynamic instability with falling cardiac output. For this reason venovenous bypass is widely, although not universally, used in liver transplantation for adult patients. Pediatric liver transplant recipients are capable of tolerating cross-clamping without the support of bypass. The conventional bypass circuit, in use since the mid 1980s, employs cannulae in the portal vein and IVC (approached via the saphenofemoral junction at the groin) and blood returned via the axillary or jugular vein. Heparin bonded tubing and a centrifugal pump are used, thereby avoiding the need for systemic heparinization.

In patients who require early acute retransplantation for primary nonfunction or early arterial thrombosis, the procedure may be very rapid and, for this reason, bypass may not be required. Before committing, however, to undertake the procedure without bypass, it is reasonable to perform a trail clamping of the IVC and portal vein in order to observe the effect on cardiac output. If cross-clamping is well-tolerated, it is reasonable to proceed without the use of bypass. If cross-clamping is poorly tolerated, the clamps can then be removed and bypass instituted prior to removing the liver.

In patients who are undergoing late retransplantation, venovenous bypass maybe beneficial. A patient who has had a functioning liver allograft for several months or years is unlikely to have portal hypertension and, therefore, will not have developed the portosystemic collateral vessels that are very frequent in patients who have cirrhosis undergoing primary liver transplantation. For this reason cross clamping of the IVC and portal vein may lead to a very substantial reduction in cardiac return with consequent hemodynamic disturbance. In addition the early institution of bypass may allow a different surgical approach to the mobilization and excision of the liver. Once the patient is placed on venovenous bypass, it is possible to divide the portal vein and infrahepatic IVC in order to enable dissection of the liver from below. This increased flexibility of approach may be helpful in a difficult dissection.

Blood loss

The requirement for blood transfusion is greater following retransplantation than after primary transplantation. This is largely because of the extensive dissection of adhesions and an operation of longer duration. There is good evidence in liver transplantation that use of aprotinin is effective in reducing blood loss, particularly in cases with high blood loss, and this is now used routinely in many units. There is also evidence that the use of tranexamic acid is effective and is substantially cheaper. In those cases in which high blood loss is expected or experienced, autotransfusion is of great benefit. Although the cost of the disposable equipment required for autotransfusion is such that it is inappropriate for low blood loss cases, the blood requirement for patients undergoing liver retransplantation is such that this procedure is justified both in terms of cost and the reduced demand on blood resources.

The use of the argon beam coagulator is now widely advocated by many liver transplant surgeons and is of particular value in those cases in which there is a large area of dissection. This device provides coagulation without contact with the tissue and enables a thin layer of coagulated tissue to be 'painted' onto extensive raw areas from which constant blood loss may occur.

IMMUNOSUPPRESSION

The immunosuppressive strategy following retransplantation is, broadly, the same as that used following primary transplantation. However, if the cause of the loss of the first graft was acute or chronic rejection, it is the practice of many units to modify the immunosuppressive regimen in an attempt to reduce the risk of further immunologically mediated graft loss. There is some evidence that the risk of chronic rejection of a second graft may be increased if the first graft was lost due to chronic rejection. For this reason, it is the practice in many units to switch to tacrolimus-based therapy following retransplantation in patients who were previously treated with a cyclosporine-based regimen. Similarly, there may be some indication for the addition of mycofenalate to the immunosuppressive regimen – this has been shown to reduce the incidence of acute rejection in primary liver transplantation. Although widely used, the place of polyclonal antilymphocyte globulin (ALG) or monoclonal antilymphocyte antibody (OKT3) induction therapy remains unproven. There is evidence that, in patients who have other complications, particularly renal dysfunction, a period of induction with OKT3 may be effective in preventing rejection while reducing the need for nephrotoxic agents, allowing renal function to recover. Otherwise, however, there is little evidence to suggest that the use of 'quadruple' induction therapy provides substantial benefit.

POSTOPERATIVE MONITORING

After retransplantation patients are monitored in the same way as after primary liver transplantation. During the immediate postoperative phase, the major complications are bleeding, primary graft nonfunction or poor function, renal dysfunction, and cardiopulmonary dysfunction. After the first 48 hours, the principal problems are of rejection and acute bacterial sepsis. After 2–3 weeks, the additional problems of opportunist infection become significant.

Other factors that should be considered in the postoperative monitoring of retransplant recipients relate to the specific risks of the individual case. If problems have been encountered with arterial reconstruction or IVC reconstruction, it may be advisable to monitor these parameters more closely than would otherwise be the case.

MANIFESTATIONS OF OVER IMMUNOSUPPRESSION

A patient who has undergone retransplantation differs from a primary transplant recipient in having been immunosuppressed before the operation. For this reason the complications of immunosuppression, which usually only occur after several weeks or months, may occur at an earlier stage. This particularly applies to the development of opportunist infections. The most common opportunist infection to cause disease is cytomegalovirus (CMV). This may present systemically with swinging fever or with localized features of hepatitis or pneumonitis. The risk of CMV disease can be reduced substantially by the use of prophylactic gancyclovir, and while this has been restricted to patients who have conventional risk factors for infection (i.e. the seronegative recipients of seropositive grafts), many centers consider retransplant recipients in the same category. In those patients who do develop clinically apparent CMV disease, gancyclovir is effective in abrogating the serious effects of CMV infection.

As in all transplant recipients, it is important that the existing microbial flora of the patient are cultured. The retransplant patient has already been immunosuppressed and may have received intensive treatment for rejection with high-dose steroids or antilymphocyte antibodies. For this reason the risk of fungal infection is even greater than normal. This may be with *Candida* species or, more ominously, with *Aspergillus*. Oral antifungal prophylaxis is given together with careful surveillance and early institution of parenteral antifungal therapy when indicated. More radically, some advocate routine intravenous antifungal therapy as prophylaxis in these patients. Antibacterial prophylaxis is given for 48 hours postoperatively (unless otherwise indicated). Antibiotic therapy must be used sparingly, prolonged treatment avoided if possible and broad-spectrum antibiotics used with great care in order to minimize the risk of fungal overgrowth. Prophylactic therapy with trimethoprim–sufamethoxazole (co-trimoxazole) against *Pneumocystisis* is given to those at significant risk, including those who have a lymphocyte count below 0.4×10^9/L.

A further complication of immunosuppression to which retransplant recipients are prone is that of post-transplant lymphoproliferative disorders (Fig. 40.8). This is also related to the extent and intensity of immunosuppression. Patients liable to a primary Epstein–Barr infection are also at greater risk. Specific antiviral treatment is not generally given specifically to reduce this risk, although the use of acyclovir is advocated by some.

OUTCOME OF RETRANSPLANTATION

In general, retransplantation has a poorer outcome than primary liver transplantation, but there is no difference between survival after the second, third, or fourth transplant (Fig. 40.9).

The results are worse in patients undergoing emergency primary transplants than in those having elective procedures (Figs 40.10 & 40.11).

Retransplantation utilizes scarce organs less efficiently. A series from the USA of 356 retransplants carried out in 299 patients showed survival rates at 1, 5, and 10 years of 62, 47, and 45%, respectively. These were substantially lower than in patients undergoing primary transplantation (83, 74, and 68%, respectively). A number of variables were shown to influence the outcome including recipient age, the interval to retransplantation, and recipient UNOS status. In a study from the UK, survival at 1 year was reduced from 80 to 50%, and indicators of poorer outcome included older age, UNOS score, bilirubin level, and creatinine level. In a further analysis of 418 retransplants in the USA, the variables found to be associated with poor outcome included recipient age (increasing over 45 years), preoperative mechanical ventilation, pretransplant serum creatinine, and preoperative serum bilirubin.

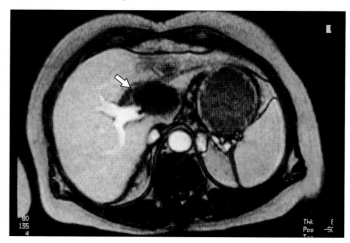

Figure 40.8 Lymphoproliferative disease. The incidence of lymphoma is increased after retransplantation. The computed tomography scan shows a mass at the hilum which proved to be a lymphoma (arrow).

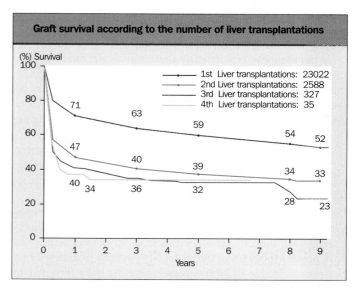

Figure 40.9 Graft survival after retransplantation. Grafts used in retransplantation have much poorer survival rates than primary transplants. (Data from European Liver Transplant Registry.)

The timing of retransplantation was also important, with the risk increasing from day 0 to day 38 and decreasing thereafter. The use of tacrolimus was also shown to be beneficial compared with cyclosporine. In children, survival rates are also lower after retransplantation. The age of the patient at the time of retransplantation (less than 3 years) and the use of a reduced size graft were found to be significant adverse factors on survival.

With increasing world experience, it is possible to identify a number of factors by which relatively better prognosis can be predicted. Indeed, in selected patients undergoing retransplantation electively for chronic rejection several months following the original operation, the outcome may be comparable to that of primary liver transplantation. Although early retransplantation is usually simpler technically, it is clear that patients who undergo urgent retransplantation early after primary transplantation have a poorer prognosis and that failure of two or more organ systems is associated with a substantially poorer outcome than patients in whom only the liver has failed. Thus patients who are retransplanted

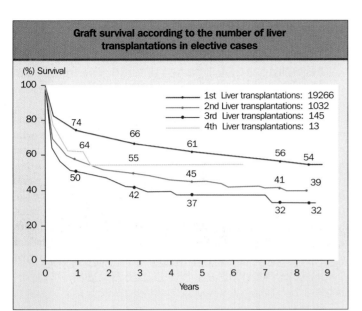

Figure 40.10 Graft survival after retransplantation. Graft survival after retransplantation following elective primary transplantation is reduced, except for the fourth transplant. (Data from European Liver Transplant Registry.)

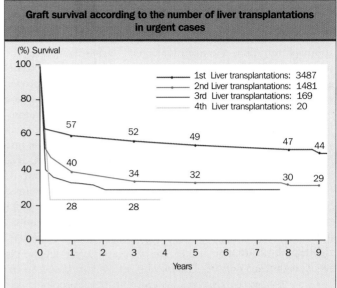

Figure 40.11 Graft survival after retransplantation. Graft survival after retransplantation following emergency primary elective transplantation is always lower than after the primary procedure. (Data from European Liver Transplant Registry.)

urgently from an intensive care unit with respiratory and possibly renal failure have an extremely poor prognosis. Patients who undergo urgent early retransplantation are, in the main, substantially more sick than those who undergo retransplantation several months later. Thus, it is likely to be not the timing of retransplantation *per se* that affects the prognosis, but rather the nature of the underlying liver dysfunction. Once it is clear that retransplantation will be required, it is usually best to proceed sooner rather than wait until the condition of the patient has deteriorated further.

IMPLICATIONS OF RETRANSPLANTATION

Prioritization of recipients

With the increase in the number of liver transplants performed in recent years and no concomitant increase in the number of liver donors available, there is now an overall shortage of livers and an appreciable risk of death for patients awaiting transplantation. This has important implications, the first being that livers should, in general, be used where transplantation is most likely to be of benefit. Thus, the retransplantation of a patient who has a prognosis of less than 10% survival could be judged to be inappropriate if this were to result in the withholding of transplantation from a patient who has an 80% chance of survival.

At the time when there were adequate donor livers available for transplantation it was possible to justify retransplantation of almost every patient in whom the first graft failed. Although the prognosis may be poor, retransplantation nonetheless offered a possibility of recovery and could, therefore, be considered to be still in the best interests of the patient. However, as the availability of donor organs is now a limiting factor in most countries, the issue has arisen of the need to use donor livers in the most effective way.

Various factors are in conflict. There is a moral obligation to a patient in whom treatment has already been initiated, coinciding with the natural wish of a clinician not to abandon a patient who has already undergone a transplant. However, if the same patient is effectively in direct competition with another patient who has not received a transplant, and who would have a substantially greater chance of long-term benefit following transplantation, there is a powerful moral pressure to transplant the liver into the latter patient in order to maximize its benefit (i.e. the utilitarian view).

The situation is complicated by the fact that it is never possible to state whether, by denying an individual patient a particular liver, this will prove to be the last opportunity for the patient to undergo transplantation. However, although an individual patient on the waiting list may survive to receive another liver, the total group of (low risk) patients on the waiting list is being denied a liver and, therefore, placed at an avoidable risk.

In the absence of national or international guidelines, these difficult decisions are made at a local level with clinicians balancing the risks and benefits to the patients who are waiting locally when deciding the priorities.

Reducing the need for retransplantation

A second implication of the shortage of donor organs is the need to reduce the demand for retransplantation. Whereas it is clearly important that the maximum number of potential organs is identified and removed for transplantation, it is important, as far as possible, to exclude from transplantation those donor livers that will not function. This assessment is notoriously difficult and, despite much effort over many years, remains imprecise.

There is much evidence now that the condition of marginal organ donors can be improved by intensive donor management. This includes attention to fluid balance, inotropes, and other factors including hormonal status. The development of University of Wisconsin preservation solution was a major technical advance in liver transplantation. However, as previously discussed, there is evidence that the incidence of medium term biliary complications is higher in those patients in whom total cold ischemia time is prolonged. Such complications increase the need for retransplantation.

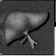
The logistics of liver transplantation must be planned such that prolonged preservation times are avoided.

Avoidance of hepatic arterial complications is an important approach to reduce the need for urgent retransplantation. The results from pediatric transplantation, particularly of segmental grafts and living donor grafts from parent to child, have improved greatly in recent years. Some of the improvement is a function of refinement of the anastomotic techniques. The use of magnification or microscopic techniques for anastomosis of very small vessels appears to have reduced the technical complication rate in this area and, thereby, the need for retransplantation. It is important to avoid iatrogenic injuries to the liver during its removal from the donor. Arterial injuries are quite easily incurred by traction on the hepatic artery during removal. Such injuries may lead to intimal dissection that does not become manifest until some time after transplantation, at which time hepatic arterial thrombosis occurs.

In the area of immunosuppression, strategies to prevent graft loss due to chronic rejection or, less commonly, intractable acute rejection, are needed. Similarly the prevention of acute cellular rejection is likely to reduce the risk of hepatic arterial thrombosis, which may occur when the arterial flow through the rejecting allograft is reduced.

Finally, it is important to consider strategies to prevent recurrence of disease. As discussed, transplantation of patients who have chronic liver failure secondary to hepatitis B has been beset by problems of recurrent hepatitis B leading to the rapid development of recurrence of chronic liver failure. The advent of novel strategies, particularly the use of antiviral agents, may reduce the serious consequences of this. Similarly hepatitis C, an increasingly frequent indication for liver transplantation, is associated with a high risk of recurrent disease. Although this leads to graft failure less commonly than with hepatitis B, again it is important that effective strategies to prevent disease recurrence are developed.

FURTHER READING

Doyle HR, Morelli F, McMichael J, et al. Hepatic retransplantation – an analysis of risk factors associated with outcome. Transplantation. 1996;61:1499–505. *An analysis of the factors predictive of outcome after retransplantation.*

Drazan K, Shaked A, Olthoff KM, et al. Etiology and management of symptomatic adult hepatic artery thrombosis after orthotopic liver transplantation (OLT). Am Surg. 1996;62:237–40. *A good account of the management of hepatic artery thrombosis in adults.*

Gane EJ, Portmann BC, Naoumov NV, et al. Long-term outcome of hepatitis C infection after liver transplantation. N Engl J Med. 1996;334:815–20. *Excellent study of the medium-term outcome after transplantation for hepatitis C.*

Gonzalez FX, Rimola A, Grande L, et al. Predictive factors of early postoperative graft function in human liver transplantation. Hepatology. 1994;20:565–73. *A study indicating important factors that are helpful in predicting early graft dysfunction.*

Goss JA, Shackleton CR, McDiarmid SV, et al. Long-term results of pediatric liver transplantation: an analysis of 569 transplants. Ann Surg. 1998;228:411–20. *A large pediatric experience including a perspective on retransplantation.*

Grellier L, Mutimer D, Ahmed M, et al. Lamivudine prophylaxis against reinfection in liver transplantation for hepatitis B cirrhosis. Lancet. 1996;348:1212–5. *An alternative approach to preventing HBV reinfection after liver transplantation – a preliminary experience.*

Ishitani M, McGory R, Dickson R, et al. Retransplantation of patients with severe posttransplant hepatitis B in the first allograft. Transplantation. 1997;64:410–4. *Valuable experience of retransplantation for reinfection with HBV.*

Langnas AN, Marujo W, Stratta RJ, Wood RP, Li SJ, Shaw BW. Hepatic allograft rescue following arterial thrombosis. Role of urgent revascularization. Transplantation. 1991;51:86–90. *Description of attempts to salvage thrombosed hepatic arteries.*

Markmann JF, Markowitz JS, Yersiz H, et al. Long-term survival after retransplantation of the liver. Ann Surg. 1997;226:408–20. *Good perspective on results of retransplantation followed by a section discussing key issues.*

Mora NP, Klintmalm GB, Cofer JB, et al. Results after liver retransplantation in a group of 50 regrafted patients: two different concepts of elective versus emergency retransplantation. Transplant Int. 1991;4:231–4. *Highlights the important difference between emergency and elective retransplantation.*

Muiesan P, Rela M, Nodari F, et al. Use of infrarenal conduits for arterial revascularization in orthotopic liver transplantation. Liver Transplant Surg. 1998;4:232–5. *A description of the use of conduits in revascularization.*

Newell KA, Millis JM, Bruce DS, et al. An analysis of hepatic retransplantation in children. Transplantation. 1998;65:1172–8. *Good outline of experience of retransplantation in a pediatric population.*

Ploeg RJ, D'Alessandro AM, Knechtle SJ, et al. Risk factors for primary dysfunction after liver transplantation – a multivariate analysis. Transplantation. 1993;55:807–13. *Another study indicating important factors that are helpful in predicting early graft dysfunction.*

Rosen HR, O'Reilly PM, Shackleton CR, et al. Graft loss following liver transplantation in patients with chronic hepatitis C. Transplantation. 1996;62:1773–6. *Another outline of the pattern of graft loss in hepatitis C virus infected liver graft recipients.*

Samuel D, Muller R, Alexander G, et al. Liver transplantation in European patients with the hepatitis B surface antigen. N Engl J Med. 1993;329:1842–7. *Excellent classification of the risk factors for HBV reinfection after liver transplantation.*

Sanchez-Urdazpal L, Gores GJ, Ward EM, et al. Ischemic-type biliary complications after orthotopic liver transplantation. Hepatology. 1992;16:49–53. *Good description of the complexities of interpreting nonanastomotic strictures.*

Sheiner PA, Schluger LK, Emre S, et al. Retransplantation for recurrent hepatitis C. Liver Transplant Surg. 1997;3:130–6. *An early report of the fairly favorable outcome of retransplantation for recurrent hepatitis C.*

van-Hoek B, Wiesner RH, Ludwig J, Paya C. Recurrence of ductopenic rejection in liver allografts after retransplantation for vanishing bile duct syndrome. Transplant Proc. 1991;23:1442–3. *One of the few studies assessing the nature and risk of recurrent ductopenia.*

Wong T, Devlin J, Rolando N, Heaton N, Williams R. Clinical characteristics affecting the outcome of liver retransplantation. Transplantation. 1997;64:878–82. *Analysis of the factors influencing outcome after retransplantation in the UK.*

Index

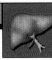

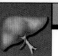

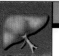

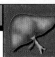

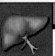